Nursing Care Planning Guides

A Nursing Diagnosis Approach

By

Susan Puderbaugh Ulrich, RN, MSN
Lane Community College
Eugene, Oregon

Suzanne Weyland Canale, RN, MSN
Lane Community College
Eugene, Oregon

Sharon Andrea Wendell, RN, MSN
Lane Community College
Eugene, Oregon

1990
W.B. SAUNDERS COMPANY
Harcourt Brace Jovanovich, Inc.
Philadelphia   London   Toronto   Montreal   Sydney   Tokyo

Nursing Care Planning Guides

A Nursing
Dia...

SECON...

W. B. SAUNDERS COMPANY
Harcourt Brace Jovanovich, Inc.

The Curtis Center
Independence Square West
Philadelphia, PA 19106

Library of Congress Cataloging-in-Publication Data

Ulrich, Susan Puderbaugh.
  Nursing care planning guides: a nursing diagnosis approach / by
Susan Puderbaugh Ulrich, Suzanne Weyland Canale, Sharon Andrea
Wendell. — 2nd ed.
    p.   cm.
  Includes bibliographical references.
  ISBN 0-7216-3091-X
  1. Nursing—Planning. 2. Nursing care plans. I. Wendell, Sharon
Andrea. II. Canale, Suzanne Weyland. III. Title.
  [DNLM: 1. Nursing Assessment—handbooks. 2. Nursing Care—
handbooks. 3. Patient Care Planning—handbooks. WY 39 U45n]
RT49.U47 1990
610.73—dc20
DNLM/DLC
for Library of Congress   90-8009

Editor: Michael Brown
Developmental Editor: Lisa Konoplisky
Designer: Terri Siegel
Production Manager: Bill Preston
Manuscript Editor: Rose Marie Klimowicz

Nursing Care Planning Guides: A Nursing Diagnosis Approach   ISBN 0-7216-3091-X

Printed in the United States of America
Last digit is the print number: 9   8   7   6   5   4   3   2

PREFACE

This book provides a comprehensive reference to guide the planning of holistic nursing care for hospitalized adults with commonly recurring medical-surgical conditions. It has been updated to reflect the current nursing diagnoses and advances in nursing and medical science. The plans provide a basic standard of care that must be individualized according to each client's history, current physiological and psychological status, medical orders, and specific response to treatment.

Each care plan utilizes the nursing process format, includes nursing and collaborative diagnoses, and reflects a format commonly used in health care settings and educational institutions. The organizational structure is based on an integrated systems approach.

With increasing specialization by health care professionals, client care is easily fragmented, making it difficult to see the interrelationships that are the basis of high-quality nursing care. These care plans integrate the various aspects of nursing care to assist the student and practitioner in seeing those interrelationships. Included in each plan are the following:

1. emphasis on psychosocial as well as physiological aspects of client care
2. etiology statements that reflect the pathophysiological basis of each nursing diagnosis
3. specific, measurable desired outcomes that can be used as a basis for evaluating the effectiveness of the nursing actions
4. integration of physical assessments, diagnostic information, and pharmacological therapy when applicable in the actions appropriate for each nursing and collaborative diagnosis
5. independent, interdependent or collaborative, and dependent nursing actions
6. selected rationales that clarify how an action relates to the nursing diagnosis statement and/or helps achieve the desired outcome
7. extensive discharge planning using terminology that most clients can understand.

There are a total of 75 care plans included in this book. In order to emphasize the use of standardized care plans as a tool in formulating individualized nursing care plans and to assist the student and practitioner to utilize the standardized care plans most effectively, the introductory chapter has been expanded in this edition. The Introduction includes specific guidelines for adapting the care plans to meet the individual client's needs. It uses a case study format to demonstrate the actual selection of pertinent diagnostic labels and the individualization of etiology statements, desired outcomes, and nursing actions.

Unit I focuses on the care of the elderly client. The care plan is directed toward the client who is hospitalized for management of a medical-surgical condition, but the biopsychosocial changes incorporated into the unit can easily be utilized in planning care for the elderly client in a variety of health care settings. Units II to V include care plans that are intended to provide standardized information regarding conditions or treatment modalities. The standardized care plans in Unit II on Preoperative and Postoperative Care should be used in conjunction with each surgical care plan in the text. The care plans on Immobility and Terminal Care (Units III and IV) are applicable to a wide range of diagnoses and should be utilized whenever appropriate. The care plans in Unit V cover treatment modalities for neoplastic disorders and are referred to when appropriate in the care plans related to neoplastic diseases. Each of the standardized care plans in these units can also be used independently and/or in planning care for clients with a condition not covered in this text. When care plans in Units VI to XVIII utilize one or more of those in Units II to V, the referral is designated in bold print by the phrase **Use in conjunction with**.

Units V to XVIII are divided according to body systems. Care plans within each unit deal with common recurring conditions that are frequently seen in an acute care setting. Each care plan includes a comprehensive listing of appropriate nursing and collaborative diagnoses with related client outcomes and pertinent actions that facilitate the achievement of each outcome.

Each care plan is organized as follows:

Introduction

The introduction provides the reader with an overview of the condition including a basic definition and discussion of the pathophysiological mechanisms involved and/ or a description of the surgical procedure or selected treatment modality. This overview is not intended to be a substitute for the information provided in either a medical-surgical nursing text or other references, but rather a quick refresher or a starting point for additional research. Within this section, the reader will also find the focus of the care plan as well as the overall goals of care.

Discharge Criteria

This section includes criteria that serve as a guide for client teaching and determinants of the client's readiness for discharge from the acute care setting. Recognizing that consumer education is a vital aspect of health care, the authors use these discharge criteria as the basis for the detailed teaching plans that are included at the end of each care plan.

Nursing Diagnosis

The nursing diagnoses describe the actual or potential health problems that a client with a particular condition may experience. The nursing diagnoses were selected from those approved by the North American Nursing Diagnosis Association (NANDA) through 1988. In a few instances the authors have included nursing diagnoses that are not currently on the NANDA list. These diagnostic categories are noted in the text by an asterisk (*) and an explanatory footnote. Nursing diagnoses that are not unique to a particular condition but may be relevant for any client (e.g. spiritual distress) have not consistently been included and should be considered when individualizing each care plan. Collaborative diagnoses have been included to incorporate potential complications and electrolyte imbalances for which there are no established nursing diagnostic labels. With the exception of "knowledge deficit," each nursing diagnosis includes a specific etiological statement pertinent to the disease condition. The etiological factor for the "knowledge deficit" diagnosis was not included because of the numerous individual variables that affect the teaching-learning process. In order to provide consistency in the care plans, the nursing and collaborative diagnosis statements have been listed in the same order for all of the care plans. This should not be construed as an attempt to set priorities for the diagnoses. Priorities will need to be established by the student and practitioner based on current client assessments and individual client needs.

Desired Outcomes

The desired outcomes for the nursing and collaborative diagnoses provide specific, measurable criteria for evaluating client progress and identifying when goals of care have been met. These outcomes identify a favorable status that can be achieved or maintained by the implementation of the identified nursing actions. The outcome criteria for the nursing diagnoses are based on the defining characteristics approved by NANDA for each nursing diagnosis. Target dates for the desired outcomes have not been included since these are determined by the client's current status.

Nursing Actions and Selected Rationales

Included in this section are the dependent, interdependent or collaborative, and independent nursing actions that are appropriate for assisting the client to achieve the desired outcomes. The actions include detailed assessments that assist the user to determine if the stated nursing diagnosis is an actual or a potential one and the priority it may assume. The interventions are specific and realistic yet global enough to allow regional and multidisciplinary variations in standards of care. Assessment criteria and interpretation of diagnostic tests are included with the appropriate nursing diagnosis rather than in a separate section in an effort to reduce fragmentation and provide the reader with a clearer understanding of why the assessments or particular tests should be performed. The selected rationales, which appear in italics, have been included to clarify actions that may not be fundamental nursing knowledge.

To facilitate the use and individualization of the standardized care plans provided here, an appendix of alphabetically arranged NANDA approved nursing diagnoses with definitions and defining characteristics has been included. An index has also been added to this edition to promote ease in locating specific care plans and nursing and collaborative diagnoses.

Ultimately, the value of a systematic approach to individualized client care is measured by its effect on the quality of care provided to the client. The authors hope that the use of the care plans in this edition will continue to facilitate implementation of the nursing process, assist with integration of the numerous aspects of health care, and provide the student and practitioner with a guide for planning high-quality client care.

ACKNOWLEDGMENTS

To our numerous readers who shared their expertise and provided valuable suggestions throughout this project.

To our students who are a continual source of inspiration.

To our friends for their support and encouragement.

Most importantly, to our families for their love, patience, and encouragement throughout this project:

Joe and Christopher Canale

Curt, Shannon, and Chad Ulrich

Steve and Traci Wendell.

Readers*

BAIRD, SANDRA R.N., Ph.D., Ed.D. Director, School of Nursing, University of Northern Colorado, Greeley, Colorado

BALLARD, NAOMI R.N., M.A., M.S. Associate Professor, Adult Health and Illness, School of Nursing, Oregon Health Sciences University, Portland, Oregon

BARKER, ELLEN R.N., M.S.N. President, Neuroscience Nursing Consultant, Newark, Delaware

BELL, SHIRLEY R.N., Ed.D. Assistant Professor, College of Nursing, Arizona State University, Tempe, Arizona

BOHNY, BARBARA R.N., D.N.S. Associate Professor, Director, Program for Theoretical Bases of Nursing Sciences, School of Nursing, New York University, New York, New York

BRILLHART, BARBARA R.N., Ph.D. Assistant Professor, School of Nursing, University of Texas at Arlington, Arlington, Texas

BROZENEC, SALLY R.N., M.S. Assistant Professor, Operating Room and Surgical Nursing, College of Nursing, Rush University, Chicago, Illinois

CAMBARERI, KATHY R.N., M.S.N., C.S. Nursing Educational Coordinator, George Washington University, Washington, D.C.

CARLOS, LETICIA B.S.N. Instructor of Nursing, Lane Community College, Eugene, Oregon (at time of review)

CASSMEYER, VIRGINIA L. R.N., M.S.N., Ph.D. Associate Professor, Medical-Surgical Nursing, School of Nursing, University of Kansas, Kansas City, Kansas

CLAYPOOL, BERNIE R.N. Certified Enterostomal Therapist, Sacred Heart General Hospital, Eugene, Oregon

DAVIDSON, SUE R.N., M.S.N. Associate Professor, Adult Health and Illness, School of Nursing, Oregon Health Sciences University, Portland, Oregon

DURHAM, JERRY R.N., Ph.D. Director, School of Nursing, Illinois Wesleyan University, Bloomington, Illinois

EARNEST, VICKI R.N., M.S.N. Associate Professor of Nursing, Community College of Denver, Denver, Colorado

EISZ, MARILYN K. R.N., M.N. Assistant Clinical Professor, Medical-Surgical Nursing, School of Nursing, University of California, Los Angeles, Los Angeles, California

---

*For the first and second editions inclusive.

ELROD, RACHEL E. R.N., M.S. Instructor of Nursing, Front Range Community College, Westminster, Colorado

ESTES, MARY ELLEN ZATOR R.N., M.S.N., C.C.R.N. Nursing Educational Coordinator for Critical Care, George Washington University, Washington, D.C.

FOSTER, ROXIE R.N., M.S. Assistant Professor of Nursing, Loretto Heights College, Denver, Colorado

GIBBS, LOU ANN R.N., B.S. Staff Nurse, Sacred Heart General Hospital Home Health Agency, Eugene, Oregon

GRECH, MARY E. R.N., M.S.N. Instructor, School of Nursing, University of California, Los Angeles, Los Angeles, California

HEATH, IRIS R.N. Charge Nurse, Orthopedic Unit, Sacred Heart General Hospital, Eugene, Oregon

HOLBROOK, NORMA B.S.N., R.N. Education Coordinator, St. Francis Hospital, Topeka, Kansas

HOWELL, DONNA R.N. Staff Nurse and Hospice Coordinator, Sacred Heart General Hospital Home Health Agency, Eugene, Oregon

ITO, DOLLY D.N.Sc., C.R.R.N., C.S. Professor of Nursing, School of Nursing, Seattle University, Seattle, Washington (at time of review)

JENNINGS, MAJOR BONNIE MOWINSKI R.N., M.S. U.S. Army Nurse Corps, Fort Gordon, Georgia (at time of review)

JOHNSON, MARY ANN B.S., M.S., Ph.D., R.N.-C., G.N.P. Clinical Assistant Professor, College of Nursing, University of Utah, Salt Lake City, Utah

KENDRICK-THOMPSON, MICHELLE R.N. Dialysis Coordinator, Home Training Program, Sacred Heart General Hospital, Eugene, Oregon

KINMAN, JAN B.S.N. Instructor of Nursing, Lane Community College, Eugene, Oregon

KLEIER, JOANN M.S.N., C.U.R.N., A.R.N.P. Instructor, Nursing Technology, Broward Community College, Ft. Lauderdale, Florida

KRUMME, URSEL R.N., M.A. Associate Professor and Adult Med-Surg Nursing Area Chair, School of Nursing, Seattle University, Seattle, Washington (at time of review)

LINVILLE, JOANN B.S.N. Instructor of Nursing, Bellingham Vocational Technical Institute, Bellingham, Washington (at time of review)

LONG, BARBARA C. R.N., M.S.N. Associate Professor Emeritus, Medical-Surgical Nursing, Frances Payne Bolton School of Nursing, Case Western Reserve University, Cleveland, Ohio

MacMULLEN, NANCY J. R.N., M.S.N. Assistant Professor, Obstetrical/Gynecological Nursing, College of Nursing, Rush University, Chicago, Illinois

MARTIN, IDA R.N. Diabetic Educator, Sacred Heart General Hospital, Eugene, Oregon (at time of review)

MARTIN, JANICE L. R.N., M.S., C.-G.N.P. Director, Geriatric Rehabilitation Project, School of Nursing, University of Northern Colorado, Greeley, Colorado

MAUER, JEAN R.N., M.S.N. Assistant Professor, College of Nursing, Villanova University, Villanova, Pennsylvania

MILLER, DEBORAH J. R.N., M.S.N. Resource Nurse, Rush-Presbyterian-St. Luke's Medical Center, Chicago, Illinois

MUNKVOLD, JULIA B.S.N., M.S. Instructor of Nursing, Lane Community College, Eugene, Oregon

NICHOLS, LYNN WEMETT R.N., M.S.N. Associate Professor of Nursing, State University of New York at Plattsburgh, Plattsburgh, New York

NULL, MARYANN R.N., M.S.N. Adjunct Professor of Nursing, Community College of the Finger Lakes, Canandaigua, New York

PAIRITZ KONSTANT, DONNA R.N., M.S. Assistant Professor, Operating Room and Surgical Nursing, College of Nursing, Rush University, Chicago, Illinois

PATRAS, ANGIE R.N., M.S. Assistant Professor, Operating and Surgical Nursing, College of Nursing, Rush University, Chicago, Illinois

PECK, MARY LOU   R.N., Ed.D.   Assistant Professor, School of Nursing, City College of New York, New York, New York (at time of review); currently Assistant Professor, Russell Sage College, Troy, New York

PFISTER, SHIRLEY   R.N., M.S., C.C.R.N., R.R.T.   Respiratory Clinical Specialist, Veterans Administration Hospital, Denver, Colorado

SABO, CAROLYN   R.N., Ed.D.   Associate Professor, Department of Nursing, University of Nevada, Las Vegas, Nevada

SCHENK, SUSAN   R.N., M.N., A.N.P.   Associate Professor, Adult Health and Illness, School of Nursing, Oregon Health Sciences University, Portland, Oregon

SCHULTZ, MARILYN DELUCA   R.N., M.A., C.N.   Clinical Specialist, Veterans Administration Medical Center, New York, New York

SIEHL, SANDRA   R.N., M.S.N.   Clinical Specialist-Oncology, The Jewish Hospital of St. Louis—Washington University Medical Center, St. Louis, Missouri

STRAUSS, MARY BETH   R.N., Ph.D.   Assistant Professor, Ohio State University College of Nursing, Columbus, Ohio

TARSITANO, BETTY J. PATTERSON   R.N., Ph.D.   Former Associate Professor and Coordinator of Adult Nursing, Graduate Program, Center for Nursing, Northwestern University, Chicago, Illinois

TENANBAUM, LINDA   R.N., M.S.N.   Oncology Nursing and Continuing Education, Broward Community College, Fort Lauderdale, Florida

TERZIAN, MAUREEN P.   R.N., M.S.N.   Assistant Professor, College of Nursing, Villanova University, Villanova, Pennsylvania

VAN VELSON, B. JANN   R.N.   Certified Enterostomal Therapist, Staff Nurse, Sacred Heart General Hospital, Eugene, Oregon (at time of review)

WALSH, MARIAN   R.N., M.S.   Assistant Professor, Operating Room and Surgical Nursing, College of Nursing—Rush University, Chicago, Illinois

WARD, SHIRLEY   R.N.   Nurse Manager, Orthopedic Unit, Sacred Heart General Hospital, Eugene, Oregon

WESTFALL, UNA BETH   R.N., M.S.N.   Assistant Professor and Faculty Clinician, Adult Health and Illness, School of Nursing, Oregon Health Sciences University, Portland, Oregon

YOUNG, M. SHELLEY   R.N., Ph.D.   Associate Professor, Adult Health and Illness, School of Nursing, Oregon Health Sciences University, Portland, Oregon (at time of review)

CONTENTS

Unit VIII
Nursing Care of the Client with Disturbances of Peripheral Vascular Function 387

Unit IX
Nursing Care of the Client with Disturbances of Respiratory Function 423

Unit X
Nursing Care of the Client with Disturbances of the Kidney and Urinary Tract 511

Unit XI
Nursing Care of the Client with Disturbances of Hematopoietic and Lymphatic Function 571

Unit XII
Nursing Care of the Client with Disturbances of the Gastrointestinal Tract 627

Unit XVIII
Nursing Care of the Client with Disturbances of the Ear,
Nose, and Throat 1051

Appendix
Nursing Diagnoses Approved by NANDA Through 1988

Bibliography

Index

INTRODUCTION
Individualizing the Care Plans

Planning nursing care is an exciting challenge and a rewarding experience when one sees positive results because of his/her efforts. However, planning care that is individualized and comprehensive can be a tedious process because of lack of time and adequate resources. This book is intended to facilitate the process by providing nursing care plans to be used in the care of adult clients with common, recurring medical-surgical conditions. Within each care plan is a list of possible diagnoses with related etiological factors, desired outcomes with measurable behavioral criteria, and a list of appropriate nursing actions with selected rationales. By utilizing this book, safe yet comprehensive care can be planned in a minimal amount of time.

To be most effective, the standard plans of care must be adapted to the client's individual needs. Using the nursing process as a framework, the authors recommend the following steps for data gathering and planning of individualized care:

1. read the admission and medication administration record of assigned client
2. review the history, current diagnostic test results, nurses' notes for the last 48 hours, physician's progress notes, and current consultations
3. interview the client and complete a physical assessment utilizing the tool provided by your nursing school or clinical setting
4. highlight abnormal data obtained
5. read about the client's diagnosis in a current medical-surgical nursing text
6. select the appropriate standardized care plan(s) from this text
7. select the nursing and collaborative diagnoses within the plan(s) that are appropriate for your particular client; choose from among the etiological factors those that are relevant for your client; add to or modify etiological factors as appropriate
8. modify the outcome criteria so that they are achievable and realistic for your client; establish appropriate target dates
9. select from the list of nursing actions those that are relevant to the client's care; add to or modify the actions to meet the needs of your particular client; include relevant medications, treatments, client preferences, and actions that will facilitate the achievement of the desired client outcomes
10. set priorities for the nursing/collaborative diagnoses using your usual system (e.g. Maslow's hierarchy, basic needs).

The following situation is used to illustrate how these standardized nursing care plans can be utilized by the student and practitioner in planning individualized care:

Mary G. is a 46-year-old woman who has been hospitalized in the terminal stages of cancer of the breast. She has been bedridden for the past 3 weeks because of severe bone pain due to metastatic lesions. She has 4 children ranging in age from 10–17. Both Mary and her husband have been trying to prepare the children for her death.

1. **Read the admission and the medication administration record of the assigned client.**

From this it is determined that Mary is a 46-year-old married woman. Her religious preference is Protestant. Her diagnosis is *Stage IV cancer of the breast.* She *needs assistance with all activities of daily living* and is *receiving morphine sulfate 15 mg every 2 hours for pain relief.* She is also receiving *Dialose 1 capsule/day, Phenergan 25 mg IM q6h prn, and Milk of Magnesia 30 cc p.o. prn.*

2. **Review the history, current diagnostic test results, nurses' notes for the last 48 hours, physician's progress notes, and current consultations.**

   From the history it is determined that Mary had a *mastectomy 5 years ago* and experienced a *disease recurrence 2 years ago.* She was treated with chemotherapeutic drugs until 3 months ago when she elected to stop treatment. She has *metastasis to the spine, hips, and sternum* and has been *bedridden for the last 3 weeks.* The progress notes indicate that Mary's *condition is steadily deteriorating* and the goal of care is to keep her comfortable.
   Diagnostic test results reveal that Mary's *RBC, Hgb., Hct., and serum protein levels are decreased.* Her *serum calcium level is moderately elevated.*
   The nurses' notes reveal that Mary *needs assistance with all personal hygiene tasks and activity.* She is able to feed herself but is only *consuming 10 percent of her meals.* She *has not had a bowel movement for 6 days.* Mary is voiding adequate amounts and her intake and output are balanced. She has been *crying frequently* and *states that neither she nor her husband is ready for her death.* It is also noted that her *husband seems uncomfortable in her room.*

3. **Interview the client and complete a physical assessment utilizing the tool provided by your nursing school or clinical setting.**

   The interview and physical assessment reveal that Mary has *persistent reddened areas on her left hip and coccyx.* Her *breath sounds are diminished in both bases* and her *respirations are 12/minute and shallow. Bowel sounds are present, but hypoactive. Abdomen is firm and distended.* She states that she usually has a bowel movement every other day. Mary is alert and oriented and able to move all extremities. She *complains of pain in her back and right hip.*

4. **Highlight abnormal data obtained.**

   Abnormal data for Mary is designated in italics in steps 1–3.

5. **Read about the client's diagnosis in a current medical-surgical nursing text.**

   Review cancer of the breast and care of the terminally ill and the immobile client.

6. **Select the appropriate standardized care plan(s) from this text.**

   Based on the physician's statement that Mary has been admitted for terminal care and will have no further palliative treatment, it is determined that the appropriate care plans for Mary are Cancer of the Breast, Terminal Care, and Immobility.

7. **Select the nursing and collaborative diagnoses within the plan(s) that are appropriate for your particular client. Choose from among the etiological factors those that are relevant for your client. Add to or modify etiological factors as appropriate.**

   It is determined that the following diagnoses and etiological factors from the Care Plans on Terminal Care and Immobility are appropriate. You will note that the etiological factors have been modified to reflect Mary's situation.

a. **Anxiety** related to separation from home and significant others, unfamiliar environment, discomfort, the unknown, loss of control over life and body functioning, changes in body image, concerns about the welfare of significant others and loss of loved ones, unfinished business, and recognition of probability of non-being.

b. **Ineffective breathing patterns** related to fear and anxiety; increased oxygen demand associated with an elevated basal metabolic rate (due to disease process); pain; depressant effects of morphine sulfate; and impaired chest expansion associated with recumbent positioning, weakness, and fatigue.

c. **Ineffective airway clearance** related to stasis of secretions associated with poor cough effort and decreased mobility.

d. **Altered electrolyte balance: hypercalcemia** related to disuse osteoporosis (a result of prolonged immobility) and breakdown of bone associated with metastatic lesions.

e. **Pain: right hip and back** related to bone metastasis.

f. **Impaired skin integrity: irritation and breakdown** related to prolonged pressure on tissues associated with decreased mobility and increased fragility of the skin associated with malnutrition.

g. **Impaired physical mobility** related to weakness and fatigue, reluctance to move because of pain, and motor deficits associated with metastasis to the spine.

h. **Self-care deficit** related to impaired physical mobility, pain, and weakness and fatigue.

i. **Constipation** related to decreased fiber and fluid intake associated with anorexia and weakness; decreased ability to respond to the urge to defecate associated with weakened abdominal and perineal muscles resulting from a generalized loss of muscle tone; and decreased gastrointestinal motility associated with decreased activity, the neuromuscular depressant effects of hypercalcemia, use of morphine sulfate, and anxiety.

j. **Sleep pattern disturbance** related to decreased physical activity, fear, anxiety, unfamiliar environment, and bone pain.

k. **Potential complication: pathologic fractures** related to disuse osteoporosis associated with prolonged immobility and the bone destruction associated with bone metastasis.

l. **Disturbance in self-concept** related to dependence on others to meet basic needs, feeling of powerlessness associated with inability to control disease process, and changes in body function.

m. **Grieving** related to loss of control over her life and usual body processes, changes in body image, loss of significant others, and imminent death.

n. **Altered family processes** related to excessive anxiety, anticipatory grief, disorganization and role changes within the family unit, an inadequate support system, and exhaustion associated with long-term home care of the dying client.

It is also determined that the following nursing and collaborative diagnoses and etiological factors from the care plan on Cancer of the Breast are appropriate. You will note that the etiological factors have been modified to reflect Mary's situation.

a. **Altered nutrition: less than body requirements** related to decreased oral intake associated with anorexia, elevated metabolic rate associated with the disease process, utilization of available nutrients by the malignant cells rather than the host, and an inefficient utilization of nutrients associated with the disease process.

b. **Activity intolerance** related to tissue hypoxia associated with anemia and decreased cardiac output (results from prolonged immobility), inadequate nutritional status, and inability to rest and sleep associated with prolonged physiological and psychological stress.

c. **Fatigue** related to inability to rest and sleep associated with discomfort; anxiety and depression associated with terminal state; and increased energy expenditure associated with an increase in the basal metabolic rate resulting from continuous, active tumor growth.

8. **Modify the outcome criteria so that they are achievable and realistic for your client. Establish appropriate target dates.**

   See the example presented on pages xxi and xxii.

9. **Select from the list of nursing actions those that are relevant to the client's care. Add to or modify the actions to meet the needs of your particular client. Include relevant medications, treatments, particular client wishes, and actions that will facilitate the achievement of the desired client outcomes.**

   See the example presented on pages xxi and xxii.

10. **Set priorities for the nursing/collaborative diagnoses using your usual system (e.g. Maslow's hierarchy, basic needs).**

    Given that Mary is terminal, the top 4 priorities are:
    1. Pain: right hip and back
    2. Grieving
    3. Constipation
    4. Altered family processes

    Based on the data presented, the following example demonstrates the individualization of the etiology, desired outcome, and nursing actions for the nursing diagnosis **Constipation**.

1. **Data available based on case study:**
   States has not had bowel movement for 6 days
   Bowel sounds present and hypoactive
   Physician's orders: MOM 30 cc qhs prn—taking every evening
                         Dialose 1 capsule q.d.
   Abdomen firm and distended
   Serum calcium moderately elevated
   Bedridden for 3 weeks
   Consuming only 10% of meals
   States usually has a bowel movement q.o.d. after breakfast
   Bedrest
   Receiving morphine sulfate every 2 hours
2. **Individualization of nursing diagnosis statement:**
   (Note that some or parts of the etiological statements from the standardized nursing care plan are omitted if they do not apply to this case study.)

STANDARDIZED	INDIVIDUALIZED
(from Immobility Care Plan)	
Constipation related to:	**Constipation** related to:
a. decreased intake of fluid and food high in fiber;	a. decreased fiber and fluid intake associated with anorexia and weakness;

STANDARDIZED	INDIVIDUALIZED
b. reluctance to use bedpan;	b. omit—etiological factor not applicable to this case study;
c. weakened abdominal and perineal muscles associated with generalized loss of muscle tone resulting from prolonged immobility;	c. weakened abdominal and perineal muscles associated with generalized loss of muscle tone resulting from prolonged immobility;
d. decreased gastrointestinal motility associated with decreased activity, the neuromuscular depressant effects of hypercalcemia if present, and increased sympathetic nervous system activity resulting from anxiety.	d. decreased gastrointestinal motility associated with decreased activity, the neuromuscular depressant effects of hypercalcemia, and increased sympathetic nervous system activity resulting from anxiety.

(from Terminal Care Plan)

Constipation related to:

STANDARDIZED	INDIVIDUALIZED
a. bedrest;	a. bedrest;
b. decreased fluid and fiber intake associated with anorexia, dysphagia, and difficulty feeding self;	b. decreased fluid and fiber intake associated with anorexia;
c. use of some medications (e.g. opiates, antacids containing aluminum or calcium);	c. use of morphine sulfate;
d. long-term use of laxatives;	d. omit—no supporting data;
e. decreased ability to respond to the urge to defecate associated with weak abdominal musculature and decreased level of consciousness;	e. decreased ability to respond to the urge to defecate associated with weak abdominal musculature;
f. increased sympathetic nervous system activity resulting from anxiety;	f. increased sympathetic nervous system activity resulting from anxiety;
g. obstruction of bowel associated with the underlying disease process.	g. omit—etiological factor not applicable to this case study.

3. **Individualization of desired outcome:**

STANDARDIZED	INDIVIDUALIZED
(from Immobility Care Plan) The client will maintain usual bowel elimination pattern.	Mary will have a soft; formed stool at least every other day.
(from Terminal Care Plan) The client will maintain a bowel routine that provides optimal comfort.	Mary will have a soft, formed stool at least every other day.

4. **Individualization of nursing actions and selected rationales:**

STANDARDIZED	INDIVIDUALIZED
(from Immobility Care Plan) a. Ascertain client's usual bowel habits.	a. Omit action—bowel habits already known.
b. Assess and record bowel movements including frequency, consistency, and shape.	b. Assess and record bowel movements including frequency, consistency, and shape.
c. Assess for signs and symptoms that may accompany constipation such as headache, anorexia, nausea, ab-	c. Assess for signs and symptoms that may accompany constipation such as headache, anorexia, nausea, ab-

STANDARDIZED	INDIVIDUALIZED
dominal distention and cramping, and feeling of fullness or pressure in abdomen or rectum.	dominal distention and cramping, or feeling of fullness or pressure in abdomen or rectum.
d. Assess bowel sounds. Report a pattern of decreasing bowel sounds.	d. Assess bowel sounds. Report a pattern of decreasing bowel sounds.
e. Implement measures *to prevent constipation:*	e. Implement measures to control Mary's constipation:
1. encourage client to defecate whenever the urge is felt	1. encourage Mary to defecate whenever the urge is felt
2. place client in high Fowler's position for bowel movements unless contraindicated; provide privacy and adequate ventilation	2. place Mary on bedpan in high Fowler's position 30 minutes after breakfast; provide privacy and open room window
3. encourage client to relax during attempts to defecate *in order to promote relaxation of the levator ani muscle and the external anal sphincter*	3. encourage relaxation during defecation attempts by turning on radio*
4. instruct client to select foods high in fiber (e.g. nuts, bran, whole grains, raw fruits and vegetables, dried fruits)	4. offer bran cereal and fresh fruit for breakfast; encourage her to select foods high in fiber for lunch and dinner
5. instruct client to maintain a minimum fluid intake of 2500 cc/day unless contraindicated	5. encourage a minimum fluid intake of 2500 cc/day; offer 200 cc of apple or orange juice or water every hour while awake
6. encourage client to drink warm liquids *to stimulate peristalsis*	6. offer hot tea with breakfast
7. perform actions to maintain serum calcium levels within normal range (see Collaborative Diagnosis 5, action b)	7. assist her to select a diet low in calcium
8. encourage client to perform isometric abdominal strengthening exercises unless contraindicated	8. omit—not applicable to case study
9. increase activity as allowed	9. omit—not applicable to case study
10. monitor for therapeutic and nontherapetutic effects of laxatives, suppositories, stool softeners, and/or enemas if administered.	10. consult physician about increasing dose of Dialose
	11. administer Milk of Magnesia 30 cc p.o. each evening.
f. Check for impaction if client has not had a bowel movement in 3 days, he/she is passing liquid stool, or if other signs and symptoms of constipation are present. Administer oil retention and/or cleansing enemas as ordered followed by digital removal of stool if necessary.	f. Check for impaction if Mary has not had a bowel movement in 3 days, is passing liquid stool, or if other signs and symptoms of constipation are present.

---

* The italicized information from the standardized action represents rationale and is omitted here. It should be placed in the rationale column of an individualized care plan.

STANDARDIZED	INDIVIDUALIZED
(from Terminal Care Plan)	
a. Establish a routine time for defecation based on client's usual bowel elimination pattern.	a. Place Mary on bedpan 30 minutes after breakfast.
b. Perform actions to reduce fear and anxiety (see Nursing Diagnosis 1, actions b and c).	b. Perform actions to reduce fear and anxiety (a few individualized actions from Nursing Diagnosis 1 in Terminal Care Plan would be included here).
c. Assist client to toilet or commode for bowel movements unless contraindicated.	c. Omit—not applicable to case study.
d. Assist with titration of laxative agents (e.g. combination of a stool softener and bulk-forming agent or lubricant wth a peristaltic stimulant).	d. Administer Dialose 1 capsule qam and Milk of Magnesia 30 cc qhs.
e. If client is on antacid therapy, consult physician about alternating those containing aluminum or calcium with those containing magnesium.	e. Omit—not applicable to case study.
f. If an oil retention enema is ordered, administer it using tap water enema equipment and technique *in order to reach a higher level in the bowel and increase effectiveness.*	f. Omit—not ordered.

5. Individualized Care Plan for Mary for the nursing diagnosis Constipation:

Data	Nursing Diagnosis	Desired Outcome	Nursing Actions

States has not had a bowel movement for 6 days
Bowel sounds present and hypoactive
Physician's order:
  MOM 30 cc qhs prn—taking every evening
  Dialose 1 capsule q.d.
Abdomen firm and distended
Serum calcium moderately elevated
Bedridden for 3 weeks
Consuming only 10% of meals
States usually has bowel movement q.o.d. after breakfast
Activity—bedrest and requires assistance with all activities
Receiving morphine sulfate every two hours
	Constipation related to:
	a. decreased fiber and fluid intake associated with anorexia and weakness;
	b. decreased ability to respond to the urge to defecate associated with weak abdominal and perineal muscles resulting from a generalized loss of muscle tone;
	c. decreased gastrointestinal motility associated with decreased activity, the neuromuscular depressant effects of hypercalcemia, use of morphine sulfate, and anxiety.
		Mary will have a soft, formed stool at least every other day.	1. Assess and record bowel movements including frequency, consistency, and shape.
			2. Assess for signs and symptoms that may accompany constipation such as headache, anorexia, nausea, abdominal distention and cramping, or feeling of fullness or pressure in abdomen or rectum.
			3. Assess bowel sounds. Report a pattern of decreasing bowel sounds.
			4. Implement measures to control Mary's constipation:
			  a. encourage Mary to defecate whenever the urge is felt
			  b. place Mary on bedpan in high Fowler's position 30 minutes after breakfast; provide privacy and open room window
			  c. encourage relaxation during defecation attempts by turning on radio
			  d. offer bran cereal and fresh fruit for breakfast; encourage her to select foods high in fiber for lunch and dinner
			  e. encourage minimum fluid intake of 2500 cc/day; offer 200 cc of apple or orange juice or water every hour while awake

Data	Nursing Diagnosis	Desired Outcome	Nursing Actions
			f. offer hot tea with breakfast
			g. assist her to select a diet low in calcium
			h. administer Dialose 1 capsule qam
			i. administer Milk of Magnesia 30 cc p.o. each evening
			j. perform actions to reduce fear and anxiety (e.g. allow family to spend time with her, control discomfort).
			5. Check for impaction if Mary has not had a bowel movement in 3 days, is passing liquid stool, or if other signs and symptoms of constipation are present.

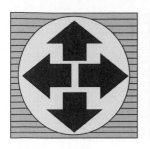 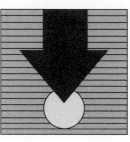 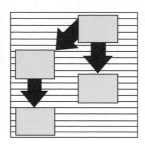 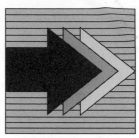 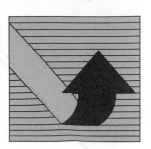

Unit I

Nursing Care of the Elderly Client

  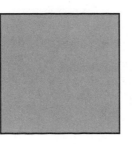 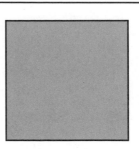 

The Elderly Client

The elderly client is a common recipient of health care in the United States today because of the marked shift in the age distribution of the population. Older persons are in the final stage of development, the stage during which many adaptations have to be made by the client because of inevitable degenerative physiological changes that occur with aging. These changes are associated with processes such as a decrease in the number and atrophy of body cells and/or deposition of substances such as lipofuscin, calcium, and collagen in certain tissues and organs. The extent or degree of changes that occur depends on genetic and environmental factors as well as on the client's previous attention to health maintenance. As a client reaches old age, there may also be many changes in roles, relationships, and ability to maintain his/her usual life style. These factors create certain unique psychosocial concerns that need to be addressed.

This care plan focuses on the elderly client hospitalized for management of a medical-surgical condition. It includes the nursing diagnoses that reflect the biopsychosocial changes that commonly occur with old age and are intensified with the stressors of acute illness and hospitalization. This care plan should be used in conjunction with the appropriate medical and/or surgical care plans in this text.

NURSING/COLLABORATIVE DIAGNOSES

1. Anxiety ☐ *3*
2. Altered systemic tissue perfusion ☐ *4*
3. Altered respiratory function:
    a. ineffective breathing patterns
    b. ineffective airway clearance
    c. impaired gas exchange ☐ *6*
4. Altered fluid volume: dehydration (usually intracellular) ☐ *7*
5A. Altered nutrition: less than body requirements ☐ *8*
5B. Altered nutrition: more than body requirements ☐ *9*
6A. Altered comfort: dyspepsia, gastric fullness, and/or gas pain ☐ *10*
6B. Altered comfort: joint pain and/or stiffness ☐ *11*
7. Sensory perceptual alterations: visual disturbances (e.g. decreased visual acuity, inability to adjust to changes in lighting, decreased peripheral vision); taste alterations; and diminished hearing, sense of smell, and tactile sensation ☐ *12*
8. Impaired skin integrity: irritation and breakdown ☐ *13*
9. Altered oral mucous membrane: dryness ☐ *14*
10. Activity intolerance ☐ *15*
11. Impaired physical mobility ☐ *16*
12. Self-care deficit ☐ *16*
13. Altered patterns of urinary elimination:
    a. frequency
    b. urgency
    c. retention
    d. incontinence ☐ *17*
14. Constipation ☐ *19*
15. Altered thought processes: slowed verbal responses, decline in memory (especially short term), and/or decline in abstract reasoning ☐ *20*
16. Sleep pattern disturbance ☐ *21*
17. Potential for infection ☐ *22*
18. Potential for trauma ☐ *23*
19. Potential for aspiration ☐ *24*

20. Potential complications:
    a. pathologic fractures
    b. thromboembolism □ 25
21. Sexual dysfunction:
    a. decreased libido
    b. dyspareunia
    c. impotence □ 27
22. Disturbance in self-concept □ 28
23. Powerlessness □ 29
24. Social isolation □ 30
25. Noncompliance □ 30
26. Altered family processes □ 31

□ ▬▬▬▬▬▬▬▬▬▬▬▬▬▬▬▬▬▬▬▬▬▬▬▬▬

1. NURSING DIAGNOSIS

Anxiety related to unfamiliar environment; signs and symptoms of current diagnosis; lack of understanding of diagnostic tests, diagnosis, and treatment plan; financial concerns; and effects of diagnosis on health status, ability to perform usual roles, and to live independently.

□ ▬▬▬▬▬▬▬▬▬▬▬▬▬▬▬▬▬▬▬▬▬▬▬▬▬

DESIRED OUTCOMES	NURSING ACTIONS AND *SELECTED RATIONALES*

1. The client will experience a reduction in fear and anxiety as evidenced by:
   a. verbalization of feeling less anxious or fearful
   b. relaxed facial expression and body movements
   c. stable vital signs
   d. usual skin color
   e. verbalization of an understanding of hospital routines, diagnostic tests, diagnosis, and treatment plan.

1.a. Assess client for signs and symptoms of fear and anxiety (e.g. verbalization of fears and concerns; tenseness; tremors; irritability; restlessness; diaphoresis; tachypnea; tachycardia; increase in blood pressure; facial tension, pallor, or flushing; noncompliance with treatment plan). Validate perceptions carefully, remembering that sympathetic responses are often diminished in the elderly.
   b. Ascertain effectiveness of current coping skills.
   c. Implement measures *to reduce fear and anxiety:*
      1. orient to hospital environment, equipment, and routines
      2. introduce staff who will be participating in his/her care; if possible, maintain consistency in staff assigned to his/her care *in order to provide feelings of stability and comfort with the environment*
      3. assure client that staff members are nearby; respond to call signal as soon as possible
      4. maintain a calm, unhurried, confident manner when interacting with client
      5. encourage verbalization of fear and anxiety; provide feedback
      6. explain all diagnostic tests
      7. reinforce physician's explanations and clarify any misconceptions client may have about his/her diagnosis, treatment plan, and prognosis
      8. allow client time to adjust psychologically to planned procedures
      9. provide a calm, restful environment
      10. perform actions to reduce discomfort (see Nursing Diagnoses 6.A, action 3 and 6.B, action 5)
      11. instruct in relaxation techniques and encourage participation in diversional activities
      12. assist client to identify specific stressors and ways to cope with them
      13. encourage significant others to project a caring, concerned attitude without obvious anxiousness
      14. if surgical intervention is indicated, begin preoperative teaching
      15. encourage client to discuss his/her concerns about the cost of health care and about future living situation; obtain a social service consult to

assist client with financial planning and finding an alternative living situation if client will be unable to live alone following discharge
16. monitor for therapeutic and nontherapeutic effects of antianxiety agents if administered; administer these agents cautiously *because the metabolism, distribution, and excretion of drugs is often altered in the elderly.*
   d. Include significant others in orientation and teaching sessions and encourage their continued support of the client.
   e. Provide information based on current needs of client and significant others at a level they can understand. Encourage questions and clarification of information provided.
   f. Consult physician if above actions fail to control fear and anxiety.

2. NURSING DIAGNOSIS

Altered systemic tissue perfusion related to:

a. decreased cardiac output associated with:
   1. decreased contractile strength of the myocardium resulting from increased stiffness and reduced compliance of the myocardium
   2. increased cardiac workload resulting from an increase in total vascular resistance and thickened and rigid cardiac valves;
b. increased total vascular resistance associated with loss of elasticity and narrowing of vessels resulting from degeneration of elastin, changes in collagen deposition, and accumulation of substances such as calcium and lipids;
c. peripheral pooling of blood associated with decreased venous return resulting from loss of muscle tone in extremities and venous dilation (due to decreased efficiency of venous valves).

DESIRED OUTCOMES	NURSING ACTIONS AND *SELECTED RATIONALES*

2. The client will maintain adequate systemic tissue perfusion as evidenced by:
a. B/P and pulse within normal range for client
b. decline in systolic B/P less than 15 mm Hg with upright position change
c. unlabored respirations at 16–20/minute
d. usual mental status
e. absence of lightheadedness or syncope
f. skin warm and usual color
g. palpable peripheral pulses
h. capillary refill time less than 3 seconds
i. BUN and serum creatinine and alkaline phosphatase within normal limits for an elderly client
j. urine output at least 30 cc/hour.
	2.a. Assess for and report the following:
	1. signs and symptoms that may specifically indicate a decrease in cardiac output:
	  a. narrowing pulse pressure (a widened pulse pressure is often present in elderly clients *because of isolated systolic hypertension*)
	  b. irregular pulse (be aware that the incidence of arrhythmias increases with age *because the myocardium is more irritable* and that arrhythmias are of concern *because of decreased cardiac reserve*)
	  c. muffled heart sounds
	  d. increase in loudness of existing systolic murmurs or presence of diastolic murmur (soft systolic murmurs are often present in elderly clients *because of sclerosed valves*)
	  e. development of or an increase in loudness of S_3 and/or S_4 gallop rhythms (an S_4 can be present in a healthy elderly client)
	  f. increased crackles and further decrease in or absent breath sounds (crackles and slightly diminished breath sounds in the morning are a usual finding in an elderly client)
	  g. peripheral edema, distended neck veins, ascites
	  h. persistent or marked weight gain
	  i. abnormal EKG readings (expected age-related changes include left axis deviation, some prolongation of all conduction intervals, and lower voltage of waves)
	  j. chest x-ray results showing cardiomegaly, pleural effusion, or pulmonary edema
	2. signs and symptoms of diminished systemic tissue perfusion:
	  a. significant decrease in B/P (elevated systolic and diastolic pressures are

often present in elderly clients *because of increased rigidity of the aorta and a generalized increase in peripheral vascular resistance*)
- b. further increase in B/P and a significant increase in pulse rate (*may indicate the body's attempt to compensate for diminished tissue perfusion*; note that pulse rate tends to be low-normal in the elderly client *because of increased vagal tone*)
- c. decline in systolic B/P of greater than 20 mm Hg when client changes from a lying to sitting or standing position (in an elderly client, there is often a decline in systolic B/P of 10–15 mm Hg with upright position change *because of a decrease in baroreceptor sensitivity*)
- d. rapid or labored respirations
- e. restlessness, confusion
- f. lightheadedness, syncope
- g. cool, pale, mottled, or cyanotic skin
- h. diminished or absent peripheral pulses
- i. capillary refill time greater than 3 seconds
- j. elevated BUN (BUN tends to be slightly elevated [21–22 mg/dl] *because of the age-related decline in renal function*)
- k. elevated serum creatinine and alkaline phosphatase
- l. urine output less than 30 cc/hour.
- b. Implement measures to *maintain adequate systemic tissue perfusion:*
  - 1. perform actions *to reduce cardiac workload:*
    - a. maintain client in a semi- to high Fowler's position if allowed
    - b. instruct client to avoid activities that create a Valsalva response (e.g. straining to have a bowel movement, bending at the waist, holding breath while moving)
    - c. implement measures to promote rest (see Nursing Diagnosis 10, action b.1)
    - d. implement measures to maintain an adequate respiratory status (see Nursing Diagnosis 3, action e) *in order to promote adequate tissue oxygenation*
    - e. discourage smoking (*smoking has a cardiostimulatory effect, causes vasoconstriction, and reduces oxygen availability*)
    - f. provide frequent, small meals rather than 3 large ones (*large meals require an increase in blood supply to gastrointestinal tract for digestion*)
    - g. discourage intake of foods/fluids high in caffeine such as coffee, tea, chocolate, and colas (*caffeine is a myocardial stimulant and increases oxygen consumption*)
    - h. increase activity gradually
  - 2. perform actions to prevent or treat dehydration (see Nursing Diagnosis 4, action c)
  - 3. perform actions *to reduce peripheral pooling of blood and increase venous return:*
    - a. instruct client in and assist with range of motion exercises at least every 4 hours
    - b. consult physician about order for antiembolic hose or elastic wraps; if applied, make sure they are not applied too tightly and remove for 30–60 minutes every shift
    - c. if client is on bedrest:
      - 1. elevate foot of bed for 20-minute intervals several times a shift unless contraindicated
      - 2. assist with intermittent venous compression using pneumatic cuffs or boots if ordered
    - d. encourage ambulation as allowed and tolerated
  - 4. instruct and assist client to change positions slowly *in order to allow autoregulatory mechanisms to adjust to position change*
  - 5. discourage positions that compromise blood flow in extremities (e.g. crossing legs, pillows under knees, use of knee gatch, sitting for long periods, prolonged standing)
  - 6. maintain a comfortable room temperature and provide client with adequate clothing and blankets (*exposure to cold causes generalized vasoconstriction*)
  - 7. instruct client in the benefits of regular isotonic exercise (e.g. walking, biking, swimming) following discharge to maintain cardiovascular health.
- c. Consult physician if signs and symptoms of diminished systemic tissue perfusion persist or worsen.

☐ ▬▬▬▬▬▬▬▬▬▬▬▬▬▬▬▬▬▬▬

3. NURSING DIAGNOSIS

Altered respiratory function:*

a. **ineffective breathing patterns** related to:
   1. fear and anxiety
   2. loss of alveolar elasticity and presence of flattened diaphragm
   3. decreased chest expansion associated with calcification of costal cartilage and weakened respiratory muscles
   4. decreased responsiveness of chemoreceptors to hypoxia and hypercapnea;
b. **ineffective airway clearance** related to stasis of secretions associated with decreased ciliary activity, reduced cough effectiveness, and decreased mobility;
c. **impaired gas exchange** related to:
   1. ineffective breathing patterns and airway clearance
   2. loss of effective lung surface associated with changes in alveolar walls and septal tissue
   3. reduced airflow associated with loss of alveolar elasticity
   4. decreased pulmonary tissue perfusion (especially in bases) associated with a decreased number of alveolar capillaries, changes in pulmonary arteries, and decreased cardiac output.

---

* This diagnostic label includes the following nursing diagnoses: ineffective breathing pattern, ineffective airway clearance, and impaired gas exchange (Carpenito, 1989).

☐ ▬▬▬▬▬▬▬▬▬▬▬▬▬▬▬▬▬▬▬

DESIRED OUTCOMES	NURSING ACTIONS AND *SELECTED RATIONALES*

3. The client will experience adequate respiratory function as evidenced by:
a. usual rate, rhythm, and depth of respirations
b. absence of dyspnea
c. usual or improved breath sounds
d. usual mental status
e. usual skin color
f. blood gases within normal range for an elderly client.
	3.a. Assess for and report signs and symptoms of altered respiratory function:
	  1. rapid, shallow, slow, or irregular respirations
	  2. dyspnea, orthopnea
	  3. use of accessory muscles when breathing
	  4. adventitious breath sounds (e.g. crackles, rhonchi); crackles may be heard especially on initial morning assessment *as a result of some alveolar collapse associated with decreased activity and the resultant hypoventilation*
	  5. diminished or absent breath sounds (diminished sounds are often present in the elderly client *because of the reduced airflow associated with loss of alveolar elasticity*)
	  6. restlessness, irritability
	  7. confusion, somnolence
	  8. dusky or cyanotic skin color.
	b. Monitor blood gases. Report abnormal results. (Be aware that oxygen saturation and PaO_2 are normally lower in the elderly client.)
	c. Monitor for and report abnormal ear oximetry and capnograph results, remembering that oxygen saturation is normally lower in the elderly client.
	d. Monitor chest x-ray results and report abnormalities.
	e. Implement measures *to maintain an adequate respiratory status:*
	  1. perform actions to reduce fear and anxiety (see Nursing Diagnosis 1, action c)
	  2. place client in a semi- to high Fowler's position; position overbed table so client can lean on it if desired
	  3. if client is on bedrest, assist him/her to turn every 2 hours
	  4. instruct client to deep breathe or use inspiratory exerciser at least every 2 hours

5. perform actions *to facilitate removal of pulmonary secretions:*
   a. instruct and assist client to cough every 1–2 hours
   b. implement measures *to liquefy secretions:*
      1. maintain a fluid intake of at least 2500 cc/day unless contraindicated
      2. consult physician about an order for humidifying air or administering mucolytic agents via nebulizer or IPPB treatment if secretions appear copious or tenacious
   c. assist with or perform postural drainage, percussion, and vibration if ordered
   d. consult physician about an order for an expectorant and/or suctioning if indicated
6. discourage smoking (*smoking irritates the respiratory tract, causes an increase in mucus production, further impairs ciliary function, and decreases oxygen availability*)
7. maintain oxygen therapy as ordered (low-flow oxygen is often ordered *because elderly clients are more susceptible to oxygen-induced respiratory depression and CO_2 narcosis as a result of their physiological adjustment to lower oxygen levels*)
8. instruct client to avoid gas-forming foods/fluids (e.g. beans, cabbage, cauliflower, onions, carbonated beverages) and large meals *in order to prevent gastric distention and pressure on the diaphragm*
9. increase activity as allowed and tolerated
10. administer central nervous system depressants (e.g. narcotic analgesics, sedatives, muscle relaxants) judiciously *because of their respiratory depressant effects* (the possibility of respiratory depression is increased in elderly clients *because of their altered metabolism, distribution, and excretion of drugs*); hold medication and consult physician if respiratory rate is less than 12/minute
11. instruct client in the benefits of a regular exercise program following discharge to maintain adequate respiratory function.

f. Consult physician if signs and symptoms of impaired respiratory function persist or worsen.

4. NURSING DIAGNOSIS

Altered fluid volume: dehydration (usually intracellular) related to:

a. a reduced number of metabolically active cells;
b. increase in body fat (fat is low in water content);
c. decreased fluid intake associated with diminished thirst sensation and attempt to avoid nocturia and/or incontinence;
d. increased water loss associated with decreased ability of kidneys to concentrate urine.

DESIRED OUTCOMES	NURSING ACTIONS AND *SELECTED RATIONALES*
4. The client will not experience dehydration as evidenced by: a. normal skin turgor for client b. moist mucous membranes c. weight loss no greater than 0.5 kg/day	4.a. Assess for factors that may precipitate dehydration (e.g. fluid restrictions, nausea, desire to avoid nocturia or incontinence, decreased level of consciousness, inability to feed self). b. Assess for and report signs and symptoms of dehydration: 1. decreased skin turgor (not always a reliable indicator *because decreased skin turgor is a normal age-related change;* turgor is best assessed over the forehead or sternum in an elderly client)

d. B/P and pulse within normal range for client with no further increase in orthostatic hypotension
e. serum osmolality, Hct., and sodium levels within normal range
f. balanced intake and output
g. urine specific gravity between 1.010 and 1.025.

2. dry mucous membranes, thirst (may not be reliable indicators *because saliva production and sensation of thirst are diminished in elderly clients*)
3. weight loss greater than 0.5 kg/day
4. low B/P and/or decline in systolic B/P of greater than 20 mm Hg when client sits up (not a reliable indicator of fluid volume unless compared with client's baseline B/P *because orthostatic hypotension often occurs in elderly clients*)
5. weak, rapid pulse
6. elevated serum osmolality, Hct., and sodium levels
7. output less than intake with urine specific gravity higher than 1.025 (reflects an actual rather than potential water deficit).

c. Implement measures *to prevent or treat dehydration:*
1. maintain a fluid intake of at least 2500 cc/day and instruct client to adhere to this at home unless contraindicated
2. maintain intravenous fluid therapy if ordered (administer intravenous fluids cautiously *because the elderly client is also at risk for fluid overload*).

d. Consult physician if signs and symptoms of dehydration persist or worsen.

5.A. NURSING DIAGNOSIS

Altered nutrition: less than body requirements related to:

1. decreased oral intake associated with:
   a. anorexia resulting from:
      1. depression, fear, and anxiety
      2. fatigue and discomfort
      3. decreased metabolic rate
      4. taste alterations due to a decreased number and/or sensitivity of taste buds and a decreased volume of saliva
      5. early satiety due to delayed esophageal and gastric emptying
      6. constipation
   b. dyspepsia
   c. dislike of prescribed diet;
2. decreased utilization of nutrients associated with:
   a. impaired digestion resulting from:
      1. decreased ability to chew foods thoroughly due to erosion or loss of teeth or ill-fitting dentures
      2. reduced secretion of digestive enzymes (e.g. salivary ptyalin, hydrochloric acid, pepsin, lipase)
   b. reduced absorption of nutrients resulting from decreased gastric acidity, atrophy of absorptive cells in the small and large intestine, and decreased intestinal blood flow
   c. decreased ability of liver to store nutrients;
3. decreased ability of liver to synthesize proteins.

DESIRED OUTCOMES	NURSING ACTIONS AND *SELECTED RATIONALES*
5.A. The client will maintain an adequate nutritional status as evidenced by: 1. weight within normal range for client's age, height, and build 2. normal BUN and serum	5.A.1. Assess client for signs and symptoms of malnutrition: a. weight below normal for client's age, height, and build b. abnormal BUN (may be elevated slightly *as a result of the age-related decline in renal function*) c. low serum albumin, protein, Hct., Hgb., cholesterol, and lymphocytes (albumin, Hct., Hgb., and lymphocytes may be low-normal *as a result of an age-related decrease in production*)

albumin, protein, Hct.,
Hgb., cholesterol, and
lymphocyte levels for
client's age
3. triceps skinfold
measurements within
normal range for client's
age
4. usual strength and
activity tolerance
5. healthy oral mucous
membrane
6. smooth nails and healthy
skin and hair.

    d. triceps skinfold measurement less than normal for build and age
    e. weakness and fatigue
    f. stomatitis
    g. smooth tongue
    h. ridged nails, scaling skin, unusual hair loss.
2. Reassess nutritional status on a regular basis and report a decline.
3. Monitor percentage of meals eaten.
4. Assess client to determine causes of inadequate intake (e.g. dyspepsia, anorexia).
5. Implement measures *to maintain an adequate nutritional status:*
    a. perform actions *to improve oral intake:*
      1. implement measures to relieve dyspepsia, gastric fullness, and gas pain (see Nursing Diagnosis 6.A, action 3)
      2. provide oral care before meals
      3. eliminate noxious stimuli from environment
      4. serve small portions of nutritious foods/fluids that are appealing to the client
      5. provide a clean, relaxed, pleasant environment
      6. obtain a dietary consult if necessary to assist client in selecting foods/fluids that meet nutritional needs as well as preferences
      7. place client in a high Fowler's position for meals *to promote gastroesophageal emptying and reduce feeling of fullness*
      8. encourage a rest period before meals *to minimize fatigue*
      9. if client has dentures, assist him/her to put them in before meals
     10. provide a soft, ground, or pureed diet if client has difficulty chewing
     11. implement measures *to compensate for taste alterations and/or dislike of prescribed diet:*
        a. serve foods warm *to stimulate sense of smell*
        b. encourage client to experiment with different flavorings and seasonings
        c. instruct client to use salt substitutes if he/she is on a low-sodium diet
        d. provide hard candy or gum before meals *to stimulate salivation and thereby improve taste sensation*
        e. encourage client to add extra sweeteners to foods unless contraindicated
     12. encourage significant others to bring in client's favorite foods and eat with him/her *to make eating more of a familiar social experience*
     13. allow adequate time for meals; reheat food if necessary
     14. increase activity as tolerated (*activity stimulates appetite*)
     15. implement measures to prevent constipation (see Nursing Diagnosis 14, action e)
    b. ensure that meals are well balanced and high in essential nutrients; offer high-protein supplements between meals if client is having difficulty maintaining an adequate caloric intake
    c. monitor for therapeutic and nontherapeutic effects of vitamins, minerals, and hematinics if administered.
6. Perform a 72-hour calorie count if nutritional status declines.
7. Consult physician regarding alternative methods of providing nutrition (e.g. parenteral nutrition, tube feedings) if client does not consume enough food or fluids to meet nutritional needs.

5.B. NURSING DIAGNOSIS

Altered nutrition: more than body requirements related to a caloric intake that exceeds metabolic needs (with advancing age, there is a decrease in basal metabolic rate and often a decline in activity, which results in decreased metabolic needs).

DESIRED OUTCOMES	NURSING ACTIONS AND *SELECTED RATIONALES*

5.B. The client will have proper balance between caloric intake and metabolic needs as evidenced by:
1. weight declining toward normal range for client's age, height, and build
2. decrease in size of triceps skinfold measurements.

5.B.1. Assess client for signs indicating that caloric intake has exceeded metabolic needs:
    a. weight at least 10–20% over ideal weight for age, height, and build
    b. triceps skinfold measurement greater than normal for build.
2. Reassess nutritional status on a regular basis (every 3–5 days) and report an increase in weight and size of triceps skinfold.
3. Monitor the amount and type of foods/fluids consumed to determine if intake appears excessive in relation to level of activity.
4. Implement measures *to maintain proper balance between caloric intake and metabolic needs:*
    a. perform actions *to assist client to reduce caloric intake:*
      1. maintain caloric restrictions if ordered
      2. obtain a dietary consult to assist client to select foods/fluids that meet caloric restrictions, nutritional needs, and personal preferences
      3. provide sugarless gum or candy and low-calorie snacks between meals
      4. if significant others are bringing client food, encourage them to select items that are low in calories and have some nutritive value
      5. encourage diversional activities between meals *to help reduce client's tendency to snack*
    b. increase activity as allowed and tolerated
    c. provide instructions regarding recommended caloric intake and exercise level following discharge.
5. Consult physician if client gains weight despite implementation of the above measures.

6.A. NURSING DIAGNOSIS

Altered comfort: dyspepsia, gastric fullness, and/or gas pain related to:

1. impaired digestion of many foods associated with reduced secretion of digestive enzymes (e.g. hydrochloric acid, pepsin, lipase);
2. irritation of gastric mucosa associated with a reduction in the number of epithelial cells and reduced secretion of alkaline mucus resulting from gastric atrophy;
3. delayed esophageal and gastric emptying.

DESIRED OUTCOMES	NURSING ACTIONS AND *SELECTED RATIONALES*

6.A. The client will experience diminished dyspepsia, gastric fullness, and gas pain as evidenced by:
1. verbalization of same
2. relaxed facial expression
3. diminished eructation.

6.A.1. Assess for nonverbal signs of dyspepsia, gastric fullness, and gas pain (e.g. clutching and guarding of abdomen, rubbing epigastric area, restlessness, reluctance to move, grimacing, frequent eructation, reluctance to eat).
2. Assess for verbal complaints of indigestion, fullness, and gas pain.
3. Implement measures *to reduce dyspepsia, gastric fullness, and gas pain:*
    a. perform actions *to reduce gastroesophageal reflux:*
      1. provide small, frequent meals rather than 3 large ones
      2. instruct client to ingest foods and fluids slowly
      3. maintain client in high Fowler's position during and for at least 30 minutes after meals and snacks
    b. instruct client to avoid foods/fluids that irritate gastric mucosa (e.g. spicy foods; citrus fruits or juices; caffeine-containing items such as chocolate, coffee, tea, or colas)
    c. perform actions *to reduce accumulation of gas in gastrointestinal tract:*

1. encourage and assist client with frequent position change and ambulation as allowed and tolerated (*activity stimulates peristalsis*)
2. instruct client to avoid activities such as gum-chewing, sucking on hard candy, and smoking *in order to reduce air swallowing*
3. encourage client to drink warm liquids *in order to stimulate peristalsis*
4. instruct client to avoid gas-producing foods/fluids (e.g. cabbage, onions, popcorn, baked beans, carbonated beverages) and fried foods
5. encourage client to eructate and expel flatus whenever the urge is felt
   d. monitor for therapeutic and nontherapeutic effects of the following medications if administered:
      1. antacids and mucosal barrier fortifiers (e.g. sucralfate) *to protect the gastric mucosa*
      2. antiflatulents *to reduce gas accumulation*
      3. gastrointestinal stimulants (e.g. metoclopramide) *to increase gastrointestinal motility.*
   4. Consult physician if signs and symptoms of dyspepsia, gastric fullness, or gas pain persist or worsen.

□ ■■■■■■■■■■■■■■■■■■■■■■■■■■■■■

6.B. NURSING DIAGNOSIS

Altered comfort:* joint pain and/or stiffness related to degenerative changes in joint cartilage.

———————————

* In this care plan, the nursing diagnosis "pain" is included under the diagnostic label of altered comfort.

□ ■■■■■■■■■■■■■■■■■■■■■■■■■■■■■

DESIRED OUTCOMES	NURSING ACTIONS AND *SELECTED RATIONALES*

6.B. The client will experience diminished joint discomfort as evidenced by:
1. verbalization of same
2. relaxed facial expression and body positioning
3. increased participation in activities.

6.B.1. Determine how the client usually responds to pain.
2. Assess for nonverbal signs of joint discomfort (e.g. wrinkled brow, clenched fists, reluctance to move, rubbing joints, restlessness). Sympathetic responses to discomfort such as diaphoresis, tachycardia, and changes in B/P are usually not present *because the joint discomfort is not severe and sympathetic responsiveness is often diminished in elderly clients.*
3. Assess verbal complaints of pain. Ask client to be specific regarding location, severity, and type of pain.
4. Assess for factors that seem to aggravate and alleviate joint discomfort.
5. Implement measures *to reduce joint discomfort:*
   a. perform actions *to protect affected joint(s) from trauma, pressure, or excessive movement:*
      1. avoid jarring the bed
      2. use a bed cradle or footboard to relieve pressure of bedding on lower extremities
      3. instruct or assist client to support affected extremity with hands or pillows when changing positions
      4. instruct client to move affected extremity slowly and cautiously
      5. apply a splint to affected joint(s) if indicated
   b. assist with mild exercise of affected joint(s) *to reduce joint stiffness;* encourage gentle circular motions beginning with proximal areas (e.g. hips, shoulders)
   c. consult physician regarding application of heat to affected joint(s)

   d. monitor for therapeutic and nontherapeutic effects of analgesics and nonsteroidal anti-inflammatory agents if administered
   e. instruct client to continue with a mild exercise program and avoid activities that stress weight-bearing joints (e.g. jogging) following discharge.
6. Consult physician if above measures fail to relieve joint discomfort.

□ ▉▉▉▉▉▉▉▉▉▉▉▉▉▉▉▉▉▉▉▉▉▉▉▉▉▉▉▉▉

7. NURSING DIAGNOSIS

Sensory-perceptual alterations: visual disturbances (e.g. decreased visual acuity, inability to adjust to changes in lighting, decreased peripheral vision); taste alterations; and diminished hearing, sense of smell, and tactile sensation related to diminished cell and sensory nerve function.

□ ▉▉▉▉▉▉▉▉▉▉▉▉▉▉▉▉▉▉▉▉▉▉▉▉▉▉▉▉▉

DESIRED OUTCOMES	NURSING ACTIONS AND *SELECTED RATIONALES*

7. The client will demonstrate adaptation to altered sensory-perceptual function as evidenced by:
   a. appropriate verbal and nonverbal responses
   b. expected level of participation in self-care activities and treatment plan
   c. safe responses to environmental stimuli.

7.a. Assess client for the following:
   1. visual disturbances
   2. decreased hearing ability (e.g. speaking loudly, staring at other person's lips during conversation, moving closer to others when they speak, acts of frustration, nodding yes with subsequent inappropriate responses)
   3. altered taste and smell (e.g. statements of same, decreased food intake, heavy use of sugar or seasonings on food)
   4. diminished tactile sensation (e.g. statements of diminished feeling in extremities, holding or touching very hot objects, use of heating pad at higher than expected temperatures).
 b. Implement measures *to assist client to adapt to changes in vision:*
   1. provide adequate lighting in room at all times
   2. avoid bright lighting (*elderly clients often have decreased tolerance of glare*)
   3. avoid sudden changes in light intensity (*elderly clients often adjust more slowly to changes in lighting*)
   4. encourage client to wear his/her glasses
   5. provide auditory rather than visual diversionary activities
   6. inform client of resources available if he/she desires additional information about visual aids (e.g. American Foundation for the Blind, publications such as Aids for the Blind).
 c. If client's hearing is impaired:
   1. assess external auditory canal for excessive cerumen accumulation
   2. implement measures *to facilitate communication:*
      a. provide adequate lighting in room *so client can read lips*
      b. reduce environmental noise
      c. speak slightly louder and more slowly; avoid lowering voice at end of sentences
      d. use simple sentences
      e. avoid overenunciation of words
      f. face client while speaking
      g. avoid chewing gum or eating while talking to client
      h. talk into the less-impaired ear
      i. rephrase sentences when client does not understand
      j. employ related nonverbal cues such as facial expressions or pointing when appropriate
      k. use alternative forms of communication (e.g. flash cards, paper and pencil, magic slate) if indicated
      l. respond to client's call signal in person rather than over intercommunication system
      m. remind client to utilize his/her hearing aid.

d. Implement measures to compensate for taste alterations if present (see Nursing Diagnosis 5.A, action 5.a.11).
e. Implement measures to prevent burns (see Nursing Diagnosis 18, action c) if client has diminished tactile sensation.
f. Instruct client and significant others in above methods of adapting to sensory-perceptual alterations.
g. Consult physician if sensory-perceptual alterations worsen.

8. NURSING DIAGNOSIS

Impaired skin integrity: irritation and breakdown related to:

a. increased fragility of the skin associated with decreased nutritional status, age-related dryness and loss of elasticity (both result from decreased hydration and vascularity of the dermis), and decreased tissue perfusion;
b. frequent contact with irritants if urinary incontinence is present;
c. prolonged pressure on tissues if mobility is decreased (particularly a risk in elderly clients because they tend to have a decreased amount of subcutaneous fat).

DESIRED OUTCOMES	NURSING ACTIONS AND *SELECTED RATIONALES*
8. The client will maintain skin integrity as evidenced by: a. absence of redness and irritation b. no skin breakdown.	8.a. Inspect the skin (especially bone prominences, dependent areas, and perineum) for pallor, redness, and breakdown. b. Implement measures *to maintain skin integrity:* 1. perform actions *to prevent skin breakdown due to decreased mobility:* a. turn client and gently massage over bone prominences and around reddened areas at least every 2 hours (elderly clients may require more frequent position change *because of decreasd tissue perfusion and reduced amounts of protective subcutaneous fat*) b. lift and move client carefully using a turn sheet and adequate assistance *to prevent the linen from shearing the skin* c. instruct or assist client to shift weight every 30 minutes d. if fade time (length of time it takes for reddened area to fade after pressure is removed) is greater than 15 minutes, increase frequency of position changes and provide more effective methods of cushioning, padding, and positioning e. keep skin clean and dry f. keep bed linens wrinkle-free g. provide alternating pressure or eggcrate mattress, flotation pad, sheepskin, and elbow and heel protectors if indicated h. perform actions to maintain an optimal level of mobility (see Nursing Diagnosis 11, action a.2) 2. perform actions *to reduce dryness of the skin:* a. avoid use of harsh soaps and hot water b. apply moisturizers or emollient creams to skin at least once/day c. assist client with total bath or shower every other day rather than daily 3. perform actions *to decrease skin irritation and prevent breakdown resulting from urinary incontinence:* a. perform actions to reduce episodes of urinary incontinence (see Nursing Diagnosis 13, action b.3) b. assist client to thoroughly cleanse and dry perineal area after each episode of incontinence; apply a protective ointment or cream (e.g. Sween cream, Desitin, Karaya gel, A & D ointment, Vaseline) c. use soft tissue to cleanse perineal area d. avoid direct contact of skin with Chux (e.g. place turn sheet or bed pad over Chux)

4. use caution with application of heat or cold to areas of sensory or circulatory impairment
5. maintain an optimal nutritional status (see Nursing Diagnosis 5.A, action 5)
6. perform actions to maintain adequate systemic tissue perfusion (see Nursing Diagnosis 2, action b).

c. If skin breakdown occurs:
1. notify physician
2. continue with above measures to prevent further irritation and breakdown
3. perform decubitus care as ordered or per standard hospital policy
4. monitor client closely and report signs and symptoms of infection (e.g. elevated temperature; redness, warmth, and edema around area of breakdown; unusual drainage from site).

9. NURSING DIAGNOSIS

Altered oral mucous membrane: dryness related to atrophy of the oral cavity epithelium, decreased salivary gland activity, and dehydration (if present).

DESIRED OUTCOMES	NURSING ACTIONS AND *SELECTED RATIONALES*
9. The client will maintain a moist, intact oral mucous membrane.	9.a. Assess client every shift for dryness of the oral mucosa.

b. Implement measures *to prevent dryness of the oral mucous membrane:*
1. instruct and assist client to perform good oral hygiene as often as needed; avoid products such as lemon-glycerin swabs and mouthwashes containing alcohol (*these products have a drying or irritating effect on the oral mucous membrane*)
2. encourage client to rinse mouth frequently with water
3. lubricate client's lips with Vaseline, K-Y jelly, ChapStick, Blistex, or mineral oil when oral care is given
4. encourage client to breathe through nose if possible
5. encourage client not to smoke (*smoking further irritates and dries the mucosa*)
6. encourage a fluid intake of at least 2500 cc/day unless contraindicated
7. perform actions *to increase salivary flow:*
   a. encourage client to chew sugarless gum or suck on sugarless, sour, hard candy
   b. offer hot tea with lemon or warm lemonade at regular intervals unless contraindicated
8. encourage client to use artificial saliva (e.g. Moi-stir, Salivart, Xero-Lube) *to lubricate the mucous membrane.*

c. If oral mucosa is irritated or cracked, implement measures to relieve discomfort and promote healing:
1. assist client to select soft, bland, and nonacidic foods
2. instruct client to avoid foods/fluids that are extremely hot or cold
3. use a soft bristle brush or low-pressure power spray for oral care
4. if client has dentures that fit poorly, remove and replace only for meals
5. monitor for therapeutic and nontherapeutic effects of topical anesthetics, oral protective pastes, and topical and systemic analgesics if administered.

d. Consult physician if dryness, irritation, and discomfort persist.

10. NURSING DIAGNOSIS

Activity intolerance related to:

a. tissue hypoxia associated with impaired alveolar gas exchange, decreased tissue perfusion, and reduced erythropoiesis (there is some decrease in hematopoietic activity as a result of the aging process);
b. increased energy expenditure required for certain activities associated with decreased muscle strength and reduced coordination;
c. decreased nutritional status and a lower glycogen reserve;
d. difficulty resting and sleeping.

DESIRED OUTCOMES	NURSING ACTIONS AND *SELECTED RATIONALES*
10. The client will demonstrate an increased tolerance for activity as evidenced by: a. verbalization of feeling less fatigued and weak b. ability to perform activities of daily living without exertional dyspnea, chest pain, diaphoresis, dizziness, or a significant change in vital signs.	10.a. Assess for signs and symptoms of activity intolerance: 1. statements of fatigue and weakness 2. exertional dyspnea, chest pain, diaphoresis, or dizziness 3. decrease in pulse rate or an increase in rate of 20 beats/minute above resting rate 4. pulse rate not returning to preactivity level within 10 minutes after stopping activity (in an elderly client, the pulse rate increases only slightly with activity and returns to preactivity level slowly) 5. decreased blood pressure or an increase in diastolic pressure of 15 mm Hg with activity. b. Implement measures *to improve activity tolerance:* 1. perform actions *to promote rest:* a. maintain activity restrictions b. minimize environmental activity and noise c. schedule nursing care and diagnostic procedures to allow periods of uninterrupted rest d. limit the number of visitors and their length of stay e. assist client with self-care activities as needed f. keep supplies and personal articles within easy reach g. implement measures to reduce fear and anxiety (see Nursing Diagnosis 1, action c) h. implement measures to promote sleep (see Nursing Diagnosis 16, action c) 2. perform actions to maintain adequate systemic tissue perfusion (see Nursing Diagnosis 2, action b) 3. perform actions to maintain an adequate respiratory status (see Nursing Diagnosis 3, action e) 4. instruct client in energy-saving techniques (e.g. using shower chair when showering, sitting to brush teeth or comb hair) 5. maintain an optimal nutritional status (see Nursing Diagnosis 5.A, action 5) 6. increase client's activity gradually as allowed and tolerated; periods of activity should be short, frequent, and interspersed with rest periods. c. Instruct client to: 1. report a decreased tolerance for activity; caution client that tolerance for vigorous activity may be diminished *because of age-related changes in thermoregulatory mechanisms and sympathetic responses* 2. stop any activity that causes chest pain, shortness of breath, dizziness, or extreme fatigue or weakness. d. Consult physician if signs and symptoms of activity intolerance persist or worsen.

☐ ▬▬▬▬▬▬▬▬▬▬▬▬▬▬▬▬

11. NURSING DIAGNOSIS

Impaired physical mobility related to:

a. decreased muscle strength and endurance associated with a decrease in the size and number of muscle fibers;
b. activity intolerance associated with less efficient respiratory and cardiac function, decreased nutritional status, and difficulty resting and sleeping;
c. slowed physical responses associated with decreased nerve conduction;
d. reduced joint mobility and joint pain associated with degenerative joint changes;
e. fear of falling;
f. activity limitations imposed by current diagnosis and/or treatment plan.

☐ ▬▬▬▬▬▬▬▬▬▬▬▬▬▬▬▬

DESIRED OUTCOMES	NURSING ACTIONS AND *SELECTED RATIONALES*

11.a. The client will maintain an optimal level of physical mobility within prescribed activity restrictions.	11.a.1. Assess for factors that impair physical mobility (e.g. weakness and fatigue, reluctance to move because of joint pain or fear of falls, restrictions imposed by treatment plan).
	 2. Implement measures *to maintain an optimal level of physical mobility:*
	   a. perform actions to reduce joint discomfort (see Nursing Diagnosis 6.B, action 5)
	   b. perform actions to improve activity tolerance (see Nursing Diagnosis 10, action b)
	   c. perform actions to prevent falls (see Nursing Diagnosis 18, action b) *ir order to reduce client's fear of injury*
	   d. instruct client in and assist with correct use of mobility aids (e.g. cane, walker) if indicated
	   e. instruct client in and assist with active and/or passive range of motion exercises at least every 4 hours unless contraindicated; inform client that he/she should begin exercises upon awakening in morning *to reduce joint stiffness*
	   f. encourage client to perform both isotonic (e.g. range of motion, walking) and isometric exercises (pressing feet against footboard, hand gripping, lifting weights) unless contraindicated; instruct client to continue a regular exercise program following discharge.
	 3. Increase activity and participation in self-care activities as allowed and tolerated.
	 4. Provide praise and encouragement for all efforts to increase physical mobility.
	 5. Encourage the support of significant others. Allow them to assist with range of motion exercises, positioning, and activity if desired.
	 6. Consult physician if client is unable to achieve expected level of mobility or range of motion becomes more restricted.

11.b. The client will not experience problems associated with immobility.	11.b. Refer to Care Plan on Immobility for actions to prevent problems associated with immobility if client is to be on bedrest longer than 48 hours.

☐ ▬▬▬▬▬▬▬▬▬▬▬▬▬▬▬▬

12. NURSING DIAGNOSIS

Self-care deficit related to impaired physical mobility, decreased activity tolerance, visual impairments, lack of motivation associated with depression, and altered thought processes (elderly clients sometimes have cognitive impairments that result in their attaching less importance to or forgetting usual grooming and hygiene practices).

□ ▬▬▬▬▬▬▬▬▬▬▬▬▬▬▬▬▬▬▬▬▬

DESIRED OUTCOMES	NURSING ACTIONS AND *SELECTED RATIONALES*

12. The client will perform self-care activities within physical limitations and activity restrictions imposed by the treatment plan.

12.a. Assess for factors that interfere with client's ability to perform self-care (e.g. visual impairments, weakness, fatigue, activity restrictions, altered thought processes).
  b. With client, develop a realistic plan for meeting daily physical needs.
  c. Encourage maximum independence within physical limitations and prescribed activity restrictions.
  d. Implement measures *to facilitate client's ability to perform self-care activities:*
    1. schedule care at a time when client is most likely to be able to participate (e.g. after rest periods, not immediately after meals or treatments)
    2. keep needed objects within easy reach and assist client to identify their location
    3. consult occupational therapist about adaptive devices available (e.g. long-handled hairbrush and shoehorn) if indicated
    4. if client has visual impairment, identify where items are placed on the plate or food tray
    5. allow adequate time for the accomplishment of self-care activities, remembering that elderly clients tend to react to stimuli and move more slowly
    6. perform actions to maintain an optimal level of mobility (see Nursing Diagnosis 11, action a.2)
    7. perform actions to facilitate client's psychological adjustment to current diagnosis and the effects of aging (see Nursing Diagnoses 22, actions c–u and 23, actions c–k) *in order to reduce depression*
    8. perform actions to maintain or improve thought processes (see Nursing Diagnosis 15, action c).
  e. Provide positive feedback for all efforts and accomplishments of self-care.
  f. Assist the client with those activities he/she is unable to perform independently.
  g. Inform significant others of client's abilities to perform own care. Explain the importance of encouraging and allowing client to maintain an optimal level of independence and allowing client to complete activities at his/her own pace.

□ ▬▬▬▬▬▬▬▬▬▬▬▬▬▬▬▬▬▬▬▬▬

13. NURSING DIAGNOSIS

Altered patterns of urinary elimination:

a. **frequency** related to decreased bladder capacity (250 cc as compared with 500–600 cc in young adult), decreased ability to concentrate urine associated with a decline in the number of functioning nephrons, and decreased central nervous system inhibition of micturition;

b. **urgency** related to decreased bladder capacity, decreased sensation of the urge to void until bladder is full, and an increase in uninhibited contractions of the detrusor muscle;

c. **retention** related to obstruction of bladder outlet by an enlarged prostate in men, pressure on the bladder outlet associated with severe constipation, reduced bladder muscle tone, and decreased neural control over micturition;

d. **incontinence:**
1. **stress** related to:
   a. an incompetent bladder outlet associated with degenerative changes in structural support (e.g. pelvic muscles)
   b. overdistention of bladder associated with loss of bladder muscle tone and decreased neural control over micturition;
2. **functional** related to inability to get to toilet in time to urinate associated with unfamiliar hospital environment, impaired physical mobility, and/or altered thought processes.

□ ▬▬▬▬▬▬▬▬▬▬▬▬▬▬▬▬▬▬▬▬▬▬▬▬

DESIRED OUTCOMES	NURSING ACTIONS AND *SELECTED RATIONALES*

13.a. The client will maintain or regain an optimal pattern of urinary elimination as evidenced by:
1. voiding at normal intervals
2. no complaints of urgency, frequency, bladder fullness, or suprapubic discomfort
3. absence of suprapubic distention
4. balanced intake and output.
	13.a.1. Gather baseline data regarding client's usual urinary elimination pattern.
	2. Assess for signs and symptoms of altered patterns of urinary elimination:
	  a. frequent voiding of small amounts (25–50 cc) of urine
	  b. nocturia
	  c. complaints of urgency, frequency, bladder fullness, or suprapubic discomfort
	  d. suprapubic distention
	  e. output less than intake.
	3. Catheterize client if ordered *to determine the amount of residual urine.*
	4. Prepare client for diagnostic tests (e.g. cystoscopy, cystometrogram) if ordered *to determine cause of altered urinary elimination pattern.*
	5. Implement measures *to maintain or regain an optimal pattern of urinary elimination:*
	  a. instruct client to urinate when the urge is first felt
	  b. perform actions *to facilitate voiding* (e.g. provide privacy, allow client to assume normal position for voiding unless contraindicated, run water, pour warm water over perineum, place client's hands in warm water)
	  c. offer bedpan or urinal or assist client to commode or bathroom every 2–3 hours
	  d. instruct and assist client to perform the Credé technique unless contraindicated *to facilitate emptying of the bladder*
	  e. instruct client to perform the Valsalva maneuver during urination unless contraindicated
	  f. consult physician regarding an order for warm sitz baths *to reduce prostate size in the male client and relax urinary sphincter*
	  g. perform actions to prevent or relieve constipation (see Nursing Diagnosis 14, actions e and f)
	  h. monitor for therapeutic and nontherapeutic effects of cholinergic drugs (e.g. bethanechol) if administered *to stimulate bladder contraction*
	  i. consult physician regarding intermittent catheterization or insertion of an indwelling catheter if above actions fail to prevent or alleviate urinary retention.

13.b. The client will experience urinary continence.	13.b.1. Assess for and report urinary incontinence.
	2. Determine from history if incontinence is established or acute.
	3. Implement measures *to prevent or treat urinary incontinence:*
	  a. offer bedpan or urinal or assist client to commode or bathroom every 2–3 hours or more frequently depending on the client's usual urinary elimination pattern
	  b. allow client to assume a normal position for voiding unless contraindicated *to promote complete bladder emptying*
	  c. instruct client to perform perineal exercises (e.g. stopping and starting stream during voiding; pressing buttocks together, then relaxing the muscles) several times a day *in order to improve urinary sphincter tone*; instruct client to continue these exercises following discharge,

emphasizing that it will take several weeks of exercise before improvement may be noted

d. limit oral fluid intake in the evening *to decrease the possibility of nighttime incontinence*

e. instruct client to avoid drinking beverages containing caffeine (*caffeine is a mild diuretic and may make urinary control more difficult*)

f. monitor for therapeutic and nontherapeutic effects of alpha-adrenergic agonists (e.g. ephedrine) if administered *to increase urinary sphincter tone*

g. if urinary incontinence persists:
1. utilize biofeedback techniques if appropriate *to assist client to regain control over the external urinary sphincter and pelvic floor musculature*
2. instruct and assist client with bladder retraining program if appropriate
3. consult physician regarding intermittent catheterization, insertion of an indwelling catheter, or use of an external catheter or penile clamp
4. provide emotional support to client and significant others.

14. NURSING DIAGNOSIS

Constipation related to:

a. decreased intake of fluids and foods high in fiber;
b. atony of intestines (may occur with chronic laxative use);
c. weakened abdominal muscles and diminished neural impulses for signal to defecate;
d. decreased gastrointestinal motility associated with decreased activity and anxiety.

DESIRED OUTCOMES	NURSING ACTIONS AND *SELECTED RATIONALES*

14. The client will maintain optimal bowel elimination pattern.	14.a. Ascertain client's usual bowel elimination habits.
	b. Monitor and record bowel movements including frequency, consistency, and shape.
	c. Assess for signs and symptoms that may accompany constipation such as headache, anorexia, nausea, abdominal distention and cramping, and feeling of fullness or pressure in abdomen or rectum.
	d. Assess bowel sounds. Report a pattern of decreasing bowel sounds.
	e. Implement measures *to prevent constipation:*
	  1. encourage client to defecate whenever the urge is felt
	  2. assist client to toilet or place in high Fowler's position or on commode for bowel movements unless contraindicated; provide privacy and adequate ventilation
	  3. encourage client to relax during attempts to defecate *in order to promote relaxation of the levator ani muscle and the external anal sphincter*
	  4. instruct client to select foods high in fiber (e.g. nuts, bran, whole grains, raw fruits and vegetables, dried fruits)
	  5. instruct client to maintain a minimum fluid intake of 2500 cc/day unless contraindicated
	  6. encourage client to drink warm liquids *to stimulate peristalsis*
	  7. increase activity as tolerated
	  8. encourage client to perform isometric abdominal strengthening exercises unless contraindicated

9. monitor for therapeutic and nontherapeutic effects of laxatives, suppositories, stool softeners, and/or enemas if administered

10. instruct client in ways to promote regular bowel function (e.g. increase fluid intake to at least 8–10 glasses/day; increase intake of foods high in fiber, particularly bran; participate in regular exercise program) following discharge.

f. Check for impaction if client has not had a bowel movement in 3 days, if he/she is passing liquid stools, or if other signs and symptoms of constipation are present. Administer oil retention and/or cleansing enemas as ordered followed by digital removal of stool if necessary.

☐ ▬▬▬▬▬▬▬▬▬▬▬▬▬▬▬▬▬▬▬▬

15. NURSING DIAGNOSIS

Altered thought processes: slowed verbal responses, decline in memory (especially short term), and/or decline in abstract reasoning related to:

a. decreased cerebral functioning associated with reduced cerebral tissue perfusion, a decrease in number of neurons, accumulation of lipofuscin and presence of senile plaque and neurofibrillary tangles in brain tissue, and neuroaxonal dystrophy;
b. disturbance in sleep pattern;
c. alteration in amounts and/or activity of chemical neurotransmitters (e.g. acetylcholine, dopamine, norepinephrine, serotonin);
d. altered metabolism, distribution, and excretion of some drugs that client may be receiving for treatment.

☐ ▬▬▬▬▬▬▬▬▬▬▬▬▬▬▬▬▬▬▬▬

DESIRED OUTCOMES	NURSING ACTIONS AND *SELECTED RATIONALES*

15. The client will experience optimal thought processes as evidenced by:
   a. usual or improved verbal response time, memory, and reasoning ability
   b. verbalization of awareness of surroundings and need to perform activities of daily living
   c. orientation to person, place, and time.

15.a. Assess client for changes in thought processes (e.g. slowed verbal response time, impaired short-term memory, poor abstract reasoning, lack of awareness of surroundings or necessary tasks to perform, confusion).
b. Ascertain from significant others client's usual level of intellectual functioning.
c. Implement measures *to maintain or improve thought processes:*
   1. perform actions to maintain adequate systemic tissue perfusion (see Nursing Diagnosis 2, action b) and keep head and neck in good alignment *in order to promote adequate cerebral blood flow*
   2. perform actions to maintain an adequate respiratory status (see Nursing Diagnosis 3, action e) *in order to maintain adequate cerebral oxygenation*
   3. perform actions to promote sleep (see Nursing Diagnosis 16, action c)
   4. administer medications, especially central nervous system depressants (e.g. narcotic analgesics, antianxiety agents, sedatives), cautiously *because of the increased risk of toxic effects resulting from age-related alterations in metabolism, distribution, and excretion of drugs.*
d. If client shows evidence of altered thought processes:
   1. allow adequate time for communication and performance of activities
   2. repeat instructions as necessary using clear, simple language
   3. write out a schedule of activities for client to refer to if desired
   4. encourage client to make lists of planned activities and questions or concerns he/she may have
   5. maintain realistic expectations of client's ability to learn, comprehend, and remember information provided
   6. reorient to person, place, and time as necessary
   7. encourage significant others to be supportive of client; instruct them in methods of dealing with the alterations in thought processes

8. discuss the physiological basis for alterations in thought processes with client and significant others
9. consult physician if alterations in thought processes worsen.

16. NURSING DIAGNOSIS

Sleep pattern disturbance related to:

a. fear, anxiety, decreased activity, unfamiliar environment, discomfort, and nocturia;
b. changes in circadian rhythm, the stages of sleep (particularly Stages III and IV), and REM sleep resulting in frequent arousal periods and an increase in the total awake time.

DESIRED OUTCOMES	NURSING ACTIONS AND *SELECTED RATIONALES*

16. The client will attain optimal amounts of sleep within the parameters of the treatment regimen as evidenced by:
a. statements of feeling well rested
b. usual behavior
c. absence of frequent yawning, thick speech, dark circles under eyes.
	16.a. Assess for signs and symptoms of a sleep pattern disturbance:
	  1. verbal complaints of difficulty falling asleep, not feeling well rested, sleep interruptions, or awakening earlier or later than desired
	  2. behavior changes (e.g. irritability, disorganization, lethargy)
	  3. frequent yawning, thick speech, dark circles under eyes, slight hand tremors.
	b. Determine the client's usual sleep habits.
	c. Implement measures *to promote sleep:*
	  1. perform actions to reduce fear and anxiety (see Nursing Diagnosis 1, action c)
	  2. perform actions to reduce dyspepsia, gastric fullness, gas pain, and joint pain and stiffness if present (see Nursing Diagnoses 6.A, action 3 and 6.B, action 5) and discomfort associated with client's diagnosis and its treatment
	  3. inform client of the normal changes in sleep pattern that occur with aging *in order to reduce concerns about quantity of sleep necessary to maintain health*
	  4. allow client to continue usual sleep practices (e.g. position, time, bedtime rituals) if possible
	  5. determine measures that have been helpful to the client in the past (e.g. milk, warm drinks, warm bath) and incorporate in plan of care
	  6. discourage long periods of sleep during the day unless sleep deprivation exists or daytime sleep is usual for client
	  7. encourage participation in relaxing diversional activities in early evening hours
	  8. provide a quiet, restful atmosphere
	  9. discourage intake of foods and fluids high in caffeine (e.g. chocolate, coffee, tea, colas) especially in the evening
	  10. satisfy basic needs such as hunger, comfort, and warmth before sleep
	  11. instruct client to limit intake of fluids in the evening and empty bladder just before bedtime *to reduce nocturia*
	  12. utilize relaxation techniques (e.g. progressive relaxation exercises, back massage, meditation, soft music) before sleep
	  13. perform actions *to provide for periods of uninterrupted sleep (90- to 120-minute periods of uninterrupted sleep are considered essential):*
	    a. restrict visitors during rest periods
	    b. group care (e.g. medications, treatments, physical care, assessments) whenever possible
	  14. monitor for therapeutic and nontherapeutic effects of sedatives and hypnotics if administered; administer these agents cautiously *because the metabolism, distribution, and excretion of drugs is often altered in the elderly.*
	d. Consult physician if signs of sleep deprivation persist or worsen.

17. NURSING DIAGNOSIS

Potential for infection related to increased susceptibility associated with:

a. stasis of respiratory secretions resulting from decreased ciliary activity, decreased cough effectiveness, and decreased mobility;

b. decreased effectiveness of alveolar macrophages;

c. decreased effectiveness of the immune system possibly resulting from reduced levels of IgA, decreased production and differentiation of T-cells, and/or decline in B-cell function associated with age-related changes in lymphatic tissue, thymus gland, and spleen;

d. malnutrition;

e. urinary stasis resulting from incomplete bladder emptying and decreased activity;

f. loss of skin integrity resulting from increased fragility of the skin (occurs due to dryness and decreased elasticity and vascularity).

DESIRED OUTCOMES	NURSING ACTIONS AND *SELECTED RATIONALES*

17. The client will remain free of infection as evidenced by:
    a. absence of chills and fever
    b. pulse within normal limits
    c. normal breath sounds
    d. voiding clear, yellow urine without complaints of burning or increased frequency or urgency
    e. absence of redness, swelling, or unusual drainage in any area where there is a break in skin integrity
    f. intact oral mucous membrane
    g. WBC and differential counts within normal range for elderly client
    h. negative results of cultured specimens.

17.a. Assess for and report signs and symptoms of infection:
    1. increase in temperature above client's usual level (be aware that normal temperature in the elderly client may be less than 37°C)
    2. chills
    3. pattern of increased pulse or pulse rate greater than 100 beats/minute (the elderly client may not demonstrate the classic elevation in pulse rate that occurs with infection *because of his/her decreased sympathetic responses*)
    4. adventitious breath sounds
    5. cloudy or foul-smelling urine
    6. complaints of burning when urinating
    7. complaints of increased urinary frequency and urgency
    8. presence of WBCs, bacteria, and/or nitrites in urine
    9. redness, swelling, or unusual drainage in any area where there is a break in skin integrity
    10. irritation or ulceration of oral mucous membrane
    11. elevated WBC count and/or significant change in differential.
  b. Obtain culture specimens (e.g. urine, vaginal, mouth, sputum, blood) as ordered. Report positive results.
  c. Implement measures *to reduce risk of infection:*
    1. maintain a fluid intake of at least 2500 cc/day unless contraindicated
    2. use good handwashing technique and encourage client to do the same
    3. maintain meticulous aseptic technique during all invasive procedures (e.g. catheterizations, venous and arterial punctures, injections)
    4. protect client from others with infection and instruct client to continue this after discharge
    5. perform actions to improve nutritional status (see Nursing Diagnosis 5.A, action 5)
    6. reinforce importance of good oral care; if client has dentures, emphasize the importance of having them checked regularly *to ensure proper fit* and having cracks, chips, or rough surfaces repaired immediately *in order to prevent trauma to the oral mucous membrane*
    7. provide the proper balance of exercise and rest
    8. perform actions to maintain an adequate respiratory status (see Nursing Diagnosis 3, action e) *in order to reduce the risk of respiratory tract infection*
    9. perform actions *to prevent urinary tract infection:*
      a. implement measures to prevent urinary retention (see Nursing Diagnosis 13, action a.5)

      b. instruct and assist female client to wipe from front to back
         following urination or defecation
      c. keep perianal area clean
    10. perform actions to maintain skin integrity (see Nursing Diagnosis 8,
        action b)
    11. instruct client to receive vaccinations for pneumococcal pneumonia and
        influenza at recommended intervals if appropriate.
  d. Monitor for therapeutic and nontherapeutic effects of anti-infectives if
    administered.

□ � ▉▉▉▉▉▉▉▉▉▉▉▉▉▉▉▉▉▉▉▉▉▉▉▉▉▉▉▉▉▉▉

18. NURSING DIAGNOSIS

Potential for trauma related to:

a. falls associated with:
    1. dizziness or syncope resulting from decreased systemic tissue perfusion and
       orthostatic hypotension (occurs as a result of loss of sensitivity of baroreceptors
       and decreased venous return)
    2. weakness and fatigue resulting from decreased muscle strength and the general
       deconditioning that occurs with reduced physical activity
    3. impaired vision
    4. slowed reflexes and reaction time to stimuli;
b. burns associated with age-related decrease in tactile sensation.

□ ▉▉▉▉▉▉▉▉▉▉▉▉▉▉▉▉▉▉▉▉▉▉▉▉▉▉▉▉▉▉▉

DESIRED OUTCOMES	NURSING ACTIONS AND *SELECTED RATIONALES*

18. The client will not experience falls or burns.	18.a. Determine whether conditions predisposing client to falls or burns (e.g. weakness, fatigue, slowed reflexes and response time, visual changes, orthostatic hypotension, diminished feeling in extremities) exist.
	  b. Implement measures *to prevent falls:*
	    1. keep bed in low position with side rails up when client is in bed
	    2. keep needed items within easy reach and assist client to identify their location
	    3. encourage client to request assistance whenever needed; have call signal within easy reach
	    4. use lap belt when client is in chair if indicated
	    5. instruct client to wear shoes with nonskid soles and low heels when ambulating
	    6. avoid unnecessary clutter in room
	    7. perform actions *to reduce dizziness associated with orthostatic drop in blood pressure:*
	      a. instruct and assist client to perform isometric exercises and put on elastic hose before getting up
	      b. encourage client to change positions slowly
	    8. accompany client during ambulation utilizing a transfer safety belt if he/she is weak or dizzy
	    9. provide ambulatory aids (e.g. walker, cane) if client is weak or unsteady on feet
	    10. if vision is impaired:
	      a. orient client to surroundings, room, and arrangement of furniture
	      b. keep room well-lit with incandescent rather than fluorescent lighting *to reduce glare*
	      c. utilize a red night light *to facilitate adaptation to a darkened environment and improve night vision*
	      d. encourage visual scanning while ambulating *to compensate for reduced peripheral vision*

   e. assist client with ambulation by walking ½ step ahead of client and describing approaching objects or obstacles; instruct client to grasp back of nurse's arm during ambulation

   11. instruct client to ambulate in well-lit areas and to utilize handrails if needed

   12. do not rush client; allow adequate time for trips to the bathroom and ambulation in hallway

   13. perform actions to improve activity tolerance and maintain an optimal level of physical mobility (see Nursing Diagnoses 10, action b and 11, action a.2).

c. Implement measures *to prevent burns:*
   1. let hot foods or fluids cool slightly before serving *to reduce the risk of burns if spills occur*
   2. supervise client while smoking if indicated
   3. assess temperature of bath water and heating pad before and during use.

d. Include client and significant others in planning and implementing measures to prevent falls and burns. Discuss need to continue with appropriate safety precautions following discharge.

e. If injury does occur, initiate appropriate first aid and notify physician.

□ ■■■■■■■■■■■■■■■■■■■■■■■■■■■■■■■■■■■■

19. NURSING DIAGNOSIS

Potential for aspiration related to depressed cough and gag reflexes, stasis of secretions or foods/fluids in esophagus associated with decreased esophageal motility, and increased esophageal reflux associated with delayed gastric emptying.

□ ■■■■■■■■■■■■■■■■■■■■■■■■■■■■■■■■■■■■

DESIRED OUTCOMES	NURSING ACTIONS AND *SELECTED RATIONALES*

19. The client will not aspirate secretions or foods/fluids as evidenced by:
   a. clear breath sounds
   b. resonant percussion note over lungs
   c. respiratory rate at 16–20/minute
   d. absence of dyspnea
   e. absence of cyanosis.

19.a. Assess for factors that indicate potential for aspiration (e.g. difficulty swallowing, choking on secretions and foods/fluids, decreased gag reflex, complaints of sour taste in throat [may indicate esophageal reflux]).

b. Assess for signs and symptoms of aspiration of secretions or foods/fluids (e.g. rhonchi, dull percussion note over lungs, tachycardia, rapid respirations, dyspnea, cyanosis).

c. Monitor chest x-ray results. Report findings of pulmonary infiltrate.

d. Implement measures *to reduce the risk of aspiration:*
   1. position client in side-lying or semi- to high Fowler's position at all times
   2. decrease environmental stimuli during meals and snacks *so client can concentrate on chewing and swallowing*
   3. allow ample time for meals
   4. instruct client to avoid laughing or talking when eating and drinking
   5. perform actions to reduce gastroesophageal reflux (see Nursing Diagnosis 6.A, action 3.a)
   6. assist client with oral hygiene after eating *to ensure that food particles do not remain in mouth*
   7. monitor for therapeutic and nontherapeutic effects of gastrointestinal stimulants (e.g. metoclopramide) if administered *to promote gastric emptying and reduce gastroesophageal reflux.*

e. If signs and symptoms of aspiration occur:
   1. perform tracheal suctioning
   2. notify physician
   3. prepare client for chest x-ray.

□ ▬▬▬▬▬▬▬▬▬▬▬▬▬▬▬▬▬▬▬▬▬▬▬▬▬

20. COLLABORATIVE DIAGNOSIS

Potential complications:

a. **pathologic fractures** related to osteoporosis associated with an imbalance between bone resorption and bone formation resulting from decreased estrogen levels in women, calcium deficiency (results from decreased dietary intake and decreased absorption due to vitamin D deficiency), and decreased activity;

b. **thromboembolism** related to:
1. venous stasis associated with decreased activity, decreased elasticity of veins, and loss of muscle tone in extremities
2. hypercoagulability associated with a possible increase in platelet adhesiveness and dehydration (if present).

□ ▬▬▬▬▬▬▬▬▬▬▬▬▬▬▬▬▬▬▬▬▬▬▬▬▬

DESIRED OUTCOMES	NURSING ACTIONS AND *SELECTED RATIONALES*

20.a. The client will not experience pathologic fractures as evidenced by:
1. maintenance of usual body movements
2. no increase in pain or swelling over skeletal structures
3. x-ray films showing absence of fractures.
	20.a.1. Determine whether conditions predisposing client to pathologic fractures (e.g. prolonged immobility, female, diagnosis of osteoporosis or osteodystrophy) exist.
	2. Assess for and report signs and symptoms of pathologic fractures (e.g. decrease in mobility and range of motion, increase in pain and swelling over skeletal structures).
	3. Monitor x-ray reports and notify physician of positive findings.
	4. Implement measures *to prevent pathologic fractures:*
	  a. caution client to avoid coughing, sneezing, and straining at stool
	  b. move client carefully; obtain adequate assistance as needed
	  c. when turning client, log roll and support all extremities
	  d. utilize smooth movements when moving client; avoid pulling or pushing on body parts
	  e. correctly apply brace, splint, or corset as ordered
	  f. instruct client in the use of correct body mechanics and the need to avoid lifting heavy objects
	  g. perform actions to prevent falls (see Nursing Diagnosis 18, action b)
	  h. perform actions *to prevent or delay bone demineralization:*
	    1. assist client to maintain maximum mobility (*weight-bearing reduces bone breakdown*)
	    2. consult physician about use of a tilt table to facilitate weight-bearing if client is immobile
	    3. administer calcium preparations, vitamin D, and medications *that promote mobilization of calcium back into bones (e.g. estrogen preparations)* if ordered.
	5. If fractures occur:
	  a. apply external stabilization device (e.g. cervical collar, brace, splint, sling) if ordered
	  b. monitor for therapeutic and nontherapeutic effects of analgesics if administered *to control pain.*

20.b.1. The client will not develop a venous thrombus as evidenced by:
a. absence of pain, tenderness, and swelling in extremities
b. usual skin color and temperature of extremities.
	20.b.1.a. Assess for and report signs and symptoms of a venous thrombus:
	  1. tenderness and pain in extremity
	  2. increase in circumference of calf or thigh (measure at the same place on leg once/shift)
	  3. unusual warmth and redness of extremity
	  4. positive Homan's sign (not always a reliable sign).
	b. Implement measures *to prevent thrombus formation:*
	  1. perform actions to reduce peripheral pooling of blood and increase venous return (see Nursing Diagnosis 2, action b.3)
	  2. maintain a minimum fluid intake of 2500 cc/day (unless

contraindicated) *to prevent dehydration and increased blood viscosity, which leads to hypercoagulability*

3. monitor for therapeutic and nontherapeutic effects of anticoagulants (e.g. heparin, warfarin) or antiplatelet agents (e.g. aspirin, dipyridamole) if administered.

c. If signs and symptoms of a venous thrombus occur:
1. maintain client on bedrest until activity orders received
2. discourage positions that compromise blood flow (e.g. pillows under knees, use of knee gatch, crossing legs, sitting for long periods)
3. prepare client for diagnostic studies (e.g. venography or phlebography, isotope studies, Doppler ultrasound, impedance plethysmography) if indicated
4. monitor for therapeutic and nontherapeutic effects of anticoagulants (e.g. heparin, warfarin) if administered (be aware that lower doses of coumarins should be administered *because of the marked sensitivity of the elderly client to oral anticoagulants*)
5. prepare client for surgical intervention (e.g. thrombectomy, insertion of an intracaval filtering device) or injection of a thrombolytic agent (e.g. urokinase, tissue plasminogen activator [tPA], streptokinase) if indicated
6. refer to Care Plan on Thrombophlebitis for additional care measures.

20.b.2. The client will not experience a pulmonary embolism as evidenced by:
a. absence of sudden chest pain, cough, hemoptysis
b. unlabored respirations
c. stable vital signs
d. usual skin color
e. usual mental status
f. blood gases within normal range for elderly client.

20.b.2.a. Assess for and report signs and symptoms of a pulmonary embolism:
1. sudden chest pain
2. cough and/or hemoptysis
3. dyspnea, tachypnea
4. tachycardia, hypotension
5. pallor, cyanosis
6. restlessness
7. low PaO_2 (be aware that the normal range for PaO_2 is lower in the elderly client).

b. Implement measures *to prevent a pulmonary embolism:*
1. perform actions to prevent the formation of a venous thrombus (see action b.1.b in this diagnosis)
2. do not exercise or massage any extremity suspected of thrombosis
3. caution client to avoid activities that create a Valsalva response (e.g. straining to have a bowel movement, bending at the waist, holding breath while moving) *in order to prevent dislodgment of existing thrombi.*

c. If signs and symptoms of a pulmonary embolism occur:
1. maintain client on strict bedrest in a semi- to high Fowler's position
2. maintain oxygen therapy as ordered
3. prepare client for diagnostic tests (e.g. blood gases, lung scan, venography, pulmonary angiography)
4. monitor for therapeutic and nontherapeutic effects of the following medications if administered:
   a. heparin
   b. thrombolytic agents (e.g. streptokinase, tissue plasminogen activator [tPA], urokinase)
   c. vasoconstrictors (*may be necessary to maintain mean arterial pressure if shock occurs*)
5. prepare client for surgical intervention (e.g. embolectomy) if indicated
6. provide emotional support to client and significant others
7. refer to Care Plan on Pulmonary Embolism for additional care measures.

21. NURSING DIAGNOSIS

Sexual dysfunction:

a. **decreased libido** related to:
   1. fear of rejection associated with feelings of loss of physical attractiveness, inadequate opportunities for sexual expression, and infrequent sexual activity
   2. misconceptions about sexual functioning in old age
   3. fear, anxiety, depression, and discomfort;
b. **dyspareunia** related to dryness of the vaginal mucosa associated with decreased estrogen levels and decreased distensibility of the vaginal vault;
c. **impotence** related to:
   1. performance anxiety, fatigue, and depression
   2. fear of rejection associated with perceived loss of sexual attractiveness and societal stereotype that the elderly do not participate in sexual intercourse
   3. increased stimulation necessary to achieve an erection
   4. increase in ratio of estrogen to testosterone associated with gonadal changes.

DESIRED OUTCOMES	NURSING ACTIONS AND *SELECTED RATIONALES*

21. The client will demonstrate beginning acceptance of changes in sexual functioning as evidenced by:
a. verbalization of a perception of self as sexually acceptable and adequate
b. maintenance of relationships with significant others.
	21.a. Assess for signs and symptoms of sexual dysfunction (e.g. verbalization of sexual concerns, failure to maintain relationships with significant others).
	b. Determine from client his/her usual pattern of sexual expression, recent changes in usual patterns, and knowledge of age-related changes in sexual functioning. Be aware that the client may be reluctant to express concerns *because of the common stereotype that the elderly are not sexually active.*
	c. Inform client of age-related changes that may occur in sexual functioning (e.g. sexual responses are slower and less intense, erections take longer to achieve but can be maintained longer). Explain that continued sexual activity may delay some of these changes. Encourage questions and clarify misconceptions.
	d. Communicate interest, understanding, and respect for the values of the client and his/her partner.
	e. Implement measures to promote a positive self-concept (see Nursing Diagnosis 22, actions c–u).
	f. Facilitate communication between client and his/her partner. Assist them to identify factors or changes that may affect their sexual relationship.
	g. Arrange for uninterrupted privacy during hospital stay if desired by the couple.
	h. Encourage female client to use a water-soluble lubricant before sexual intercourse *to decrease vaginal dryness.*
	i. If impotence is a problem:
	  1. encourage client to discuss it with physician *(impotence may be due to reversible factors such as medication therapy, alcohol, or poorly controlled chronic disease conditions)*
	  2. assure client that occasional episodes of impotence are normal
	  3. suggest alternative modes of sexual gratification and use of assistive devices if appropriate
	  4. discuss ways to be creative in expressing sexuality (e.g. massage, fantasies, cuddling)
	  5. encourage client to discuss the possibility of a penile prosthesis with physician if desired.
	j. Include partner in above discussions and encourage his/her continued support of the client.
	k. Consult physician if counseling appears indicated.

22. NURSING DIAGNOSIS

Disturbance in self-concept* related to:

a. changes in appearance and body functioning (e.g. graying and thinning of hair; increase in length and width of nose and ears; dry, wrinkled skin; reduced height; increase and change in distribution of body fat; reduction in lean body mass; impotence; decreased bladder control; diminished visual acuity, hearing, taste sensation, sense of smell, and tactile sensation);
b. increased dependence on others to meet basic needs;
c. feelings of powerlessness;
d. changes in usual life style and roles associated with decreased strength and endurance and sensory-perceptual alterations.

_____

* This diagnostic label includes the nursing diagnoses of body image disturbance and self-esteem disturbance.

DESIRED OUTCOMES	NURSING ACTIONS AND *SELECTED RATIONALES*
22. The client will demonstrate beginning adaptation to changes in appearance, body functioning, life style, and roles as evidenced by: a. verbalization of feelings of self-worth and sexual adequacy b. maintenance of relationships with significant others c. active participation in activities of daily living d. active interest in personal appearance e. willingness to participate in social activities f. verbalization of a beginning plan for adapting life style to meet restrictions imposed by the aging process and current diagnosis.	22.a. Determine the meaning of changes in appearance, body functioning, life style, and roles to the client by encouraging him/her to verbalize feelings and by noting nonverbal responses to the changes experienced. b. Assess for signs and symptoms of a disturbance in self-concept (e.g. verbal or nonverbal cues denoting a negative response to changes in body functioning and appearance such as denial of or preoccupation with the changes that have occurred or withdrawal from significant others). c. Be aware that the client will grieve the changes that have occurred. Assist him/her through the stages of denial, anger, bargaining, and depression. d. Assist client to identify strengths and qualities that have a positive effect on self-concept. e. Implement measures to assist client *to increase self-esteem* (e.g. limit negative self-criticism, encourage positive comments about self, give positive feedback about accomplishments). f. Assist client to identify and utilize coping techniques that have been helpful in the past. g. Reinforce measures that may assist client to adjust to altered sexual functioniong (see Nursing Diagnosis 21, actions c–j). h. Implement measures to assist client to adapt to sensory-perceptual alterations (see Nursing Diagnosis 7, actions b–f) and altered thought processes (see Nursing Diagnosis 15, actions c and d). i. If client is incontinent, instruct in ways to minimize the problem (e.g. placing disposable liners in underwear, wearing absorbent undergarments such as Attends). j. Assist client with usual grooming and makeup habits if necessary. k. Implement measures to reduce client's feelings of powerlessness (see Nursing Diagnosis 23, actions c–k). l. Demonstrate acceptance of client using techniques such as therapeutic touch and frequent visits. Encourage significant others to do the same. m. Assess for and support behaviors suggesting positive adaptation to changes experienced (e.g. interest in personal appearance, maintenance of relationships with significant others). n. Encourage significant others to allow client to do what he/she is able *so that independence can be re-established and/or self-esteem redeveloped.* o. Assist client's and significant others' adjustment by listening, facilitating communication, and providing information. p. If appropriate, discuss with client ways to modify environment of his/her living situation *so that he/she will be able to maintain maximum independence.*

q. Ensure that client and significant others have similar expectations and understanding of future life style. Assist them to identify ways that personal and family goals can be adjusted rather than abandoned.
r. Encourage visits and support from significant others.
s. Encourage client to continue involvement in social activities and to pursue interests if able. If previous interests and hobbies cannot be pursued, encourage development of new ones.
t. Instruct client in ways to promote and maintain optimal body functioning (e.g. maintain good nutritional status, participate in an active exercise program).
u. Provide information about and encourage utilization of community agencies or support groups (e.g. senior centers; family, individual, and/or financial counseling).
v. Consult physician about psychological counseling if client desires or if he/she seems unwilling or unable to adapt to changes resulting from the aging process.

□ ▰▰▰▰▰▰▰▰▰▰▰▰▰▰▰▰▰▰▰▰▰▰▰▰▰

23. NURSING DIAGNOSIS

Powerlessness related to:

a. increased dependence on others to meet basic needs;
b. inability to pursue usual life activities associated with decreased strength and activity tolerance, age-related changes in body functioning, current diagnosis and its treatment, and inadequate financial resources;
c. feeling of loss of control over changes in body functioning.

□ ▰▰▰▰▰▰▰▰▰▰▰▰▰▰▰▰▰▰▰▰▰▰▰▰▰

DESIRED OUTCOMES	NURSING ACTIONS AND *SELECTED RATIONALES*
23. The client will demonstrate increasing feelings of control over his/her situation as evidenced by: a. verbalization of same b. active participation in the planning of care c. participation in self-care activities within physical limitations.	23.a. Assess for behaviors that may indicate feelings of powerlessness (e.g. verbalization of lack of control; unexplained anger, apathy, and hostility; excessive dependency; lack of participation in self-care or care planning). b. Obtain information from client and significant others regarding client's usual response to situations in which client has had limited control (e.g. loss of job, financial stress). c. Encourage client to verbalize feelings about self and current situation. d. Reinforce physician's explanations about the aging process, disease condition or injury, and treatment plan. Clarify any misconceptions. e. Remind client of his/her right to ask questions about changes that are occurring, current condition, and plan of care. f. Support client's efforts to increase knowledge of and control over condition. Provide relevant pamphlets and audiovisual materials. g. Include client in the planning of care, encourage maximum participation in the treatment plan, and allow choices whenever possible *to enable him/her to maintain a sense of control.* h. Consult physical or occupational therapist if indicated about adaptive devices that would allow client more independence in performing activities of daily living. i. Encourage significant others to allow client to do as much as he/she is able *so that a feeling of independence can be maintained.* j. Encourage client to be as active as possible in making decisions about his/her living situation. Assist client to establish realistic short- and long-term goals. k. Encourage client's participation in self-help groups if indicated. l. Provide continuity of care through written individualized care plans *to ensure that client can maintain appropriate control over his/her environment.*

☐ ▬▬▬▬▬▬▬▬▬▬▬▬▬▬▬▬

24. NURSING DIAGNOSIS

Social isolation related to:

a. decreased sensory and motor functioning;
b. reduced opportunities for socialization associated with inadequate financial resources, death or disability of friends and family members, and reluctance to establish new relationships and try new activities;
c. fear of injury in unfamiliar surroundings;
d. withdrawal from others associated with fear of embarrassment due to functional changes such as incontinence, hearing loss, or impaired memory.

☐ ▬▬▬▬▬▬▬▬▬▬▬▬▬▬▬▬

DESIRED OUTCOMES	NURSING ACTIONS AND *SELECTED RATIONALES*
24. The client will experience a decreased sense of isolation as evidenced by: a. maintenance of relationships with significant others and casual acquaintances b. verbalization of decreasing loneliness and feelings of rejection.	24.a. Ascertain client's usual degree of social interaction. b. Assess for and report behaviors indicative of social isolation (e.g. decreased interaction with significant others and staff; expression of feelings of rejection, abandonment, or being different from others; hostility; sad affect). c. Encourage client to express feelings of rejection and aloneness. Provide feedback and support. d. Implement measures *to decrease social isolation:* 　1. set up a schedule of visiting times so that client will not go for long periods without visitors 　2. encourage telephone contact with others 　3. schedule time each day to sit and talk with client 　4. assist client to identify a few persons he/she feels comfortable with and encourage interactions with them 　5. change room assignments as feasible *to provide client with roommate with similar interests* 　6. instruct family in behavior modification techniques if indicated *to assist client to develop more social types of behaviors* 　7. emphasize the importance of maintaining active friendships and seeking out new relationships 　8. support any appropriate movement away from social isolation 　9. encourage client to participate in structured activity programs following discharge; provide information about community senior centers and the programs they offer.

☐ ▬▬▬▬▬▬▬▬▬▬▬▬▬▬▬▬

25. NURSING DIAGNOSIS

Noncompliance* related to:

a. lack of motivation, impaired memory, inadequate support and supervision, insufficient financial resources;
b. confusion about appropriate health care practices and a decreased level of trust associated with conflicting advice from multiple health care providers;
c. conflicting values between client and health care providers;
d. knowledge deficit regarding current diagnosis, medications prescribed, and consequences of failure to comply with treatment plan.

---

* This diagnostic label includes both an informed decision by client not to comply and an inability to comply due to circumstances beyond the client's control.

☐ ▬▬▬▬▬▬▬▬▬▬▬▬▬▬▬▬

DESIRED OUTCOMES	NURSING ACTIONS AND *SELECTED RATIONALES*

25. The client will demonstrate the probability of future compliance with the prescribed treatment plan as evidenced by:
    a. a willingness to learn about and participate in treatments and care
    b. statements reflecting ways to modify personal habits and integrate treatments into life style
    c. statements reflecting an understanding of the implications of not following the prescribed treatment plan.

25.a. Assess for indications that the client may be unwilling or unable to comply with the prescribed treatment plan:
    1. statements reflecting that he/she was unable to manage care at home
    2. failure to adhere to treatment plan while in hospital (e.g. not adhering to dietary modifications, refusing medications, refusing to ambulate)
    3. statements reflecting a lack of understanding of the factors that will cause further progression of current illness and/or accelerate aging process
    4. statements reflecting an unwillingness or inability to modify personal habits and integrate necessary treatments into life style
    5. statements reflecting view that his/her situation is hopeless and that efforts to comply are useless.
  b. Implement measures *to improve client compliance:*
    1. discuss with client the specific factors that may be inhibiting compliance (e.g. inadequate financial resources, religious or cultural conflicts, lack of support systems)
    2. explain the aging process and current diagnosis in terms the client can understand; stress the fact that adherence to the treatment plan is essential *in order to delay and/or prevent complications associated with the diagnosis and minimize some of the changes that occur with aging*
    3. assist client to clarify his/her values and to identify ways to incorporate the therapeutic goals and priorities into value system
    4. encourage questions and clarify any misconceptions the client has about aging and current diagnosis and their effects
    5. perform actions to assist client to cope with the aging process and current condition and their effects
    6. perform actions to promote trust in caregivers (e.g. validate conflicting advice, explain reasons for treatment plan)
    7. assist client to identify ways he/she can incorporate treatments into life style; focus on modifications of life style rather than complete change if possible
    8. obtain a social service consult to assist client with financial planning and to obtain financial aid if indicated
    9. encourage client to attend follow-up educational classes if appropriate.
  c. Assess for and reinforce behaviors suggesting future compliance with prescribed treatments (e.g. statements reflecting plans for integrating treatments into life style, active participation in exercise program, changes in personal habits).
  d. Include significant others in explanations and teaching sessions and encourage their support.
  e. Reinforce the need for client to assume responsibility for managing as much of care as possible.
  f. Consult physician about referrals to community health agencies if continued instruction, support, or supervision is needed.

□ ▬▬▬▬▬▬▬▬▬▬▬▬▬▬▬▬▬▬▬▬

26. NURSING DIAGNOSIS

Altered family processes related to:

a. financial, physical, and psychological stresses associated with illness and/or progressive disability of client;
b. inadequate knowledge about the normal aging process and client's current diagnosis;
c. inadequate support services;
d. decreased ability of client to fulfill usual family roles;
e. guilt associated with need to institutionalize client resulting from inability of family to manage client's care at home.

□ ▬▬▬▬▬▬▬▬▬▬▬▬▬▬▬▬▬▬▬▬

DESIRED OUTCOMES	NURSING ACTIONS AND *SELECTED RATIONALES*

26. The family members* will demonstrate beginning adjustment to changes in family roles and structure as evidenced by:
   a. verbalization of ways to adapt to required role and life-style changes
   b. active participation in decision making and client's rehabilitation
   c. positive interactions with one another.

26.a. Identify components of the family and their pattern of communication and role expectations.
   b. Assess for signs and symptoms of altered family processes (e.g. statements of not being able to accept client's physical impairments and changes in intellectual functioning or to make necessary role and life-style changes, inability to make decisions, inability or refusal to participate in client's care, negative family interactions).
   c. Implement measures *to facilitate family members' adjustment to age- or diagnosis-related changes in client and resultant changes in family roles and structure:*
      1. instruct client and family about normal aging processes (e.g. sensory deficits, short-term memory loss, slowed response time)
      2. reinforce physician's explanation of the effects of the current diagnosis and planned treatment and rehabilitation
      3. encourage verbalization of feelings about changes in client and the effect of these on family structure
      4. provide privacy so that family members can share their feelings with one another; stress the importance and facilitate the use of good communication techniques
      5. assist family members to progress through their own grieving process; explain that during this progression, they may encounter times when they need to focus on meeting their own rather than the client's needs
      6. emphasize the need for family members to obtain adequate rest and nutrition and to identify and utilize stress management techniques *so they are better able to emotionally and physically deal with the changes and losses experienced*
      7. encourage and assist family members to identify coping strategies for dealing with client's age-related functional changes and changes in health status and their effect on the family
      8. include family members in decision making about client and his/her care; convey appreciation for their input and continued support of client
      9. encourage and allow family members to participate in client's care; provide necessary instruction and stress the importance of allowing the client to use adaptive devices, mobility aids, and techniques to improve thought processes if appropriate *so that he/she can maintain as much independence as possible*
      10. assist family members to identify resources that could assist them in coping with their feelings and meeting their immediate and long-term needs (e.g. counseling and social services; pastoral care; service, church, and support groups); initiate a referral if indicated.
   d. Consult physician if family members continue to demonstrate difficulty adapting to changes in roles, family structure, and aging of a family member.

* The term family members is being used here to include client's significant others.

☐ ▬▬▬▬▬▬▬▬▬▬▬▬▬▬▬▬▬▬▬▬▬▬▬▬▬▬▬▬▬▬▬▬▬▬▬

Reference

Carpenito, LJ. Handbook of nursing diagnosis (3rd ed.). Philadelphia: J.B. Lippincott Company, 1989.

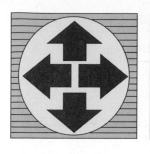
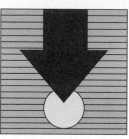
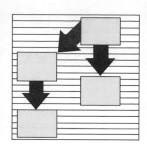
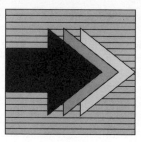
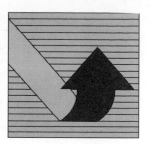

Unit II

Nursing Care of the Client Having Surgery

Preoperative Care

This care plan focuses on the adult client who is scheduled for a surgical procedure. The goals of preoperative care are to prepare the client physically and psychologically for the surgery and for the postoperative period. Good preoperative preparation greatly reduces the client's postoperative fear and anxiety and the risk of postoperative complications. Basic preoperative care is discussed here. In order to individualize this care plan, the client's emotional and physiological status, type of anesthesia to be used, and planned surgical procedure must be considered. This care plan is to be used in conjunction with each surgical care plan.

PREOPERATIVE CRITERIA

Prior to surgery, the client will:

- share thoughts and feelings about the impending surgery and its anticipated effects
- verbalize an understanding of usual preoperative and postoperative care and routines
- demonstrate the ability to perform techniques designed to prevent postoperative complications.

NURSING DIAGNOSES

1. Anxiety □ *34*
2. Sleep pattern disturbance □ *35*
3. Grieving □ *36*
4. Knowledge deficit regarding hospital routines associated with surgery, physical preparation for the surgical procedure, and postoperative care □ *37*

1. NURSING DIAGNOSIS

Anxiety related to:

a. unfamiliar environment;
b. separation from significant others;
c. lack of understanding of diagnostic tests and planned surgical procedure;
d. economic factors associated with hospitalization;
e. potential embarrassment or loss of dignity associated with body exposure;
f. effects of anesthesia;
g. anticipated discomfort, mutilation, limitations, and changes in usual life style and roles;
h. possibility of death.

DESIRED OUTCOMES

1. The client will experience a reduction in fear and anxiety as evidenced by:
   a. verbalization of feeling less anxious or fearful
   b. relaxed facial expression and body movements
   c. stable vital signs
   d. usual skin color
   e. verbalization of an understanding of hospital routines, diagnostic tests, preoperative procedures, and the surgery and its anticipated effects.

NURSING ACTIONS AND *SELECTED RATIONALES*

1.a. Gather the following data from the client during the preoperative period:
   1. fears, misconceptions, and level of understanding of planned surgical procedure
   2. perception of anticipated results of surgery
   3. significance of the surgical procedure and hospitalization
   4. previous surgical and hospital experiences
   5. availability of adequate support systems.

b. Assess client for signs and symptoms of fear and anxiety (e.g. verbalization of fears and concerns; tenseness; tremors; irritability; restlessness; diaphoresis; tachypnea; tachycardia; elevated blood pressure; facial tension, pallor, or flushing; noncompliance with treatment plan).

c. Ascertain effectiveness of current coping skills.

d. Implement measures *to reduce fear and anxiety:*
   1. orient to hospital environment, equipment, and routines
   2. introduce staff who will be participating in his/her care; if possible, maintain consistency in staff assigned to his/her care *to provide feelings of stability and comfort with the environment*
   3. assure client that staff members are nearby; respond to call signal as soon as possible
   4. maintain a calm, confident manner when interacting with client
   5. encourage verbalization of fear and anxiety; provide feedback
   6. reinforce the physician's explanations and clarify any misconceptions the client may have about the surgical procedure (e.g. purpose, size and location of incision, outcome)
   7. explain all presurgical diagnostic tests
   8. instruct client regarding planned preoperative procedures and postoperative care (see Nursing Diagnosis 4, actions a.1–4 and b.1)
   9. enable client *to maintain a sense of control by:*
      a. including him/her in planning of preoperative care
      b. allowing choices whenever possible
      c. explaining purpose and importance of the written consent form (e.g. indicates voluntary and informed consent, protects against unsanctioned surgery)
   10. provide a calm, restful environment
   11. instruct in relaxation techniques and encourage participation in diversional activities
   12. assist client to identify specific stressors and ways to cope with them
   13. assure client that pain relief needs will be met postoperatively
   14. encourage significant others to project a caring, concerned attitude without obvious anxiousness
   15. arrange for a visit from clergy if client desires
   16. monitor for therapeutic and nontherapeutic effects of antianxiety agents if administered.

e. Include significant others in orientation and teaching sessions and encourage their continued support of client.

f. Provide information based on current needs of client and significant others at a level they can understand. Encourage questions and clarification of information provided.

g. Consult physician if above actions fail to control fear and anxiety.

2. NURSING DIAGNOSIS

Sleep pattern disturbance related to fear, anxiety, and unfamiliar environment.

DESIRED OUTCOMES	NURSING ACTIONS AND *SELECTED RATIONALES*

2. The client will attain optimal amounts of sleep within the parameters of the treatment regimen as evidenced by:
   a. statements of feeling well rested
   b. usual behavior
   c. absence of frequent yawning, thick speech, dark circles under eyes.

2.a. Assess for signs and symptoms of a sleep pattern disturbance:
   1. verbal complaints of difficulty falling asleep, not feeling well rested, sleep interruptions, or awakening earlier or later than desired
   2. behavior changes (e.g. irritability, disorganization, lethargy)
   3. frequent yawning, thick speech, dark circles under eyes, slight hand tremors.
   b. Determine the client's usual sleep habits.
   c. Implement measures *to promote sleep:*
      1. perform actions to reduce fear and anxiety (see Nursing Diagnosis 1, action d)
      2. allow client to continue usual sleep practices (e.g. position, time, bedtime rituals) if possible
      3. determine measures that have been helpful to the client in the past (e.g. milk, warm drinks, warm bath) and incorporate in plan of care
      4. discourage long periods of sleep during the day unless sleep deprivation exists or daytime sleep is usual for client
      5. encourage participation in relaxing diversional activities in early evening hours
      6. provide a quiet, restful atmosphere
      7. discourage intake of foods and fluids high in caffeine (e.g. chocolate, coffee, tea, colas), especially in the evening
      8. satisfy basic needs such as hunger, comfort, and warmth before sleep
      9. have client empty bladder just before bedtime
      10. utilize relaxation techniques (e.g. progressive relaxation exercises, back massage, meditation, soft music) before sleep
      11. perform actions *to provide for periods of uninterrupted sleep (90- to 120-minute periods of uninterrupted sleep are considered essential):*
         a. restrict visitors during rest periods
         b. group care (e.g. medications, treatments, physical care, assessments) whenever possible
      12. monitor for therapeutic and nontherapeutic effects of sedatives and hypnotics if administered.
   d. Consult physician if signs of sleep deprivation persist or worsen.

☐ ▬▬▬▬▬▬▬▬▬▬▬▬▬▬▬▬▬▬▬▬▬▬▬▬

3. NURSING DIAGNOSIS

Grieving* related to potential loss of or change in a body part and/or usual body functioning.

---

* This diagnostic label includes anticipatory grieving and grieving following the actual losses/changes.

☐ ▬▬▬▬▬▬▬▬▬▬▬▬▬▬▬▬▬▬▬▬▬▬▬▬

DESIRED OUTCOMES	NURSING ACTIONS AND *SELECTED RATIONALES*

3. The client will demonstrate beginning progression through the grieving process as evidenced by:
   a. verbalization of feelings about anticipated change in body image and usual body functioning
   b. expression of grief

3.a. Determine the client's perception of the impact of surgery on his/her future.
   b. Determine how the client usually expresses grief.
   c. Observe for signs of grieving (e.g. changes in eating habits, insomnia, anger, noncompliance, denial).
   d. Implement measures *to facilitate the grieving process:*
      1. assist client to acknowledge the losses and changes experienced *so grief work can begin*; assess for factors that may hinder or facilitate acknowledgment
      2. discuss the grieving process and assist client to accept the stages of grieving as an expected response to anticipated losses and/or changes

c. participation in preoperative care and self-care activities
d. utilization of available support systems.

3. allow time for client to progress through the stages of grieving (denial, anger, bargaining, depression, acceptance [Kübler-Ross, 1969]); be aware that not every stage is experienced or expressed by all individuals
4. provide an atmosphere of care and concern (e.g. provide privacy, be available and nonjudgmental, display empathy and respect) *so that client will feel free to verbalize both positive and negative feelings and concerns*
5. perform actions *to promote trust* (e.g. answer questions honestly, provide requested information)
6. encourage the expression of anger and sadness about the losses and changes that may be experienced
7. encourage client to express his/her feelings in whatever ways are comfortable (e.g. writing, drawing, conversation)
8. assist client to identify personal strengths that have helped him/her to cope in previous situations of loss or change
9. support realistic hope about changes/losses that may result from surgery.
e. Assess for and support behaviors suggesting successful resolution of grief (e.g. verbalizing feelings about anticipated losses, expressing sorrow, focusing on ways to adapt to changes/losses that will occur).
f. Explain stages of grieving process to significant others. Encourage their support and understanding.
g. Assist significant others in their adjustment to losses or changes that will be experienced by the client by encouraging them to voice their concerns and preparing them for anticipated changes in the client.
h. Provide information regarding counseling services and support groups that might assist client and significant others in working through grief.
i. Arrange for a visit from clergy if desired by client.
j. Monitor for therapeutic and nontherapeutic effects of antidepressants if administered.
k. Consult physician regarding a referral for counseling if signs of dysfunctional grieving (e.g. persistent denial of the situation being experienced, excessive anger or sadness, hysteria, suicidal behaviors) occur.

□ ▬▬▬▬▬▬▬▬▬▬▬▬▬▬▬▬▬▬▬▬▬▬▬▬▬▬▬▬▬▬▬▬▬▬

4. NURSING DIAGNOSIS

Knowledge deficit regarding hospital routines associated with surgery, physical preparation for the surgical procedure, and postoperative care.

□ ▬▬▬▬▬▬▬▬▬▬▬▬▬▬▬▬▬▬▬▬▬▬▬▬▬▬▬▬▬▬▬▬▬▬

DESIRED OUTCOMES	NURSING ACTIONS AND *SELECTED RATIONALES*

4.a. The client will verbalize an understanding of usual preoperative and postoperative care and routines.	4.a.1. Provide information about usual preoperative routines for the surgery to be performed (e.g. blood work, EKG, urinalysis, chest x-ray, insertion of urinary catheter and/or nasogastric tube, bowel and skin preparation, removal of prosthetic devices).
	2. Provide information related to:
	  a. scheduled time and estimated length of surgery
	  b. reasons for food and fluid restrictions before surgery
	  c. preoperative medications
	  d. body position during surgical procedure
	  e. induction and recovery room (e.g. purpose and estimated length of stay).
	3. Reinforce teaching and information provided by the anesthesiologist and the surgeon.
	4. Inform client of the anticipated postoperative care:
	  a. equipment (e.g. dressings, intravenous lines, drainage tubes, traction devices)

   b. activity limitations and expectations
   c. dietary modifications
   d. treatments (e.g. respiratory care, circulatory management, wound care) and expected frequency
   e. assessments (e.g. intake and output, chest sounds, vital signs, neurological checks, bowel sounds) and expected frequency
   f. medications (e.g. antiemetics, analgesics, anti-infectives)
   g. methods for controlling pain (e.g. positioning, medications, transcutaneous electrical nerve stimulation, progressive relaxation exercises, patient-controlled analgesia [PCA]).
5. Allow time for questions and clarification. Provide feedback.

4.b. The client will demonstrate the ability to perform techniques designed to prevent postoperative complications.

4.b.1. Demonstrate actions or techniques that the client will be expected to perform postoperatively. These may include:
   a. effective coughing and deep breathing techniques
   b. correct use of the inspiratory exerciser
   c. active foot and leg exercises
   d. correct methods for changing position and increasing activity (e.g. moving slowly, keeping body in proper alignment, using good body mechanics, requesting assistance when needed).
2. Allow time for questions, clarification, and return demonstration.

Reference

Kübler-Ross, E. On death and dying. New York: Macmillan, 1969.

Postoperative Care

The postoperative period begins immediately after surgery. This care plan focuses on the postoperative care of an adult client who has received a general anesthetic. The goals of care are to prevent complications and assist the client to attain an optimal health status postoperatively.

This care plan should be used in conjunction with any surgical care plan.

DISCHARGE CRITERIA

Prior to discharge, the client will:

- identify ways to prevent postoperative infection
- demonstrate the ability to perform wound care
- state signs and symptoms of complications to report to the health care provider
- share thoughts and feelings about the surgery, diagnosis, prognosis, and treatment plan
- verbalize an understanding of and a plan for adhering to recommended follow-up care including future appointments with health care provider, dietary modifications, activity level, treatments, and medications prescribed.

NURSING/COLLABORATIVE DIAGNOSES

1. Anxiety □ 39
2. Altered systemic tissue perfusion □ 40
3. Ineffective breathing patterns □ 41
4. Ineffective airway clearance □ 42
5. Altered fluid and electrolyte balance:
   a. fluid volume deficit, hyponatremia, hypokalemia, hypochloremia, and metabolic alkalosis
   b. fluid volume excess or water intoxication □ 43
6. Altered nutrition: less than body requirements □ 44
7A. Altered comfort: pain □ 45
7B. Altered comfort: abdominal discomfort (distention and gas pain) □ 46
7C. Altered comfort: nausea and vomiting □ 47
7D. Altered comfort: hiccoughs □ 48
8. Altered oral mucous membrane: dryness □ 48
9. Impaired skin integrity:
   a. surgical incision
   b. impaired wound healing
   c. irritation or breakdown □ 49
10. Activity intolerance □ 51
11. Impaired physical mobility □ 52
12. Self-care deficit □ 52
13. Urinary retention □ 53
14. Constipation □ 54
15. Sleep pattern disturbance □ 55
16. Potential for infection:
    a. pneumonia
    b. wound infection
    c. urinary tract infection □ 56
17. Potential for trauma □ 57
18. Potential for aspiration □ 58
19. Potential complications:
    a. hypovolemic shock
    b. atelectasis
    c. thromboembolism
    d. paralytic ileus
    e. dehiscence □ 59
20. Knowledge deficit regarding follow-up care □ 62

1. NURSING DIAGNOSIS

Anxiety related to unfamiliar environment; lack of understanding of diagnosis, surgical procedure performed, and postoperative management; pain; temporary or permanent change in life style; financial concerns; and alterations in self-concept.

DESIRED OUTCOMES	NURSING ACTIONS AND *SELECTED RATIONALES*

1. The client will experience a reduction in fear and anxiety as evidenced by:
   a. verbalization of feeling less anxious or fearful
   b. relaxed facial expression and body movements
   c. stable vital signs
   d. usual skin color
   e. verbalization of an understanding of hospital routines, diagnosis, surgical procedure performed, and treatments.

1.a. Assess client for signs and symptoms of fear and anxiety (e.g. verbalization of fears and concerns; tenseness; tremors; irritability; restlessness; diaphoresis; tachycardia; tachypnea; elevated blood pressure; facial tension, pallor, or flushing; noncompliance with treatment plan). Validate perceptions carefully, remembering that some behavior may result from factors such as pain, impaired gas exchange, and infection.
   b. Ascertain effectiveness of current coping skills.
   c. Implement measures *to reduce fear and anxiety:*
      1. orient to hospital environment, equipment, and routines
      2. introduce staff who will be participating in his/her care; if possible, maintain consistency in staff assigned to his/her care *to provide feelings of stability and comfort with the environment*
      3. assure client that staff members are nearby; respond to call signal as soon as possible
      4. maintain a calm, confident manner when interacting with client
      5. encourage verbalization of fear and anxiety; provide feedback
      6. reinforce the physician's explanations and clarify any misconceptions the client may have about the diagnosis, surgical procedure performed, treatment plan, and prognosis
      7. perform actions to reduce pain (see Nursing Diagnosis 7.A, action 5)
      8. provide a calm, restful environment
      9. instruct in relaxation techniques and encourage participation in diversional activities
      10. assist client to identify specific stressors and ways to cope with them
      11. arrange for visit from clergy if client desires
      12. initiate financial and/or social service referrals if indicated
      13. encourage significant others to project a caring, concerned attitude without obvious anxiousness
      14. monitor for therapeutic and nontherapeutic effects of antianxiety agents if administered.
   d. Include significant others in orientation and teaching sessions and encourage their continued support of the client.
   e. Provide information based on current needs of client and significant others at a level they can understand. Encourage questions and clarification of information provided.
   f. Consult physician if above actions fail to control fear and anxiety.

---

2. NURSING DIAGNOSIS

Altered systemic tissue perfusion related to:

a. hypovolemia resulting from fluid loss and decreased fluid intake;
b. peripheral pooling of blood associated with decreased venous return resulting from a loss of vasomotor tone associated with anesthesia, some medications (e.g. narcotic analgesics, muscle relaxants), and decreased activity;
c. vasoconstriction associated with hypothermia resulting from cool operating and recovery room temperatures (the rooms are kept cool to decrease the client's basal metabolic rate).

DESIRED OUTCOMES	NURSING ACTIONS AND *SELECTED RATIONALES*

2. The client will maintain adequate systemic tissue perfusion as evidenced by:

2.a. Assess for and report signs and symptoms of diminished systemic tissue perfusion:
   1. significant decrease in B/P

a. B/P and pulse within normal range for client and stable with position change
b. unlabored respirations at 16–20/minute
c. usual mental status
d. skin warm and usual color
e. palpable peripheral pulses
f. capillary refill time less than 3 seconds
g. urine output at least 30 cc/hour.

2. resting pulse rate greater than 100 beats/minute
3. decline in systolic B/P of at least 15 mm Hg with a concurrent rise in pulse when client changes from lying to sitting or standing position
4. rapid or labored respirations
5. restlessness, slow responses, confusion
6. cool, pale, mottled, or cyanotic skin
7. diminished or absent peripheral pulses
8. capillary refill time greater than 3 seconds
9. urine output less than 30 cc/hour.

b. Implement measures *to maintain adequate systemic tissue perfusion:*
1. monitor for therapeutic and nontherapeutic effects of fluid and/or blood replacement therapy if administered
2. maintain a minimum fluid intake of at least 2500 cc/day unless contraindicated
3. perform actions *to prevent peripheral pooling of blood:*
   a. instruct client in and assist with active foot and leg exercises for 5–10 minutes every 1–2 hours
   b. encourage and assist with ambulation as soon as ordered (client should be instructed to pick up instead of shuffle feet *in order to maximize muscular contraction*)
   c. discourage positions that compromise blood flow in lower extremities (e.g. crossing legs, pillows under knees, use of knee gatch, sitting for long periods)
   d. consult physician regarding order for antiembolic hose or elastic wraps if prolonged activity restriction is expected; if these are applied, remove for 30–60 minutes every shift
   e. assist with intermittent venous compression using pneumatic cuffs or boots if ordered
4. instruct client to change positions slowly *to allow time for autoregulatory mechanisms to adjust to position changes*
5. discourage smoking (*smoking decreases oxygen availability and causes vasoconstriction*)
6. maintain a comfortable room temperature and provide client with adequate clothing and blankets (*exposure to cold causes generalized vasoconstriction*).
c. Consult physician if signs and symptoms of decreased systemic tissue perfusion persist or worsen.

□ ▬▬▬▬▬▬▬▬▬▬▬▬▬▬▬▬▬▬▬▬▬▬▬▬

3. NURSING DIAGNOSIS

Ineffective breathing patterns related to fear, anxiety, pain, depressant effects of anesthesia and some medications (e.g. narcotic analgesics, muscle relaxants), abdominal distention, positioning, weakness, and fatigue.

□ ▬▬▬▬▬▬▬▬▬▬▬▬▬▬▬▬▬▬▬▬▬▬▬▬

DESIRED OUTCOMES	NURSING ACTIONS AND *SELECTED RATIONALES*
3. The client will maintain an effective breathing pattern as evidenced by: a. normal rate, rhythm, and depth of respirations b. blood gases within normal range.	3.a. Assess for signs and symptoms of ineffective breathing patterns (e.g. shallow or slow respirations, hyperventilation, dyspnea, use of accessory muscles for breathing). b. Monitor blood gases. Report abnormal results. c. Monitor for and report significant changes in ear oximetry and capnograph results. d. Implement measures *to improve breathing pattern:* 　1. perform actions to decrease fear and anxiety (see Nursing Diagnosis 1, action c) 　2. perform actions to decrease pain (see Nursing Diagnosis 7.A, action 5)

3. perform actions to reduce the accumulation of gastrointestinal gas and fluid (see Nursing Diagnosis 7.B, action 3) *in order to decrease pressure on the diaphragm*
4. perform actions to increase strength and improve activity tolerance (see Nursing Diagnosis 10, action b)
5. encourage deep breathing and use of inspiratory exerciser at least every 2 hours
6. administer or assist with IPPB treatments as ordered
7. place client in a semi- to high Fowler's position unless contraindicated
8. instruct client to breathe slowly if he/she is hyperventilating
9. if client is on bedrest, assist him/her to turn at least every 2 hours
10. increase activity as allowed and tolerated
11. administer central nervous system depressants (e.g. narcotic analgesics, sedatives, muscle relaxants) judiciously; hold medication and consult physician if respiratory rate is less than 12/minute.

e. Consult physician if:
1. ineffective breathing patterns continue
2. signs and symptoms of impaired gas exchange (e.g. confusion, restlessness, irritability, cyanosis, decreased PaO_2 and increased $PaCO_2$ levels) are present.

☐ ▆▆▆▆▆▆▆▆▆▆▆▆▆▆▆▆▆▆▆▆▆▆▆▆▆▆▆▆▆▆▆▆

4. NURSING DIAGNOSIS

Ineffective airway clearance related to:

a. stasis of secretions associated with decreased activity and poor cough effort resulting from depressant effects of anesthesia and some medications (e.g. narcotic analgesics, muscle relaxants), pain, weakness, and fatigue;
b. increased secretions associated with irritation of the respiratory tract (can result from inhalation anesthetics and endotracheal intubation);
c. tenacious secretions associated with fluid loss and decreased fluid intake.

☐ ▆▆▆▆▆▆▆▆▆▆▆▆▆▆▆▆▆▆▆▆▆▆▆▆▆▆▆▆▆▆▆▆

DESIRED OUTCOMES	NURSING ACTIONS AND *SELECTED RATIONALES*
4. The client will maintain clear, open airways as evidenced by: a. normal breath sounds b. normal rate and depth of respirations c. absence of dyspnea d. absence of cyanosis.	4.a. Assess for signs and symptoms of ineffective airway clearance (e.g. adventitious breath sounds; rapid, shallow respirations; dyspnea; cyanosis). b. Implement measures *to promote effective airway clearance:* 　1. perform actions to decrease pain (see Nursing Diagnosis 7.A, action 5) 　2. increase activity as allowed and tolerated 　3. perform actions *to facilitate removal of pulmonary secretions:* 　　a. implement measures *to liquefy tenacious secretions:* 　　　1. maintain a fluid intake of at least 2500 cc/day unless contraindicated 　　　2. humidify inspired air as ordered 　　　3. assist with administration of mucolytic agents via nebulizer or IPPB treatment 　　b. instruct and assist client with effective coughing techniques every 1–2 hours unless contraindicated 　　c. assist with or perform postural drainage, percussion, and vibration if ordered 　　d. perform tracheal suctioning if needed 　　e. monitor for therapeutic and nontherapeutic effects of expectorants if administered 　4. discourage smoking (*smoking causes an increase in mucus production and impairs ciliary function*).

    c. Consult physician if:
      1. signs and symptoms of ineffective airway clearance persist
      2. signs and symptoms of impaired gas exchange (e.g. confusion, restlessness, irritability, cyanosis, decreased PaO_2 and increased $PaCO_2$ levels) are present.

5. NURSING/COLLABORATIVE DIAGNOSIS

Altered fluid and electrolyte balance:

a. **fluid volume deficit, hyponatremia, hypokalemia, hypochloremia, and metabolic alkalosis** related to excessive loss of fluid and electrolytes associated with vomiting, nasogastric tube drainage, and profuse wound drainage;

b. **fluid volume excess or water intoxication** related to vigorous fluid therapy during and immediately following surgery and increased production of antidiuretic hormone (ADH) and aldosterone (output of these hormones is stimulated by trauma, pain, anesthetic agents, and narcotic analgesics).

DESIRED OUTCOMES	NURSING ACTIONS AND *SELECTED RATIONALES*

5.a. The client will maintain fluid and electrolyte balance as evidenced by:
  1. normal skin turgor
  2. moist mucous membranes
  3. stable weight
  4. B/P and pulse within normal range for client and stable with position change
  5. urine specific gravity between 1.010 and 1.030
  6. no evidence of confusion, irritability, lethargy, excessive thirst, ileus, cardiac arrhythmias, muscle weakness
  7. normal serum osmolality, electrolytes, and blood gases.

5.a.1. Assess for and report signs and symptoms of:
  a. fluid volume deficit:
    1. decreased skin turgor, dry mucous membranes, thirst
    2. weight loss greater than 0.5 kg/day
    3. low B/P and/or decline in B/P of at least 15 mm Hg with concurrent rise in pulse when client sits up
    4. weak, rapid pulse
    5. urine specific gravity higher than 1.030 (reflects an actual rather than a potential fluid volume deficit)
  b. hyponatremia (e.g. nausea and vomiting, abdominal cramps, weakness, twitching, lethargy, confusion, seizures)
  c. hypokalemia (e.g. irregular pulse, muscle weakness and cramping, paresthesias, nausea and vomiting, hypoactive or absent bowel sounds, drowsiness)
  d. hypochloremia (e.g. twitching, tetany, depressed respirations)
  e. metabolic alkalosis (e.g. dizziness; confusion; bradypnea; tingling of fingers, toes, and circumoral area; muscle twitching; seizures).
2. Monitor serum osmolality, electrolyte, and blood gas results. Report abnormal values.
3. Implement measures *to prevent and treat fluid and electrolyte imbalances:*
  a. perform actions to prevent vomiting (see Nursing Diagnosis 7.C, action 2)
  b. if irrigation of the nasogastric tube is indicated, use normal saline rather than water
  c. monitor for therapeutic and nontherapeutic effects of fluid and electrolyte replacements if administered
  d. maintain a fluid intake of at least 2500 cc/day unless contraindicated
  e. when oral intake is allowed and tolerated, assist client to select foods/fluids high in potassium (e.g. bananas, oranges, potatoes, raisins, figs, apricots, dates, tomatoes, Gatorade, fruit juices) and sodium (e.g. cured meats, processed cheese, soups, catsup, tomato juice, canned vegetables, pickles, bouillon).
4. Consult physician if signs and symptoms of fluid and electrolyte imbalances persist or worsen.

5.b. The client will not experience fluid volume excess or water intoxication as evidenced by:
1. stable weight
2. stable B/P and pulse
3. absence of gallop rhythms
4. balanced intake and output within 48 hours following surgery
5. usual mental status
6. normal breath sounds
7. serum osmolality, Hct., and sodium levels within normal range
8. urine specific gravity between 1.010 and 1.030
9. absence of dyspnea, edema, distended neck veins
10. CVP within normal range.

5.b.1. Assess for and report signs and symptoms of fluid volume excess and water intoxication:
a. significant weight gain (greater than 0.5 kg/day)
b. elevated B/P and pulse (B/P may not be elevated if fluid has shifted out of vascular space)
c. development of an S_3 and/or S_4 gallop rhythm
d. intake that continues to be greater than output 48 hours postoperatively (for the first 48 hours after surgery, output is expected to be less than intake *due to increased secretion of ADH and aldosterone*)
e. change in mental status
f. crackles and diminished or absent breath sounds
g. low serum sodium and osmolality (indicates water intoxication)
h. decreased Hct. (may also indicate blood loss)
i. urine specific gravity less than 1.010
j. dyspnea, orthopnea
k. edema (peripheral edema reflects fluid volume excess; cellular edema reflects water intoxication)
l. distended neck veins
m. elevated CVP (use internal jugular vein pulsation method to estimate CVP if monitoring device not present).
2. Monitor chest x-ray results. Report findings of vascular congestion, pleural effusion, or pulmonary edema.
3. Implement measures *to prevent and treat fluid volume excess and water intoxication:*
a. administer fluid replacement therapy judiciously especially within first 48 hours after surgery
b. maintain fluid restrictions as ordered
c. restrict sodium intake as ordered
d. encourage client to lie flat periodically as tolerated *(lying flat promotes reshifting of fluid into the vascular space, which allows for diuresis of excess fluid)*
e. monitor for therapeutic and nontherapeutic effects of the following medications if administered:
1. diuretics *to increase excretion of water*
2. positive inotropic agents and arterial vasodilators *to increase cardiac output and subsequently improve renal blood flow.*
4. Consult physician if signs and symptoms of fluid volume excess or water intoxication persist or worsen.

6. NURSING DIAGNOSIS

Altered nutrition: less than body requirements related to:

a. decreased oral intake associated with:
1. anorexia resulting from discomfort, fatigue, constipation, and decreased activity
2. nausea
3. dislike of prescribed diet
4. prescribed dietary modifications;
b. inadequate nutritional replacement therapy;
c. loss of nutrients associated with vomiting;
d. increased nutritional needs associated with increased metabolic rate that occurs during wound healing.

DESIRED OUTCOMES	NURSING ACTIONS AND *SELECTED RATIONALES*

6. The client will maintain an adequate nutritional status as evidenced by:
   a. weight within normal range for client's age, height, and build
   b. normal BUN and serum albumin, protein, Hct., Hgb., cholesterol, and lymphocyte levels
   c. triceps skinfold measurements within normal range
   d. usual strength and activity tolerance
   e. healthy oral mucous membrane.

6.a. Assess the client for signs and symptoms of malnutrition:
1. weight below normal for client's age, height, and build
2. abnormal BUN and low serum albumin, protein, Hct., Hgb., cholesterol, and lymphocyte levels (decreased Hct. and Hgb. may also result from blood loss)
3. triceps skinfold measurement less than normal for build
4. weakness and fatigue
5. stomatitis.
   b. Reassess nutritional status on a regular basis and report decline.
   c. Assess for return of normal bowel function every 2–4 hours. Notify physician when client has normal bowel sounds and is expelling flatus *so that oral intake can be resumed as soon as possible.*
   d. When oral intake is allowed, monitor percentage of meals eaten.
   e. Assess client to determine the causative factors of inadequate intake (e.g. prescribed dietary modifications, inadequate nutritional replacement therapy, nausea, pain, fatigue).
   f. Implement measures *to maintain and improve nutritional status:*
1. when food and fluids are allowed, perform actions *to improve oral intake:*
   a. implement measures to prevent nausea and vomiting (see Nursing Diagnosis 7.C, action 2)
   b. implement measures to reduce discomfort (see Nursing Diagnoses 7.A, action 5; 7.B, action 3; and 7.D)
   c. implement measures to prevent constipation (see Nursing Diagnosis 14, action e)
   d. provide a clean, relaxed, pleasant atmosphere
   e. increase activity as allowed and tolerated (*activity stimulates appetite*)
   f. encourage a rest period before meals *to minimize fatigue*
   g. encourage significant others to bring in client's favorite foods in accordance with prescribed dietary modifications
   h. allow adequate time for meals; reheat food if necessary
2. perform actions *to meet increased nutritional needs:*
   a. provide foods and fluids high in protein, calories, vitamins, and minerals as allowed and tolerated; obtain a dietary consult if necessary to assist client in selecting items that meet nutritional needs, prescribed dietary modifications, and preferences
   b. monitor for therapeutic and nontherapeutic effects of vitamins, minerals, and hematinics if administered.
   g. Perform a 72-hour calorie count if nutritional status declines or fails to improve.
   h. Consult physician regarding alternative methods of providing nutrition (e.g. parenteral nutrition, tube feedings) if client does not consume enough food or fluids to meet nutritional needs.

□ ▬▬▬▬▬▬▬▬▬▬▬▬▬▬▬▬▬▬▬▬▬▬▬

7.A. NURSING DIAGNOSIS

Altered comfort:* pain related to tissue trauma and reflex muscle spasm associated with the surgical procedure.

---

* In this care plan, the nursing diagnosis "pain" is included under the diagnostic label of altered comfort.

□ ▬▬▬▬▬▬▬▬▬▬▬▬▬▬▬▬▬▬▬▬▬▬▬

DESIRED OUTCOMES	NURSING ACTIONS AND *SELECTED RATIONALES*

7.A. The client will experience diminished pain as evidenced by:
  1. verbalization of pain relief
  2. relaxed facial expression and body positioning
  3. increased participation in activities
  4. stable vital signs.

7.A.1. Determine how the client usually responds to pain.
  2. Assess for nonverbal signs of pain (e.g. wrinkled brow, clenched fists, reluctance to move, restlessness, diaphoresis, facial pallor or flushing, change in B/P, tachycardia).
  3. Assess verbal complaints of pain. Ask client to be specific about location, severity, and type of pain.
  4. Assess for factors that seem to aggravate and alleviate pain.
  5. Implement measures *to reduce pain:*
      a. perform actions to reduce fear and anxiety about the pain experience (e.g. assure client that his/her need for pain relief will be met)
      b. medicate prior to any painful treatments or procedures and before pain is severe
      c. provide or assist with nonpharmacological measures for pain relief (e.g. back rub, position change, relaxation techniques, transcutaneous electrical nerve stimulation, guided imagery, quiet conversation, restful environment, diversional activities)
      d. instruct and assist client to support abdominal or chest incision with a pillow or hands when turning, coughing, and deep breathing
      e. encourage client to use patient-controlled analgesia (PCA) device as instructed
      f. monitor for therapeutic and nontherapeutic effects of analgesics and muscle relaxants if administered.
  6. Consult physician if above measures fail to provide adequate pain relief.

☐ ██████████████████████████████████

7.B. NURSING DIAGNOSIS

Altered comfort: abdominal discomfort (distention and gas pain) related to accumulation of gas and fluid associated with decreased peristalsis resulting from manipulation of the bowel during abdominal surgery, depressant effects of anesthesia and some medications (e.g. narcotic analgesics, muscle relaxants, antiemetics), and decreased activity.

☐ ██████████████████████████████████

DESIRED OUTCOMES	NURSING ACTIONS AND *SELECTED RATIONALES*

7.B. The client will experience diminished abdominal distention and gas pain as evidenced by:
  1. verbalization of decreased abdominal fullness and pain
  2. relaxed facial expression and body positioning
  3. decrease in abdominal distention.

7.B.1. Assess for nonverbal signs of abdominal distention and gas pain (e.g. clutching and guarding of abdomen, restlessness, reluctance to move, grimacing, increasing abdominal girth, dyspnea).
  2. Assess verbal complaints of abdominal discomfort (e.g. increasing feeling of abdominal fullness, gas pain).
  3. Implement measures *to reduce the accumulation of gastrointestinal gas and fluid:*
      a. encourage and assist client with frequent position changes and ambulation as soon as allowed and tolerated (*activity stimulates peristalsis and expulsion of flatus*)
      b. instruct the client to avoid activities such as chewing gum, sucking on hard candy, and smoking *in order to reduce air swallowing*
      c. maintain patency of gastric or intestinal tube if present
      d. maintain food and fluid restrictions as ordered
      e. when oral intake is allowed:
          1. encourage client to drink warm liquids *to stimulate peristalsis*
          2. instruct client to avoid gas-producing foods/fluids (e.g. carbonated beverages, cabbage, onions, popcorn, baked beans)

f. encourage client to expel flatus whenever the urge is felt
g. apply heat to the abdomen for 20 minutes every 2–3 hours unless contraindicated
h. consult physician regarding insertion of a rectal tube or administration of a return flow enema if indicated
i. encourage use of nonnarcotic analgesics once the period of severe pain has subsided (*narcotic analgesics depress gastrointestinal activity*)
j. monitor for therapeutic and nontherapeutic effects of gastrointestinal stimulants (e.g. metoclopramide, bisacodyl) if administered *to increase gastrointestinal motility.*

4. Inform client that although the increased movement of accumulated gas is often quite painful, it does signal return of peristalsis.
5. Consult physician if abdominal discomfort persists or worsens.

7.C. NURSING DIAGNOSIS

Altered comfort: nausea and vomiting related to stimulation of the vomiting center associated with:

1. vagal and/or sympathetic stimulation resulting from visceral irritation associated with abdominal distention;
2. cortical stimulation due to pain and stress.

DESIRED OUTCOMES	NURSING ACTIONS AND *SELECTED RATIONALES*

7.C. The client will experience relief of nausea and vomiting as evidenced by:
1. verbalization of relief of nausea
2. absence of vomiting.
	7.C.1. Assess client to determine factors that contribute to nausea and vomiting (e.g. abdominal distention, pain, anxiety, certain foods and medications).
	2. Implement measures *to prevent nausea and vomiting:*
	  a. perform actions to decrease the accumulation of gastrointestinal gas and fluid (see Nursing Diagnosis 7.B, action 3)
	  b. perform actions to reduce pain (see Nursing Diagnosis 7.A, action 5)
	  c. perform actions to reduce fear and anxiety (see Nursing Diagnosis 1, action c)
	  d. eliminate noxious sights and smells from the environment (*noxious stimuli cause cortical stimulation of the vomiting center*)
	  e. encourage client to take deep, slow breaths when nauseated
	  f. instruct client to change positions slowly (*movement stimulates the chemoreceptor trigger zone*)
	  g. provide oral hygiene every 2 hours or before meals if oral intake is allowed and after each emesis
	  h. when oral intake is allowed:
	    1. advance diet slowly (usually beginning with clear liquids and progressing to solid food)
	    2. provide small, frequent meals rather than 3 large ones
	    3. instruct client to ingest foods and fluids slowly
	    4. instruct client to avoid foods/fluids that irritate the gastric mucosa (e.g. spicy foods; citrus fruits or juices; caffeine-containing items such as chocolate, coffee, tea, and colas)
	    5. encourage client to eat dry foods (e.g. toast, crackers) and avoid drinking liquids with meals if nauseated
	    6. instruct client to rest after eating with head of bed elevated
	  i. monitor for therapeutic and nontherapeutic effects of antiemetics and gastrointestinal stimulants (e.g. metoclopramide) if administered.
	3. Consult physician if above measures fail to control nausea and vomiting.

7.D. NURSING DIAGNOSIS

Altered comfort: hiccoughs related to irritation of the phrenic or vagus nerve associated with gastric and abdominal distention and/or presence of gastric or abdominal drainage tubes.

DESIRED OUTCOMES	NURSING ACTIONS AND *SELECTED RATIONALES*
7.D. The client will not experience persistent hiccoughs.	7.D.1. Implement measures *to prevent irritation of the phrenic and vagus nerves:* a. perform actions to reduce the accumulation of gastrointestinal gas and fluid (see Nursing Diagnosis 7.B, action 3) b. instruct client to avoid drinking very hot or cold liquids *to prevent reflex irritation of the phrenic and vagus nerves* c. securely anchor gastric and abdominal drainage tubes if present *in order to minimize movement of the tubes and subsequent irritation of the phrenic or vagus nerve.* 2. Implement measures *to control hiccoughs if they occur:* a. instruct client to perform techniques such as breathing deeply, rebreathing into a paper bag, holding breath, applying finger pressure on the eyeballs through closed lids for several minutes, eating a teaspoon of sugar, or drinking water while holding breath unless contraindicated b. monitor for therapeutic and nontherapeutic effects of sedatives and/or phenothiazines if administered. 3. Consult physician if hiccoughs persist. Be prepared to assist with the following treatments for intractable hiccoughs if ordered: a. gastric lavage or suction *to decrease abdominal distention* b. removal of gastric or abdominal tubes (*these may be irritating the phrenic or vagus nerve*) c. inhalation of carbon dioxide (*the depressant effect of CO_2 reduces spasm of the diaphragm*) d. gentle rotation of a suction catheter after inserting it into the pharynx (*this movement can interrupt impulses from the vagus nerve*) e. phrenic nerve block or phrenic nerve crushing.

8. NURSING DIAGNOSIS

Altered oral mucous membrane: dryness related to:

a. fluid volume deficit associated with fluid loss and fluid restrictions;
b. decreased salivation associated with fluid volume deficit, food and fluid restrictions, and some medications (e.g. anesthetic agents, narcotic analgesics).

DESIRED OUTCOMES	NURSING ACTIONS AND *SELECTED RATIONALES*
8. The client will maintain a moist, intact oral mucous membrane.	8.a. Assess client for dryness of the oral mucosa. b. Assure client that dry mouth and thirst are temporary conditions that will resolve as fluid intake increases and medications are decreased. c. Implement measures *to relieve dryness of the oral mucous membrane:* 　1. instruct and assist client to perform good oral hygiene as often as needed; avoid use of products such as lemon-glycerin swabs and commercial mouthwashes containing alcohol (*these products have a drying or irritating effect on the mucous membrane*) 　2. lubricate client's lips with Vaseline, K-Y jelly, Chapstick, Blistex, or mineral oil when oral care is given 　3. encourage client to breathe through nose if possible 　4. encourage client not to smoke (*smoking further irritates and dries the mucosa*) 　5. maintain intravenous fluid therapy as ordered *to improve hydration* 　6. provide sips of water frequently if allowed 　7. encourage client to suck on sour, hard candy unless contraindicated *in order to stimulate salivation* 　8. advance oral intake as soon as allowed and tolerated *to improve hydration and stimulate salivation.* d. Consult physician if signs and symptoms of parotitis (e.g. swelling of the parotid glands, ear pain, difficulty swallowing, fever) occur.

□ ▬▬▬▬▬▬▬▬▬▬▬▬▬▬▬▬▬▬▬▬▬▬

9. NURSING DIAGNOSIS

Impaired skin integrity:

a. **surgical incision**;
b. **impaired wound healing** related to inadequate nutritional status, inadequate blood supply to wound area, stress on wound area, infection, and increased levels of glucocorticoids (levels usually rise with stress);
c. **irritation or breakdown** related to contact of skin with wound drainage, pressure from drainage tubes, and use of tape.

□ ▬▬▬▬▬▬▬▬▬▬▬▬▬▬▬▬▬▬▬▬▬▬

DESIRED OUTCOMES	NURSING ACTIONS AND *SELECTED RATIONALES*
9.a. The client will experience normal healing of surgical wounds as evidenced by: 　1. gradual reduction in redness and swelling at wound site 　2. presence of granulation tissue if healing is by secondary and tertiary intention 　3. intact, approximated wound edges if healing is by primary intention.	9.a.1. Assess for and report signs and symptoms of impaired wound healing (e.g. increasing redness and swelling at wound site, pale or necrotic tissue in wounds healing by secondary and tertiary intention, separation of wound edges in wounds healing by primary intention). 　2. Implement measures *to promote normal wound healing:* 　a. perform actions to maintain an optimal nutritional status (see Nursing Diagnosis 6, action f) 　b. perform actions *to maintain adequate circulation to wound area:* 　　1. implement measures to maintain adequate systemic tissue perfusion (see Nursing Diagnosis 2, action b) 　　2. do not apply dressings tightly unless ordered (*excessive pressure impairs circulation to the area*) 　　3. implement measures *to decrease swelling in wound area:*

a. apply cold compresses as ordered
b. elevate wound area if feasible
c. administer anti-inflammatory drugs as ordered

c. perform actions *to protect the wound from mechanical injury:*
1. ensure that dressings are secure enough to keep them from rubbing and irritating wound
2. carefully remove tape and dressings when performing wound care
3. remind client to keep hands away from wound area
4. implement measures to prevent falls (see Nursing Diagnosis 17, action b)

d. perform actions *to decrease stress on wound area:*
1. instruct and assist client to support the involved area when moving
2. instruct and assist client to splint abdominal and chest wounds when coughing; consult physician regarding an order for antitussive if persistent cough is present
3. apply an abdominal binder during periods of activity if ordered *for additional support following abdominal surgery*
4. implement measures to reduce the accumulation of gastrointestinal gas and fluid (see Nursing Diagnosis 7.B, action 3) in clients who have had abdominal surgery
5. implement measures to prevent nausea and vomiting (see Nursing Diagnosis 7.C, action 2) in clients who have had chest, back, or abdominal surgery

e. perform actions to prevent wound infection (see Nursing Diagnosis 16, action b.4)

f. perform actions to reduce fear and anxiety (see Nursing Diagnosis 1, action c) *in order to prevent a continued increase in glucocorticoid level.*

3. If signs and symptoms of impaired wound healing occur:
a. assist with wound debridement if performed
b. provide emotional support to client and significant others.

9.b. The client will maintain skin integrity as evidenced by:
1. absence of redness and irritation
2. no skin breakdown.

9.b.1. Inspect skin areas that are in contact with wound drainage, tape, and drainage tubings for signs of irritation and breakdown.
2. Implement measures *to prevent skin irritation and breakdown:*
a. perform actions *to prevent wound drainage from contacting or remaining on skin:*
1. inspect dressings, wounds, and areas around drains or puncture sites; cleanse skin and change dressings if appropriate
2. maintain patency of drainage tubes *to decrease risk of leakage around the tubes*
3. apply a collection pouch over drains or incisions that are draining copiously
4. apply a protective paste to skin areas that are likely to be in contact with drainage

b. when positioning client, ensure that he/she is not lying on drainage tubings (*the pressure from the tubing can compromise circulation to the area and can also occlude the tubing*)

c. secure all tubings *to prevent excessive movement, which can irritate mucous membranes or skin*

d. apply a water-soluble lubricant to external nares every 2–4 hours *to decrease irritation from nasogastric tube and nasal airway or cannula*

e. perform actions *to decrease skin irritation resulting from the use of tape:*
1. use only necessary amount of tape
2. use hypoallergenic tape whenever possible to secure tubings and dressings
3. utilize Montgomery straps or elastic netting *to avoid repeated application and removal of tape if frequent dressing changes are anticipated*
4. apply skin sealants or barriers before application of tape if necessary *to prevent irritation and provide additional skin protection*
5. when removing tape, pull it in the direction of hair growth; use adhesive solvents if necessary.

3. If skin irritation or breakdown occurs:
a. notify physician

b. continue with above measures to prevent further irritation and breakdown
c. perform wound care as ordered or per standard hospital policy
d. monitor client closely and report signs and symptoms of infection (e.g. elevated temperature; redness, warmth, and edema around incision or area of breakdown; unusual drainage from site).

10. NURSING DIAGNOSIS

Activity intolerance related to:

a. tissue hypoxia associated with diminished tissue perfusion and anemia resulting from blood loss during surgery;
b. inadequate nutritional status;
c. inability to rest and sleep associated with discomfort, fear, and anxiety.

DESIRED OUTCOMES	NURSING ACTIONS AND *SELECTED RATIONALES*

10. The client will demonstrate an increased tolerance for activity as evidenced by:
a. verbalization of feeling less fatigued and weak
b. ability to perform activities of daily living without exertional dyspnea, chest pain, diaphoresis, dizziness, or a significant change in vital signs.

10.a. Assess for signs and symptoms of activity intolerance:
  1. statements of fatigue and weakness
  2. exertional dyspnea, chest pain, diaphoresis, or dizziness
  3. decrease in pulse rate or an increase in rate of 20 beats/minute above resting rate
  4. pulse rate not returning to preactivity level within 5 minutes after stopping activity
  5. decreased blood pressure or an increase in diastolic pressure of 15 mm Hg with activity.
b. Implement measures *to improve activity tolerance:*
  1. perform actions *to promote rest:*
    a. maintain activity restrictions if ordered
    b. minimize environmental activity and noise
    c. schedule nursing care to allow for periods of uninterrupted rest
    d. limit the number of visitors and their length of stay
    e. assist client with self-care activities as needed
    f. keep supplies and personal articles within easy reach
    g. implement measures to reduce fear and anxiety (see Nursing Diagnosis 1, action c)
    h. implement measures to promote sleep (see Nursing Diagnosis 15, action c)
    i. implement measures to reduce discomfort (see Nursing Diagnoses 7.A, action 5; 7.B, action 3; 7.C, action 2; and 7.D)
  2. perform actions to maintain adequate systemic tissue perfusion (see Nursing Diagnosis 2, action b)
  3. instruct client in energy-saving techniques (e.g. using shower chair when showering, sitting to brush teeth or comb hair)
  4. perform actions to improve nutritional status (see Nursing Diagnosis 6, action f)
  5. monitor for therapeutic and nontherapeutic effects of whole blood or packed red cells if administered
  6. increase client's activity gradually as allowed and tolerated.
c. Instruct client to:
  1. report a decreased tolerance for activity
  2. stop any activity that causes chest pain, shortness of breath, dizziness, or extreme fatigue or weakness.
d. Consult physician if signs and symptoms of activity intolerance persist or worsen.

☐ ▬▬▬▬▬▬▬▬▬▬▬▬▬▬▬▬▬▬

11. NURSING DIAGNOSIS

Impaired physical mobility related to:

a. decreased activity tolerance associated with tissue hypoxia, inadequate nutritional status, and inability to rest and sleep;
b. pain and nausea;
c. depressant effects of anesthesia and some medications (e.g. narcotic analgesics, muscle relaxants, antiemetics);
d. fear of falling, dislodging tubes, and compromising surgical wound;
e. activity restrictions imposed by the treatment plan.

☐ ▬▬▬▬▬▬▬▬▬▬▬▬▬▬▬▬▬▬

DESIRED OUTCOMES	NURSING ACTIONS AND *SELECTED RATIONALES*

11. The client will achieve maximum physical mobility within the limitations imposed by the surgical procedure and postoperative management.	11.a. Assess for factors that impair physical mobility (e.g. decreased activity tolerance; pain and/or nausea; fear of falling, dislodging tubes, and compromising surgical wound; prescribed activity restrictions).
	b. Implement measures *to increase mobility:*
	  1. perform actions to improve activity tolerance (see Nursing Diagnosis 10, action b)
	  2. perform actions to reduce pain (see Nursing Diagnosis 7.A, action 5)
	  3. perform actions to prevent nausea and vomiting (see Nursing Diagnosis 7.C, action 2)
	  4. schedule attempts to increase activity when analgesics and/or antiemetics are at peak action
	  5. encourage use of nonnarcotic analgesics once severe pain has subsided
	  6. perform actions *to decrease client's fear of injury:*
	    a. implement measures to prevent falls (see Nursing Diagnosis 17, action b)
	    b. secure all dressings and tubings *to decrease risk of inadvertent removal during activity*
	  7. assure client that level of activity ordered will enhance rather than compromise healing process.
	c. Increase activity and participation in self-care activities as allowed and tolerated.
	d. Provide praise and encouragement for all efforts to increase physical mobility.
	e. Encourage the support of significant others. Allow them to assist client with increased activity if desired.
	f. Consult physician if client is unable to achieve expected level of mobility.

☐ ▬▬▬▬▬▬▬▬▬▬▬▬▬▬▬▬▬▬

12. NURSING DIAGNOSIS

Self-care deficit related to impaired physical mobility associated with activity intolerance, pain, nausea, depressant effects of some medications, fear of dislodging tubes and compromising surgical wound, and activity restrictions.

☐ ▬▬▬▬▬▬▬▬▬▬▬▬▬▬▬▬▬▬

DESIRED OUTCOMES	NURSING ACTIONS AND *SELECTED RATIONALES*

12. The client will perform self-care activities within physical limitations and postoperative activity restrictions.	12.a. Assess for factors that interfere with the client's ability to perform self-care (e.g. weakness and fatigue, pain, fear of dislodging tubes or compromising surgical incision, activity restrictions imposed by treatment plan).
	b. With client, develop a realistic plan for meeting daily physical needs.
	c. Encourage maximum independence within physical limitations and postoperative activity restrictions.
	d. Implement measures *to facilitate the client's ability to perform self-care activities:*
	  1. schedule care at a time when client is most likely to be able to participate (e.g. when analgesics are at peak action, after rest periods, not immediately after meals or treatments)
	  2. keep needed objects within easy reach
	  3. allow adequate time for accomplishment of self-care activities
	  4. perform actions to increase physical mobility (see Nursing Diagnosis 11, action b).
	e. Provide positive feedback for all efforts and accomplishments of self-care.
	f. Assist client with those activities he/she is unable to perform independently.
	g. Inform significant others of client's abilities to perform own care. Explain the importance of encouraging and allowing client to maintain an optimal level of independence within prescribed activity restrictions and his/her activity tolerance level.

□ ▬▬▬▬▬▬▬▬▬▬▬▬▬▬▬▬▬

13. NURSING DIAGNOSIS

Urinary retention related to:

a. pooling of urine in kidney and bladder associated with horizontal positioning;
b. stimulation of the sympathetic nervous system associated with pain, fear, and anxiety;
c. depressant effects of some medications (e.g. anesthetic agents, narcotic analgesics) on bladder muscle tone.

□ ▬▬▬▬▬▬▬▬▬▬▬▬▬▬▬▬▬

DESIRED OUTCOMES	NURSING ACTIONS AND *SELECTED RATIONALES*

13. The client will not experience urinary retention as evidenced by:
a. voiding adequate amounts at normal intervals
b. no complaints of urgency, bladder fullness, or suprapubic discomfort
c. absence of suprapubic distention
d. balanced intake and output within 48 hours following surgery.
	13.a. Gather baseline data regarding client's usual urinary elimination pattern.
	b. Assess for signs and symptoms of urinary retention:
	  1. frequent voiding of small amounts (25–50 cc) of urine
	  2. complaints of urgency, bladder fullness, or suprapubic discomfort
	  3. suprapubic distention.
	c. Monitor intake and output. Consult physician if there is no urine output within 6–12 hours after surgery or if intake and output are not balanced within 48 hours after surgery (for first 48 hours postoperatively, urine output is expected to be less than intake *due to blood loss and increased secretion of ADH and aldosterone*).
	d. Implement measures *to prevent urinary retention:*
	  1. instruct client to urinate when the urge is first felt
	  2. perform actions *to facilitate voiding* (e.g. provide privacy, allow client to assume normal position for voiding unless contraindicated, run water, pour warm water over perineum, place client's hands in warm water)
	  3. offer bedpan or urinal or assist client to commode or bathroom every 2–3 hours

    4. instruct and assist client to perform the Credé technique unless contraindicated *in order to facilitate emptying of bladder*
    5. perform actions to reduce postoperative pain (see Nursing Diagnosis 7.A, action 5)
    6. encourage use of nonnarcotic analgesics once period of severe pain has subsided
    7. monitor for therapeutic and nontherapeutic effects of cholinergic drugs (e.g. bethanechol) if administered *to stimulate bladder contraction.*
e. Consult physician regarding intermittent catheterization or insertion of an indwelling catheter if above actions fail to alleviate urinary retention.
f. If urinary catheter is present, prevent urinary retention by maintaining patency of catheter (e.g. keep tubing free of kinks, irrigate as ordered).

14. NURSING DIAGNOSIS

Constipation related to:

a. decreased gastrointestinal motility associated with anesthesia, manipulation of bowel during abdominal surgery, narcotic analgesics, and decreased activity;
b. decreased fluid intake;
c. decreased intake of foods high in fiber.

DESIRED OUTCOMES	NURSING ACTIONS AND *SELECTED RATIONALES*

14. The client will resume usual bowel elimination pattern.	14.a. Ascertain client's usual bowel elimination habits.
	b. Assess bowel sounds. Report diminishing sounds or sounds that do not return to normal when expected.
	c. Monitor and record bowel movements including frequency, consistency, and shape.
	d. Assess for signs and symptoms that may accompany constipation such as headache, anorexia, nausea, abdominal distention and cramping, and feeling of fullness or pressure in abdomen or rectum.
	e. Implement measures *to prevent constipation:*
	  1. increase activity as allowed and tolerated
	  2. encourage client to defecate whenever the urge is felt
	  3. assist client to toilet or place in high Fowler's position or on commode for bowel movements unless contraindicated; provide privacy and adequate ventilation
	  4. encourage client to relax during attempts to defecate *in order to promote relaxation of the levator ani muscle and the external anal sphincter*
	  5. encourage use of nonnarcotic analgesics once period of severe pain has subsided
	  6. when oral intake is allowed:
	    a. instruct client to maintain a minimum fluid intake of 2500 cc/day unless contraindicated
	    b. encourage client to drink warm liquids *to stimulate peristalsis*
	    c. when diet advances, instruct client to select high-fiber foods (e.g. bran, whole grains, raw fruits and vegetables, dried fruits) unless contraindicated

7. monitor for therapeutic and nontherapeutic effects of laxatives, suppositories, stool softeners, and/or enemas if administered.
   f. Consult physician if signs and symptoms of constipation persist.

□ ▇▇▇▇▇▇▇▇▇▇▇▇▇▇▇▇▇▇▇▇▇▇▇▇▇▇▇▇▇▇

15. NURSING DIAGNOSIS

Sleep pattern disturbance related to fear, anxiety, discomfort, decreased physical activity, inability to assume usual sleep position, and frequent assessments and treatments.

□ ▇▇▇▇▇▇▇▇▇▇▇▇▇▇▇▇▇▇▇▇▇▇▇▇▇▇▇▇▇▇

DESIRED OUTCOMES	NURSING ACTIONS AND *SELECTED RATIONALES*

15. The client will attain optimal amounts of sleep within the parameters of the treatment regimen as evidenced by:
a. statements of feeling well rested
b. usual behavior
c. absence of frequent yawning, thick speech, dark circles under eyes.

15.a. Assess for signs and symptoms of a sleep pattern disturbance:
1. verbal complaints of difficulty falling asleep, not feeling well rested, sleep interruptions, or awakening earlier or later than desired
2. behavior changes (e.g. irritability, disorganization, lethargy)
3. frequent yawning, thick speech, dark circles under eyes, slight hand tremors.
b. Determine the client's usual sleep habits.
c. Implement measures *to promote rest and sleep:*
1. satisfy needs such as comfort, warmth, thirst, and hunger whenever possible
2. perform actions to reduce fear and anxiety (see Nursing Diagnosis 1, action c)
3. perform actions to reduce discomfort (see Nursing Diagnoses 7.A, action 5; 7.B, action 3; 7.C, action 2; and 7.D)
4. minimize environmental activity and noise
5. allow client to resume usual sleep practices (e.g. position, time, bedtime rituals) if possible
6. utilize relaxation techniques (e.g. progressive relaxation exercises, back massage, meditation, soft music) before rest and sleep
7. determine measures that have been helpful to the client in the past (e.g. milk, warm drinks) and incorporate in plan of care unless contraindicated
8. discourage long periods of sleep during the day unless sleep is interrupted frequently during the night or daytime sleep is usual for client
9. when oral intake is allowed, discourage intake of foods and fluids high in caffeine (e.g. chocolate, coffee, tea, colas) before rest periods and sleep
10. have client empty bladder just before bedtime
11. perform actions *to provide for periods of uninterrupted sleep (90- to 120-minute periods of uninterrupted sleep are considered essential):*
    a. restrict visitors during rest periods
    b. group care (e.g. medications, treatments, physical care, assessments) whenever possible
12. monitor for therapeutic and nontherapeutic effects of sedatives and hypnotics if administered.
d. Consult physician if signs of sleep deprivation persist or worsen.

16. NURSING DIAGNOSIS

Potential for infection:

a. **pneumonia** related to stasis of pulmonary secretions and aspiration;
b. **wound infection** related to wound contamination and decreased resistance to infection associated with decreased tissue perfusion and malnutrition;
c. **urinary tract infection** related to urinary retention, fluid volume deficit, and urinary catheterization.

DESIRED OUTCOMES	NURSING ACTIONS AND *SELECTED RATIONALES*

16.a. The client will not develop pneumonia as evidenced by:
1. normal breath sounds
2. resonant percussion note over lungs
3. respiratory rate at 16–20/minute
4. cough productive of clear mucus only
5. afebrile status
6. absence of pleuritic pain
7. WBC count returning toward normal
8. blood gases within normal range for client
9. negative sputum culture.
	16.a.1. Assess for and report signs and symptoms of pneumonia:
	  a. adventitious breath sounds (e.g. crackles, pleural friction rub, tubular breath sounds)
	  b. diminished or absent breath sounds with a dull percussion note over affected area
	  c. increase in respiratory rate
	  d. cough productive of purulent, green, or rust-colored sputum
	  e. chills and fever
	  f. pleuritic pain
	  g. persistent elevation or increase in WBC count.
	2. Monitor blood gases. Report abnormal results.
	3. Monitor chest x-ray results. Report findings indicative of pneumonia.
	4. Monitor for and report significant changes in ear oximetry and capnograph results.
	5. Obtain sputum specimen for culture as ordered. Report abnormal results.
	6. Implement measures *to prevent pneumonia:*
	  a. perform actions to maintain an effective breathing pattern and airway clearance (see Nursing Diagnoses 3, action d and 4, action b)
	  b. perform actions to reduce risk of aspiration (see Nursing Diagnosis 18, action d)
	  c. encourage and assist client to perform good oral hygiene *in order to reduce the number of microorganisms in the oropharynx*
	  d. protect client from persons with respiratory tract infections.
	7. If signs and symptoms of pneumonia occur:
	  a. continue with above measures
	  b. administer oxygen as ordered
	  c. monitor for therapeutic and nontherapeutic effects of anti-infectives, bronchodilators, expectorants, and mucolytics if administered
	  d. refer to Care Plan on Pneumonia for additional care measures.

16.b. The client will remain free of wound infection as evidenced by:
1. absence of chills and fever
2. absence of redness, warmth, and swelling around incisions or open wounds
3. usual drainage from wounds
4. WBC count returning toward normal
5. negative cultures of wound drainage.
	16.b.1. Assess for and report signs and symptoms of wound infection (e.g. chills; fever; redness, warmth, and swelling of wound area; unusual wound drainage; foul odor from wound area).
	2. Monitor WBC count. Report persistent elevation or increasing values.
	3. Obtain cultures of wound drainage as ordered. Report positive results.
	4. Implement measures *to prevent wound infection:*
	  a. perform actions to promote normal wound healing (see Nursing Diagnosis 9, action a.2)
	  b. use good handwashing technique and encourage client to do the same
	  c. instruct client to avoid touching incisions, dressings, drainage tubings, and open wounds
	  d. maintain meticulous aseptic technique during all dressing changes and wound care
	  e. protect client from others with infections

      f. monitor for therapeutic and nontherapeutic effects of anti-infectives if administered prophylactically.

5. If signs and symptoms of infection are present:
    a. continue with above actions
    b. monitor for therapeutic and nontherapeutic effects of anti-infectives if administered.

16.c. The client will remain free of urinary tract infection as evidenced by:
1. clear urine
2. no unusual odor to urine
3. absence of frequency, urgency, or burning on urination
4. absence of chills and fever
5. absence of nitrites, bacteria, and/or WBCs in urine
6. negative urine culture.

16.c.1. Assess for and report signs and symptoms of urinary tract infection (e.g. cloudy, foul-smelling urine; complaints of frequency, urgency, and/or burning on urination; elevated temperature; chills).

2. Monitor urinalysis and report presence of nitrites, bacteria, and/or WBCs.

3. Obtain a urine specimen for culture and sensitivity if ordered. Report abnormal results.

4. Implement measures *to prevent urinary tract infection:*
    a. perform actions to prevent urinary retention (see Nursing Diagnosis 13, actions d and f)
    b. instruct female client to wipe from front to back after urinating or defecating
    c. assist client with perineal care every shift and after each bowel movement
    d. maintain fluid intake of at least 2500 cc/day unless contraindicated
    e. maintain sterile technique during urinary catheterizations and irrigations
    f. if an indwelling urinary catheter is present:
        1. secure the catheter tubing to abdomen or thigh on males or to thigh on females *to minimize risk of accidental traction and subsequent trauma to the bladder and urethra*
        2. perform catheter care as often as needed *to prevent accumulation of mucus around the meatus*
        3. keep urine collection container lower than level of the bladder at all times *to prevent reflux or stasis of urine*
    g. when oral intake is permitted and tolerated, perform actions *to maintain urine acidity:*
        1. monitor for therapeutic and nontherapeutic effects of ascorbic acid if administered
        2. instruct client to increase intake of foods/fluids that form an acid ash (e.g. cranberry and prune juice, meats, eggs, poultry, fish, grapes, whole grains)
        3. instruct client to decrease intake of milk, most fruits and vegetables, and carbonated beverages (*these tend to alkalinize the urine*).

5. If signs and symptoms of urinary tract infection are present:
    a. continue with the above actions
    b. monitor for therapeutic and nontherapeutic effects of anti-infectives if administered.

17. NURSING DIAGNOSIS

Potential for trauma related to falls associated with:

a. weakness and fatigue;
b. orthostatic hypotension resulting from peripheral pooling of blood and blood loss during surgery;
c. central nervous system depressant effects of some medications;
d. presence of drainage tubings or equipment that must accompany client.

DESIRED OUTCOMES	NURSING ACTIONS AND *SELECTED RATIONALES*

17. The client will not experience falls.

17.a. Determine whether conditions predisposing client to falls (e.g. weakness; fatigue; orthostatic hypotension; use of narcotic analgesics, sedatives, or muscle relaxants; presence of long tubings and equipment) exist.
  b. Implement measures *to prevent falls:*
    1. keep bed in low position with side rails up when client is in bed
    2. keep needed items within easy reach
    3. encourage client to request assistance whenever needed; have call signal within easy reach
    4. use lap belt when client is in chair if indicated
    5. instruct client to wear shoes with nonskid soles and low heels when ambulating
    6. avoid unnecessary clutter in room
    7. carefully position tubings and equipment attached to client *so that they will not interfere with ambulation*
    8. instruct and assist client to change positions slowly *to reduce dizziness associated with orthostatic drop in B/P*
    9. accompany client during ambulation utilizing a transfer safety belt if he/she is weak or dizzy
    10. instruct client to ambulate in well-lit areas and to utilize handrails if needed
    11. do not rush client; allow adequate time for trips to the bathroom and ambulation in hallway
    12. perform actions to increase strength and improve activity tolerance (see Nursing Diagnosis 10, action b).
  c. Include client and significant others in planning and implementing measures to prevent falls.
  d. If falls occur, initiate appropriate first aid measures and notify physician.

☐ ▬▬▬▬▬▬▬▬▬▬▬▬▬▬▬

18. NURSING DIAGNOSIS

Potential for aspiration related to:

a. decreased level of consciousness and absent or diminished gag reflex associated with effects of anesthesia;
b. flat, supine positioning.

☐ ▬▬▬▬▬▬▬▬▬▬▬▬▬▬▬

DESIRED OUTCOMES	NURSING ACTIONS AND *SELECTED RATIONALES*

18. The client will not aspirate secretions or foods/fluids as evidenced by:
  a. clear breath sounds
  b. resonant percussion note over lungs
  c. respiratory rate at 16–20/ minute
  d. absence of dyspnea
  e. absence of cyanosis.

18.a. Assess for factors that indicate potential for aspiration (e.g. decreased level of consciousness, absent gag reflex, choking on secretions and foods/fluids).
  b. Assess for signs and symptoms of aspiration of secretions or foods/fluids (e.g. rhonchi, dull percussion note over lungs, tachycardia, rapid respirations, dyspnea, cyanosis).
  c. Monitor chest x-ray results. Report findings of pulmonary infiltrate.
  d. Implement measures *to reduce the risk of aspiration:*
    1. position client in side-lying position unless contraindicated until he/she is awake and alert
    2. have suction equipment readily available for use
    3. perform oropharyngeal suctioning and provide oral care as often as needed *to remove secretions*
    4. perform actions to prevent vomiting (see Nursing Diagnosis 7.C, action 2)
    5. withhold oral foods/fluids if gag reflex is absent or client is not alert

6. place client in semi- to high Fowler's position during and for at least 30 minutes after eating or drinking unless contraindicated.
    e. If signs and symptoms of aspiration occur:
        1. perform tracheal suctioning
        2. notify physician
        3. prepare client for chest x-ray.

19. COLLABORATIVE DIAGNOSIS

Potential complications:

a. **hypovolemic shock** related to hemorrhage and fluid volume deficit associated with excessive fluid loss and inadequate fluid replacement;
b. **atelectasis** related to hypoventilation and obstruction of the bronchioles associated with retained secretions;
c. **thromboembolism** related to:
    1. venous stasis associated with decreased activity, positioning during and following surgery, and abdominal distention (the distended intestine may put pressure on the abdominal vessels)
    2. hypercoagulability associated with fluid volume deficit
    3. trauma to vein walls during surgery;
d. **paralytic ileus** related to manipulation of intestines during abdominal surgery, effects of anesthesia and some medications (e.g. central nervous system depressants), hypokalemia, peritonitis or abdominal wound infection, toxemia, and hypovolemia (can cause decreased blood supply to the intestine);
e. **dehiscence** related to:
    1. inadequate wound closure
    2. stress on incision line associated with persistent coughing, distention, or vomiting
    3. poor wound healing associated with decreased tissue perfusion, malnutrition, and infection.

DESIRED OUTCOMES	NURSING ACTIONS AND *SELECTED RATIONALES*

19.a. The client will not develop hypovolemic shock as evidenced by:
1. usual mental status
2. stable vital signs
3. skin warm and usual color
4. palpable peripheral pulses
5. capillary refill time less than 3 seconds
6. urine output at least 30 cc/hour.
	19.a.1. Assess for and report excessive bleeding and gastrointestinal and wound drainage, persistent vomiting, and/or difficulty maintaining intravenous or oral fluid intake as ordered.
	2. Monitor RBC, Hct., and Hgb. levels. Report declining values.
	3. Assess for and report signs and symptoms of hypovolemic shock:
	  a. restlessness, agitation, confusion
	  b. significant decrease in B/P
	  c. decline in B/P of at least 15 mm Hg with concurrent rise in pulse when client changes from lying to sitting or standing position
	  d. resting pulse rate greater than 100 beats/minute
	  e. rapid or labored respirations
	  f. cool, pale, or cyanotic skin
	  g. diminished or absent peripheral pulses
	  h. capillary refill time greater than 3 seconds
	  i. urine output less than 30 cc/hour.
	4. Implement measures *to prevent hypovolemic shock:*
	  a. administer fluid volume replacements as ordered
	  b. perform actions to prevent nausea and vomiting (see Nursing Diagnosis 7.C, action 2)

    c. when oral intake is allowed, maintain a fluid intake of at least 2500 cc/day unless contraindicated

    d. if bleeding occurs, apply firm, prolonged pressure to area if possible.

5. If signs and symptoms of hypovolemic shock occur:

    a. continue with above measures to control bleeding and prevent fluid volume deficit

    b. place client flat in bed with legs elevated unless contraindicated

    c. monitor vital signs frequently

    d. administer oxygen as ordered

    e. monitor for therapeutic and nontherapeutic effects of the following if administered:

        1. blood products and/or volume expanders

        2. vasopressors (may be given for short periods *to maintain mean arterial pressure*)

    f. assist with the application of military antishock trousers (MAST) if indicated

    g. provide emotional support to client and significant others.

19.b. The client will not develop atelectasis as evidenced by:
1. normal breath sounds
2. resonant percussion note over lungs
3. pulse and respiratory rates within normal limits for client
4. afebrile status.

19.b.1. Assess for and report signs and symptoms of atelectasis (e.g. diminished or absent breath sounds, dull percussion note over a particular area, increased pulse and respiratory rates, elevated temperature).

2. Monitor chest x-ray results. Report findings of atelectasis.

3. Implement measures *to prevent and treat atelectasis:*

    a. perform actions to maintain an effective breathing pattern (see Nursing Diagnosis 3, action d)

    b. perform actions to maintain effective airway clearance (see Nursing Diagnosis 4, action b).

4. If signs and symptoms of atelectasis occur:

    a. increase frequency of turning, coughing, deep breathing, and use of inspiratory exerciser

    b. consult physician if signs and symptoms of atelectasis persist or worsen.

19.c.1. The client will not develop a venous thrombus as evidenced by:
    a. absence of pain, tenderness, and swelling in extremities
    b. usual skin color and temperature of extremities.

19.c.1.a. Assess for and report signs and symptoms of a venous thrombus:
1. tenderness and pain in extremity
2. increase in circumference of calf or thigh (measure at the same place on leg once a shift)
3. unusual warmth and redness of extremity
4. positive Homan's sign (not always a reliable indicator).

    b. Implement measures *to prevent thrombus formation:*

        1. perform actions to prevent peripheral pooling of blood (see Nursing Diagnosis 2, action b.3)

        2. maintain a minimum fluid intake of 2500 cc/day unless contraindicated *to prevent fluid volume deficit and increased blood viscosity, which leads to hypercoagulability*

        3. monitor for therapeutic and nontherapeutic effects of anticoagulants (e.g. heparin, Embolex, warfarin) or antiplatelet agents (e.g. aspirin, dipyridamole) if administered.

    c. If signs and symptoms of a venous thrombus occur:

        1. maintain client on bedrest until activity orders received

        2. discourage positions that compromise blood flow (e.g. pillows under knees, use of knee gatch, crossing legs, sitting for long periods)

        3. prepare client for diagnostic studies (e.g. venography or phlebography, isotope studies, Doppler ultrasound, impedance plethysmography) if indicated

        4. monitor for therapeutic and nontherapeutic effects of anticoagulants (e.g. heparin, warfarin) if administered

        5. prepare client for surgical intervention (e.g. thrombectomy, insertion of an intracaval filtering device) or injection of a thrombolytic agent (e.g. urokinase, tissue plasminogen activator [tPA], streptokinase) if indicated

        6. refer to Care Plan on Thrombophlebitis for additional care measures.

19.c.2. The client will not experience a pulmonary embolism as evidenced by:

19.c.2.a. Assess for and report signs and symptoms of a pulmonary embolism:
1. sudden chest pain
2. cough and/or hemoptysis
3. dyspnea, tachypnea

a. absence of sudden chest pain, cough, hemoptysis
b. unlabored respirations
c. stable vital signs
d. usual skin color
e. usual mental status
f. blood gases within normal range.

4. tachycardia, hypotension
5. pallor, cyanosis
6. restlessness
7. low PaO_2.

b. Implement measures *to prevent a pulmonary embolism:*
   1. perform actions to prevent the formation of a venous thrombus (see action c.1.b in this diagnosis)
   2. do not exercise or massage any extremity suspected of thrombosis
   3. caution client to avoid activities that create a Valsalva response (e.g. straining to have a bowel movement, bending at the waist, holding breath while moving) *in order to prevent dislodgment of existing thrombi.*

c. If signs and symptoms of a pulmonary embolism occur:
   1. maintain client on strict bedrest in a semi- to high Fowler's position
   2. maintain oxygen therapy as ordered
   3. prepare client for diagnostic tests (e.g. blood gases, lung scan, venography, pulmonary angiography)
   4. monitor for therapeutic and nontherapeutic effects of the following medications if administered:
      a. heparin
      b. thrombolytic agents (e.g. streptokinase, tissue plasminogen activator [tPA], urokinase)
      c. vasoconstrictors *(may be necessary to maintain mean arterial pressure if shock occurs)*
   5. prepare client for surgical intervention (e.g. embolectomy) if indicated
   6. provide emotional support to client and significant others
   7. refer to Care Plan on Pulmonary Embolism for additional care measures.

19.d. The client will not develop a paralytic ileus as evidenced by:
1. resolution of abdominal pain and cramping
2. soft, nondistended abdomen
3. gradual return of bowel sounds
4. passage of flatus.

19.d.1. Assess for and report signs and symptoms of paralytic ileus (e.g. persistent or worsening abdominal pain and cramping; firm, distended abdomen; absent bowel sounds; failure to pass flatus).
2. Implement measures *to prevent paralytic ileus:*
   a. increase activity as soon as allowed and tolerated
   b. perform actions to maintain fluid and electrolyte balance (see Nursing Diagnosis 5, action a.3)
   c. perform actions to prevent wound infection (see Nursing Diagnosis 16, action b.4)
   d. monitor for therapeutic and nontherapeutic effects of blood and/or volume expanders if administered *(decreased blood supply to the bowel can cause paralytic ileus)*
   e. monitor for therapeutic and nontherapeutic effects of gastrointestinal stimulants if administered.
3. If signs and symptoms of paralytic ileus occur:
   a. continue with above measures to promote bowel activity
   b. withhold all oral intake
   c. insert nasogastric tube and maintain suction as ordered
   d. monitor for and report signs of bowel necrosis (e.g. fever, increased or persistent elevation of WBCs, shock).

19.e. The client will not experience dehiscence as evidenced by intact, approximated wound edges.

19.e.1. Assess for factors that may predispose client to dehiscence (e.g. advanced age, decreased nutritional status, decreased tissue perfusion, wound infection, general debilitation, obesity, diseases such as diabetes and cancer).
2. Assess for and report evidence of dehiscence (separation of edges of the wound).
3. Implement measures to promote normal wound healing (see Nursing Diagnosis 9, action a.2) *in order to decrease the risk of dehiscence.*
4. If dehiscence occurs:
   a. apply skin closures (e.g. butterfly bandages, Steri-Strips) to the incision line and/or assist with resuturing the wound if indicated
   b. if client has an abdominal incision, assess for and immediately report signs and symptoms of evisceration (e.g. client statements that "something popped" or "gave way," sudden drainage of serosanguineous peritoneal fluid from wound, protrusion of intestinal contents).

☐ ▓▓

20. NURSING DIAGNOSIS

Knowledge deficit regarding follow-up care.

☐ ▓▓

DESIRED OUTCOMES	NURSING ACTIONS AND *SELECTED RATIONALES*
20.a. The client will identify ways to prevent postoperative infection.	20.a. Instruct client in ways *to prevent postoperative infection:* 1. continue with coughing (if allowed) and deep breathing every 2 hours while awake 2. reinforce continued use of inspiratory exerciser if indicated 3. increase activity as ordered 4. avoid contact with persons who have infections 5. avoid crowds during flu or cold season 6. decrease or stop smoking 7. drink at least 10 glasses of liquid/day 8. maintain a balanced nutritional intake 9. maintain a proper balance of rest and activity 10. maintain good personal hygiene (especially oral care, handwashing, perineal care) 11. avoid touching any wound unless it is completely healed 12. maintain sterile or clean technique as ordered during wound care.
20.b. The client will demonstrate the ability to perform wound care.	20.b.1. Discuss the rationale for, frequency of, and equipment necessary for the prescribed wound care. 2. Provide client with the necessary equipment (e.g. dressings, irrigating solution, tape) for wound care and with names and addresses of places where additional equipment can be obtained. 3. Demonstrate wound care and proper cleansing of any reusable equipment. Allow time for questions, clarification, and return demonstration.
20.c. The client will state signs and symptoms of complications to report to the health care provider.	20.c. Instruct the client to report the following signs and symptoms: 1. persistent low-grade or significantly elevated (38.3°C [101°F]) temperature 2. difficulty breathing 3. chest pain 4. cough productive of purulent, green, or rust-colored sputum 5. increasing weakness or inability to tolerate prescribed activity level 6. increasing discomfort or discomfort not controlled by prescribed medications and treatments 7. continued nausea or vomiting 8. increasing abdominal distention and/or discomfort 9. separation of wound edges 10. increasing redness, warmth, and swelling around wound 11. unusual or excessive drainage from any wound site 12. pain, redness, or swelling in calf of one or both legs 13. urine retention 14. frequency, urgency, or burning on urination 15. cloudy, foul-smelling urine.
20.d. The client will verbalize an understanding of and a plan for adhering to recommended follow-up care including future appointments with health	20.d.1. Reinforce importance of keeping scheduled follow-up appointments with the health care provider. 2. Reinforce physician's instructions about dietary modifications. Obtain a dietary consult for client if needed. 3. Reinforce physician's instructions on suggested activity level and treatment plan.

care provider, dietary modifications, activity level, treatments, and medications prescribed.

4. Explain the rationale for, side effects of, and importance of taking medications prescribed.
5. Implement measures *to improve client compliance:*
   a. include significant others in teaching sessions if possible
   b. encourage questions and allow time for reinforcement or clarification of information provided
   c. provide written instructions on scheduled appointments with health care provider, dietary modifications, activity level, treatment plan, medications prescribed, and signs and symptoms to report.

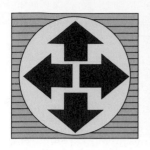 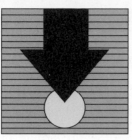 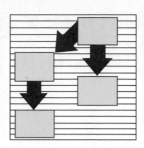 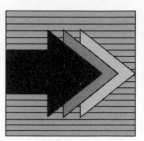 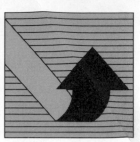

Unit III

Nursing Care of the Immobile Client (Immobility)

   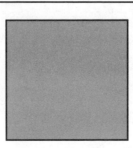 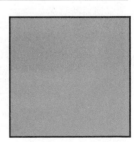

Immobility

Immobility refers to a limitation of physical activity as a result of a disease process, trauma, or therapeutic intervention. Immobility for periods greater than 48 hours will result in changes in all body systems. This care plan focuses on the adult client who is physically immobilized for a prolonged period during hospitalization. Goals of care are to maintain comfort, prevent complications, and educate the client regarding follow-up care. The nursing diagnoses of impaired physical mobility and potential for disuse syndrome are assumed diagnoses in this care plan. Many of the actions included in the care plan will help prevent the disuse syndrome, which is a deterioration of body systems as a result of prescribed or unavoidable musculoskeletal inactivity.

DISCHARGE CRITERIA

Prior to discharge, the client will:

- verbalize an understanding of ways to prevent complications associated with continued decreased mobility
- demonstrate techniques for meeting self-care needs
- state signs and symptoms to report to the health care provider
- identify community agencies that may provide assistance with home care and transportation
- verbalize an understanding of and a plan for adhering to recommended follow-up care including future appointments with health care provider and physical therapist, exercise regimen, and medications prescribed.

NURSING/COLLABORATIVE DIAGNOSES

1. Anxiety □ 67
2. Altered systemic tissue perfusion □ 68
3. Ineffective breathing pattern: hypoventilation □ 69
4. Ineffective airway clearance □ 69
5. Altered electrolyte balance: hypercalcemia □ 70
6. Altered nutrition: less than body requirements □ 71
7. Impaired skin integrity: irritation and breakdown □ 72
8. Activity intolerance □ 73
9. Self-care deficit □ 74
10. Urinary retention □ 74
11. Constipation □ 75
12. Sleep pattern disturbance □ 76
13. Potential for infection:
    a. pneumonia
    b. urinary tract infection □ 77
14. Potential complications:
    a. thromboembolism
    b. atelectasis
    c. renal calculi
    d. contractures
    e. pathologic fractures □ 78
15. Sexual dysfunction:
    a. alteration in usual sexual activities
    b. impotence □ 81

1. NURSING DIAGNOSIS

Anxiety related to unfamiliar environment; lack of understanding of diagnosis, diagnostic tests, and treatments; and feelings of confinement.

DESIRED OUTCOMES	NURSING ACTIONS AND *SELECTED RATIONALES*

1. The client will experience a reduction in fear and anxiety as evidenced by:
   a. verbalization of feeling less anxious or fearful
   b. relaxed facial expression and body movements
   c. stable vital signs
   d. usual skin color
   e. verbalization of an understanding of hospital routines, diagnosis, diagnostic procedures, and treatments.

1.a. Assess client for signs and symptoms of fear and anxiety (e.g. verbalization of fears and concerns; tenseness; tremors; irritability; restlessness; diaphoresis; tachypnea; tachycardia; elevated blood pressure; facial tension, pallor, or flushing; noncompliance with treatment plan).
   b. Ascertain effectiveness of current coping skills.
   c. Implement measures *to reduce fear and anxiety:*
      1. orient to hospital environment, equipment, and routines; explain the purpose for and operation of a kinetic bed if indicated
      2. introduce staff who will be participating in his/her care; if possible, maintain consistency in staff assigned to his/her care *to provide feelings of stability and comfort with the environment*
      3. assure client that staff members are nearby; respond to call signal as soon as possible
      4. keep door and bed and window curtains open as much as possible *to reduce feeling of confinement*
      5. maintain a calm, confident manner when interacting with client
      6. encourage verbalization of fear and anxiety; provide feedback
      7. reinforce physician's explanations and clarify any misconceptions client may have about his/her diagnosis, treatment plan, and prognosis
      8. explain all diagnostic tests
      9. provide a calm, restful environment
      10. instruct in relaxation techniques and encourage participation in diversional activities
      11. assist client to identify specific stressors and ways to cope with them
      12. encourage significant others to project a caring, concerned attitude without obvious anxiousness
      13. monitor for therapeutic and nontherapeutic effects of antianxiety agents if administered.
   d. Include significant others in orientation and teaching sessions and encourage their continued support of the client.
   e. Provide information based on current needs of client and significant others at a level they can understand. Encourage questions and clarification of information provided.
   f. Consult physician if above actions fail to control fear and anxiety.

☐ ▬▬▬▬▬▬▬▬▬▬▬▬▬▬▬▬▬▬▬▬▬▬▬▬▬▬▬▬▬

2. NURSING DIAGNOSIS

Altered systemic tissue perfusion related to:

a. decreased cardiac output associated with:
   1. hypovolemia resulting from positional diuresis
   2. decreased venous return
   3. cardiac deconditioning resulting from prolonged immobility;
b. peripheral pooling of blood associated with decreased venous return resulting from a loss of muscle tone in extremities.

☐ ▬▬▬▬▬▬▬▬▬▬▬▬▬▬▬▬▬▬▬▬▬▬▬▬▬▬▬▬▬

DESIRED OUTCOMES	NURSING ACTIONS AND *SELECTED RATIONALES*

2. The client will maintain adequate systemic tissue perfusion as evidenced by:
a. B/P and pulse within normal range for client and stable with position change
b. absence of syncope when changing to an upright position
c. unlabored respirations at 16–20/minute
d. usual mental status
e. skin warm and usual color
f. palpable peripheral pulses
g. capillary refill time less than 3 seconds
h. urine output at least 30 cc/hour.
	2.a. Assess for and report signs and symptoms of diminished systemic tissue perfusion:
	1. significant decrease in B/P
	2. resting pulse rate greater than 100 beats/minute
	3. decline in systolic B/P of at least 15 mm Hg with a concurrent rise in pulse when client changes from lying to sitting or upright position
	4. syncope when changing to an upright position
	5. rapid or labored respirations
	6. restlessness, slow responses, confusion
	7. cool, pale, mottled, or cyanotic skin
	8. diminished or absent peripheral pulses
	9. capillary refill time greater than 3 seconds
	10. urine output less than 30 cc/hour.
	b. Implement measures *to maintain adequate systemic tissue perfusion:*
	1. perform actions *to reduce cardiac workload:*
	  a. place client in a semi- to high Fowler's position if allowed
	  b. instruct client to avoid activities that create a Valsalva response (e.g. straining to have a bowel movement, bending at the waist, holding breath while moving)
	  c. promote physical and emotional rest
	  d. implement measures to ensure adequate oxygenation (see Nursing Diagnosis 3, action d and Nursing Diagnosis 4, action b for measures to improve breathing pattern and promote effective airway clearance)
	  e. provide frequent, small meals rather than 3 large ones *(large meals require an increased blood supply to gastrointestinal tract for digestion)*
	  f. increase activity gradually as allowed
	2. perform actions *to prevent peripheral pooling of blood and increase venous return:*
	  a. instruct client in and assist with range of motion exercises at least every 4 hours
	  b. consult physician about order for antiembolic hose or elastic wraps; if applied, remove for 30–60 minutes every shift
	  c. assist with intermittent venous compression using pneumatic cuffs or boots if ordered
	  d. elevate foot of bed for 20-minute intervals several times a shift unless contraindicated
	3. instruct and assist client to change positions slowly *in order to allow autoregulatory mechanisms to adjust to position change*
	4. discourage positions that compromise blood flow in lower extremities (e.g. crossing legs, pillows under knees, use of knee gatch, sitting for long periods)
	5. discourage smoking *(smoking decreases oxygen availability and causes vasoconstriction)*

6. maintain a comfortable room temperature and provide client with adequate clothing and blankets *(exposure to cold causes generalized vasoconstriction).*

c. Consult physician if signs and symptoms of diminished tissue perfusion persist or worsen.

3. NURSING DIAGNOSIS

Ineffective breathing pattern: hypoventilation related to:

a. depressant effects of some medications (e.g. narcotic analgesics, sedatives, muscle relaxants) that may be given for treatment of current diagnosis;
b. impaired chest expansion associated with recumbent positioning, weakness, and eventual fixation of intercostal joints in an expiratory state (joints become fixed as a result of a prolonged lack of usual inspiratory movement).

DESIRED OUTCOMES	NURSING ACTIONS AND *SELECTED RATIONALES*

3. The client will maintain an effective breathing pattern as evidenced by:
a. normal rate, rhythm, and depth of respirations
b. blood gases within normal range.
	3.a. Assess for signs and symptoms of an ineffective breathing pattern (e.g. shallow or slow respirations).
	b. Monitor blood gases. Report abnormal results.
	c. Monitor for and report significant changes in ear oximetry and capnograph results.
	d. Implement measures *to improve breathing pattern:*
	  1. place client in a semi- to high Fowler's position unless contraindicated
	  2. turn client at least every 2 hours
	  3. instruct client to deep breathe or use inspiratory exerciser at least every 2 hours
	  4. administer or assist with IPPB treatments as ordered
	  5. instruct client to avoid intake of gas-forming foods/fluids (e.g. beans, cauliflower, cabbage, onions, carbonated beverages) and large meals *in order to prevent gastric distention and pressure on the diaphragm*
	  6. increase activity as allowed and tolerated
	  7. administer central nervous system depressants (e.g. narcotic analgesics, sedatives, muscle relaxants) judiciously; hold medication and consult physician if respiratory rate is less than 12/minute.
	e. Consult physician if:
	  1. ineffective breathing pattern continues
	  2. signs and symptoms of impaired gas exchange (e.g. confusion, restlessness, irritability, cyanosis, decreased PaO_2 and increased $PaCO_2$ levels) are present.

4. NURSING DIAGNOSIS

Ineffective airway clearance related to stasis of secretions resulting from poor cough effort and decreased mobility.

DESIRED OUTCOMES	NURSING ACTIONS AND *SELECTED RATIONALES*

4. The client will maintain clear, open airways as evidenced by:
   a. normal breath sounds
   b. normal rate and depth of respirations
   c. absence of dyspnea
   d. absence of cyanosis.

4.a. Assess for signs and symptoms of ineffective airway clearance (e.g. adventitious breath sounds; rapid, shallow respirations; dyspnea; cyanosis).
  b. Implement measures *to promote effective airway clearance:*
    1. instruct and assist client to turn, cough, and deep breathe every 1–2 hours
    2. reinforce correct use of inspiratory exerciser at least every 2 hours
    3. perform actions *to facilitate removal of secretions:*
      a. implement measures *to liquefy tenacious secretions:*
        1. maintain a fluid intake of at least 2500 cc/day unless contraindicated
        2. humidify inspired air as ordered
        3. assist with administration of mucolytic agents via nebulizer or IPPB treatment
      b. assist with or perform postural drainage, percussion, and vibration if ordered
      c. perform nasal, oral, pharyngeal, or tracheal suctioning if needed
      d. monitor for therapeutic and nontherapeutic effects of expectorants if administered
    4. discourage smoking (*smoking causes an increase in mucus production and impairs ciliary function*)
    5. increase activity as allowed and tolerated.
  c. Consult physician if:
    1. signs and symptoms of ineffective airway clearance persist
    2. signs and symptoms of impaired gas exchange (e.g. confusion, restlessness, irritability, cyanosis, decreased PaO_2 and increased $PaCO_2$ levels) are present.

□ ▬▬▬▬▬▬▬▬▬▬▬▬▬▬▬▬▬▬▬▬▬▬▬▬▬▬▬▬▬▬

5. COLLABORATIVE DIAGNOSIS

Altered electrolyte balance: hypercalcemia related to disuse osteoporosis (an actual elevation of serum calcium level occurs only in clients whose kidneys cannot compensate by excreting the increased calcium that results from bone breakdown).

□ ▬▬▬▬▬▬▬▬▬▬▬▬▬▬▬▬▬▬▬▬▬▬▬▬▬▬▬▬▬▬

DESIRED OUTCOMES	NURSING ACTIONS AND *SELECTED RATIONALES*

5. The client will maintain a safe serum calcium level as evidenced by:
   a. usual mental status
   b. usual strength and muscle tone
   c. absence of nausea, vomiting, anorexia
   d. regular pulse at 60–100 beats/minute
   e. serum calcium within normal range.

5.a. Assess for and report signs and symptoms of hypercalcemia (e.g. change in mental status, muscle weakness and flaccidity, nausea, vomiting, anorexia, constipation, cardiac arrhythmias, polyuria, elevated serum calcium level).
  b. Implement measures *to prevent or treat hypercalcemia:*
    1. instruct client to avoid excessive intake of foods high in calcium (e.g. dairy products)
    2. maintain dietary restrictions of calcium as ordered
    3. avoid giving calcium-containing antacids (e.g. Os-Cal, Tums, Titralac)
    4. consult physician regarding increasing dietary sodium (*sodium inhibits tubular reabsorption of calcium*)
    5. mobilize client as possible or consult physician about use of a tilt table (*weight-bearing reduces calcium loss from the bones*)
    6. maintain a minimum fluid intake of 2500 cc/day unless contraindicated (*hydrating the client lowers serum calcium by dilution*)
    7. monitor for therapeutic and nontherapeutic effects of the following if administered:
      a. saline infusions *to increase urinary calcium excretion*
      b. inorganic phosphates *to decrease gastrointestinal absorption of*

*calcium (phosphates bind with calcium in intestines and both are then
excreted in stool)*
   c. calcitonin *to inhibit bone resorption and increase renal clearance of
calcium*
   d. loop diuretics (e.g. ethacrynic acid, furosemide) *to increase renal
excretion of calcium*
   e. corticosteroids *to promote urinary calcium excretion and decrease
absorption of calcium from the intestine*
   f. mithramycin *to inhibit loss of calcium from bones*
   g. etidronate *to decrease bone resorption.*
  c. Consult physician if serum calcium levels remain above a safe level.

□ ▬▬▬▬▬▬▬▬▬▬▬▬▬▬▬▬▬▬▬▬▬▬▬

6. NURSING DIAGNOSIS

Altered nutrition: less than body requirements related to decreased oral intake
associated with:

a. anorexia resulting from:
   1. boredom, depression, constipation, and slowed metabolic rate (results from
decreased activity)
   2. early satiety associated with decreased gastrointestinal motility (slowed motility is a result of hypercalcemia and decreased activity);
b. difficulty feeding self as a result of impaired or limited physical mobility.

□ ▬▬▬▬▬▬▬▬▬▬▬▬▬▬▬▬▬▬▬▬▬▬▬

DESIRED OUTCOMES	NURSING ACTIONS AND *SELECTED RATIONALES*

6. The client will maintain an adequate nutritional status as evidenced by:
a. weight within normal range for client's age, height, and build
b. normal BUN and serum albumin, protein, Hct., Hgb., cholesterol, and lymphocyte levels
c. triceps skinfold measurements within normal range
d. increased strength and activity tolerance
e. healthy oral mucous membrane.
	6.a. Assess the client for signs and symptoms of malnutrition:
	  1. weight below normal for client's age, height, and build
	  2. abnormal BUN and low serum albumin, protein, Hct., Hgb., cholesterol, and lymphocyte levels
	  3. triceps skinfold measurement less than normal for build
	  4. weakness and fatigue
	  5. stomatitis.
	b. Reassess nutritional status on a regular basis and report a decline.
	c. Monitor percentage of meals eaten.
	d. Assess client to determine causes of inadequate intake (e.g. anorexia, inability to feed self, fatigue).
	e. Implement measures *to maintain an adequate nutritional status:*
	  1. perform actions *to improve oral intake:*
	    a. provide oral care before meals
	    b. provide a clean, relaxed, pleasant atmosphere
	    c. serve small portions of nutritious foods/fluids that are appealing to client
	    d. obtain a dietary consult if necessary to assist client in selecting foods/fluids that meet nutritional needs as well as preferences
	    e. eliminate noxious stimuli from environment
	    f. encourage a rest period before meals *to minimize fatigue*
	    g. implement measures to reduce boredom (see Nursing Diagnosis 18, action c)
	    h. implement measures to prevent constipation (see Nursing Diagnosis 11, action e)
	    i. implement measures to decrease serum calcium if serum levels are elevated (see Collaborative Diagnosis 5, action b)
	    j. encourage significant others to bring in client's favorite foods unless contraindicated and eat with him/her *to make eating more of a familiar social experience*

      k. encourage significant others to be present to assist client with meals if needed

      l. allow adequate time for meals; reheat food if necessary

     m. increase activity as allowed (*activity stimulates appetite*)

   2. ensure that meals are well balanced and high in essential nutrients

   3. monitor for therapeutic and nontherapeutic effects of vitamins and minerals if administered.

  f. Perform a 72-hour calorie count if nutritional status declines.

  g. Consult physician regarding alternative methods of providing nutrition (e.g. parenteral nutrition, tube feedings) if client does not consume enough food or fluids to meet nutritional needs.

---

7. NURSING DIAGNOSIS

Impaired skin integrity: irritation and breakdown related to:

a. prolonged pressure on tissues associated with decreased mobility;

b. increased fragility of the skin associated with dependent edema, decreased tissue perfusion, and malnutrition.

DESIRED OUTCOMES	NURSING ACTIONS AND *SELECTED RATIONALES*

7. The client will maintain skin integrity as evidenced by:
  a. absence of redness and irritation
  b. no skin breakdown.
	7.a. Inspect the skin, especially bone prominences and dependent areas, for pallor, redness, and breakdown.
	  b. Implement measures *to prevent skin breakdown:*
	    1. turn client and gently massage over bone prominences and around reddened areas at least every 2 hours (if turning is contraindicated, lift and gently massage back, buttocks, and heels every 2 hours)
	    2. lift and move client carefully using a turn sheet and adequate assistance *to prevent the linen from shearing the skin*
	    3. instruct or assist client to shift weight every 30 minutes
	    4. if fade time (length of time it takes for reddened area to fade after pressure is removed) is greater than 15 minutes, increase frequency of position changes and/or provide more effective methods of cushioning, padding, and positioning
	    5. keep skin clean and dry
	    6. keep bed linens wrinkle-free
	    7. provide alternating pressure or eggcrate mattress, flotation pad, sheepskin, and elbow and heel protectors if indicated
	    8. perform actions *to prevent drying of the skin:*
	      a. avoid use of harsh soaps and hot water
	      b. apply skin moisturizers or emollient creams to skin at least once a day
	    9. perform actions to maintain an adequate nutritional status (see Nursing Diagnosis 6, action e)
	    10. perform actions to promote adequate tissue perfusion (see Nursing Diagnosis 2, action b)
	    11. increase activity as allowed.
	  c. If skin breakdown occurs:
	    1. notify physician
	    2. continue with above measures to prevent further irritation and breakdown

3. perform decubitus care as ordered or per standard hospital policy
4. monitor client closely and report signs and symptoms of infection (e.g. elevated temperature; redness, warmth, and edema around area of breakdown; unusual drainage from site).

□ ▄▄▄▄▄▄▄▄▄▄▄▄▄▄▄▄▄▄▄▄▄▄▄▄▄▄▄▄▄▄▄▄▄▄▄▄▄▄▄

8. NURSING DIAGNOSIS

Activity intolerance related to:

a. inadequate nutritional status;
b. cardiac deconditioning associated with prolonged immobility;
c. difficulty resting and sleeping associated with inability to assume usual sleep position, frequent assessments and treatments, fear, anxiety, and unfamiliar environment.

□ ▄▄▄▄▄▄▄▄▄▄▄▄▄▄▄▄▄▄▄▄▄▄▄▄▄▄▄▄▄▄▄▄▄▄▄▄▄▄▄

DESIRED OUTCOMES	NURSING ACTIONS AND *SELECTED RATIONALES*

8. The client will demonstrate an increased tolerance for activity as evidenced by:
a. verbalization of feeling less fatigued and weak
b. ability to perform activities of daily living within physical limitations/restrictions without exertional dyspnea, chest pain, diaphoresis, dizziness, or a significant change in vital signs.
	8.a. Assess for signs and symptoms of activity intolerance:
	1. statements of fatigue and weakness
	2. exertional dyspnea, chest pain, diaphoresis, or dizziness
	3. decrease in pulse rate or an increase in rate of 20 beats/minute above resting rate
	4. pulse rate not returning to preactivity level within 5 minutes after stopping activity
	5. decreased blood pressure or an increase in diastolic pressure of 15 mm Hg with activity.
	b. Implement measures *to improve activity tolerance:*
	  1. perform actions *to promote rest:*
	    a. minimize environmental activity and noise
	    b. schedule nursing care and diagnostic procedures to allow periods of uninterrupted rest
	    c. limit the number of visitors and their length of stay
	    d. assist client with self-care activities as needed
	    e. keep supplies and personal articles within easy reach
	    f. implement measures to reduce fear and anxiety (see Nursing Diagnosis 1, action c)
	    g. implement measures to promote sleep (see Nursing Diagnosis 12, action c)
	  2. perform actions to maintain an adequate nutritional status (see Nursing Diagnosis 6, action e)
	  3. when activity can be increased:
	    a. increase activity gradually
	    b. instruct client in energy-saving techniques (e.g. using shower chair when showering, sitting to brush teeth or comb hair).
	c. Instruct client to:
	  1. report a decreased tolerance for activity
	  2. stop any activity that causes chest pain, shortness of breath, dizziness, or extreme fatigue or weakness.
	d. Consult physician if signs and symptoms of activity intolerance persist or worsen.

■

9. NURSING DIAGNOSIS

Self-care deficit related to:

a. limitations in movement associated with the reason for immobility;
b. activity intolerance associated with cardiac deconditioning, malnutrition, and rest and sleep deficit;
c. muscle weakness associated with prolonged disuse and the neuromuscular depressant effects of hypercalcemia if present.

■

DESIRED OUTCOMES	NURSING ACTIONS AND *SELECTED RATIONALES*

9. The client will perform self-care activities within physical limitations and activity restrictions imposed by treatment plan.	9.a. Assess for factors that interfere with the client's ability to perform self-care (e.g. sensory and motor deficits, activity restrictions, weakness, fatigue).
	 b. With client, develop a realistic plan for meeting daily physical needs.
	 c. Encourage client to perform as much of self-care as possible within physical limitations and activity restrictions imposed by the treatment plan.
	 d. Implement measures *to facilitate client's ability to perform self-care activities:*
	   1. schedule care at a time when client is most likely to be able to participate (e.g. when analgesics are at peak action, after rest periods, not immediately after meals or treatments)
	   2. keep needed objects within easy reach
	   3. perform actions to increase activity tolerance (see Nursing Diagnosis 8, action b)
	   4. perform actions to maintain serum calcium levels within normal range (see Collaborative Diagnosis 5, action b)
	   5. instruct client in and assist with range of motion exercises at least every 4 hours *to maintain muscle strength*
	   6. consult occupational therapist about adaptive devices available if indicated
	   7. allow adequate time for accomplishment of self-care activities.
	 e. Provide positive feedback for all efforts and accomplishments of self-care.
	 f. Assist the client with those activities he/she is unable to perform independently.
	 g. Inform significant others of client's abilities to perform own care. Explain importance of encouraging and allowing client to maintain an optimal level of independence within prescribed activity restrictions and physical capabilities.

■

10. NURSING DIAGNOSIS

Urinary retention related to:

a. pooling of urine in kidney and bladder associated with prolonged horizontal positioning;
b. decreased bladder muscle tone associated with the generalized loss of muscle tone resulting from prolonged immobility.

■

DESIRED OUTCOMES	NURSING ACTIONS AND *SELECTED RATIONALES*

10. The client will not experience urinary retention as evidenced by:
  a. voiding adequate amounts at normal intervals
  b. no complaints of urgency, bladder fullness, or suprapubic discomfort
  c. absence of suprapubic distention
  d. balanced intake and output.

10.a. Gather baseline data regarding client's usual urinary elimination pattern.
  b. Assess for signs and symptoms of urinary retention:
   1. frequent voiding of small amounts (25–50 cc) of urine
   2. complaints of urgency, bladder fullness, or suprapubic discomfort
   3. suprapubic distention
   4. output less than intake.
  c. Catheterize client if ordered *to determine the amount of residual urine.*
  d. Implement measures *to prevent urinary retention:*
   1. instruct client to urinate when the urge is first felt
   2. perform actions *to facilitate voiding* (e.g. provide privacy, allow client to assume normal position for voiding unless contraindicated, run water, pour warm water over perineum, place client's hands in warm water)
   3. offer bedpan or urinal every 2–3 hours
   4. instruct and assist client to perform the Credé technique unless contraindicated *to facilitate emptying of bladder*
   5. monitor for therapeutic and nontherapeutic effects of cholinergic drugs (e.g. bethanechol) if administered *to stimulate bladder contraction.*
  e. Consult physician about intermittent catheterization or insertion of an indwelling catheter if above actions fail to alleviate urinary retention.

11. NURSING DIAGNOSIS

Constipation related to:

a. decreased intake of fluid and foods high in fiber;
b. reluctance to use a bedpan;
c. weakened abdominal and perineal muscles associated with generalized loss of muscle tone resulting from prolonged immobility;
d. decreased gastrointestinal motility associated with decreased activity, the neuromuscular depressant effects of hypercalcemia if present, and increased sympathetic nervous system activity resulting from anxiety.

DESIRED OUTCOMES	NURSING ACTIONS AND *SELECTED RATIONALES*

11. The client will maintain usual bowel elimination pattern.

11.a. Ascertain client's usual bowel elimination habits.
  b. Monitor and record bowel movements including frequency, consistency, and shape.
  c. Assess for signs and symptoms that may accompany constipation such as headache, anorexia, nausea, abdominal distention and cramping, and feeling of fullness or pressure in abdomen or rectum.
  d. Assess bowel sounds. Report a pattern of decreasing bowel sounds.
  e. Implement measures *to prevent constipation:*
   1. encourage client to defecate whenever the urge is felt
   2. place client in high Fowler's position for bowel movements unless contraindicated; provide privacy and adequate ventilation
   3. encourage client to relax during attempts to defecate *in order to promote relaxation of the levator ani muscle and the external anal sphincter*
   4. instruct client to select foods high in fiber (e.g. nuts, bran, whole grains, raw fruits and vegetables, dried fruits)

5. instruct client to maintain a minimum fluid intake of 2500 cc/day unless contraindicated
6. encourage client to drink warm liquids *to stimulate peristalsis*
7. perform actions to maintain serum calcium levels within normal range (see Collaborative Diagnosis 5, action b)
8. encourage client to perform isometric abdominal strengthening exercises unless contraindicated
9. increase activity as allowed
10. monitor for therapeutic and nontherapeutic effects of laxatives, suppositories, stool softeners, and/or enemas if administered.

    f. Check for impaction if client has not had a bowel movement in 3 days, he/ she is passing liquid stool, or if other signs and symptoms of constipation are present. Administer oil retention and/or cleansing enemas as ordered followed by digital removal of stool if necessary.

☐ ▬▬▬▬▬▬▬▬▬▬▬▬▬▬▬▬▬▬▬▬▬

12. NURSING DIAGNOSIS

Sleep pattern disturbance related to decreased physical activity, fear, anxiety, inability to assume usual sleep position, frequent assessments or treatments, and unfamiliar environment.

☐ ▬▬▬▬▬▬▬▬▬▬▬▬▬▬▬▬▬▬▬▬▬

DESIRED OUTCOMES	NURSING ACTIONS AND *SELECTED RATIONALES*

12. The client will attain optimal amounts of sleep within the parameters of the treatment regimen as evidenced by:
    a. statements of feeling well rested
    b. usual behavior
    c. absence of frequent yawning, thick speech, dark circles under eyes.

12.a. Assess for signs and symptoms of a sleep pattern disturbance:
    1. verbal complaints of difficulty falling asleep, not feeling well rested, sleep interruptions, or awakening earlier or later than desired
    2. behavior changes (e.g. irritability, disorganization, lethargy)
    3. frequent yawning, thick speech, dark circles under eyes, slight hand tremors.
  b. Determine the client's usual sleep habits.
  c. Implement measures *to promote sleep:*
    1. perform actions to reduce fear and anxiety (see Nursing Diagnosis 1, action c)
    2. allow client to continue usual sleep practices (e.g. position, time, bedtime rituals) if possible
    3. determine measures that have been helpful to the client in the past (e.g. milk, warm drinks) and incorporate in plan of care
    4. discourage long periods of sleep during the day unless sleep deprivation exists or daytime sleep is usual for client
    5. encourage participation in relaxing diversional activities in early evening hours
    6. provide a quiet, restful atmosphere
    7. discourage intake of foods and fluids high in caffeine (e.g. chocolate, coffee, tea, colas) especially in the evening
    8. satisfy basic needs such as hunger, comfort, and warmth before sleep
    9. have client empty bladder just before bedtime
    10. utilize relaxation techniques (e.g. progressive relaxation exercises, back massage, meditation, soft music) before sleep
    11. perform actions *to provide for periods of uninterrupted sleep (90- to 120-minute periods of uninterrupted sleep are considered essential):*
      a. restrict visitors during rest periods
      b. group care (e.g. medications, treatments, physical care, assessments) whenever possible
    12. monitor for therapeutic and nontherapeutic effects of sedatives and hypnotics if administered.
  d. Consult physician if signs of sleep deprivation persist or worsen.

13. NURSING DIAGNOSIS

Potential for infection:

a. **pneumonia** related to stasis of secretions in the lungs;
b. **urinary tract infection** related to urinary stasis, alkaline urine associated with hypercalciuria, tears in the bladder mucosa due to distention, and indwelling catheter if present.

DESIRED OUTCOMES	NURSING ACTIONS AND *SELECTED RATIONALES*
13.a. The client will not develop pneumonia as evidenced by: 1. normal breath sounds 2. resonant percussion note over lungs 3. respiratory rate at 16–20/minute 4. cough productive of clear mucus only 5. afebrile status 6. absence of pleuritic pain 7. blood gases and WBC count within normal range for client 8. negative sputum culture.	13.a.1. Assess for and report signs and symptoms of pneumonia: a. adventitious breath sounds (e.g. crackles, pleural friction rub, tubular breath sounds) b. diminished or absent breath sounds with a dull percussion note over affected area c. tachypnea d. cough productive of purulent, green, or rust-colored sputum e. chills and fever f. pleuritic pain g. elevated WBC count. 2. Monitor blood gases. Report abnormal results. 3. Monitor for and report significant changes in ear oximetry and capnograph results. 4. Obtain sputum specimen for culture as ordered. Report abnormal results. 5. Monitor chest x-ray results. Report findings indicative of pneumonia. 6. Implement measures *to prevent pneumonia:* a. perform actions to improve breathing pattern (see Nursing Diagnosis 3, action d) and promote effective airway clearance (see Nursing Diagnosis 4, action b) b. protect client from persons with respiratory tract infections c. encourage and assist client to perform good oral care *in order to reduce the number of microorganisms in the oropharynx.* 7. If signs and symptoms of pneumonia occur: a. continue with above measures b. administer oxygen as ordered c. monitor for therapeutic and nontherapeutic effects of anti-infectives if administered d. refer to Care Plan on Pneumonia for additional care measures.
13.b. The client will remain free of urinary tract infection as evidenced by: 1. clear urine 2. no unusual odor to urine 3. absence of frequency, urgency, or burning on urination 4. absence of chills and fever 5. absence of nitrites, bacteria, and/or WBCs in urine 6. negative urine culture.	13.b.1. Assess for and report signs and symptoms of urinary tract infection (e.g. cloudy, foul-smelling urine; complaints of frequency, urgency, and/or burning on urination; elevated temperature; chills). 2. Monitor urinalysis and report presence of nitrites, bacteria, and/or WBCs. 3. Obtain a urine specimen for culture and sensitivity if ordered. Report abnormal results. 4. Implement measures *to prevent urinary tract infection:* a. perform actions to prevent urinary stasis (see Collaborative Diagnosis 14, action c.4.a) and retention (see Nursing Diagnosis 10, action d) b. perform actions to maintain urine acidity (see Collaborative Diagnosis 14, action c.4.d) c. instruct female client to wipe from front to back after urinating or defecating d. assist client with perineal care every shift and after each bowel movement e. maintain sterile technique during urinary catheterization and irrigations f. use silicone catheter rather than latex for long-term catheterization

g. if an indwelling urinary catheter is present:
 1. secure the catheter tubing to abdomen or thigh on males or to thigh on females *to minimize risk of accidental traction and subsequent trauma to the bladder and urethra*
 2. perform catheter care as often as needed *to prevent accumulation of mucus around the meatus*
 3. keep urine collection container below bladder level at all times *to prevent reflux or stasis of urine*
 4. change catheter every 3 weeks or per hospital policy.
 5. If signs and symptoms of urinary tract infection are present:
 a. continue with above actions
 b. monitor for therapeutic and nontherapeutic effects of anti-infectives if administered.

☐ ■■■■■■■■■■■■■■■■■■■■■■■■■■■■■■■■■■■■■■

14. COLLABORATIVE DIAGNOSIS

Potential complications:

a. **thromboembolism** related to venous stasis resulting from decreased mobility;
b. **atelectasis** related to hypoventilation, obstruction of bronchioles with mucus, and decreased surfactant production associated with reduced pulmonary blood flow (can result from decreased tissue perfusion);
c. **renal calculi** related to urinary stasis and increased renal calcium excretion associated with disuse osteoporosis;
d. **contractures** related to prolonged immobility of joints;
e. **pathologic fractures** related to disuse osteoporosis associated with prolonged immobility.

☐ ■■■■■■■■■■■■■■■■■■■■■■■■■■■■■■■■■■■■■■

DESIRED OUTCOMES	NURSING ACTIONS AND *SELECTED RATIONALES*

14.a.1. The client will not develop a venous thrombus as evidenced by:
a. absence of pain, tenderness, and swelling in extremities
b. usual skin color and temperature of extremities.
	14.a.1.a. Assess for and report signs and symptoms of a venous thrombus:
	  1. tenderness and pain in extremity
	  2. increase in circumference of calf or thigh (measure at the same place on leg once a shift)
	  3. unusual warmth and redness of extremity
	  4. positive Homan's sign (not always a reliable indicator).
	 b. Implement measures *to prevent thrombus formation:*
	  1. encourage and assist client to perform active foot and leg exercises for 5–10 minutes every 1–2 hours while awake
	  2. assist client to change positions at least every 2 hours
	  3. instruct client to avoid positions that compromise blood flow (e.g. pillows under knees, use of knee gatch, crossing legs, sitting for long periods)
	  4. elevate foot of bed for 20-minute intervals several times a shift unless contraindicated
	  5. consult physician about order for antiembolic hose or elastic wraps; if applied, remove for 30–60 minutes every shift
	  6. assist with intermittent venous compression using pneumatic cuffs or boots if ordered
	  7. maintain a minimum fluid intake of 2500 cc/day unless contraindicated *to prevent dehydration and increased blood viscosity, which leads to hypercoagulability*
	  8. monitor for therapeutic and nontherapeutic effects of anticoagulants (e.g. heparin, Embolex) or antiplatelet agents (e.g. aspirin, dipyridamole) if administered
	  9. progress activity as allowed.

c. If signs and symptoms of a venous thrombus occur:
1. maintain client on bedrest
2. discourage positions that compromise blood flow (e.g. pillows under knees, use of knee gatch, crossing legs, sitting for long periods)
3. prepare client for diagnostic studies (e.g. venography or phlebography, isotope studies, Doppler ultrasound, impedance plethysmography) if indicated
4. monitor for therapeutic and nontherapeutic effects of anticoagulants (e.g. heparin, warfarin) if administered
5. prepare client for surgical intervention (e.g. thrombectomy, insertion of an intracaval filtering device) or injection of a thrombolytic agent (e.g. urokinase, tissue plasminogen activator [tPA], streptokinase) if indicated
6. refer to Care Plan on Thrombophlebitis for additional care measures.

14.a.2. The client will not experience a pulmonary embolism as evidenced by:
a. absence of sudden chest pain, cough, hemoptysis
b. unlabored respirations
c. stable vital signs
d. usual skin color
e. usual mental status
f. blood gases within normal range.

14.a.2.a. Assess for and report signs and symptoms of pulmonary embolism:
1. sudden chest pain
2. cough and/or hemoptysis
3. dyspnea, tachypnea
4. tachycardia, hypotension
5. pallor, cyanosis
6. restlessness
7. low PaO_2.
b. Implement measures *to prevent a pulmonary embolism:*
1. perform actions to prevent formation of a venous thrombus (see action a.1.b. in this diagnosis)
2. do not exercise or massage any extremity suspected of thrombosis
3. caution client to avoid activities that create a Valsalva response (e.g. straining to have a bowel movement, bending at the waist, holding breath while moving) *in order to prevent dislodgment of existing thrombi.*
c. If signs and symptoms of a pulmonary embolism occur:
1. maintain client on strict bedrest in a semi- to high Fowler's position
2. maintain oxygen therapy as ordered
3. prepare client for diagnostic tests (e.g. blood gases, lung scan, venography, pulmonary angiography)
4. monitor for therapeutic and nontherapeutic effects of the following medications if administered:
   a. heparin
   b. thrombolytic agents (e.g. streptokinase, tissue plasminogen activator [tPA], urokinase)
   c. vasoconstrictors (*may be necesssary to maintain mean arterial pressure if shock occurs*)
5. prepare client for surgical intervention (e.g. embolectomy) if indicated
6. provide emotional support to client and significant others
7. refer to Care Plan on Pulmonary Embolism for additional care measures.

14.b. The client will not develop atelectasis as evidenced by:
1. normal breath sounds
2. resonant percussion note over lungs
3. pulse and respiratory rates within normal limits for client
4. afebrile status.

14.b.1. Assess for and report signs and symptoms of atelectasis (e.g. diminished or absent breath sounds, dull percussion note over a particular area, increased pulse and respiratory rates, elevated temperature).
2. Monitor chest x-ray results. Report findings of atelectasis.
3. Implement measures *to prevent and treat atelectasis:*
   a. perform actions to maintain an effective breathing pattern (see Nursing Diagnosis 3, action d)
   b. perform actions to maintain effective airway clearance (see Nursing Diagnosis 4, action b).
4. If signs and symptoms of atelectasis occur:
   a. increase frequency of turning, coughing, deep breathing, and use of inspiratory exerciser
   b. consult physician if signs and symptoms of atelectasis persist or worsen.

14.c. The client will not develop renal calculi as evidenced by:

14.c.1. Assess for and report signs and symptoms of renal calculi (e.g. dull, aching or severe, colicky flank pain; hematuria; urinary frequency or urgency; nausea; vomiting).

1. absence of flank pain, hematuria, urinary frequency or urgency, nausea, vomiting
2. clear urine without calculi.

2. Monitor serum calcium levels and report elevations.
3. Obtain a urine specimen for analysis if ordered. Report the presence of calcium crystals and/or high levels of calcium.
4. Implement measures *to prevent calcium stone formation:*
   a. perform actions *to prevent urinary stasis:*
      1. encourage a minimum fluid intake of 2500 cc/day unless contraindicated
      2. assist client to change positions at least every 2 hours
      3. progress activity as allowed
      4. maintain patency of urinary catheter if present
      5. implement measures to prevent urinary retention (see Nursing Diagnosis 10, action d)
   b. perform actions to maintain serum calcium levels within normal range (see Collaborative Diagnosis 5, action b)
   c. monitor pH of urine every shift; report levels above 6 (*calcium salts are more likely to precipitate in an alkaline urine*)
   d. perform actions *to maintain urine acidity:*
      1. assist the client with active-resistive exercises (*muscle activity produces an acid end product*)
      2. encourage client to increase intake of foods/fluids that form an acid ash (e.g. cranberry and prune juice, meat, eggs, poultry, fish, grapes, whole grains)
      3. instruct client to decrease intake of milk, most fruits and vegetables, and carbonated beverages (*these tend to alkalinize urine*)
      4. administer medications as ordered *to acidify the urine* (e.g. ascorbic acid)
      5. prevent urinary tract infections (*urea-splitting organisms tend to alkalinize urine*)
      6. irrigate urinary catheter with acetic acid or Renacidin if ordered
   e. instruct client to reduce intake of foods/fluids high in oxalate (e.g. tea, instant coffee, colas, chocolate, rhubarb, spinach) *to help prevent precipitation of calcium stones.*
5. If signs and symptoms of renal calculi occur:
   a. strain all urine carefully and save any calculi for analysis; report finding to physician
   b. encourage maximum fluid intake allowed
   c. administer analgesics as ordered
   d. refer to Care Plan on Renal Calculi for additional care measures.

14.d. The client will regain or maintain normal range of motion.

14.d.1. Assess for and report limitations in range of motion.
2. Implement general measures *to prevent contractures:*
   a. maintain proper body alignment at all times
   b. instruct client in and assist with range of motion exercises to all joints at least every 4 hours unless contraindicated
   c. encourage client to perform as much of self-care as possible
   d. progress activity as allowed.
3. Implement measures *to prevent hip and knee flexion contractures:*
   a. place client in a flat, supine position at least every 4 hours
   b. limit length of time client is in high Fowler's position (usually no longer than an hour at a time)
   c. avoid use of the knee gatch or pillows under knees
   d. instruct client to do quadriceps- and gluteal-setting exercises if able
   e. when client is in supine position, place trochanter roll or sandbag along outer aspect of each thigh *to prevent external rotation of the hips.*
4. Implement measures *to prevent footdrop:*
   a. instruct and assist the client to flex, extend, and rotate feet for 5–10 minutes every 1–2 hours
   b. use a footboard, sandbags, pillows, high-topped tennis shoes, foam boots, or foot positioners *to keep feet in a neutral or slightly dorsiflexed position*
   c. keep bed linen from exerting excessive pressure on toes and feet.
5. Implement measures *to prevent contractures in upper extremities:*
   a. encourage client to use upper extremities to perform self-care and assist in moving unless contraindicated

b. reposition upper extremities at least every 2 hours
c. use handroll and wrist splints if indicated
d. place foam ball in hand and encourage client to squeeze *in order to exercise hand.*

6. Consult physician if range of motion becomes more restricted.

14.e. The client will not experience pathologic fractures as evidenced by:
1. maintenance of usual body movements
2. no pain or swelling over skeletal structures
3. x-ray films showing absence of fractures.
	14.e.1. Determine whether conditions predisposing client to pathologic fractures (e.g. prolonged immobility, advanced age, female, diagnosis of osteoporosis or osteodystrophy) exist.
	2. Assess for and report signs and symptoms of pathologic fractures (e.g. further decrease in mobility and range of motion, pain or swelling over skeletal structures).
	3. Monitor x-ray reports and notify physician of positive findings.
	4. Implement measures *to prevent pathologic fractures:*
	  a. caution client to avoid coughing, sneezing, and straining at stool
	  b. move client carefully; obtain adequate assistance as needed
	  c. when turning client, log roll and support all extremities
	  d. utilize smooth movements when moving client; avoid pulling or pushing on body parts
	  e. correctly apply brace, splint, or corset as ordered
	  f. perform actions *to prevent or delay bone demineralization:*
	   1. consult physician about the use of a tilt table while client is immobile
	   2. assist client with weight-bearing activities as soon as allowed and tolerated (*weight-bearing reduces bone breakdown*)
	   3. administer medications *that promote mobilization of calcium back into bones* (e.g. calcitonin, estrogen preparations) if ordered.
	5. If fractures occur:
	  a. apply external stabilization device (e.g. cervical collar, brace, splint, sling) if ordered
	  b. monitor for therapeutic and nontherapeutic effects of analgesics if administered *to control pain.*

□ ▬▬▬▬▬▬▬▬▬▬▬▬▬▬▬▬▬▬▬▬▬▬▬▬▬

15. NURSING DIAGNOSIS

Sexual dysfunction:

a. **alteration in usual sexual activities** related to disease condition and immobility;
b. **impotence** related to depression, fear, anxiety, and disturbance in self-concept.

□ ▬▬▬▬▬▬▬▬▬▬▬▬▬▬▬▬▬▬▬▬▬▬▬▬▬

DESIRED OUTCOMES	NURSING ACTIONS AND *SELECTED RATIONALES*
15. The client will perceive self as sexually adequate and acceptable as evidenced by: a. verbalization of same b. maintenance of relationships with significant others.	15.a. Assess for signs and symptoms of sexual dysfunction (e.g. verbalization of sexual concerns, failure to maintain relationships with significant others, limitations imposed by disease and/or treatment). b. Determine attitudes, knowledge, and concerns about disease condition and immobility in relation to sexual functioning. c. Communicate interest, understanding, and respect for the values of the client and his/her partner. d. Facilitate communication between the client and his/her partner. Assist them to identify factors that may affect their sexual relationship. e. Implement measures to improve client's self-concept (see Nursing Diagnosis 16, actions c–m). f. Implement measures to reduce fear and anxiety (see Nursing Diagnosis 1, action c).

g. If impotence is a problem:
  1. encourage client to discuss it with physician (impotence may be due to reversible factors such as medication therapy or a poorly controlled health problem)
  2. suggest alternative methods of sexual gratification and use of assistive devices if appropriate.
h. Discuss ways to be creative in expressing sexuality (e.g. massage, fantasies, cuddling).
i. Arrange for uninterrupted privacy during hospital stay if desired by the couple.
j. Include partner in above discussions and encourage his/her support of the client.
k. Consult physician if counseling appears indicated.

□ ▬▬▬▬▬▬▬▬▬▬▬▬▬▬▬▬▬▬▬▬▬

16. NURSING DIAGNOSIS

Disturbance in self-concept* related to dependence on others to meet basic needs; feelings of powerlessness; and change in body functioning, appearance, sexual functioning, and usual roles and life style.

---

* This diagnostic label includes the nursing diagnoses of body image disturbance and self-esteem disturbance.

□ ▬▬▬▬▬▬▬▬▬▬▬▬▬▬▬▬▬▬▬▬▬

DESIRED OUTCOMES	NURSING ACTIONS AND *SELECTED RATIONALES*
16. The client will demonstrate beginning adaptation to changes in body functioning, appearance, life style, roles, and level of independence as evidenced by: a. verbalization of feelings of self-worth and sexual adequacy b. maintenance of relationships with significant others c. active participation in activities of daily living d. active interest in personal appearance.	16.a. Determine the meaning of feelings of dependency and changes in appearance, body functioning, life style, and roles to the client by encouraging him/her to verbalize feelings and by noting nonverbal responses to the changes experienced. b. Assess for signs and symptoms of a disturbance in self-concept (e.g. verbal or nonverbal cues denoting a negative response to changes in body functioning or appearance such as denial of or preoccupation with changes that have occurred or withdrawal from significant others). c. Assist client to identify strengths and qualities that have a positive effect on self-concept. d. Implement measures *to assist client to increase self-esteem* (e.g. limit negative self-criticism, encourage positive comments about self, give positive feedback about accomplishments). e. Assist client to identify and utilize coping techniques that have been helpful in the past. f. Assist client with usual grooming and makeup habits if necessary. g. Implement measures to assist client to adjust to alterations in sexual functioning (see Nursing Diagnosis 15, actions c–j). h. Implement measures to reduce client's feelings of powerlessness (see Nursing Diagnosis 17, actions c–k). i. Assess for and support behaviors suggesting positive adaptation to changes experienced (e.g. verbalization of feelings of self-worth, maintenance of relationships with significant others). j. Assist client's and significant others' adjustment by listening, facilitating communication, and providing information. k. Encourage visits and support from significant others. l. Encourage client to continue involvement in social activities and to pursue interests. If previous interests and hobbies cannot be pursued, encourage development of new ones.

m. Provide information about and encourage utilization of community agencies or support groups (e.g. vocational rehabilitation; sexual, family, individual, and/or financial counseling).

n. Consult physician about psychological counseling if client desires or if he/she seems unwilling or unable to adapt to changes that have occurred as a result of the disease and its treatment.

17. NURSING DIAGNOSIS

Powerlessness related to:

a. physical limitations and/or prescribed activity restrictions;
b. dependence on others to meet basic needs;
c. feeling of loss of control over life;
d. alterations in roles, relationships, and future plans.

DESIRED OUTCOMES	NURSING ACTIONS AND *SELECTED RATIONALES*

17. The client will demonstrate increasing feelings of control over his/her situation as evidenced by:
   a. verbalization of same
   b. active participation in planning of care
   c. participation in self-care activities within physical limitations.

17.a. Assess for behaviors that may indicate a feeling of powerlessness (e.g. verbalization of lack of control, anger, apathy, hostility, lack of participation in self-care or care planning).

b. Obtain information from client and significant others regarding client's usual response to situations in which client has had limited control (e.g. loss of job, financial stress).

c. Encourage client to verbalize feelings about self and current situation.

d. Reinforce physician's explanations about the disease, injury, and treatment plan. Clarify any misconceptions.

e. Remind client of his/her right to ask questions about condition and treatment regimen.

f. Support client's efforts to increase knowledge of and control over condition; provide relevant pamphlets and audiovisual materials.

g. Include client in the planning of care, encourage maximum participation in the treatment plan, and allow choices whenever possible *to enable him/her to maintain a sense of control.*

h. Consult physical or occupational therapist if indicated about adaptive devices that would allow client more independence in performing activities of daily living.

i. Encourage significant others to allow client to do as much as he/she is able *so that a feeling of independence can be maintained.*

j. Assist client to establish realistic short- and long-term goals.

k. Encourage client's participation in self-help groups if indicated.

l. Provide continuity of care through written individualized care plans *to ensure that client can maintain appropriate control over his/her environment.*

18. NURSING DIAGNOSIS

Diversional activity deficit related to inability to participate in usual recreational or leisure activities due to physical limitations and/or prescribed activity restrictions.

DESIRED OUTCOMES	NURSING ACTIONS AND *SELECTED RATIONALES*

18. The client will have needs for diversional activity met as evidenced by:
    a. no statements of boredom
    b. participation in diversional activities.

18.a. Assess for symptoms of diversional activity deficit (e.g. statements of boredom, verbalization of being unable to pursue usual hobbies in the hospital).
  b. Gather information from the client regarding his/her usual diversional activities. Discuss how these may be adapted to meet current activity restrictions.
  c. Implement measures *to decrease boredom:*
     1. schedule periods each day to sit and talk with client
     2. set up a schedule of visiting times *so that client does not go for long periods of time without visitors*
     3. encourage telephone contact with others
     4. consult occupational therapist regarding diversional activities that are appropriate for and of interest to the client
     5. contact significant others, volunteer services, and/or social services to obtain objects or projects that interest the client (e.g. books, magazines, puzzles, needlework, art or writing supplies, radio).

19. NURSING DIAGNOSIS

Knowledge deficit regarding follow-up care.

DESIRED OUTCOMES	NURSING ACTIONS AND *SELECTED RATIONALES*

19.a. The client will verbalize an understanding of ways to prevent complications associated with continued decreased mobility.

19.a.1. Provide instructions regarding ways *to prevent respiratory tract infection:*
  a. avoid contact with persons having respiratory tract infections
  b. drink at least 10 glasses of liquid/day
  c. continue with respiratory care (e.g. postural drainage, inspiratory exerciser, coughing and deep breathing) as long as mobility is impaired
  d. take expectorants, mucolytics, and prophylactic anti-infectives as prescribed.
2. Provide instructions regarding ways *to prevent urinary tract infection:*
  a. drink at least 10 glasses of liquid/day
  b. avoid urinary retention by:
     1. voiding whenever the urge is felt
     2. performing the Credé technique unless contraindicated *to facilitate bladder emptying*
  c. maintain urine acidity by:
     1. increasing intake of foods/fluids that form an acid ash (e.g. cranberry or prune juice, meat, eggs, poultry, fish, grapes, whole grains)
     2. limiting intake of dairy products, carbonated beverages, and citrus fruits
     3. taking acidifying agents (e.g. ascorbic acid) as prescribed
  d. take prophylactic anti-infectives as prescribed.
3. Provide instructions regarding ways *to prevent urinary calcium stone formation:*
  a. drink at least 10 glasses of liquid/day
  b. avoid urinary retention (see action a.2.b in this diagnosis)
  c. maintain urine acidity (see action a.2.c in this diagnosis)
  d. avoid excessive intake of foods high in calcium and vitamin D (e.g. dairy products)

  e. avoid excessive intake of foods/fluids high in oxalate (e.g. instant coffee, colas, tea, chocolate, rhubarb, spinach)
  f. take calcium-binding resins and thiazide diuretics as prescribed.
4. Provide instructions regarding ways *to prevent a thromboembolism:*
  a. drink at least 10 glasses of liquid/day
  b. avoid placing pillows under knees, crossing legs, and prolonged sitting
  c. perform active foot and leg exercises every 1–2 hours during periods of inactivity
  d. wear antiembolic hose or elastic wraps as prescribed
  e. do not massage extremities.
5. Provide instructions regarding ways *to prevent fainting spells associated with position change:*
  a. wear antiembolic hose or elastic wraps as prescribed
  b. change from a lying to sitting or standing position slowly.
6. Provide instructions regarding ways *to prevent skin breakdown:*
  a. change positions at least every 2 hours
  b. avoid pressure on any reddened or irritated area
  c. keep skin lubricated, clean, and dry
  d. use alternating pressure pad or eggcrate mattress on bed if prone to skin breakdown or activity is severely limited.
7. Provide instructions regarding ways *to prevent constipation:*
  a. drink at least 10 glasses of liquid/day
  b. increase intake of foods high in fiber (e.g. nuts, bran, whole grains, raw fruits and vegetables, dried fruits)
  c. defecate whenever the urge is felt
  d. assume a natural position for defecation if possible.

19.b. The client will demonstrate techniques for meeting self-care needs.	19.b.1. Assist the client to identify techniques that will allow him/her to perform as much self-care as possible. 2. Reinforce physical or occupational therapist's instructions about use of adaptive devices. 3. Allow time for return demonstration of self-care techniques and use of adaptive devices.
19.c. The client will state signs and symptoms to report to the health care provider.	19.c. Instruct client to report the following signs and symptoms: 1. temperature elevation lasting longer than 3 days 2. skin breakdown 3. cough productive of purulent, green, or rust-colored sputum 4. pain and swelling in any extremity 5. chest pain 6. flank pain 7. frequency, urgency, or burning on urination 8. cloudy, foul-smelling urine 9. nausea and vomiting 10. increased restriction of any joint motion.
19.d. The client will identify community agencies that may provide assistance with home care and transportation.	19.d.1. Provide information about community agencies that might provide assistance to client with home care or transportation (e.g. Visiting Nurse Association, home health agencies, Meals on Wheels, church groups, transportation agencies). 2. Initiate a referral if indicated.

19.e. The client will verbalize an understanding of and a plan for adhering to recommended follow-up care including future appointments with health care provider and physical therapist, exercise regimen, and medications prescribed.	19.e.1. Reinforce the importance of keeping follow-up appointments with health care provider and physical therapist.
	2. Reinforce physician's instructions regarding exercises and activity limitations.
	3. Explain the rationale for, side effects of, and importance of taking medications prescribed.
	4. Implement measures *to improve client compliance:*
	  a. include significant others in teaching sessions if possible
	  b. encourage questions and allow time for reinforcement or clarification of information provided
	  c. provide written instructions regarding scheduled appointments with health care provider and physical therapist, medications prescribed, and signs and symptoms to report.

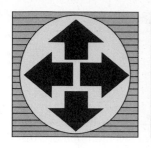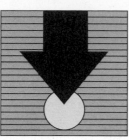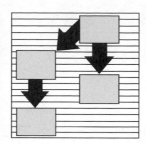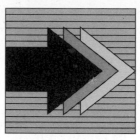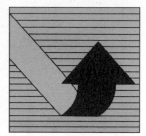

Unit IV

Nursing Care of the Client Who Is Dying (Terminal Care)

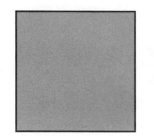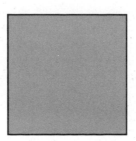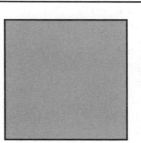

Terminal Care

This care plan focuses on care of the hospitalized adult client who is facing death in the very near future. The major goals of nursing care are to maintain an optimal level of comfort; facilitate progression through the grieving process; and provide for a peaceful, dignified death. The nurse also plays an important role in assisting the significant others to provide effective support to the dying person and adjust to their loss of that person.

This care plan does not deal with any particular medical diagnosis. The nursing diagnoses included are those that are relatively common to all persons facing death. Causal statements and actions for each nursing diagnosis will need to be individualized for each client and his/her underlying disease process. Care plans that pertain to the client's particular medical diagnosis will provide additional specific guidelines for nursing care during the terminal stages of that illness.

Use in conjunction with the Care Plan on Immobility and care plans that pertain to the client's medical diagnosis.

NURSING DIAGNOSES

1. Anxiety ☐ 89
2. Altered respiratory function:
   a. ineffective breathing patterns
   b. ineffective airway clearance
   c. impaired gas exchange ☐ 89
3. Fluid volume deficit ☐ 91
4. Impaired swallowing ☐ 91
5A. Altered comfort: pain ☐ 92
5B. Altered comfort: nausea and vomiting ☐ 93
5C. Altered comfort: pruritus ☐ 94
5D. Altered comfort: abdominal distention and gas pain ☐ 94
5E. Altered comfort: hiccoughs ☐ 95
6. Impaired skin integrity: irritation or breakdown ☐ 96
7. Altered oral mucous membrane: dryness ☐ 97
8. Impaired physical mobility ☐ 98
9. Self-care deficit ☐ 98
10. Altered pattern of urinary elimination: incontinence ☐ 99
11. Constipation ☐ 99
12. Diarrhea ☐ 100
13. Bowel incontinence ☐ 101
14. Altered thought processes: impaired memory, shortened attention span, slowed verbal response time, restlessness, agitation, and confusion ☐ 101
15. Sleep pattern disturbance ☐ 102
16. Potential for trauma ☐ 103
17. Potential for aspiration ☐ 103
18. Grieving ☐ 104
19. Hopelessness ☐ 106
20. Altered family processes ☐ 107

1. NURSING DIAGNOSIS

Anxiety related to separation from home, significant others, and familiar environment; feelings of abandonment; the unknown; loss of control over life and body functioning; discomfort; dyspnea; changes in body image; concern about the welfare of significant others and loss of loved ones; unfinished business; recognition of nonbeing; and religious conflicts.

DESIRED OUTCOMES	NURSING ACTIONS AND *SELECTED RATIONALES*

1. The client will experience a reduction in fear and anxiety as evidenced by:
a. verbalization of feeling less anxious or fearful
b. relaxed facial expression and body movements
c. statements reflecting resolution of unfinished business, conflicts, and concerns
d. verbalization of an understanding of hospital routines and treatment measures.
	1.a. Determine client's and significant others' perception of the reason for hospital admission.
	b. Refer to Care Plan on Immobility, Nursing Diagnosis 1, for measures related to assessment and reduction of fear and anxiety.
	c. Implement additional measures *to reduce fear and anxiety:*
	  1. perform actions to reduce discomfort (see Nursing Diagnoses 5.A, action 5; 5.B, action 2; 5.C, actions 2 and 3; 5.D, action 3; and 5.E)
	  2. perform actions to improve respiratory status (see Nursing Diagnosis 2, action d) *in order to relieve dyspnea*
	  3. encourage client to verbalize feelings about changes in body image
	  4. assist client to formulate plans for completing unfinished business and providing for care of significant others if appropriate
	  5. encourage client and significant others to share feelings of anxiety and loss with one another
	  6. encourage significant others to stay with client and participate in his/her care if their presence seems to relieve the client's fear and anxiety; offer support to significant others as necessary
	  7. arrange for a visit with clergy if desired by client or significant others.

2. NURSING DIAGNOSIS

Altered respiratory function:[*]

a. **ineffective breathing patterns** related to:
1. fear and anxiety
2. pain
3. cerebral hypoxia
4. depressant effects of some medications (e.g. narcotic analgesics, muscle relaxants)
5. impaired chest expansion associated with decreased mobility and weakened abdominal, intercostal, and diaphragm muscles
6. restricted lung expansion associated with abdominal distention and/or pleural effusion (may occur as a result of particular disease processes);

b. **ineffective airway clearance** related to:
1. fluid accumulation in the alveoli and bronchioles associated with pulmonary edema and poor cough effort
2. accumulation of tenacious secretions associated with fluid volume deficit
3. airway obstruction associated with underlying disease process and/or aspiration;

[*] This diagnostic label includes the following nursing diagnoses: ineffective breathing pattern, ineffective airway clearance, and impaired gas exchange (Carpenito, 1989).

   c. **impaired gas exchange** related to:
1. ineffective breathing patterns and airway clearance
2. loss of effective lung tissue associated with the underlying disease process
3. a thickened alveolar-capillary membrane associated with pulmonary edema.

☐ ▪▪▪

DESIRED OUTCOMES	NURSING ACTIONS AND *SELECTED RATIONALES*

2. The client will experience adequate respiratory function as evidenced by:
   a. usual rate, rhythm, and depth of respirations
   b. decreased dyspnea
   c. usual or improved breath sounds
   d. usual mental status
   e. usual skin color
   f. blood gases within normal range for client.

2.a. Assess for signs and symptoms of altered respiratory function:
1. shallow, rapid, slow, or irregular respirations
2. dyspnea, orthopnea
3. use of accessory muscles when breathing
4. adventitious breath sounds (e.g. crackles, rhonchi)
5. diminished or absent breath sounds
6. restlessness, irritability
7. confusion, somnolence
8. dusky or cyanotic skin color.
  b. Monitor blood gases. Report values that worsen.
  c. Monitor for and report significant changes in ear oximetry and capnograph results.
  d. Implement measures *to improve respiratory status:*
1. perform actions to reduce pain (see Nursing Diagnosis 5.A, action 5)
2. perform actions to decrease accumulation of gastrointestinal gas and fluid (see Nursing Diagnosis 5.D, action 3) *in order to reduce pressure on the diaphragm*
3. perform actions to decrease fear and anxiety (see Nursing Diagnosis 1, actions b and c)
4. place client in a semi- to high Fowler's position; position overbed table so client can lean on it if desired
5. maintain oxygen therapy as ordered
6. instruct client to breathe slowly if he/she is hyperventilating
7. assist client to turn at least every 2 hours
8. instruct client to deep breathe and, if able, to use inspiratory exerciser at least every 2 hours
9. perform actions to reduce the risk of aspiration (see Nursing Diagnosis 17, action e)
10. perform actions *to facilitate removal of secretions:*
    a. instruct and assist client to cough every 1–2 hours
    b. implement measures *to liquefy tenacious secretions:*
       1. maintain a fluid intake of at least 2500 cc/day unless contraindicated
       2. humidify inspired air as ordered
       3. assist with administration of mucolytic agents via nebulizer or IPPB treatment
    c. perform nasal, oral, pharyngeal, and/or tracheal suctioning only if necessary (deep suctioning should be avoided in final stage of dying process)
    d. monitor for therapeutic and nontherapeutic effects of expectorants if administered
11. protect client from exposure to irritating substances (e.g. smoke, flowers, perfume)
12. encourage as much activity as tolerated
13. monitor for therapeutic and nontherapeutic effects of the following medications if administered:
    a. diuretics *to decrease pulmonary fluid accumulation*
    b. morphine sulfate *to decrease pulmonary vascular congestion (its vasodilatory action reduces cardiac workload and eventually improves left ventricular emptying, which results in increased blood return from the pulmonary veins) and reduce apprehension associated with dyspnea*
    c. bronchodilators

14. prepare client for thoracentesis or paracentesis if performed *to facilitate lung expansion.*

   e. Consult physician about an order for an anticholinergic medication (e.g. atropine) *to reduce bronchial secretions if the final stage of dying process is prolonged, frequent suctioning is necessary, or the sound of excessive secretions is disturbing to significant others.*

   f. Consult physician if dyspnea persists or worsens and the client appears uncomfortable despite implementation of above actions.

3. NURSING DIAGNOSIS

Fluid volume deficit related to:

a. decreased oral fluid intake associated with dysphagia, nausea, anorexia, fatigue, weakness, dyspnea, and/or decreased level of consciousness;

b. increased fluid loss associated with vomiting, diarrhea, and hyperventilation (may result from fear, anxiety, and respiratory acidosis).

DESIRED OUTCOMES	NURSING ACTIONS AND *SELECTED RATIONALES*

3. The client will not experience a fluid volume deficit as evidenced by:
a. normal skin turgor
b. moist mucous membranes
c. weight loss no greater than 0.5 kg/day
d. B/P and pulse within normal range for client and stable with position change
e. balanced intake and output
f. urine specific gravity between 1.010 and 1.030.
	3.a. Assess for and report signs and symptoms of fluid volume deficit:
	1. decreased skin turgor
	2. dry mucous membranes, thirst
	3. weight loss greater than 0.5 kg/day
	4. low B/P and or decline in systolic B/P of at least 15 mm Hg with concurrent rise in pulse when client sits up
	5. weak, rapid pulse
	6. output less than intake with urine specific gravity higher than 1.030 (reflects an actual rather than potential water deficit).
	b. Implement measures *to prevent or treat fluid volume deficit:*
	1. perform actions to prevent nausea and vomiting (see Nursing Diagnosis 5.B, action 2)
	2. perform actions to control diarrhea (see Nursing Diagnosis 12, action d)
	3. perform actions *to prevent hyperventilation:*
	  a. implement measures to reduce fear and anxiety (see Nursing Diagnosis 1, actions b and c)
	  b. implement measures to improve respiratory status (see Nursing Diagnosis 2, action d) *in order to prevent respiratory acidosis, which can cause hyperventilation*
	4. encourage maximum fluid intake allowed and tolerated
	5. if client cannot tolerate drinking from a glass and/or is too weak to drink through a straw:
	  a. give frequent sips of water or juice using an eye dropper or syringe
	  b. use a spoon to provide small amounts of ice chips.
	c. Consult physician if signs and symptoms of fluid volume deficit persist or worsen and the client is uncomfortable. Encourage significant others and client to discuss the positive and negative aspects of intravenous therapy with physician.

4. NURSING DIAGNOSIS

Impaired swallowing related to impaired tongue movement and coordination associated with weakness and fatigue, depressed pharyngeal reflexes, and dry mouth.

UNIT
IV

DESIRED OUTCOMES	NURSING ACTIONS AND *SELECTED RATIONALES*

4. The client will experience an improvement in swallowing as evidenced by:
   a. verbalization of same
   b. absence of coughing or choking when eating and drinking.

4.a. Assess for and report signs and symptoms of impaired swallowing (e.g. coughing or choking when eating or drinking, stasis of food in the oral cavity).
   b. Implement measures *to improve ability to swallow:*
      1. perform actions to reduce dryness of the oral mucous membrane (see Nursing Diagnosis 7, action b)
      2. perform actions *to stimulate salivation at mealtime in order to further reduce dry mouth:*
         a. provide oral care before meals
         b. provide sour, hard candy for client to suck just before meals unless contraindicated
         c. serve foods that are visually pleasing
         d. place a piece of lemon or sour pickle on plate
      3. place client in high Fowler's position for meals and snacks; head should be erect with chin tilted forward *to facilitate elevation of the larynx and posterior movement of the tongue*
      4. assist client to select foods that are easily chewed and swallowed (e.g. custard, flavored gelatin, cottage cheese, ground meat)
      5. avoid serving foods that are sticky (e.g. peanut butter, soft bread, bananas)
      6. serve foods/fluids that are hot or cold instead of room temperature (*the more extreme temperatures stimulate the sensory receptors and swallowing reflex*)
      7. moisten dry foods with gravy or sauces (e.g. sour cream, salad dressing).
   c. Consult physician if swallowing difficulties persist or worsen.

☐ ▬▬▬▬▬▬▬▬▬▬▬▬▬▬▬▬▬▬▬▬▬▬▬▬▬▬▬▬▬▬▬▬

5.A. NURSING DIAGNOSIS

Altered comfort:* **pain** related to advancing disease process.

---

* In this care plan, the nursing diagnosis "pain" is included under the diagnostic label of altered comfort.

☐ ▬▬▬▬▬▬▬▬▬▬▬▬▬▬▬▬▬▬▬▬▬▬▬▬▬▬▬▬▬▬▬▬

DESIRED OUTCOMES	NURSING ACTIONS AND *SELECTED RATIONALES*

5.A. The client will experience diminished pain as evidenced by:
   1. verbalization of pain relief
   2. relaxed facial expression and body positioning
   3. increased participation in activities
   4. stable vital signs.

5.A.1. Determine how client usually responds to pain.
   2. Assess for nonverbal signs of pain (e.g. social withdrawal, wrinkled brow, clenched fists, reluctance to move, guarding of affected body part, restlessness, diaphoresis, facial pallor or flushing, change in B/P, tachycardia).
   3. Assess verbal complaints of pain. Ask client to be specific about location, severity, and type of pain. Ascertain if pain experienced is of an acute or chronic nature *in order to determine the most effective means of control.*
   4. Assess for factors that seem to aggravate and alleviate pain.
   5. Implement measures *to reduce pain:*
      a. assure client that his/her needs for pain relief will be met *in order to reduce fear and anxiety about the pain experience*
      b. medicate prior to any painful treatments or procedures and before pain is severe
      c. plan methods for achieving pain relief (e.g. nonpharmacological measures, scheduled or "as necessary" administration of analgesics, methods of alternating or combining medications, medications at bedside [e.g. morphine elixir] to take as needed, patient-controlled

analgesia [PCA]) with the client *in order to assist him/her to maintain a sense of control over the pain experience*
   d. provide or assist with nonpharmacological measures for pain relief (e.g. cutaneous stimulation techniques such as pressure, massage, heat and cold applications, transcutaneous electrical nerve stimulation, or vibration; relaxation techniques such as progressive relaxation exercises or meditation; distraction by quiet conversation, rhythmic massage, or diversional activities; guided imagery; position change)
   e. monitor for therapeutic and nontherapeutic effects of analgesics if administered; assist with titration of prescribed medications *in order to achieve adequate pain relief with minimal side effects;* assure client that drug addiction is not a concern.
  6. Consult physician if above measures fail to provide adequate pain relief.

□ ▬▬▬▬▬▬▬▬▬▬▬▬▬▬▬▬▬▬▬▬▬▬▬▬▬▬

5.B. NURSING DIAGNOSIS

Altered comfort: nausea and vomiting related to stimulation of the vomiting center associated with:

1. vagal and/or sympathetic stimulation resulting from visceral irritation associated with abdominal distention;
2. cortical stimulation due to pain and stress;
3. stimulation of the chemoreceptor trigger zone by some medications (e.g. morphine sulfate, meperidine hydrochloride).

□ ▬▬▬▬▬▬▬▬▬▬▬▬▬▬▬▬▬▬▬▬▬▬▬▬▬▬

DESIRED OUTCOMES	NURSING ACTIONS AND *SELECTED RATIONALES*

5.B. The client will experience relief of nausea and vomiting as evidenced by:
1. verbalization of relief of nausea
2. absence of vomiting.
	5.B.1. Assess client to determine factors that contribute to nausea and vomiting (e.g. abdominal distention, movement or body position, pain, anxiety, certain foods, some medications).
	  2. Implement measures *to prevent nausea and vomiting:*
	    a. perform actions to decrease accumulation of gastrointestinal gas and fluid (see Nursing Diagnosis 5.D, action 3)
	    b. perform actions to reduce pain (see Nursing Diagnosis 5.A, action 5)
	    c. perform actions to reduce fear and anxiety (see Nursing Diagnosis 1, actions b and c)
	    d. eliminate noxious sights and smells from the environment (*noxious stimuli cause cortical stimulation of the vomiting center*)
	    e. encourage client to take deep, slow breaths when nauseated
	    f. instruct client to change positions slowly (*movement stimulates the chemoreceptor trigger zone*)
	    g. provide oral hygiene after each emesis and before meals
	    h. if oral intake is allowed:
	      1. provide small, frequent meals rather than 3 large ones
	      2. instruct client to ingest foods and fluids slowly
	      3. instruct client to avoid foods/fluids that irritate gastric mucosa (e.g. spicy foods; citrus fruits or juices; caffeine-containing items such as chocolate, coffee, tea, and colas)
	      4. encourage client to eat dry foods (e.g. toast, crackers) and avoid drinking liquids with meals if nauseated
	      5. instruct client to rest after eating with head of bed elevated
	    i. monitor for therapeutic and nontherapeutic effects of antiemetics or gastrointestinal stimulants (e.g. metoclopramide) if administered.
	  3. If above measures fail to control nausea and vomiting:
	    a. consult physician
	    b. be prepared to insert a nasogastric tube and maintain suction as ordered.

☐ ▬▬▬▬▬▬▬▬▬▬▬▬▬▬▬▬▬▬▬

5.C. NURSING DIAGNOSIS

Altered comfort: pruritus related to dry skin associated with fluid volume deficit.

☐ ▬▬▬▬▬▬▬▬▬▬▬▬▬▬▬▬▬▬▬

DESIRED OUTCOMES	NURSING ACTIONS AND *SELECTED RATIONALES*

5.C. The client will experience relief of pruritus as evidenced by:
1. verbalization of same
2. no scratching or rubbing of skin.
	5.C.1. Assess pruritus including onset, characteristics, location, factors that aggravate or alleviate it, and client tolerance.
	2. Instruct client in and/or implement measures *to relieve pruritus:*
	  a. perform actions *to promote capillary constriction:*
	    1. apply cool, moist compresses to pruritic areas
	    2. maintain a cool environment
	  b. apply emollients to skin *to help alleviate dryness*
	  c. add emollients, cornstarch, baking soda, or oatmeal to bath water
	  d. use tepid water and mild soaps for bathing
	  e. pat skin dry, making sure to dry thoroughly
	  f. encourage participation in diversional activity
	  g. utilize relaxation techniques
	  h. encourage client to wear loose cotton garments
	  i. utilize cutaneous stimulation techniques (e.g. pressure, massage, vibration, stroking with a soft brush) at site of itching or acupressure points.
	3. Monitor for therapeutic and nontherapeutic effects of antihistamines and antipruritic lotions if administered.
	4. Consult physician if above measures fail to alleviate pruritus or if the skin becomes excoriated.

☐ ▬▬▬▬▬▬▬▬▬▬▬▬▬▬▬▬▬▬▬

5.D. NURSING DIAGNOSIS

Altered comfort: abdominal distention and gas pain related to an accumulation of gas and fluid associated with decreased peristalsis resulting from depressant effects of some medications (e.g. narcotic analgesics, muscle relaxants) and decreased activity.

☐ ▬▬▬▬▬▬▬▬▬▬▬▬▬▬▬▬▬▬▬

DESIRED OUTCOMES	NURSING ACTIONS AND *SELECTED RATIONALES*

5.D. The client will experience diminished abdominal distention and gas pain as evidenced by:
1. verbalization of decreased abdominal fullness and pain
2. relaxed facial expression and body positioning
3. decrease in abdominal distention.
	5.D.1. Assess for nonverbal signs of abdominal distention and gas pain (e.g. clutching and guarding of abdomen, restlessness, reluctance to move, grimacing, increasing abdominal girth, dyspnea).
	2. Assess verbal complaints of abdominal discomfort (e.g. increasing feeling of abdominal fullness, gas pain).
	3. Implement measures *to reduce the accumulation of gastrointestinal gas and fluid:*
	  a. encourage and assist client with frequent position changes and ambulation as tolerated (*activity stimulates peristalsis and expulsion of flatus*)
	  b. instruct client to avoid activities such as chewing gum, sucking on hard candy, and smoking *in order to reduce air swallowing*

c. maintain patency of gastric or intestinal tube if present
d. maintain food and fluid restrictions as ordered
e. encourage client to drink warm liquids *to stimulate peristalsis*
f. instruct client to avoid gas-producing foods/fluids (e.g. carbonated beverages, cabbage, onions, baked beans)
g. apply heat to the abdomen for 20 minutes every 3–4 hours unless contraindicated
h. encourage client to expel flatus whenever the urge is felt
i. consult physician about insertion of a rectal tube or administration of a return flow enema if indicated
j. encourage use of nonnarcotic analgesics if possible (*narcotic analgesics depress gastrointestinal activity*)
k. monitor for therapeutic and nontherapeutic effects of gastrointestinal stimulants (e.g. metoclopramide, bisacodyl) if administered *to increase gastrointestinal motility.*
4. Consult physician if abdominal discomfort persists or worsens.

5.E. NURSING DIAGNOSIS

Altered comfort: hiccoughs related to irritation of the phrenic or vagus nerve associated with such things as gastric and abdominal distention, abdominal tumors, and gastric or abdominal drainage tubes.

DESIRED OUTCOMES	NURSING ACTIONS AND *SELECTED RATIONALES*
5.E. The client will not experience persistent hiccoughs.	5.E.1. Implement measures *to prevent irritation of the phrenic and vagus nerves:* a. perform actions to reduce the accumulation of gastrointestinal gas and fluid (see Nursing Diagnosis 5.D, action 3) b. instruct client to avoid drinking very hot or cold liquids *to avoid reflex irritation of phrenic and vagus nerves* c. if gastric and abdominal drainage tubes are present, anchor them securely *in order to minimize movement of the tubes and subsequent phrenic or vagus nerve irritation.* 2. Implement measures *to control hiccoughs if they occur:* a. instruct client to perform techniques such as breathing deeply, rebreathing into a paper bag, holding breath, applying finger pressure on the eyeballs through closed lids for several minutes, eating a teaspoon of sugar, or drinking water while holding breath unless contraindicated b. monitor for therapeutic and nontherapeutic effects of sedatives and/or phenothiazines if administered. 3. Consult physician if hiccoughs persist. Be prepared to assist with the following treatments for intractable hiccoughs if ordered: a. gastric lavage or suction *to decrease abdominal distention* b. removal of gastric or abdominal tubes (*these may be irritating the phrenic or vagus nerve*) c. inhalation of carbon dioxide (*the depressant effect of CO_2 reduces spasm of the diaphragm*) d. gentle rotation of a suction catheter after inserting it into pharynx (*this movement can interrupt impulses from the vagus nerve*) e. phrenic nerve block or phrenic nerve crushing.

☐ ▬▬▬▬▬▬▬▬▬▬▬▬▬▬▬▬

6. NURSING DIAGNOSIS

Impaired skin integrity: irritation or breakdown related to:

a. prolonged pressure on tissues associated with decreased mobility;
b. frequent contact with irritants associated with persistent diarrhea or incontinence of urine or stool;
c. increased fragility of skin associated with malnutrition, fluid volume deficit, and dependent edema;
d. excessive scratching associated with pruritus resulting from dry skin.

☐ ▬▬▬▬▬▬▬▬▬▬▬▬▬▬▬▬

DESIRED OUTCOMES	NURSING ACTIONS AND *SELECTED RATIONALES*

6. The client will maintain skin integrity as evidenced by:
  a. absence of redness and irritation
  b. no skin breakdown.
	6.a. Inspect the skin (especially bone prominences; dependent, edematous, and pruritic areas; and perianal area) for pallor, redness, and breakdown.
	b. Implement measures *to maintain skin integrity:*
	  1. refer to Care Plan on Immobility, Nursing Diagnosis 7, action b, for measures to prevent skin breakdown associated with decreased mobility
	  2. perform actions *to decrease skin irritation and prevent breakdown resulting from diarrhea and incontinence of urine or stool:*
	    a. implement measures to control diarrhea and reduce the risk of bowel incontinence (see Nursing Diagnoses 12, action d and 13, action b)
	    b. provide soft toilet tissue for wiping after urination or defecation
	    c. instruct and assist client to thoroughly cleanse and dry perineal area after each episode of diarrhea and incontinence; apply a protective ointment or cream (e.g. Sween cream, Desitin, Karaya gel, A & D ointment, Vaseline)
	    d. apply a perianal pouch if bowel incontinence is a persistent problem
	    e. implement measures to maintain or regain urinary continence (see Nursing Diagnosis 10, action b)
	    f. consult physician about placement of external or indwelling catheter if urinary incontinence persists
	    g. avoid direct contact of skin with Chux (e.g. place turn sheet or bed pad over Chux)
	  3. perform actions *to prevent skin breakdown associated with scratching:*
	    a. implement measures to relieve pruritus (see Nursing Diagnosis 5.C, actions 2 and 3)
	    b. keep nails trimmed and/or apply mittens if necessary
	    c. instruct client to apply firm pressure to pruritic areas rather than scratching
	  4. perform actions *to prevent skin breakdown associated with edema:*
	    a. implement measures *to reduce fluid accumulation in dependent areas:*
	      1. assist with range of motion exercises
	      2. turn client at least every 2 hours
	      3. elevate lower extremities
	      4. apply elastic wraps or hose to lower extremities as ordered
	      5. apply a scrotal support if scrotal edema is present
	    b. handle edematous areas carefully
	  5. perform actions to prevent or treat fluid volume deficit (see Nursing Diagnosis 3, action b) *in order to reduce risk of skin breakdown associated with dehydration.*
	c. If skin breakdown occurs:
	  1. notify physician
	  2. continue with above measures to prevent further irritation and breakdown
	  3. perform decubitus care as ordered or per standard hospital policy (extensiveness of treatment is usually limited to that necessary to maintain comfort in the final stages of life)

4. monitor client closely and report signs and symptoms of infection (e.g. elevated temperature; redness, warmth, and edema around area of breakdown; unusual drainage from site).

7. NURSING DIAGNOSIS

Altered oral mucous membrane: dryness related to:

a. decreased salivation associated with fluid volume deficit, decreased oral intake, and some medications (e.g. tricyclic antidepressants, anticholinergics, narcotic analgesics, phenothiazines);
b. prolonged oxygen therapy;
c. chronic mouth breathing.

DESIRED OUTCOMES	NURSING ACTIONS AND *SELECTED RATIONALES*

7. The client will maintain a moist, intact oral mucous membrane.	7.a. Assess client frequently for dryness of the oral mucosa.
	b. Implement measures *to relieve dryness of the oral mucous membrane:*
	  1. provide or assist client to perform good oral hygiene as often as needed:
	    a. use a soft bristle brush, gauze wrapped around tongue blade, or Toothettes to cleanse mouth and remove encrustations (soften with water-soluble lubricant if difficult to remove)
	    b. rinse mouth with water, saline solution, or dilute mouthwash
	    c. avoid products such as lemon-glycerin swabs and commercial mouthwashes containing alcohol (*these have a drying or irritating effect on oral mucous membrane*)
	  2. lubricate client's lips with Vaseline, K-Y jelly, ChapStick, Blistex, or mineral oil when oral care is given
	  3. encourage client to breathe through nose if possible
	  4. encourage client not to smoke (*smoking further irritates and dries the mucosa*)
	  5. perform actions to prevent or treat fluid volume deficit (see Nursing Diagnosis 3, action b)
	  6. if salivary production is diminished:
	    a. perform actions *to increase salivary flow:*
	      1. encourage client to suck on sour, hard candy if allowed
	      2. offer hot tea with lemon or warm lemonade at regular intervals unless contraindicated
	      3. apply pressure to sternal notch and massage back of neck at regular intervals
	    b. use artificial saliva (e.g. Moi-stir, Salivart, Xero-Lube) *to lubricate mucosa.*
	c. If oral mucosa is irritated or cracked, implement measures *to relieve discomfort and promote healing:*
	  1. if client is alert and able to take nourishment by mouth, assist him/her to select soft, bland, and nonacidic foods
	  2. instruct client to avoid extremely hot or cold foods/fluids
	  3. use a low-pressure power spray for oral care
	  4. apply carbamide peroxide (e.g. Gly-Oxide, Proxigel) to irritated areas
	  5. monitor for therapeutic and nontherapeutic effects of topical anesthetics, oral protective pastes, and topical and systemic analgesics if administered.
	d. Consult physician if dryness, irritation, and discomfort persist.

8. NURSING DIAGNOSIS

Impaired physical mobility related to weakness, fatigue, dyspnea, sensory and motor deficits, reluctance to move because of pain, and/or decreased level of consciousness.

DESIRED OUTCOMES	NURSING ACTIONS AND *SELECTED RATIONALES*

8.a. The client will achieve maximum physical mobility within limitations imposed by terminal state.	8.a.1. Assess for factors that impair physical mobility (e.g. weakness, fatigue, pain, sensory and motor deficits, decreased level of consciousness).
	 2. Implement measures *to increase mobility:*
	   a. perform actions to maintain or improve activity tolerance (see Care Plan on Immobility, Nursing Diagnosis 8, action b)
	   b. perform actions to control pain (see Nursing Diagnosis 5.A, action 5)
	   c. perform actions to improve respiratory status (see Nursing Diagnosis 2, action d) *in order to relieve dyspnea*
	   d. instruct client in and assist with active and/or passive range of motion exercises
	   e. instruct client in and assist with correct use of mobility aids (e.g. cane, walker) if appropriate.
	 3. Increase activity and participation in self-care activities as tolerated.
	 4. Provide praise and encouragement for all efforts to maintain or increase physical mobility.
	 5. Encourage the support of significant others. Allow them to assist with range of motion exercises, positioning, and activity if desired.

8.b. The client will not experience problems associated with immobility.	8.b. Refer to Care Plan on Immobility for actions to prevent problems associated with immobility.

9. NURSING DIAGNOSIS

Self-care deficit related to altered thought processes and impaired physical mobility associated with sensory and motor deficits, pain, weakness, fatigue, dyspnea, and decreased level of consciousness.

DESIRED OUTCOMES	NURSING ACTIONS AND *SELECTED RATIONALES*
9. The client will perform self-care activities within physical limitations.	9.a. Refer to Care Plan on Immobility, Nursing Diagnosis 9, for measures related to assessment of, planning for, and meeting client's self-care needs. b. Implement measures to increase mobility (see Nursing Diagnosis 8, action a.2) *in order to further facilitate client's ability to perform self-care.*

□ ▬▬▬▬▬▬▬▬▬▬▬▬▬▬▬▬▬▬▬▬▬▬▬▬▬▬▬▬▬▬

10. NURSING DIAGNOSIS

Altered pattern of urinary elimination: incontinence related to poor urinary sphincter control associated with a decreased level of consciousness and/or neurological deficits resulting from the underlying disease process.

□ ▬▬▬▬▬▬▬▬▬▬▬▬▬▬▬▬▬▬▬▬▬▬▬▬▬▬▬▬▬▬

DESIRED OUTCOMES	NURSING ACTIONS AND *SELECTED RATIONALES*

10. The client will maintain or regain urinary continence.	10.a. Assess for and report urinary incontinence.
	b. Implement measures *to maintain or regain urinary continence:*
	  1. offer bedpan or urinal or assist client to commode or bathroom every 2–3 hours
	  2. allow client to assume a normal position for voiding unless contraindicated *in order to promote complete bladder emptying*
	  3. instruct client to perform perineal exercises (e.g. stopping and starting stream during voiding; pressing buttocks together, then relaxing the muscles) *in order to improve urinary sphincter tone*
	  4. limit oral fluid intake in the evening *to decrease possibility of nighttime incontinence*
	  5. instruct client to avoid drinking beverages containing caffeine (*caffeine is a mild diuretic and may make urinary control more difficult*)
	  6. monitor for therapeutic and nontherapeutic effects of alpha-adrenergic agonists (e.g. ephedrine) if administered *to increase urinary sphincter tone.*
	c. If urinary incontinence persists:
	  1. consult physician about intermittent catheterization, insertion of indwelling catheter, or use of external catheter or penile clamp
	  2. provide emotional support to client and significant others.

□ ▬▬▬▬▬▬▬▬▬▬▬▬▬▬▬▬▬▬▬▬▬▬▬▬▬▬▬▬▬▬

11. NURSING DIAGNOSIS

Constipation related to:

a. decreased activity;
b. decreased fluid and fiber intake associated with anorexia, dysphagia, and difficulty feeding self;
c. use of some medications (e.g. opiates, antacids containing aluminum or calcium);
d. long-term use of laxatives;
e. decreased ability to respond to the urge to defecate associated with weak abdominal musculature and decreased level of consciousness;
f. increased sympathetic nervous system activity resulting from anxiety;
g. obstruction of the bowel associated with the underlying disease process.

□ ▬▬▬▬▬▬▬▬▬▬▬▬▬▬▬▬▬▬▬▬▬▬▬▬▬▬▬▬▬▬

DESIRED OUTCOMES	NURSING ACTIONS AND *SELECTED RATIONALES*
11. The client will maintain a bowel routine that provides optimal comfort.	11.a. Refer to Care Plan on Immobility, Nursing Diagnosis 11, for measures related to assessment, prevention, and management of constipation. b. Implement additional measures *to prevent constipation:*

1. establish a routine time for defecation based on client's usual bowel elimination pattern
2. perform actions to reduce fear and anxiety (see Nursing Diagnosis 1, actions b and c)
3. assist client to toilet or place in high Fowler's position or on commode for bowel movements unless contraindicated; provide privacy and adequate ventilation
4. assist with titration of laxative agents (e.g. combination of a stool softener and bulk-forming agent or lubricant with a peristaltic stimulant)
5. if client is on antacid therapy, consult physician about alternating those containing aluminum or calcium with those containing magnesium
6. if an oil retention enema is ordered, administer it using tap water enema equipment and technique *in order to reach a higher level in the bowel and increase effectiveness.*

☐ ▐██▌

12. NURSING DIAGNOSIS

Diarrhea related to:

a. increased intestinal motility associated with extreme fear and anxiety;
b. reduction in usual bowel flora associated with anti-infective therapy;
c. increased water in the bowel associated with high osmolarity supplemental feedings;
d. use of antacids containing magnesium sulfate;
e. excessive use of cathartics and stool softeners.

☐ ▐██▌

DESIRED OUTCOMES	NURSING ACTIONS AND *SELECTED RATIONALES*

12. The client will have fewer bowel movements and more formed stool.	12.a. Ascertain client's usual bowel elimination habits.
	 b. Assess for and report signs and symptoms of diarrhea (e.g. frequent, loose stools; abdominal pain and cramping).
	 c. Assess bowel sounds regularly. Report an increase in frequency of and/or high-pitched bowel sounds.
	 d. Implement measures *to control diarrhea:*
	   1. perform actions to reduce fear and anxiety (see Nursing Diagnosis 1, actions b and c)
	   2. instruct client to avoid foods/fluids that are poorly digested or could act as irritants to the bowel:
	     a. those high in fat (e.g. butter, cream, oils, whole milk, ice cream, pork, fried foods, gravies, nuts)
	     b. those with high fiber content (e.g. whole-grain cereals, nuts, raw fruits and vegetables)
	     c. those known to cause diarrhea or be gas-producers (e.g. cabbage, onions, prunes, baked beans, carbonated beverages)
	     d. those high in caffeine (e.g. coffee, tea, chocolate, colas)
	     e. spicy foods
	     f. extremely hot or cold foods/fluids
	   3. encourage consumption of low-residue foods/fluids (e.g. apple or grape juice, ripe bananas, cooked vegetables, chicken, fish, ground beef, white rice or bread, cooked cereals, pasta)
	   4. provide small, frequent meals
	   5. discourage smoking (*nicotine has a stimulant effect on gastrointestinal tract*)
	   6. if diarrhea is related to anti-infective therapy, encourage intake of flora-containing foods (e.g. yogurt, buttermilk)

7. if client is receiving a commercial dietary supplement, dilute it and instruct him/her to drink it slowly; consult physician about use of a low-osmolarity preparation (e.g. Osmolite)
8. if client is on antacid therapy, consult physician about alternating those containing magnesium with one containing aluminum or calcium
9. monitor for therapeutic and nontherapeutic effects of the following medications if administered:
   a. opiate or opiate-like substances (e.g. loperamide, diphenoxylate hydrochloride) *to decrease gastrointestinal motility*
   b. bulk-forming agents (e.g. methylcellulose, psyllium hydrophilic mucilloid, calcium polycarbophil) *to absorb water in the bowel and produce a soft, formed stool.*
e. Consult physician if diarrhea persists.

☐ ▬▬▬▬▬▬▬▬▬▬▬▬▬▬▬▬▬▬▬▬▬▬▬▬

13. NURSING DIAGNOSIS

Bowel incontinence related to poor sphincter control associated with a decreased level of consciousness and/or neurological deficits resulting from the underlying disease process.

☐ ▬▬▬▬▬▬▬▬▬▬▬▬▬▬▬▬▬▬▬▬▬▬▬▬

DESIRED OUTCOMES	NURSING ACTIONS AND *SELECTED RATIONALES*

13. The client will maintain optimal bowel control as evidenced by absence of or decreased episodes of incontinence.	13.a. Assess for episodes of bowel incontinence.
	b. Implement measures *to reduce risk of bowel incontinence:*
	   1. perform actions to control diarrhea (see Nursing Diagnosis 12, action d)
	   2. instruct client to perform perineal exercises (e.g. relaxing and tightening perineal and gluteal muscles) if able *in order to strengthen anal sphincter*
	   3. have commode or bedpan readily available to client
	   4. with client, establish a routine time for defecation; try to schedule it 20–30 minutes after a meal *to take advantage of the gastrocolic reflex.*
	c. If bowel incontinence persists:
	   1. consult physician about use of a rectal tube or perianal pouch if client is experiencing constant drainage of liquid stool
	   2. provide emotional support to client and significant others.

☐ ▬▬▬▬▬▬▬▬▬▬▬▬▬▬▬▬▬▬▬▬▬▬▬▬

14. NURSING DIAGNOSIS

Altered thought processes: impaired memory, shortened attention span, slowed verbal response time, restlessness, agitation, and confusion related to:

a. drug toxicity associated with organ failure;
b. fluid and electrolyte imbalances;
c. cerebral hypoxia or neurological disorders associated with the underlying disease process;
d. uncontrolled pain.

☐ ▬▬▬▬▬▬▬▬▬▬▬▬▬▬▬▬▬▬▬▬▬▬▬▬

DESIRED OUTCOMES	NURSING ACTIONS AND *SELECTED RATIONALES*

14. The client will maintain usual thought processes as evidenced by:
a. usual attention span
b. usual verbal response time
c. absence of restlessness and agitation
d. orientation to person, place, time, and others.
	14.a. Assess client for altered thought processes (e.g. impaired memory, shortened attention span, slowed verbal response time, restlessness, agitation, confusion).
	b. Ascertain from significant others client's usual level of intellectual functioning.
	c. If client shows evidence of altered thought processes:
	  1. assess for possible causes (e.g. drug toxicity, pain, hypoxia, fluid and electrolyte imbalances) and treat accordingly
	  2. implement measures to protect client from injury (see Nursing Diagnosis 16, actions b–e)
	  3. allow adequate time for communication and performance of activities
	  4. repeat instructions as necessary using clear, simple language
	  5. reorient client to person, place, time, and others as necessary
	  6. encourage significant others to be supportive of client; instruct them to reorient client as necessary
	  7. encourage significant others to bring in client's favorite objects and place in room
	  8. leave a light on at night *to facilitate client's orientation to surroundings*
	  9. implement measures *to ease restlessness:*
	    a. spend time with client and urge significant others to do the same
	    b. increase activity if possible
	    c. perform actions to reduce pain (see Nursing Diagnosis 5.A, action 5)
	    d. perform actions to improve respiratory status (see Nursing Diagnosis 2, action d) *in order to improve tissue oxygenation.*

15. NURSING DIAGNOSIS

Sleep pattern disturbance related to decreased physical activity, fear, anxiety, unfamiliar environment, discomfort, diarrhea, and inability to assume usual sleep position due to orthopnea.

DESIRED OUTCOMES	NURSING ACTIONS AND *SELECTED RATIONALES*

15. The client will attain optimal amounts of sleep (see Care Plan on Immobility, Nursing Diagnosis 12, for outcome criteria).	15.a. Refer to Care Plan on Immobility, Nursing Diagnosis 12, for measures related to assessment and promotion of sleep.
	b. Implement additional measures *to promote sleep:*
	  1. perform actions to reduce fear and anxiety (see Nursing Diagnosis 1, actions b and c)
	  2. perform actions to reduce discomfort (see Nursing Diagnoses 5.A, action 5; 5.B, action 2; 5.C, actions 2 and 3; 5.D, action 3; and 5.E)
	  3. perform actions to control diarrhea (see Nursing Diagnosis 12, action d)
	  4. assist client to assume a comfortable sleep position (e.g. bed in reverse Trendelenburg position with client in usual recumbent sleep position, head of bed elevated with arms supported on pillows, resting forward on overbed table with good pillow support, sitting in chair) if he/she has orthopnea
	  5. maintain oxygen therapy during sleep if indicated
	  6. ensure good room ventilation.

16. NURSING DIAGNOSIS

Potential for trauma related to falls, burns, and cuts associated with weakness, confusion, and decreased level of consciousness.

DESIRED OUTCOMES	NURSING ACTIONS AND *SELECTED RATIONALES*

16. The client will not experience falls, burns, or cuts.

16.a. Determine whether conditions predisposing client to falls, burns, and cuts (e.g. weakness, confusion) exist.
b. Implement measures *to prevent falls:*
  1. keep bed in low position with side rails up when client is in bed
  2. keep needed items within easy reach
  3. encourage client to request assistance whenever needed; have call signal within easy reach
  4. use lap belt when client is in chair if indicated
  5. instruct client to wear shoes with nonskid soles and low heels when ambulating
  6. avoid unnecessary clutter in room
  7. accompany client during ambulation utilizing a transfer safety belt
  8. provide ambulatory aids (e.g. walker, cane) if the client is weak or unsteady on feet
  9. reinforce instructions from physical therapist on correct transfer and ambulation techniques
  10. instruct client to ambulate in well-lit areas and to utilize handrails if needed
  11. do not rush client; allow adequate time for trips to the bathroom and ambulation in hallways.
c. Implement measures *to prevent burns:*
  1. let hot foods or fluids cool slightly before serving *to reduce risk of burns if spills occur*
  2. supervise client while smoking if indicated
  3. assess temperature of bath water and heating pad before and during use.
d. Assist client with tasks that require fine motor skills (e.g. shaving) *in order to prevent cuts.*
e. If client is confused, implement additional measures *to reduce the risk of injury:*
  1. reorient frequently to surroundings and necessity of adhering to safety precautions
  2. provide constant supervision (e.g. staff member, significant other) if indicated
  3. use jacket or wrist restraints or safety alarm device if necessary *to reduce risk of client's getting out of bed or chair unattended*
  4. monitor for therapeutic and nontherapeutic effects of antianxiety and antipsychotic medications if administered.
f. Include client and significant others in planning and implementing measures to prevent injury.
g. If injury does occur, initiate appropriate first aid and notify physician.

17. NURSING DIAGNOSIS

Potential for aspiration related to impaired swallowing, depressed cough and gag reflexes, and decreased level of consciousness.

DESIRED OUTCOMES	NURSING ACTIONS AND *SELECTED RATIONALES*

17. The client will not aspirate secretions or foods/fluids as evidenced by:
   a. clear or usual breath sounds
   b. resonant percussion note over lungs
   c. respiratory rate at 16–20/ minute
   d. absence of dyspnea
   e. absence of cyanosis.

17.a. Assess for factors that indicate potential for aspiration (e.g. difficulty swallowing, choking on secretions and foods/fluids, decreased level of consciousness, depressed cough and/or gag reflexes).
   b. Assess for signs and symptoms of aspiration of secretions or foods/fluids (e.g. rhonchi, dull percussion note over lungs, tachycardia, rapid respirations, dyspnea, cyanosis, presence of tube feeding in tracheal aspirate).
   c. Monitor chest x-ray results. Report findings of pulmonary infiltrate.
   d. If client is receiving tube feedings, add food coloring to the solution *so that it can be readily identified in tracheal aspirate.*
   e. Implement measures *to reduce the risk of aspiration:*
      1. position client in side-lying or semi- to high Fowler's position at all times
      2. have suction equipment readily available for use; perform oropharyngeal suctioning as often as needed *to remove secretions*
      3. withhold foods/fluids if gag reflex is absent or if client is experiencing severe dysphagia
      4. perform actions to prevent nausea and vomiting (see Nursing Diagnosis 5.B, action 2)
      5. if client is receiving tube feedings:
         a. check tube placement before each feeding or on a routine basis if continuous feeding
         b. administer solution slowly
         c. maintain client in semi- to high Fowler's position during and for at least 30 minutes after feeding
      6. if client is taking foods/fluids orally:
         a. perform actions to improve ability to swallow (see Nursing Diagnosis 4, action b)
         b. decrease environmental stimuli during meals and snacks *so client can concentrate on chewing and swallowing*
         c. provide small, frequent meals rather than 3 large ones *to decrease the risk of gastric distention and regurgitation*
         d. allow ample time for meals
         e. instruct client to avoid laughing or talking while eating or drinking
         f. maintain client in high Fowler's position during and for at least 30 minutes after meals and snacks
         g. assist client with oral hygiene after eating *to ensure that food particles do not remain in mouth*
      7. monitor for therapeutic and nontherapeutic effects of gastrointestinal stimulants (e.g. metoclopramide) if administered *to decrease risk of gastric distention and regurgitation.*
   f. If signs and symptoms of aspiration occur:
      1. perform tracheal suctioning
      2. notify physician
      3. prepare client for chest x-ray if ordered.

☐ ▄▄▄▄▄▄▄▄▄▄▄▄▄▄▄▄▄▄▄▄▄▄▄▄▄▄▄▄▄▄▄

18. NURSING DIAGNOSIS

Grieving* related to loss of control over his/her life and usual body processes, changes in body image, loss of significant others, and imminent death.

---

* This diagnostic label includes anticipatory grieving and grieving following the actual losses/changes.

☐ ▄▄▄▄▄▄▄▄▄▄▄▄▄▄▄▄▄▄▄▄▄▄▄▄▄▄▄▄▄▄▄

DESIRED OUTCOMES	NURSING ACTIONS AND *SELECTED RATIONALES*

18. The client will demonstrate progression through the grieving process as evidenced by:
    a. verbalization of feelings about dying
    b. expression of grief
    c. utilization of available support systems.

18.a. Ascertain how the client has responded in previous situations of loss.
   b. Observe for verbal and nonverbal cues indicative of the following stages of grieving according to Kübler-Ross:
      1. denial (e.g. noncompliance with treatment plan, avoidance of the words "dying" or "death," making long-range plans, hyperactivity, relating symptoms experienced to a minor problem)
      2. anger (e.g. abusive language; negative remarks about staff, family, and hospital; overcompliance; inappropriate responses to unpleasant procedures or current circumstances)
      3. bargaining (e.g. magical thinking, making personal sacrifices, verbalizing renewed spiritual faith)
      4. depression (e.g. expression of sadness, crying, withdrawal, change in sleep patterns and activity level)
      5. acceptance (e.g. decreasing interest in the environment and visitors except for a significant few, decreased interest in talking or in treatment plan, increased desire to rest and sleep, verbalization of acceptance of death).
   c. Implement measures *to facilitate the grieving process:*
      1. assist client to acknowledge that death is imminent *so grief work can begin;* assess for factors that hinder or facilitate acknowledgment
      2. assist client to identify personal strengths that have helped him/her to cope in previous situations of loss
      3. allow time for client to progress through the stages of grieving; be aware that not every stage is experienced or expressed by each person, stages do not necessarily occur in sequential order, and stages can recur during the course of an illness and the dying process
      4. perform actions *to support the client and facilitate movement through each stage of the grieving process:*
         a. denial:
            1. do not reinforce denial of terminal state, yet be aware that a period of denial is essential for client to mobilize inner strengths and resources
            2. reinforce what client has been told about his/her current status
            3. allow client to move toward the reality of the situation at his/her own pace
            4. do not provide false reassurances, but support expressions or feelings of hope
            5. perform actions *to promote trust* (e.g. answer questions honestly, provide requested information)
         b. anger:
            1. recognize displacement of anger and assist client to see actual cause of angry feelings and resentment
            2. encourage expression of thoughts and anger but establish limits on abusive behavior
            3. include client in planning of care, encourage maximum participation in treatment plan, and allow choices whenever possible *to enable him/her to maintain a sense of control*
         c. bargaining:
            1. assist client to look at available options realistically; discuss expectations and treatment options with him/her
            2. monitor for possible guilt feelings; encourage verbalization and provide feedback
            3. encourage significant others to spend time with client
            4. provide accurate information and reinforce teaching about the disease process and grieving *in order to help the client see the reality of the situation*
         d. depression:
            1. allow client to express feelings of sadness and to cry; acknowledge his/her expressions of grief
            2. listen empathetically if client chooses to verbalize feelings; emphasize that his/her response to impending death is normal

3. sit quietly with client; utilize therapeutic touch if appropriate
4. encourage those most significant to client to spend time with him/her; explain that depression facilitates the process of detachment that is essential to the client in adjusting to death
    e. acceptance:
       1. follow client cues in relation to desire for conversation, presence of others, and involvement in care
       2. accept lack of interest in environment, world events, people, and treatments; recognize that client is detaching from life and avoid false cheer and hope
       3. sit with the client when there are no tasks to perform; use touch as appropriate *to demonstrate caring*
       4. recognize that the client may be experiencing feelings of isolation and loneliness if he/she has reached the stage of acceptance and the significant others have not
       5. encourage client to express his/her feelings in whatever ways are comfortable (e.g. writing, drawing, conversation)
       6. if desired by client, assist with after-death arrangements (e.g. funeral, religious service, who should be called); be careful not to interject your own beliefs.
  d. Implement measures *to assist the client to maintain a positive self-concept and feel good about the life he/she has experienced:*
     1. visit frequently and encourage verbalization about past events, interests, and feelings
     2. help client to focus on positive rather than negative aspects of his/her life experience
     3. maintain a nonjudgmental attitude about the kind of life client has led and his/her beliefs
     4. encourage participation in decisions about care
     5. encourage and assist client with good physical hygiene and grooming; suggest use of personal rather than hospital clothing *to assist client to maintain his/her identity.*
  e. Explain the stages of the grieving process to significant others. Encourage their support and understanding.
  f. Provide information about counseling services and support groups that might be of assistance to client and significant others in working through grief.
  g. Arrange for visit from clergy if desired by client.
  h. Monitor for therapeutic and nontherapeutic effects of antidepressants if administered.
  i. Consult physician regarding referral for counseling if signs of dysfunctional grieving (e.g. persistent denial of losses or changes, excessive anger or sadness, hysteria, suicidal behaviors, phobias) occur.

☐ ▬▬▬▬▬▬▬▬▬▬▬▬▬▬▬▬▬▬▬▬▬▬▬▬

19. NURSING DIAGNOSIS

Hopelessness related to deteriorating physical condition, feelings of abandonment, and inability to reach self-fulfillment associated with terminal state.

☐ ▬▬▬▬▬▬▬▬▬▬▬▬▬▬▬▬▬▬▬▬▬▬▬▬

DESIRED OUTCOMES	NURSING ACTIONS AND *SELECTED RATIONALES*
19. The client will maintain hope as evidenced by: a. verbal and nonverbal expression of same	19.a. Assess client for signs and symptoms of hopelessness (e.g. verbal and nonverbal cues indicating feelings of despondency such as passivity, decreased response to significant others, decreased verbalization, or flat affect).

b. maintenance of satisfying relationships with others
c. participation in self-care as able
d. identification of realistic goals.

b. Implement measures *to assist client to maintain hope:*
  1. perform actions to facilitate the grieving process (see Nursing Diagnosis 18, action c)
  2. if client has religious beliefs, encourage the use of them as a support system; support his/her renewal of spiritual being by creating an environment in which these beliefs can be openly acknowledged and practiced
  3. allow client to retain as much control as possible over activities of daily living; involve him/her in as much self-care and decision making as feasible
  4. develop an atmosphere of hopefulness by assisting client to identify goals that are achievable in the time that he/she has left or ways to continue working toward goals previously set even if not possible to achieve them totally.
c. Consult physician if client demonstrates increased feelings of hopelessness.

☐ ▉▉▉▉▉▉▉▉▉▉▉▉▉▉▉▉▉▉▉▉▉▉▉▉▉▉▉▉▉▉▉▉

20. NURSING DIAGNOSIS

Altered family processes related to excessive anxiety, anticipatory grief, disorganization and role changes within the family unit, inadequate support system, and exhaustion associated with long-term care of the dying client.

☐ ▉▉▉▉▉▉▉▉▉▉▉▉▉▉▉▉▉▉▉▉▉▉▉▉▉▉▉▉▉▉▉▉

DESIRED OUTCOMES	NURSING ACTIONS AND *SELECTED RATIONALES*

20. The significant others will demonstrate beginning adjustment to loss of client and changes in family roles and structure as evidenced by:
  a. verbalization of ways to adapt to required role and life-style changes
  b. active participation in decision making and care of client
  c. ability to effectively support client
  d. positive interactions with one another.

20.a. Identify components of the family and their patterns of communication and role expectations.
b. Assess for signs and symptoms of alterations in family processes (e.g. statements of not being able to accept client's imminent death or to make necessary role and life-style changes, inability to make decisions, infrequent visits, inappropriate response to client's situation, verbalization of guilt, preoccupation with other aspects of life, client statements about lack of support).
c. Implement measures *to facilitate significant others' adjustment to imminent loss of client and resulting changes in family roles and structure:*
  1. explain the process of grieving that all experience in adjusting to a loss
  2. assist significant others to progress through their own grieving process; recognize that they may be unable to provide adequate support to the client because of their own needs
  3. encourage and assist significant others to verbalize their needs, fears, feelings, and concerns
  4. allow significant others to express their anger about expectations and demands being placed on them, being left to cope with problems alone, and/or the necessity of assuming a different and perhaps difficult family role
  5. assist significant others to confront the reality of the client's imminent death when they are ready; encourage them to imagine life after death of the client and to set some personal goals if appropriate
  6. assist significant others to make necessary postmortem arrangements for client (e.g. funeral home, clergy visitation)
  7. assist significant others to identify effective coping strategies for dealing with the client's death and its effect on those left behind
  8. provide accurate information to significant others about:
    a. the current status of client

      b. behaviors to expect as the client progresses through terminal stages of disease and his/her own grieving

      c. ways they can best assist in meeting client's needs

9. instruct significant others in signs of approaching death (e.g. reduced level of consciousness; reduced urine output; cool, mottled extremities; labored breathing or periods of no breathing)

10. prepare significant others for the sound of a "death rattle" associated with accumulation of secretions in major airways when death is imminent; describe the sound and explain that it is usually not disturbing or uncomfortable for the client

11. include significant others in decision making about client and his/her care; convey appreciation for their input and continued support of client

12. encourage and allow significant others to participate in physical care of the client if desired by both client and significant others; provide necessary instruction if indicated

13. emphasize the need for significant others to obtain adequate rest and nutrition; assure them that the client will be well cared for in their absence

14. when appropriate, help and encourage significant others to "let go" of client and say goodbye

15. provide privacy so that client and significant others can share their feelings and grief with one another

16. assist significant others to identify sources of support in the community that could assist them in coping with feelings and in meeting their immediate needs (e.g. counseling and social services, pastoral care, church groups, Hospice); initiate a referral if indicated

17. assist significant others to contact appropriate persons (e.g. funeral home director, clergy) when death occurs.

d. Consult physician if significant others continue to demonstrate difficulty in adjusting to the loss of the client and changes in their roles and family structure.

□ ▮▬▬▬▬▬▬▬▬▬▬▬▬▬▬▬▬▬▬▬▬▬▬▬▬▬▬▬▬

References

Carpenito, LJ. Handbook of nursing diagnosis (3rd ed.). Philadelphia: J.B. Lippincott Company, 1989.

Kübler-Ross, E. On death and dying. New York: Macmillan, 1969.

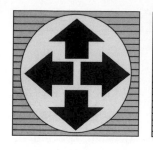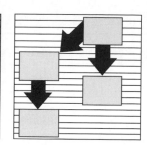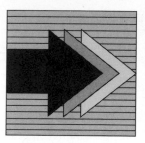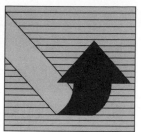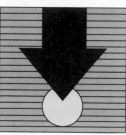

Unit XIV

Nursing Care of the Client with Disturbances of Metabolic Function

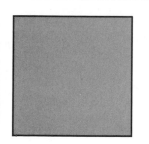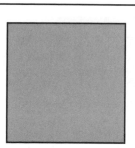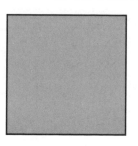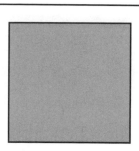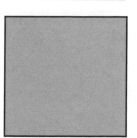

Brachytherapy

Brachytherapy is a method of delivering a high dose of radiation to a specific body surface, tissue, or organ while causing minimal damage to the surrounding area. It can be systemic or local, sealed or unsealed, and temporary or permament. The type of application selected depends on the size, location, and cell type of the tumor, in addition to the age and general physical condition of the client. The isotope used depends on availability, type of radiation emitted, half-life, and financial and safety concerns.

The most common types of brachytherapy are sealed, temporary intracavitary and interstitial implants using iridium 192 (^{192}Ir), cesium 137 (^{137}Cs), gold grains (^{198}Au), or cobalt 60 (^{60}C). Interstitial implants are used in the treatment of breast, skin, brain, and oral cavity lesions, whereas intracavitary insertions are used primarily in treating gynecological malignancies. With both types, varying kinds of applicators are surgically placed in the tissue or cavity to be treated and the radioactive source is usually "after-loaded" when the client returns to his/her room. Another type of brachytherapy, surface brachytherapy, is accomplished by putting a radioactive source in a mold, which is then placed on or adjacent to an external body surface.

Unsealed brachytherapy can be ingested, injected, or implanted in a body part such as the bladder or the prostate. A common type of unsealed brachytherapy is iodine 131 (^{131}I), which is used in the treatment of cancer of the thyroid or Graves' disease. It is ingested orally and metabolized by the body before being concentrated in the thyroid gland in 3–5 days. Although not in common use, colloidal forms of phosphorus 32 (^{32}P) or gold 198 (^{198}Au) can be injected into the pleural or peritoneal cavity to treat effusions or ascites associated with malignant disease. Both unsealed and sealed types are frequently used adjunctively to external radiation therapy.

This care plan focuses on the adult client hospitalized for brachytherapy. The nursing care required will depend on the type of isotope used, its method of administration, and the general physiological condition of the client. Before the initiation of brachytherapy, the goals of care are to reduce fear and anxiety by educating the client regarding therapy and expected side effects. During and following the treatment, the goals of care are to maintain comfort and educate the client regarding follow-up care.

DISCHARGE CRITERIA

Prior to discharge, the client will:

- verbalize appropriate safety precautions related to a radioactive implant
- identify measures to increase comfort and prevent complications associated with vaginal irradiation
- identify common sensations that may be felt and measures to prevent complications associated with breast irradiation
- share thoughts and feelings about the diagnosis and need for radiation therapy
- state signs and symptoms to report to the health care provider
- identify community resources that can assist with adjustment to the effects of the diagnosis and its treatment
- verbalize an understanding of and a plan for adhering to recommended follow-up care including future appointments with health care provider and radiologist and medications prescribed.

NURSING DIAGNOSES

Preradiation Care
1. Knowledge deficit □ *111*

Radiation and Postradiation Care
1. Pain:
   a. muscle aches
   b. pain at or around implant site □ *114*
2. Impaired physical mobility □ *114*
3. Self-care deficit □ *115*
4. Knowledge deficit regarding follow-up care □ *115*

Preradiation Care

Use in conjunction with the Standardized Preoperative Care Plan.

1. NURSING DIAGNOSIS

Knowledge deficit regarding:

a. hospital routines associated with brachytherapy;
b. implant procedures;
c. precautions necessary to protect staff and significant others from exposure to radiation and prevent dislodgment of the radioactive source;
d. effects of the implant on usual physiological functioning.

DESIRED OUTCOMES	NURSING ACTIONS AND *SELECTED RATIONALES*

1.a. The client will verbalize an understanding of usual preradiation and postradiation care and routines.	1.a.1. Refer to Standardized Preoperative Care Plan, Nursing Diagnosis 4, actions a.1–4, for teaching related to routine preoperative and postoperative care.
	2. Provide additional information regarding care associated with the type of brachytherapy the client will be receiving:
	  a. if the client is to receive a sealed, temporary interstitial or intracavitary implant:
	    1. reinforce preoperative teaching (a general anesthetic may be used)
	    2. explain that localization x-rays will be done following insertion of tubes, needles, template, or applicators *in order to determine accuracy of placement and dosimetry*
	    3. explain the loading procedure; reassure client that it is not painful
	    4. assure client that redness and drainage around insertion sites of tubes, needles, or template are normal
	    5. explain that a minimum fluid intake of 2500 cc/day will be encouraged *to prevent fluid volume deficit and promote elimination of the byproducts of tumor breakdown*
	    6. explain the purpose of temporary isolation procedures; emphasize that these precautions are necessary only for a limited time
	    7. assure client that personal belongings will not be contaminated
	    8. explain that body fluids are not contaminated

9. explain the time and distance precautions that must be followed by all who come in contact with client particularly during the first 24–72 hours after the implant
10. explain that only essential care will be given (e.g. change of soiled linen, basic hygiene) *in order to decrease staff exposure*
11. inform client that each visitor should be limited to 30–60 minutes/day and that children and pregnant women will not be permitted to visit
12. if a perineal or vaginal implant is planned:
    a. inform client that sensations of rectal fullness, lower abdominal pressure, and low back pain may be experienced *due to pressure of applicator and vaginal packing* (vaginal packing is inserted *to separate the bladder and rectum from the radioactive source and to maintain applicator position*)
    b. instruct client in isometric exercises that should be performed at regular intervals while on bedrest
    c. explain the purpose for the thigh-high antiembolic hose or elastic wraps the client will wear while on bedrest
    d. inform client that applicator will be checked for correct position at least twice/shift *to monitor for dislodgment*
    e. explain the safety precautions that will be taken *to prevent dislodgment of the implant:*
       1. complete bedrest with head of bed slightly elevated
       2. only minimal movement will be allowed (some physicians allow client to logroll from side to side 3–4 times/day)
       3. a Foley catheter will be inserted *to reduce the need for frequent use of bedpan (the catheter also maintains bladder decompression and inhibits close contact of bladder with radioactive source)*
       4. an enema will be given and a liquid or low-residue diet may be prescribed *to cleanse the bowel and decrease the chance that the client will have a bowel movement after implant insertion;* fracture pan will be used if bowel movement is necessary
       5. no perineal care will be given unless absolutely necessary
13. if a breast implant is planned:
    a. explain that radioactivity is limited to the catheters implanted in the breast and that body fluids are not considered to be hazardous
    b. inform client that ambulation in room is encouraged *to prevent the respiratory and circulatory complications of bedrest*
14. if a brain implant is planned:
    a. reinforce physician's explanation about the procedure for implanting the radioactive source (usually 2–5 catheters are placed, depending on tumor size); and stereotactic equipment if it will be used to implant radioactive source:
       1. describe the stereotactic frame using pictures or diagrams and explain how it will be applied
       2. discuss the use of the CT scanner in conjunction with the stereotactic frame (*this is done to facilitate precise placement of the radioactive source*)
       3. explain that local anesthesia will be used during the procedure
       4. explain that while the frame is being applied, pressure from the ear bars may cause a temporary ear discomfort; emphasize that the bars will be removed once the frame is in place
       5. clarify the physician's explanation about the amount of scalp hair that will be removed for the procedure
    b. explain the safety precautions that will be followed while the radioactive source is in place (these will vary depending on the isotope used)
    c. explain that self-care will be encouraged *to minimize staff exposure to the radioactive source*

            d. arrange for a visit to the intensive care unit if client is expected
               to be there following implant insertion

      b. if the client is to receive oral ^{131}I:

         1. explain that the isotope will be mixed with water and that he/she
            should drink it through a straw (may also be given in capsule form)

         2. instruct client to notify staff if nauseated; emphasize the
            importance of not vomiting, particularly during first 4 hours after
            ingestion of the isotope *in order to retain it and prevent*
            contamination of others

         3. reinforce physician's explanation that stool, urine, sweat, saliva,
            and other body fluids will be highly contaminated for about 4 days

         4. emphasize the need to wear hospital clothing *to prevent*
            contamination of personal articles

         5. instruct client in good handwashing technique; stress the need to
            wash hands carefully, particularly after contact with urine, for 14
            days after ingestion of the isotope

         6. instruct client to flush toilet 3 times after each voiding for 14 days
            after ingestion of the isotope *in order to dilute the excreted*
            isotope

         7. assure client that body fluids are no longer contaminated once the
            isotope is metabolized and excreted

      c. if the client is to receive an intracavitary injection of colloidal ^{32}P or
        ^{198}Au:

         1. explain that there are no isolation requirements *(the isotope emits*
            beta particles and is hazardous only if the colloidal substance leaks
            from body) but that staff will wear gloves when handling dressings
            or linens in case leakage has occurred

         2. explain that he/she will be assisted to turn frequently *in order to*
            ensure equal distribution of the colloid within body cavity

         3. explain that colloidal substance is dyed so that leakage is easily
            recognized by stains on dressings or linens

      d. if the client is receiving a permanent implant of ^{125}I in a tumor or body
        part (e.g. bladder, prostate, lung, head, neck):

         1. explain that neither client nor his/her body fluids are contaminated
            because the range of radiation for ^{125}I *is only about 2 cm*

         2. caution client to notify staff immediately if a seed is found in urine
            or wound dressing

         3. inform client that time and distance precautions will be followed
            while he/she is hospitalized

      e. if client is receiving a permanent implant of ^{198}Au seeds into the
        prostate:

         1. explain that ^{198}Au seeds have a very short half-life (2.7 days) and
            safety precautions will be necessary during that time

         2. inform client that his urine will need to be filtered before being
            disposed of in the toilet *in order to monitor for seed dislodgment.*

    3. Allow adequate time for questions and clarification of information
      provided.

1.b. The client will demonstrate the ability to perform techniques designed to prevent postoperative complications.	1.b. Refer to Standardized Preoperative Care Plan, Nursing Diagnosis 4, action b, for teaching related to techniques to prevent postoperative complications.

Radiation and Postradiation Care

Use in conjunction with the Standardized Postoperative Care Plan and the Care Plan on Immobility.

1. NURSING DIAGNOSIS

Pain:

a. **muscle aches** related to prescribed activity restrictions associated with intra-cavitary and some interstitial implants;
b. **pain at or around implant site** related to:
 1. contractions of hollow organs if an intracavitary implant has been done
 2. tissue trauma associated with placement of tubes, catheters, template, needles, or applicator used to hold the radioactive source in place.

DESIRED OUTCOMES	NURSING ACTIONS AND *SELECTED RATIONALES*

1. The client will experience diminished muscle aches and pain as evidenced by:
a. verbalization of same
b. relaxed facial expression and body positioning
c. stable vital signs.
	1.a. Determine how client usually responds to pain.
	b. Assess for nonverbal signs of discomfort (e.g. wrinkled brow; clenched fists; guarding of implant site; reluctance to move; restlessness; rubbing hips, shoulders, and lower back; diaphoresis; facial pallor or flushing; change in B/P; tachycardia).
	c. Assess verbal complaints of discomfort. Ask client to be specific regarding location, severity, and type of discomfort.
	d. Assess for factors that seem to aggravate and alleviate discomfort.
	e. Implement measures *to reduce discomfort:*
	  1. support body parts with pillows if a particular body position needs to be maintained
	  2. provide or assist with nonpharmacological measures for relief of discomfort (e.g. back rub, position change as allowed, relaxation techniques, guided imagery, quiet conversation, restful environment, diversional activities), being careful to adhere to time and distance requirements
	  3. place an alternating pressure or eggcrate mattress or sheepskin on bed *to reduce discomfort associated with restricted body movement*
	  4. monitor for therapeutic and nontherapeutic effects of analgesics and muscle relaxants if administered.
	f. Consult physician if above measures fail to provide adequate relief of pain and muscle aches.

2. NURSING DIAGNOSIS

Impaired physical mobility related to:

a. prescribed activity restrictions associated with the need to maintain accurate placement of the radioactive source;
b. reluctance to move associated with pain; muscle aches; and fear of dislodging template, applicator, needles, catheters, or tubes.

DESIRED OUTCOMES	**NURSING ACTIONS AND *SELECTED RATIONALES***

2.a. The client will achieve maximum physical mobility within prescribed activity restrictions.

2.a.1. Assess for factors that impair physical mobility (e.g. prescribed activity restrictions; reluctance to move because of pain, muscle aches, and fear of dislodging radioactive implant device).
2. Implement measures *to increase mobility if allowed:*
   a. perform actions to reduce discomfort (see Radiation and Postradiation Nursing Diagnosis 1, action e)
   b. assure client that the device containing the radioactive source will not dislodge if activity restrictions are adhered to (mobility restrictions will depend on the type of applicator and/or location of the implant)
   c. instruct client in exercises that can be performed in bed without affecting implant and encourage him/her to do them frequently.
3. Encourage activity and participation in self-care activities as allowed.
4. Provide praise and encouragement for all efforts to maintain level of mobility allowed.

2.b. The client will not experience problems associated with immobility.

2.b. Refer to Care Plan on Immobility for actions to prevent problems associated with immobility if client is immobilized for longer than 48 hours.

UNIT V

□ ▬▬▬▬▬▬▬▬▬▬▬▬▬▬▬▬▬▬▬▬▬

3. NURSING DIAGNOSIS

Self-care deficit related to reluctance to move prescribed activity restrictions during the time that the radioactive source is in place.

□ ▬▬▬▬▬▬▬▬▬▬▬▬▬▬▬▬▬▬▬▬▬

DESIRED OUTCOMES	**NURSING ACTIONS AND *SELECTED RATIONALES***

3. The client will perform self-care activities within restrictions imposed by the treatment plan.

3.a. Refer to Care Plan on Immobility, Nursing Diagnosis 9, for measures related to assessment of, planning for, and meeting the client's self-care needs.
b. Reinforce that because of the time and distance precautions for the isotope, the nursing staff will assist only with necessary hygiene activities that the client is unable to perform independently.

□ ▬▬▬▬▬▬▬▬▬▬▬▬▬▬▬▬▬▬▬▬▬

4. NURSING DIAGNOSIS

Knowledge deficit regarding follow-up care.

□ ▬▬▬▬▬▬▬▬▬▬▬▬▬▬▬▬▬▬▬▬▬

DESIRED OUTCOMES	**NURSING ACTIONS AND *SELECTED RATIONALES***

4.a. The client will verbalize appropriate safety precautions related to a radioactive implant.

4.a.1. If client has received systemic ^{131}I, instruct him/her to:
   a. flush toilet 3 times after voiding *in order to dilute the excreted isotope*
   b. perform good handwashing after toileting
   c. sleep alone and avoid kissing, sexual intercourse, and prolonged physical contact particularly with children and pregnant women
   d. avoid sharing eating utensils
   e. avoid sharing towels and washcloths; launder items separately

f. drink at least 10 glasses of liquid/day *to facilitate more rapid excretion of the isotope*

g. if breastfeeding, stop until permission to resume is given by physician (*radioiodine is excreted in breast milk*).

2. Reinforce physician's instructions regarding the length of time precautions should be adhered to following systemic ^{131}I (usually a few days to 2 weeks after implant).

3. If client has had a temporary interstitial or intracavitary implant, reinforce the fact that no precautions are necessary after discharge.

4. If client has had a permanent implant, inform him/her that no particular precautions need to be observed unless a seed is excreted. If one is found, instruct client to handle it with a spoon and dispose of it according to radiologist's instructions (the seed is usually flushed down the toilet).

4.b. The client will identify measures to increase comfort and prevent complications associated with vaginal irradiation.	**4.b.1.** If client has received vaginal irradiation:
	a. instruct in correct douche technique if appropriate (betadine or vinegar douche may be ordered *to cleanse the vagina and decrease inflammation*)
	b. explain that a pink to tan vaginal discharge is normal for 7–10 days after removal of the implant
	c. instruct client to avoid using tampons and to change sanitary napkins every 4 hours
	d. reinforce physician's explanation about the possibility of vaginal stenosis occurring and ways to prevent permanent sealing of vaginal walls (e.g. intercourse 3 times/week as soon as allowed, use of vaginal dilator [obturator] for 5–10 minutes 3 times/week)
	e. if client is sexually active:
	  1. explain that intercourse can be resumed in 2–3 weeks
	  2. encourage her to try various positions for intercourse *to compensate for shortening and narrowing of the vagina* (some clients may lose the upper ⅔ of the vaginal vault)
	  3. explain that having male partner use a condom will prevent the burning sensation that may result when semen comes in contact with the fragile vaginal tissue
	  4. explain that a water-soluble lubricant can be used *to reduce discomfort if dryness associated with decreased vaginal secretions is problematic.*
	2. Allow time for questions, clarification, and demonstration of techniques.

4.c. The client will identify common sensations that may be felt and measures to prevent complications associated with breast irradiation.	**4.c.** If client has received breast irradiation:
	1. explain that minor painful sensations throughout the treatment area may occur at times *because of irritation of the pectoral muscles*; assure client that this is expected to resolve in approximately 1 year or less
	2. instruct her regarding ways *to prevent complications:*
	  a. avoid having venipunctures or blood pressure measurements taken on arm on affected side
	  b. protect treatment area by minimizing exposure of area to ultraviolet rays for at least a year and using a strong sunscreen (SPF-15)
	  c. perform range of motion exercises of affected hand and arm daily *to prevent axillary discomfort and tightening.*

4.d. The client will state signs and symptoms to report to the health care provider.	**4.d.** Instruct client to report the following: 1. unusual discharge, odor, or excessive bleeding from irradiated area 2. signs and symptoms of radiation cystitis (e.g. blood in urine, pain on urination, urinary frequency or urgency) 3. signs and symptoms of tissue fibrosis within the treatment area (e.g. BOWEL: inability to move bowels, distended abdomen, loss of appetite, alternating diarrhea and constipation; SKIN: uneven texture, changes in appearance of surface blood vessels; VAGINA: pain or difficulty with sexual intercourse) 4. increasing pain in irradiated area 5. significant, unexplained weight loss 6. excessive depression or difficulty coping 7. persistent urgency, frequency, or burning on urination and/or increased temperature after removal of a gynecological implant. (Although these symptoms are an expected response to inflammation that will occur 8–10

days after removal of the radioactive source, the health care provider should be notified if symptoms do not diminish by day 15.)

4.e. The client will identify community resources that can assist with adjustment to the effects of the diagnosis and its treatment.	**4.e.1.** Provide information about and encourage utilization of community resources that can assist the client and significant others with adjustment to effects of the diagnosis and radiation therapy (e.g. local support groups, American Cancer Society, counselors, social service agencies, Make Today Count, Hospice). **2.** Initiate a referral if indicated.

4.f. The client will verbalize an understanding of and a plan for adhering to recommended follow-up care including future appointments with health care provider and radiologist and medications prescribed.	**4.f.1.** Reinforce the importance of keeping follow-up appointments with the health care provider and radiologist.
	2. Teach the client the rationale for, side effects of, and importance of taking prescribed medications (e.g. anti-infectives).
	3. Implement measures *to improve client compliance:*
	  a. include significant others in teaching sessions if possible
	  b. encourage questions and allow time for reinforcement or clarification of information provided
	  c. provide written instructions on future appointments with health care provider and radiologist, medications prescribed, and signs and symptoms to report.

UNIT
V

■ ■

Chemotherapy

This care plan focuses on the use of cytotoxic drugs in the treatment of cancer. The drugs are used alone or with surgery and/or radiation therapy to achieve a cure or to relieve symptoms associated with advanced disease.

The goal of curative chemotherapy is to eliminate all malignant cells without causing permanent damage to normal ones. Success of the therapy depends on the duration, size, type, and location of the tumor in addition to the client's physiological condition, prior treatment with radiation and/or chemotherapy, and the status of his/her immune system.

Cytotoxic drugs are classified according to their chemical structure or their effect on the cell life cycle. Some are cell cycle nonspecific (e.g. alkylating agents, nitrosoureas, some antibiotics) and will destroy a cell regardless of its phase of replication. Others are cell cycle specific (e.g. antimetabolites, vinca alkaloids) and are only effective against the actively dividing cell.

Cytotoxic drugs are thought to kill a fixed percentage of the tumor cells with each dose because only a fraction of the tumor cell mass is in the process of dividing and therefore is sensitive to the drugs. Cells in the resting phase are less responsive to chemotherapeutic agents and are better able to repair themselves if damaged during treatment.

Clients with cancer are usually treated with a combination of drugs given simultaneously or in a particular sequence or protocol. The additive and sometimes synergistic effects that occur when drugs are used together allow an increased percentage of tumor cell kill without a concomitant increase in drug-induced toxicities. Drugs are selected for combination based on their effectiveness, action on the cell cycle, toxic effects, and nadir.

Cytotoxic drugs do not discriminate between the normal and the cancerous cell, and as a result, the client will experience certain side effects and/or toxic effects following their administration. The drugs have the greatest effect on rapidly dividing cancerous and normal cells (e.g. bone marrow, skin, hair follicles, lining of the gastrointestinal tract). Because of lack of selectivity between the cancerous and the normal cell, nursing care of the recipient of the drugs is indeed a challenge.

This care plan focuses on the adult client hospitalized for chemotherapy. The major goals of care include assessing the client for drug side effects and toxic effects; teaching the client to recognize and effectively manage the expected drug side effects and toxic effects; and assisting the client and significant others to cope with changes that may occur in body image, life style, and roles as a result of cancer and chemotherapy.

DISCHARGE CRITERIA

Prior to discharge, the client will:

- identify ways to prevent infection during periods of lowered immunity
- demonstrate the ability to correctly take an oral and axillary temperature
- demonstrate appropriate oral hygiene techniques
- identify techniques to control nausea and vomiting
- verbalize ways to improve appetite and nutritional status
- verbalize ways to manage and cope with persistent fatigue
- verbalize ways to prevent urinary calculi
- verbalize ways to prevent bleeding when platelet counts are low
- demonstrate the ability to care for a central venous catheter, a peritoneal catheter, or an implanted infusion device if in place
- verbalize an understanding of the care and precautions necessary if an Ommaya reservoir is in place
- verbalize an understanding of an implanted infusion pump and precautions necessary if one is in place
- state signs and symptoms of complications to report to the health care provider
- share thoughts and feelings about changes in body image resulting from chemotherapy
- identify community resources that can assist with home management and adjustment to the diagnosis of cancer and chemotherapy and its effects
- verbalize an understanding of and a plan for adhering to recommended follow-up care including schedule for chemotherapy, laboratory studies, and future appointments with health care provider and medications prescribed.

NURSING/COLLABORATIVE DIAGNOSES

1. Anxiety ☐ 119
2. Altered fluid and electrolyte balance:
   a. fluid volume deficit, hyponatremia, hypokalemia, and hypochloremia
   b. metabolic acidosis
   c. metabolic alkalosis ☐ 120
3. Altered nutrition: less than body requirements ☐ 121
4. Impaired swallowing ☐ 123
5A. Altered comfort: oral, pharyngeal, esophageal, and abdominal pain ☐ 124
5B. Altered comfort: perianal and vulvar pain ☐ 124
5C. Altered comfort: abdominal discomfort and distention ☐ 125
5D. Altered comfort: nausea and vomiting ☐ 126
5E. Altered comfort: pruritus ☐ 127
6. Sensory-perceptual alteration: auditory: tinnitus and/or unilateral or bilateral hearing loss ☐ 127
7. Impaired verbal communication ☐ 128
8. Impaired skin integrity:
   a. irritation or breakdown
   b. ulcerations in perianal and vulvar area ☐ 129
9. Altered oral mucous membrane:
   a. dryness
   b. stomatitis ☐ 130
10. Fatigue ☐ 131
11. Activity intolerance ☐ 132
12. Impaired physical mobility ☐ 133

13. Self-care deficit □ *133*
14. Diarrhea □ *134*
15. Constipation □ *135*
16. Sleep pattern disturbance □ *136*
17. Potential for infection □ *136*
18. Potential for trauma □ *138*
19. Potential complications:
    a. bleeding
    b. renal calculi
    c. impaired renal function
    d. hemorrhagic cystitis
    e. local tissue irritation and sloughing
    f. arrhythmias
    g. congestive heart failure (CHF)
    h. inflammation and fibrosis of lung tissue
    i. neurotoxicity (e.g. paresthesias, proprioceptive and reflex losses, muscle weakness, footdrop, visual disturbances)
    j. herpes zoster
    k. anaphylactic reaction
    l. shock
    m. peritonitis □ *139*
20. Sexual dysfunction:
    a. decreased libido
    b. dyspareunia
    c. impotence □ *146*
21. Disturbance in self-concept □ *147*
22. Ineffective individual coping □ *149*
23. Grieving □ *150*
24. Knowledge deficit regarding follow-up care □ *151*

□ ▬▬▬▬▬▬▬▬▬▬▬▬▬▬▬▬▬▬▬▬▬▬▬

1. NURSING DIAGNOSIS

Anxiety related to unfamiliar environment; lack of knowledge about chemotherapy including administration procedure, expected side effects, and impact on usual life style and roles; and diagnosis of cancer with potential for premature death.

□ ▬▬▬▬▬▬▬▬▬▬▬▬▬▬▬▬▬▬▬▬▬▬▬

DESIRED OUTCOMES	NURSING ACTIONS AND *SELECTED RATIONALES*
1. The client will experience a reduction in fear and anxiety as evidenced by: a. verbalization of feeling less anxious or fearful b. relaxed facial expression and body movements c. stable vital signs d. usual skin color	1.a. Assess client on admission for: 　1. fears, misconceptions, and level of understanding of chemotherapy and its effects on body functioning, life style, and roles 　2. perception of anticipated results or success of planned chemotherapeutic regimen 　3. feelings about past experiences with chemotherapy or other treatments for cancer 　4. availability of an adequate support system 　5. signs and symptoms of fear and anxiety (e.g. verbalization of fears and

e. verbalization of an understanding of hospital routines and drugs prescribed, expected side effects, and protocol to be followed.

concerns; tenseness; tremors; irritability; restlessness; diaphoresis; tachypnea; tachycardia; elevated blood pressure; facial tension, pallor, or flushing; noncompliance with treatment plan). Validate perceptions carefully, remembering that some behavior may be a result of physiological changes associated with the disease process.

b. Ascertain effectiveness of current coping skills.

c. Implement measures *to reduce fear and anxiety:*
1. orient to hospital environment, equipment, and routines
2. introduce staff who will be participating in his/her care; if possible, maintain consistency in staff assigned to his/her care *to provide feelings of stability and comfort with the environment*
3. assure client that staff members are nearby; respond to call signal as soon as possible
4. maintain a calm, confident manner when interacting with client
5. encourage verbalization of fear and anxiety; provide feedback
6. explain all tests to be done before the initiation of chemotherapy (e.g. blood and urine studies, chest x-ray, EKG)
7. reinforce physician's explanation about how prescribed drugs work, expected side effects and ways of effectively managing them, and potential drug toxicities
8. provide a calm, restful environment
9. instruct in relaxation techniques and encourage participation in diversional activities
10. perform actions to assist the client to cope with the diagnosis of cancer and chemotherapy and its effects (see Nursing Diagnosis 22, action d)
11. encourage significant others to project a caring, concerned attitude without obvious anxiousness
12. initiate preoperative teaching if placement of a peritoneal or central venous catheter, Ommaya reservoir, or implanted infusion device is planned
13. monitor for therapeutic and nontherapeutic effects of antianxiety agents if administered.

d. Include significant others in orientation and teaching sessions and encourage their continued support of the client.

e. Provide information based on current needs of client and significant others at a level they can understand. Encourage questions and clarification of information provided.

f. Consult physician if above actions fail to control fear and anxiety.

☐ ▉▉▉▉▉▉▉▉▉▉▉▉▉▉▉▉▉▉▉▉▉▉▉▉▉▉▉▉

2. NURSING/COLLABORATIVE DIAGNOSIS

Altered fluid and electrolyte balance:

a. **fluid volume deficit, hyponatremia, hypokalemia, and hypochloremia** related to:
1. decreased oral intake associated with nausea; anorexia; and oral, pharyngeal, and esophageal pain
2. excessive loss of fluid and electrolytes associated with persistent vomiting and diarrhea;

b. **metabolic acidosis** related to hyponatremia and persistent diarrhea associated with the effects of cytotoxic agents on the gastrointestinal mucosa;

c. **metabolic alkalosis** related to persistent vomiting, hypokalemia, and hypochloremia.

☐ ▉▉▉▉▉▉▉▉▉▉▉▉▉▉▉▉▉▉▉▉▉▉▉▉▉▉▉▉

DESIRED OUTCOMES	NURSING ACTIONS AND *SELECTED RATIONALES*
2.a. The client will maintain fluid and electrolyte balance as evidenced by:	2.a.1. Assess for and report signs and symptoms of: a. fluid volume deficit: 1. decreased skin turgor, dry mucous membranes, thirst

1. normal skin turgor
2. moist mucous membranes
3. stable weight
4. B/P and pulse within normal range for client and stable with position change
5. balanced intake and output
6. urine specific gravity between 1.010 and 1.030
7. no evidence of confusion, irritability, lethargy, excessive thirst, ileus, cardiac arrhythmias, muscle weakness
8. normal serum osmolality and electrolytes.

2. weight loss greater than 0.5 kg/day
3. low B/P and/or decline in systolic B/P of at least 15 mm Hg with concurrent rise in pulse when client sits up
4. weak, rapid pulse
5. output less than intake with urine specific gravity higher than 1.030 (reflects an actual rather than potential fluid volume deficit)
  b. hyponatremia (e.g. nausea and vomiting, abdominal cramps, weakness, twitching, lethargy, confusion, seizures)
  c. hypokalemia (e.g. irregular pulse, muscle weakness and cramping, paresthesias, nausea and vomiting, hypoactive or absent bowel sounds, drowsiness)
  d. hypochloremia (e.g. twitching, tetany, depressed respirations).
2. Monitor serum osmolality and electrolyte results. Report abnormal values.
3. Implement measures *to prevent and treat fluid and electrolyte imbalances:*
  a. perform actions to control diarrhea (see Nursing Diagnosis 14, action d)
  b. perform actions to reduce vomiting (see Nursing Diagnosis 5.D, action 2)
  c. perform actions to improve oral intake (see Nursing Diagnosis 3, action f.1)
  d. monitor for therapeutic and nontherapeutic effects of fluid and electrolyte replacements if administered
  e. maintain a fluid intake of at least 2500 cc/day unless contraindicated
  f. assist client to select foods/fluids high in potassium (e.g. bananas, potatoes, raisins, figs, apricots, dates, Gatorade) and sodium (e.g. cured meats, processed cheese, soups, catsup, pickles, canned vegetables, bouillon) if serum levels of sodium and potassium are low.
4. Consult physician if signs and symptoms of fluid and electrolyte imbalances persist or worsen.

2.b. The client will maintain acid-base balance as evidenced by:
1. usual mental status
2. unlabored respirations at 16–20/minute
3. absence of dizziness, confusion, headache, nausea, vomiting, paresthesias, muscle twitching, seizure activity
4. blood gases within normal range.

2.b.1. Assess for and report signs and symptoms of:
  a. metabolic acidosis (e.g. drowsiness; disorientation; stupor; rapid, deep respirations; headache; nausea; vomiting; low pH and CO_2 content and negative base excess)
  b. metabolic alkalosis (e.g. dizziness; confusion; bradypnea; tingling of fingers, toes, and circumoral area; muscle twitching; seizures; elevated pH and CO_2 content and a positive base excess).
2. Implement measures *to prevent or treat metabolic acidosis:*
  a. perform actions to control diarrhea (see Nursing Diagnosis 14, action d)
  b. monitor for therapeutic and nontherapeutic effects of sodium bicarbonate if administered (reserved for use in severe acidosis when pH is less than 7.1)
  c. perform actions to maintain serum sodium within normal range (see action a.3 in this diagnosis).
3. Implement measures *to prevent or treat metabolic alkalosis:*
  a. perform actions to reduce vomiting (see Nursing Diagnosis 5.D, action 2)
  b. perform actions to maintain serum potassium and chloride within normal range (see action a.3 in this diagnosis).
4. Consult physician if signs and symptoms of acid-base imbalance persist or worsen.

□ ▬▬▬▬▬▬▬▬▬▬▬▬▬▬▬▬▬▬▬▬▬▬▬▬

3. NURSING DIAGNOSIS

Altered nutrition: less than body requirements related to:*

a. decreased oral intake associated with:
  1. dysphagia and oral, pharyngeal, and esophageal pain resulting from mucositis associated with effects of cytotoxic drugs on the gastrointestinal mucosa
  2. anorexia resulting from:
    a. depression, fear, and anxiety

---

* Some of the etiologic factors presented here are currently under investigation.

   b. fatigue and discomfort
   c. taste alteration associated with:
      1. change in the sense of smell and the threshold for bitter, sweet, sour, and salt taste (particularly red meat, coffee, tea, tomatoes, and chocolate) related to the release of tumor byproducts into the bloodstream
      2. zinc, copper, nickel, niacin, and vitamin A deficiency and increased serum levels of calcium and lactate resulting from the disease process
   d. alteration in the metabolism of proteins, fats, and carbohydrates
   e. early satiety associated with abdominal distention (if client receiving peritoneal chemotherapy) and direct stimulation of the satiety center by anorexigenic factors (e.g. peptides) secreted by tumor cells
   f. increased concentration of neurotransmitters in the brain and/or derangements in the serotoninergic system associated with the disease process
3. nausea;
b. loss of nutrients associated with persistent vomiting;
c. malabsorption associated with loss of absorptive surface of the intestinal mucosa resulting from mucositis;
d. elevated metabolic rate associated with an increased and continuous energy utilization by rapidly proliferating malignant cells;
e. utilization of available nutrients by the malignant cells rather than the host;
f. failure of feeding center to induce a sufficient increase in the intake of food to match metabolic needs;
g. inefficient and accelerated metabolism of proteins, fats, and carbohydrates associated with the disease process.

DESIRED OUTCOMES	NURSING ACTIONS AND *SELECTED RATIONALES*

3. The client will maintain an adequate nutritional status as evidenced by:
   a. weight within normal range for client's age, height, and build
   b. normal BUN and serum albumin, protein, Hct., Hgb., B_{12}, and cholesterol levels
   c. triceps skinfold measurements within normal range
   d. usual strength and activity tolerance
   e. healthy oral mucous membrane.

3.a. Assess the client for signs and symptoms of malnutrition:
   1. weight below normal for client's age, height, and build
   2. abnormal BUN and low serum albumin, protein, Hct., Hgb., B_{12}, and cholesterol levels
   3. triceps skinfold measurement less than normal for build
   4. weakness and fatigue
   5. stomatitis.
b. Monitor for and report:
   1. declining zinc, copper, nickel, and niacin levels
   2. increasing calcium and lactate levels.
c. Reassess nutritional status on a regular basis and report decline.
d. Monitor percentage of meals eaten.
e. Assess the client to determine causes of inadequate intake (e.g. fatigue, nausea, taste distortion, stomatitis).
f. Implement measures *to maintain an adequate nutritional status:*
   1. perform actions *to improve oral intake:*
      a. implement measures to reduce nausea and vomiting (see Nursing Diagnosis 5.D, action 2)
      b. implement measures to reduce discomfort associated with mucositis of gastrointestinal tract and abdominal distention (see Nursing Diagnoses 5.A, action 2 and 5.C, action 3)
      c. implement measures *to compensate for taste alteration:*
         1. encourage the client to select fish, cold chicken, eggs, and cheese as protein sources if beef or pork tastes bitter or rancid
         2. provide meat for breakfast if aversion to meat tends to increase as day progresses
         3. add extra sweeteners to foods if acceptable to client
         4. experiment with different flavorings, seasonings, and textures
         5. serve food warm *to stimulate sense of smell*
         6. provide sour, hard candy or gum before meals *to stimulate salivation*

7. monitor for therapeutic and nontherapeutic effects of trace elements if administered *to correct abnormalities of taste*
d. implement measures to improve client's ability to swallow (see Nursing Diagnosis 4, action b)
e. avoid serving liquids with meals *to minimize early satiety and nausea*
f. serve small portions of nutritious foods/fluids that are appealing to client
g. provide a clean, relaxed, pleasant atmosphere
h. encourage significant others to bring in client's favorite foods and eat with him/her *to make eating more of a familiar social experience*
i. encourage a rest period before meals *to minimize fatigue*
j. allow adequate time for meals; reheat food if necessary
k. increase activity as tolerated *(activity stimulates appetite)*
l. implement measures to assist client to progress through the grieving process (see Nursing Diagnosis 23, action d) and to cope effectively (see Nursing Diagnosis 22, action d)
m. obtain a dietary consult if necessary to assist the client in selecting foods/fluids that meet nutritional needs (high-calorie, high-protein) as well as preferences
2. ensure that meals are well balanced and high in essential nutrients
3. provide snacks of sweetened, high-calorie, high-protein foods (e.g. milk shakes, puddings, or eggnog made with cream or powdered milk reconstituted with whole milk)
4. monitor for therapeutic and nontherapeutic effects of vitamins, minerals, and hematinics if administered.
g. Perform a 72-hour calorie count if nutritional status declines or fails to improve.
h. Consult physician regarding alternative methods of providing nutrition (e.g. parenteral nutrition, tube feedings) if client does not consume enough food or fluids to meet nutritional needs.

□ ▅▅▅▅▅▅▅▅▅▅▅▅▅▅▅▅▅▅▅▅▅▅▅▅▅

4. NURSING DIAGNOSIS

Impaired swallowing related to:

a. oral, pharyngeal, and esophageal pain associated with mucositis resulting from the effects of cytotoxic drugs;
b. dry mouth and viscous oral secretions associated with the changes in the quantity and quality of saliva resulting from stomatitis and decreased oral intake.

□ ▅▅▅▅▅▅▅▅▅▅▅▅▅▅▅▅▅▅▅▅▅▅▅▅▅

DESIRED OUTCOMES	NURSING ACTIONS AND *SELECTED RATIONALES*
4. The client will experience an improvement in swallowing as evidenced by: a. verbalization of same b. absence of coughing or choking when eating or drinking.	4.a. Assess for and report signs and symptoms of impaired swallowing (e.g. coughing or choking when eating or drinking, stasis of food in oral cavity). b. Implement measures *to improve ability to swallow:* 1. perform actions to reduce discomfort associated with mucositis of the gastrointestinal tract (see Nursing Diagnosis 5.A, action 2) 2. assist client to select foods that are easily chewed and swallowed (e.g. custard, flavored gelatin, cottage cheese, ground meat) 3. avoid serving foods that are sticky (e.g. peanut butter, soft bread, bananas) 4. serve foods/fluids that are hot or cold instead of room temperature *(the more extreme temperatures stimulate the sensory receptors and swallowing reflex)* 5. moisten dry foods with gravy or sauces (e.g. sour cream, salad dressing) 6. perform actions *to stimulate salivation:* a. serve foods that are visually pleasing

UNIT V

      b. provide oral care before meals

      c. place a piece of lemon or sour pickle on plate

      d. provide sour, hard candy for client to suck just before meals unless contraindicated

   7. perform actions *to reduce and/or liquefy viscous oral secretions:*

      a. encourage a fluid intake of 2500 cc/day unless contraindicated

      b. encourage client to avoid milk and milk products (unless boiled) and chocolate *(when combined with saliva, these produce very thick secretions).*

   c. Consult physician if swallowing difficulties persist or worsen.

☐ ▐██▌

5.A. NURSING DIAGNOSIS

Altered comfort:* oral, pharyngeal, esophageal, and abdominal pain related to mucositis associated with effects of cytotoxic drugs on the rapidly dividing cells of gastrointestinal (GI) mucosa.

* In this care plan, the nursing diagnosis "pain" is included under the diagnostic·label of altered comfort.

☐ ▐██▌

DESIRED OUTCOMES	NURSING ACTIONS AND *SELECTED RATIONALES*

5.A. The client will experience diminished GI discomfort as evidenced by:
1. verbalization of pain relief
2. less difficulty swallowing.

5.A.1. Assess client for complaints of oral, pharyngeal, esophageal, and abdominal pain; inability to tolerate spicy, acidic, or hot foods/fluids; and difficulty swallowing.

   2. Implement measures *to reduce GI discomfort:*

      a. perform actions to prevent or reduce the severity of stomatitis (see Nursing Diagnosis 9, actions d and e)

      b. instruct client to avoid substances that might further irritate the gastrointestinal mucosa (e.g. alcoholic beverages; extremely hot, spicy, or acidic foods/fluids; smoke; dry or hard foods; raw fruits and vegetables)

      c. offer cool, soothing liquids such as nonacidic juices, ices, and ice cream

      d. instruct client to gargle with a saline solution every 2 hours *to soothe the mucous membrane*

      e. monitor for therapeutic and nontherapeutic effects of topical anesthetics, oral protective pastes, topical or systemic analgesics, and antacids if administered.

   3. Consult physician if discomfort persists or worsens.

☐ ▐██▌

5.B. NURSING DIAGNOSIS

Altered comfort:* perianal and vulvar pain related to inflammation and ulceration of the mucous membranes associated with the effects of cytotoxic drugs on tissues composed of rapidly dividing cells.

* In this care plan, the nursing diagnosis "pain" is included under the diagnostic label of altered comfort.

☐ ▐██▌

DESIRED OUTCOMES	**NURSING ACTIONS AND *SELECTED RATIONALES***

5.B. The client will experience diminished perianal and vulvar pain as evidenced by:
 1. verbalization of pain relief
 2. relaxed facial expression and body positioning
 3. increased participation in activities
 4. stable vital signs.

5.B.1. Determine how the client usually responds to pain.
 2. Assess for nonverbal signs of pain (e.g. wrinkled brow, clenched fists, reluctance to sit or move, awkward ambulation, restlessness, diaphoresis, facial pallor or flushing, change in B/P, tachycardia).
 3. Assess verbal complaints of pain. Ask client to be specific about location, severity, and type of pain.
 4. Assess for factors that seem to aggravate and alleviate pain.
 5. Assess perianal and vulvar area every shift for signs of inflammation and ulceration.
 6. Implement measures *to reduce perianal and vulvar pain:*
　a. apply warm, moist compresses and/or assist with sitz baths after bowel movements and whenever necessary
　b. expose perineal area to air for 30 minutes each shift *to facilitate healing*
　c. consult physician about the application of soothing ointments and creams to perianal and/or vulvar area
　d. avoid use of rectal thermometer or suppositories
　e. encourage client to wear cotton underwear
　f. provide or assist with nonpharmacological measures for pain relief (e.g. position change, relaxation techniques, guided imagery, diversional activities)
　g. monitor for therapeutic and nontherapeutic effects of analgesics and topical anesthetics if administered.
 7. Consult physician if above measures fail to provide adequate relief of perianal and vulvar pain.

□ ▬▬▬▬▬▬▬▬▬▬▬▬▬▬▬▬▬▬▬

5.C. NURSING DIAGNOSIS

Altered comfort: abdominal discomfort and distention related to peritoneal irritation associated with presence of peritoneal catheter and inadequate drainage of dialysate solution used for peritoneal chemotherapy (inadequate drainage may occur as a result of the formation of a fibrous sheath around catheter tip, kinking of the catheter, and/or obstruction of fluid flow due to adhesions).

□ ▬▬▬▬▬▬▬▬▬▬▬▬▬▬▬▬▬▬▬

DESIRED OUTCOMES	**NURSING ACTIONS AND *SELECTED RATIONALES***

5.C. The client will experience relief of abdominal discomfort and distention as evidenced by:
 1. verbalization of decreased abdominal fullness and discomfort
 2. relaxed facial expression and body positioning
 3. decrease in abdominal girth.

5.C.1. Assess for signs and symptoms of abdominal discomfort and distention (e.g. complaints of persistent feeling of abdominal fullness or pain, clutching and guarding of abdomen, restlessness, dyspnea, reluctance to move, increased abdominal girth).
 2. Assess for adequate drainage of dialysate solution. Report a significant imbalance between intake and output.
 3. Implement measures *to reduce abdominal discomfort and distention:*
　a. use the minimum volume of solution recommended to infuse the cytotoxic agent
　b. encourage and assist client with frequent position changes *to permit even distribution of fluid within the peritoneal cavity*
　c. perform actions *to facilitate drainage of the dialysate solution:*
　　1. keep exit tubing free of kinks
　　2. keep drainage catheter and collection device below access point
　　3. if inadequate volume of dialysate solution returns:
　　　a. reposition client *to redistribute fluid within the peritoneal cavity*

    b. instruct client to perform a Valsalva maneuver *to increase intra-abdominal pressure and promote dialysate drainage*

    c. irrigate peritoneal catheter with 10 cc normal saline *to clear catheter and move the fibrous sheath away from the catheter tip*

    d. aspirate remaining solution if possible

  d. monitor for therapeutic and nontherapeutic effects of analgesics if administered.

4. Assure client that fluid remaining in the peritoneal cavity will be absorbed in 7–10 days.

5. Consult physician if abdominal distention and discomfort persist or worsen.

5.D. NURSING DIAGNOSIS

Altered comfort: nausea and vomiting related to stimulation of the vomiting center associated with:

1. direct stimulation and stimulation of the chemoreceptor trigger zone resulting from cytotoxic drugs and absorption of toxic waste products from cellular destruction;

2. vagal and/or sympathetic stimulation resulting from visceral irritation associated with inflammation of the gastrointestinal mucosa due to effects of cytotoxic drugs on rapidly dividing epithelial cells;

3. cortical stimulation due to discomfort and stress.

DESIRED OUTCOMES	NURSING ACTIONS AND *SELECTED RATIONALES*

5.D. The client will experience a reduction in nausea and vomiting as evidenced by:
1. verbalization of decreased nausea
2. reduction in the number of episodes of vomiting.
	5.D.1. Assess client to determine factors that contribute to nausea and vomiting (e.g. administration of cytotoxic drugs, fear, anxiety).
	2. Implement measures *to reduce nausea and vomiting:*
	  a. initiate antiemetic drug therapy 4 to 24 hours before administering chemotherapy and give routinely for at least 24 hours after cessation of therapy
	  b. administer intravenous cytotoxic drugs slowly unless contraindicated *to decrease stimulation of the vomiting center*
	  c. if feasible, administer the cytotoxic drugs at night *so client will sleep and experience less nausea*
	  d. display a positive attitude about nausea and vomiting not occurring (*not every client experiences nausea and vomiting every time*)
	  e. provide sour, hard candy for client to suck if he/she can taste the drug
	  f. eliminate noxious sights and smells from the environment (*noxious stimuli cause cortical stimulation of the vomiting center*)
	  g. encourage client to take deep, slow breaths when nauseated
	  h. provide oral hygiene after each emesis and before meals
	  i. provide small, frequent, low-fat meals (*fat delays gastric emptying*) rather than 3 large ones
	  j. instruct client to ingest foods and fluids slowly
	  k. instruct client to avoid foods/fluids that irritate the gastric mucosa (e.g. spicy foods; citrus fruits or juices; caffeine-containing items such as chocolate, coffee, tea, and colas)
	  l. encourage client to eat dry foods (e.g. toast, crackers) and avoid drinking liquids with meals if nauseated
	  m. provide carbonated beverages for client to sip if nauseated
	  n. instruct client to rest with head of bed elevated after eating
	  o. encourage client to change positions slowly (*movement stimulates the chemoreceptor trigger zone*)

p. administer antiemetics or gastrointestinal stimulants (e.g. metoclopramide) on a routine schedule before meals as ordered
q. perform actions to reduce fear and anxiety (see Nursing Diagnosis 1, action c)
r. perform actions to reduce discomfort (see Nursing Diagnoses 5.A, action 2; 5.B, action 6; and 5.C, action 3).
3. Consult physician if above measures fail to control nausea and vomiting.

□ ▉▉▉▉▉▉▉▉▉▉▉▉▉▉▉▉▉▉▉▉▉▉▉▉▉▉▉▉

5.E. NURSING DIAGNOSIS

Altered comfort: pruritus related to:

1. accumulation of bile salts under the skin associated with bile flow obstruction resulting from effects of cytotoxic drugs on hepatic function;
2. dry skin associated with the effects of cytotoxic drugs on sebaceous and sweat glands.

□ ▉▉▉▉▉▉▉▉▉▉▉▉▉▉▉▉▉▉▉▉▉▉▉▉▉▉▉▉

DESIRED OUTCOMES	NURSING ACTIONS AND *SELECTED RATIONALES*

5.E. The client will experience relief of pruritus as evidenced by:
1. verbalization of same
2. no scratching or rubbing of skin.
	5.E.1. Assess pruritus including onset, characteristics, location, factors that aggravate or alleviate it, and client tolerance.
	2. Instruct client in and/or implement measures *to relieve pruritus:*
	  a. perform actions *to promote capillary constriction:*
	    1. apply cool, moist compresses to pruritic areas
	    2. maintain a cool environment
	  b. apply emollients to skin *to help alleviate dryness*
	  c. add emollients, cornstarch, baking soda, or oatmeal to bath water
	  d. use tepid water and mild soaps for bathing
	  e. pat skin dry, making sure to dry thoroughly
	  f. encourage participation in diversional activity
	  g. utilize relaxation techniques
	  h. utilize cutaneous stimulation techniques (e.g. pressure, massage, vibration, stroking with a soft brush) at the sites of itching or acupressure points
	  i. encourage client to wear loose cotton garments.
	3. Monitor for therapeutic and nontherapeutic effects of antihistamines and antipruritic lotions if administered.
	4. Consult physician if above measures fail to alleviate pruritus or if the skin becomes excoriated.

□ ▉▉▉▉▉▉▉▉▉▉▉▉▉▉▉▉▉▉▉▉▉▉▉▉▉▉▉▉

6. NURSING DIAGNOSIS

Sensory-perceptual alteration: auditory: tinnitus and/or unilateral or bilateral hearing loss (usually high-frequency range) related to loss of hair cells in the organ of Corti associated with use of cytotoxic drugs (e.g. cisplatin, nitrogen mustard).

□ ▉▉▉▉▉▉▉▉▉▉▉▉▉▉▉▉▉▉▉▉▉▉▉▉▉▉▉▉

DESIRED OUTCOMES	NURSING ACTIONS AND *SELECTED RATIONALES*

6. The client will maintain usual hearing as evidenced by:
   a. verbalization of same
   b. absence of tinnitus
   c. appropriate responses.

6.a. Assess client's ability to hear by:
   1. observing for cues indicative of decreased hearing ability (e.g. speaking loudly, staring at other person's lips during conversation, moving closer to others when they speak, acts of frustration, nodding yes with subsequent inappropriate responses)
   2. noting client's verbal complaints of not being able to hear or understand what others are saying.
   b. Instruct client to report tinnitus immediately. Reinforce that auditory damage is usually reversible if the cytotoxic drugs are discontinued.
   c. Be particularly alert for auditory changes if other ototoxic drugs (e.g. furosemide, gentamicin, neomycin) are given concurrently with cytotoxic drugs.
   d. Instruct client to listen to music with earphones or to utilize a radio for "white noise" if tinnitus is problematic.
   e. Implement measures *to facilitate communication if hearing loss occurs:*
      1. provide adequate lighting in room *so client can read lips*
      2. reduce environmental noise
      3. speak slightly louder and more slowly; avoid lowering voice at end of sentences
      4. use simple sentences
      5. avoid overenunciation of words
      6. face client while speaking
      7. avoid chewing gum or eating while talking to client
      8. rephrase sentences when client does not understand
      9. employ related nonverbal cues such as facial expressions or pointing when appropriate
      10. use alternative forms of communication (e.g. flash cards, paper and pencil, magic slate) if indicated
      11. respond to client's call signal in person rather than over intercommunication system.
   f. Instruct significant others regarding communication techniques effective with client.
   g. Reinforce physician's explanation about permanency of tinnitus and hearing loss.
   h. Consult physician if hearing impairment or tinnitus worsens.

☐ ▬▬▬▬▬▬▬▬▬▬▬▬▬▬▬▬▬▬▬▬▬▬▬▬

7. NURSING DIAGNOSIS

Impaired verbal communication related to:

a. dry mouth and accumulation of secretions associated with changes in the quality and quantity of saliva;
b. discomfort associated with stomatitis.

☐ ▬▬▬▬▬▬▬▬▬▬▬▬▬▬▬▬▬▬▬▬▬▬▬▬

DESIRED OUTCOMES	NURSING ACTIONS AND *SELECTED RATIONALES*

7. The client will communicate needs and desires effectively.

7.a. Assess for factors that may impair verbal communication (e.g. painful lesions in or around mouth; dry mouth; thick, tenacious saliva).
   b. Implement measures *to facilitate communication:*
      1. perform actions to reduce the severity of stomatitis and relieve oral dryness (see Nursing Diagnosis 9, actions d and e)
      2. remove tenacious secretions using gentle suction

3. maintain a patient, calm approach; avoid interrupting client and allow ample time for communication
4. maintain a quiet environment *so that client does not have to raise voice to be heard*
5. ask questions that require short answers or nod of head
6. provide materials necessary for communication (e.g. magic slate, pad and pencil, flash cards)
7. ensure that intravenous therapy does not interfere with client's ability to write
8. answer call signal promptly and in person rather than using intercommunication system
9. make frequent rounds *to ascertain needs*
10. if client is frustrated or fatigued, try to anticipate needs *in order to minimize the necessity of verbal communication.*
  c. Reassure client that verbal impairment is temporary.
  d. Inform significant others and health care personnel of approaches being used to maximize the client's ability to communicate.

8. NURSING DIAGNOSIS

Impaired skin integrity:

a. **irritation or breakdown** related to:
  1. continued exposure to irritants associated with persistent diarrhea
  2. excessive scratching associated with pruritus
  3. prolonged pressure on tissues associated with decreased mobility
  4. increased skin fragility associated with malnutrition and tissue hypoxia resulting from anemia
  5. dry skin associated with effects of cytotoxic drugs on sebaceous and sweat glands;
b. **ulcerations in perianal and vulvar area** related to cytotoxic drug effects on rapidly dividing cells of the mucous membranes.

DESIRED OUTCOMES	NURSING ACTIONS AND *SELECTED RATIONALES*

8. The client will maintain skin integrity as evidenced by:
  a. absence of redness and irritation
  b. no skin breakdown.
	8.a. Inspect the skin (especially bone prominences, dependent and pruritic areas, and perineum) for pallor, redness, and breakdown.
	  b. Implement measures *to maintain skin integrity:*
	    1. perform actions *to prevent skin breakdown due to decreased mobility:*
	      a. turn client and gently massage over bone prominences and around reddened areas at least every 2 hours
	      b. lift and move client carefully using a turn sheet and adequate assistance *to prevent the linen from shearing skin*
	      c. instruct or assist client to shift weight every 30 minutes
	      d. if fade time (length of time it takes for reddened area to fade after pressure is removed) is greater than 15 minutes, increase frequency of position changes
	      e. keep skin clean and dry
	      f. keep bed linens wrinkle-free
	      g. provide alternating pressure or eggcrate mattress, flotation pad, sheepskin, and elbow and heel protectors if indicated
	      h. increase activity as tolerated

2. perform actions *to prevent drying of the skin:*
   a. avoid use of harsh soaps and hot water
   b. apply skin moisturizers or emollient creams to skin at least once a day
3. perform actions *to decrease skin irritation and prevent breakdown resulting from diarrhea:*
   a. implement measures to control diarrhea (see Nursing Diagnosis 14, action d)
   b. assist client to thoroughly cleanse and dry perineal area after each bowel movement; apply a protective ointment or cream (e.g. Sween cream, Desitin, Karaya gel, A & D ointment, Vaseline)
   c. use soft tissue to cleanse perianal area
   d. apply a perianal pouch if diarrhea is a persistent problem
   e. avoid direct contact of skin with Chux (e.g. place turn sheet or bed pad over Chux)
4. perform actions *to prevent skin breakdown associated with scratching:*
   a. implement measures to relieve pruritus (see Nursing Diagnosis 5.E, actions 2 and 3)
   b. keep nails trimmed and/or apply mittens if necessary
   c. instruct client to apply firm pressure to pruritic areas instead of scratching
5. maintain an optimal nutritional status (see Nursing Diagnosis 3, action f).
c. If skin breakdown occurs:
1. notify physician
2. continue with above measures to prevent further irritation and breakdown
3. perform meticulous decubitus care as ordered or per standard hospital policy
4. monitor client closely and report signs and symptoms of infection (e.g. elevated temperature; redness, warmth, and edema around area of breakdown; unusual drainage from site).

☐ ▬▬▬▬▬▬▬▬▬▬▬▬▬▬▬▬▬▬▬▬▬▬▬▬▬▬

9. NURSING DIAGNOSIS

Altered oral mucous membrane:

a. **dryness** related to fluid volume deficit and decreased salivary flow associated with a reduction in oral intake and stomatitis;
b. **stomatitis** related to malnutrition, fluid volume deficit, poor oral hygiene, and disruption in the normal renewal process of rapidly dividing mucosal epithelial cells associated with use of cytotoxic drugs.

☐ ▬▬▬▬▬▬▬▬▬▬▬▬▬▬▬▬▬▬▬▬▬▬▬▬▬▬

DESIRED OUTCOMES	NURSING ACTIONS AND *SELECTED RATIONALES*

9. The client will maintain a healthy oral cavity as evidenced by:
a. absence of inflammation and ulcerations
b. pink, moist, intact mucosa
c. absence of oral dryness or burning
d. ability to swallow without discomfort
e. usual consistency of saliva.
	9.a. Assess client every shift for dryness of the oral mucosa.
	b. Assess client for and report signs and symptoms of stomatitis (e.g. inflamed and/or ulcerated oral mucosa, leukoplakia, complaints of oral dryness and burning, changes in quality of voice, dysphagia, viscous saliva).
	c. Obtain cultures from suspicious oral lesions as ordered. Report positive results.
	d. Implement measures *to prevent or reduce the severity of stomatitis and relieve dryness of the oral mucous membrane:*
	  1. reinforce importance of and assist client with oral hygiene after meals and snacks
	  2. have client rinse mouth frequently with warm saline or baking soda and water
	  3. instruct client to avoid products such as lemon-glycerin swabs and

commercial mouthwashes containing alcohol (*these have a drying or irritating effect on oral mucous membrane*)
4. encourage client to breathe through nose *in order to reduce mouth dryness*
5. if stomatitis is not severe, encourage client to use artificial saliva (e.g. Moi-stir, Salivart, Xero-Lube) *to lubricate the mucous membrane*
6. encourage a fluid intake of at least 2500 cc/day unless contraindicated
7. encourage client not to smoke (*smoking irritates and dries the mucosa*)
8. instruct client to avoid substances that might further irritate the oral mucosa (e.g. extremely hot, spicy, or acidic foods/fluids)
9. lubricate client's lips with Vaseline, K-Y jelly, ChapStick, Blistex, or mineral oil when oral care is given
10. use a soft bristle brush or low-pressure power spray for oral care
11. maintain an optimal nutritional status (see Nursing Diagnosis 3, action f)
12. consult physician regarding an order for an antifungal or antibacterial agent.
  e. If stomatitis is not controlled:
    1. increase frequency of oral hygiene
    2. if client has dentures, remove and replace only for meals.
  f. Monitor for therapeutic and nontherapeutic effects of topical anesthetics, oral protective pastes, and topical or systemic analgesics if administered.
  g. Consult physician if signs and symptoms of stomatitis persist or worsen.

10. NURSING DIAGNOSIS

Fatigue related to:

a. accumulation of cellular waste products associated with rapid lysis of cancerous and normal cells exposed to cytotoxic drugs;
b. inability to rest and sleep;
c. anxiety and depression associated with the diagnosis, the treatment regimen and its effects, the need to alter usual activities, and the inability to fulfill usual roles;
d. increased energy expenditure associated with an increase in the basal metabolic rate resulting from continuous, active tumor growth.

DESIRED OUTCOMES	NURSING ACTIONS *AND SELECTED RATIONALES*

10. The client will experience a reduction in fatigue as evidenced by:
  a. verbalization of feelings of increased energy
  b. increased interest in surroundings and ability to concentrate
  c. decreased emotional lability.
	10.a. Assess for signs and symptoms of fatigue (e.g. verbalization of continuous, overwhelming lack of energy; lack of interest in surroundings; decreased ability to concentrate; increased emotional lability).
	  b. Inform client that a feeling of persistent fatigue is expected as a result of the disease itself and as a side effect of chemotherapy.
	  c. Encourage client to view fatigue as a protective mechanism rather than a problematic limitation *in order to enable him/her to feel a sense of control over the situation.*
	  d. Assist client to identify personal patterns of fatigue (e.g. time of day, after certain activities) and to plan activities so that times of greatest fatigue are avoided.
	  e. Implement measures *to reduce fatigue:*
	    1. perform actions *to promote rest:*
	      a. schedule several short rest periods during the day
	      b. minimize environmental activity and noise
	      c. schedule nursing care and diagnostic procedures to allow periods of uninterrupted rest
	      d. limit the number of visitors and their length of stay
	      e. assist client with self-care activities as needed

UNIT V

      f. keep needed supplies and personal articles within easy reach

      g. perform actions to reduce fear and anxiety (see Nursing Diagnosis 1, action c)

      h. perform actions to promote sleep (see Nursing Diagnosis 16, action c)

      i. perform actions to reduce discomfort (see Nursing Diagnoses 5.A, action 2; 5.B, action 6; 5.C, action 3; 5.D, action 2; and 5.E, actions 2 and 3)

      j. perform actions to control diarrhea (see Nursing Diagnosis 14, action d)

  2. instruct client in energy-saving techniques (e.g. using shower chair when showering, sitting to brush teeth or comb hair)

  3. keep room temperature below 75°F and instruct client to avoid using hot water for showers and baths (*increased body temperature increases the basal metabolic rate*)

  4. perform actions to maintain an adequate nutritional status (see Nursing Diagnosis 3, action f)

  5. encourage client to maintain a fluid intake of at least 2500 cc/day *to promote elimination of the byproducts of cellular breakdown*

  6. perform actions to facilitate client's psychological adjustment to the diagnosis of cancer and the treatment regimen and its effects (see Nursing Diagnoses 21, actions d–q; 22, action d; and 23, action d).

f. Consult physician if signs and symptoms of fatigue worsen.

11. NURSING DIAGNOSIS

Activity intolerance related to:

a. malnutrition;

b. tissue hypoxia associated with anemia resulting from chemotherapy-induced bone marrow suppression and nutritional deficits;

c. inability to rest and sleep associated with discomfort, diarrhea, and prolonged physiological and psychological stress.

DESIRED OUTCOMES	NURSING ACTIONS AND *SELECTED RATIONALES*
11. The client will demonstrate an increased tolerance for activity as evidenced by: a. verbalization of feeling less fatigued and weak b. ability to perform activities of daily living without exertional dyspnea, chest pain, diaphoresis, dizziness, or a significant change in vital signs.	11.a. Assess for signs and symptoms of activity intolerance: 1. statements of fatigue and weakness 2. exertional dyspnea, chest pain, diaphoresis, or dizziness 3. decrease in pulse rate or an increase in rate of 20 beats/minute above resting rate 4. pulse rate not returning to preactivity level within 5 minutes after stopping activity 5. decreased blood pressure or an increase in diastolic pressure of 15 mm Hg with activity. b. Implement measures *to improve activity tolerance:* 1. perform actions to promote rest (see Nursing Diagnosis 10, action e.1) 2. perform actions to maintain an adequate nutritional status (see Nursing Diagnosis 3, action f) 3. monitor for therapeutic and nontherapeutic effects of whole blood or packed red cells if administered 4. increase client's activity gradually as tolerated. c. Instruct client to: 1. report a decreased tolerance for activity 2. stop any activity that causes chest pain, shortness of breath, dizziness, or extreme fatigue or weakness. d. Consult physician if signs and symptoms of activity intolerance persist or worsen.

12. NURSING DIAGNOSIS

Impaired physical mobility related to:

a. sensory and motor deficits associated with interference with normal nerve conduction patterns resulting from fluid and electrolyte imbalances and administration of some cytotoxic drugs (e.g. vinca alkaloids, cisplatin);
b. discomfort associated with the disease process and/or side effects of cytotoxic drugs;
c. fatigue, weakness;
d. reluctance to move associated with fear of falls.

DESIRED OUTCOMES	NURSING ACTIONS AND *SELECTED RATIONALES*
12.a. The client will maintain an optimal level of physical mobility.	12.a.1. Assess for factors that impair physical mobility (e.g. paresthesias, impaired proprioception, muscle weakness, foot and wrist drop, fatigue, weakness, nausea, vomiting). 2. Implement measures *to increase mobility:* a. perform actions to reduce fatigue and improve activity tolerance (see Nursing Diagnoses 10, action e and 11, action b) b. perform actions to reduce discomfort (see Nursing Diagnoses 5.A, action 2; 5.B, action 6; 5.C, action 3; and 5.D, action 2) c. instruct client in and assist with correct use of mobility aids (e.g. cane, walker, crutches) if appropriate d. instruct client in and assist with active and/or passive range of motion exercises every 4 hours unless contraindicated e. reinforce instructions, activities, and exercise plan recommended by physical and occupational therapists f. perform actions to prevent falls (see Nursing Diagnosis 18, action b) *in order to reduce fear of injury.* 3. Increase activity and participation in self-care activities as tolerated. 4. Provide praise and encouragement for all efforts to increase or maintain physical mobility. 5. Encourage the support of significant others. Allow them to assist with activity if desired.
12.b. The client will not experience problems associated with immobility.	12.b. Refer to Care Plan on Immobility for actions to prevent problems associated with immobility if client is on bedrest for longer than 48 hours.

13. NURSING DIAGNOSIS

Self-care deficit related to impaired physical mobility associated with fatigue, weakness, fear of falls, sensory and motor deficits, and discomfort.

DESIRED OUTCOMES	NURSING ACTIONS AND *SELECTED RATIONALES*
13. The client will perform self-care activities within physical limitations.	13.a. Assess for factors that interfere with client's ability to perform self-care (e.g. fatigue, weakness, nausea, vomiting, sensory and motor deficits). b. With client, develop a realistic plan for meeting daily physical needs.

c. Encourage maximum independence within limitations imposed by fatigue, discomfort, weakness, and sensory or motor deficits.
d. Implement measures *to facilitate client's ability to perform self-care activities:*
   1. perform actions to increase mobility (see Nursing Diagnosis 12, action a.2)
   2. schedule care at a time when client is most likely to be able to participate (e.g. following rest periods, not immediately after meals or treatments)
   3. allow adequate time for accomplishment of self-care activities.
e. Provide positive feedback for all self-care efforts and accomplishments.
f. Assist the client with those activities he/she is unable to perform independently.
g. Inform significant others of client's abilities to perform own care. Explain the importance of encouraging and allowing client to maintain optimal level of independence within his/her activity tolerance level.

☐ ▬▬▬▬▬▬▬▬▬▬▬▬▬▬▬▬▬▬▬▬▬▬

14. NURSING DIAGNOSIS

Diarrhea related to increased intestinal motility associated with extreme fear and anxiety and inflammation and ulceration of the gastrointestinal mucosa resulting from effects of cytotoxic drugs on rapidly dividing epithelial cells.

☐ ▬▬▬▬▬▬▬▬▬▬▬▬▬▬▬▬▬▬▬▬▬▬

DESIRED OUTCOMES	NURSING ACTIONS AND *SELECTED RATIONALES*

14. The client will maintain usual bowel elimination pattern.

14.a. Ascertain client's usual bowel elimination habits.
 b. Assess for signs and symptoms of diarrhea (e.g. frequent, loose stools; abdominal pain and cramping).
 c. Assess bowel sounds regularly. Report an increase in frequency of and/or high-pitched bowel sounds.
 d. Implement measures *to control diarrhea:*
   1. perform actions *to rest the bowel:*
      a. instruct client to avoid foods/fluids that are poorly digested or act as irritants to the inflamed bowel:
         1. those high in fat (e.g. butter, cream, oils, whole milk, fried foods, gravies, nuts)
         2. those with high fiber content (e.g. whole-grain cereals; raw vegetables and fruit except ripe bananas, peeled apples, and avocados; nuts)
         3. those known to cause diarrhea or be gas-producers (e.g. cabbage, onions, popcorn, licorice, prunes, chili, baked beans, carbonated beverages)
         4. spicy foods
         5. foods/fluids high in caffeine (e.g. coffee, tea, chocolate, colas)
         6. extremely hot or cold foods/fluids
      b. provide small, frequent meals that are low in residue but still supply the needed protein and carbohydrates (e.g. eggs; smooth peanut butter; baked fish or poultry; cooked cereal; white rice or breads; bland, cooked vegetables)
      c. season appropriate foods with nutmeg *to decrease motility of the gastrointestinal tract*
      d. implement measures to reduce fear and anxiety (see Nursing Diagnosis 1, action c)

e. discourage smoking (*nicotine has a stimulant effect on the gastrointestinal tract*)
2. monitor for therapeutic and nontherapeutic effects of the following medications if administered:
    a. opiate or opiate-like substances (e.g. loperamide, diphenoxylate hydrochloride) *to decrease gastrointestinal motility*
    b. bulk-forming agents (e.g. methylcellulose, psyllium hydrophilic mucilloid, calcium polycarbophil) *to absorb water in the bowel and produce a soft, formed stool.*
e. Consult physician if diarrhea persists.

15. NURSING DIAGNOSIS

Constipation related to autonomic nerve dysfunction (associated primarily with the vinca alkaloids), decreased intake of fluids and foods high in fiber, anxiety, and decreased activity.

DESIRED OUTCOMES	NURSING ACTIONS AND *SELECTED RATIONALES*

15. The client will maintain usual bowel elimination pattern.

15.a. Ascertain client's usual bowel elimination habits.
  b. Monitor and record bowel movements including frequency, consistency, and shape particularly during the first 3–5 days after drug administration (constipation is one of the earliest manifestations of neurotoxicity associated with use of vinca alkaloids).
  c. Assess for signs and symptoms that may accompany constipation such as headache, anorexia, nausea, abdominal distention and cramping, and feeling of fullness or pressure in abdomen or rectum.
  d. Assess bowel sounds. Report a pattern of decreasing bowel sounds.
  e. Implement measures *to prevent constipation:*
    1. encourage client to defecate whenever the urge is felt
    2. assist client to toilet or place in high Fowler's position or on commode for bowel movements unless contraindicated; provide privacy and adequate ventilation
    3. encourage client to relax during attempts to defecate *in order to promote relaxation of the levator ani muscle and the external anal sphincter*
    4. instruct client to select foods high in fiber (e.g. nuts, bran, whole grains, raw fruits and vegetables, dried fruits) if mucositis is not severe
    5. instruct client to maintain a minimum fluid intake of 2500 cc/day unless contraindicated
    6. encourage client to drink warm liquids *to stimulate peristalsis*
    7. increase activity as tolerated
    8. encourage client to perform isometric abdominal strengthening exercises unless contraindicated
    9. monitor for therapeutic and nontherapeutic effects of laxatives, suppositories, stool softeners, and/or enemas if administered.
  f. If client has not had a bowel movement in 3 days or if other signs and symptoms of constipation are present:
    1. check for impaction and administer oil retention and/or cleansing enemas as ordered if the client's WBC count is adequate
    2. consult physician about alternative bowel care orders that do not involve invasive procedures if the client's WBC count is inadequate.
  g. Instruct client to monitor elimination pattern throughout entire course of therapy if being treated with vinca alkaloids and to report any difficulty with bowel elimination immediately.

16. NURSING DIAGNOSIS

Sleep pattern disturbance related to:

a. discomfort associated with nausea, vomiting, pain, and other side effects of che-motherapy;
b. anxiety, fear, and depression;
c. frequent need to defecate associated with diarrhea.

DESIRED OUTCOMES	NURSING ACTIONS AND *SELECTED RATIONALES*
16. The client will attain optimal amounts of sleep within the parameters of the treatment regimen as evidenced by: a. statements of feeling well rested b. usual behavior c. absence of frequent yawning, thick speech, dark circles under eyes.	16.a. Assess for signs and symptoms of a sleep pattern disturbance: 1. verbal complaints of difficulty falling asleep, not feeling well rested, sleep interruptions, or awakening earlier or later than desired 2. behavior changes (e.g. irritability, disorganization, lethargy) 3. frequent yawning, thick speech, dark circles under eyes, slight hand tremors. b. Determine the client's usual sleep habits. c. Implement measures *to promote sleep:* 1. perform actions to reduce discomfort (see Nursing Diagnoses 5.A, action 2; 5.B, action 6; 5.C, action 3; 5.D, action 2; and 5.E, actions 2 and 3) 2. perform actions to control diarrhea (see Nursing Diagnosis 14, action d) 3. perform actions to reduce fear and anxiety (see Nursing Diagnosis 1, action c) 4. allow client to continue usual sleep practices (e.g. position, time, bedtime rituals) if possible 5. determine measures that have been helpful to client in the past (e.g. milk, warm drinks, warm bath) and incorporate in plan of care 6. discourage long periods of sleep during the day unless sleep deprivation exists or daytime sleep is usual for client 7. encourage participation in relaxing diversional activities in early evening hours 8. provide a quiet, restful atmosphere 9. discourage intake of foods and fluids high in caffeine (e.g. chocolate, coffee, tea, colas) especially in the evening 10. satisfy basic needs such as hunger, comfort, and warmth before sleep 11. have client empty bladder just before bedtime 12. utilize relaxation techniques (e.g. progressive relaxation exercises, back massage, meditation, soft music) before sleep 13. perform actions *to provide for periods of uninterrupted sleep (90- to 120-minute periods of uninterrupted sleep are considered essential):* a. restrict visitors during rest periods b. group care (e.g. medications, treatments, physical care, assessments) whenever possible 14. monitor for therapeutic and nontherapeutic effects of sedatives and hypnotics if administered. d. Consult physician if signs of sleep deprivation persist or worsen.

17. NURSING DIAGNOSIS

Potential for infection related to:

a. immunosuppression associated with chemotherapy-induced bone marrow suppression and long-term treatment with corticosteroids;

b. lowered natural resistance associated with malnutrition, anemia, general debilitation, and disruption of normal bacterial flora (results from antibiotic therapy);
c. break in integrity of the skin associated with placement of a central venous catheter (e.g. Groshong), implanted infusion device (e.g. Port-a-Cath), or peritoneal catheter (e.g. Tenckhoff).

□ ▬▬▬▬▬▬▬▬▬▬▬▬▬▬▬▬▬▬▬▬▬▬▬▬

DESIRED OUTCOMES	NURSING ACTIONS AND *SELECTED RATIONALES*
17. The client will remain free of infection as evidenced by: a. absence of chills and fever b. pulse within normal limits c. normal breath sounds d. voiding clear, yellow urine without complaints of frequency, urgency, or burning e. absence of redness, swelling, or unusual drainage in any area where there is a break in skin integrity f. intact oral mucous membrane g. absence of perianal abscesses h. absence of painful, pruritic skin lesions i. WBC and differential counts within normal range for client j. negative results of cultured specimens.	17.a. Assess for and report signs and symptoms of infection (be aware of subtle changes in client as signs of infection may be very minimal due to immunosuppression): 　1. increase in temperature above client's usual level 　2. chills 　3. pattern of increased pulse or pulse rate greater than 100 beats/minute 　4. adventitious breath sounds 　5. cloudy or foul-smelling urine 　6. complaints of frequency, urgency, or burning when urinating 　7. presence of WBCs, bacteria, and/or nitrites in urine 　8. redness, change in skin temperature, swelling, or unusual drainage in any area where there is a break in skin integrity including previous and current puncture sites 　9. irritation or ulceration of oral mucous membrane 　10. complaints of perineal or rectal pain and any unusual vaginal or rectal discharge 　11. increased hemorrhoidal pain, redness, or bleeding 　12. painful, pruritic skin lesions (herpes zoster) particularly in cervical or thoracic area 　13. change in WBC count, especially an increase in immature neutrophils. b. Obtain culture specimens (e.g. urine, vaginal, rectal, mouth, sputum, blood, skin lesions) as ordered. Report positive results. c. Implement measures *to reduce the risk of infection:* 　1. protect client from others with infection and those who have recently been vaccinated (*a person may have a subclinical infection after a vaccination*) 　2. use good handwashing technique and encourage client to do the same 　3. instruct client to avoid use of shared eating utensils 　4. maintain a fluid intake of at least 2500 cc/day unless contraindicated 　5. maintain an optimal nutritional status (see Nursing Diagnosis 3, action f) 　6. encourage a low-bacteria diet (e.g. cooked foods, no fresh fruit) if the client is immunosuppressed 　7. perform actions to prevent or reduce severity of stomatitis (see Nursing Diagnosis 9, actions d and e) 　8. perform actions to maintain skin integrity (see Nursing Diagnosis 8, action b) 　9. avoid invasive procedures (e.g. urinary catheterizations, arterial or venous punctures, injections) whenever possible; if such procedures are necessary, maintain meticulous aseptic technique 　10. give meticulous attention to any break in the skin; cleanse carefully with antiseptic solution at least twice daily or as ordered 　11. initiate measures to prevent constipation (see Nursing Diagnosis 15, action e) in order to avoid damage *to rectal mucosa from hard or impacted stool* 　12. avoid unnecessary rectal invasion (e.g. temperature taking, enemas, suppositories, rectal tube) *to prevent trauma to rectal mucosa and possible abscess formation* 　13. provide proper balance of exercise and rest 　14. perform actions *to prevent a respiratory tract infection:* 　　a. instruct and assist client to turn, cough, and deep breathe at least every 2 hours if his/her activity is limited 　　b. instruct and assist client in use of inspiratory exerciser at least every 2 hours if indicated

    c. encourage client to stop smoking
    d. increase activity as tolerated
15. perform actions *to prevent a urinary tract infection:*
    a. instruct and assist client to wash his/her perianal area every shift and after each bowel movement
    b. instruct female client to wipe from front to back following urination or defecation
16. instruct and assist client in proper care of the exit site of a central venous catheter or insertion site of an implanted infusion device and/or peritoneal catheter (see Nursing Diagnosis 24, actions i.1–3).
d. Monitor for therapeutic and nontherapeutic effects of anti-infectives and granulocyte transfusions if administered (the latter may be used if client is not responsive to anti-infective therapy or if the period of leukopenia is prolonged).

☐ ▬▬▬▬▬▬▬▬▬▬▬▬▬▬▬▬▬▬▬▬▬▬▬

18. NURSING DIAGNOSIS

Potential for trauma related to falls associated with:

a. weakness resulting from anemia, fluid and electrolyte imbalances, and malnutrition;
b. motor and sensory disturbances or changes (e.g. gait disturbances, blurred vision, impaired proprioception) resulting from damage to the nervous system associated with the use of neurotoxic drugs (e.g. vinca alkaloids, cisplatin).

☐ ▬▬▬▬▬▬▬▬▬▬▬▬▬▬▬▬▬▬▬▬▬▬▬

DESIRED OUTCOMES	NURSING ACTIONS AND *SELECTED RATIONALES*

18. The client will not experience falls.	18.a. Determine whether conditions predisposing client to falls (e.g. weakness, fatigue, blurred vision, impaired proprioception, gait disturbances) exist.
	b. Implement measures *to prevent falls:*
	  1. keep bed in low position with side rails up when client is in bed
	  2. keep needed items within easy reach
	  3. encourage client to request assistance whenever needed; have call signal within easy reach
	  4. use lap belt when client is in chair if indicated
	  5. instruct client to wear shoes with nonskid soles and low heels when ambulating
	  6. avoid unnecessary clutter in room
	  7. accompany client during ambulation utilizing a transfer safety belt if he/she is weak or dizzy
	  8. provide ambulatory aids (e.g. walker, cane) if client is weak or unsteady on feet
	  9. reinforce instructions from physical therapist regarding correct transfer and ambulation techniques
	  10. if vision is impaired:
	    a. orient client to surroundings, room, and arrangement of furniture
	    b. assist client with ambulation by walking 1/2 step ahead of client and describing approaching objects or obstacles; instruct client to grasp back of nurse's arm during ambulation
	  11. instruct client to ambulate in well-lit areas and to utilize handrails if needed
	  12. do not rush client; allow adequate time for trips to the bathroom and ambulation in hallway
	  13. perform actions to reduce fatigue and improve activity tolerance (see Nursing Diagnoses 10, action e and 11, action b)

14. perform actions to maintain fluid and electrolyte balance (see Nursing Diagnosis 2, actions a.3 and b.2 and 3).
  c. Include client and significant others in planning and implementing measures to prevent falls.
  d. If falls occur, initiate appropriate first aid measures and notify physician.

19. COLLABORATIVE DIAGNOSIS

Potential complications:

a. **bleeding** related to thrombocytopenia associated with bone marrow depression;
b. **renal calculi** related to hyperuricemia associated with rapid lysis of tumor cells;
c. **impaired renal function** related to toxic effects of cytotoxic drugs on glomeruli and tubules and/or nephropathy associated with uric acid accumulation;
d. **hemorrhagic cystitis** related to irritation of the bladder mucosa by cyclophosphamide;
e. **local tissue irritation and sloughing** related to extravasation of vesicant drugs (e.g. doxorubicin, daunorubicin, vinblastine, vincristine);
f. **arrhythmias** related to the cardiotoxic effects of cytotoxic drugs (primarily doxorubicin and daunorubicin);
g. **congestive heart failure (CHF)** related to arrhythmias, cardiotoxic effects of cytotoxic drugs (e.g. doxorubicin, daunorubicin), and cor pulmonale if pulmonary fibrosis develops;
h. **inflammation and fibrosis of lung tissue** related particularly to the administration of bleomycin and the nitrosoureas;
i. **neurotoxicity (e.g. paresthesias, proprioceptive and reflex losses, muscle weakness, footdrop, visual disturbances)** related to demyelination of nerve fibers (occurs primarily with the vinca alkaloids and cisplatin);
j. **herpes zoster** related to an increased susceptibility to infection associated with decreased immunological functioning;
k. **anaphylactic reaction** related to a hypersensitivity response to a cytotoxic drug (occurs primarily with cisplatin and L-asparaginase);
l. **shock** related to hemorrhage, fluid volume deficit, and anaphylaxis;
m. **peritonitis** related to chemical irritation by cytotoxic agent(s) used for intraperitoneal chemotherapy and contamination of dialysate solution, peritoneal catheter, or implanted infusion device.

DESIRED OUTCOMES	NURSING ACTIONS AND *SELECTED RATIONALES*
19.a. The client will not experience unusual bleeding as evidenced by: 1. skin and mucous membranes free of bleeding, petechiae, and ecchymosis 2. absence of unusual joint pain or swelling 3. absence of frank or occult blood in stool, urine, and vomitus 4. no increase in abdominal girth 5. usual menstrual flow	19.a.1. Assess client for and report signs and symptoms of unusual bleeding: a. petechiae b. multiple ecchymotic areas c. bleeding gums d. frequent or uncontrollable episodes of epistaxis e. unusual oozing from injection sites f. unusual joint pain or swelling g. hematemesis, melena, red or smoke-colored urine h. increase in abdominal girth i. hypermenorrhea j. significant drop in B/P accompanied by an increased pulse rate k. decline in Hct. and Hgb. levels l. restlessness, confusion. 2. Monitor coagulation test results (e.g. platelet count, bleeding time). Report abnormal values.

6. vital signs within normal range for client
7. stable or improved Hct. and Hgb.
8. usual mental status.

3. If coagulation test results are abnormal or Hct. and Hgb. levels decline, test all stools, urine, and vomitus for occult blood. Report positive results.
4. Implement measures *to prevent bleeding:*
   a. use the smallest gauge needle possible when giving injections and performing venous or arterial punctures
   b. apply gentle, prolonged pressure after injections and venous or arterial punctures
   c. take B/P only when necessary and avoid overinflating the cuff
   d. caution client to avoid activities that increase potential for trauma (e.g. shaving with a straight-edge razor, cutting nails, using stiff bristle toothbrush or dental floss)
   e. pad side rails if client is confused or restless
   f. perform actions to prevent falls (see Nursing Diagnosis 18, action b)
   g. instruct client to avoid blowing nose forcefully or straining to have a bowel movement; consult physician about order for decongestants, stool softeners, and/or laxatives if indicated
   h. avoid taking temperatures rectally and administering rectal suppositories
   i. monitor for therapeutic and nontherapeutic effects of the following if administered:
      1. estrogen-progestin preparations *to suppress menses*
      2. platelets
      3. plasma or whole blood.
5. If bleeding occurs and does not subside spontaneously:
   a. apply firm, prolonged pressure to bleeding area if possible
   b. if epistaxis occurs, place client in high Fowler's position and apply pressure and ice packs to nasal area
   c. maintain oxygen therapy as ordered
   d. perform iced water or saline lavage as ordered *to control gastric bleeding*
   e. administer blood products as ordered
   f. provide emotional support to client and significant others.

19.b. The client will not develop renal calculi as evidenced by:
1. absence of flank pain, hematuria, urinary frequency or urgency, nausea, vomiting
2. clear urine without calculi.

19.b.1. Assess for and report signs and symptoms of renal calculi (e.g. dull, aching or severe, colicky flank pain; hematuria; urinary frequency or urgency; nausea; vomiting).
2. Monitor serum uric acid levels and report elevations.
3. Obtain a urine specimen for analysis if ordered. Report increases in numbers of crystals or high levels of uric acid.
4. Implement measures *to prevent uric acid stone formation:*
   a. perform actions *to prevent urinary stasis:*
      1. encourage a minimum fluid intake of 2500 cc/day unless contraindicated
      2. instruct and assist client to change positions at least every 2 hours
      3. encourage activity as tolerated
      4. implement measures *to facilitate voiding* (e.g. provide privacy, allow client to assume normal voiding position unless contraindicated, run warm water over perineum)
      5. instruct client to void whenever the urge is felt
      6. maintain patency of urinary catheter if present
   b. monitor pH of urine every shift and report levels below 6 (*uric acid precipitates in an acidic environment*)
   c. perform actions *to maintain an alkaline urine:*
      1. encourage client to increase intake of foods/fluids that leave an alkaline ash (e.g. milk; vegetables, especially legumes and green vegetables; fruits except prunes, plums, and cranberries)
      2. administer medications that alkalinize the urine (e.g. sodium bicarbonate, citrate preparations) as ordered
   d. instruct client to reduce intake of foods high in purine content (e.g. liver, kidney, goose, venison, seafood, meat soups and gravies, anchovies) *in order to prevent a further increase in uric acid*
   e. monitor for therapeutic and nontherapeutic effects of xanthine oxidase inhibitor (allopurinol) if administered *to decrease uric acid production.*
5. If signs and symptoms of renal calculi occur:
   a. strain all urine carefully and save any calculi for analysis; report finding to physician

b. encourage a minimum fluid intake of 2500 cc/day unless contraindicated
c. administer analgesics as ordered
d. refer to Care Plan on Renal Calculi for additional care measures.

19.c. The client will maintain adequate renal function as evidenced by:
1. urine output at least 30 cc/hour
2. urine specific gravity between 1.010–1.030
3. BUN and serum creatinine levels within normal range.
	19.c.1. Assess for and report a urine output below 100 cc/hour during and for 24 hours after administration of nephrotoxic drugs (consult physician about insertion of a urinary catheter if output cannot be monitored accurately).
	2. Assess for and report signs and symptoms of impaired renal function (e.g. urine output less than 30 cc/hour, urine specific gravity fixed at/or less than 1.010, elevated BUN and serum creatinine levels).
	3. Collect a 24-hour urine specimen if ordered. Report decreased creatinine clearance.
	4. Implement measures *to maintain adequate renal function:*
	    a. hydrate client with 200 cc fluid/hour unless contraindicated for 6–24 hours before administration of drugs known to be nephrotoxic (e.g. cisplatin, methotrexate, mitomycin)
	    b. maintain intravenous fluids as ordered during administration of drugs and for 24 hours after therapy *to maintain a high rate of glomerular blood flow*
	    c. monitor for therapeutic and nontherapeutic effects of diuretics if administered concurrently with cytotoxic agent(s) *to promote a more rapid plasma clearance of the drug(s)*
	    d. perform actions to prevent uric acid stone formation (see action b.4 in this diagnosis).
	5. If signs and symptoms of impaired renal function occur:
	    a. continue with above actions
	    b. administer diuretics as ordered
	    c. monitor for and report signs of acute renal failure (e.g. oliguria or anuria; weight gain; edema; elevated B/P; lethargy and confusion; increasing BUN and serum creatinine, phosphorus, and potassium levels)
	    d. prepare client for dialysis if indicated
	    e. refer to Care Plan on Renal Failure for additional care measures.

19.d. The client will not develop hemorrhagic cystitis as evidenced by absence of dysuria, urinary frequency or urgency, and hematuria.	19.d.1. Assess for and report signs and symptoms of hemorrhagic cystitis (e.g. dysuria, urinary frequency and/or urgency, frank or occult blood in urine).
	2. Implement measures *to prevent hemorrhagic cystitis:*
	    a. encourage a minimum fluid intake of 2500 cc/day; if client is unable to tolerate oral fluids, consult physician about an order for intravenous fluids *to ensure adequate hydration*
	    b. administer cyclophosphamide early in the day and encourage client to void every 2 hours and before going to bed *in order to prevent stasis of drug in the bladder.*
	3. If signs and symptoms of hemorrhagic cystitis occur:
	    a. continue with above actions
	    b. administer diuretics as ordered *to increase urine output and thereby decrease urinary concentration of cyclophosphamide*
	    c. monitor for therapeutic and nontherapeutic effects of continuous bladder irrigations with silver nitrate solution if performed *to stop bleeding*
	    d. assist with or perform bladder irrigations as ordered *to facilitate removal of drug and flush clots from the bladder*
	    e. provide emotional support to client and significant others.

19.e. The client will not experience drug extravasation as evidenced by: 1. absence of swelling around drug administration site 2. no complaints of stinging or burning pain at needle site 3. absence of erythema at infusion site.	19.e.1. Assess for signs and symptoms of drug extravasation (e.g. swelling around drug administration site, client complaints of stinging or burning pain at needle site, erythema at infusion site several hours after drug administration). 2. Differentiate between a flare reaction and extravasation if giving doxorubicin. (With a flare reaction, swelling and erythema occur within minutes, usually along vein line, and disappear in 60–90 minutes. A good blood return is also present and the client experiences itching rather than pain at the infusion site.) 3. Ensure that the insertion site and surrounding tissue are visible at all times. 4. Implement measures *to prevent drug extravasation:*

a. select the best vein possible for vesicant drug administration:
   1. do not use a vein that has been previously used for vesicant agents
   2. avoid antecubital fossa and small veins in the hand
   3. do not use an existing intravenous site unless no other site is available and blood return is excellent
   4. avoid extremities with compromised circulation
b. tape needle securely
c. perform actions *to ensure that the drug is infusing into the vein:*
   1. test patency of vein with a minimum of 5 cc of normal saline before administration of cytotoxic drug
   2. check blood return after every 3–4 cc if giving the drug by direct push
   3. stay with client while a vesicant drug is infusing; check site every 2–3 minutes
d. perform actions *to prevent increased irritation of the vein:*
   1. dilute drug according to manufacturer's recommendations
   2. administer drug at recommended rate of infusion
e. stop infusion if there is any indication that the drug is not infusing properly (e.g. poor or absent blood return, client complaints of pain at infusion site)
f. when the drug infusion is complete, flush needle with a minimum of 30 cc of normal saline; apply pressure to site for at least 4 minutes after needle removal *to minimize oozing.*

5. If signs and symptoms of drug extravasation occur:
   a. stop infusion immediately
   b. treat area of extravasation as ordered or per standard hospital policy
   c. monitor the site closely every shift for signs of inflammation or necrosis
   d. provide emotional support to client and significant others.

19.f. The client will experience resolution of cardiac arrhythmias if they occur as evidenced by:
1. regular apical pulse at 60–100 beats/minute
2. equal apical and radial pulses
3. absence of syncope and palpitations
4. EKG reading showing normal sinus rhythm.

19.f.1. Assess closely for and report signs and symptoms of arrhythmias (e.g. irregular apical pulse; pulse rate below 60 or above 100 beats/minute; apical-radial pulse deficit; syncope; palpitations; abnormal rate, rhythm, or configurations on EKG).
2. Monitor liver and kidney function studies and report abnormal results (*cardiotoxicity can result from delayed metabolism or excretion of cytotoxic drugs by the liver and/or kidneys*).
3. If arrhythmias occur:
   a. initiate cardiac monitoring if not already being done
   b. monitor for therapeutic and nontherapeutic effects of the following medications if administered:
      1. Class I antiarrhythmics (e.g. phenytoin, tocainide, lidocaine, flecainide, procainamide, disopyramide, quinidine) *to interfere directly with depolarization*
      2. Class II antiarrhythmics (e.g. propranolol) *to block beta-adrenergic stimulation*
      3. Class III antiarrhythmics (e.g. bretylium, amiodarone) *to prolong the duration of the action potential*
      4. Class IV antiarrhythmics (e.g. verapamil, diltiazem) *to block the slow inward depolarizing current*
      5. anticholinergic agents (e.g. atropine) or sympathomimetics (e.g. ephedrine, isoproterenol) *to increase heart rate*
      6. cardiac glycosides (e.g. digitalis) *to decrease the heart rate*
   c. restrict client's activity based on his/her tolerance and severity of arrhythmia
   d. maintain oxygen therapy as ordered
   e. assist with cardioversion if performed
   f. monitor cardiovascular status closely and report signs and symptoms of inadequate tissue perfusion (e.g. decline in B/P; cool, clammy, mottled skin; cyanosis; diminished peripheral pulses; declining urine output; restlessness and agitation; shortness of breath)
   g. have emergency cart readily available for cardiopulmonary resuscitation.

19.g. The client will not develop CHF as evidenced by:

19.g.1. Assess for and report signs and symptoms of CHF:
   a. tachycardia

1. vital signs within normal range for client
2. audible heart sounds without an S_3 or S_4 or softening of pre-existing murmurs
3. normal breath sounds
4. absence of dyspnea and orthopnea
5. palpable peripheral pulses and normal carotid pulse amplitude
6. balanced intake and output
7. stable weight
8. CVP within normal range
9. absence of peripheral edema; distended neck veins; enlarged, tender liver
10. BUN and serum creatinine and alkaline phosphatase levels within normal range.

b. softened or muffled heart sounds
c. development of or intensified S_3 and/or S_4 gallop rhythm
d. crackles and diminished or absent breath sounds
e. dyspnea, orthopnea
f. displaced apical impulse
g. diminished or absent peripheral pulses
h. decreased amplitude of carotid pulse
i. intake greater than output
j. weight gain
k. elevated CVP
l. peripheral edema
m. distended neck veins
n. enlarged, tender liver
o. elevated BUN and serum creatinine and alkaline phosphatase levels.

2. Monitor chest x-ray results. Report findings of cardiomegaly, pleural effusion, or pulmonary edema.
3. Implement measures *to prevent CHF:*
   a. consult physician before administering cytotoxic drugs if liver and kidney function studies are abnormal (*cardiotoxicity can result from delayed metabolism or excretion of cytotoxic drugs by liver and/or kidneys*)
   b. perform actions to treat arrhythmias (see action f.3 in this diagnosis)
   c. perform actions to treat pulmonary inflammation and fibrosis (see action h.5. in this diagnosis)
   d. perform actions *to reduce cardiac workload:*
      1. place client in a semi- to high Fowler's position
      2. implement measures to promote physical and emotional rest
      3. instruct client to avoid activities that create a Valsalva response (e.g. straining to have a bowel movement, bending at the waist, holding breath while moving)
      4. discourage smoking (*smoking has a cardiostimulatory effect, causes vasoconstriction, and reduces myocardial oxygen availability*)
      5. discourage intake of foods/fluids high in caffeine such as coffee, tea, chocolate, and colas (*caffeine is a myocardial stimulant and increases myocardial oxygen consumption*)
      6. provide small, frequent meals rather than 3 large ones (*large meals require an increased blood supply to gastrointestinal tract for digestion*).
4. If signs and symptoms of CHF occur:
   a. continue with above actions
   b. monitor for therapeutic and nontherapeutic effects of medications that may be administered *to reduce vascular congestion and/or cardiac workload* (e.g. cardiotonics, diuretics, vasodilators, morphine sulfate)
   c. apply rotating tourniquets according to hospital policy if ordered *to reduce pulmonary vascular congestion*
   d. refer to Care Plan on Congestive Heart Failure for additional care measures.

19.h. The client will experience decreased signs and symptoms of pulmonary inflammation and fibrosis if they occur as evidenced by:
1. absence of cough
2. afebrile status
3. absence of tachypnea and exertional dyspnea
4. increased strength
5. improved skin color
6. improved breath sounds
7. blood gases returning toward normal range
8. improved chest x-ray and pulmonary function studies.

19.h.1. Assess for signs and symptoms of pulmonary inflammation and fibrosis (e.g. dry, hacking, persistent cough; fever; tachypnea; dyspnea on exertion; weakness; cyanosis; crackles; rhonchi).
2. Monitor blood gas values. Report abnormal results.
3. Monitor for and report significant changes in ear oximetry and capnograph results.
4. Monitor for and report changes in chest x-ray reports and pulmonary function studies.
5. If signs and symptoms of pulmonary inflammation and fibrosis occur:
   a. monitor for therapeutic and nontherapeutic effects of the following medications if administered:
      1. anti-infectives *to prevent respiratory infection*
      2. corticosteroids *to reduce inflammatory response*
      3. bronchodilators
   b. implement measures *to improve gas exchange:*
      1. place client in a semi- to high Fowler's position unless contraindicated

UNIT V

2. instruct and assist client to turn, cough, and deep breathe at least every 2 hours
3. reinforce correct use of inspiratory exerciser at least every 2 hours
4. assist with chest physiotherapy (e.g. IPPB, postural drainage, percussion, vibration) if ordered
5. maintain oxygen therapy as ordered
6. administer central nervous system depressants (e.g. narcotic analgesics, sedatives, muscle relaxants) judiciously; hold medication and consult physician if respiratory rate is less than 12/minute
   c. provide emotional support to client and significant others
   d. consult physician if signs and symptoms of pulmonary inflammation and fibrosis worsen.

19.i. The client will experience resolution of signs and symptoms of neurotoxicity if they occur as evidenced by usual motor and sensory function.

19.i.1. Assess for and report signs and symptoms of neurotoxicity (e.g. ataxia, numbness and tingling of extremities, unusual muscle weakness, gait disturbances, difficulty with fine motor movements, foot or wrist drop, blurred vision, impaired color perception or discrimination).
2. Assure client that most changes in neurological function may be reversible if reported immediately and medication is discontinued.
3. If signs and symptoms of neurotoxicity occur:
   a. implement measures to prevent falls (see Nursing Diagnosis 18, action b)
   b. implement measures *to maintain optimal muscle tone and joint flexibility:*
      1. instruct client to flex, extend, and rotate feet for 5–10 minutes every 1–2 hours
      2. use a footboard, sandbags, pillows, high-topped tennis shoes, foam boots, or foot positioners if necessary *to keep feet in a neutral or slightly dorsiflexed position*
      3. utilize devices such as splints if indicated *to maintain wrist in correct alignment*
      4. instruct client in and assist with range of motion exercises at least every 4 hours unless contraindicated
   c. implement measures *to reduce risk of tissue trauma and breakdown in areas of paresthesias:*
      1. perform actions to prevent skin irritation and breakdown due to decreased mobility (see Nursing Diagnosis 8, action b.1)
      2. perform actions *to prevent burns:*
         a. let hot foods or fluids cool slightly before serving *in order to reduce risk of burns if spills occur*
         b. assess temperature of bath water and heating pad before and during use
      3. avoid use of cold applications on areas of decreased sensation
      4. assist client with tasks that require fine motor skills (e.g. shaving) *to prevent cuts*
   d. consult physician if signs and symptoms of neurotoxicity persist or worsen.

19.j. The client will experience a reduction in herpes zoster lesions if they occur.

19.j.1. Assess for and report signs and symptoms of herpes zoster (e.g. groups of painful nodules or vesicles along the course of a nerve, malaise, fever).
2. If herpes zoster occurs:
   a. assess skin every shift for characteristics and distribution of lesions
   b. note color, amount, and consistency of drainage from lesions
   c. implement measures *to relieve discomfort:*
      1. apply cool, moist compresses or therapeutic soaks to affected area(s) as ordered
      2. splint affected area(s) with soft elastic bandages if possible
   d. monitor for therapeutic and nontherapeutic effects of analgesics, corticosteroids, and/or anti-infectives if administered
   e. maintain isolation precautions per hospital policy while vesicular lesions are present
   f. assess for and report signs and symptoms of complications of herpes zoster:
      1. infected lesions (e.g. increased erythema, fever, purulent drainage)
      2. ophthalmic damage (e.g. keratitis, corneal ulcerations, blindness)

3. Ramsey-Hunt syndrome (e.g. facial paralysis, vertigo, tinnitus, hearing loss)
4. postherpetic neuralgia.

19.k. The client will not develop an anaphylactic reaction as evidenced by:
1. usual skin color
2. absence of urticaria and pruritus
3. no complaints of headache
4. unlabored respirations at 16–20/minute
5. absence of wheezing and stridor
6. stable vital signs
7. absence of facial and peripheral edema
8. usual speaking ability.

19.k.1. Assess for and report signs and symptoms of an anaphylactic reaction (usually some or all of the signs and symptoms will occur within minutes of drug administration):
  a. flushing of skin
  b. generalized urticaria and pruritus
  c. headache
  d. dyspnea, wheezing, stridor
  e. irregular and/or increased pulse rate, decline in B/P
  f. edema of face, hands, and feet
  g. inability to speak.
2. Implement measures *to prevent an anaphylactic reaction:*
  a. consult physician before giving any drug that is the same as or similar to one client has reacted to previously
  b. administer a skin test before giving drug if appropriate.
3. If signs and symptoms of an anaphylactic reaction occur:
  a. discontinue the cytotoxic drug but keep intravenous line open with a normal saline solution
  b. administer oxygen as ordered
  c. monitor for therapeutic and nontherapeutic effects of the following drugs if administered:
    1. sympathomimetics (e.g. epinephrine) *to stimulate peripheral vasoconstriction and bronchodilation*
    2. antihistamines (e.g. diphenhydramine) *to reduce the sensitivity reaction and control urticaria*
    3. bronchodilators (e.g. theophylline) *to relieve bronchospasm*
    4. corticosteroids *to reduce the allergic response and maintain usual vascular wall permeability*
  d. provide emotional support to client and significant others.

19.l. The client will not develop shock as evidenced by:
1. usual mental status
2. stable vital signs
3. skin warm and usual color
4. palpable peripheral pulses
5. capillary refill time less than 3 seconds
6. urine output at least 30 cc/hour.

19.l.1. Assess for and report the following:
  a. significant abnormalities in coagulation test results
  b. signs and symptoms of bleeding (see action a.1 in this diagnosis)
  c. signs and symptoms of anaphylaxis (see action k.1 in this diagnosis)
  d. signs and symptoms of fluid volume deficit (see Nursing Diagnosis 2, action a.1.a)
  e. signs and symptoms of shock:
    1. restlessness, agitation, confusion
    2. significant decrease in B/P
    3. decline in B/P of at least 15 mm Hg with concurrent rise in pulse when client changes from lying to sitting or standing position
    4. resting pulse rate greater than 100 beats/minute
    5. rapid or labored respirations
    6. cool, pale, or cyanotic skin
    7. diminished or absent peripheral pulses
    8. capillary refill time greater than 3 seconds
    9. urine output less than 30 cc/hour.
2. Implement measures *to prevent shock:*
  a. perform actions to prevent and control bleeding (see actions a.4 and 5 in this diagnosis)
  b. perform actions to prevent and treat an anaphylactic reaction (see actions k.2 and 3 in this diagnosis)
  c. perform actions to maintain fluid and electrolyte balance (see Nursing Diagnosis 2, action a.3).
3. If signs and symptoms of shock occur:
  a. continue with above measures
  b. place client flat in bed with legs elevated unless contraindicated
  c. monitor vital signs frequently
  d. administer oxygen as ordered
  e. monitor for therapeutic and nontherapeutic effects of the following if administered:
    1. blood products and/or volume expanders

2. vasopressors (may be given for a short period *to maintain mean arterial pressure*)

f. assist with application of military antishock trousers (MAST) if indicated

g. provide emotional support to client and significant others.

19.m. The client will not develop peritonitis as evidenced by:
1. no complaints of an increase in abdominal pain and tenderness
2. soft, nondistended abdomen after dialysate has drained
3. afebrile status
4. stable vital signs
5. normal bowel sounds
6. WBC count within normal range for client.

19.m.1. Assess for and report signs and symptoms of peritonitis (e.g. increase in severity of abdominal pain; rebound tenderness; tense, rigid abdomen after drainage of dialysate; elevated temperature; tachycardia; tachypnea; hypotension; diminished or absent bowel sounds).
2. Monitor WBC counts. Report increasing levels.
3. Implement measures *to prevent peritonitis:*
   a. dilute cytotoxic agent as recommended
   b. maintain patency of peritoneal catheter if present (e.g. keep tubing free of kinks, flush as ordered, keep collection device below level of abdomen)
   c. maintain aseptic technique during peritoneal catheter dressing changes and when accessing implanted infusion device
   d. keep peritoneal catheter dressings clean and dry
   e. monitor for therapeutic and nontherapeutic effects of anti-infectives if administered.
4. If signs and symptoms of peritonitis occur:
   a. discontinue infusion of cytotoxic drugs if ordered
   b. withhold all food and fluid as ordered
   c. place client on bedrest in a semi-Fowler's position *to assist in pooling or localizing drainage in the pelvis rather than under the diaphragm*
   d. insert a nasogastric or intestinal tube and maintain suction as ordered
   e. monitor for therapeutic and nontherapeutic effects of anti-infectives if administered
   f. monitor for therapeutic and nontherapeutic effects of intravenous fluids and/or blood volume expanders if administered *to prevent or treat shock* (*shock can occur as a result of the escape of protein, fluid, and electrolytes into the peritoneal cavity*)
   g. provide emotional support to client and significant others.

20. NURSING DIAGNOSIS

Sexual dysfunction:

a. **decreased libido** related to:
1. disturbance in self-concept
2. anxiety, pain, weakness, and fatigue
3. fear of rejection by partner associated with perceived loss of sexual appeal resulting from changes in physical appearance
4. ovarian and/or testicular failure associated with extensive therapy with cytotoxic drugs, particularly alkylating agents;
b. **dyspareunia** related to:
1. mucositis and ulceration of the vaginal mucosa associated with effects of cytotoxic drugs on the rapidly dividing epithelial cells
2. dryness of vaginal mucosa associated with decreased estrogen levels (may occur due to ovarian failure resulting from extensive chemotherapy);
c. **impotence** related to psychological factors and/or hormone imbalance associated with testicular failure that may result from treatment with cytotoxic drugs, particularly alkylating agents.

DESIRED OUTCOMES	**NURSING ACTIONS AND *SELECTED RATIONALES***

20. The client will demonstrate beginning acceptance of changes in sexual functioning as evidenced by:
   a. verbalization of a perception of self as sexually acceptable and adequate
   b. statements reflecting beginning adjustment to the effects of chemotherapy on sexual functioning
   c. maintenance of relationships with significant others.

20.a. Assess for signs and symptoms of sexual dysfunction (e.g. verbalization of sexual concerns, failure to maintain relationships with significant others).
   b. Determine attitudes, knowledge, and concerns about effects of chemotherapy on sexual functioning.
   c. Communicate interest, understanding, and respect for the values of the client and his/her partner.
   d. Provide accurate information about effects of chemotherapy on sexual functioning (e.g. decreased libido, dyspareunia, impotence). Encourage questions and clarify misconceptions.
   e. Assure client that many of the side effects of chemotherapy are temporary or can be treated.
   f. Facilitate communication between the client and his/her partner. Assist them to identify factors that may affect their sexual relationship.
   g. Arrange for uninterrupted privacy during hospital stay if desired by the couple.
   h. Implement measures to improve self-concept (see Nursing Diagnosis 21, actions c–q).
   i. Implement measures to reduce fear and anxiety (see Nursing Diagnosis 1, action c).
   j. Instruct client in measures *to decrease discomfort associated with decreased vaginal secretions and mucositis:*
      1. use an ample amount of a water-soluble lubricant *to prevent trauma to vaginal mucosa and increase lubrication during intercourse*
      2. utilize a vaginal steroid cream as ordered *to ease dryness and inflammation if present*
      3. take a sitz bath 2–3 times a day
      4. avoid intercourse until mucositis of the vaginal canal resolves.
   k. Instruct client to allow for adequate rest periods before and after sexual activity.
   l. If impotence is a problem:
      1. encourage client to discuss it with physician (impotence usually resolves after cessation of therapy)
      2. suggest alternative methods of sexual gratification and use of assistive devices if appropriate
      3. discuss ways to be creative in expressing sexuality (e.g. massage, fantasies, cuddling)
      4. encourage client to discuss the possibility of a penile prosthesis with physician if impotence will be permanent.
   m. Monitor for therapeutic and nontherapeutic effects of hormone replacements (e.g. estrogen, testosterone) if administered *to relieve symptoms.*
   n. Include partner in above discussions and encourage his/her continued support of the client.
   o. Consult physician if counseling appears indicated.

□ ▮▮▮▮▮▮▮▮▮▮▮▮▮▮▮▮▮▮▮▮▮▮▮▮▮▮▮▮▮▮▮▮

21. NURSING DIAGNOSIS

Disturbance in self-concept* related to:

a. changes in appearance (e.g. alopecia, excessive weight loss, skin changes) associated with side effects of chemotherapy and presence of external catheter;
b. possible alteration in usual sexual activities associated with weakness, fatigue, ovarian or testicular failure, and vaginal discomfort;

---

* This diagnostic label includes the nursing diagnoses of body image disturbance and self-esteem disturbance.

c. temporary or permanent sterility associated with gonadal dysfunction resulting from extensive therapy with cytotoxic drugs (particularly alkylating agents);
d. increased dependence on others to meet self-care needs;
e. changes in life style and roles associated with effects of the disease process and its treatment.

DESIRED OUTCOMES	NURSING ACTIONS AND *SELECTED RATIONALES*

21. The client will demonstrate beginning adaptation to changes in appearance, body functioning, life style, and roles as evidenced by:
a. verbalization of feelings of self-worth and sexual adequacy
b. maintenance of relationships with significant others
c. active participation in activities of daily living
d. active interest in personal appearance
e. willingness to participate in social activities
f. verbalization of a beginning plan for adapting life style to meet restrictions imposed by the residual effects of chemotherapy.
	21.a. Determine the meaning of changes in appearance, body functioning, life style, and roles to the client by encouraging him/her to verbalize feelings and by noting nonverbal responses to changes experienced.
	b. Assess for signs and symptoms of a disturbance in self-concept (e.g. verbal or nonverbal cues denoting a negative response to changes in body functioning or appearance such as denial of or preoccupation with changes that have occurred or withdrawal from significant others).
	c. Reinforce actions to facilitate the grieving process (see Nursing Diagnosis 23, action d).
	d. Assist client to identify strengths and qualities that have a positive effect on his/her self-concept.
	e. Implement measures *to assist client to increase self-esteem* (e.g. limit negative self-criticism, encourage positive comments about self, give positive feedback about accomplishments).
	f. Reinforce actions to assist client to cope with effects of chemotherapy (see Nursing Diagnosis 22, action d).
	g. Reinforce actions that may assist client to adjust to alteration in sexual functioning (see Nursing Diagnosis 20, actions c–n).
	h. Implement measures *to assist client to adapt to the following changes in body functioning and appearance if appropriate:*
	  1. alopecia:
	    a. inform client that hair loss can be expected approximately 2 weeks after initiation of chemotherapy; may be sudden, gradual, partial, or complete; and can extend to other parts of the body such as pubic hair, beard, eyebrows, and eyelashes
	    b. reassure client that hair loss is temporary (regrowth sometimes occurs before cessation of treatment but usually occurs 2–3 months after it)
	    c. inform client that hair regrowth may be a different color, texture, and consistency
	    d. encourage client to cut long hair *to decrease the debris and anxiety related to seeing large quantities of hair fall out*
	    e. inform client that he/she *can reduce rate of scalp hair loss by:*
	      1. brushing hair gently using a soft bristle brush
	      2. avoiding use of harsh shampoos
	      3. wearing an ice cap or scalp tourniquet if offered during drug administration to *reduce blood supply and therefore contact of the cytotoxic agent with hair follicles*
	    f. encourage client to use a wig, scarf, false eyelashes, or makeup if desired *to camouflage hair loss*; contact the American Cancer Society for a wig if client desires one but is unable to obtain it
	    g. encourage use of the wig before hair loss *to facilitate adjustment to wig and its integration into self-image*
	  2. skin and vein hyperpigmentation:
	    a. inform client that skin and vein hyperpigmentation may occur if he/she is receiving cytotoxic drugs such as bleomycin, busulfan, methotrexate, and 5-fluorouracil
	    b. inform client that skin and vein discoloration is usually temporary

      c. instruct client to avoid exposure to sunlight and to use sun screens *to prevent increase in hyperpigmentation and photosensitivity reactions*

      d. assist client to identify types of clothing that can be worn to camouflage hyperpigmented areas

    3. nail changes:

      a. inform client that his/her nails may thicken and stop growing, develop ridges, darken, and detach from nail bed during treatment with certain cytotoxic drugs (e.g. cyclophosphamide, doxorubicin, bleomycin, 5-fluorouracil)

      b. reassure client that normal nail growth will resume when chemotherapy is completed

    4. sterility or decreased fertility:

      a. clarify physician's explanation that sterility is a possible permanent effect of chemotherapy; caution the female client that ovarian failure during therapy may result in decreased libido, irritability, hot flashes, and other symptoms of premature menopause

      b. encourage client in the childbearing years to use contraception (*many cytotoxic drugs cause genetic abnormalities in the developing fetus*)

      c. discuss alternative methods of becoming a parent (e.g. artificial insemination, adoption) if of concern to client

      d. before chemotherapy is begun, suggest the possibility of sperm-banking to the male client if sperm is of good concentration and motility

      e. reinforce the need to take hormone replacements (e.g. estrogen, testosterone) as prescribed.

  i. Assist client with usual grooming and makeup habits if necessary.

  j. Assess for and support behaviors suggesting positive adaptation to changes that have occurred (e.g. interest in personal appearance, maintenance of relationships with significant others).

  k. Assist client's and significant others' adjustment to changes by listening, facilitating communication, and providing information.

  l. Encourage significant others to allow client to do what he/she is able *so that independence can be re-established and/or self-esteem redeveloped.*

  m. Encourage client contact with others *so that he/she can test and establish a new self-image.*

  n. Ensure that client and significant others have similar expectations and understanding of future life style. Assist them to identify ways that personal and family goals can be adjusted rather than abandoned.

  o. Encourage visits and support from significant others.

  p. Encourage client to continue involvement in social activities and to pursue interests. If previous interests and hobbies cannot be pursued, encourage development of new ones.

  q. Provide information about and encourage utilization of community agencies or support groups (e.g. vocational rehabilitation; sexual, family, individual, and/or financial counseling).

  r. Consult physician about psychological counseling if client desires or if he/she seems unwilling or unable to adapt to changes that have occurred as a result of cancer and its treatment.

22. NURSING DIAGNOSIS

Ineffective individual coping related to an inadequate support system, persistent discomfort associated with the side effects of chemotherapy, fear, anxiety, chronic fatigue, and uncertainty of the effectiveness of chemotherapy.

DESIRED OUTCOMES	NURSING ACTIONS AND *SELECTED RATIONALES*

22. The client will demonstrate the use of effective coping skills as evidenced by:
    a. willingness to participate in treatment plan and self-care activities
    b. verbalization of ability to cope with chemotherapy and its effects
    c. identification of stressors
    d. utilization of appropriate problem-solving techniques
    e. recognition and utilization of available support systems.

22.a. Assess effectiveness of client's coping strategies by observing behavior and noting strengths, weaknesses, ability to express feelings and concerns, and willingness to participate in the treatment plan.
   b. Assess for and report signs and symptoms that may indicate ineffective coping (e.g. sleep disturbances, increasing fatigue, difficulty concentrating, irritability, decreased tolerance for pain, verbalization of inability to cope, inability to problem-solve).
   c. Allow time for client to adjust psychologically to diagnosis, need for chemotherapy, side effects of drugs administered, and anticipated changes in life style and roles.
   d. Implement measures *to promote effective coping*:
      1. arrange for a visit with another who has been successfully treated for cancer with cytotoxic drugs
      2. perform actions to reduce fear and anxiety (see Nursing Diagnosis 1, action c)
      3. perform actions to reduce discomfort (see Nursing Diagnoses 5.A, action 2; 5.B, action 6; 5.C, action 3; 5.D, action 2; and 5.E, actions 2 and 3)
      4. perform actions to reduce fatigue (see Nursing Diagnosis 10, action e)
      5. include client in planning of care, encourage maximum participation in treatment plan, and allow choices when possible *to enable him/her to maintain a sense of control*
      6. instruct client in effective problem-solving techniques (e.g. accurate identification of stressors, determination of various options to solve problem)
      7. assist client to maintain usual daily routines whenever possible
      8. assist client as he/she starts to plan for necessary life-style and role changes; provide input related to realistic prioritization of problems that need to be dealt with
      9. assist the client and significant others to identify ways that personal and family goals can be adjusted rather than abandoned
      10. assist client to identify and utilize available support systems; provide information regarding available community resources that can assist client and significant others in coping with effects of chemotherapy and diagnosis of cancer (e.g. American Cancer Society; support groups; individual, family, and financial counselors).
   e. Encourage continued emotional support from significant others.
   f. Encourage client to share with significant others the kind of support that would be most beneficial to him/her (e.g. listening, inspiring hope, providing reassurance and accurate information).
   g. Assess for and support behaviors suggesting positive adaptation to changes experienced (e.g. willingness to care for central venous catheter, compliance with treatment plan, verbalization of ability to cope, utilization of effective problem-solving strategies).
   h. Consult physician about psychological counseling if appropriate. Initiate a referral if necessary.

□ ▬▬▬▬▬▬▬▬▬▬▬▬▬▬▬▬▬▬▬▬▬▬▬

23. NURSING DIAGNOSIS

Grieving* related to:

a. changes in body image and usual roles and life style;
b. diagnosis of cancer with potential for premature death.

---

* This diagnostic label includes anticipatory grieving and grieving following the actual losses/changes.

□ ▬▬▬▬▬▬▬▬▬▬▬▬▬▬▬▬▬▬▬▬▬▬▬

DESIRED OUTCOMES	**NURSING ACTIONS AND *SELECTED RATIONALES***

23. The client will demonstrate beginning progression through the grieving process as evidenced by:
    a. verbalization of feelings about the diagnosis of cancer and chemotherapy
    b. expression of grief
    c. participation in the treatment plan and self-care activities
    d. utilization of available support systems
    e. verbalization of a plan for integrating prescribed follow-up care into life style.

23.a. Determine the client's perception of the impact of the diagnosis of cancer and chemotherapy on his/her future.
   b. Determine how client usually expresses grief.
   c. Observe for signs of grieving (e.g. changes in eating habits, insomnia, anger, noncompliance, denial).
   d. Implement measures *to facilitate the grieving process:*
      1. assist client to acknowledge the losses and changes experienced *so grief work can begin*; assess for factors that may hinder or facilitate acknowledgment
      2. discuss the grieving process and assist client to accept the stages of grieving as an expected response to actual and/or anticipated changes or losses
      3. allow time for client to progress through the stages of grieving (denial, anger, bargaining, depression, acceptance [Kübler-Ross, 1969]); be aware that not every stage is experienced or expressed by all individuals
      4. provide an atmosphere of care and concern (e.g. provide privacy, be available and nonjudgmental, display empathy and respect) *so that client will feel free to verbalize both positive and negative feelings and concerns*
      5. perform actions *to promote trust* (e.g. answer questions honestly, provide requested information)
      6. encourage the expression of anger and sadness about the losses/changes experienced
      7. encourage client to express his/her feelings in whatever ways are comfortable (e.g. writing, drawing, conversation)
      8. perform actions to facilitate effective coping (see Nursing Diagnosis 22, action d)
      9. support realistic hope about the prognosis and the temporary nature of most of the physical changes.
   e. Assess for and support behaviors suggesting successful resolution of grief (e.g. verbalizing feelings about losses, expressing sorrow, focusing on ways to adapt to changes/losses).
   f. Explain the stages of the grieving process to significant others. Encourage their support and understanding.
   g. Provide information regarding counseling services and support groups that might assist client in working through grief.
   h. Arrange for visit from clergy if desired by client.
   i. Monitor for therapeutic and nontherapeutic effects of antidepressants if administered.
   j. Consult physician regarding referral for counseling if signs of dysfunctional grieving (e.g. persistent denial of losses or changes, excessive anger or sadness, hysteria, suicidal behaviors, phobias) occur.

□ ▬▬▬▬▬▬▬▬▬▬▬▬▬▬▬▬▬▬▬▬▬▬▬▬

24. NURSING DIAGNOSIS

Knowledge deficit regarding follow-up care.

□ ▬▬▬▬▬▬▬▬▬▬▬▬▬▬▬▬▬▬▬▬▬▬▬▬

DESIRED OUTCOMES	**NURSING ACTIONS AND *SELECTED RATIONALES***

24.a. The client will identify ways to prevent infection during periods of lowered immunity.

24.a.1. Explain to client that his/her resistance to infection is reduced when WBC counts are low. Emphasize the need to adhere closely to recommended techniques to prevent infection.
   2. Instruct the client in ways *to prevent infection:*

a. avoid crowds, persons with any sign of infection, and persons recently vaccinated
b. avoid any trauma to skin or mucous membranes
c. take axillary rather than oral temperature if stomatitis is present
d. lubricate skin frequently *to prevent dryness and subsequent cracking*
e. cleanse any breaks in the skin with a recommended antiseptic solution as directed
f. use excellent handwashing technique
g. maintain sterile technique in caring for a central venous or peritoneal catheter, Ommaya reservoir, or implanted infusion device (e.g. MediPort) if in place
h. avoid any unnecessary rectal invasion (e.g. temperature taking, enemas, suppositories, sexual activity) *to prevent rectal trauma and subsequent infection, fistula, or abscess formation*
i. if hemorrhoids are present, avoid situations that could aggravate them (e.g. constipation, sitting for prolonged periods)
j. avoid constipation *to prevent damage to the rectal mucosa from hard or impacted stool*
k. wash perianal area thoroughly with soap and water after each bowel movement; instruct female client to always wipe from front to back after urination and defecation
l. drink at least 10 glasses of liquid/day
m. cough and deep breathe or use inspiratory exerciser every 2 hours until usual activity is resumed
n. stop smoking
o. perform meticulous oral hygiene
p. avoid douching unless ordered (*douching disturbs normal vaginal flora, thereby increasing susceptibility to infection*)
q. maintain an optimal nutritional status (e.g. diet high in protein, calories, vitamins, and minerals)
r. avoid intake of foods with a high bacterial content (e.g. fresh fruit, uncooked foods)
s. avoid sharing eating utensils
t. maintain an adequate balance between activity and rest.

24.b. The client will demonstrate the ability to correctly take an oral and axillary temperature.

24.b.1. Demonstrate the proper way to take an oral and axillary temperature.
2. Allow time for questions, clarification, and return demonstration.

24.c. The client will demonstrate appropriate oral hygiene techniques.

24.c.1. Explain rationale for and importance of frequent oral hygiene.
2. Provide instructions regarding oral hygiene techniques:
a. cleanse mouth after eating and at bedtime; increase frequency to every 2 hours if stomatitis is present
b. use a soft bristle toothbrush *to prevent trauma to fragile mucous membranes*
c. rinse mouth frequently with the following types of solutions as necessary:
1. hydrogen peroxide (1 tbsp/cup of water) if crusting and/or debris are present; mix just before use (*hydrogen peroxide rapidly decomposes when mixed with water*)
2. baking soda (½ tsp/cup of water) if hardened mucus and crusts need to be removed
3. salt (1 tsp/quart of water) after use of either of above solutions and as a routine mouthwash
d. avoid commercial mouthwashes that have an alcohol base (*these are drying to oral mucosa*).

24.d. The client will identify techniques to control nausea and vomiting.

24.d. Instruct client in methods *to control nausea and vomiting:*
1. eat foods that are cool or room temperature (*hot foods frequently have an overpowering aroma that stimulates nausea*)
2. eat dry foods (e.g. toast, crackers) or sour foods (e.g. lemon drops, pickles, lemon ice) or sip cold carbonated beverages if nausea is present
3. eat several small meals instead of 3 large ones

4. avoid liquids at mealtime
5. select bland foods (e.g. mashed potatoes, applesauce, cottage cheese) rather than fatty, spicy foods (e.g. fried potatoes, chili)
6. rest after eating
7. if feasible, have someone else prepare the food
8. avoid offensive odors and sights
9. cleanse mouth frequently
10. take deep, slow breaths when nauseated
11. take antiemetics on a regular basis if nausea is persistent.

24.e. The client will verbalize ways to improve appetite and nutritional status.

24.e. Instruct client in ways *to improve appetite and maintain an adequate nutritional status:*
1. try fish, cheese, and eggs as protein sources instead of beef and pork if taste distortion is a problem
2. increase amount of sugar or sweeteners and seasonings usually used in foods or beverages
3. eat in a pleasant environment with company if possible
4. perform frequent meticulous oral hygiene *to eliminate disagreeable tastes in mouth*
5. try recommended methods of controlling nausea (see action d in this diagnosis)
6. eat high-caloric, high-protein, nutritious snacks rather than 3 meals/day
7. take vitamins, minerals, and hematinics as prescribed.

24.f. The client will verbalize ways to manage and cope with persistent fatigue.

24.f. Instruct client in ways *to manage and cope with persistent fatigue:*
1. view fatigue as a protective mechanism rather than a problematic limitation
2. determine ways in which daily patterns of activity can be modified *to conserve energy and prevent excessive fatigue* (e.g. spread light and heavy tasks throughout the day, take short rests during an activity whenever possible, sit during an activity whenever possible, take several short rest periods during the day instead of one long one)
3. determine if life demands are realistic in light of physical state and adjust short- and long-term goals accordingly
4. avoid situations that are particularly fatiguing such as those that are boring, frustrating, or require prolonged or strenuous physical activity
5. participate in a regular aerobic exercise program *to improve cardiovascular and respiratory fitness, reduce anxiety and stress, and build up tolerance for activity.*

24.g. The client will verbalize ways to prevent urinary calculi.

24.g. Instruct the client in ways *to prevent urinary uric acid stone formation:*
1. avoid foods high in purine (e.g. liver, kidney, goose, venison, seafood, meat soups and gravies, anchovies)
2. increase intake of foods/fluids that leave an alkaline ash (e.g. milk; vegetables, especially legumes and green vegetables; fruits except prunes, plums, and cranberries)
3. drink at least 10 glasses of liquid/day
4. increase activity as tolerated and void whenever the urge is felt *to prevent urinary stasis*
5. take medication to decrease uric acid production as prescribed.

24.h. The client will verbalize ways to prevent bleeding when platelet counts are low.

24.h.1. Instruct client in ways *to minimize risk of bleeding:*
a. avoid taking aspirin, aspirin-containing compounds, and ibuprofen
b. use an electric rather than a straight-edge razor
c. floss and brush teeth gently
d. cut nails and cuticles carefully
e. use caution when ambulating *to prevent falls or bumps*
f. avoid situations that could result in injury (e.g. contact sports)
g. avoid straining to have a bowel movement
h. avoid blowing nose forcefully
i. avoid constrictive clothing.
2. Instruct client to control any bleeding by applying firm, prolonged pressure to the area if possible.

UNIT V

24.i. The client will demonstrate the ability to care for a central venous cathether, peritoneal catheter, or an implanted infusion device if in place.

24.i.1. Provide instructions related to care of a central venous catheter (e.g. Groshong) if appropriate:
   a. change dressing if present according to protocol utilizing aseptic technique
   b. observe exit site for changes in appearance, redness, swelling, or unusual drainage
   c. flush catheter according to protocol *to maintain patency* (syringe should be attached directly to connector hub rather than injection cap)
   d. replace injection cap as directed
   e. tape catheter securely to the chest wall *to prevent accidental dislodgment*
   f. notify physician if unable to flush catheter, if signs and symptoms of infection occur at exit site, or if catheter appears to be leaking.
2. Provide instructions related to care of a peritoneal catheter if in place:
   a. change dressing daily according to protocol utilizing aseptic technique
   b. keep catheter capped between treatments
   c. keep water below the level of the catheter when taking a tub bath (a tub bath may be taken 7–10 days after catheter insertion)
   d. observe for and notify physician if any of the following occur:
      1. change in appearance, redness, swelling, or unusual drainage from exit site
      2. increasing abdominal pain
      3. chills and fever
      4. increased abdominal distention between treatments
      5. persistent nausea and vomiting
      6. dyspnea.
3. Provide instructions related to care of an implanted infusion device (e.g. MediPort, Port-a-Cath) if in place:
   a. keep appointment to have device flushed or flush as instructed
   b. avoid trauma to insertion site
   c. notify physician if area around infusion device becomes reddened or painful.
4. Allow time for questions, clarification, and return demonstration of procedures.

24.j. The client will verbalize an understanding of the care and precautions necessary if an Ommaya reservoir is in place.

24.j. Provide instructions related to care and precautions necessary if an Ommaya reservoir is in place:
   1. wash site daily with soap and water
   2. observe for and report redness, drainage, and discomfort at insertion site; stiff neck; and persistent headache
   3. avoid any activities that could result in trauma to the head and damage to reservoir.

24.k. The client will verbalize an understanding of an implanted infusion pump and precautions necessary if one is in place.

24.k.1. Reinforce physician's explanation about the purpose of the pump and how it works.
2. Instruct client to avoid any activities that could result in abdominal trauma and dislodgment of pump.
3. Caution client to notify physician if:
   a. air travel is planned (*client should carry an explanatory letter since pump may trigger airport weapon security devices; flow rate may also need to be adjusted if the flight time is lengthy*)
   b. body temperature is elevated more than 2°F for more than 24 hours (*increase in vapor pressure would increase flow rate*)
   c. he/she plans to move to an area of greater or lesser altitude (*alterations in flow rate would need to be made*)
   d. redness, swelling, or drainage occurs at incisional or refilling site.
4. Emphasize importance of keeping appointments to have pump refilled (*permanent blockage of the catheter will occur if pump is allowed to empty completely*).

24.l. The client will state signs and symptoms of complications to report to the health care provider.

24.l. Instruct client to observe for and report the following:
   1. signs and symptoms of infection (stress that usual signs of infection are lacking in people with altered bone marrow function and/or a suppressed immune system and that it is necessary to monitor closely for the following signs and symptoms):

    a. temperature above 38°C (100.4°F)
    b. changes in odor, color, or consistency of urine or pain on urination
    c. white patches in mouth or vagina
    d. crusted ulcerations around or in oral cavity
    e. swollen, reddened, coated tongue
    f. painful rectal or vaginal area
    g. redness, increased pain, or bleeding of hemorrhoids
    h. changes in the appearance or temperature of skin particularly around injection sites
    i. appearance of painful, pruritic skin lesions particularly in cervical or thoracic area
    j. persistent productive or nonproductive cough

2. signs and symptoms of bleeding (e.g. excessive bruising, black stools, persistent nose bleeds or bleeding from gums, sudden swelling and pain in joints, red or smoke-colored urine, blood in vomitus)
3. signs and symptoms of urinary calculi (e.g. dull, aching or sharp, colicky flank pain; urinary urgency or frequency; unusual appearance of urine)
4. signs and symptoms of hemorrhagic cystitis (e.g. blood in urine, pain on urination, urinary frequency or urgency)
5. signs and symptoms of extravasation (e.g. redness, pain, swelling, and/or skin changes at infusion site)
6. signs and symptoms of pulmonary dysfunction (e.g. shortness of breath; persistent dry, hacking cough; fever)
7. signs and symptoms of dehydration (e.g. dry mouth, weight loss, concentrated urine, lightheadedness)
8. signs and symptoms of sodium deficit (e.g. nausea, vomiting, abdominal cramps, weakness, muscle twitching, seizures)
9. signs and symptoms of potassium deficit (e.g. irregular pulse, muscle weakness, cramps, numbness and tingling of extremities)
10. signs and symptoms of cardiotoxicity (e.g. irregular or rapid heart rate, increased weakness and fatigue, shortness of breath, unexplained weight gain, swelling of extremities); emphasize that cardiotoxicity can occur several days to months after administration of drugs known to cause it
11. signs and symptoms of neurotoxicity (e.g. numbness and tingling of extremities, change in hearing acuity, blurred vision or change in ability to perceive and discriminate color, constipation, change in motor function and coordination)
12. inability to eat
13. significant weight loss
14. inability to cope with the effects of the diagnosis and treatment.

24.m. The client will identify community resources that can assist with home management and adjustment to the diagnosis of cancer and chemotherapy and its effects.

24.m.1. Provide information about and encourage utilization of community resources that can assist client and significant others with home management and adjustment to diagnosis of cancer and chemotherapy and its effects (e.g. American Cancer Society, Visiting Nurse Association, counselors, social service agencies, Meals on Wheels, Make Today Count, Hospice, local community support groups).
    2. Initiate a referral if indicated.

24.n. The client will verbalize an understanding of and a plan for adhering to recommended follow-up care including schedule for chemotherapy, laboratory studies, and future appointments with health care provider and medications prescribed.

24.n.1. Reinforce physician's explanation of planned chemotherapy schedule (varies according to protocol used).
    2. Discuss with client any difficulties he/she might have adhering to the schedule and assist in planning ways to overcome these.
    3. Reinforce importance of keeping appointments for chemotherapy and laboratory studies.
    4. Reinforce importance of keeping follow-up appointments with health care provider.
    5. Thoroughly explain rationale for, side effects of, and importance of taking medications prescribed.
    6. Implement measures *to improve client compliance:*
      a. include significant others in teaching sessions
      b. encourage questions and allow time for reinforcement and clarification of information provided

    c. provide written instructions regarding ways to maintain nutritional status, future appointments with health care provider and laboratory, medications prescribed, and signs and symptoms to report.

Reference

Kübler-Ross, E. On death and dying. New York: Macmillan, 1969.

External Radiation Therapy

Radiation therapy is one of the four major modes of treatment for cancer. It is used alone or in combination with surgery, chemotherapy, or immunotherapy to achieve palliative or curative results. Radiation therapy can be either external or internal (brachytherapy) and is a local treatment with cellular destruction occurring only at the treatment site. Radiation therapy is effective because it stimulates change in both the structure and function of the cell. Unfortunately, it is not a selective process and similar changes will occur in both the cancerous and the normal cell. The normal cell, however, has a greater capacity for self-repair.

Radiation therapy is a complex process with the effect on the cell beginning immediately and continuing for an unlimited time period. The time of cellular death and the side effects experienced by the client depend on the radiation absorbed dose (rad), whether or not both strands of DNA are broken, the condition of the cellular membrane, the mitotic rate of the cell, and the damage to the cell's reproductive abilities. The side effects that all clients receiving external radiation may experience are a skin reaction at the radiation entry and/or exit sites, fatigue, malaise, and anorexia. Other side effects experienced depend on the anatomical site being radiated, fractionation of the dose, total dose delivered, and general condition of the client.

This care plan focuses on the adult client hospitalized for initiation of external radiation therapy. The major goals of care are to maintain comfort; prevent complications; and educate the client about radiation therapy, expected side effects, and toxic effects to be reported. The nurse also plays a major role in supporting and assisting the client and significant others to cope with changes that may occur in body image, life style, and roles as a result of cancer and radiation therapy.

DISCHARGE CRITERIA

Prior to discharge, the client will:

- demonstrate the ability to give appropriate skin care at radiation entry and exit sites
- identify techniques to control nausea and vomiting
- verbalize ways to improve appetite and nutritional status
- demonstrate appropriate oral hygiene techniques
- identify ways to prevent urinary calculi
- identify ways to prevent bleeding if platelet counts are low
- identify ways to prevent infection if WBC counts are low
- verbalize an understanding of the effects of radiation therapy on reproductive function

- verbalize ways to manage and cope with persistent fatigue
- state signs and symptoms of complications to report to the health care provider
- share feelings and thoughts about the effects of radiation therapy on body image
- identify community resources that can assist with home management and adjustment to the diagnosis of cancer and radiation therapy and its effects
- verbalize an understanding of and a plan for adhering to recommended follow-up care including future appointments with health care provider, radiation department, and laboratory and medications prescribed.

NURSING/COLLABORATIVE DIAGNOSES

1. Anxiety □ *158*
2. Altered fluid and electrolyte balance:
   a. fluid volume deficit, hyponatremia, hypokalemia, and hypochloremia
   b. metabolic acidosis
   c. metabolic alkalosis □ *159*
3. Altered nutrition: less than body requirements □ *161*
4. Impaired swallowing □ *162*
5A. Altered comfort:
   1. pain within the irradiated area
   2. perianal pain
   3. oral, pharyngeal, and esophageal pain
   4. headache □ *163*
5B. Altered comfort: nausea and vomiting □ *164*
5C. Altered comfort: pruritus □ *165*
6. Impaired verbal communication □ *166*
7. Impaired skin integrity: irritation and breakdown □ *167*
8. Altered oral mucous membrane:
   a. dryness
   b. stomatitis □ *169*
9. Fatigue □ *170*
10. Activity intolerance □ *171*
11. Self-care deficit □ *172*
12. Diarrhea □ *172*
13. Sleep pattern disturbance □ *173*
14. Potential for infection □ *174*
15. Potential for trauma □ *175*
16. Potential complications:
   a. bleeding
   b. dental caries and periodontal disease
   c. acute or chronic pericarditis
   d. radiation cystitis
   e. renal calculi □ *176*
17. Sexual dysfunction:
   a. decreased libido
   b. temporary or permanent impotence
   c. dyspareunia □ *179*
18. Disturbance in self-concept □ *180*
19. Ineffective individual coping □ *182*
20. Grieving □ *183*
21. Knowledge deficit regarding follow-up care □ *184*

1. NURSING DIAGNOSIS

Anxiety related to:

a. unfamiliar environment;
b. lack of knowledge and preconceived ideas about radiation therapy and its potential effects on physiological functioning and usual life style and roles;
c. diagnosis of cancer with potential for premature death.

DESIRED OUTCOMES	NURSING ACTIONS AND *SELECTED RATIONALES*

1. The client will experience a reduction in fear and anxiety as evidenced by:
a. verbalization of feeling less anxious or fearful
b. relaxed facial expression and body movements
c. stable vital signs
d. usual skin color
e. verbalization of an understanding of hospital routines and radiation therapy and its effects.
	1.a. Assess client on admission for:
	  1. fears, misconceptions, and level of understanding of radiation therapy and its therapeutic and nontherapeutic effects
	  2. concerns about particular side effects of radiation and their effect on his/her life style
	  3. significance of the site to be irradiated
	  4. perception of the impact of daily radiation therapy for several weeks on usual life style and personal relationships
	  5. availability of an adequate support system
	  6. past experiences with radiation therapy or other treatments for cancer
	  7. signs and symptoms of fear and anxiety (e.g. verbalization of fears and concerns; tenseness; tremors; irritability; restlessness; diaphoresis; tachypnea; tachycardia; elevated blood pressure; facial tension, pallor, or flushing; noncompliance with treatment plan); validate perceptions carefully, remembering that some behavior may be a result of physiological changes associated with the disease process.
	b. Ascertain effectiveness of current coping skills.
	c. Implement measures *to reduce fear and anxiety:*
	  1. orient to hospital environment, equipment, and routines
	  2. introduce staff who will be participating in his/her care; if possible, maintain consistency in staff assigned to his/her care *to provide feelings of stability and comfort with the environment*
	  3. assure client that staff members are nearby; respond to call signal as soon as possible
	  4. maintain a calm, confident manner when interacting with client
	  5. encourage verbalization of fear and anxiety; provide feedback
	  6. reinforce physician's explanation of expected therapeutic effects of radiation therapy
	  7. provide instructions about radiation therapy:
	    a. explain how radiation therapy works and why total radiation dose prescribed is fractionated
	    b. inform client that he/she will be alone in the room during the few minutes of therapy but will be observed continuously via a television monitor; explain that he/she will be able to communicate by means of an intercommunication system
	    c. inform client that the machine may click or make a whirring noise but that no discomfort will be felt during treatment
	    d. assure client that his/her body, excreta, and clothing will not be radioactive
	    e. instruct client about the expected general side effects of radiation therapy (e.g. fatigue; anorexia; itchy, dry, reddened skin; dry or moist desquamation and increase in skin pigmentation at radiation site) and anticipated side effects for the particular site being irradiated; explain when they can be expected to occur and disappear

      f. explain the treatment simulation process the client will experience before initiation of therapy

      g. inform client that vital organs within the radiation treatment field(s) are shielded during treatment *to prevent unnecessary exposure to radiation*; assure client that the treatment field(s) will include the smallest amount of normal tissue possible and that field(s) may be changed or reduced as the tumor shrinks in size

      h. explain to client how treatment field(s) will be outlined (e.g. skin markings with an indelible dye, ink, or felt tip marker; plaster casts or molds; lead blocks); inform client that ink markings must not be washed off or altered between treatments

    8. arrange for client and significant others to visit the radiation department, see equipment and machines, and meet those responsible for his/her care

    9. prepare client for his/her waiting room experiences with others receiving therapy; emphasize that each is an individual with different treatment plans, responses, and prognoses and that comparison should be avoided

   10. reinforce physician's explanations and clarify any misconceptions client may have about the diagnosis of cancer, treatment plan, and prognosis

   11. allow time for client to adjust psychologically to the idea of radiation therapy and its effects

   12. provide a calm, restful environment

   13. instruct in relaxation techniques and encourage participation in diversional activities

   14. perform actions to assist client to cope with radiation therapy and its effects (see Nursing Diagnosis 19, action d)

   15. encourage significant others to project a caring, concerned attitude without obvious anxiousness

   16. monitor for therapeutic and nontherapeutic effects of antianxiety agents if administered.

  d. Include significant others in orientation and teaching sessions and encourage their continued support of client.

  e. Provide information based on current needs of client and significant others at a level they can understand. Encourage questions and clarification of information provided.

  f. Consult physician if above actions fail to control fear and anxiety.

2. NURSING/COLLABORATIVE DIAGNOSIS

Altered fluid and electrolyte balance:

a. **fluid volume deficit, hyponatremia, hypokalemia, and hypochloremia** related to:
  1. decreased oral intake associated with:
    a. anorexia
    b. oral, pharyngeal, and esophageal pain and dysphagia resulting from mucositis (occurs with radiation to head, neck, and upper chest)
    c. nausea
  2. excessive loss of fluid and electrolytes associated with persistent vomiting and diarrhea resulting from the effects of radiation on gastrointestinal tract;

b. **metabolic acidosis** related to hyponatremia and persistent radiation-induced diarrhea;

c. **metabolic alkalosis** related to persistent vomiting, hypokalemia, and hypochloremia.

DESIRED OUTCOMES	NURSING ACTIONS AND *SELECTED RATIONALES*

2.a. The client will maintain fluid and electrolyte balance as evidenced by:
1. normal skin turgor
2. moist mucous membranes
3. stable weight
4. B/P and pulse within normal range for client and stable with position change
5. balanced intake and output
6. urine specific gravity between 1.010 and 1.030
7. no evidence of irritability, confusion, lethargy, excessive thirst, ileus, cardiac arrhythmias, muscle weakness
8. normal serum osmolality and electrolytes.

2.a.1. Assess for and report signs and symptoms of:
  a. fluid volume deficit:
    1. decreased skin turgor, dry mucous membranes, thirst
    2. weight loss greater than 0.5 kg/day
    3. low B/P and/or decline in systolic B/P of at least 15 mm Hg with concurrent rise in pulse when client sits up
    4. weak, rapid pulse
    5. output less than intake with urine specific gravity higher than 1.030 (reflects an actual rather than potential fluid volume deficit)
  b. hyponatremia (e.g. nausea and vomiting, abdominal cramps, weakness, twitching, lethargy, confusion, seizures)
  c. hypokalemia (e.g. irregular pulse, muscle weakness and cramping, paresthesias, nausea and vomiting, hypoactive or absent bowel sounds, drowsiness)
  d. hypochloremia (e.g. twitching, tetany, depressed respirations).
2. Monitor serum osmolality and electrolyte results. Report abnormal values.
3. Implement measures *to prevent and treat fluid and electrolyte imbalances:*
  a. perform actions to control diarrhea (see Nursing Diagnosis 12, action d)
  b. perform actions to reduce vomiting (see Nursing Diagnosis 5.B, action 2)
  c. perform actions to improve oral intake (see Nursing Diagnosis 3, action f.1)
  d. monitor for therapeutic and nontherapeutic effects of fluid and electrolyte replacements if administered
  e. maintain a fluid intake of at least 2500 cc/day unless contraindicated
  f. assist client to select foods/fluids high in potassium (e.g. bananas, potatoes, raisins, figs, apricots, dates, Gatorade) and sodium (e.g. cured meats, processed cheese, soups, catsup, pickles, canned vegetables, bouillon) if serum sodium and potassium levels are low.
4. Consult physician if signs and symptoms of fluid and electrolyte imbalances persist or worsen.

2.b. The client will maintain acid-base balance as evidenced by:
1. usual mental status
2. unlabored respirations at 16–20/minute
3. absence of dizziness, confusion, headache, nausea, vomiting, paresthesias, muscle twitching, seizure activity
4. blood gases within normal range.

2.b.1. Assess for and report signs and symptoms of:
  a. metabolic acidosis (e.g. drowsiness; disorientation; stupor; rapid, deep respirations; headache; nausea; vomiting; low pH and CO_2 content and negative base excess)
  b. metabolic alkalosis (e.g. dizziness; confusion; bradypnea; tingling of fingers, toes, and circumoral area; muscle twitching; seizures; elevated pH and CO_2 content and positive base excess).
2. Implement measures *to prevent or treat metabolic acidosis:*
  a. perform actions to control diarrhea (see Nursing Diagnosis 12, action d)
  b. monitor for therapeutic and nontherapeutic effects of sodium bicarbonate if administered (reserved for use in severe acidosis when pH is less than 7.1)
  c. perform actions to maintain serum sodium within normal range (see action a.3 in this diagnosis).
3. Implement measures *to prevent or treat metabolic alkalosis:*
  a. perform actions to reduce vomiting (see Nursing Diagnosis 5.B, action 2)
  b. perform actions to maintain serum potassium and chloride within normal range (see action a.3 in this diagnosis).
4. Consult physician if signs and symptoms of acid-base imbalance persist or worsen.

3. NURSING DIAGNOSIS

Altered nutrition: less than body requirements related to:*

a. decreased oral intake associated with:
   1. anorexia resulting from:
      a. depression, fear, and anxiety
      b. fatigue and discomfort
      c. taste alteration associated with:
         1. destruction of microvilli of the taste cells, reduced salivation (food must be in solution to be dissolved and tasted) related to salivary gland damage, and destruction of nerve fibers that innervate the tongue if the radiation field includes head and neck area
         2. change in sense of smell and threshold for bitter, sweet, sour, and salt taste (particularly red meat, coffee, tea, tomatoes, and chocolate) related to the release of tumor byproducts into the bloodstream
         3. zinc, copper, nickel, niacin, and vitamin A deficiency and increased serum levels of calcium and lactate related to the disease process
      d. alteration in metabolism of proteins, fats, and carbohydrates
      e. early satiety associated with direct stimulation of the satiety center by anorexigenic factors (e.g. peptides) secreted by tumor cells
      f. increased concentration of neurotransmitters in the brain and/or derangements in the serotoninergic system associated with the disease process
   2. oral pain resulting from stomatitis
   3. dysphagia resulting from pharyngitis, esophagitis, and dry mouth
   4. nausea and dyspepsia;
b. loss of nutrients associated with vomiting;
c. malabsorption associated with loss of the absorptive surface of the intestinal mucosa resulting from ulceration and damage to the villi and microvilli of the intestine if the treatment field includes the abdomen or lower back;
d. elevated metabolic rate associated with an increased and continuous energy utilization by rapidly proliferating malignant cells;
e. utilization of available nutrients by the malignant cells rather than the host;
f. failure of feeding center to induce a sufficient increase in the intake of food to match metabolic needs;
g. inefficient and accelerated metabolism of proteins, fats, and carbohydrates associated with the disease process.

---

* Some of the etiologic factors presented here are currently under investigation.

DESIRED OUTCOMES	NURSING ACTIONS AND *SELECTED RATIONALES*
3. The client will maintain an adequate nutritional status as evidenced by: a. weight within normal range for client's age, height, and build b. normal BUN and serum albumin, protein, Hct., Hgb., B_{12}, and cholesterol levels	3.a. Assess the client for signs and symptoms of malnutrition: 1. weight below normal for client's age, height, and build 2. abnormal BUN and low serum albumin, protein, Hct., Hgb., B_{12}, and cholesterol levels 3. triceps skinfold measurement less than normal for build 4. weakness and fatigue 5. stomatitis. b. Monitor for and report: 1. declining serum zinc, copper, nickel, and niacin levels 2. increasing calcium and lactate levels.

c. triceps skinfold measurements within normal range
d. usual strength and activity tolerance
e. healthy oral mucous membrane.

c. Reassess nutritional status on a regular basis and report decline.
d. Monitor percentage of meals eaten.
e. Assess client to determine causes of inadequate intake (e.g. nausea, dyspepsia, dysphagia, fatigue, taste alteration, stomatitis).
f. Implement measures *to maintain an adequate nutritional status:*
  1. perform actions *to improve oral intake:*
    a. implement measures to relieve nausea and vomiting (see Nursing Diagnosis 5.B, action 2)
    b. implement measures to reduce oral, pharyngeal, and esophageal discomfort (see Nursing Diagnosis 5.A, action 5.d)
    c. implement measures to improve client's ability to swallow (see Nursing Diagnosis 4, action b)
    d. implement measures *to compensate for taste alteration* (loss of sense of taste occurs within 2 weeks of initiation of radiation treatment to head and neck, persists for 4–6 weeks after completion of therapy, and usually is not permanent):
      1. encourage client to select fish, cold cooked chicken, eggs, and cheese as protein sources if beef or pork tastes bitter or rancid
      2. provide meat for breakfast if aversion to meat tends to increase during day
      3. add extra sweeteners to foods if acceptable to client
      4. experiment with different flavorings, seasonings, and textures
      5. serve food warm *to stimulate the sense of smell*
      6. monitor for therapeutic and nontherapeutic effects of trace elements if administered *to correct abnormalities of taste*
    e. avoid serving liquids with meals *to minimize early satiety and nausea*
    f. serve small portions of nutritious foods/fluids that are appealing to the client
    g. provide a clean, relaxed, pleasant atmosphere
    h. encourage significant others to bring in client's favorite foods and eat with him/her *to make eating more of a familiar social experience*
    i. encourage a rest period before meals *to minimize fatigue*
    j. allow adequate time for meals; reheat food if necessary
    k. increase activity as tolerated (*activity stimulates appetite*)
    l. implement measures to assist client to progress through the grieving process (see Nursing Diagnosis 20, action d) and to cope effectively (see Nursing Diagnosis 19, action d)
    m. obtain a dietary consult if necessary to assist client in selecting foods/ fluids that meet nutritional needs (high-calorie, high-protein) as well as preferences
  2. ensure that meals are well balanced and high in essential nutrients
  3. monitor for therapeutic and nontherapeutic effects of vitamins, minerals, and hematinics if administered.
g. Perform a 72-hour calorie count if nutritional status declines or fails to improve.
h. Consult physician about alternative methods of providing nutrition (e.g. parenteral nutrition, tube feedings) if client does not consume enough food or fluids to meet nutritional needs.

□ ▬▬▬▬▬▬▬▬▬▬▬▬▬▬▬▬▬▬▬▬▬▬▬▬

4. NURSING DIAGNOSIS

Impaired swallowing related to:

a. oral, pharyngeal, and esophageal pain associated with inflammation and/or ulceration of the mucosa resulting from radiation to the head, neck, and upper chest;
b. dry mouth and viscous oral secretions associated with destruction of the salivary glands within the treatment field and reduced oral intake.

□ ▬▬▬▬▬▬▬▬▬▬▬▬▬▬▬▬▬▬▬▬▬▬▬▬

DESIRED OUTCOMES	NURSING ACTIONS AND *SELECTED RATIONALES*

4. The client will experience an improvement in swallowing as evidenced by:
   a. verbalization of same
   b. absence of coughing or choking when eating or drinking.

4.a. Assess for and report signs and symptoms of impaired swallowing (e.g. coughing or choking when eating or drinking, stasis of food in the oral cavity).
   b. Implement measures *to improve ability to swallow:*
      1. perform actions to reduce oral, pharyngeal, and esophageal pain (see Nursing Diagnosis 5.A, action 5.d)
      2. perform actions to decrease dryness of the oral mucous membrane (see Nursing Diagnosis 8, action a.2)
      3. assist client to select foods that are easily chewed and swallowed (e.g. custard, flavored gelatin, cottage cheese, ground meat)
      4. avoid serving foods that are sticky (e.g. peanut butter, soft bread, bananas)
      5. serve foods/fluids that are hot or cold instead of room temperature (*the more extreme temperatures stimulate the sensory receptors and swallowing reflex*)
      6. moisten dry foods with gravy or sauces (e.g. sour cream, salad dressing)
      7. perform actions *to stimulate salivation:*
         a. serve foods that are visually pleasing
         b. provide oral care before meals
         c. place a piece of lemon or sour pickle on plate
         d. if some saliva is present, provide sour, hard candy for client to suck just before meals unless contraindicated
      8. perform actions *to reduce and/or liquefy viscous oral secretions:*
         a. encourage a fluid intake of 2500 cc/day unless contraindicated
         b. encourage client to avoid milk and milk products (unless boiled) and chocolate (*when combined with saliva, these produce very thick secretions*)
         c. dissolve a papain product (e.g. papase tablet, meat tenderizer made from papaya) under tongue 10 minutes before eating (*papain contains a proteolytic enzyme that will liquefy secretions*)
      9. provide an oily liquid such as chicken or beef broth at the beginning of a meal.
   c. Consult physician if swallowing difficulties persist or worsen.

□ ▬▬▬▬▬▬▬▬▬▬▬▬▬▬▬▬▬▬▬▬▬▬▬▬

5.A. NURSING DIAGNOSIS

Altered comfort:*

1. **pain within the irradiated area** related to:
   a. inflammation associated with high cumulative doses of radiation (this level will vary depending on the site being irradiated)
   b. exposed nerve endings associated with moist desquamation;
2. **perianal pain** related to skin irritation and breakdown associated with diarrhea;
3. **oral, pharyngeal, and esophageal pain** related to inflammation and/or ulceration of the mucosa associated with a radiation exposure of approximately 3000 rads to head, neck, and upper chest (discomfort usually begins about 2 weeks after therapy is begun and persists for approximately a month after cessation of treatment);
4. **headache** related to cerebral edema associated with the inflammatory process if the brain is included within treatment field.

---

* In this care plan, the nursing diagnosis "pain" is included under the diagnostic label of altered comfort.

□ ▬▬▬▬▬▬▬▬▬▬▬▬▬▬▬▬▬▬▬▬▬▬▬▬

DESIRED OUTCOMES	NURSING ACTIONS AND *SELECTED RATIONALES*

5.A. The client will experience diminished pain as evidenced by:
1. verbalization of decreased pain
2. relaxed facial expression and body positioning
3. increased participation in activities
4. stable vital signs.

5.A.1. Determine how client usually responds to pain.
2. Assess for nonverbal signs of pain (e.g. guarding of irradiated area, wrinkled brow, clenched fists, reluctance to move, restlessness, diaphoresis, facial pallor or flushing, change in B/P, tachycardia).
3. Assess verbal complaints of pain. Ask client to be specific about location, severity, and type of pain.
4. Assess for factors that seem to aggravate and alleviate pain.
5. Implement measures *to reduce discomfort:*
   a. monitor for therapeutic and nontherapeutic effects of corticosteroids if administered *to reduce pain resulting from inflammation of irradiated area*
   b. perform actions *to reduce pain associated with moist desquamation:*
      1. keep irradiated site clean and dry
      2. apply dressings if ordered or position a covered bed cradle over affected area *to reduce airflow over exposed nerve endings*
   c. perform actions *to reduce perianal pain:*
      1. provide a foam pad for client to sit on
      2. consult physician about an order for sitz bath
      3. implement measures to decrease skin irritation and prevent breakdown associated with diarrhea (see Nursing Diagnosis 7, action c.3)
      4. avoid taking rectal temperature or administering suppositories
   d. perform actions *to reduce oral, pharyngeal, and esophageal pain:*
      1. implement measures to reduce severity of and discomfort of stomatitis (see Nursing Diagnosis 8, actions b.3–5)
      2. instruct client to avoid substances that might further irritate gastrointestinal mucosa (e.g. alcoholic beverages; extremely hot, spicy, or acidic foods/fluids; smoke; dry or hard foods; raw fruits and vegetables)
      3. encourage client to swallow antacids every 2 hours *to coat and protect inflamed tissues*
      4. offer cool, soothing liquids such as nonacidic juices, ices, and ice cream
      5. instruct client to gargle with a saline solution every 2 hours *to soothe the oral mucous membrane*
   e. perform actions *to relieve headache:*
      1. implement measures *to minimize environmental stimuli* (e.g. provide a calm environment, restrict visitors, dim lights)
      2. avoid jarring bed or startling client *to minimize risk of sudden movements*
   f. provide or assist with nonpharmacological measures for pain relief (e.g. cool cloth to forehead, back rub, position change, relaxation techniques, guided imagery, quiet conversation, restful environment, diversional activities)
   g. plan methods for achieving pain relief with client *in order to assist him/her to maintain a sense of control over the pain experience*
   h. monitor for therapeutic and nontherapeutic effects of analgesics if administered.
6. Consult physician if above measures fail to provide adequate pain relief.

☐ ▬▬▬▬▬▬▬▬▬▬▬▬▬▬▬▬▬

5.B. NURSING DIAGNOSIS

Altered comfort: nausea and vomiting related to stimulation of the vomiting center associated with:

1. stimulation of the chemoreceptor trigger zone resulting from absorption of toxic waste products from cellular destruction;
2. vagal and/or sympathetic stimulation resulting from visceral irritation associated

with inflammation of gastrointestinal mucosa (occurs when areas of chest, back, abdomen, and pelvis are irradiated);
3. direct stimulation resulting from:
   a. cerebral inflammation (occurs with radiation to the brain)
   b. absorption of toxic waste products from cellular destruction if receiving large daily dose of radiation or daily treatments over a period of several weeks;
4. cortical stimulation due to discomfort and stress.

DESIRED OUTCOMES	NURSING ACTIONS AND *SELECTED RATIONALES*

5.B. The client will experience a reduction in nausea and vomiting as evidenced by:
1. verbalization of decreased nausea
2. reduction in the number of episodes of vomiting.

5.B.1. Assess client to determine factors that contribute to nausea and vomiting (e.g. radiation to brain, chest, back, abdomen, or pelvis; daily radiation dose greater than 250 rads; prolonged treatment; fear; anxiety). Nausea and vomiting tend to occur within 6 hours and peak 12 hours after treatment or may be continuous.
2. Implement measures *to reduce nausea and vomiting:*
   a. eliminate noxious sights and smells from environment (*noxious stimuli cause cortical stimulation of the vomiting center*)
   b. encourage client to take deep, slow breaths when nauseated
   c. encourage client to change positions slowly (*movement stimulates the chemoreceptor trigger zone*)
   d. provide oral hygiene after each emesis and before meals
   e. maintain food and fluid restrictions if ordered (client may be placed on a clear liquid or bland diet for short periods *to reduce severe nausea*)
   f. instruct client to avoid foods/fluids for 3 hours before and after treatments
   g. provide small, frequent, low-fat meals (*fat delays emptying of the stomach*)
   h. instruct client to ingest foods and fluids slowly
   i. if nausea tends to peak and recede after each treatment, instruct client to eat his/her major meal of the day about 3 hours before treatment and to eat lightly for the rest of the day
   j. instruct client to avoid foods/fluids that irritate gastric mucosa (e.g. spicy foods; citrus fruits or juices; caffeine-containing items such as chocolate, coffee, tea, and colas)
   k. encourage client to eat dry foods (e.g. toast, crackers) and avoid drinking liquids with meals if nauseated
   l. provide carbonated beverages for client to sip if nauseated
   m. instruct client to rest after eating with head of bed elevated
   n. perform actions to reduce fear and anxiety (see Nursing Diagnosis 1, action c)
   o. perform actions to reduce pain (see Nursing Diagnosis 5.A, action 5)
   p. monitor for therapeutic and nontherapeutic effects of antiemetics if administered (these are often given 1–2 hours before radiation therapy and every 4–6 hours for 12 hours after treatment).
3. Consult physician if above measures fail to reduce nausea and vomiting.

5.C. NURSING DIAGNOSIS

Altered comfort: pruritus related to dry skin associated with impaired function of sebaceous and sweat glands within the treatment field resulting from a cumulative dose of 2000–2800 rads.

DESIRED OUTCOMES	NURSING ACTIONS AND *SELECTED RATIONALES*

5.C. The client will experience relief of pruritus as evidenced by:
1. verbalization of same
2. no scratching or rubbing of skin.
	5.C.1. Assess skin within the treatment field, particularly body folds and thin epidermal areas (e.g. face, axilla, perineum), for dryness and itching.
	2. Assess pruritus including onset, characteristics, location, factors that aggravate or alleviate it, and client tolerance.
	3. Instruct client in and/or implement measures *to relieve pruritus in the treatment area:*
	   a. perform actions *to prevent further skin dryness:*
	     1. lubricate skin frequently with water-soluble emollients (lanolin lotions and A & D ointment can also be used but must be removed before treatments)
	     2. instruct client to avoid frequent hot baths and harsh alkaline soaps
	     3. encourage a fluid intake of at least 2500 cc/day unless contraindicated
	   b. perform actions *to promote capillary constriction:*
	     1. apply cool, moist compresses to pruritic areas
	     2. maintain a cool environment
	   c. add emollients, cornstarch, baking soda, or oatmeal to bath water
	   d. apply powdered cornstarch to areas of dry desquamation and between skin folds
	   e. pat skin dry, making sure to dry thoroughly
	   f. encourage participation in diversional activity
	   g. utilize relaxation techniques
	   h. utilize cutaneous stimulation techniques (e.g. pressure, stroking with a soft brush) at sites of itching or acupressure points (skin within the treatment field should never be rubbed or massaged)
	   i. encourage client to wear loose cotton garments.
	4. Monitor for therapeutic and nontherapeutic effects of antihistamines and antipruritic lotions if administered. (Topical corticosteroids should be avoided *because of the possibility of diffuse thinning of the skin related to atrophy of epidermis and dermal collagen.*)
	5. Consult physician if above measures fail to reduce pruritus or if the skin becomes excoriated.

☐ ▄▄▄▄▄▄▄▄▄▄▄▄▄▄▄▄▄▄▄▄▄▄▄▄▄▄▄▄▄

6. NURSING DIAGNOSIS

Impaired verbal communication related to mucositis of the oropharynx and dryness of the oral mucous membrane associated with radiation to the head and neck.

☐ ▄▄▄▄▄▄▄▄▄▄▄▄▄▄▄▄▄▄▄▄▄▄▄▄▄▄▄▄▄

DESIRED OUTCOMES	NURSING ACTIONS AND *SELECTED RATIONALES*

6. The client will communicate needs and desires effectively.	6.a. Assess for factors that may impair verbal communication (e.g. painful lesions in mouth and pharynx; dry mouth; thick, tenacious saliva).
	   b. Implement measures *to facilitate communication:*
	     1. perform actions to relieve oral dryness and reduce severity of stomatitis (see Nursing Diagnosis 8, actions a.2 and b.3)
	     2. maintain a patient, calm approach; avoid interrupting client and allow ample time for communication
	     3. maintain a quiet environment *so that client need not raise voice to be heard*
	     4. ask questions that require short answers or nod of head
	     5. provide materials necessary for communication (e.g. magic slate, pad and pencil, flash cards)

6. ensure that intravenous therapy does not interfere with client's ability to write
7. answer call signal promptly and in person rather than using intercommunication system
8. make frequent rounds *to ascertain needs*
9. if client is frustrated or fatigued, try to anticipate needs *in order to minimize the necessity of verbal communication.*

   c. Reassure client that verbal impairment is temporary.
   d. Inform significant others and health care personnel of approaches being used to maximize the client's ability to communicate.
   e. Consult physician if client experiences increasing impairment of verbal communication.

7. NURSING DIAGNOSIS

Impaired skin integrity: irritation and breakdown related to:

a. dry desquamation at sites of entry and exit of radiation associated with destruction of rapidly dividing epithelial cells of the skin and increased sensitivity of certain body parts (e.g. opposing skin surfaces, face, axilla, perineum) resulting from a cumulative dose of 2000–2800 rads;
b. moist desquamation at sites of entry and exit of radiation associated with inability of basal cells to provide sufficient differentiated, cornified cells resulting from doses above 3600 rads or lower cumulative doses if client is receiving concurrent chemotherapy (Hassey and Rose, 1982);
c. increased skin fragility associated with:
   1. tissue edema resulting from vascular changes following radiation exposure
   2. malnutrition
   3. tissue hypoxia resulting from anemia associated with bone marrow suppression if the treatment field includes more than 25% of the active bone marrow;
d. excessive scratching associated with pruritus;
e. prolonged pressure on tissues associated with decreased mobility;
f. continued exposure to irritants associated with persistent diarrhea.

DESIRED OUTCOMES	NURSING ACTIONS AND *SELECTED RATIONALES*

7. The client will maintain or regain skin integrity as evidenced by:
a. minimal redness and irritation within the treatment field
b. absence of redness and irritation in other body areas
c. no skin breakdown.
	7.a. Assess radiation entry and exit sites every shift for changes in color, scaling, drainage, increased temperature, and discomfort.
	b. Inspect the skin (especially areas within the treatment field[s] that are considered to be high risk [e.g. opposing skin surfaces such as buttocks, groin, axilla, and breast]; bone prominences; dependent, pruritic, and edematous areas; and the perineum) for pallor, redness, and breakdown.
	c. Implement measures *to maintain or regain skin integrity*:
	  1. perform actions *to prevent or treat skin irritation or breakdown within the treatment field(s)*:
	    a. cleanse irradiated area(s) gently each shift with tepid water and mild soap *to reduce incidence of localized skin infections* (may be contraindicated if skin markings rather than tattoos are used)
	    b. pat skin dry using soft materials, paying particular attention to opposing skin surfaces within the treatment field
	    c. expose irradiated area to the air as much as possible, avoiding extremes in temperature
	    d. avoid use of tape within irradiated area

    e. instruct client to:
1. wear loose cotton clothing
2. avoid use of perfumed lotions or soaps, cosmetics, and deodorants *to prevent chemical irritation* (*many of these products contain heavy metals that will potentiate a skin reaction resulting from radiation*)
3. apply cornstarch to areas of dry desquamation *to reduce friction*
4. use water-based (hydrophilic), mild, lubricant lotions (e.g. Lubriderm, Eucerin, Aquaphor) *to ease dry skin and prevent cracking*
5. avoid use of hydrophobic products (e.g. petroleum jelly) *because they are difficult to remove and are poorly absorbed*
6. use an electric rather than a straight-edge razor if it is necessary to shave in irradiated area(s)
7. avoid applications of heat or cold to irradiated area(s)

    f. implement measures to relieve pruritus (see Nursing Diagnosis 5.C, actions 3 and 4)

    g. implement measures to treat a moist desquamation reaction if it has occurred:
1. keep involved areas clean and free of drainage if open method treatment is prescribed (the area remains exposed to the air as much as possible with this method)
2. assist with or administer hydrotherapy (e.g. whirlpool, shower) *to remove skin debris*
3. if semi-open treatment method is used:
    a. monitor for therapeutic and nontherapeutic effects of saline, hydrogen peroxide, or calcium acetate soaks if ordered
    b. apply dressings (e.g. wet to dry, nonadhering, hydrophilic, occlusive) as ordered *to protect or debride wound, absorb exudate, and promote client comfort*
    c. change dressings frequently *to prevent maceration of the skin and bacterial growth*

2. perform actions *to prevent skin breakdown due to decreased mobility:*
    a. turn client and gently massage over bone prominences and around reddened areas at least every 2 hours
    b. lift and move client carefully using a turn sheet and adequate assistance *to prevent the linen from shearing the skin*
    c. instruct or assist client to shift weight every 30 minutes
    d. if fade time (length of time it takes for reddened area to fade after pressure is removed) is greater than 15 minutes, increase frequency of position changes
    e. keep skin lubricated, clean, and dry
    f. keep bed linens wrinkle-free
    g. provide alternating pressure or eggcrate mattress, flotation pad, sheepskin, and elbow and heel protectors if indicated
    h. increase activity as tolerated

3. perform actions *to decrease skin irritation and prevent breakdown associated with diarrhea:*
    a. implement measures to control diarrhea (see Nursing Diagnosis 12, action d)
    b. assist client to thoroughly cleanse and dry perineal area after each bowel movement; apply a protective ointment or cream (e.g. Sween cream, Desitin, Karaya gel, A & D ointment, Vaseline), being sure to remove it before treatments if rectal area is within treatment field(s)
    c. avoid direct contact of skin with Chux (e.g. place turn sheet or bed pad over Chux)

4. perform actions *to prevent skin breakdown associated with scratching:*
    a. implement measures to relieve pruritus (see Nursing Diagnosis 5.C, actions 3 and 4)
    b. keep nails trimmed and/or apply mittens if necessary
    c. instruct client to apply firm pressure to pruritic areas instead of scratching

5. perform actions to maintain an optimal nutritional status (see Nursing Diagnosis 3, action f).

d. If unexpected skin irritation or breakdown occurs:
1. notify physician
2. continue with above measures to prevent further irritation and breakdown
3. perform decubitus and other wound care as ordered or per standard hospital policy
4. monitor client closely and report signs and symptoms of infection (e.g. elevated temperature; redness, warmth, and edema around area of breakdown; unusual drainage from site).

UNIT
V

---

8. NURSING DIAGNOSIS

Altered oral mucous membrane:

a. **dryness** related to:
   1. fluid volume deficit associated with fluid loss and decreased oral intake
   2. decreased salivary flow associated with a reduction in oral intake, stomatitis, and destruction of salivary glands within treatment field;
b. **stomatitis** related to malnutrition, fluid volume deficit, poor oral hygiene, and disruption in the normal renewal process of mucosal epithelial cells associated with radiation to the oral cavity.

DESIRED OUTCOMES	NURSING ACTIONS AND *SELECTED RATIONALES*
8.a. The client will maintain a moist, intact oral mucous membrane.	8.a.1. Assess client every shift for dryness of the oral mucosa (reduction in salivary flow will occur after cumulative dose of 2500–3000 rads to the head and neck area and may persist for many months after treatment; dryness will be permanent after a radiation exposure of 5000–6000 rads).
	2. Implement measures *to decrease dryness of oral mucous membrane:*
	a. instruct and assist client to perform oral hygiene after eating and as often as needed
	b. encourage client to rinse or spray mouth frequently with water
	c. instruct client to avoid products such as lemon-glycerin swabs and commercial mouthwashes containing alcohol (*these products have a drying or irritating effect on oral mucous membrane*)
	d. lubricate client's lips with Vaseline, K-Y jelly, ChapStick, Blistex, or mineral oil when oral care is given
	e. encourage client to breathe through nose if possible
	f. encourage client not to smoke (*smoking further irritates and dries the mucosa*)
	g. encourage a fluid intake of at least 2500 cc/day unless contraindicated
	h. if stomatitis is not severe, encourage client to use artificial saliva (e.g. Moi-stir, Salivart, Xero-Lube) *to lubricate mucous membrane*
	i. if some salivary production is occurring, encourage the client to suck on sour, hard candy or chew gum *to stimulate salivation.*
8.b. The client will maintain oral cavity integrity as evidenced by:	8.b.1. Assess client for and report signs and symptoms of stomatitis such as inflamed and/or ulcerated oral mucosa, leukoplakia, complaints of oral dryness or burning, changes in quality of voice, dysphagia, and viscous saliva. (Stomatitis will usually begin by the end of the second week of therapy and persist for up to 4 weeks following the cessation of treatments. Signs and symptoms initially appear on the buccal surfaces and/or palate.)
1. absence of inflammation and ulcerations	
2. pink, intact mucosa	
3. absence of oral dryness or burning	2. Obtain cultures from suspicious oral lesions as ordered. Report positive results.
4. ability to swallow without discomfort	3. Implement measures *to prevent or reduce the severity of stomatitis:*

5. usual consistency of saliva.

   a. perform actions to reduce dryness (see action a.2 in this diagnosis)
   b. reinforce the importance of and assist client with oral hygiene after meals and snacks
   c. have client rinse mouth frequently with warm saline or baking soda and water
   d. instruct client to avoid substances that might further irritate the oral mucosa (e.g. extremely hot, spicy, or acidic foods/fluids)
   e. use a soft bristle brush or low-pressure power spray for oral care
   f. maintain an optimal nutritional status (see Nursing Diagnosis 3, action f)
   g. consult physician regarding an order for an antifungal or antibacterial agent.

4. If stomatitis is not controlled:
   a. increase frequency of oral hygiene
   b. if client has dentures, remove and replace only for meals.
5. Monitor for therapeutic and nontherapeutic effects of topical anesthetics, oral protective pastes, and topical and systemic analgesics if administered.
6. Consult physician if signs and symptoms of stomatitis persist or worsen.

---

9. NURSING DIAGNOSIS

Fatigue related to:

a. accumulation of cellular waste products associated with rapid lysis of cancerous and normal cells exposed to radiation;
b. inability to rest and sleep;
c. anxiety and depression associated with the diagnosis, the treatment regimen and its effects, the need to alter usual activities, and the inability to fulfill usual roles;
d. increased energy expenditure associated with an increase in the basal metabolic rate resulting from continuous, active tumor growth.

DESIRED OUTCOMES	NURSING ACTIONS AND *SELECTED RATIONALES*

9. The client will experience a reduction in fatigue as evidenced by:
   a. verbalization of feelings of increased energy
   b. increased interest in surroundings and ability to concentrate
   c. decreased emotional lability.

9.a. Assess for signs and symptoms of fatigue (e.g. verbalization of continuous, overwhelming lack of energy; lack of interest in surroundings; decreased ability to concentrate; increased emotional lability).
  b. Inform client that a feeling of persistent fatigue is expected as a result of the disease itself and side effect of radiation therapy.
  c. Encourage client to view fatigue as a protective mechanism rather than a problematic limitation *in order to enable him/her to feel a sense of control over the situation.*
  d. Assist client to identify personal patterns of fatigue (e.g. time of day, after certain activities) and to plan activities so that times of greatest fatigue are avoided.
  e. Implement measures *to reduce fatigue:*
    1. perform actions *to promote rest:*
      a. schedule several short rest periods during the day
      b. minimize environmental activity and noise
      c. schedule nursing care and diagnostic procedures to allow periods of uninterrupted rest
      d. limit the number of visitors and their length of stay
      e. assist client with self-care activities as needed
      f. keep needed supplies and personal articles within easy reach
      g. implement measures to promote sleep (see Nursing Diagnosis 13, action c)

>   h. implement measures to reduce discomfort (see Nursing Diagnoses 5.A,
>   action 5; 5.B, action 2; and 5.C, actions 3 and 4)
>   i. implement measures to control diarrhea (see Nursing Diagnosis 12,
>   action d)
>   2. instruct client in energy-saving techniques (e.g. using shower chair when
>   showering, sitting to brush teeth or comb hair)
>   3. keep room temperature below 75°F and instruct client to avoid using hot
>   water for showers and baths (*increased body temperature increases the
>   basal metabolic rate*)
>   4. perform actions to maintain an adequate nutritional status (see Nursing
>   Diagnosis 3, action f)
>   5. encourage client to maintain a fluid intake of at least 2500 cc/day *to
>   promote elimination of the byproducts of cellular breakdown*
>   6. perform actions to facilitate client's psychological adjustment to the
>   diagnosis of cancer and the treatment regimen and its effects (see
>   Nursing Diagnoses 1, action c; 18, actions d–q; 19, action d; and 20,
>   action d).
> f. Consult physician if signs and symptoms of fatigue worsen.

10. NURSING DIAGNOSIS

Activity intolerance related to:

a. malnutrition;

b. inability to rest and sleep associated with discomfort, diarrhea, and prolonged physiological and psychological stress;

c. tissue hypoxia associated with anemia resulting from nutritional deficits and bone marrow suppression if treatment field includes more than 25% of the active bone marrow (would occur only if the total body or entire pelvis is irradiated).

DESIRED OUTCOMES	NURSING ACTIONS AND *SELECTED RATIONALES*

10. The client will demonstrate an increased tolerance for activity as evidenced by:
a. verbalization of feeling less fatigued and weak
b. ability to perform activities of daily living without exertional dyspnea, chest pain, diaphoresis, dizziness, or a significant change in vital signs.
	10.a. Assess for signs and symptoms of activity intolerance:
	  1. statements of fatigue and weakness
	  2. exertional dyspnea, chest pain, diaphoresis, or dizziness
	  3. decrease in pulse rate or an increase in rate of 20 beats/minute above resting rate
	  4. pulse rate not returning to preactivity level within 5 minutes after stopping activity
	  5. decreased blood pressure or an increase in diastolic pressure of 15 mm Hg with activity.
	  b. Implement measures *to improve activity tolerance:*
	    1. perform actions to promote rest (see Nursing Diagnosis 9, action e.1)
	    2. perform actions to maintain an adequate nutritional status (see Nursing Diagnosis 3, action f)
	    3. monitor for therapeutic and nontherapeutic effects of whole blood or packed red cells if administered
	    4. increase client's activity gradually as tolerated.
	  c. Instruct client to:
	    1. report a decreased tolerance for activity
	    2. stop any activity that causes chest pain, shortness of breath, dizziness, or extreme fatigue or weakness.
	  d. Consult physician if signs and symptoms of activity intolerance persist or worsen.

11. NURSING DIAGNOSIS

Self-care deficit related to discomfort, fatigue, and decreased activity tolerance.

DESIRED OUTCOMES	NURSING ACTIONS AND *SELECTED RATIONALES*
11. The client will demonstrate increased participation in self-care activities.	11.a. Assess for factors that interfere with client's ability to perform self-care (e.g. fatigue, weakness, nausea, vomiting, pain).
	b. With client, develop a realistic plan for meeting daily physical needs.
	c. Encourage maximum independence within limitations imposed by weakness, fatigue, nausea, vomiting, and pain.
	d. Implement measures *to facilitate client's ability to perform self-care activities:*
	1. perform actions to reduce fatigue and improve activity tolerance (see Nursing Diagnoses 9, action e and 10, action b)
	2. perform actions to reduce pain and nausea (see Nursing Diagnosis 5.A, action 5 and 5.B, action 2)
	3. schedule care at a time when client is most likely to be able to participate (e.g. when analgesics are at peak action, after rest periods, not immediately after treatments or meals)
	4. allow adequate time for accomplishment of self-care activities.
	e. Provide positive feedback for all efforts and accomplishments of self-care.
	f. Assist client with those activities he/she is unable to perform independently.
	g. Inform significant others of client's abilities to perform own care. Explain the importance of encouraging and allowing client to maintain an optimal level of independence within his/her activity tolerance level.

12. NURSING DIAGNOSIS

Diarrhea related to:

a. decreased absorption of water from the intestines as a result of destruction of the villi and microvilli associated with radiation to abdomen or lower back (the intestinal villi have a high mitotic rate and are quite susceptible to damage);
b. increased intestinal motility associated with extreme fear and anxiety and inflammation, denuding, and ulceration of the gastrointestinal mucosa (occurs with radiation to abdomen or lower back).

DESIRED OUTCOMES	NURSING ACTIONS AND *SELECTED RATIONALES*
12. The client will have fewer bowel movements and more formed stool.	12.a. Ascertain client's usual bowel elimination habits.
	b. Assess for signs and symptoms of diarrhea (e.g. frequent, loose stools; abdominal pain and cramping). Diarrhea will usually begin about 2 weeks after initiation of therapy and end 2–3 weeks after cessation of treatment.
	c. Assess bowel sounds regularly. Report an increase in frequency of and/or high-pitched bowel sounds.
	d. Implement measures *to control diarrhea:*
	1. perform actions *to rest the bowel:*
	a. instruct client to avoid foods and fluids that are poorly digested or act as irritants to the inflamed bowel:

1. milk and milk products (*a lactase deficiency results from destruction of intestinal villi and may cause milk intolerance*)
2. those high in fat (e.g. butter, cream, oils, whole milk, fried foods, gravies, nuts)
3. those with high fiber content (e.g. whole-grain cereals; raw vegetables and fruit except ripe bananas, peeled apples, and avocados; nuts)
4. those known to cause diarrhea or be gas-producers (e.g. cabbage, onions, popcorn, licorice, prunes, chili, baked beans, carbonated beverages)
5. spicy foods
6. those high in caffeine (e.g. coffee, tea, chocolate, colas)
7. extremely hot or cold foods/fluids

b. provide small, frequent meals that are low in residue but still supply the needed protein and carbohydrates (e.g. eggs; smooth peanut butter; baked fish or poultry; cooked cereal; white rice or breads; pasta; bland, cooked vegetables)

c. season appropriate foods with nutmeg *to decrease motility of the gastrointestinal tract*

d. implement measures to reduce fear and anxiety (see Nursing Diagnosis 1, action c)

e. discourage smoking (*nicotine has a stimulant effect on gastrointestinal tract*)

2. monitor for therapeutic and nontherapeutic effects of the following medications if administered:
   a. opiate or opiate-like substances (e.g. loperamide, diphenoxylate hydrochloride) *to decrease gastrointestinal motility*
   b. bulk-forming agents (e.g. methylcellulose, psyllium hydrophilic mucilloid, calcium polycarbophil) *to absorb water in bowel and produce a soft, formed stool.*

e. Consult physician if diarrhea persists despite implementation of above actions.

UNIT V ·

□ ▬▬▬▬▬▬▬▬▬▬▬▬▬▬▬▬▬▬▬▬▬▬▬▬▬▬▬

13. NURSING DIAGNOSIS

Sleep pattern disturbance related to:

a. discomfort associated with nausea, vomiting, pruritus, xerostomia, and pain resulting from effects of radiation therapy on body tissues;
b. anxiety, fear, and depression;
c. frequent need to defecate associated with diarrhea if present.

□ ▬▬▬▬▬▬▬▬▬▬▬▬▬▬▬▬▬▬▬▬▬▬▬▬▬▬▬

DESIRED OUTCOMES	NURSING ACTIONS AND *SELECTED RATIONALES*

13. The client will attain optimal amounts of sleep within parameters of the treatment regimen as evidenced by:
   a. statements of feeling well rested
   b. usual behavior
   c. absence of frequent yawning, thick speech, dark circles under eyes.

13.a. Assess for signs and symptoms of a sleep pattern disturbance:
   1. verbal complaints of difficulty falling asleep, not feeling well rested, sleep interruptions, or awakening earlier or later than desired
   2. behavior changes (e.g. irritability, disorganization, lethargy)
   3. frequent yawning, thick speech, dark circles under eyes, slight hand tremors.

b. Determine the client's usual sleep habits.

c. Implement measures *to promote sleep:*
   1. perform actions to reduce fear and anxiety (see Nursing Diagnosis 1, action c)
   2. perform actions to reduce discomfort (see Nursing Diagnoses 5.A, action 5; 5.B, action 2; and 5.C, actions 3 and 4)

3. perform actions to control diarrhea (see Nursing Diagnosis 12, action d)
4. if client has xerostomia, instruct him/her to use artificial saliva (e.g. Moi-stir, Xero-Lube) before sleep *to prevent dry, choking sensation that often occurs*
5. allow client to continue usual sleep practices (e.g. position, time, bedtime rituals) if possible
6. determine measures that have been helpful to client in the past (e.g. milk, warm drinks, warm bath) and incorporate in plan of care
7. discourage long periods of sleep during the day unless sleep deprivation exists or daytime sleep is usual for client
8. encourage participation in relaxing diversional activities in early evening hours
9. provide a quiet, restful atmosphere
10. discourage intake of foods/fluids high in caffeine (e.g. chocolate, coffee, tea, colas) especially in the evening
11. satisfy basic needs such as hunger, comfort, and warmth before sleep
12. have client empty bladder just before bedtime
13. utilize relaxation techniques (e.g. progressive relaxation exercises, back massage, meditation, soft music) before sleep
14. perform actions *to provide for periods of uninterrupted sleep* (*90- to 120-minute periods of uninterrupted sleep are considered essential*):
    a. restrict visitors during rest periods
    b. group care (e.g. medications, treatments, physical care, assessments) whenever possible
15. monitor for therapeutic and nontherapeutic effects of sedatives and hypnotics if administered.
   d. Consult physician if signs of sleep deprivation persist or worsen.

14. NURSING DIAGNOSIS

Potential for infection related to:

a. break in the integrity of the skin associated with dry or moist desquamation;
b. lowered natural resistance associated with:
   1. malnutrition, anemia
   2. neutropenia resulting from slow recovery rate of myeloblasts and bone marrow suppression associated with irradiation of more than 25% of the body's bone marrow (would occur only if the total body or entire pelvis is irradiated).

DESIRED OUTCOMES	NURSING ACTIONS AND *SELECTED RATIONALES*
14. The client will remain free of infection as evidenced by: a. absence of chills and fever b. pulse within normal limits c. normal breath sounds d. voiding clear, yellow urine without complaints of frequency, urgency, or burning e. absence of redness, swelling, or unusual drainage in any area where there is a break in skin integrity	14.a. Assess for and report signs and symptoms of infection: 1. elevated temperature 2. chills 3. pattern of increased pulse or pulse rate greater than 100 beats/minute 4. adventitious breath sounds 5. cloudy or foul-smelling urine 6. complaints of frequency, urgency, or burning when urinating 7. presence of WBCs, bacteria, and/or nitrites in urine 8. redness, change in skin temperature, swelling, or unusual drainage in any area where there has been a break in skin integrity 9. irritation or ulceration of oral mucous membrane 10. complaints of perineal or rectal pain or any unusual vaginal or rectal discharge 11. increased hemorrhoidal pain, redness, or bleeding

f. intact oral mucous membrane
g. absence of perianal abscesses
h. WBC and differential counts within normal range for client
i. negative results of cultured specimens.

12. elevated WBC count and/or significant change in differential.
b. Obtain culture specimens (e.g. urine, vaginal, rectal, mouth, sputum, blood, moist desquamation sites, lesions) as ordered. Report positive results.
c. Implement measures *to reduce risk of infection:*
  1. protect client from others with infection and those who have recently been vaccinated (*a person may have a subclinical infection after a vaccination*)
  2. use good handwashing technique and encourage client to do the same
  3. instruct client to avoid use of shared eating utensils
  4. maintain a fluid intake of at least 2500 cc/day unless contraindicated
  5. maintain an optimal nutritional status (see Nursing Diagnosis 3, action f)
  6. encourage a low-bacteria diet (e.g. cooked foods, no fresh fruit) if client is immunosuppressed
  7. perform actions to prevent or reduce severity of stomatitis (see Nursing Diagnosis 8, actions b.3 and 4)
  8. perform actions to maintain or regain skin integrity (see Nursing Diagnosis 7, action c)
  9. give meticulous attention to any break in skin integrity; provide wound care as ordered
  10. avoid invasive procedures (e.g. urinary catheterizations, arterial or venous punctures, injections) whenever possible; if such procedures are necessary, maintain meticulous aseptic technique
  11. initiate measures to prevent constipation *in order to avoid damage to rectal mucosa from hard or impacted stool*
  12. avoid unnecessary rectal invasion (e.g. temperature taking, enemas, suppositories, rectal tube) *to prevent trauma to rectal mucosa and possible abscess formation*
  13. provide proper balance of exercise and rest
  14. perform actions *to prevent a respiratory tract infection:*
    a. instruct and assist client to turn, cough, and deep breathe at least every 2 hours if activity is limited
    b. instruct and assist client in use of inspiratory exerciser at least every 2 hours if indicated
    c. encourage client to stop smoking
    d. increase activity as tolerated
  15. perform actions *to prevent urinary tract infection:*
    a. instruct and assist female client to wipe from front to back following urination or defecation
    b. keep perianal area clean.
d. Monitor for therapeutic and nontherapeutic effects of anti-infectives if administered.

15. NURSING DIAGNOSIS

Potential for trauma related to falls associated with weakness resulting from anemia, malnutrition, and fluid and electrolyte imbalances.

DESIRED OUTCOMES	NURSING ACTIONS AND *SELECTED RATIONALES*
15. The client will not experience falls.	15.a. Determine whether conditions predisposing client to falls (e.g. weakness, fatigue) exist. b. Implement measures *to prevent falls:* 1. keep bed in low position with side rails up when client is in bed 2. keep needed items within easy reach

3. encourage client to request assistance whenever needed; have call signal within easy reach
4. use lap belt when client is in chair if indicated
5. instruct client to wear shoes with nonskid soles and low heels when ambulating
6. avoid unnecessary clutter in room
7. accompany client during ambulation utilizing a transfer safety belt if he/she is weak
8. provide ambulatory aids (e.g. walker, cane) if the client is weak or unsteady on feet
9. instruct client to ambulate in well-lit areas and to utilize handrails if needed
10. do not rush client; allow adequate time for trips to the bathroom and ambulation in hallway
11. perform actions to reduce fatigue and improve activity tolerance (see Nursing Diagnoses 9, action e and 10, action b)
12. perform actions to maintain fluid, electrolyte, and acid-base balance (see Nursing Diagnosis 2, actions a.3 and b.2 and 3).
c. Include client and significant others in planning and implementing measures to prevent falls.
d. If falls occur, initiate appropriate first aid measures and notify physician.

☐ ▬▬▬▬▬▬▬▬▬▬▬▬▬▬▬▬▬▬▬▬▬▬▬▬▬▬▬

16. COLLABORATIVE DIAGNOSIS

Potential complications:

a. **bleeding** related to thrombocytopenia associated with slow recovery rate of platelet precursors and bone marrow suppression resulting from radiation to more than 25% of the body's active bone marrow (would occur only if the total body or entire pelvis is irradiated);
b. **dental caries and periodontal disease** related to:
1. destruction of tooth enamel occurring with radiation to head and neck (causes a drop in the usual pH of saliva and results in an inability of the saliva to buffer lactic acid in the mouth [Bersani and Carl, 1983])
2. inadequate oral hygiene
3. damage to the periodontal membrane associated with direct radiation resulting in alveolar bone destruction and eventual loss of teeth;
c. **acute or chronic pericarditis** related to damage to the pericardium associated with exposure of the heart to greater than 4000 rads;
d. **radiation cystitis** related to thinning and ulceration of the bladder epithelial lining after radiation exposure of the bladder to more than 7000 rads;
e. **renal calculi** related to hyperuricemia associated with rapid lysis of tumor cells.

☐ ▬▬▬▬▬▬▬▬▬▬▬▬▬▬▬▬▬▬▬▬▬▬▬▬▬▬▬

DESIRED OUTCOMES	NURSING ACTIONS AND *SELECTED RATIONALES*
16.a. The client will not experience unusual bleeding as evidenced by: 1. skin and mucous membranes free of bleeding, petechiae, and ecchymosis 2. absence of unusual joint pain or swelling	16.a.1. Assess client for and report signs and symptoms of unusual bleeding: a. petechiae b. multiple ecchymotic areas c. bleeding gums d. frequent or uncontrollable episodes of epistaxis e. unusual oozing from injection sites f. unusual joint pain or swelling g. increase in abdominal girth h. hematemesis, melena, red or smoke-colored urine

3. no increase in abdominal girth
4. absence of frank or occult blood in stool, urine, and vomitus
5. usual menstrual flow
6. vital signs within normal range for client
7. stable or improved Hct. and Hgb.
8. usual mental status.

    i. hypermenorrhea
    j. significant drop in B/P accompanied by an increased pulse rate
    k. decline in Hct. and Hgb. levels
    l. restlessness, confusion.
2. Monitor coagulation test results (e.g. platelet count, bleeding time). Report abnormal values.
3. If coagulation test results are abnormal or Hct. and Hgb. levels decline, test all stools, urine, and vomitus for occult blood. Report positive results.
4. Implement measures *to prevent bleeding:*
    a. use the smallest gauge needle possible when giving injections and performing venous or arterial punctures
    b. apply gentle, prolonged pressure after injections and venous or arterial punctures
    c. take B/P only when necessary and avoid overinflating the cuff
    d. caution client to avoid activities that increase the potential for trauma (e.g. shaving with a straight-edge razor, cutting nails, using stiff bristle toothbrush or dental floss)
    e. pad side rails if client is confused or restless
    f. perform actions to prevent falls (see Nursing Diagnosis 15, action b)
    g. instruct client to avoid blowing nose forcefully or straining to have a bowel movement; consult physician regarding order for decongestants, stool softeners, and/or laxatives if indicated
    h. avoid taking temperatures rectally and administering rectal suppositories
    i. monitor for therapeutic and nontherapeutic effects of the following if administered:
        1. estrogen-progestin preparations *to suppress menses*
        2. platelets
        3. plasma or whole blood.
5. If bleeding occurs and does not subside spontaneously:
    a. apply firm, prolonged pressure to bleeding area if possible
    b. if epistaxis occurs, place client in a high Fowler's position and apply pressure and ice packs to nasal area
    c. administer blood products as ordered
    d. maintain oxygen therapy as ordered
    e. perform iced water or saline lavage as ordered *to control gastric bleeding*
    f. provide emotional support to client and significant others.

16.b. The client will not experience dental caries or periodontal disease as evidenced by:
1. intact tooth enamel
2. no loosening or loss of teeth
3. absence of inflamed gingivae.

16.b.1. Assess oral cavity for evidence of tooth decay or periodontal disease (e.g. loose teeth; reddened, receding gingivae).
2. Inform client that dental caries and periodontal disease can occur months to years after radiation to the jaw, neck, or oral cavity. Emphasize that a meticulous oral hygiene program is essential, particularly if salivary flow is permanently reduced.
3. Implement measures *to reduce risk of radiation-induced dental caries and periodontal disease:*
    a. instruct and/or assist client to:
        1. brush teeth thoroughly with a fluoridated toothpaste several times a day, particularly after eating (if thrombocytopenia or severe stomatitis is present, irrigate mouth rather than brushing *in order to prevent trauma to oral mucous membrane*)
        2. use a small, soft, flexible brush to cleanse the teeth and gingival crevices
        3. rinse mouth with a topical fluoride solution after each brushing
        4. use a molded dental carrier and fluoride gel if ordered (should be used for 1–2 minutes each day until salivary function has returned to normal)
        5. irrigate the mouth with a 10% solution of hydrogen peroxide and water or baking soda and water ($\frac{1}{2}$ tsp/cup of water) if gingivae are infected *to facilitate healing*
    b. perform actions to prevent or treat stomatitis (see Nursing Diagnosis 8, actions b.3 and 4).
4. Consult physician if signs and symptoms of tooth decay and periodontal disease develop.

16.c. The client will experience resolution of pericarditis if it occurs as evidenced by:
1. decreasing complaints of substernal or precordial pain
2. resolution of pericardial friction rub
3. unlabored respirations at 16–20/minute
4. temperature returning toward normal
5. WBC count and sedimentation rate returning toward normal range.

16.c.1. Assess for and report signs and symptoms of pericarditis (may occur several weeks to months following treatment):
a. substernal or precordial pain that frequently radiates to left shoulder, neck, and arm; is intensified during deep inspiration; and usually is relieved by sitting up
b. pericardial friction rub (may be transient)
c. dyspnea, tachypnea
d. elevated temperature
e. elevated WBC count and sedimentation rate
f. chest x-ray and echocardiography results showing cardiomegaly and pericardial effusion.
2. If signs and symptoms of pericarditis occur:
a. allay client's anxiety (client may believe that symptoms indicate a heart attack)
b. monitor for therapeutic and nontherapeutic effects of medications that may be administered *to reduce inflammation* (e.g. aspirin, indomethacin, ibuprofen, corticosteroids)
c. monitor for and immediately report signs of cardiac tamponade (e.g. rapid and continual decline in B/P; narrowed pulse pressure; pulsus paradoxus; weak rapid pulse; distant or muffled heart sounds; neck vein distention on inspiration; decreased amplitude of waves on EKG; increased CVP and pulmonary pressures)
d. prepare client for and assist with pericardiocentesis if performed.

16.d. The client will experience resolution of radiation cystitis if it occurs as evidenced by:
1. decreasing complaints of dysuria, urinary frequency or urgency
2. absence of hematuria.

16.d.1. Assess for and report signs and symptoms of radiation cystitis (e.g. dysuria, urinary frequency and/or urgency, frank or occult blood in the urine). Acute symptoms may appear toward the end of treatment regimen and persist about 3 weeks.
2. If signs and symptoms of radiation cystitis occur:
a. implement measures *to reduce discomfort associated with cystitis:*
1. encourage a minimum fluid intake of 2500 cc/day *to keep urine dilute and reduce irritation of the bladder lining*
2. instruct client to avoid foods/fluids that may further irritate the bladder lining (e.g. those containing caffeine such as coffee, chocolate, and colas; alcoholic beverages; spicy foods)
3. monitor for therapeutic and nontherapeutic effects of urinary anesthetics and antispasmodics if administered
b. assist with or perform bladder irrigations *to remove clots and maintain urinary flow*
c. monitor for therapeutic and nontherapeutic effects of continuous bladder irrigations with silver nitrate solution if performed *to stop bleeding*
d. implement the following measures if bleeding is persistent or severe:
1. monitor for therapeutic and nontherapeutic effects of vasoconstrictors, volume expanders, blood products, and/or hemostatic agents (e.g. aminocaproic acid) if administered
2. prepare client for electrocoagulation if appropriate
e. provide emotional support to client and significant others.

16.e. The client will not develop renal calculi as evidenced by:
1. absence of flank pain, hematuria, urinary frequency or urgency, nausea, vomiting
2. clear urine without calculi.

16.e.1. Assess for and report signs and symptoms of renal calculi (e.g. dull, aching or severe, colicky flank pain; hematuria; urinary frequency or urgency; nausea; vomiting).
2. Monitor serum uric acid levels and report elevations.
3. Obtain a urine specimen for analysis if ordered. Report increases in numbers of crystals or high levels of uric acid.
4. Implement measures *to prevent uric acid stone formation:*
a. perform actions *to prevent urinary stasis:*
1. encourage a minimum fluid intake of 2500 cc/day unless contraindicated
2. assist client to change positions at least every 2 hours
3. progress activity as tolerated
4. implement measures *to facilitate voiding* (e.g. provide privacy, allow client to assume normal voiding position unless contraindicated, run warm water over perineum)
5. instruct client to void whenever the urge is felt
6. maintain patency of urinary catheter if present

    b. monitor pH of urine every shift and report levels below 6 (*uric acid precipitates in an acidic environment*)

    c. perform actions *to maintain an alkaline urine:*

       1. encourage client to increase intake of foods/fluids that leave an alkaline ash (e.g. milk; vegetables, especially legumes and green vegetables; fruits except prunes, plums, and cranberries)

       2. administer medications *that alkalinize the urine* (e.g. sodium bicarbonate, citrate preparations) as ordered

    d. instruct client to reduce intake of foods high in purine content (e.g. liver, kidney, goose, venison, seafood, meat soups and gravies, anchovies) *in order to prevent a further increase in uric acid*

    e. monitor for therapeutic and nontherapeutic effects of xanthine oxidase inhibitor (allopurinol) if administered *to decrease uric acid production.*

  5. If signs and symptoms of renal calculi occur:

    a. strain all urine carefully and save any calculi for analysis; report finding to physician

    b. encourage a minimum fluid intake of 2500 cc/day unless contraindicated

    c. administer analgesics as ordered

    d. refer to Care Plan on Renal Calculi for additional care measures.

☐ ▬▬▬▬▬▬▬▬▬▬▬▬▬▬▬▬▬▬▬▬▬

17. NURSING DIAGNOSIS

Sexual dysfunction:

a. **decreased libido** related to fatigue, weakness, discomfort, anxiety, fear, grieving, altered self-esteem, and altered hormone balance (occurs if gonads are located within treatment field);

b. **temporary or permanent impotence** related to psychological factors (e.g. fear of uncontrolled diarrhea, anxiety, depression) and decreased testosterone levels associated with Leydig cell destruction if the testes are included in treatment field;

c. **dyspareunia** related to:

  1. decrease in lubrication of the vagina associated with decreased estrogen levels resulting from radiation to ovarian tissue

  2. mucositis and ulceration of vaginal mucosa related to the effect of radiation on the rapidly dividing epithelial cells

  3. shortening of vagina associated with fibrosis and stenosis of vagina as a result of cellular repair after radiation exposure

  4. contact of fragile tissue of vagina and external genitalia with semen.

☐ ▬▬▬▬▬▬▬▬▬▬▬▬▬▬▬▬▬▬▬▬▬

DESIRED OUTCOMES	NURSING ACTIONS AND *SELECTED RATIONALES*
17. The client will demonstrate beginning acceptance of changes in sexual functioning as evidenced by: a. verbalization of a perception of self as sexually acceptable and adequate b. statements reflecting beginning acceptance of and adjustment to effects of radiation therapy on sexual functioning	17.a. Assess for signs and symptoms of sexual dysfunction (e.g. verbalization of sexual concerns, failure to maintain relationships with significant others). b. Determine attitudes, knowledge, and concerns about effects of radiation therapy on sexual functioning. c. Communicate interest, understanding, and respect for the values of the client and his/her partner. d. Provide accurate information about the effects of radiation therapy on sexual functioning. Encourage questions and clarify misconceptions. e. Assure client that many side effects of radiation therapy (e.g. decreased libido, dyspareunia, impotence) are temporary or can be treated. f. Facilitate communication between the client and his/her partner. Assist them to identify issues that may affect their sexual relationship. g. Arrange for uninterrupted privacy during hospital stay if desired by the couple.

c. maintenance of relationships with significant others.

h. Implement measures to improve self-concept (see Nursing Diagnosis 18, actions c–q).

i. Implement measures to reduce fear and anxiety (see Nursing Diagnosis 1, action c).

j. Instruct client in measures *to reduce or prevent dyspareunia:*
   1. insert an ample amount of water-soluble lubricant into the vagina before intercourse *to prevent mechanical trauma to vaginal mucosa and increase comfort*
   2. avoid intercourse if mucositis of vaginal tract is a problem
   3. utilize a vaginal steroid cream as ordered *to ease dryness and inflammation if present*
   4. emphasize the need for frequent intercourse or vaginal dilatation *to prevent stenosis of the vaginal canal* (may occur several weeks or months after cessation of treatment)
   5. have partner use a condom *to prevent contact of vaginal area with semen* (*semen can cause a burning sensation in the early months after radiation therapy*).

k. Instruct the client to allow adequate rest periods before and after sexual activity.

l. If impotence is a problem:
   1. encourage client to discuss it with physician; reinforce physician's explanation about its temporary or permanent nature
   2. suggest alternative methods of sexual gratification and use of assistive devices if appropriate
   3. discuss ways to be creative in expressing sexuality (e.g. massage, fantasies, cuddling)
   4. encourage client to discuss the possibility of a penile prosthesis with physician if impotence will be permanent.

m. Instruct client to take antidiarrheal medication before sexual activity if indicated.

n. Include partner in above discussions and encourage his/her continued support of the client.

o. Monitor for therapeutic and nontherapeutic effects of hormone replacements (e.g. estrogen, testosterone) if administered *to relieve symptoms and discomfort.*

p. Consult physician if counseling appears indicated.

☐ ▮▮▮

18. NURSING DIAGNOSIS

Disturbance in self-concept* related to:

a. changes in appearance (e.g. temporary or permanent hair loss within the treatment field; skin changes such as erythema, telangiectasia, or uneven skin texture; excessive weight loss);
b. changes in sexual functioning;
c. altered reproductive function:
   1. temporary or permanent sterility associated with exposure of testes and ovaries to significant doses of radiation (500 rads or more to testes, 2000 rads over several weeks in a young female, or 500 rads in a woman over 40 will cause permanent sterility)
   2. potential genetic mutations associated with sperm and ova chromosomal damage resulting from radiation exposure to the gonads (oophoropexy is frequently done in a woman of childbearing age to prevent ovarian exposure);
d. increased dependence on others to meet self-care needs;
e. changes in life style and roles associated with the effects of the disease process and its treatment.

---

* This diagnostic label includes the nursing diagnoses of body image disturbance and self-esteem disturbance.

☐ ▮▮▮

DESIRED OUTCOMES	NURSING ACTIONS AND *SELECTED RATIONALES*

18. The client will demonstrate beginning adaptation to changes in appearance, body functioning, life style, and roles as evidenced by:
    a. verbalization of feelings of self-worth and sexual adequacy
    b. maintenance of relationships with significant others
    c. active participation in activities of daily living
    d. active interest in personal appearance
    e. willingness to participate in social activities
    f. verbalization of a beginning plan for adapting life style to meet restrictions imposed by the residual effects of radiation therapy.

18.a. Determine the meaning to the client of changes in appearance, body functioning, life style, and roles by encouraging him/her to verbalize feelings and by noting nonverbal responses to changes experienced.
   b. Assess for signs and symptoms of a disturbance in self-concept (e.g. verbal or nonverbal cues denoting a negative response to changes in body functioning or appearance such as denial of or preoccupation with changes that have occurred or withdrawal from significant others).
   c. Reinforce actions to facilitate the grieving process (see Nursing Diagnosis 20, action d).
   d. Assist client to identify strengths and qualities that have a positive effect on self-concept.
   e. Implement measures *to assist client to increase self-esteem* (e.g. limit negative self-criticism, encourage positive comments about self, give positive feedback about accomplishments).
   f. Reinforce actions to assist client to cope with effects of radiation therapy (see Nursing Diagnosis 19, action d).
   g. Reinforce actions that may assist the client to adjust to alteration in sexual functioning (see Nursing Diagnosis 17, actions c–o).
   h. Implement measures *to assist client to adapt to the following changes in appearance and body functioning if appropriate:*
      1. alopecia:
         a. inform client that hair loss usually occurs 2–3 weeks after initiation of therapy
         b. reassure client that regrowth of hair will occur within 1–3 months after cessation of therapy if the loss is temporary (temporary or patchy loss will usually occur with a radiation dose of 1500–3000 rads; response of the hair follicle will vary among clients exposed to 3000–4500 rads; delayed hair growth or complete, permanent hair loss within the treatment field will result from a radiation exposure above 4500 rads); explain that regrowth may be a different color, texture, and thickness
         c. instruct the client in ways *to minimize scalp hair loss if thinning or partial hair loss is anticipated:*
            1. brush and comb hair gently
            2. wash hair only when necessary and avoid harsh shampoo, cream rinse, and other hair products
            3. do not use hair dryers, curling irons, curlers, or constrictive decorations (e.g. clips, rubber bands) on hair
         d. encourage the client to wear a wig, scarf, or turban if desired *to conceal hair loss*; contact the American Cancer Society for a wig if client is unable to obtain one but desires to do so
         e. encourage use of the wig before hair loss *to facilitate adjustment to wig and integration into body image*
      2. skin changes:
         a. reinforce physician's explanation about skin changes that will occur and when they can be expected
         b. assist client with usual grooming and makeup habits if necessary
         c. suggest possible clothing styles that will make changes in skin texture and pigmentation less obvious
      3. decreased fertility, sterility, or chromosomal damage:
         a. clarify physician's explanation about probable effects of radiation therapy on the gonads
         b. discuss alternative methods of becoming a parent (e.g. artificial insemination, adoption) if of concern to client
         c. reinforce the need to take hormone replacements (e.g. estrogen, testosterone) as prescribed.
   i. Assess for and support behaviors suggesting positive adaptation to changes that have occurred (e.g. interest in personal appearance, maintenance of relationships with significant others).
   j. Encourage significant others to allow client to do what he/she is able *so that independence can be re-established and/or self-esteem redeveloped.*
   k. Encourage client contact with others *so that he/she can test and establish a new self-image.*

UNIT
V

l. Assist client's and significant others' adjustment by listening, facilitating communication, and providing information.

m. Ensure that client and significant others have similar expectations and understanding of future life style.

n. Assist client and significant others to identify ways that personal and family goals can be adjusted rather than abandoned.

o. Encourage visits and support from significant others.

p. Encourage client to continue involvement in social activities and to pursue interests. If previous interests and hobbies cannot be pursued, encourage development of new ones.

q. Provide information about and encourage use of community agencies or support groups (e.g. vocational rehabilitation; sexual, family, individual, and/or financial counseling).

r. Consult physician about psychological counseling if client desires or if he/she seems unwilling or unable to adapt to changes resulting from cancer and radiation therapy.

☐ ▬▬▬▬▬▬▬▬▬▬▬▬▬▬▬▬▬▬▬▬▬▬

19. NURSING DIAGNOSIS

Ineffective individual coping related to discomfort associated with side effects of radiation therapy, chronic fatigue, fear, anxiety, uncertainty of the effectiveness of radiation therapy, and an inadequate support system.

☐ ▬▬▬▬▬▬▬▬▬▬▬▬▬▬▬▬▬▬▬▬▬▬

DESIRED OUTCOMES	NURSING ACTIONS AND *SELECTED RATIONALES*

19. The client will demonstrate the use of effective coping skills as evidenced by:
a. willingness to participate in treatment plan and self-care activities
b. verbalization of ability to cope with radiation therapy and its effects
c. identification of stressors
d. utilization of appropriate problem-solving techniques
e. recognition and utilization of available support systems.
	19.a. Assess effectiveness of client's coping strategies by observing behavior and noting strengths, weaknesses, ability to express feelings and concerns, and willingness to participate in the treatment plan.
	b. Assess for and report signs and symptoms that may indicate ineffective coping (e.g. sleep disturbances, increasing fatigue, difficulty concentrating, irritability, decreased tolerance for pain, verbalization of inability to cope, inability to problem-solve).
	c. Allow time for client to adjust psychologically to the diagnosis, need for radiation therapy, side effects experienced, and anticipated changes in life style and roles.
	d. Implement measures *to promote effective coping:*
	  1. arrange for a visit with another who has been successfully treated with radiation therapy
	  2. perform actions to reduce pain, nausea, vomiting, and pruritus (see Nursing Diagnoses 5.A, action 5; 5.B, action 2; and 5.C, actions 3 and 4)
	  3. perform actions to reduce fear and anxiety (see Nursing Diagnosis 1, action c)
	  4. include client in planning of care, encourage maximum participation in treatment plan, and allow choices when possible *to enable him/her to maintain a sense of control*
	  5. instruct client in effective problem-solving techniques (e.g. accurate identification of stressors, determination of various options to solve problem)
	  6. perform actions to reduce fatigue (see Nursing Diagnosis 9, action e)
	  7. assist client to maintain usual daily routines whenever possible
	  8. provide diversional activities according to client's interests
	  9. assist client as he/she starts to plan for necessary life-style and role changes after discharge; provide input on realistic prioritization of problems that need to be dealt with
	  10. assist the client and significant others to identify ways that personal and family goals can be adjusted rather than abandoned

11. assist client to identify and utilize available support systems; provide information regarding available community resources that can assist client and significant others in coping with effects of radiation therapy and the diagnosis of cancer (e.g. American Cancer Society; support groups; individual, family, and financial counselors)

12. discuss any difficulties client may have in meeting the schedule for radiation treatments (usually 5 days/week for 3–8 weeks depending on site, dose, and desired therapeutic effect); refer to community agencies or support groups if transportation is a problem.

e. Encourage continued emotional support from significant others.

f. Encourage the client to share with significant others the kind of support that would be most beneficial (e.g. listening, inspiring hope, providing reassurance and accurate information).

g. Assess for and support behaviors suggesting positive adaptation to changes experienced (e.g. compliance with treatment plan, maintenance of personal appearance, verbalization of ability to cope, utilization of effective problem-solving strategies).

h. Consult physician about psychological counseling if appropriate. Initiate a referral if necessary.

20. NURSING DIAGNOSIS

Grieving* related to:

a. changes in body image and usual life style and roles;
b. diagnosis of cancer with the potential for premature death.

---

* This diagnostic label includes anticipatory grieving and grieving following the actual losses/changes.

DESIRED OUTCOMES	NURSING ACTIONS AND *SELECTED RATIONALES*
20. The client will demonstrate beginning progression through the grieving process as evidenced by: a. verbalization of feelings about the diagnosis of cancer and radiation treatment and its effects b. expression of grief c. participation in treatment plan and self-care activities d. utilization of available support systems e. verbalization of a plan for integrating prescribed follow-up care into life style.	20.a. Determine client's perception of the impact of the diagnosis of cancer and radiation therapy on his/her future. b. Determine how client usually expresses grief. c. Observe for signs of grieving (e.g. changes in eating habits, insomnia, anger, noncompliance, denial). d. Implement measures *to facilitate the grieving process:* 　1. assist client to acknowledge the losses and changes experienced *so grief work can begin*; assess for factors that may hinder or facilitate acknowledgment 　2. discuss the grieving process and assist client to accept the stages of grieving as an expected response to actual and/or anticipated changes or losses 　3. allow time for client to progress through the stages of grieving (denial, anger, bargaining, depression, acceptance [Kübler-Ross, 1969]); be aware that not every stage is experienced or expressed by all individuals 　4. provide an atmosphere of care and concern (e.g. provide privacy, be available and nonjudgmental, display empathy and respect) *so that client will feel free to verbalize both positive and negative feelings and concerns* 　5. perform actions *to promote trust* (e.g. answer questions honestly, provide requested information) 　6. encourage the expression of anger and sadness about the losses/changes experienced 　7. encourage client to express his/her feelings in whatever ways are comfortable (e.g. writing, drawing, conversation)

8. perform actions to facilitate effective coping (see Nursing Diagnosis 19, action d)
9. support realistic hope about the prognosis and the temporary nature of most of the changes in body image.
   e. Assess for and support behaviors suggesting successful resolution of grief (e.g. verbalizing feelings about changes, expressing sorrow, focusing on ways to adapt to changes/losses that have occurred).
   f. Explain stages of the grieving process to significant others. Encourage their support and understanding.
   g. Provide information regarding counseling services and support groups that might assist client in working through grief.
   h. Arrange for visit from clergy if desired by client.
   i. Monitor for therapeutic and nontherapeutic effects of antidepressants if administered.
   j. Consult physician about referral for counseling if signs of dysfunctional grieving (e.g. persistent denial of losses or changes, excessive anger or sadness, hysteria, suicidal behaviors, phobias) occur.

□ ▓▓▓▓▓▓▓▓▓▓▓▓▓▓▓▓▓▓▓▓▓▓▓▓▓▓▓▓▓▓▓

21. NURSING DIAGNOSIS

Knowledge deficit regarding follow-up care.

□ ▓▓▓▓▓▓▓▓▓▓▓▓▓▓▓▓▓▓▓▓▓▓▓▓▓▓▓▓▓▓▓

DESIRED OUTCOMES	NURSING ACTIONS AND *SELECTED RATIONALES*

21.a. The client will demonstrate the ability to give appropriate skin care at radiation entry and exit sites.	21.a.1. Reinforce teaching about the expected skin reaction to radiation therapy (e.g. redness, tanned appearance, peeling, itching, loss of hair, decreased perspiration).
	2. Instruct the client to:
	  a. cleanse irradiated area(s) gently using a mild soap and tepid water, being careful not to wash off skin markings
	  b. pat skin dry with a soft cotton towel
	  c. avoid rubbing, scratching, or massaging irradiated skin
	  d. relieve itching by:
	    1. applying powdered cornstarch to areas of dry desquamation and between skin folds
	    2. adding emollients, cornstarch, baking soda, or oatmeal to bath water
	  e. relieve dryness by applying A & D ointment, baby oil, or lanolin cream as prescribed
	  f. avoid use of deodorant if treatment field includes axilla
	  g. check with physician before using cosmetics or perfumed lotions or creams in treatment area
	  h. protect irradiated skin from exposure to temperature extremes and wind
	  i. avoid exposure to the sun after therapy is complete (*burns can occur easily because melanin production in new epidermal cells is slowed*)
	  j. wear soft cotton garments next to treatment area
	  k. avoid wearing tight or constrictive clothing over irradiated area *in order to reduce mechanical irritation*
	  l. avoid shaving and using tape within treatment field; use an electric razor if shaving is absolutely necessary
	  m. care for a moist desquamation reaction by:
	    1. performing wound irrigations and applying sterile dressings as prescribed (stretchable netting should be used to hold dressings in place)
	    2. exposing area to the air as much as possible.

3. Demonstrate care of radiation entry and exit sites.
4. Allow time for questions, clarification, and return demonstration of skin and wound care.

21.b. The client will identify techniques to control nausea and vomiting.

21.b. Instruct client in the following techniques *to control nausea and vomiting:*
  1. cleanse mouth frequently
  2. avoid offensive odors and sights
  3. avoid eating and food aromas 3 hours before and after treatments
  4. eat several small meals instead of 3 large ones
  5. eat the largest meal 3–4 hours before treatments and eat lightly for the rest of the day if nausea peaks after treatments
  6. eat foods that are cool or at room temperature (*hot foods frequently have an overpowering aroma that stimulates nausea*)
  7. eat dry foods (e.g. toast, crackers) or sour foods (e.g. lemon drops, pickles, lemon ice) or sip cold carbonated beverages if nausea is present
  8. select bland foods (e.g. mashed potatoes, applesauce, cottage cheese) rather than fatty, spicy foods (e.g. fried potatoes, chili)
  9. if feasible, have someone else prepare the food
  10. avoid liquids at mealtime
  11. rest after eating
  12. take deep, slow breaths when nauseated
  13. follow prescribed antiemetic regimen if nausea is continuous.

21.c. The client will verbalize ways to improve appetite and nutritional status.

21.c. Instruct client in ways *to improve appetite and maintain an adequate nutritional status:*
  1. try chicken, fish, cheese, and eggs as protein sources instead of beef and pork if taste distortion is a problem
  2. increase the amount of sweeteners and seasonings usually used in foods or beverages
  3. moisten dry foods with sauces, salad dressing, or sour cream
  4. eat in a pleasant environment with company if possible
  5. perform frequent oral hygiene *to eliminate disagreeable tastes in mouth*
  6. try recommended methods of controlling nausea (see action b in this diagnosis)
  7. increase intake of high-protein, high-caloric foods
  8. eat several high-caloric, nutritious, small meals rather than 3 large ones
  9. take vitamins, minerals, and hematinics as prescribed.

21.d. The client will demonstrate appropriate oral hygiene techniques.

21.d.1. Instruct client in appropriate techniques for cleansing his/her teeth:
  a. brush teeth with a fluoridated toothpaste several times a day for 3–4 minutes, particularly after eating
  b. use a small, soft, flexible toothbrush
  c. brush all aspects of teeth and gingival crevices
  d. rinse with a topical fluoride solution (e.g. Phos-Flur, Nafrinse) after brushing.
  2. Emphasize the importance of using dental carrier and fluoride gel daily as ordered until salivary gland function has returned to normal.
  3. If stomatitis is present, instruct client to:
    a. irrigate mouth and cleanse teeth frequently with a gentle power spray instead of brushing
    b. rinse mouth frequently with baking soda and water or a 10% solution of hydrogen peroxide and water.
  4. Allow time for questions, clarification, and practice of oral hygiene techniques.
  5. Instruct client to discuss any planned dental care with the radiologist and to inform the dentist that he/she is receiving or has had radiation to the oral cavity.

21.e. The client will identify ways to prevent urinary calculi.

21.e. Instruct the client regarding ways *to prevent urinary uric acid stone formation:*
  1. avoid foods high in purine (e.g. liver, kidney, goose, venison, seafood, meat soups and gravies, anchovies)
  2. increase intake of foods/fluids that leave an alkaline ash (e.g. milk; vegetables, especially legumes and green vegetables; fruits except prunes, plums, and cranberries)

3. drink at least 10 glasses of liquid/day
4. prevent stasis of urine by:
   a. voiding whenever the urge is felt
   b. increasing activity as tolerated
5. take medication to decrease uric acid production as prescribed.

21.f. The client will identify ways to prevent bleeding if platelet counts are low.	21.f.1. Instruct client in ways *to minimize risk of bleeding:*

      a. avoid taking aspirin, aspirin-containing compounds, and ibuprofen
      b. use an electric rather than a straight-edge razor
      c. floss and brush teeth gently
      d. cut nails carefully
      e. use caution when ambulating *to prevent falls or bumps*
      f. avoid blowing nose forcefully
      g. avoid situations that could result in injury (e.g. contact sports)
      h. avoid straining to have a bowel movement
      i. avoid constrictive clothing.
  2. Instruct client to control any bleeding by applying firm, prolonged pressure to the area if possible.

21.g. The client will identify ways to prevent infection if WBC counts are low.

21.g.1. Explain to client that his/her resistance to infection is reduced when WBC counts are low. Emphasize the need to adhere closely to recommended techniques to prevent infection.
  2. Instruct client in ways *to prevent infection:*
      a. avoid crowds, persons with any sign of infection, and persons who have been recently vaccinated
      b. avoid trauma to the skin or mucous membranes
      c. take an axillary rather than an oral temperature if stomatitis is present
      d. lubricate the skin outside irradiated area frequently *to prevent dryness and subsequent cracking*
      e. cleanse and care for skin within treatment field as recommended (see action a.2 in this diagnosis)
      f. use excellent handwashing technique
      g. avoid any unnecessary rectal invasion (e.g. temperature taking, enemas, suppositories, sexual activity) *to prevent rectal trauma and subsequent rectal infection, fistula, or abscess formation*
      h. if hemorrhoids are present, avoid situations that could aggravate them (e.g. constipation, sitting for prolonged periods)
      i. avoid constipation *to prevent trauma to the rectal mucosa from hard or impacted stool*
      j. wash perianal area thoroughly with soap and water after each bowel movement; caution female client to always wipe from front to back after defecation and urination
      k. avoid douching unless ordered (*douching disturbs the normal vaginal flora, thereby increasing susceptibility to infection*)
      l. drink at least 10 glasses of liquid/day
      m. cough and deep breathe or use inspiratory exerciser every 2 hours until usual activity level is resumed
      n. stop smoking
      o. perform meticulous oral hygiene
      p. maintain an optimal nutritional status (e.g. diet high in protein, calories, vitamins, and minerals)
      q. avoid intake of foods with a high bacteria content (e.g. fresh fruit, uncooked foods)
      r. avoid sharing eating utensils
      s. maintain an adequate balance between activity and rest.

21.h. The client will verbalize an understanding of the effects of radiation therapy on reproductive function.

21.h.1. Clarify physician's explanation about the possible effects of radiation on the gonads if included in the treatment field(s).
  2. Caution the female client that ovarian failure during therapy may result in decreased libido, irritability, hot flashes, and other symptoms of premature menopause.
  3. Inform the female client that her usual menstrual cycle will resume within 6 months to a year after treatment if sterility is temporary.
  4. Emphasize the need for both the male and female client to practice birth control during treatment and for at least 2 years after it.

5. Encourage both the male and female client to seek genetic counseling before attempting conception *to ascertain the risk of chromosomal anomalies.*

21.i. The client will verbalize ways to manage and cope with persistent fatigue.

21.i. Instruct client in ways *to manage and cope with persistent fatigue:*
1. view fatigue as a protective mechanism rather than a problematic limitation
2. determine ways that daily patterns of activity can be modified *to conserve energy and prevent excessive fatigue* (e.g. spread light and heavy tasks throughout the day, take short rests during an activity whenever possible, take several short rest periods during the day instead of one long one)
3. determine if life demands are realistic in light of physical state and adjust short- and long-term goals accordingly
4. avoid situations that are particularly fatiguing such as those that are boring, frustrating, or require prolonged or strenuous physical activity
5. participate in a regular aerobic exercise program *to improve cardiovascular and respiratory fitness, reduce anxiety and stress, and build up tolerance for activity.*

21.j. The client will state signs and symptoms of complications to report to the health care provider.

21.j. Instruct the client to observe for and report the following:
1. signs and symptoms of infection (stress that the usual signs of infection are absent in people with altered bone marrow function and/or a suppressed immune system and that it is necessary to monitor closely for the following signs and symptoms):
   a. temperature above 38°C (100.4°F)
   b. changes in odor, color, or consistency of urine or pain on urination
   c. white patches in mouth or vagina
   d. crusted ulcerations around or in oral cavity
   e. swollen, reddened, coated tongue
   f. painful rectal or vaginal area
   g. redness, increased pain, or bleeding of hemorrhoids
   h. changes in appearance or temperature of the skin, particularly around injection sites
   i. persistent or productive cough
   j. unusual odor or drainage from treatment area
2. signs and symptoms of bleeding (e.g. excessive bruising, black stools, persistent nose bleeds or bleeding from gums, sudden swelling and pain in joints, red or smoke-colored urine, blood in vomitus)
3. signs and symptoms of urinary calculi (e.g. dull, aching or sharp, colicky flank pain; urinary urgency or frequency; unusual appearance of urine)
4. signs and symptoms of radiation cystitis (e.g. blood in the urine, pain on urination, urinary frequency or urgency)
5. signs and symptoms of radiation pneumonitis (e.g. shortness of breath; persistent, dry, hacking cough; fever)
6. signs and symptoms of tissue fibrosis within treatment field (e.g. LUNG: increasing shortness of breath, cough, hemoptysis; BOWEL: inability to move bowels, distended abdomen, loss of appetite, alternating diarrhea and constipation; ESOPHAGUS: difficulty swallowing; SKIN: uneven texture; VAGINA: pain during intercourse)
7. excessive tooth decay
8. signs and symptoms of dehydration (e.g. dry mouth, weight loss, concentrated urine, lightheadedness)
9. inability to eat
10. significant weight loss
11. persistent vomiting and/or diarrhea
12. increase in pain in irradiated area
13. excessive depression or difficulty coping with the effects of the diagnosis and treatment.

21.k. The client will identify community resources that can assist with home management and adjustment to the diagnosis of cancer and radiation therapy and its effects.

21.k.1. Provide information about and encourage utilization of community resources that can assist the client and significant others with home management and adjustment to cancer and the effects of radiation therapy (e.g. local support groups, American Cancer Society, Visiting Nurse Association, counselors, social service agencies, Dial-a-Bus, Meals on Wheels, Make Today Count, Hospice).
2. Initiate a referral if indicated.

UNIT V

21.l. The client will verbalize an understanding of and a plan for adhering to recommended follow-up care including future appointments with health care provider, radiation department, and laboratory and medications prescribed.

21.l.1. Reinforce physician's explanation of planned radiation therapy schedule.
2. Discuss with client any difficulties he/she might have adhering to the schedule and assist in planning ways to overcome these.
3. Reinforce the importance of keeping appointments for radiation treatments and follow-up laboratory studies.
4. Reinforce the importance of keeping follow-up appointments with health care provider.
5. Explain the rationale for, side effects of, and importance of taking medications prescribed.
6. Implement measures *to improve client compliance:*
   a. include significant others in teaching sessions
   b. encourage questions and allow time for reinforcement or clarification of information provided
   c. provide written instructions regarding future appointments with health care provider, radiation department, and laboratory; medications prescribed; and signs and symptoms to report.

☐ ███

References

Bersani, G, and Carl, W. Oral care for cancer patients. American Journal of Nursing, *83*(4):533–536, 1983.
Hassey, KM, and Rose, CM. Altered skin integrity in patients receiving radiation therapy. Oncology Nursing Forum, *9*(4):44–50, 1982.
Kübler-Ross, F. On death and dying. New York: Macmillan, 1969.

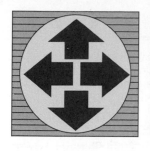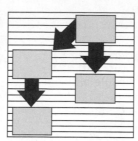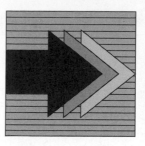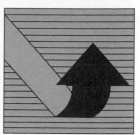

Unit VI

Nursing Care of the Client with Disturbances of Neurological Function

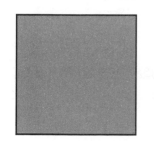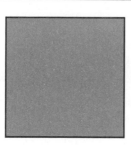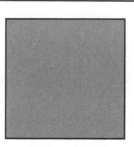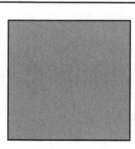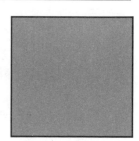

Cerebrovascular Accident

A cerebrovascular accident (CVA) is the result of an interruption in the blood supply to certain parts of the brain and is characterized by the sudden development of focal neurological deficits. These deficits range from mild transient symptoms such as tingling, weakness, and slight speech impairment to severe permanent symptoms such as hemiplegia, aphasia, visual field cuts, and loss of consciousness. CVAs are classified according to etiology. Thrombosis is the most common cause and can result from atherosclerotic changes, arteritis, and conditions of hypercoagulability. Thrombotic CVAs are further classified according to their stage of development: transient ischemic attack (brief temporary episode of neurological deficits), stroke in evolution (neurological deficits that continue to worsen over a period of a few days), and completed stroke (neurological deficits that remain unchanged after 2–3 days). Other causes of a CVA include embolus, cerebral hemorrhage, generalized hypoxia, and, less frequently, vasospasm and compression of the cerebral vessels. The manifestations of a CVA depend upon the area of the brain involved, the size of the lesion, and the effectiveness of collateral circulation. Treatment is dependent upon the etiology and extensiveness of the deficits.

This care plan focuses on the adult client hospitalized with signs and symptoms of a CVA. In the acute phase, goals of care are to improve cerebral tissue perfusion, prevent life-threatening complications, and perform or assist the client with those activities he/she is unable to accomplish independently. The goals of care in the rehabilitation phase are to prevent complications and assist the client to attain an optimal level of independence. This care plan focuses on the most common deficits that occur as a result of a CVA. The reader should refer to neurological texts for further information about the numerous speech, motor, and sensory deficits that can occur.

DISCHARGE CRITERIA

Prior to discharge, the client will:

- communicate an awareness of ways to decrease the risk of a recurrent CVA
- identify ways to manage sensory and verbal communication impairments and alterations in thought processes
- identify ways to manage urinary and bowel incontinence
- demonstrate techniques to facilitate performance of activities of daily living and increase physical mobility
- communicate an awareness of signs and symptoms to report to the health care provider
- share thoughts and feelings about the effects of the CVA on life style, roles, and self-concept
- communicate knowledge of community agencies that can assist with home management and the adjustment to changes resulting from the CVA
- communicate an understanding of and a plan for adhering to recommended follow-up care including future appointments with health care provider and therapists and medications prescribed.

Use in conjunction with the Care Plan on Immobility.

NURSING/COLLABORATIVE DIAGNOSES

1. Anxiety □ *191*
2. Altered cerebral tissue perfusion □ *192*
3. Ineffective breathing patterns □ *193*
4. Ineffective airway clearance □ *193*
5. Altered nutrition: less than body requirements □ *194*
6. Impaired swallowing □ *194*
7. Unilateral neglect □ *195*
8. Impaired verbal communication:
   a. dysarthria
   b. aphasia or dysphasia □ *196*
9. Impaired skin integrity: irritation or breakdown □ *197*
10. Impaired physical mobility □ *197*
11. Self-care deficit □ *198*
12. Altered pattern of urinary elimination: incontinence □ *199*
13. Constipation □ *200*
14. Bowel incontinence □ *200*
15. Altered thought processes: shortened attention span, impaired memory, confusion, slowed or quick and impulsive responses, and aggressive and/or inappropriate responses □ *201*
16. Potential for infection: pneumonia □ *202*
17. Potential for trauma □ *202*
18. Potential for aspiration □ *204*
19. Potential complications:
   a. increased intracranial pressure (IICP)
   b. seizures
   c. gastrointestinal (GI) bleeding
   d. corneal irritation and abrasion
   e. subluxation of shoulder □ *204*
20. Sexual dysfunction:
   a. alteration in usual activities
   b. decreased libido and/or impotence □ *207*
21. Disturbance in self-concept □ *208*
22. Ineffective individual coping □ *209*
23. Powerlessness □ *211*
24. Grieving □ *211*
25. Social isolation □ *212*
26. Knowledge deficit regarding follow-up care □ *213*

1. NURSING DIAGNOSIS

Anxiety related to unfamiliar environment; lack of understanding of diagnosis, diagnostic tests, and treatments; uncertain prognosis; impaired verbal communication and motor and sensory function; altered thought processes; and anticipated effect of the CVA on future life style and roles.

DESIRED OUTCOMES	NURSING ACTIONS AND *SELECTED RATIONALES*

1. The client will experience a reduction in fear and anxiety (see Care Plan on Immobility, Nursing Diagnosis 1, for outcome criteria).

1.a. Assess client for signs and symptoms of fear and anxiety (e.g. communication of fears and concerns; tenseness; tremors; irritability; restlessness; diaphoresis; tachypnea; elevated blood pressure; tachycardia; facial tension, pallor, or flushing; noncompliance with treatment plan). Validate perceptions carefully, remembering that some behaviors may be due to neurological changes resulting from the CVA.
   b. Ascertain effectiveness of current coping skills.
   c. Refer to Care Plan on Immobility, Nursing Diagnosis 1, action c, for measures to reduce fear and anxiety.
   d. Implement additional measures *to reduce fear and anxiety:*
      1. if speech or comprehension has been affected, establish an effective communication system (e.g. paper and pencil, letter or picture board, magic slate, gestures) as soon as possible
      2. assure client that staff members are nearby; check client frequently and respond to call signal as soon as possible
      3. if client is experiencing homonymous hemianopsia, approach on unaffected side within his/her visual field
      4. simplify environment as much as possible
      5. explain that motor, sensory, and speech impairments and alterations in thought processes are often more extensive initially and gradually improve
      6. explain all diagnostic procedures (e.g. neurological examination, computed tomography, magnetic resonance imaging [MRI], EEG, cerebral angiography, visual field examination)
      7. perform actions to assist client to cope with diagnosis and its implications (see Nursing Diagnosis 22, action d).

□ ▮▮

2. NURSING DIAGNOSIS

Altered cerebral tissue perfusion related to an interruption of cerebral blood flow associated with thrombus, embolus, cerebral hemorrhage, and spasm or compression of cerebral vessels.

□ ▮▮

DESIRED OUTCOMES	NURSING ACTIONS AND *SELECTED RATIONALES*

2. The client will experience improved cerebral tissue perfusion as evidenced by:
   a. absence of or reduction in dizziness, syncope, visual disturbances
   b. improved mental status
   c. pupils equal and normally reactive to light
   d. improved motor and sensory function.

2.a. Assess the client for signs and symptoms of decreased cerebral tissue perfusion:
   1. dizziness, syncope
   2. blurred or dimmed vision, diplopia, change in visual field
   3. irritability and restlessness
   4. decreased level of consciousness
   5. unequal pupils or a sluggish or absent pupillary reaction to light
   6. paresthesias, motor weakness, paralysis
   7. seizures.
   b. Implement measures *to improve cerebral tissue perfusion:*
      1. if a thrombus or embolus is present, monitor for therapeutic and nontherapeutic effects of the following medications if administered:
         a. anticoagulants (e.g. warfarin, heparin) or antiplatelet agents (e.g. aspirin, dipyridamole)
         b. peripheral vasodilators (e.g. cyclandelate, papaverine, isoxsuprine)
      2. if intracerebral hemorrhage has occurred as a result of cerebral aneurysm rupture, monitor for therapeutic and nontherapeutic effects of

hemostatic agents (e.g. aminocaproic acid) if administered *to prevent lysis of formed clots and subsequent rebleeding*
3. monitor for therapeutic and nontherapeutic effects of medications administered *to decrease spasm of cerebral vessels* (e.g. papaverine)
4. perform actions *to reduce cerebral edema in order to decrease pressure on the blood vessels:*
   a. maintain fluid restrictions as ordered
   b. administer fluids at an even rate
   c. elevate head of bed 20–30° unless contraindicated *to promote adequate cerebral venous drainage*
   d. monitor for therapeutic and nontherapeutic effects of osmotic diuretics (e.g. mannitol), loop diuretics (e.g. furosemide), and corticosteroids (e.g. methylprednisolone, dexamethasone) if administered
5. keep head and neck in proper alignment
6. perform actions to prevent and treat increased intracranial pressure (see Collaborative Diagnosis 19, actions a.2 and 3).
   c. Consult physician if signs and symptoms of decreased cerebral tissue perfusion worsen.

3. NURSING DIAGNOSIS

Ineffective breathing patterns related to fear, anxiety, impaired chest expansion associated with decreased mobility and weakened muscles of respiration on the affected side, and possible ischemia of the respiratory center in the brain stem.

DESIRED OUTCOMES	NURSING ACTIONS AND *SELECTED RATIONALES*

3. The client will maintain an effective breathing pattern (see Care Plan on Immobility, Nursing Diagnosis 3, for outcome criteria).	3.a. Refer to Care Plan on Immobility, Nursing Diagnosis 3, for measures related to assessment and improvement of ineffective breathing patterns.
	b. Implement additional measures *to improve breathing pattern:*
	  1. perform actions to improve cerebral tissue perfusion (see Nursing Diagnosis 2, action b)
	  2. if client has weakened muscles of respiration:
	    a. instruct him/her in and assist with methods *to increase amount of air exhaled* (e.g. place towel around abdomen and gently tighten it during expiration while client does pursed-lip breathing)
	    b. encourage and assist client to perform exercises that can help strengthen the accessory muscles used in breathing (e.g. shoulder shrugs *to strengthen the trapezius muscles*, progressive application of weights to the upper abdomen during diaphragmatic breathing *to strengthen abdominal muscles*) when allowed and tolerated.

4. NURSING DIAGNOSIS

Ineffective airway clearance related to:

a. stasis of secretions associated with decreased mobility and poor cough effort;
b. airway obstruction resulting from tongue falling back in throat.

DESIRED OUTCOMES	NURSING ACTIONS AND *SELECTED RATIONALES*
4. The client will maintain clear, open airways (see Care Plan on Immobility, Nursing Diagnosis 4, for outcome criteria).	4.a. Refer to Care Plan on Immobility, Nursing Diagnosis 4, for measures related to assessment and promotion of effective airway clearance. b. Position client on side and/or insert an artificial airway if necessary *to prevent obstruction of airway by tongue.*

☐ ▬▬▬▬▬▬▬▬▬▬▬▬▬▬▬▬▬▬▬▬▬

5. NURSING DIAGNOSIS

Altered nutrition: less than body requirements related to decreased oral intake associated with:

a. anorexia resulting from fear, anxiety, depression, decreased activity, and constipation;
b. dysphagia and difficulty chewing resulting from muscular impairment on the affected side;
c. difficulty feeding self as a result of impaired motor function and visual and spatial-perceptual deficits.

☐ ▬▬▬▬▬▬▬▬▬▬▬▬▬▬▬▬▬▬▬▬▬

DESIRED OUTCOMES	NURSING ACTIONS AND *SELECTED RATIONALES*
5. The client will maintain an adequate nutritional status (see Care Plan on Immobility, Nursing Diagnosis 6, for outcome criteria).	5.a. Refer to Care Plan on Immobility, Nursing Diagnosis 6, for measures related to assessment and maintenance of an adequate nutritional status. b. Implement additional measures *to improve oral intake and maintain an adequate nutritional status:* 1. perform actions to reduce fear and anxiety (see Nursing Diagnosis 1, actions c and d) 2. perform actions to prevent constipation (see Nursing Diagnosis 13, actions a and b) 3. perform actions to facilitate client's psychological adjustment to the effects of the CVA (see Nursing Diagnoses 21, actions d–w; 22, action d; 23; and 24, action d) 4. assist client to select foods that require little or no chewing (e.g. custards, applesauce, pureed foods) 5. perform actions to improve ability to swallow (see Nursing Diagnosis 6, action b) 6. perform actions to enable client to feed self (see Nursing Diagnosis 11, action d.6) 7. encourage significant others to bring in client's favorite foods that are easily chewed and swallowed.

☐ ▬▬▬▬▬▬▬▬▬▬▬▬▬▬▬▬▬▬▬▬▬

6. NURSING DIAGNOSIS

Impaired swallowing related to weakened muscles of deglutition and decreased swallowing reflex.

☐ ▬▬▬▬▬▬▬▬▬▬▬▬▬▬▬▬▬▬▬▬▬

DESIRED OUTCOMES	NURSING ACTIONS AND *SELECTED RATIONALES*

6. The client will experience an improvement in swallowing as evidenced by:
a. communication of same
b. absence of coughing and choking when eating and drinking.
	6.a. Assess for and report signs and symptoms of impaired swallowing (e.g. coughing or choking when eating and drinking, stasis of food in oral cavity).
	b. Implement measures *to improve ability to swallow:*
	  1. place client in high Fowler's position for meals and snacks; head should be erect with chin tilted forward *to facilitate elevation of the larynx and posterior movement of the tongue*
	  2. assist client to select foods that have a distinct texture and are easy to swallow (e.g. applesauce, custard, cottage cheese, ground meat)
	  3. instruct client to avoid mixing foods of different texture in his/her mouth at the same time
	  4. avoid serving foods that are sticky (e.g. peanut butter, soft bread, bananas)
	  5. serve foods/fluids that are hot or cold instead of room temperature (*the more extreme temperatures stimulate the sensory receptors and swallowing reflex*)
	  6. utilize adaptive devices (e.g. long-handled spoon, "pusher" spoon) to place food in back of mouth on unaffected side if tongue movement is impaired
	  7. moisten dry foods with gravy or sauces (e.g. catsup, salad dressing, sour cream)
	  8. encourage client to concentrate on the act of swallowing
	  9. if client is retaining food/fluid in mouth, instruct him/her to tilt head to unaffected side when eating or drinking
	  10. gently stroke client's throat when he/she is swallowing if indicated
	  11. encourage client to drink through a straw *in order to decrease risk of choking and strengthen facial and swallowing muscles*
	  12. consult speech pathologist about methods for dealing with impaired swallowing; reinforce exercises and techniques prescribed.
	c. Consult physician if swallowing difficulties persist or worsen.

□ ▬▬▬▬▬▬▬▬▬▬▬▬▬▬▬▬▬▬▬▬

7. NURSING DIAGNOSIS

Unilateral neglect related to:

a. homonymous hemianopsia associated with ischemia of visual pathways;
b. ischemia of portions of the nondominant hemisphere.

□ ▬▬▬▬▬▬▬▬▬▬▬▬▬▬▬▬▬▬▬▬

DESIRED OUTCOMES	NURSING ACTIONS AND *SELECTED RATIONALES*

7. The client will experience a gradual reduction in and/or demonstrate beginning adaptation to unilateral neglect as evidenced by:
a. awareness of stimuli on affected side
b. awareness of the affected side of body.
	7.a. Assess client for presence of unilateral neglect (e.g. leaving food on plate on the affected side, not looking toward affected side, no response to stimuli on affected side, lack of awareness of affected extremities).
	b. Implement measures to maintain adequate cerebral tissue perfusion (see Nursing Diagnosis 2, action b) *in order to prevent further cerebral ischemia.*
	c. If unilateral neglect is present:
	  1. ensure that affected extremities are positioned properly at all times
	  2. protect affected extremities from injury
	  3. encourage client to handle affected extremities when bathing, dressing, and positioning *in order to increase awareness of his/her whole body*
	  4. as condition stabilizes, place some items (e.g. television, clock) on affected side *to increase the frequency of viewing affected extremities and promote environmental scanning*

      5. consult physical and occupational therapists about additional ways to facilitate client's adaptation to unilateral neglect

      6. inform significant others and health care personnel of approaches being used to increase client's awareness of affected side; encourage their use of these techniques.

  d. Consult physician if unilateral neglect becomes more severe or client is unable to begin to adapt to it.

☐ ▬▬▬▬▬▬▬▬▬▬▬▬▬▬▬▬▬▬▬▬▬▬

8. NURSING DIAGNOSIS

Impaired verbal communication:

a. **dysarthria** related to loss of motor function of the muscles of speech articulation;
b. **aphasia or dysphasia** related to ischemia of the dominant hemisphere (ischemia of Wernicke's area of the temporal lobe will result in receptive aphasia; ischemia of Broca's area of the frontal lobe will result in expressive aphasia).

☐ ▬▬▬▬▬▬▬▬▬▬▬▬▬▬▬▬▬▬▬▬▬▬

DESIRED OUTCOMES	NURSING ACTIONS AND *SELECTED RATIONALES*

8. The client will communicate needs and desires effectively.	8.a. Assess for difficulties in verbal communication (e.g. inability to speak, difficulty with articulation, incorrect ordering of words, inability to find or name words and objects). Consult speech pathologist for assistance in determining types of aphasia or dysphasia present.
	b. Implement measures *to facilitate communication:*
	  1. answer call signal in person rather than using the intercommunication system
	  2. make frequent rounds *to ascertain needs*
	  3. maintain a patient, calm approach; listen carefully, avoid interrupting client, and allow ample time for communication
	  4. if client is frustrated or fatigued, try to anticipate needs and ask questions that require short answers or nod of head *in order to minimize the necessity of verbal communication*
	  5. schedule rest periods before visiting hours and speech therapy sessions *to maximize communication ability during those times*
	  6. decrease environmental stimuli *so client can better concentrate on efforts to communicate*
	  7. when speaking to client, face him/her; speak slowly; use direct, short statements; repeat key words; and avoid using unrelated gestures
	  8. provide and/or utilize appropriate aids to communication (e.g. related gestures, pictures, letter board, magic slate)
	  9. ensure that intravenous therapy does not interfere with the client's ability to write
	  10. encourage client to perform exercises and utilize techniques identified by speech pathologist.
	c. Do not focus on automatic speech (e.g. cursing, singing, use of exclamatory remarks). Inform client and significant others that this speech is uncontrollable and should diminish.
	d. Validate verbal responses with an assessment of nonverbal behavior *(the ability to speak does not necessarily indicate the ability to comprehend).*
	e. Inform significant others and health care personnel of approaches being used to maximize client's ability to communicate. Encourage their use of these techniques.
	f. Encourage significant others and staff to talk to client even if he/she is unresponsive or unable to communicate.
	g. Consult physician if client experiences increasing impairment of verbal communication.

9. NURSING DIAGNOSIS

Impaired skin integrity: irritation or breakdown related to:

a. prolonged pressure on tissues associated with decreased mobility;
b. frequent contact with irritants associated with urinary and/or bowel incontinence;
c. increased fragility of skin associated with dependent edema and malnutrition.

DESIRED OUTCOMES	NURSING ACTIONS AND *SELECTED RATIONALES*

9. The client will maintain skin integrity as evidenced by:
a. absence of redness and irritation
b. no skin breakdown.
	9.a. Inspect the skin (especially bone prominences, dependent areas, perineum, and areas of decreased sensation and edema) for pallor, redness, and breakdown.
	b. Refer to Care Plan on Immobility, Nursing Diagnosis 7, action b, for measures to prevent skin breakdown associated with decreased mobility.
	c. Implement measures *to prevent skin breakdown associated with edema:*
	  1. perform actions *to reduce fluid accumulation in dependent areas:*
	    a. instruct client in and assist with range of motion exercises
	    b. assist client to turn at least every 2 hours (most resources recommend that client remain on affected side for only 20 minutes at a time)
	    c. elevate affected extremities whenever possible
	    d. apply elastic wraps or hose to lower extremities as ordered
	  2. handle edematous areas carefully.
	d. Implement measures *to decrease skin irritation and prevent breakdown resulting from incontinence of urine or stool:*
	  1. perform actions to prevent urinary and bowel incontinence (see Nursing Diagnoses 12, action b and 14, action b)
	  2. provide soft toilet tissue for wiping after urination and defecation
	  3. assist client to thoroughly cleanse and dry perineal area after each episode of incontinence; apply a protective ointment or cream (e.g. Sween cream, Desitin, A & D ointment, Vaseline)
	  4. avoid direct contact of skin with Chux (e.g. place turn sheet or bed pad over Chux).
	e. If skin breakdown occurs:
	  1. notify physician
	  2. continue with above measures to prevent further irritation and breakdown
	  3. perform decubitus care as ordered or per standard hospital policy
	  4. monitor client closely and report signs and symptoms of infection (e.g. elevated temperature; redness, warmth, and edema around area of breakdown; unusual drainage from site).

10. NURSING DIAGNOSIS

Impaired physical mobility related to decreased motor function, spatial-perceptual impairments, and fear of injury.

DESIRED OUTCOMES	NURSING ACTIONS AND *SELECTED RATIONALES*

10.a. The client will achieve maximum physical mobility within limitations imposed by the CVA.

10.a.1. Assess for factors that impair physical mobility (e.g. loss of motor function, spatial-perceptual impairments, fear of injury).
   2. Implement measures *to increase mobility:*
     a. instruct client in and assist with active and active-resistive exercises of unaffected extremities at least every 4 hours unless contraindicated
     b. perform passive range of motion exercises of affected extremities at least every 4 hours unless contraindicated
     c. provide adequate rest periods before activity sessions
     d. monitor for therapeutic and nontherapeutic effects of muscle relaxants (e.g. baclofen, dantrolene) if administered *to relieve spasticity in affected extremities* (spasticity usually follows initial period of flaccidity)
     e. perform actions to prevent falls (see Nursing Diagnosis 17, action b) *in order to decrease client's fear of injury*
     f. instruct client in and assist with correct use of mobility aids (e.g. cane, walker) if appropriate
     g. if spatial-perceptual impairments are present, place client in front of a full-length mirror *in order to assist him/her to identify vertical and horizontal planes*
     h. reinforce instructions, activities, and exercise plan recommended by physical and/or occupational therapists.
   3. Increase activity and participation in self-care activities as tolerated.
   4. Provide praise and encouragement for all efforts to increase physical mobility.
   5. Encourage the support of significant others. Allow them to assist with range of motion exercises, positioning, and activity if desired.
   6. Consult physician if client is unable to achieve expected level of mobility or range of motion becomes restricted.

10.b. The client will not experience problems associated with immobility.

10.b. Refer to Care Plan on Immobility for actions to prevent problems associated with immobility.

11. NURSING DIAGNOSIS

Self-care deficit related to impaired physical mobility, visual impairments, apraxia, unilateral neglect, and alteration in thought processes.

DESIRED OUTCOMES	NURSING ACTIONS AND *SELECTED RATIONALES*

11. The client will perform self-care activities within physical limitations.

11.a. Assess for factors that interfere with client's ability to perform self-care (e.g. visual and motor deficits, apraxia, alteration in thought processes).
  b. With client, develop a realistic plan for meeting daily physical needs.
  c. Encourage maximum independence within limitations imposed by impairments resulting from the CVA.
  d. Implement measures *to facilitate client's ability to perform self-care activities:*
   1. schedule care at a time when client is most likely to be able to participate (e.g. after rest periods, not immediately after meals or treatments)
   2. keep needed objects within easy reach and within visual field
   3. if apraxia is present, explain and demonstrate use of items such as toothbrush, comb, and washcloth as often as necessary

4. encourage client's efforts to use nondominant hand if dominant one has been affected
5. encourage client to wear eyepatch or frosted lens if diplopia is present
6. perform actions *to enable client to feed self:*
   a. place foods/fluids within client's visual field until he/she learns to effectively utilize scanning techniques
   b. place only a few items on the tray at one time if spatial-perceptual deficits are present
   c. identify where items are placed on the plate or tray and open containers, cut meat, or butter bread as indicated
   d. consult with occupational therapist about adaptive devices available (e.g. broad-handled utensils, rocker knives, plate guards); reinforce use of these devices
7. perform actions *to enable client to dress self when condition stabilizes:*
   a. encourage use of adaptive devices such as button hooks, long-handled shoehorns, and pull loops for pants
   b. encourage client to select clothing that is easy to put on and remove (e.g. clothing with zippers rather than buttons, loose-fitting clothing, shoes with Velcro fasteners rather than laces)
   c. if client has difficulty distinguishing right from left, mark outer aspect of shoes with tape or label with *R* or *L*
8. reinforce exercises and activities prescribed by physical and occupational therapists to improve fine motor skills
9. allow adequate time for accomplishment of self-care activities.

e. Provide positive feedback for all efforts and accomplishments of self-care.
f. Assist client with those activities he/she is unable to perform independently.
g. Inform significant others of client's abilities to perform own care. Explain importance of encouraging and allowing client to maintain an optimal level of independence within physical limitations.

□ ▉▉

12. NURSING DIAGNOSIS

Altered pattern of urinary elimination: incontinence related to:

a. loss of voluntary control of urinary elimination associated with upper motor neuron involvement;
b. decreased ability to respond to the urge to urinate associated with decreased level of consciousness, inability to communicate need to urinate, and impaired physical mobility.

□ ▉▉

DESIRED OUTCOMES	NURSING ACTIONS AND *SELECTED RATIONALES*

12. The client will experience urinary continence.	12.a. Monitor for and report urinary incontinence.
	b. Implement measures *to prevent urinary incontinence:*
	  1. offer bedpan or urinal or assist client to commode or bathroom every 2–3 hours
	  2. allow client to assume a normal position for voiding unless contraindicated *to promote complete bladder emptying*
	  3. instruct client to perform perineal exercises (e.g. stopping and starting stream during voiding; pressing buttocks together, then relaxing the muscles) *in order to improve urinary sphincter tone*
	  4. limit oral fluid intake in the evening *to decrease possibility of nighttime incontinence*

5. instruct client to avoid drinking beverages containing caffeine *(caffeine is a mild diuretic and may make urinary control more difficult)*
6. monitor for therapeutic and nontherapeutic effects of alpha-adrenergic agonists (e.g. ephedrine) if administered *to increase tone of the urinary sphincter.*

c. If urinary incontinence persists:
1. consult physician about intermittent catheterization, insertion of indwelling catheter, or use of external catheter or penile clamp
2. provide emotional support to client and significant others.

13. NURSING DIAGNOSIS

Constipation related to:

a. decreased activity;
b. decreased intake of fluid and foods high in fiber associated with dysphagia, anorexia, and difficulty feeding self;
c. decreased ability to respond to the urge to defecate associated with decreased level of consciousness, inability to communicate need to defecate, and impaired physical mobility;
d. increased sympathetic nervous system activity associated with anxiety.

DESIRED OUTCOMES	NURSING ACTIONS AND *SELECTED RATIONALES*

13. The client will maintain usual bowel elimination pattern.	13.a. Refer to Care Plan on Immobility, Nursing Diagnosis 11, for measures related to assessment, prevention, and management of constipation.
	b. Implement additional measures *to prevent constipation* (the measures to prevent constipation are the basis for the bowel training program):
	  1. establish a routine time for defecation based on client's usual bowel elimination pattern
	  2. perform or, as the rehabilitation program progresses, assist client with digital stimulation of the rectum if indicated
	  3. if client is dysphasic, establish an effective method for him/her to communicate the urge to defecate.
	c. If constipation persists, review and revise bowel training program as needed.

14. NURSING DIAGNOSIS

Bowel incontinence related to:

a. loss of control of bowel elimination associated with upper motor neuron involvement;
b. decreased ability to respond to the urge to defecate associated with decreased level of consciousness, inability to communicate need to defecate, and impaired physical mobility.

DESIRED OUTCOMES	**NURSING ACTIONS AND *SELECTED RATIONALES***

14. The client will not experience bowel incontinence.

14.a. Monitor for episodes of bowel incontinence.
  b. Implement measures *to reduce the risk of bowel incontinence:*
    1. establish and adhere to a bowel training program *so that the client will evacuate the rectum at regularly scheduled intervals*
    2. have commode or bedpan readily available to client
    3. if client is dysphasic, establish an effective method for him/her to communicate the urge to defecate
    4. instruct client to perform perineal exercises (e.g. relaxing and tightening perineal and gluteal muscles) *to strengthen the anal sphincter.*
  c. If bowel incontinence persists:
    1. review and revise bowel training program as needed
    2. provide client with liners for underwear or disposable undergarments such as Attends
    3. utilize room deodorizers as necessary
    4. provide emotional support to client and significant others.

□ ▰▰▰▰▰▰▰▰▰▰▰▰▰▰▰▰▰▰▰▰▰

15. NURSING DIAGNOSIS

Altered thought processes: shortened attention span, impaired memory, confusion, slowed or quick and impulsive responses, and aggressive and/or inappropriate responses related to cerebral ischemia.

□ ▰▰▰▰▰▰▰▰▰▰▰▰▰▰▰▰▰▰▰▰▰

DESIRED OUTCOMES	**NURSING ACTIONS AND *SELECTED RATIONALES***

15. The client will have gradual improvement of and/or demonstrate beginning adaptation to alterations in thought processes as evidenced by:
a. usual or improved attention span and problem-solving abilities
b. improved level of orientation
c. reduction in episodes of aggressive or inappropriate responses
d. utilization of techniques to aid memory.

15.a. Assess client for alterations in thought processes (e.g. shortened attention span, impaired memory, decreased ability to problem-solve, confusion, aggressive and/or inappropriate responses).
  b. Ascertain from significant others client's usual level of intellectual functioning and whether personality changes have occurred.
  c. Implement measures to maintain adequate cerebral tissue perfusion (see Nursing Diagnosis 2, action b) *in order to prevent further cerebral ischemia.*
  d. If client shows evidence of altered thought processes:
    1. reorient to person, place, and time as necessary
    2. allow adequate time for communication and performance of activities
    3. implement measures *to assist client to adapt to his/her shortened attention span and impaired memory:*
      a. encourage client to make lists of planned activities and questions or concerns he/she may have
      b. provide written or taped instructions and information whenever possible for client to review as often as necessary
    4. implement measures *to assist client to adapt to impaired reasoning ability:*
      a. allow adequate time for client to clarify information
      b. keep environmental stimuli to a minimum during treatments, conversations, and teaching sessions
      c. assist client to problem-solve as necessary
    5. implement measures *to stop emotional outbursts, aggressive behavior, and inappropriate responses* (e.g. provide distraction by clapping hands or whistling loudly, instruct client to hold mouth open if he/she is crying inappropriately)
    6. maintain realistic expectations of client's ability to learn, comprehend, and remember information provided

UNIT
VI

7. encourage significant others to be supportive of client; instruct them in methods of dealing with alterations in client's thought processes.
   e. Consult physician if client demonstrates increased alterations in thought processes or is unable to adapt to existing ones.

16. NURSING DIAGNOSIS

Potential for infection: pneumonia related to:

a. aspiration associated with difficulty swallowing, depressed cough and gag reflexes, and decreased level of consciousness;
b. stasis of secretions in the lungs associated with poor cough effort and decreased mobility.

DESIRED OUTCOMES	NURSING ACTIONS AND *SELECTED RATIONALES*
16. The client will not develop pneumonia (see Care Plan on Immobility, Nursing Diagnosis 13, outcome a, for outcome criteria).	16.a. Refer to Care Plan on Immobility, Nursing Diagnosis 13, action a, for measures related to assessment, prevention, and treatment of pneumonia. b. Implement additional measures *to prevent pneumonia*: 1. perform actions to improve breathing pattern and promote effective airway clearance (see Nursing Diagnoses 3 and 4) 2. perform actions to reduce the risk of aspiration (see Nursing Diagnosis 18, action e).

17. NURSING DIAGNOSIS

Potential for trauma related to:

a. falls associated with motor, visual, and spatial-perceptual impairments; weakness resulting from prolonged immobility; spasticity; altered thought processes; decreased level of consciousness; and seizure activity;
b. burns and cuts associated with motor, sensory, and spatial-perceptual impairments and quick, impulsive behavior (occurs primarily with involvement of the nondominant hemisphere).

DESIRED OUTCOMES	NURSING ACTIONS AND *SELECTED RATIONALES*
17. The client will not experience falls, burns, or cuts.	17.a. Determine whether conditions predisposing the client to falls, burns, or cuts exist: 1. weakness and fatigue 2. motor and spatial-perceptual impairments

    3. decreased level of consciousness
    4. previous seizure activity and/or abnormal EEG
    5. decreased sensation in extremities
    6. altered thought processes
    7. visual disturbances.
  b. Implement measures *to prevent falls:*
    1. keep bed in low position with side rails up when client is in bed
    2. keep needed items within easy reach and assist client to identify their location
    3. encourage client to request assistance whenever needed; have call signal within easy reach
    4. if vision is impaired:
      a. orient client to surroundings, room, and arrangement of furniture
      b. provide an eyepatch or frosted lens for client to wear if diplopia is present
      c. encourage visual scanning if homonymous hemianopsia is present
    5. use lap belt when client is in chair if indicated
    6. instruct client to wear shoes with nonskid soles and low heels when ambulating
    7. avoid unnecessary clutter in room
    8. accompany client during ambulation utilizing a transfer safety belt
    9. provide ambulatory aids (e.g. walker, cane) if client is weak or unsteady on feet
    10. reinforce instructions from physical therapist on correct transfer and ambulation techniques
    11. instruct client to ambulate in well-lit areas and to utilize handrails if needed
    12. do not rush client; allow adequate time for trips to the bathroom and ambulation in hallway
    13. perform actions *to reduce weakness:*
      a. maintain an adequate nutritional status (see Nursing Diagnosis 5)
      b. implement measures to improve activity tolerance (see Care Plan on Immobility, Nursing Diagnosis 8, action b)
    14. stabilize client's affected arm with a sling when he/she is out of bed *in order to improve balance.*
  c. Implement measures *to prevent burns:*
    1. let hot foods/fluids cool slightly before serving *to reduce risk of burns if spills occur*
    2. supervise client while smoking if indicated
    3. assess temperature of bath water and heating pad before and during use.
  d. Assist client with tasks that require fine motor skills (e.g. shaving) *in order to prevent cuts.*
  e. If neglect of affected extremities is severe, tie a ribbon or bell on extremities *to remind client to protect them from injury* (affected foot may get caught under wheelchair or in door *because it is not recognized as being part of his/her body).*
  f. Assist with all activities if proprioception is severely impaired.
  g. If client is confused or irrational, implement additional measures *to reduce risk of injury:*
    1. reorient frequently to surroundings and necessity of adhering to safety precautions
    2. provide constant supervision (e.g. staff member, significant other) if indicated
    3. use jacket or wrist restraints or safety alarm device if necessary *to reduce the risk of client's getting out of bed or chair unattended*
    4. monitor for therapeutic and nontherapeutic effects of antianxiety and antipsychotic medications if administered.
  h. Monitor for therapeutic and nontherapeutic effects of muscle relaxants if administered *to reduce spasticity of affected muscles.*
  i. Implement measures to prevent seizures and resultant injury (see Collaborative Diagnosis 19, actions b.2–4).
  j. Include client and significant others in planning and implementing measures to prevent injury.
  k. If injury does occur, initiate appropriate first aid and notify physician.

☐ ▬▬▬▬▬▬▬▬▬▬▬▬▬▬▬▬▬▬▬▬

18. NURSING DIAGNOSIS

Potential for aspiration related to impaired swallowing, depressed cough and gag reflexes, and decreased level of consciousness.

☐ ▬▬▬▬▬▬▬▬▬▬▬▬▬▬▬▬▬▬▬▬

DESIRED OUTCOMES	NURSING ACTIONS AND *SELECTED RATIONALES*

18. The client will not aspirate secretions and foods/fluids as evidenced by:
   a. clear breath sounds
   b. resonant percussion note over lungs
   c. respiratory rate at 16-20/minute
   d. absence of dyspnea
   e. absence of cyanosis.

18.a. Assess for factors that indicate potential for aspiration (e.g. difficulty swallowing, choking on secretions and foods/fluids, pocketing of food between gingivae and cheek on affected side, decreased level of consciousness, absent gag reflex).
   b. Assess for signs and symptoms of aspiration of secretions or foods/fluids (e.g. rhonchi, dull percussion note over lungs, tachycardia, rapid respirations, dyspnea, cyanosis, presence of tube feeding in tracheal aspirate).
   c. Monitor chest x-ray results. Report findings of pulmonary infiltrate.
   d. If client is receiving tube feedings, add food coloring to the solution *so that it can readily be identified in tracheal aspirate.*
   e. Implement measures *to reduce the risk of aspiration:*
      1. position client in side-lying or semi- to high Fowler's position at all times
      2. have suction equipment readily available for use
      3. perform oropharyngeal suctioning, encourage client to use tonsil-tip suction, and provide oral care as often as needed *to remove secretions*
      4. withhold foods/fluids if gag reflex is absent, client is not alert, or he/she is experiencing severe dysphagia
      5. if client is receiving tube feedings:
         a. check tube placement before each feeding or on a routine basis if feeding is continuous
         b. administer solution slowly
         c. maintain client in a semi- to high Fowler's position during and for at least 30 minutes after feeding
      6. if oral intake is allowed:
         a. perform actions to improve ability to swallow (see Nursing Diagnosis 6, action b)
         b. decrease environmental stimuli during meals and snacks *so client can concentrate on chewing and swallowing*
         c. provide small, frequent meals rather than 3 large ones *to decrease risk of gastric distention and regurgitation*
         d. allow ample time for meals
         e. instruct client to avoid laughing or talking while eating and drinking
         f. maintain client in high Fowler's position during and for at least 30 minutes after meals and snacks
         g. assist client with oral hygiene after eating *to ensure that food particles do not remain in mouth.*
   f. If signs and symptoms of aspiration occur:
      1. perform tracheal suctioning
      2. notify physician
      3. prepare client for chest x-ray.

☐ ▬▬▬▬▬▬▬▬▬▬▬▬▬▬▬▬▬▬▬▬

19. COLLABORATIVE DIAGNOSIS

Potential complications:

a. **increased intracranial pressure (IICP)** related to cerebral hemorrhage, edema, and vasodilation and seizures;

b. **seizures** related to increased irritability of neurons and disruption of nerve transmission associated with cerebral hypoxia and IICP;

c. **gastrointestinal (GI) bleeding** related to:

1. development of a stress (Cushing's) ulcer (cerebral injury and continued stress cause vagal stimulation that results in gastric hyperacidity and multiple diffuse erosions of the gastric and duodenal mucosa)
2. irritation of gastric mucosa associated with side effects of some medications (e.g. corticosteroids, aspirin, phenytoin);

d. **corneal irritation and abrasion** related to inability to close eye as a result of facial nerve paresis or paralysis;

e. **subluxation of shoulder** related to muscle weakness and gravity pull on affected arm.

DESIRED OUTCOMES	NURSING ACTIONS AND *SELECTED RATIONALES*

19.a. The client will not develop IICP as evidenced by:
1. usual or improved level of consciousness
2. stable or improved motor and sensory function
3. usual pupillary size and reactivity
4. no complaints of headache
5. absence of vomiting
6. absence of papilledema and seizure activity
7. stable vital signs.

19.a.1. Assess for and report:
a. early signs and symptoms of IICP:
1. restlessness, agitation, confusion, lethargy
2. decreasing motor and sensory function
3. change in pupil size or shape
4. sluggish pupillary response to light
5. altered vision (e.g. blurred vision, diplopia, decreased visual acuity)
6. headache
b. later signs and symptoms of IICP:
1. vomiting (frequently projectile)
2. papilledema
3. seizures
4. dilated, nonreactive pupils
5. stupor, coma
6. rise in systolic B/P with widening pulse pressure
7. full, bounding, slow pulse
8. altered respiratory pattern (e.g. Cheyne-Stokes, central neurogenic hyperventilation)
9. decerebrate or decorticate posturing.

2. Implement measures *to prevent IICP:*
a. perform actions to maintain adequate cerebral tissue perfusion (see Nursing Diagnosis 2, action b) *in order to prevent cerebral vasodilation that occurs as a result of cerebral hypoxia*
b. observe for and control conditions that could cause increasing restlessness and agitation (e.g. distended bladder, constipation, hypoxia, headache, fear, anxiety)
c. monitor for therapeutic and nontherapeutic effects of laxatives, stool softeners, antitussives, and antiemetics if administered *to prevent straining to have a bowel movement, coughing, and vomiting (these conditions cause an increase in intrathoracic pressure that impedes venous return from the brain)*
d. instruct client to avoid activities such as pushing feet against footboard or tightly gripping side rails *(isometric muscle contractions raise systemic blood pressure)*
e. monitor for therapeutic and nontherapeutic effects of anticonvulsants (e.g. phenytoin, carbamazepine, phenobarbital) if administered *to prevent seizure activity*
f. schedule care so activities that could raise intracranial pressure (e.g. suctioning, bathing, repositioning) are not grouped together
g. assist with mechanical hyperventilation that may be done *to decrease arterial CO_2 and prevent vasodilation.*

3. If signs and symptoms of IICP are present:
a. continue with above actions to help decrease and prevent a further rise in intracranial pressure
b. initiate seizure precautions

c. assist with lumbar or ventricular puncture or placement of shunt if performed *to remove some cerebral spinal fluid*

d. prepare client for insertion of continuous intracranial monitoring device (e.g. intraventricular catheter, subarachnoid screw or bolt) if indicated

e. prepare client for surgical intervention (e.g. ligation of bleeding vessel, removal of space-occupying lesion) if indicated

f. provide emotional support to client and significant others.

19.b. The client will not experience seizure activity or associated injury.

19.b.1. Assess for and report signs and symptoms of seizure activity (e.g. twitching, clonic-tonic movements).

2. Implement measures *to prevent seizures:*
   a. perform actions to prevent and treat IICP (see actions a.2 and 3 in this diagnosis)
   b. monitor for therapeutic and nontherapeutic effects of anticonvulsants (e.g. phenytoin, carbamazepine, phenobarbital) if administered.

3. Initiate and maintain seizure precautions:
   a. have plastic airway readily available
   b. pad side rails with blankets or soft pads
   c. keep bed in low position with side rails up when client is in bed.

4. If seizures do occur:
   a. implement measures *to decrease risk of injury:*
      1. ease client to the floor if he/she is sitting in chair or ambulating at onset of seizure
      2. remain with and do not restrain client during seizure activity
      3. turn client on his/her side and insert an airway if possible during clonic phase *to prevent obstruction of airway by tongue or secretions*
      4. do not force any object between clenched teeth or try to pry mouth open
      5. remove from area items that may cause injury
      6. place towel or pillow under head
   b. observe for and report characteristics of seizures (e.g. progression, time elapsed)
   c. monitor for therapeutic and nontherapeutic effects of intravenous anticonvulsants (e.g phenytoin, phenobarbital) if administered
   d. provide emotional support to client and significant others.

19.c. The client will not experience GI bleeding as evidenced by:
1. no complaints of epigastric discomfort and fullness
2. absence of occult or frank blood in stool and gastric contents
3. B/P and pulse within normal range for client
4. RBC, Hct., and Hgb. levels within normal range.

19.c.1. Assess for and report signs and symptoms of GI bleeding (e.g. complaints of epigastric discomfort or fullness, frank or occult blood in stool or gastric contents, decreased B/P, increased pulse).

2. Monitor RBC, Hct., and Hgb. levels. Report declining values.

3. Implement measures *to prevent ulceration of gastric or duodenal mucosa:*
   a. perform actions to decrease fear and anxiety (see Nursing Diagnosis 1, actions c and d)
   b. encourage client to reduce intake of foods/fluids that are acidic, spicy, or high in caffeine (e.g. chocolate, colas, coffee, tea)
   c. administer ulcerogenic medications (e.g. corticosteroids, aspirin, phenytoin) with meals or snacks *to decrease gastric irritation*
   d. monitor for therapeutic and nontherapeutic effects of histamine$_2$ receptor antagonists (e.g. cimetidine, ranitidine, famotidine), antacids, and mucosal barrier fortifiers (e.g. sucralfate) if administered.

4. If signs and symptoms of GI bleeding occur:
   a. insert nasogastric tube and maintain suction as ordered
   b. assist with iced water or saline gastric lavage, transendoscopic electrocoagulation, selective arterial embolization, endoscopic laser photocoagulation, and/or intra-arterial administration of vasopressors (e.g. vasopressin) if ordered
   c. monitor for therapeutic and nontherapeutic effects of blood products and/or volume expanders if administered
   d. prepare client for surgery (e.g. ligation of bleeding vessels, partial gastrectomy) if indicated
   e. provide emotional support to client and significant others
   f. refer to Care Plan on Peptic Ulcer for additional care measures.

19.d. The client will not experience corneal irritation or abrasion as evidenced by:
1. absence of eye redness and excessive tearing
2. no complaints of eye discomfort
3. usual visual acuity.

19.d.1. Assess for and report signs and symptoms of corneal irritation and abrasion (e.g. excessive tearing; reddened, itchy eye; sensation of foreign body in eye; eye pain; blurred vision).
2. Implement measures *to prevent corneal irritation and abrasion:*
   a. reduce exposure to irritants such as powder, dust, and smoke
   b. have client wear his/her glasses *to protect affected eye*
   c. lubricate conjunctivae with isotonic eyedrops frequently
   d. tape affected eyelid shut if client is unable to close eye completely.
3. If signs and symptoms of irritation or abrasion occur:
   a. continue with above measures
   b. assist with removal of any foreign body in the eye
   c. instruct client to avoid rubbing eye
   d. apply warm compresses to the eye *to promote comfort*
   e. monitor for therapeutic and nontherapeutic effects of anesthetic, anti-infective, and anti-inflammatory ophthalmic ointments or solutions if administered
   f. consult physician if signs and symptoms of corneal irritation or abrasion persist or worsen.

19.e. The client will not experience subluxation of affected shoulder as evidenced by:
1. absence of shoulder pain, tenderness, and swelling
2. maintenance of full range of motion of shoulder.

19.e.1. Assess for and report signs and symptoms of subluxation of the shoulder (e.g. shoulder pain and tenderness, swelling of soft tissues in region of the shoulder joint, decreased range of motion of shoulder).
2. Implement measures *to prevent subluxation of the affected shoulder:*
   a. instruct client in and assist with active or passive range of motion to affected upper extremity *in order to improve muscle tone*
   b. when client is in bed or chair, position arm in correct alignment using pillows or lap board for support if necessary
   c. assist client with application of an arm support before getting out of bed or sitting up
   d. use turn sheet or transfer belt when assisting client to move; never pull on axilla, shoulder, or arm.
3. If signs and symptoms of shoulder subluxation occur:
   a. continue with above actions
   b. apply heat to area as ordered
   c. monitor for therapeutic and nontherapeutic effects of anti-inflammatory medications and analgesics if administered.

20. NURSING DIAGNOSIS

Sexual dysfunction:

a. **alteration in usual sexual activities** related to impaired motor function and lengthy hospitalization;
b. **decreased libido and/or impotence** related to:
   1. depression, anxiety, and fatigue
   2. impaired motor and sensory function
   3. fear of urinary and bowel incontinence
   4. alteration in self-concept
   5. fear of rejection by desired partner.

DESIRED OUTCOMES	NURSING ACTIONS AND *SELECTED RATIONALES*

20. The client will perceive self as sexually adequate and acceptable as evidenced by:
a. communication of same

20.a. Refer to Care Plan on Immobility, Nursing Diagnosis 15, for measures related to assessment and management of sexual dysfunction.
b. Implement additional measures *to assist the client to promote optimal sexual functioning:*

b. maintenance of relationships with significant others.

1. perform actions to reduce fear and anxiety (see Nursing Diagnosis 1, actions c and d)
2. perform actions to improve self-concept (see Nursing Diagnosis 21, actions c–w)
3. perform actions *to decrease the possibility of rejection by partner:*
   a. assist the partner to acknowledge both positive and negative feelings
   b. if appropriate, involve partner in care (e.g. bathing, dressing, transfer activities) *to facilitate adjustment to and integration of the changes in client's body image*
4. clarify misconceptions about future limitations on sexual activity; discuss positions that may facilitate sexual activity (e.g. lying on affected side, client in supine position) if appropriate
5. instruct client to establish a relaxed, unhurried atmosphere for sexual activity
6. if incontinence of urine or stool is a problem:
   a. reinforce adherence to bowel and bladder training programs *to decrease risk of incontinence*
   b. encourage client to void and/or defecate just before intercourse or other sexual activity.

□ ▬▬▬▬▬▬▬▬▬▬▬▬▬▬▬▬▬▬▬▬▬▬▬

21. NURSING DIAGNOSIS

Disturbance in self-concept* related to:

a. change in appearance (e.g. hemiplegia, facial droop, ptosis) and sexual functioning;
b. life-style and role changes associated with motor and spatial-perceptual impairments and alteration in thought processes;
c. impaired verbal communication;
d. loss of self-control (e.g. automatic speech, emotional lability);
e. urinary and bowel incontinence;
f. dependence on others to meet basic needs;
g. feeling of powerlessness.

---

* This diagnostic label includes the nursing diagnoses of body image disturbance and self-esteem disturbance.

□ ▬▬▬▬▬▬▬▬▬▬▬▬▬▬▬▬▬▬▬▬▬▬▬

DESIRED OUTCOMES	NURSING ACTIONS AND *SELECTED RATIONALES*
21. The client will demonstrate beginning adaptation to changes in appearance, physical and mental functioning, life style, and roles as evidenced by: a. communication of feelings of self-worth and sexual adequacy b. maintenance of relationships with significant others c. active participation in activities of daily living d. active interest in personal appearance	21.a. Determine the meaning of changes in appearance, physical and mental functioning, life style, and roles to the client by encouraging him/her to communicate feelings and by noting nonverbal responses to the changes experienced. b. Assess for signs and symptoms of a disturbance in self-concept (e.g. verbal or nonverbal cues denoting a negative response to changes in body functioning or appearance such as denial of or preoccupation with changes that have occurred, refusal to look at or touch a body part, or withdrawal from significant others). c. Implement measures to facilitate the grieving process (see Nursing Diagnosis 24, action d). d. Assist the client to identify strengths and qualities that have a positive effect on self-concept. e. Implement measures *to assist client to increase self-esteem* (e.g. limit negative self-criticism, encourage positive comments about self, give positive feedback about accomplishments).

e. willingness to participate in social activities
f. communication of a beginning plan for adapting life style to meet changes in physical and mental functioning.

f. Reinforce measures to assist client to cope with effects of CVA (see Nursing Diagnosis 22, action d).
g. Reinforce measures to promote optimal sexual functioning (see Nursing Diagnosis 20).
h. Implement measures to reduce client's sense of powerlessness (see Nursing Diagnosis 23).
i. Discuss techniques the client can utilize *to adapt to alterations in thought processes:*
   1. encourage client to make lists and jot down messages and refer to these notes rather than relying on his/her memory
   2. instruct client to place self in a calm environment when making decisions
   3. encourage client to validate decisions, clarify information, and seek assistance in problem-solving if indicated.
j. Instruct significant others in ways to manage client's emotional lability and inappropriate laughing, crying, or swearing (e.g. provide privacy; tell client to open mouth if crying; distract client by clapping hands, singing, or whistling loudly).
k. Implement measures to prevent urinary and bowel incontinence (see Nursing Diagnoses 12, action b and 14, action b).
l. Implement measures *to assist client to adapt to changes in appearance:*
   1. instruct and assist client to position self with affected extremities well supported and in proper alignment *(if extremities are positioned awkwardly, the impairment is more obvious)*
   2. assist client with usual grooming and makeup habits.
m. Demonstrate acceptance of client using techniques such as therapeutic touch and frequent visits. Encourage significant others to do the same.
n. Implement measures to facilitate communication (see Nursing Diagnosis 8, action b).
o. Reinforce use of adaptive devices (e.g. plate guards, broad-handled utensils, universal cuff, button hook, long-handled shoehorn) and mobility aids (e.g. walker, cane) *to increase client's independence.*
p. Encourage significant others to allow client to do what he/she is able *so that independence can be re-established and/or self-esteem redeveloped.*
q. Use adjectives such as weak, affected, or right- or left-sided rather than "bad" when referring to side of hemiplegia.
r. Assess for and support behaviors suggesting positive adaptation to changes experienced (e.g. increased participation in care, compliance with treatment plan).
s. Assist client's and significant others' adjustment by listening, facilitating communication, and providing information.
t. Ensure that client and significant others have similar expectations and understanding of future life style.
u. Encourage visits and support from significant others.
v. Encourage client to continue involvement in social activities and to pursue interests. If previous interests and hobbies cannot be pursued, encourage development of new ones.
w. Provide information about and encourage utilization of community agencies or support groups (e.g. stroke support groups; vocational rehabilitation; sexual, family, individual, and/or financial counseling).
x. Consult physician about psychological counseling if client desires or if he/she seems unwilling or unable to adapt to changes resulting from CVA.

22. NURSING DIAGNOSIS

Ineffective individual coping related to fear; anxiety; decreased ability to communicate verbally; feeling of powerlessness; changes in motor and sensory function, thought processes, and future life style and roles; and need for lengthy rehabilitation.

DESIRED OUTCOMES	NURSING ACTIONS AND *SELECTED RATIONALES*

22. The client will demonstrate the use of effective coping skills as evidenced by:
    a. willingness to participate in treatment plan and self-care activities
    b. communication of ability to cope with the effects of the CVA
    c. identification of stressors
    d. utilization of appropriate problem-solving techniques
    e. recognition and utilization of available support systems.

22.a. Assess effectiveness of client's coping strategies by observing behavior and noting strengths, weaknesses, ability to express feelings and concerns, and willingness to participate in treatment plan.
   b. Assess for and report signs and symptoms that may indicate ineffective coping (e.g. sleep disturbances, increasing fatigue, increased difficulty concentrating, irritability, communication of inability to cope).
   c. Allow time for client to adjust psychologically to diagnosis and planned treatment, residual effects of CVA, and anticipated life-style and role changes.
   d. Implement measures *to promote effective coping:*
      1. perform actions to facilitate communication (see Nursing Diagnosis 8, action b)
      2. assist client to relearn or communicate names of significant others if memory loss or dysphasia is present
      3. perform actions to reduce fear and anxiety (see Nursing Diagnosis 1, actions c and d)
      4. arrange for a visit with another who has successfully adjusted to effects of a CVA
      5. include client in the planning of care, encourage maximum participation in treatment plan, and allow choices when possible *to enable him/her to maintain a sense of control*
      6. instruct client in effective problem-solving techniques (e.g. accurate identification of stressors, determination of various options to solve problem)
      7. assist client to maintain usual daily routines whenever possible
      8. provide diversional activities according to client's interests and abilities
      9. assist client as he/she starts to plan for necessary life-style and role changes after discharge; provide input related to realistic prioritization of problems that need to be dealt with
      10. assist client through methods such as role playing to prepare for negative reactions from others because of altered appearance and neurological impairments
      11. if client is incontinent, instruct in ways to minimize the problem *so that socialization with others is possible* (e.g. placing disposable liners in underwear, wearing absorbent undergarments such as Attends)
      12. set up a home evaluation appointment with occupational and physical therapists before client's discharge *so that changes in home environment (e.g. installation of ramps and handrails, widening doorways, altering kitchen facilities) can be completed by discharge*
      13. assist client and significant others to identify ways that personal and family goals can be adjusted rather than abandoned
      14. inform client that he/she will have times when impairments worsen; assure client that this is usually temporary and the result of physical and/or emotional stress or fatigue rather than an indication of deteriorating neurological status
      15. assist client to identify and utilize available support systems; provide information regarding available community resources that can assist client and significant others in coping with effects of CVA (e.g. stroke support groups, local chapter of the American Heart Association).
   e. Encourage continued emotional support from significant others.
   f. Encourage the client to share with significant others the kind of support that would be most beneficial (e.g. listening, inspiring hope, providing reassurance and accurate information).
   g. Assess for and support behaviors suggesting positive adaptation to changes experienced (e.g. participation in treatment plan and self-care activities, communication of ability to cope, utilization of effective problem-solving strategies).
   h. Consult physician about psychological or vocational rehabilitation counseling if appropriate.

□ ▬▬▬▬▬▬▬▬▬▬▬▬▬▬▬▬▬▬▬

23. NURSING DIAGNOSIS

Powerlessness related to:

a. physical limitations, impaired verbal communication, and sensory-perceptual alterations;
b. dependence on others to meet basic needs;
c. feeling of loss of control over life;
d. alterations in usual roles, relationships, and future plans associated with residual impairments and need for lengthy rehabilitation.

□ ▬▬▬▬▬▬▬▬▬▬▬▬▬▬▬▬▬▬▬

DESIRED OUTCOMES	NURSING ACTIONS AND *SELECTED RATIONALES*
23. The client will demonstrate increasing feelings of control over his/her situation (see Care Plan on Immobility, Nursing Diagnosis 17, for outcome criteria).	23.a. Refer to Care Plan on Immobility, Nursing Diagnosis 17, for measures related to assessment of feelings of powerlessness and measures to promote client's feeling of control over his/her situation. b. Implement additional measures *to reduce client's feeling of powerlessness:* 1. perform actions to facilitate communication (see Nursing Diagnosis 8, action b) as soon as client's condition allows *in order to enable him/her to interact meaningfully with others* 2. perform actions to promote effective coping (see Nursing Diagnosis 22, action d) *in order to promote an increased sense of control over his/her situation* 3. support realistic hope about effects of rehabilitation on future independence 4. discuss with significant others the client's need to maintain as much control over his/her life as possible; stress the necessity of their encouraging and allowing the client to actively participate in rehabilitation program scheduling and discharge planning.

□ ▬▬▬▬▬▬▬▬▬▬▬▬▬▬▬▬▬▬▬

24. NURSING DIAGNOSIS

Grieving* related to changes in motor and sensory function and thought processes and the effect of these changes on future life style and roles.

---

* This diagnostic label includes anticipatory grieving and grieving following the actual losses/changes.

□ ▬▬▬▬▬▬▬▬▬▬▬▬▬▬▬▬▬▬▬

DESIRED OUTCOMES	NURSING ACTIONS AND *SELECTED RATIONALES*
24. The client will demonstrate beginning progression through the grieving process as evidenced by: a. communication of feelings about the CVA and its effects b. expression of grief c. participation in treatment	24.a. Determine client's perception of impact of CVA on his/her future. b. Determine how the client usually expresses grief. c. Observe for signs of grieving (e.g. changes in eating habits, insomnia, anger, noncompliance, denial). d. Implement measures *to facilitate the grieving process:* 1. assist client to acknowledge the changes experienced *so grief work can begin*; assess for factors that may hinder or facilitate acknowledgment 2. discuss the grieving process and assist client to accept the stages of grieving as an expected response to changes that have occurred

plan and self-care
activities
d. utilization of available
support systems
e. communication of a plan
for integrating prescribed
follow-up care into life
style.

3. allow time for client to progress through the stages of grieving (denial, anger, bargaining, depression, acceptance [Kübler-Ross, 1969]); be aware that not every stage is experienced or expressed by all individuals
4. provide an atmosphere of care and concern (e.g. provide privacy, be available and nonjudgmental, display empathy and respect) *so that client will feel free to communicate both positive and negative feelings and concerns*
5. perform actions *to promote trust* (e.g. answer questions honestly, provide requested information)
6. encourage the expression of anger and sadness about the changes experienced
7. encourage client to express his/her feelings in whatever ways are comfortable (e.g. writing, drawing, conversation)
8. perform actions to facilitate effective coping (see Nursing Diagnosis 22, action d)
9. perform actions *to support realistic hope about the effects of treatment on the residual impairments:*
   a. focus on what the client is able to accomplish independently and with the use of adaptive devices
   b. reinforce knowledge that impairments may improve with time
   c. reinforce positive effects of speech, physical, and occupational therapies; medication therapy; and control of underlying cause of CVA (e.g. hypertension, diabetes).
e. Assess for and support behaviors suggesting successful resolution of grief (e.g. communicating feelings about losses, expressing sorrow, focusing on ways to adapt to losses that have occurred).
f. Explain the stages of the grieving process to significant others. Encourage their support and understanding.
g. Provide information regarding counseling services and support groups that might assist client in working through grief.
h. Arrange for visit from clergy if desired by client.
i. Monitor for therapeutic and nontherapeutic effects of antidepressants if administered.
j. Consult physician regarding referral for counseling if signs of dysfunctional grieving (e.g. persistent denial of losses or changes, excessive anger or sadness, hysteria, suicidal behaviors, phobias) occur.

☐ ▬▬▬▬▬▬▬▬▬▬▬▬▬▬▬▬

25. NURSING DIAGNOSIS

Social isolation related to:

a. inability to participate in usual activities associated with hemiplegia and spatial-perceptual impairments;
b. impaired ability to communicate verbally;
c. prolonged hospitalization;
d. depression associated with feeling of powerlessness and the anticipated effects of altered motor and sensory function on life style.

☐ ▬▬▬▬▬▬▬▬▬▬▬▬▬▬▬▬

DESIRED OUTCOMES	NURSING ACTIONS AND *SELECTED RATIONALES*
25. The client will experience a decreased sense of isolation as evidenced by: a. maintenance of relationships with	25.a. Ascertain the client's usual degree of social interaction. b. Assess for and report behaviors indicative of social isolation (e.g. decreased interaction with significant others and staff; expression of feelings of rejection, abandonment, or being different from others; hostility; sad affect).

significant others and
casual acquaintances
b. communication of
decreasing loneliness and
feelings of rejection.

c. Encourage client to express feelings of rejection and aloneness. Provide feedback and support.
d. Implement measures *to decrease social isolation:*
   1. schedule time each day to be with client; encourage staff and significant others to talk to client even if he/she is unresponsive or unable to communicate verbally
   2. make objects such as clocks, TV, radio, and greeting cards accessible to client (be sure to place them within his/her visual field)
   3. have significant others bring client's favorite objects from home and place in room
   4. set up a schedule of visiting times so that client will not go for long periods of time without visitors
   5. position bed in room so that client receives the greatest amount of visual stimuli (e.g. when client is lying in bed, the door or rest of the room rather than the wall should be within visual field)
   6. instruct visitors and staff to stand or sit within client's visual field when talking with him/her
   7. make a telephone accessible to client if he/she is able to communicate verbally
   8. perform actions to facilitate communication (see Nursing Diagnosis 8, action b)
   9. perform actions to decrease sense of powerlessness (see Nursing Diagnosis 23)
   10. routinely move client to more stimulating environments (e.g. hall, lounge, nurses' station, garden) when condition allows
   11. assist client to identify a few persons he/she feels comfortable with and encourage interactions with them
   12. change room assignments as feasible *to provide client with roommate with similar interests*
   13. support any appropriate movement away from social isolation.
e. Consult physician if signs and symptoms of social isolation persist or worsen.

☐ ▬▬▬▬▬▬▬▬▬▬▬▬▬▬▬▬▬▬▬▬▬

26. NURSING DIAGNOSIS

Knowledge deficit regarding follow-up care.

☐ ▬▬▬▬▬▬▬▬▬▬▬▬▬▬▬▬▬▬▬▬▬

DESIRED OUTCOMES	NURSING ACTIONS AND *SELECTED RATIONALES*
26.a. The client will communicate an awareness of ways to decrease the risk of a recurrent CVA.	26.a.1. Assist client to recognize factors that may have contributed to CVA (e.g. hypertension, diabetes, obesity, atrial fibrillation, use of oral contraceptives). 2. Identify appropriate actions client can take *to decrease risk of a recurrent CVA* (e.g. take medications on schedule, decrease stress, lose weight, stop smoking, alter diet, use another form of birth control if taking oral contraceptives). 3. Provide the names and phone numbers of resources that can help client to control risk factors (e.g. stop smoking clinics, weight reduction and stress management programs).
26.b. The client will identify ways to manage sensory and verbal communication impairments and alterations in thought processes.	26.b.1. Reinforce instructions regarding ways *to adapt to visual impairments if present:* a. utilize scanning techniques if visual field cut is present b. arrange home setting so that when in favorite chair or in bed, stimuli rather than wall or furniture are within visual field c. wear eyepatch or frosted lens if double vision persists.

2. Reinforce use of established communication techniques and continuation with speech therapy if indicated.
3. If spatial-perceptual deficits and/or unilateral neglect are present, stress need for assistance with usual daily activities and strict adherence to safety measures *to prevent injury.*
4. Reinforce methods of managing impaired memory and shortened attention span (e.g. make lists of planned activities, review taped information or written instructions frequently).
5. Instruct client to request assistance when problem-solving and setting priorities and to seek validation of decisions if reasoning ability is impaired.

26.c. The client will identify ways to manage urinary and bowel incontinence.

26.c.1. Reinforce instructions regarding client's bladder and bowel training programs. Stress the importance of adhering to the programs *in order to reduce the risk of incontinence.*
2. Demonstrate intermittent catheterization, application of a penile clamp or external catheter, insertion of a rectal suppository, and administration of an enema if indicated. Allow time for questions, clarification, and return demonstration.

26.d. The client will demonstrate techniques to facilitate the performance of activities of daily living and increase physical mobility.

26.d.1. Reinforce techniques that the client is using to improve his/her ability to perform activities of daily living and increase physical mobility (e.g. participation in exercise program; use of adaptive devices and mobility aids; continued concentration on body positioning, balance, and movement).
2. Allow time for questions, clarification, and return demonstration of the techniques.

26.e. The client will communicate an awareness of signs and symptoms to report to the health care provider.

26.e.1. Refer to Care Plan on Immobility, Nursing Diagnosis 19, action c, for signs and symptoms to report to health care provider.
2. Instruct client to report these additional signs and symptoms:
   a. increased weakness or loss of sensation in extremities
   b. increase in or development of visual disturbances such as tunnel vision, blurred vision, transient blindness
   c. increased lethargy, irritability, or confusion
   d. loss of emotional control
   e. increased difficulty chewing or swallowing
   f. increased difficulty speaking or understanding verbal and nonverbal communication
   g. increased difficulty maintaining balance
   h. seizures.

26.f. The client will communicate knowledge of community agencies that can assist with home management and the adjustment to changes resulting from the CVA.

26.f.1. Provide information about community resources that can assist client and significant others with home management and adjustment to impairments in motor and sensory function and thought processes resulting from CVA (e.g. home health agencies, Visiting Nurse Association, Meals on Wheels, social and financial services, local chapter of the American Heart Association, local service groups that can help obtain adaptive devices, public health agencies, individual and family counselors).
2. Initiate a referral if indicated.

26.g. The client will communicate an understanding of and a plan for adhering to recommended follow-up care including future appointments with health care provider and therapists and medications prescribed.

26.g.1. Reinforce the importance of keeping follow-up appointments with health care provider and physical, occupational, and speech therapists.
2. Teach client the rationale for, side effects of, and importance of taking prescribed medications (e.g. anticoagulants, antihypertensives, anticonvulsants, corticosteroids).
3. Implement measures *to improve client compliance:*
   a. include significant others in teaching sessions if possible
   b. encourage questions and allow time for reinforcement or clarification of information provided
   c. provide written instructions on scheduled appointments with health care provider and occupational, physical, and speech therapists; medications prescribed; signs and symptoms to report; and exercise program.

Reference

Kübler-Ross, E. On death and dying. New York: Macmillan, 1969.

Craniocerebral Trauma

Craniocerebral trauma (head injury) can be the result of a variety of factors including motor vehicle accidents, falls, sports injuries, and acts of violence. The types of injury that may occur include scalp laceration; skull fracture; dural tear; cerebral contusion, concussion, or laceration; brain stem damage; and intracranial hemorrhage. The severity of trauma ranges from mild or minor (usually a concussion) to severe, in which extensive contusion and/or laceration of brain tissue and possibly brain stem injury occurred. Severe craniocerebral trauma usually involves a period of prolonged unconsciousness and results in permanent physical impairments and alterations in thought processes that require extensive rehabilitation and long-term care. Craniocerebral trauma can be classified by type and severity of injury, as open (penetrating) or closed (impact), and/or as direct (e.g. acceleration, deceleration, coup, contrecoup) or indirect. Brain damage can occur during the initial injury or as a result of subsequent cerebral tissue ischemia, seizure activity, cerebral hemorrhage or hematoma, cerebral edema, and/or interruption in the flow of cerebral spinal fluid. The location and extensiveness of cerebral tissue trauma are the primary determinants of the prognosis.

Generally, clients who have experienced craniocerebral trauma have headache, some degree of irritability, and disruption in thought processes. Additional signs and symptoms vary depending on the area of the brain that has been affected. For example, tissue damage in the frontal lobe could result in loss of voluntary motor control, personality changes, and/or expressive aphasia; damage to the occipital lobe could result in visual disturbances; and damage to the temporal lobe could result in receptive aphasia and/or hearing impairment.

This care plan focuses on the adult client hospitalized after craniocerebral trauma. Goals of care in the acute phase are to prevent life-threatening complications and perform or assist the client with those activities he/she is unable to do independently. After the client's condition has stabilized, care is focused on assisting him/her to adapt to any residual neurological impairments. This care plan will deal mainly with those nursing and collaborative diagnoses appropriate for a client with a moderate degree of brain injury. Additional care objectives and discharge teaching will need to be established on the basis of the area of the brain affected and the extensiveness of tissue damage. If the client has sustained more severe craniocerebral trauma, refer also to the Care Plans on Immobility and Cerebrovascular Accident.

DISCHARGE CRITERIA

Prior to discharge, the client will:

- identify ways to adapt to neurological deficits that may persist following craniocerebral trauma
- identify ways to reduce headache
- state signs and symptoms of complications to report to the health care provider
- share thoughts and feelings about any residual neurological impairments
- identify community agencies that can assist with home management and adjustment to changes resulting from the injury
- verbalize an understanding of and a plan for adhering to recommended follow-up care including future appointments with health care provider and therapists and medications prescribed.

NURSING/COLLABORATIVE DIAGNOSES

1. Anxiety □ *216*
2. Altered cerebral tissue perfusion □ *217*
3. Altered nutrition: less than body requirements □ *218*
4. Impaired swallowing □ *219*
5. Pain: headache □ *220*
6. Impaired physical mobility □ *220*
7. Self-care deficit □ *221*
8. Altered thought processes: shortened attention span, slowness in thinking and perceiving, impaired memory, confusion, irritability, aggressiveness, inappropriate responses, and personality changes □ *222*
9. Sleep pattern disturbance □ *223*
10. Potential for trauma □ *223*
11. Potential for aspiration □ *225*
12. Potential altered body temperature: increased □ *225*
13. Potential complications:
    a. increased intracranial pressure (IICP)
    b. meningitis
    c. seizures
    d. diabetes insipidus
    e. syndrome of inappropriate antidiuretic hormone (SIADH)
    f. gastrointestinal (GI) bleeding □ *226*
14. Disturbance in self-concept □ *230*
15. Ineffective individual coping □ *232*
16. Grieving □ *233*
17. Altered family processes □ *234*
18. Knowledge deficit regarding follow-up care □ *235*

1. NURSING DIAGNOSIS

Anxiety related to unfamiliar environment; impaired motor and/or sensory function; altered thought processes; uncertainty as to permanence of neurological deficits; and lack of understanding of diagnostic tests, diagnosis, and treatments.

DESIRED OUTCOMES	NURSING ACTIONS AND *SELECTED RATIONALES*
1. The client will experience a reduction in fear and anxiety as evidenced by: a. verbalization of feeling less anxious or fearful b. relaxed facial expression and body movements c. stable vital signs d. usual skin color	1.a. Assess client for signs and symptoms of fear and anxiety (e.g. verbalization of fears and concerns; tenseness; tremors; irritability; restlessness; diaphoresis; tachypnea; elevated blood pressure; tachycardia; facial tension, pallor, or flushing; noncompliance with treatment plan). Validate perceptions carefully, remembering that some behavior may be due to neurological changes resulting from craniocerebral trauma. b. Ascertain effectiveness of current coping skills. c. Implement measures *to reduce fear and anxiety:* 1. orient client to person, place, and situation if necessary

e. verbalization of an understanding of hospital routines, diagnostic tests, diagnosis, and treatments.

2. explain necessity of frequent neurological assessments and importance of cooperating during assessments
3. avoid leaving client alone if he/she is agitated, extremely frightened, or confused
4. maintain a calm, confident manner when interacting with client
5. if client is left alone, assure him/her that staff members are nearby; check client frequently and respond to call signal as soon as possible
6. as agitation and confusion subside:
   a. orient to hospital environment, equipment, and routines
   b. introduce staff who will be participating in his/her care; if possible, maintain consistency in staff assigned to his/her care *to provide feelings of stability and comfort with the environment*
   c. encourage verbalization of fear and anxiety; provide feedback
   d. explain all diagnostic tests (e.g. skull x-rays, computed tomography, magnetic resonance imaging [MRI], cerebral spinal fluid analysis, echoencephalogram, brain scan, EEG, visual field examination)
   e. reinforce physician's explanations and clarify any misconceptions client may have about extent of injury, treatment plan, and prognosis
   f. if surgical intervention is indicated, begin preoperative teaching
   g. instruct in relaxation techniques and encourage participation in diversional activities
   h. perform actions to assist the client to cope with the effects of the injury (see Nursing Diagnosis 15, action d)
7. encourage significant others to project a caring, concerned attitude without obvious anxiousness
8. monitor for therapeutic and nontherapeutic effects of antianxiety agents if administered.

d. Include significant others in orientation and teaching sessions and encourage their continued support of the client.
e. Provide information based on current needs of client and significant others at a level they can understand. Encourage questions and clarification of information provided.
f. Consult physician if above actions fail to control fear and anxiety.

2. NURSING DIAGNOSIS

Altered cerebral tissue perfusion related to an interruption of cerebral blood flow associated with cerebral hemorrhage, hematoma, and/or edema.

DESIRED OUTCOMES

2. The client will experience improved cerebral tissue perfusion as evidenced by:
   a. decrease in or absence of dizziness, syncope, visual disturbances
   b. improved mental status
   c. pupils equal and normally reactive to light
   d. improved or normal motor and sensory function.

NURSING ACTIONS AND *SELECTED RATIONALES*

2.a. Assess client for signs and symptoms of decreased cerebral tissue perfusion:
   1. dizziness, syncope
   2. blurred or dimmed vision, diplopia, change in visual field
   3. irritability and restlessness
   4. decreased level of consciousness
   5. unequal pupils or a sluggish or absent pupillary reaction to light
   6. paresthesias, motor weakness, paralysis
   7. seizures.

b. Implement measures *to improve cerebral tissue perfusion:*
   1. perform actions *to reduce cerebral edema in order to prevent pressure on the blood vessels:*
      a. maintain fluid restrictions as ordered
      b. administer fluids at an even rate

   c. elevate head of bed 20–30° unless contraindicated *to promote adequate cerebral venous drainage*
   d. monitor for therapeutic and nontherapeutic effects of osmotic diuretics (e.g. mannitol), loop diuretics (e.g. furosemide), and corticosteroids (e.g. dexamethasone, methylprednisolone) if administered
2. keep head and neck in proper alignment
3. perform actions to prevent and treat increased intracranial pressure (see Collaborative Diagnosis 13, actions a.2 and 3).
   c. Consult physician if signs and symptoms of decreased cerebral tissue perfusion worsen.

---

3. NURSING DIAGNOSIS

Altered nutrition: less than body requirements related to:

a. decreased oral intake associated with:
   1. anorexia resulting from fear, anxiety, pain, fatigue, and anosmia (loss of sense of smell occurs frequently following craniocerebral trauma because the olfactory nerves are very sensitive to pressure)
   2. dysphagia resulting mainly from damage to cranial nerves IX and X
   3. difficulty feeding self if motor function is impaired or visual disturbances are present
   4. prescribed dietary restrictions if conditions such as decreased level of consciousness, absent gag reflex, or severe dysphagia are present;
b. increased nutritional needs associated with increased metabolic rate that occurs following craniocerebral trauma.

DESIRED OUTCOMES	NURSING ACTIONS AND *SELECTED RATIONALES*
3. The client will maintain an adequate nutritional status as evidenced by: a. weight within normal range for client's age, height, and build b. normal BUN and serum albumin, protein, Hct., Hgb., cholesterol, and lymphocyte levels c. triceps skinfold measurements within normal range d. usual strength and activity tolerance e. healthy oral mucous membrane.	3.a. Assess the client for signs and symptoms of malnutrition: 1. weight below normal for client's age, height, and build 2. abnormal BUN and low serum albumin, protein, Hct., Hgb., cholesterol, and lymphocyte levels 3. triceps skinfold measurement less than normal for build 4. weakness and fatigue 5. stomatitis. b. Reassess nutritional status on a regular basis and report a decline. c. Monitor percentage of meals eaten. d. Assess client to determine causes of inadequate intake (e.g. anorexia, dietary restrictions, difficulty swallowing and/or feeding self). e. Implement measures *to maintain an adequate nutritional status:* 1. when oral intake is allowed, perform actions *to improve oral intake:* a. implement measures to reduce headache (see Nursing Diagnosis 5, action e) b. implement measures to reduce fear and anxiety (see Nursing Diagnosis 1, action c) c. provide oral care before meals d. eliminate noxious stimuli from environment e. serve small portions of nutritious foods/fluids that are appealing to the client (visual appeal is very important if client has lost his/her sense of smell) f. provide a clean, relaxed, pleasant atmosphere

g. obtain a dietary consult if necessary to assist client in selecting foods/fluids that meet nutritional needs as well as preferences
h. encourage a rest period before meals *to minimize fatigue*
i. encourage significant others to bring in client's favorite foods and eat with him/her *to make eating more of a familiar social experience*
j. allow adequate time for meals; reheat food if necessary
k. if client is experiencing dysphagia, implement measures to improve ability to swallow (see Nursing Diagnosis 4, action b)
l. reinforce use of adaptive devices to enable client to feed self (e.g. broad-handled utensils, plate guards) or feed client if necessary
m. increase activity as allowed and tolerated *(activity stimulates appetite)*

2. ensure that meals are well balanced and high in essential nutrients
3. monitor for therapeutic and nontherapeutic effects of vitamins and minerals if administered.

f. Perform a 72-hour calorie count if nutritional status declines.
g. Consult physician regarding alternative methods of providing nutrition (e.g. parenteral nutrition, tube feedings) if client does not consume enough food or fluids to meet nutritional needs.

4. NURSING DIAGNOSIS

Impaired swallowing related to damage to cranial nerves IX and X.

DESIRED OUTCOMES	NURSING ACTIONS AND *SELECTED RATIONALES*
4. The client will experience an improvement in swallowing as evidenced by: a. verbalization of same b. absence of coughing and choking when eating and drinking.	4.a. Assess for and report signs and symptoms of impaired swallowing (e.g. coughing or choking when eating and drinking, stasis of food in oral cavity). b. Implement measures *to improve ability to swallow:* 　1. place client in high Fowler's position for meals and snacks; head should be erect with chin tilted forward *to facilitate elevation of the larynx and posterior movement of the tongue* 　2. assist client to select foods that have a distinct texture and are easy to swallow (e.g. applesauce, custard, cottage cheese, ground meat) 　3. instruct client to avoid mixing foods of different texture in his/her mouth at the same time 　4. avoid serving foods that are sticky (e.g. peanut butter, soft bread, bananas) 　5. serve foods/fluids that are hot or cold instead of room temperature *(the more extreme temperatures stimulate the sensory receptors and swallowing reflex)* 　6. utilize adaptive devices (e.g. long-handled spoon, "pusher" spoon) to place food in back of mouth if tongue movement is impaired 　7. moisten dry foods with gravy or sauces (e.g. catsup, salad dressing, sour cream) 　8. encourge client to concentrate on the act of swallowing 　9. gently stroke client's throat when he/she is swallowing if indicated 　10. encourage client to drink through a straw *in order to decrease risk of choking and strengthen swallowing muscles* 　11. consult speech pathologist about methods for dealing with impaired swallowing; reinforce exercises and techniques prescribed. c. Consult physician if swallowing difficulties persist or worsen.

☐ ▬▬▬▬▬▬▬▬▬▬▬▬▬▬▬▬▬▬▬▬▬▬▬▬

5. NURSING DIAGNOSIS

Pain: headache related to:

a. cerebral tissue irritation and stretching or compression of pain-sensitive dura and cerebral vascular structures associated with bleeding and/or edema and increased intracranial pressure;
b. meningeal irritation associated with presence of blood in the subarachnoid space and/or inflammation of the meninges.

☐ ▬▬▬▬▬▬▬▬▬▬▬▬▬▬▬▬▬▬▬▬▬▬▬▬

DESIRED OUTCOMES	NURSING ACTIONS AND *SELECTED RATIONALES*

5. The client will obtain relief from headache as evidenced by:
  a. verbalization of headache relief
  b. relaxed facial expression and body positioning
  c. increased participation in activities.
	5.a. Determine how the client usually responds to pain.
	  b. Assess for nonverbal signs of headache (e.g. reluctance to move head, wrinkled brow, clenched fists, squinting, rubbing head, avoidance of bright lights and noises).
	  c. Assess verbal complaints of pain. Ask client to be specific about type, location, and severity of headache.
	  d. Assess for factors that seem to aggravate and alleviate headache.
	  e. Implement measures *to relieve headache:*
	    1. perform actions *to minimize environmental stimuli* (e.g. provide a quiet environment, restrict visitors, dim lights)
	    2. avoid jarring bed or startling client *to minimize risk of sudden movements*
	    3. perform actions to prevent and treat increased intracranial pressure and meningitis (see Collaborative Diagnosis 13, actions a.2 and 3 and b.5 and 6)
	    4. provide nonpharmacological measures for headache relief (e.g. cool cloth to forehead, back rub, distraction)
	    5. monitor for therapeutic and nontherapeutic effects of nonnarcotic analgesics or codeine (other narcotic analgesics are usually contraindicated *because they have a greater depressant effect on the central nervous system)* if administered.
	  f. Consult physician if above actions fail to relieve headache.

☐ ▬▬▬▬▬▬▬▬▬▬▬▬▬▬▬▬▬▬▬▬▬▬▬▬

6. NURSING DIAGNOSIS

Impaired physical mobility related to:

a. neuromuscular impairments (e.g. paresis, paralysis);
b. activity restrictions imposed by the treatment plan;
c. reluctance to move because of pain and fear of injury.

☐ ▬▬▬▬▬▬▬▬▬▬▬▬▬▬▬▬▬▬▬▬▬▬▬▬

DESIRED OUTCOMES	NURSING ACTIONS AND *SELECTED RATIONALES*

6.a. The client will achieve maximum physical mobility within limitations imposed by the treatment plan and the effects of the injury.	6.a.1. Assess for factors that impair physical mobility (e.g. loss of motor function, restrictions imposed by treatment plan, reluctance to move because of headache and fear of injury).
	    2. Implement measures *to increase mobility when allowed:*
	      a. instruct client in and assist with active and active-resistive exercises of unaffected extremities unless contraindicated

   b. instruct client in and assist with passive range of motion exercises of affected extremities at least every 4 hours unless contraindicated
   c. provide adequate rest periods before activity sessions
   d. instruct client in and assist with correct use of mobility aids (e.g. cane, walker) if appropriate
   e. reinforce instructions, activities, and exercise plan recommended by physical and/or occupational therapists
   f. perform actions to relieve headache (see Nursing Diagnosis 5, action e)
   g. perform actions to prevent falls (see Nursing Diagnosis 10, action b) *in order to decrease client's fear of injury.*
3. Increase activity and participation in self-care activities as allowed and tolerated.
4. Provide praise and encouragement for all efforts to increase physical mobility.
5. Encourage the support of significant others. Allow them to assist with range of motion exercises, positioning, and activity if desired.
6. Consult physician if client is unable to achieve expected level of mobility or range of motion becomes restricted.

UNIT VI

6.b. The client will not experience problems associated with immobility.

6.b. Refer to Care Plan on Immobility for actions to prevent problems associated with immobility if client remains on bedrest for longer than 48 hours.

---

7. NURSING DIAGNOSIS

Self-care deficit related to impaired physical mobility, sensory alterations (e.g. paresthesias, visual impairments such as diplopia or visual field cut), and alteration in thought processes.

DESIRED OUTCOMES	NURSING ACTIONS AND *SELECTED RATIONALES*
7. The client will perform self-care activities within physical limitations and prescribed activity restrictions.	7.a. Assess for factors that interfere with client's ability to perform self-care (e.g. sensory and motor deficits, activity restrictions, headache, alteration in thought processes).

   b. With client, develop a realistic plan for meeting daily physical needs.
   c. Encourage client to perform as much of self-care as possible within physical limitations and activity restrictions imposed by the treatment plan.
   d. Implement measures *to facilitate client's ability to perform self-care activities:*
   1. perform actions to increase mobility when allowed (see Nursing Diagnosis 6, action a.2)
   2. schedule care at a time when client is most likely to be able to participate (e.g. when analgesics are at peak action, after rest periods, not immediately after meals or treatments)
   3. keep needed objects within easy reach
   4. allow adequate time for accomplishment of self-care activities
   5. if visual impairments are present:
      a. identify where items are placed on his/her plate and tray
      b. keep needed objects within visual field
      c. instruct client to visually scan his/her environment to locate needed items
      d. encourage client to wear alternating eyepatch or frosted lens if diplopia is present
   6. if client is having difficulty feeding self, consult occupational therapist about adaptive devices available (e.g. broad-handled utensils, rocker knives, plate guards); reinforce use of these devices
   7. perform actions *to assist or enable client to dress self when condition stabilizes:*
      a. encourage use of adaptive devices such as button hooks, long-handled shoehorns, and pull loops for pants

    b. encourage client to select clothing that is easy to put on and remove (e.g. clothing with zippers rather than buttons, loose-fitting clothing, shoes with Velcro fasteners rather than laces)

    8. reinforce exercises and activities prescribed by the physical and occupational therapists to improve fine motor skills.

e. Provide positive feedback for all efforts and accomplishments of self-care.

f. Assist client with those activities he/she is unable to perform independently.

g. Inform significant others of client's abilities to perform own care. Explain importance of encouraging and allowing client to maintain an optimal level of independence within prescribed activity restrictions and physical limitations.

8. NURSING DIAGNOSIS

Altered thought processes: shortened attention span, slowness in thinking and perceiving, impaired memory, confusion, irritability, aggressiveness, inappropriate responses, and personality changes related to cerebral hypoxia and cerebral irritation associated with the craniocerebral trauma.

DESIRED OUTCOMES	NURSING ACTIONS AND *SELECTED RATIONALES*

8. The client will have gradual improvement of and/or demonstrate beginning adaptation to alterations in thought processes as evidenced by:
a. usual or improved attention span and problem-solving abilities
b. decreased irritability and aggressiveness
c. improved level of orientation
d. utilization of techniques to aid memory.
	8.a. Assess client for alterations in thought processes (e.g. shortened attention span, impaired memory, decreased ability to problem-solve, irritability, aggressiveness, inappropriate responses, confusion).
	b. Ascertain from significant others client's usual level of intellectual functioning and whether personality changes have occurred.
	c. Implement measures to improve cerebral tissue perfusion (see Nursing Diagnosis 2, action b) *in order to prevent further cerebral hypoxia.*
	d. If client shows evidence of altered thought processes:
	  1. reorient to person, place, and time as necessary
	  2. allow adequate time for communication and performance of activities
	  3. repeat instructions as necessary using clear, simple language
	  4. keep environmental stimuli to a minimum (clients who have more severe alterations in mental functioning are sometimes put in floor beds [floor mattresses surrounded by "walls" of mattresses or padding] *in order to reduce environmental stimuli and the risk of injury)*
	  5. write out schedule of activities for client to refer to if desired
	  6. encourage client to make lists of planned activities and questions or concerns he/she may have
	  7. assist client to problem-solve as necessary
	  8. implement measures *to stop emotional outbursts, aggressive behavior, and inappropriate responses* (e.g. provide distraction by clapping hands or whistling loudly, instruct client to hold mouth open if he/she is crying inappropriately, decrease environmental stimuli by turning off television or radio and/or requesting that visitors leave for a short while)
	  9. maintain realistic expectations of client's ability to learn, comprehend, and remember information provided
	  10. encourage significant others to be supportive of client; instruct them in methods of dealing with alterations in client's thought processes
	  11. inform client and significant others that intellectual and emotional functioning usually improve as the cerebral irritation decreases, but caution them that "postconcussional syndrome" (a post–head injury syndrome manifested by persistent headache and alterations in thought processes) may persist for a few months to a year or more depending on the severity of the head injury
	  12. assist with neuropsychological testing if indicated
	  13. consult physician if client demonstrates increased alterations in thought processes or is unable to adapt to existing ones.

9. NURSING DIAGNOSIS

Sleep pattern disturbance related to frequent assessments, decreased physical activity, fear, anxiety, headache, and inability to assume usual sleep position (usually need to have head of bed elevated).

DESIRED OUTCOMES	NURSING ACTIONS AND *SELECTED RATIONALES*

9. The client will attain optimal amounts of sleep within the parameters of the treatment regimen as evidenced by:
   a. statements of feeling well rested
   b. no increase in irritability, lethargy, or confusion
   c. absence of frequent yawning, thick speech, dark circles under eyes.

9.a. Assess for signs and symptoms of a sleep pattern disturbance:
   1. verbal complaints of difficulty falling asleep, not feeling well rested, sleep interruptions, or awakening earlier or later than desired
   2. increased irritability, lethargy, or confusion
   3. frequent yawning, thick speech, dark circles under eyes, slight hand tremors.
   b. Determine client's usual sleep habits.
   c. Implement measures *to promote sleep:*
      1. perform actions to reduce fear and anxiety (see Nursing Diagnosis 1, action c)
      2. perform actions to relieve headache (see Nursing Diagnosis 5, action e)
      3. allow client to continue usual sleep practices (e.g. position, time, bedtime rituals) if possible
      4. determine measures that have been helpful to client in the past (e.g. milk, warm drinks) and incorporate in plan of care
      5. discourage long periods of sleep during the day unless sleep deprivation exists or daytime sleep is usual for client
      6. encourage participation in relaxing diversional activities in early evening hours
      7. provide a quiet, restful atmosphere
      8. discourage intake of foods and fluids high in caffeine (e.g. chocolate, coffee, tea, colas), especially in the evening
      9. satisfy basic needs such as hunger, comfort, and warmth before sleep
      10. have client empty bladder just before bedtime
      11. utilize relaxation techniques (e.g. progressive relaxation exercises, back massage, meditation, soft music) before sleep
      12. perform actions *to provide for periods of uninterrupted sleep (90- to 120-minute periods of uninterrupted sleep are considered essential):*
         a. restrict visitors during rest periods
         b. group care (e.g. medications, treatments, physical care, assessments) whenever possible
         c. consult physician regarding the possibility of reducing the frequency of neurological assessments once client's condition stabilizes
      13. monitor for therapeutic and nontherapeutic effects of sedatives and hypnotics if administered.
   d. Consult physician if signs of sleep deprivation persist or worsen.

10. NURSING DIAGNOSIS

Potential for trauma related to:

a. falls associated with motor and sensory impairments, altered thought processes, and seizure activity;
b. burns and cuts associated with motor and sensory impairments.

DESIRED OUTCOMES	NURSING ACTIONS AND *SELECTED RATIONALES*

10. The client will not experience falls, burns, or cuts.

10.a. Determine whether conditions predisposing client to falls, burns, or cuts exist:
   1. motor and sensory impairments
   2. decreased level of consciousness
   3. previous seizure activity and/or abnormal EEG
   4. altered thought processes.
  b. Implement measures *to prevent falls:*
   1. keep bed in low position with side rails up when client is in bed
   2. keep needed items within easy reach and assist client to identify their location
   3. encourage client to request assistance whenever needed; have call signal within easy reach
   4. use lap belt when client is in chair if indicated
   5. instruct client to wear shoes with nonskid soles and low heels when ambulating
   6. avoid unnecessary clutter in room
   7. accompany client during ambulation utilizing a transfer safety belt
   8. provide ambulatory aids (e.g. walker, cane) if client is weak or unsteady on feet
   9. reinforce instructions from physical therapist on correct transfer and ambulation techniques
   10. instruct client to ambulate in well-lit areas and to utilize handrails if needed
   11. do not rush client; allow adequate time for trips to the bathroom and ambulation in hallway
   12. if vision is impaired:
     a. orient client to surroundings, room, arrangement of furniture, and placement of personal belongings
     b. instruct client to wear an eyepatch or frosted lens if diplopia is present
     c. reinforce the need to visually scan the environment if a visual field cut is present
     d. assist with ambulation by walking a half step ahead of client and describing approaching objects or obstacles; instruct client to grasp back of nurse's arm during ambulation.
  c. Implement measures *to prevent burns:*
   1. let hot foods or fluids cool slightly before serving *to reduce risk of burns if spills occur*
   2. supervise client while smoking if indicated
   3. assess temperature of bath water and heating pad before and during use.
  d. Assist client with tasks that require fine motor skills (e.g. shaving) *in order to prevent cuts.*
  e. If client is confused or irrational, implement additional measures *to reduce risk of injury:*
   1. reorient frequently to surroundings and necessity of adhering to safety precautions
   2. provide constant supervision (e.g. staff member, significant other) if indicated
   3. use jacket or wrist restraints or safety alarm device if necessary *to reduce the risk of client's getting out of bed or chair unattended* or, in cases of more severe head injury, place client in a floor bed (mattresses on floor with surrounding "wall" of mattresses or padding) if indicated
   4. monitor for therapeutic and nontherapeutic effects of antianxiety and antipsychotic medications if administered.
  f. Implement measures to prevent seizures and resultant injury (see Collaborative Diagnosis 13, actions c.2–4).
  g. Include client and significant others in planning and implementing measures to prevent injury.
  h. If injury does occur, initiate appropriate first aid and notify physician.

11. NURSING DIAGNOSIS

Potential for aspiration related to decreased level of consciousness, absent gag reflex, and/or impaired swallowing.

DESIRED OUTCOMES	NURSING ACTIONS AND *SELECTED RATIONALES*

11. The client will not aspirate secretions and foods/fluids as evidenced by:
a. clear breath sounds
b. resonant percussion note over lungs
c. respiratory rate at 16–20/ minute
d. absence of dyspnea
e. absence of cyanosis.
	11.a. Assess for factors that indicate potential for aspiration (e.g. decreased level of consciousness, absent gag reflex, choking on secretions and foods/fluids).
	b. Assess for signs and symptoms of aspiration of secretions or foods/fluids (e.g. rhonchi, dull percussion note over lungs, tachycardia, rapid respirations, dyspnea, cyanosis).
	c. Monitor chest x-ray results. Report findings of pulmonary infiltrate.
	d. Implement measures *to reduce the risk of aspiration:*
	  1. position client in side-lying or semi- to high Fowler's position at all times
	  2. have suction equipment readily available for use
	  3. perform oropharyngeal suctioning and provide oral care as often as needed *to remove secretions*
	  4. withhold oral foods/fluids if gag reflex is absent, if client is not alert, or if he/she is experiencing severe dysphagia
	  5. if oral intake is allowed:
	    a. perform actions to improve ability to swallow (see Nursing Diagnosis 4, action b)
	    b. decrease environmental stimuli during meals and snacks *so client can concentrate on chewing and swallowing*
	    c. allow ample time for meals
	    d. instruct client to avoid laughing or talking while eating and drinking
	    e. maintain client in high Fowler's position during and for at least 30 minutes after meals and snacks
	    f. assist client with oral hygiene after eating *to ensure that food particles do not remain in mouth.*
	e. If signs and symptoms of aspiration occur:
	  1. perform tracheal suctioning
	  2. notify physician
	  3. prepare client for chest x-ray.

12. NURSING DIAGNOSIS

Potential altered body temperature: increased related to trauma to the hypothalamus.

DESIRED OUTCOMES	NURSING ACTIONS AND *SELECTED RATIONALES*
12. The client will maintain a normal body temperature.	12.a. Assess for and report signs and symptoms of increased body temperature resulting from trauma to the hypothalamus (e.g. elevated temperature; pale or mottled skin color; absence of perspiration; hot, dry trunk and cool extremities).

b. Monitor for therapeutic and nontherapeutic effects of corticosteroids if administered *to reduce edema of and around hypothalamus in order to prevent increased body temperature.*
c. If increased body temperature occurs:
1. continue with above action
2. implement measures *to gradually reduce client's body temperature toward normal* (e.g. hypothermia blanket, tepid water bath)
3. monitor for therapeutic and nontherapeutic effects of antipyretics if administered.

13. COLLABORATIVE DIAGNOSIS

Potential complications:

a. **increased intracranial pressure (IICP)** related to cerebral hypoxia, hemorrhage, hematoma, and edema; meningitis; and seizures;
b. **meningitis** related to bleeding into the meninges and/or contamination of the cerebral spinal fluid or the meninges during or after the injury (especially with frontal or temporal bone fractures);
c. **seizures** related to cerebral irritation associated with the injury and disruption of nerve transmission resulting from cerebral hypoxia and IICP;
d. **diabetes insipidus** related to trauma to the hypothalamus and/or pituitary gland resulting in decreased production and/or secretion of antidiuretic hormone (ADH);
e. **syndrome of inappropriate antidiuretic hormone (SIADH)** related to:
1. trauma to the hypothalamus and/or pituitary gland resulting in increased production and/or secretion of ADH
2. stimulation of ADH output associated with pain, trauma, and acute stress;
f. **gastrointestinal (GI) bleeding** related to:
1. development of a stress (Cushing's) ulcer (cerebral injury and continued stress cause vagal stimulation that results in gastric hyperacidity and multiple diffuse erosions of the gastric and duodenal mucosa)
2. irritation of gastric mucosa associated with side effects of some medications (e.g. corticosteroids, phenytoin).

DESIRED OUTCOMES	NURSING ACTIONS AND *SELECTED RATIONALES*
13.a. The client will not develop IICP as evidenced by: 1. usual or improved level of consciousness 2. stable or improved motor and sensory function 3. usual pupillary size and reactivity 4. no complaints of increased headache 5. absence of vomiting 6. absence of papilledema and seizure activity 7. stable vital signs.	13.a.1. Assess for and report: a. early signs and symptoms of IICP: 1. development of or increased restlessness, agitation, confusion, lethargy 2. decreasing motor and sensory function 3. change in pupil size or shape 4. sluggish pupillary response to light 5. altered vision (e.g. blurred vision, diplopia, decreased visual acuity) 6. increased headache b. later signs and symptoms of IICP: 1. vomiting (frequently projectile) 2. papilledema 3. seizures 4. dilated, nonreactive pupils 5. stupor, coma 6. rise in systolic B/P with widening pulse pressure 7. full, bounding, slow pulse

8. altered respiratory pattern (e.g. Cheyne-Stokes, central neurogenic hyperventilation)
9. decerebrate or decorticate posturing.

2. Implement measures *to prevent IICP:*
   a. perform actions to improve cerebral tissue perfusion (see Nursing Diagnosis 2, action b) *in order to prevent cerebral vasodilation that occurs as a result of cerebral hypoxia*
   b. observe for and control conditions that could cause increasing restlessness and agitation (e.g. distended bladder, constipation, hypoxia, headache, fear, anxiety)
   c. monitor for therapeutic and nontherapeutic effects of laxatives, stool softeners, antitussives, and antiemetics if administered *to prevent straining to have a bowel movement, coughing, and vomiting (these conditions cause an increase in intrathoracic pressure that impedes venous return from the brain)*
   d. instruct client to avoid activities such as pushing feet against footboard or tightly gripping side rails *(isometric muscle contractions raise systemic blood pressure)*
   e. monitor for therapeutic and nontherapeutic effects of anticonvulsants (e.g. phenytoin, phenobarbital, carbamazepine) if administered *to prevent seizure activity*
   f. perform actions to prevent and treat increased body temperature (see Nursing Diagnosis 12, actions b and c) *in order to prevent cerebral hypoxia and subsequent vasodilation (hypoxia occurs in response to the increased metabolic rate and oxygen utilization)*
   g. perform actions to prevent and treat meningitis (see actions b.5 and 6 in this diagnosis)
   h. schedule care so activities that could raise intracranial pressure (e.g. suctioning, bathing, repositioning) are not grouped together
   i. assist with mechanical hyperventilation that may be done *to decrease arterial CO_2 and prevent vasodilation.*

3. If signs and symptoms of IICP are present:
   a. continue with above actions to help decrease and prevent a further rise in intracranial pressure
   b. initiate seizure precautions
   c. assist with a lumbar or ventricular puncture if performed *to remove some cerebral spinal fluid*
   d. prepare client for insertion of continuous intracranial monitoring device (e.g. intraventricular catheter, subarachnoid screw or bolt) if indicated
   e. prepare client for surgical intervention (e.g. ligation of bleeding vessel, aspiration of hematoma) if indicated
   f. provide emotional support to client and significant others.

13.b. The client will not develop meningitis as evidenced by:
1. absence of fever and chills
2. gradual resolution of headache
3. absence of nuchal rigidity and photophobia
4. negative Kernig's and Brudzinski's signs
5. normal cerebral spinal fluid (CSF) analysis.

13.b.1. Assess for and report signs and symptoms of a CSF leak:
   a. presence of glucose in nasal, ear, or wound drainage as shown by positive Tes-Tape or Dextrostix results; be aware that any drainage containing blood will also test positive for glucose
   b. clear halo or watery, pale ring around bloody or serosanguineous drainage on dressing or pillowcase
   c. complaints of postnasal drip
   d. constant swallowing.
2. Assess for and report signs and symptoms of meningitis:
   a. fever, chills
   b. increasing or persistent headache
   c. photophobia
   d. nuchal rigidity
   e. positive Kernig's sign (inability to straighten knee when hip is flexed)
   f. positive Brudzinski's sign (flexion of hip and knee in response to forward flexion of the neck).
3. Assist with lumbar puncture if indicated. Document appearance of CSF (a milky appearance indicates elevated WBC levels) and CSF pressure (pressure is usually elevated with meningitis).
4. Monitor results of the CSF analysis and report increased WBC and protein levels.

5. Implement measures *to prevent meningitis:*
   a. use sterile technique when changing dressings and working with intracranial pressure monitoring device
   b. instruct client to keep hands away from dressing; use restraints or mittens if necessary
   c. if a CSF leak is present:
      1. instruct client to avoid excessive movement and activity (bedrest is usually ordered *to prevent further stress on the torn dura)*
      2. instruct client to avoid coughing, sneezing, blowing nose, or straining to have a bowel movement *(these activities raise intracranial pressure and can cause increased CSF leakage and/or extension of the dural tear)*; consult physician regarding an order for antitussives, decongestants, stool softeners, and laxatives if indicated
      3. if CSF is leaking from nose:
         a. position client with head of bed elevated 20° unless contraindicated *to allow free drainage of fluid*
         b. instruct client to avoid putting finger in nose
         c. do not perform nasal suctioning or insert a nasogastric tube
         d. do not attempt to clean nose unless ordered by physician
      4. if CSF is leaking from ear:
         a. position client on back or on side of CSF leakage unless contraindicated *to allow free drainage of fluid*
         b. instruct client to avoid putting finger in ear
         c. do not attempt to clean ear unless ordered by physician
      5. do not pack dressing into area of CSF leakage (nose, ear, or wound) *because it will interfere with free flow of fluid;* place a sterile pad over area of CSF leakage to absorb drainage and change pad as soon as it becomes damp
      6. prepare client for surgical repair of the torn dura if the leak does not heal spontaneously
   d. monitor for therapeutic and nontherapeutic effects of anti-infectives if administered prophylactically.
6. If signs and symptoms of meningitis occur:
   a. continue with above measures
   b. initiate seizure precautions *(cerebral irritation can cause seizures)*
   c. maintain activity restrictions as ordered
   d. provide a quiet environment with dim lighting *to reduce discomfort associated with headache and photophobia*
   e. monitor for therapeutic and nontherapeutic effects of the following medications if administered:
      1. corticosteroids *to reduce inflammation*
      2. anti-infectives
   f. monitor for signs and symptoms of IICP (see action a.1 in this diagnosis)
   g. provide emotional support to client and significant others.

13.c. The client will not experience seizure activity or associated injury.

13.c.1. Assess for and report signs and symptoms of seizure activity (e.g. twitching, clonic-tonic movements).
2. Implement measures *to prevent seizures:*
   a. perform actions to prevent and treat IICP (see actions a.2 and 3 in this diagnosis)
   b. perform actions to prevent and treat meningitis (see actions b.5 and 6 in this diagnosis)
   c. monitor for therapeutic and nontherapeutic effects of anticonvulsants (e.g. phenytoin, phenobarbital, carbamazepine) if administered.
3. Initiate and maintain seizure precautions:
   a. have plastic airway readily available
   b. pad side rails with blankets or soft pads
   c. keep bed in low position with side rails up when client is in bed.
4. If seizures do occur:
   a. implement measures *to decrease risk of injury:*
      1. ease client to the floor if he/she is sitting in chair or ambulating at onset of seizure
      2. remain with and do not restrain client during seizure activity

    3. turn client on his/her side and insert an airway if possible during clonic phase *to prevent obstruction of airway by tongue or secretions*

    4. do not force any object between clenched teeth or try to pry mouth open

    5. remove from area items that may cause injury

    6. place towel or pillow under client's head

  b. observe for and report characteristics of seizures (e.g. progression, time elapsed)

  c. monitor for therapeutic and nontherapeutic effects of intravenous anticonvulsants (e.g. phenytoin, phenobarbital) if administered

  d. provide emotional support to client and significant others.

13.d. The client will not experience diabetes insipidus as evidenced by:
1. absence of polyuria and polydipsia
2. urine specific gravity between 1.010 and 1.030.

13.d.1. Assess for and report signs and symptoms of diabetes insipidus:
  a. polyuria (urine output can range from 4–10 or more liters/day)
  b. polydipsia (if the client is able to tolerate oral liquids, he/she may drink 4–10 or more liters of fluid/day)
  c. urine specific gravity less than 1.005.
  2. Monitor for therapeutic and nontherapeutic effects of corticosteroids if administered *to reduce inflammation of and around hypothalamus and pituitary gland.*
  3. If signs and symptoms of diabetes insipidus occur:
    a. maintain fluid intake equal to output *in order to prevent dehydration*
    b. monitor for therapeutic and nontherapeutic effects of the following medications if administered:
      1. ADH replacements (e.g. vasopressin, lypressin, desmopressin acetate [DDAVP])
      2. medications that enhance the action of available ADH (e.g. chlorpropamide, clofibrate, carbamazepine)
    c. assess closely for and report signs and symptoms of dehydration (e.g. decreased skin turgor, significant weight loss, dry mucous membranes, decreased B/P, increased pulse, elevated serum sodium and osmolality).

13.e. The client will not develop SIADH as evidenced by:
1. stable weight
2. balanced intake and output
3. stable or improved mental status
4. stable or improved muscle strength
5. decreased complaints of headache
6. absence of cellular edema, abdominal cramping, nausea, vomiting, seizure activity
7. serum and urine sodium and osmolality levels within normal limits.

13.e.1. Assess for and report signs and symptoms of SIADH:
  a. sudden weight gain
  b. intake greater than output
  c. increased irritability, confusion, or personality change
  d. increasing muscle weakness
  e. complaints of persistent or increased headache
  f. fingerprint edema over sternum (reflects cellular edema)
  g. abdominal cramping, nausea, vomiting
  h. seizures
  i. urine specific gravity greater than 1.012
  j. elevated urine sodium and osmolality levels
  k. low serum sodium and osmolality levels.
  2. Implement measures *to prevent development of SIADH:*
    a. perform actions to reduce pain (see Nursing Diagnosis 5, action e)
    b. perform actions to reduce fear and anxiety (see Nursing Diagnosis 1, action c)
    c. monitor for therapeutic and nontherapeutic effects of corticosteroids if administered *to reduce inflammation of and around hypothalamus and pituitary gland.*
  3. If signs and symptoms of SIADH occur:
    a. maintain fluid restrictions if ordered (usually 500–1000 cc/day) *to prevent further fluid retention*
    b. encourage intake of foods/fluids high in sodium (e.g. cured meats, processed cheese, soups, catsup, canned vegetables, pickles, bouillon)
    c. continue to adhere to seizure precautions (see action c.3 in this diagnosis) until sodium levels return to normal
    d. monitor for therapeutic and nontherapeutic effects of the following if administered:
      1. diuretics (usually furosemide) *to aid in water excretion*
      2. infusions of normal or hypertonic saline solutions *to treat hyponatremia*

3. lithium carbonate and demeclocycline *to promote water excretion (inhibit the action of ADH at the renal tubular level)*
4. urea *to promote osmotic diuresis*

e. provide emotional support to client and significant others.

13.f. The client will not experience GI bleeding as evidenced by:
1. no complaints of epigastric discomfort and fullness
2. absence of occult or frank blood in stool and gastric contents
3. B/P and pulse within normal range for client
4. RBC, Hct., and Hgb. levels within normal range.
	13.f.1. Assess for and report signs and symptoms of GI bleeding (e.g. complaints of epigastric discomfort or fullness, frank or occult blood in stool or gastric contents, decreased B/P, increased pulse).
	2. Monitor RBC, Hct., and Hgb. levels. Report declining values.
	3. Implement measures *to prevent ulceration of gastric or duodenal mucosa:*
	  a. perform actions to decrease fear and anxiety (see Nursing Diagnosis 1, action c)
	  b. encourage client to reduce intake of foods/fluids that are acidic, spicy, or high in caffeine (e.g. chocolate, colas, coffee, tea)
	  c. administer ulcerogenic medications (e.g. corticosteroids, phenytoin) with meals or snacks *to decrease gastric irritation*
	  d. monitor for therapeutic and nontherapeutic effects of histamine₂ receptor antagonists (e.g. cimetidine, ranitidine, famotidine), antacids, and mucosal barrier fortifiers (e.g. sucralfate) if administered.
	4. If signs and symptoms of GI bleeding occur:
	  a. insert nasogastric tube and maintain suction as ordered
	  b. assist with iced water or saline gastric lavage, transendoscopic electrocoagulation, selective arterial embolization, endoscopic laser photocoagulation, and/or intra-arterial administration of vasopressors (e.g. vasopressin) if ordered
	  c. monitor for therapeutic and nontherapeutic effects of blood products and/or volume expanders if administered
	  d. prepare client for surgery (e.g. ligation of bleeding vessels, partial gastrectomy) if indicated
	  e. provide emotional support to client and significant others
	  f. refer to Care Plan on Peptic Ulcer for additional care measures.

☐ ▄▄

14. NURSING DIAGNOSIS

Disturbance in self-concept* related to:

a. changes in appearance (e.g. periocular edema and ecchymosis, loss of hair on head if an area is shaved to repair lacerations or perform cranial surgery);
b. changes in motor and sensory function;
c. increased dependence on others to meet basic needs;
d. anticipated changes in life style and roles associated with sensory and motor impairments and alteration in thought processes.

---

* This diagnostic label includes the nursing diagnoses of body image disturbance and self-esteem disturbance.

☐ ▄▄

DESIRED OUTCOMES	NURSING ACTIONS AND *SELECTED RATIONALES*
14. The client will demonstrate beginning adaptation to changes in appearance, physical and mental functioning, life style, and roles as evidenced by:	14.a. Determine the meaning of changes in appearance, physical and mental functioning, life style, and roles to the client by encouraging him/her to verbalize feelings and by noting nonverbal responses to the changes experienced. b. Assess for signs and symptoms of a disturbance in self-concept (e.g. verbal or nonverbal cues denoting a negative response to changes in body

a. verbalization of feelings of self-worth
b. maintenance of relationships with significant others
c. active participation in activities of daily living
d. active interest in personal appearance
e. willingness to participate in social activities
f. verbalization of a beginning plan for adapting life style to meet changes in physical and mental functioning.

functioning and appearance such as denial of or preoccupation with changes that have occurred, refusal to look at or touch affected body part, or withdrawal from significant others).
c. Implement measures to facilitate the grieving process (see Nursing Diagnosis 16, action d).
d. Assist the client to identify strengths and qualities that have a positive effect on self-concept.
e. Implement measures *to assist client to increase self-esteem* (e.g. limit negative self-criticism, encourage positive comments about self, give positive feedback about accomplishments).
f. Implement measures to assist the client to cope with the effects of craniocerebral trauma (see Nursing Diagnosis 15, action d).
g. Clarify misconceptions about changes in motor and sensory function and thought processes. If appropriate, assure client that these residual effects are usually temporary but caution him/her that recovery is slow (may take months to years).
h. If periocular edema and ecchymosis are present:
   1. reinforce that it is temporary and will begin to subside within 48–72 hours after injury
   2. instruct and assist client with measures *to reduce swelling* (e.g. cold compresses to affected area, lying on unaffected side, keeping head of bed elevated 20–30°).
i. Implement measures *to reduce client's embarrassment about loss of hair* (e.g. assist with hair styling that makes shaved area less obvious, provide a scarf or surgical cap if desired). Reinforce the fact that the hair will grow back.
j. Assist client with usual grooming and makeup habits if necessary.
k. Discuss techniques the client can utilize *to adapt to alterations in thought processes:*
   1. encourage client to make lists and jot down messages and to refer to these rather than relying on his/her memory
   2. instruct the client to place self in a calm environment when making decisions
   3. encourage client to validate decisions, clarify information, and seek assistance to problem-solve if indicated
   4. encourage client to schedule adequate rest periods and reduce stressors *in order to decrease irritability.*
l. Instruct significant others in ways to deal with client's emotional lability and inappropriate laughing, crying, or swearing (e.g. provide privacy; tell client to open mouth if crying; distract client by clapping hands, singing, or whistling loudly).
m. Reinforce use of adaptive devices (e.g. plate guards, broad-handled utensils, universal cuff, button hook, long-handled shoehorn) and mobility aids (e.g. walker, cane) *to increase client's independence.*
n. Encourage significant others to allow client to do what he/she is able *so that independence can be re-established and/or self-esteem redeveloped.*
o. Demonstrate acceptance of client using techniques such as therapeutic touch and frequent visits. Encourage significant others to do the same.
p. Encourage client contact with others *so that he/she can test and establish a new self-image.*
q. Assist client's and significant others' adjustment by listening, facilitating communication, and providing information.
r. Assess for and support behaviors suggesting positive adaptation to changes experienced (e.g. scanning environment or wearing eyepatch if visual disturbances are present, utilizing alternative methods of communicating if speech is impaired, using adaptive devices to perform self-care activities).
s. Ensure that client and significant others have similar expectations and understanding of future life style.
t. Encourage visits and support from significant others.
u. Encourage client to continue involvement in social activities and to pursue interests. If previous interests and hobbies cannot be pursued, encourage development of new ones.
v. Provide information about and encourage utilization of community agencies or support groups (e.g. head injury support groups, vocational rehabilitation, family and individual counseling) if appropriate.

UNIT VI

w. Consult physician about psychological counseling if client desires or if he/she seems unwilling or unable to adapt to changes resulting from craniocerebral trauma.

☐ �███

15. NURSING DIAGNOSIS

Ineffective individual coping related to fear, anxiety, persistent headache, changes in motor and sensory function, alterations in thought processes, and possibility of lengthy rehabilitation.

☐ ▇▇▇

DESIRED OUTCOMES	NURSING ACTIONS AND *SELECTED RATIONALES*

15. The client will demonstrate the use of effective coping skills as evidenced by:
   a. willingness to participate in treatment plan and self-care activities
   b. verbalization of ability to cope with the effects of craniocerebral trauma
   c. identification of stressors
   d. utilization of appropriate problem-solving techniques
   e. recognition and utilization of available support systems.

15.a. Assess effectiveness of client's coping strategies by observing behavior and noting strengths, weaknesses, ability to express feelings and concerns, and willingness to participate in treatment plan.
   b. Assess for and report signs and symptoms that may indicate ineffective coping (e.g. sleep disturbances; increased fatigue, difficulty concentrating, and irritability; decreased tolerance for pain; verbalization of inability to cope; inability to problem-solve).
   c. Allow time for client to adjust psychologically to planned treatment, residual effects of craniocerebral trauma, and anticipated life-style and role changes.
   d. Implement measures *to promote effective coping:*
      1. establish a communication system as quickly as possible if speech is affected
      2. assist client to relearn or communicate the names of significant others if memory loss or dysphasia is present
      3. perform actions to reduce fear and anxiety (see Nursing Diagnosis 1, action c)
      4. perform actions to reduce headache (see Nursing Diagnosis 5, action e)
      5. arrange for a visit with another who has successfully recovered from craniocerebral trauma
      6. include client in the planning of care, encourage maximum participation in treatment plan, and allow choices when possible *to enable him/her to maintain a sense of control*
      7. instruct client in effective problem-solving techniques (e.g. accurate identification of stressors, determination of various options to solve problem)
      8. assist client to maintain usual daily routines whenever possible
      9. provide diversional activities according to client's interests and abilities
      10. assist client as he/she starts to plan for necessary life-style and role changes after discharge; provide input related to realistic prioritization of problems that need to be dealt with
      11. set up a home evaluation appointment with occupational and physical therapists before client's discharge if indicated *so that changes in the home environment (e.g. installation of ramps and handrails, widening doorways, altering kitchen facilities) can be completed by discharge*
      12. assist the client and significant others to identify ways that personal and family goals can be adjusted rather than abandoned
      13. inform client that he/she will have days when impairments worsen; assure client that this is usually temporary and the result of physical and/or emotional stress or fatigue rather than an indication of deteriorating neurological status
      14. assist client to identify and utilize available support systems; provide information regarding available community resources that can assist client and significant others in coping with effects of craniocerebral

trauma (e.g. head injury support groups; individual, family, and financial counseling services)

15. monitor for therapeutic and nontherapeutic effects of antidepressants if administered.

e. Encourage continued emotional support from significant others.

f. Encourage the client to share with significant others the kind of support that would be most beneficial (e.g. listening, inspiring hope, providing reassurance and accurate information).

g. Assess for and support behaviors suggesting positive adaptation to changes experienced (e.g. participation in treatment plan and self-care activities, communication of ability to cope, utilization of effective problem-solving strategies).

h. Consult physician about psychological or vocational rehabilitation counseling if appropriate. Initiate a referral if necessary.

□ ▬▬▬▬▬▬▬▬▬▬▬▬▬▬▬▬▬▬▬

16. NURSING DIAGNOSIS

Grieving* related to changes in motor and sensory function and thought processes and the effect of these changes on future life style and roles.

———————

* This diagnostic label includes anticipatory grieving and grieving following the actual losses/changes.

□ ▬▬▬▬▬▬▬▬▬▬▬▬▬▬▬▬▬▬▬

DESIRED OUTCOMES	NURSING ACTIONS AND *SELECTED RATIONALES*

16. The client will demonstrate beginning progression through the grieving process as evidenced by:
a. verbalization of feelings about the craniocerebral trauma and its effects
b. expression of grief
c. participation in treatment plan and self-care activities
d. utilization of support systems
e. verbalization of a plan for integrating prescribed follow-up care into life style.
	16.a. Determine client's perception of impact of craniocerebral trauma on his/her future.
	b. Determine how the client usually expresses grief.
	c. Observe for signs of grieving (e.g. changes in eating habits, insomnia, anger, noncompliance, denial).
	d. Implement measures *to facilitate the grieving process:*
	  1. assist client to acknowledge the changes experienced *so grief work can begin*; assess for factors that may hinder or facilitate acknowledgment
	  2. discuss the grieving process and assist client to accept the stages of grieving as an expected response to changes that have occurred
	  3. allow time for client to progress through the stages of grieving (denial, anger, bargaining, depression, acceptance [Kübler-Ross, 1969]); be aware that not every stage is experienced or expressed by all individuals
	  4. provide an atmosphere of care and concern (e.g. provide privacy, be available and nonjudgmental, display empathy and respect) *so that client will feel free to verbalize both positive and negative feelings and concerns*
	  5. perform actions *to promote trust* (e.g. answer questions honestly, provide requested information)
	  6. encourage the expression of anger and sadness about the changes experienced
	  7. encourage client to express his/her feelings in whatever ways are comfortable (e.g. writing, drawing, conversation)
	  8. perform actions to facilitate effective coping (see Nursing Diagnosis 15, action d)
	  9. perform actions *to support realistic hope about the effects of treatment on the residual impairments:*
	    a. focus on what the client is able to accomplish independently and with the use of adaptive devices
	    b. reinforce knowledge that impairments may improve with time
	    c. reinforce positive effects of speech, physical, and occupational therapies.

e. Assess for and support behaviors suggesting resolution of grief (e.g. verbalizing feelings about losses or changes, expressing sorrow, focusing on ways to adapt to losses).
f. Explain the stages of the grieving process to significant others. Encourage their support and understanding.
g. Provide information regarding counseling services and support groups that might assist client in working through grief.
h. Arrange for visit from clergy if desired by client.
i. Monitor for therapeutic and nontherapeutic effects of antidepressants if administered.
j. Consult physician about referral for counseling if signs of dysfunctional grieving (e.g. persistent denial of losses or changes, excessive anger or sadness, hysteria, suicidal behaviors, phobias) occur.

☐ ▬▬▬▬▬▬▬▬▬▬▬▬▬▬▬▬▬▬▬▬▬▬▬▬▬▬▬▬▬▬▬▬

17. NURSING DIAGNOSIS

Altered family processes related to change in family roles and structure associated with the motor and sensory impairments and alterations in thought processes of a family member and the need for lengthy rehabilitation (especially with moderate to severe head injury).

☐ ▬▬▬▬▬▬▬▬▬▬▬▬▬▬▬▬▬▬▬▬▬▬▬▬▬▬▬▬▬▬▬▬

DESIRED OUTCOMES	NURSING ACTIONS AND *SELECTED RATIONALES*

17. The family members* will demonstrate beginning adjustment to changes in family roles and structure as evidenced by:
   a. verbalization of ways to adapt to required role and life-style changes
   b. active participation in decision making and client's rehabilitation
   c. positive interactions with one another.

17.a. Identify components of the family and their patterns of communication and role expectations.
b. Assess for signs and symptoms of alterations in family processes (e.g. statements of not being able to accept client's physical impairments and changes in thought processes or to make necessary role and life-style changes, inability to make decisions, inability or refusal to participate in client's rehabilitation, negative family interactions).
c. Implement measures *to facilitate family members' adjustment to changes in family roles and structure:*
   1. encourage verbalization of feelings about client's disabilities and the effect of these on the family structure
   2. reinforce physician's explanations of the effects of craniocerebral trauma and planned treatment and rehabilitation
   3. provide privacy *so that family members and client can share their feelings with one another;* stress the importance and facilitate the use of good communication techniques
   4. assist family members to progress through their own grieving process; explain that during this progression, they may encounter times when they need to focus on meeting their own rather than the client's needs
   5. emphasize the need for family members to obtain adequate rest and nutrition and to identify and utilize stress management techniques *so that they are better able to emotionally and physically deal with the changes and losses experienced*
   6. encourage and assist family members to identify coping strategies for dealing with the client's disabilities and their effects on the family
   7. include family members in decision making about client and his/her care; convey appreciation for their input and continued support of client
   8. encourage and allow family members to participate in client's care; provide necessary instruction and stress the importance of allowing the

---
* The term "family members" is being used here to include client's significant others.

client to utilize adaptive devices, mobility aids, and techniques to improve thought processes *so that he/she can maintain as much independence as possible*

9. assist family members to identify sources that could assist them in coping with their feelings and meeting their immediate and long-term needs (e.g. counseling and social services; pastoral care; service, church, and head injury support groups); initiate a referral if indicated.

d. Consult physician if family members continue to demonstrate difficulty adapting to changes in roles and family structures.

□

18. NURSING DIAGNOSIS

Knowledge deficit regarding follow-up care.

□

DESIRED OUTCOMES	NURSING ACTIONS AND *SELECTED RATIONALES*
18.a. The client will identify ways to adapt to neurological deficits that may persist following craniocerebral trauma.	18.a.1. Instruct client in ways *to adapt to neurological deficits* resulting from the craniocerebral trauma:* a. wear an eyepatch or frosted lens if double vision is a problem b. utilize scanning techniques if visual field cut is present c. utilize paper and pencil, magic slate, computer, pictures, and pantomiming to express self if verbal communication is impaired d. write down messages and reminders and refer to written instructions repeatedly if experiencing difficulty concentrating or remembering e. instruct client to request assistance when problem-solving and setting priorities and to seek validation of decisions if reasoning ability is impaired f. continue with techniques and exercises to improve swallowing if indicated g. prepare meals that are visually appealing *to help stimulate appetite if sense of smell is lost* h. reduce alcohol intake *(intolerance to usual amounts of alcohol often occurs for a few months after injury)* i. utilize adaptive devices (e.g. wheelchair, cane, walker, broad-handled eating utensils, plate guard) if motor function is impaired j. plan daily activities to allow for adequate rest periods *in order to reduce irritability that often occurs after craniocerebral trauma.* 2. Allow time for questions, clarification, and return demonstration of techniques.
18.b. The client will identify ways to reduce headache.	18.b. Instruct client in ways *to reduce headache* (headache may persist for months following injury): 1. dim environmental lighting if possible or wear sunglasses when light is bright 2. reduce environmental noise whenever possible (e.g. lower volume on TV and radio) 3. avoid situations that increase stress 4. take analgesics as prescribed.
18.c. The client will state signs and symptoms of	18.c. Instruct client to report the following signs and symptoms: 1. increasing drowsiness or difficulty awakening

---

* Neurological deficits can range from a temporary increase in irritability or a slight facial droop to hemiplegia, aphasia, or permanent alterations in thought processes depending on the extensiveness and location of cerebral injury. Ways of adapting to a few of the more common deficits are included here. For more specific rehabilitative measures and a more extensive discussion of deficits, refer to textbooks on neurological nursing and the Care Plan on Cerebrovascular Accident.

complications to report to the health care provider.

2. increased irritability and restlessness
3. changes in behavior, increased difficulty remembering or concentrating, loss of emotional control
4. new or increased weakness of extremities
5. decreased sensation in extremities
6. severe headache
7. increased difficulty speaking or comprehending what others are saying
8. increased difficulty chewing or swallowing
9. increase in or development of changes in vision (e.g. double vision, blurred vision, visual field cuts)
10. increase in size of one pupil
11. dizziness, difficulty maintaining balance
12. bloody or clear drainage from nose or ears
13. stiff neck
14. sudden weight gain or loss
15. excessive thirst
16. unexplained fever
17. seizures.

18.d. The client will identify community agencies that can assist with home management and adjustment to changes resulting from the injury.

18.d.1. Inform client and significant others of community resources that can assist with home management and the adjustment to changes resulting from craniocerebral trauma (e.g. home health agencies, Visiting Nurse Association, Meals on Wheels, social and financial services, head injury support groups, local service groups that can help obtain adaptive devices, individual and family counseling services).
2. Initiate a referral if indicated.

18.e. The client will verbalize an understanding of and a plan for adhering to recommended follow-up care including future appointments with health care provider and therapists and medications prescribed.

18.e.1. Reinforce the importance of keeping follow-up appointments with health care provider and physical, occupational, and speech therapists.
2. Teach client the rationale for, side effects of, schedule for taking, and importance of taking medications prescribed (e.g. phenytoin, corticosteroids, anti-infectives).
3. Implement measures *to improve client compliance:*
   a. include significant others in teaching sessions if possible
   b. encourage questions and allow time for reinforcement or clarification of information provided
   c. provide written instructions on scheduled appointments with health care provider and occupational, physical, and speech therapists; medications prescribed; and signs and symptoms to report.

■ ■

Intracranial Surgery

Intracranial surgery may be done to remove space-occupying lesions and abscesses, repair vascular abnormalities such as aneurysms and arteriovenous malformations, improve ventricular drainage, treat certain injuries following craniocerebral trauma, and facilitate definitive diagnosis of some neurological conditions. Intracranial surgery may also be performed to disrupt various nerve fiber tracts in order to provide relief from intractable pain or alleviate unmanageable neurological symptoms such as spasm, tremors, or seizure activity. Surgery is accomplished by a craniotomy. The portion

of the skull involved may be replaced after surgery, left out permanently, or removed and replaced at a later date with a synthetic or metal plate.

Intracranial surgery is described in relation to the tentorium (supratentorial, infratentorial) or by the operative approach (e.g. transmastoidal, anterior, posterior, transorbital, cerebellar, suboccipital). Residual neurological deficits depend largely on the approach used (e.g. ataxia is expected after the cerebellar approach, speech may be impaired after a temporal approach).

This care plan focuses on the adult client hospitalized

for intracranial surgery. Preoperative goals of care are to decrease fear and anxiety and educate the client about postoperative expectations and management. Postoperatively, goals of care are to maintain comfort, prevent complications, assist the client to adjust to any residual effects of the surgery, and educate the client regarding follow-up care. Objectives of care and discharge teaching will need to be individualized according to the client's diagnosis, area of the brain affected, neurological deficits, and prognosis.

DISCHARGE CRITERIA

Prior to discharge, the client will:

- identify ways to adapt to neurological deficits resulting from the underlying disease condition and/or the surgical procedure
- state signs and symptoms to report to the health care provider
- share thoughts and feelings about the diagnosis and neurological deficits that may be the result of the underlying disease process and/or the surgery
- identify community resources that can assist with home management and adjustment to changes resulting from the diagnosis and/or the surgery
- verbalize an understanding of and a plan for adhering to recommended follow-up care including future appointments with health care provider, activity level, pain management, medications prescribed, and wound care.

UNIT VI

NURSING/COLLABORATIVE DIAGNOSES

Preoperative
1. Anxiety □ *238*
Postoperative
1. Pain: headache □ *239*
2. Potential altered body temperature: increased □ *239*
3. Potential complications:
   a. increased intracranial pressure (IICP)
   b. meningitis
   c. seizures
   d. diabetes insipidus
   e. gastrointestinal (GI) bleeding □ *240*
4. Disturbance in self-concept □ *244*
5. Knowledge deficit regarding follow-up care □ *246*

☐ ▬▬▬▬▬▬▬▬▬▬▬▬▬▬▬▬▬▬▬▬▬▬▬▬▬▬▬▬

Preoperative

Use in conjunction with the Standardized Preoperative Care Plan.

☐ ▬▬▬▬▬▬▬▬▬▬▬▬▬▬▬▬▬▬▬▬▬▬▬▬▬▬▬▬

1. NURSING DIAGNOSIS

Anxiety related to:

a. unfamiliar environment and separation from significant others;
b. lack of understanding of diagnostic tests and planned surgical procedure;
c. economic factors associated with hospitalization;
d. possibility of residual neurological impairments;
e. anticipated postoperative discomfort and changes in appearance (e.g. shaved head, scalp indentation) and usual life style and roles;
f. possibility of death.

☐ ▬▬▬▬▬▬▬▬▬▬▬▬▬▬▬▬▬▬▬▬▬▬▬▬▬▬▬▬

DESIRED OUTCOMES	NURSING ACTIONS AND *SELECTED RATIONALES*

1. The client will experience a reduction in fear and anxiety (see Standardized Preoperative Care Plan, Nursing Diagnosis 1, for outcome criteria).	1.a. Refer to Standardized Preoperative Care Plan, Nursing Diagnosis 1, for measures related to assessment and reduction of fear and anxiety.
	b. Implement additional measures *to reduce fear and anxiety:*
	  1. explain all diagnostic tests (e.g. skull x-rays, computed tomography, magnetic resonance imaging [MRI], EEG, cerebral angiography)
	  2. assure client that there is usually very little pain associated with intracranial surgery
	  3. explain the necessity for intensive care monitoring after some intracranial surgeries; orient to the intensive care unit and equipment that may be used (e.g. intracranial pressure monitoring device, ventricular drains, wound catheters, respirator) if appropriate
	  4. identify and practice alternative forms of communication (e.g. magic slate, word or picture board, hand signals) if client is expected to be intubated or speech impairment is anticipated following surgery
	  5. perform actions *to reduce fear and anxiety about anticipated changes in physical appearance:*
	    a. assure client that when head dressing is removed, he/she can wear a surgical cap or scarf if desired (most physicians advise clients to avoid wearing a wig until sutures are removed)
	    b. inform client that incision lines are usually behind normal hairline and will not be apparent when hair grows back
	    c. if a craniectomy is planned, discuss the possibility of having a cranioplasty in a few months if appropriate
	    d. discuss alternative hair styles that might make incision lines or cranial defect less apparent
	    e. inform client that periocular edema and ecchymosis usually begin to subside 2–3 days postoperatively
	  6. reinforce physician's explanations about anticipated effects of the surgery on neurological function (this depends on the diagnosis and extensiveness and site of surgery); discuss resources available to assist client to adapt to anticipated impairments (e.g. speech, occupational, and physical therapists).

Postoperative

Use in conjunction with the Standardized Postoperative Care Plan.

1. NURSING DIAGNOSIS

Pain: headache related to:

a. cerebral tissue trauma associated with the surgical procedure;
b. stretching or compression of the pain-sensitive dura and cerebral vascular structures associated with cerebral bleeding and/or edema and increased intracranial pressure;
c. meningeal irritation associated with the presence of blood in the subarachnoid space and/or inflammation of the meninges.

DESIRED OUTCOMES	NURSING ACTIONS AND *SELECTED RATIONALES*

1. The client will obtain relief from headache as evidenced by:
a. verbalization of headache relief
b. relaxed facial expression and body positioning.
	1.a. Determine how the client usually responds to pain.
	b. Assess for nonverbal signs of headache (e.g. reluctance to move head, wrinkled brow, clenched fists, squinting, rubbing head, avoidance of bright lights and noises).
	c. Assess verbal complaints of pain. Ask client to be specific about type, location, and severity of headache.
	d. Assess for factors that seem to aggravate and alleviate headache.
	e. Implement measures *to relieve headache:*
	  1. perform actions *to minimize environmental stimuli* (e.g. provide a quiet environment, restrict visitors, dim lights)
	  2. avoid jarring bed or startling client *to minimize risk of sudden movements*
	  3. perform actions to prevent and treat increased intracranial pressure and meningitis (see Postoperative Collaborative Diagnosis 3, actions a.2 and 3 and b.5 and 6)
	  4. provide nonpharmacological measures for headache relief (e.g. cool cloth to forehead, back rub, distraction)
	  5. monitor for therapeutic and nontherapeutic effects of nonnarcotic analgesics or codeine (other narcotic analgesics are usually contraindicated *because they have a greater depressant effect on the central nervous system)* if administered.
	f. Consult physician if above actions fail to relieve headache.

2. NURSING DIAGNOSIS

Potential altered body temperature: increased related to trauma to the hypothalamus during surgery or as a result of postoperative cerebral edema, hematoma, or hemorrhage.

DESIRED OUTCOMES	NURSING ACTIONS AND *SELECTED RATIONALES*

2. The client will maintain a normal body temperature.	2.a. Assess for and report signs and symptoms of increased body temperature resulting from trauma to the hypothalamus (e.g. elevated temperature; pale or mottled skin color; absence of perspiration; hot, dry trunk and cool extremities).
	b. Monitor for therapeutic and nontherapeutic effects of corticosteroids if administered *to reduce edema of and around hypothalamus in order to prevent increased body temperature.*
	c. If increased body temperature occurs:
	  1. continue with above action
	  2. implement measures *to gradually reduce client's body temperature toward normal* (e.g. hypothermia blanket, tepid water bath)
	  3. monitor for therapeutic and nontherapeutic effects of antipyretics if administered.

☐ ▉▉▉▉▉▉▉▉▉▉▉▉▉▉▉▉▉▉▉▉▉▉▉▉▉▉▉▉▉▉▉▉

3. COLLABORATIVE DIAGNOSIS

Potential complications:

a. **increased intracranial pressure (IICP)** related to cerebral bleeding, hematoma, edema, and/or hypoxia; obstructed flow of cerebral spinal fluid; meningitis; and seizures;

b. **meningitis** related to bleeding into the meninges and/or contamination of the meninges or cerebral spinal fluid (can occur as a result of initial injury, surgery, or postoperative wound infection);

c. **seizures** related to cerebral irritation associated with the surgical procedure and disruption of nerve transmission as a result of IICP and meningitis;

d. **diabetes insipidus** related to surgical trauma and/or inflammation in the region of the hypothalamus or pituitary gland (can result in decreased production and/or secretion of antidiuretic hormone [ADH]);

e. **gastrointestinal (GI) bleeding** related to:
1. development of a stress (Cushing's) ulcer (cerebral injury and continued stress cause vagal stimulation that results in gastric hyperacidity and multiple diffuse erosions of the gastric and duodenal mucosa)
2. irritation of gastric mucosa associated with side effects of some medications (e.g. phenytoin, corticosteroids).

☐ ▉▉▉▉▉▉▉▉▉▉▉▉▉▉▉▉▉▉▉▉▉▉▉▉▉▉▉▉▉▉▉▉

DESIRED OUTCOMES	NURSING ACTIONS AND *SELECTED RATIONALES*

3.a. The client will not develop IICP as evidenced by:
  1. usual or improved level of consciousness
  2. stable or improved motor and sensory function
  3. usual pupillary size and reactivity
  4. no complaints of increased headache
  5. absence of vomiting
  6. absence of papilledema and seizure activity
	3.a.1. Assess for and report:
	  a. early signs and symptoms of IICP:
	    1. restlessness, agitation, confusion, lethargy
	    2. decreasing motor and sensory function
	    3. change in pupil size or shape
	    4. sluggish pupillary response to light
	    5. altered vision (e.g. blurred vision, diplopia, decreased visual acuity)
	    6. increased headache
	    7. elevation of bone flap or bulging in area where bone flap has been removed
	  b. later signs and symptoms of IICP:
	    1. vomiting (frequently projectile)
	    2. papilledema

7. stable vital signs.

3. seizures
4. dilated, nonreactive pupils
5. stupor, coma
6. rise in systolic B/P with widening pulse pressure
7. full, bounding, slow pulse
8. altered respiratory pattern (e.g. Cheyne-Stokes, central neurogenic hyperventilation)
9. decerebrate or decorticate posturing.

2. Implement measures *to prevent IICP:*
   a. observe for and control conditions that could cause increasing restlessness and agitation (e.g. distended bladder, constipation, hypoxia, headache, fear, anxiety)
   b. monitor for therapeutic and nontherapeutic effects of laxatives, stool softeners, antitussives, and antiemetics if administered *to prevent straining to have a bowel movement, coughing, and vomiting (these conditions cause an increase in intrathoracic pressure that impedes venous return from the brain)*
   c. instruct client to avoid activities such as pushing feet against footboard or tightly gripping side rails *(isometric muscle contractions raise systemic blood pressure)*
   d. perform actions to prevent and treat meningitis (see actions b.5 and 6 in this diagnosis)
   e. monitor for therapeutic and nontherapeutic effects of anticonvulsants (e.g. phenytoin, phenobarbital, carbamazepine) if administered *to prevent seizure activity*
   f. schedule care so activities that could raise intracranial pressure (e.g. suctioning, bathing, repositioning) are not grouped together
   g. perform actions *to prevent cerebral edema:*
      1. maintain fluid restrictions as ordered
      2. administer fluids at an even rate
      3. position client with head of bed elevated 20–30° unless contraindicated and keep head and neck in proper alignment *to promote adequate cerebral venous drainage*
      4. monitor for therapeutic and nontherapeutic effects of osmotic diuretics (e.g. mannitol), loop diuretics (e.g. furosemide), and corticosteroids (e.g. dexamethasone, methylprednisolone) if administered
   h. perform actions *to prevent cerebral hypoxia and subsequent vasodilation:*
      1. implement measures *to maintain a patent airway* (e.g. position client on side, suction if necessary)
      2. administer central nervous system depressants (e.g. narcotic analgesics, sedatives) judiciously; hold medication and consult physician if respiratory rate is less than 12/minute
      3. administer oxygen as ordered and before and after tracheal suctioning
      4. implement measures to prevent and treat increased body temperature (see Postoperative Nursing Diagnosis 2, actions b and c) *in order to prevent the increased metabolic rate and oxygen utilization that occur with hyperthermia*
   i. assist with mechanical hyperventilation that may be done *to decrease arterial* CO_2 *and prevent vasodilation*
   j. position client on unoperative side if bone flap and/or large mass was removed *(this helps prevent increased pressure and venous congestion in the operative area)*
   k. if client has an internal shunt, perform actions *to maintain its patency* (e.g. avoid pressure on the shunt, tubing, and reservoir site; pump shunt as ordered)
   l. if client has an external shunt, perform actions *to maintain its patency* (e.g. avoid kinks in tubing, keep client's head and drainage receptacle at the prescribed levels).

3. If signs and symptoms of IICP are present:
   a. continue with above actions to help decrease and prevent a further rise in intracranial pressure
   b. initiate seizure precautions

UNIT
VI

    c. assist with lumbar or ventricular puncture if performed *to remove some cerebral spinal fluid*

    d. prepare client for insertion of continuous intracranial monitoring device (e.g. intraventricular catheter, subarachnoid screw or bolt) if indicated

    e. prepare client for surgical intervention (e.g. ligation of bleeding vessel, repair of blocked shunt, removal of bone flap or hematoma) if indicated

    f. provide emotional support to client and significant others.

3.b. The client will not develop meningitis as evidenced by:
1. absence of fever and chills
2. absence of nuchal rigidity and photophobia
3. gradual resolution of headache
4. negative Kernig's and Brudzinski's signs
5. normal cerebral spinal fluid (CSF) analysis.

3.b.1. Assess for and report signs and symptoms of a CSF leak:
    a. presence of glucose in nasal, ear, or wound drainage as shown by positive Tes-Tape or Dextrostix results; be aware that any drainage containing blood will also test positive for glucose
    b. clear halo or a watery, pale ring around bloody or serosanguineous drainage on dressing or pillowcase
    c. complaints of postnasal drip
    d. constant swallowing.

2. Assess for and report signs and symptoms of meningitis:
    a. fever, chills
    b. nuchal rigidity
    c. photophobia
    d. increasing or persistent headache
    e. positive Kernig's sign (inability to straighten knee when hip is flexed)
    f. positive Brudzinski's sign (flexion of hip and knee in response to forward flexion of the neck).

3. Assist with lumbar puncture if indicated. Document appearance of CSF (a milky appearance indicates elevated WBC levels) and CSF pressure (pressure is usually elevated with meningitis).

4. Monitor results of CSF analysis and report increased WBC and protein levels.

5. Implement measures *to prevent meningitis:*
    a. use sterile technique when changing dressings and when working with external ventricular shunts, wound drains, and intracranial monitoring device
    b. instruct client to keep hands away from drains and dressings; use restraints or mittens if necessary
    c. if a CSF leak is present:
      1. instruct client to avoid excessive movement and activity (bedrest is usually ordered *to prevent further stress on the torn dura)*
      2. instruct client to avoid coughing, sneezing, blowing nose, and straining to have a bowel movement *(these activities raise intracranial pressure and can cause increased CSF leakage and/or extension of the dural tear)*; consult physician about an order for antitussives, decongestants, laxatives, and stool softeners if indicated
      3. if CSF is leaking from nose:
        a. position client with head of bed elevated 20° unless contraindicated *to allow free drainage of fluid*
        b. instruct client to avoid putting finger in nose
        c. do not perform nasal suctioning or insert a nasogastric tube
        d. do not attempt to clean nose unless ordered by physician
      4. if CSF is leaking from ear:
        a. position client on back or on side of CSF leakage unless contraindicated *to allow free drainage of fluid*
        b. instruct client to avoid putting finger in ear
        c. do not attempt to clean ear unless ordered by physician
      5. do not pack dressing into area of CSF leakage (nose, ear, or wound) *because it will interfere with free flow of fluid*; place a sterile pad over area of CSF leakage to absorb drainage and change pad as soon as it becomes damp
      6. prepare client for surgical repair of the torn dura if leak does not heal spontaneously (the area usually heals without surgical intervention within 10–14 days)
    d. monitor for therapeutic and nontherapeutic effects of anti-infectives if administered prophylactically.

6. If signs and symptoms of meningitis occur:
    a. continue with above measures

b. initiate seizure precautions *(cerebral irritation can cause seizures)*
c. maintain activity restrictions as ordered
d. provide a quiet environment with dim lighting *to reduce discomfort associated with headache and photophobia*
e. monitor for therapeutic and nontherapeutic effects of the following medications if administered:
   1. anti-infectives
   2. corticosteroids *to reduce inflammation*
f. monitor for and report signs and symptoms of IICP (see action a.1 in this diagnosis)
g. provide emotional support to client and significant others.

3.c. The client will not experience seizure activity or associated injury.

3.c.1. Assess for and report signs and symptoms of seizure activity (e.g. twitching, clonic-tonic movements).
  2. Implement measures *to prevent seizures:*
    a. perform actions to prevent and treat IICP (see actions a.2 and 3 in this diagnosis)
    b. perform actions to prevent and treat meningitis (see actions b.5 and 6 in this diagnosis)
    c. monitor for therapeutic and nontherapeutic effects of anticonvulsants (e.g. phenytoin, phenobarbital, carbamazepine) if administered.
  3. Initiate and maintain seizure precautions:
    a. have plastic airway readily available
    b. pad side rails with blankets or soft pads
    c. keep bed in low position with side rails up when client is in bed.
  4. If seizures do occur:
    a. implement measures *to decrease risk of injury:*
      1. ease client to the floor if he/she is sitting in chair or ambulating at onset of seizure
      2. remain with and do not restrain client during seizure activity
      3. turn client on his/her side and insert an airway if possible during clonic phase *to prevent obstruction of airway by tongue or secretions*
      4. do not force any object between clenched teeth or try to pry mouth open
      5. remove from area items that may cause injury
      6. place towel or pillow under client's head
    b. observe for and report characteristics of seizures (e.g. progression, time elapsed)
    c. monitor for therapeutic and nontherapeutic effects of intravenous anticonvulsants (e.g. phenytoin, phenobarbital) if administered
    d. provide emotional support to client and significant others.

3.d. The client will not experience diabetes insipidus as evidenced by:
  1. absence of polyuria and polydipsia
  2. urine specific gravity between 1.010 and 1.030.

3.d.1. Assess for and report signs and symptoms of diabetes insipidus:
    a. polyuria (urine output can range from 4–10 or more liters/day)
    b. polydipsia (if the client is able to tolerate oral liquids, he/she may drink 4–10 or more liters of fluid/day)
    c. urine specific gravity less than 1.005.
  2. Monitor for therapeutic and nontherapeutic effects of corticosteroids if administered *to reduce inflammation of and around hypothalamus and pituitary gland.*
  3. If signs and symptoms of diabetes insipidus occur:
    a. maintain fluid intake equal to output *in order to prevent dehydration*
    b. monitor for therapeutic and nontherapeutic effects of the following medications if administered:
      1. ADH replacements (e.g. vasopressin, lypressin, desmopressin acetate [DDAVP])
      2. medications that enhance the action of available ADH (e.g. chlorpropamide, clofibrate, carbamazepine)
    c. assess closely for and report signs and symptoms of dehydration (e.g. decreased skin turgor, significant weight loss, dry mucous membranes, decreased B/P, increased pulse, elevated serum sodium and osmolality).

3.e. The client will not experience GI bleeding as evidenced by:

3.e.1. Assess for and report signs and symptoms of GI bleeding (e.g. complaints of epigastric discomfort or fullness, frank or occult blood in stool or gastric contents, decreased B/P, increased pulse).

UNIT
VI

1. no complaints of epigastric discomfort and fullness
2. absence of occult or frank blood in stool and gastric contents
3. B/P and pulse within normal range for client
4. gradual return of RBC, Hct., and Hgb. levels toward normal range.

2. Monitor RBC, Hct., and Hgb. levels. Report values that continue to decline or fail to improve.
3. Implement measures *to prevent ulceration of gastric or duodenal mucosa:*
   a. perform actions to decrease fear and anxiety (see Standardized Postoperative Care Plan, Nursing Diagnosis 1, action c)
   b. encourage client to reduce intake of foods/fluids that are acidic, spicy, or high in caffeine (e.g. chocolate, colas, coffee, tea)
   c. administer ulcerogenic medications (e.g. corticosteroids, phenytoin) with meals or snacks *to decrease gastric irritation*
   d. monitor for therapeutic and nontherapeutic effects of histamine$_2$ receptor antagonists (e.g. cimetidine, ranitidine, famotidine), antacids, and mucosal barrier fortifiers (e.g. sucralfate) if administered.
4. If signs and symptoms of GI bleeding occur:
   a. insert nasogastric tube and maintain suction as ordered
   b. assist with iced water or saline gastric lavage, transendoscopic electrocoagulation, selective arterial embolization, endoscopic laser photocoagulation, and/or intra-arterial administration of vasopressors (e.g. vasopressin) if ordered
   c. monitor for therapeutic and nontherapeutic effects of blood products and/or volume expanders if administered
   d. prepare client for surgery (e.g. ligation of bleeding vessels, partial gastrectomy) if indicated
   e. provide emotional support to client and significant others
   f. refer to Care Plan on Peptic Ulcer for additional care measures.

□ ▬▬▬▬▬▬▬▬▬▬▬▬▬▬▬▬▬▬▬▬▬

4. NURSING DIAGNOSIS

Disturbance in self concept* related to:

a. changes in appearance (e.g. periocular edema and ecchymosis, loss of scalp hair);
b. dependence on others to meet basic needs;
c. anticipated changes in life style and roles associated with alterations in motor and sensory function (e.g. hemiplegia, visual disturbances such as diplopia or visual field cut, speech impairment) and usual thought processes (changes may occur as a result of cerebral tissue injury).

---

* This diagnostic label includes the nursing diagnoses of body image disturbance and self-esteem disturbance.

□ ▬▬▬▬▬▬▬▬▬▬▬▬▬▬▬▬▬▬▬▬▬

DESIRED OUTCOMES	NURSING ACTIONS AND *SELECTED RATIONALES*
4. The client will demonstrate beginning adaptation to changes in appearance, physical and mental functioning, life style, and roles as evidenced by: a. verbalization of feelings of self-worth b. maintenance of	4.a. Determine the meaning of the changes in appearance, physical and mental functioning, life style, and roles to the client by encouraging him/her to verbalize feelings and by noting nonverbal responses to the changes experienced. b. Assess for signs and symptoms of a disturbance in self-concept (e.g. verbal or nonverbal cues denoting a negative response to changes in body functioning and appearance such as denial of or preoccupation with changes that have occurred, refusal to look in the mirror, or withdrawal from significant others).

relationships with significant others
c. active participation in activities of daily living
d. active interest in personal appearance
e. willingness to participate in social activities
f. verbalization of a beginning plan for adapting life style to meet changes resulting from the underlying disease process and/or residual effects of the surgery.

c. Be aware that the client may recognize and grieve the changes or losses experienced. Assist him/her through the stages of denial, anger, bargaining, and depression when appropriate.
d. Assist client to identify strengths and qualities that have a positive effect on self-concept.
e. Implement measures *to assist client to increase self-esteem* (e.g. limit negative self-criticism, encourage positive comments about self, give positive feedback about accomplishments).
f. Assist the client to identify and utilize coping techniques that have been helpful in the past.
g. Clarify misconceptions about changes in motor and sensory function and thought processes. If appropriate, assure client that these residual effects are usually temporary but caution him/her that recovery is slow (may take months to years). Offer hope of total recovery (depending on diagnosis and success of surgery) but do not predict exactly when or promise that it will occur.
h. If periocular edema and ecchymosis are present:
   1. reinforce that it is temporary and will begin to subside within 48–72 hours after surgery
   2. instruct client in and assist with measures *to reduce swelling* (e.g. cold compresses to affected area, lying on unoperative side, keeping head of bed elevated 20–30°).
i. Implement measures *to reduce client's embarrassment about partial or total loss of hair and misshapen skull if bone flap was removed* (e.g. provide client with a surgical cap or scarf if desired, assist client to obtain a wig when allowed). Reinforce the fact that the hair will grow back and, if indicated, a cranioplasty can be performed in a few months to restore original shape of the skull.
j. Assist client with usual grooming and makeup habits if necessary.
k. Discuss techniques the client can utilize *to adapt to alterations in thought processes if they have occurred:*
   1. encourage client to make lists and jot down messages and to refer to these rather than relying on his/her memory
   2. instruct the client to place self in a calm environment when making decisions
   3. encourage client to validate decisions, clarify information, and seek assistance to problem-solve if indicated
   4. encourage client to schedule adequate rest periods and reduce stressors *in order to decrease irritability.*
l. Demonstrate acceptance of client using techniques such as therapeutic touch and frequent visits. Encourage significant others to do the same.
m. Assess for and support behaviors suggesting positive adaptation to changes experienced (e.g. scanning environment or wearing eyepatch if visual disturbances are present, utilizing alternative methods of communicating if speech is impaired, utilizing adaptive devices to perform self-care activities).
n. Encourage significant others to allow client to do what he/she is able *so that independence can be re-established and/or self-esteem redeveloped.*
o. Encourage client contact with others *so that he/she can test and establish a new self-image.*
p. Assist client's and significant others' adjustment by listening, facilitating communication, and providing information.
q. Ensure that client and significant others have similar expectations and understanding of future life style.
r. Assist the client and significant others to identify ways that personal and family goals can be adjusted rather than abandoned.
s. Teach client the rationale for treatments and encourage maximum participation in treatment regimen *to enable him/her to maintain a sense of control over life.*
t. Encourage visits and support from significant others.
u. Encourage client to continue involvement in social activities and to pursue interests. If previous interests and hobbies cannot be pursued, encourage development of new ones.
v. Provide information about and encourage utilization of community agencies or support groups (e.g. head injury support groups; vocational

rehabilitation; American Cancer Society; family, individual, and/or financial counseling) if appropriate.

w. Consult physician about psychological counseling if client desires or if he/she seems unwilling or unable to adapt to changes resulting from the disease and the surgery.

5. NURSING DIAGNOSIS

Knowledge deficit regarding follow-up care.

DESIRED OUTCOMES	NURSING ACTIONS AND *SELECTED RATIONALES*
5.a. The client will identify ways to adapt to neurological deficits resulting from the underlying disease condition and/or the surgical procedure.	5.a.1. Instruct client in ways *to adapt to neurological deficits* resulting from the underlying disease condition and/or the surgical procedure:* a. wear an eyepatch or frosted lens if double vision is a problem b. utilize scanning techniques if visual field cut is present c. utilize pencil and paper, magic slate, computer, pictures, and pantomiming to express self if verbal communication is impaired d. write down messages and reminders and refer to written instructions repeatedly if experiencing difficulty concentrating or memory is impaired e. instruct client to request assistance when problem-solving and setting priorities and to seek validation of decisions if reasoning ability is impaired f. prepare meals that are visually appealing *to help stimulate appetite if sense of smell is lost* (anosmia sometimes occurs after surgery but is usually temporary) g. reduce alcohol intake (intolerance to usual amounts of alcohol may occur for a few months following the surgical cerebral trauma) h. utilize adaptive devices (e.g. wheelchair, cane, walker, broad-handled eating utensils, plate guard) if motor function is impaired i. plan daily activities to allow for adequate rest periods *in order to reduce the irritability that often occurs after cerebral tissue trauma.* 2. Allow time for questions, clarification, and return demonstration of techniques.
5.b. The client will state signs and symptoms to report to the health care provider.	5.b.1. Refer to Standardized Postoperative Care Plan, Nursing Diagnosis 20, action c, for signs and symptoms to report to the health care provider. 2. Instruct client to report these additional signs and symptoms: a. increasing drowsiness or difficulty awakening b. increased irritability and restlessness c. changes in behavior, increased difficulty remembering or concentrating, loss of emotional control d. decreased sensation in extremities e. new or increased weakness of extremities f. difficulty speaking or comprehending what others are saying g. changes in vision (e.g. double vision, blurred vision, visual field cuts) h. increase in size of one pupil i. dizziness, difficulty maintaining balance j. elevation of bone flap or bulging in area where bone flap has been removed

---

* Neurological deficits can range from a temporary increase in irritability or a slight facial droop to hemiplegia, aphasia, or confusion depending on the extensiveness and location of cerebral injury. Ways of adapting to a few of the more common deficits are included here. For more specific rehabilitative measures and a more extensive discussion of deficits, refer to textbooks on neurological and neurosurgical nursing and the Care Plan on Cerebrovascular Accident.

k. bloody or clear drainage from ears, nose, or incision
l. stiff neck
m. excessive thirst
n. severe or persistent headache
o. seizures.

5.c. The client will identify community resources that can assist with home management and adjustment to changes resulting from the diagnosis and/or the surgery.	5.c.1. Inform client and significant others of community resources that can assist with home management and adjustment to temporary or permanent neurological changes resulting from the diagnosis and/or surgery (e.g. physical, occupational, and speech therapists; Meals on Wheels; social services; home health agencies; Visiting Nurse Association; American Cancer Society; head injury support groups).
	2. Initiate a referral if indicated.
5.d. The client will verbalize an understanding of and a plan for adhering to recommended follow-up care including future appointments with health care provider, activity level, pain management, medications prescribed, and wound care.	5.d.1. Refer to Standardized Postoperative Care Plan, Nursing Diagnosis 20, for routine postoperative instructions and measures to improve client compliance.
	2. Instruct client in ways to reduce headache if present (e.g. reduce environmental lighting and noise whenever possible, avoid situations that increase stress, take analgesics as prescribed).
	3. Explain the rationale for, side effects of, schedule for taking, and importance of taking the prescribed medications (e.g. phenytoin, corticosteroids, anti-infectives).

Multiple Sclerosis

Multiple sclerosis (MS) is a disseminating, degenerative disease of the long fiber tracts of the white matter of the central nervous system. The exact etiology of the disease is unknown but it is believed that a virus or an abnormal immunological response may be the causative factor. The disease process involves the demyelinization of the nerve sheath with eventual formation of plaque or sclerotic tissue that causes the slowing or blocking of impulses along the nerve fibers. Signs and symptoms such as weakness, visual disturbances, mood changes, and sensory and motor impairment vary from person to person depending on the sites of the lesions, degree of myelin loss, and extent of plaque formation. There are two categories of MS. The most common is relapsing, remitting MS, which is characterized by periods of remission and exacerbation and has an unpredictable progression. It is believed that increases in signs and symptoms during an exacerbation are caused by inflammation of the sheath of previously affected and unaffected nerves. Treatment during an exacerbation usually consists of decreasing the client's activity and administering parenteral adrenocorticotropic hormone (ACTH) and corticosteroids for 7–14 days to reduce inflammation of and around the nerves. The signs and symptoms evident during exacerbation typically diminish or resolve during and following treatment. Rehabilitation may be indicated to assist the client to manage any residual impairments.

The other category of MS is characterized by a chronic progression of signs and symptoms that result in severe debilitation. There is no period of disease remission with this type. Treatment is primarily directed at helping the client and significant others adapt to the client's increasing impairments in motor, sensory, and mental functioning. Over the past few years, however, antineoplastic agents (particularly cyclophosphamide) have been administered in an effort to delay the disease progression. In some instances, this treatment has been effective for about one year and efforts are now directed toward identifying methods for extending that length of time. Unfortunately, not all persons with chronic progressive MS are candidates for this treatment because of the side effects of the medication therapy.

This care plan focuses on the adult client with relapsing, remitting MS who is hospitalized with exacerbation of the disease.* The goals of care are to prevent complications, provide emotional support, and educate the client in ways to maintain an optimal level of independence and decrease the risk of recurrent exacerbations.

---

* If the client has chronic progressive MS and is being admitted for treatment with an antineoplastic agent, use in conjunction with the Care Plan on Chemotherapy.

DISCHARGE CRITERIA

Prior to discharge, the client will:

- identify ways to maintain an optimal level of independence
- identify ways to decrease the risk of disease exacerbation
- identify ways to manage incontinence
- verbalize ways to manage and cope with fatigue
- identify appropriate safety measures
- state signs and symptoms to report to the health care provider
- share thoughts and feelings about multiple sclerosis and its effects on self-concept, life style, and roles
- identify community resources that can assist with home management and adjustment to changes in life style, body functioning, and roles
- verbalize an understanding of and a plan for adhering to recommended follow-up care including future appointments with health care provider and physical and occupational therapists and medications prescribed.

□ ▬▬▬▬▬▬▬▬▬▬▬▬▬▬▬▬▬▬▬▬▬▬▬▬▬▬▬▬▬▬▬▬▬▬▬▬▬

Use in conjunction with the Care Plan on Immobility.

□ ▬▬▬▬▬▬▬▬▬▬▬▬▬▬▬▬▬▬▬▬▬▬▬▬▬▬

NURSING DIAGNOSES

1. Anxiety □ *249*
2. Altered nutrition: less than body requirements □ *249*
3. Impaired swallowing □ *250*
4. Altered comfort:
   a. trigeminal neuralgia
   b. paresthesias (especially burning sensation) of the extremities
   c. low back pain □ *250*
5. Sensory-perceptual alteration: visual □ *251*
6. Impaired verbal communication □ *252*
7. Impaired skin integrity: irritation or breakdown □ *253*
8. Fatigue □ *254*
9. Impaired physical mobility □ *255*
10. Self-care deficit □ *256*
11. Altered patterns of urinary elimination:
    a. retention
    b. incontinence
    c. urgency and frequency □ *256*
12. Constipation □ *257*
13. Bowel incontinence □ *257*
14. Altered thought processes: impaired memory, decreased ability to problem-solve, and inappropriate emotional responses □ *258*
15. Potential for infection:
    a. pneumonia
    b. urinary tract infection □ *259*
16. Potential for trauma □ *259*
17. Potential for aspiration □ *260*

□

1. NURSING DIAGNOSIS

Anxiety related to unfamiliar environment; lack of understanding of the disease process, diagnostic tests, and treatments; uncertainty as to whether the intensified or new symptoms will persist following treatment; and anticipated effects of impairments on future life style and roles.

□

DESIRED OUTCOMES	NURSING ACTIONS AND *SELECTED RATIONALES*

1. The client will experience a reduction in fear and anxiety (see Care Plan on Immobility, Nursing Diagnosis 1, for outcome criteria).	1.a. Refer to Care Plan on Immobility, Nursing Diagnosis 1, for measures related to assessment and reduction of fear and anxiety.
	b. Implement additional measures *to reduce fear and anxiety:*
	  1. assure client that staff members are nearby; respond to call signal as soon as possible (provide a pressure-sensitive pad if client is unable to use traditional call signal because of upper extremity motor deficits)
	  2. explain all tests performed to confirm the diagnosis or determine extensiveness of the disease process (e.g. computed tomography; magnetic resonance imaging [MRI]; cerebral spinal fluid analysis; visual, somatosensory, and auditory evoked responses; EEG)
	  3. perform actions to assist the client to cope with the diagnosis and its implications (see Nursing Diagnosis 20, action d)
	  4. assure client that signs and symptoms resulting from the disease exacerbation should diminish with treatment.

□

2. NURSING DIAGNOSIS

Altered nutrition: less than body requirements related to decreased oral intake associated with:

a. anorexia resulting from fear, anxiety, pain, fatigue, depression, constipation, and decreased activity;

b. dysphagia resulting from cerebellar lesions;

c. difficulty feeding self as a result of tremors, weakness, spasticity, and impaired coordination resulting from cerebellar and corticospinal tract lesions.

□

UNIT
VI

DESIRED OUTCOMES	NURSING ACTIONS AND *SELECTED RATIONALES*
2. The client will maintain an adequate nutritional status (see Care Plan on Immobility, Nursing Diagnosis 6, for outcome criteria).	2.a. Refer to Care Plan on Immobility, Nursing Diagnosis 6, for measures related to assessment and maintenance of nutritional status. b. Implement additional measures *to improve oral intake and maintain an adequate nutritional status:* 1. perform actions to decrease fear and anxiety (see Nursing Diagnosis 1) 2. perform actions to reduce discomfort (see Nursing Diagnosis 4, action e) 3. perform actions to reduce fatigue (see Nursing Diagnosis 8, action b) 4. perform actions to improve ability to swallow (see Nursing Diagnosis 3, action b) 5. perform actions to enable client to feed self (see Nursing Diagnosis 10, action b.2).

3. NURSING DIAGNOSIS

Impaired swallowing related to ataxia, spasticity, and tremors of the muscles of swallowing associated with cerebellar lesions.

DESIRED OUTCOMES	NURSING ACTIONS AND *SELECTED RATIONALES*
3. The client will experience an improvement in swallowing as evidenced by: a. verbalization of same b. absence of coughing and choking when eating and drinking.	3.a. Assess for and report signs and symptoms of impaired swallowing (e.g. coughing or choking when eating and drinking, stasis of food in oral cavity). b. Implement measures *to improve ability to swallow:* 1. place client in high Fowler's position for meals and snacks; head should be erect with chin tilted forward *to facilitate elevation of the larynx and posterior movement of the tongue* 2. assist client to select foods that have a distinct texture and are easy to swallow (e.g. applesauce, custard, cottage cheese, ground meat) 3. avoid serving foods that are sticky (e.g. peanut butter, soft bread, bananas) 4. utilize adaptive devices (e.g. long-handled spoon, "pusher" spoon) to place food in back of mouth if tongue movement is impaired 5. moisten dry foods with gravy or sauces (e.g. catsup, salad dressing, sour cream) 6. encourage client to concentrate on the act of swallowing 7. gently stroke client's throat when he/she is swallowing if indicated 8. consult speech pathologist about methods for dealing with impaired swallowing; reinforce exercises and techniques prescribed 9. monitor for therapeutic and nontherapeutic effects of ACTH and/or corticosteroids if administered *to control signs and symptoms associated with exacerbation or disease progression.* c. Consult physician if swallowing difficulties persist or worsen.

4. NURSING DIAGNOSIS

Altered comfort:*

a. **trigeminal neuralgia** related to lesions of the sensory portion of the facial nerve;
b. **paresthesias (especially burning sensation) of the extremities** related to involvement of the sensory nerves;

---

* In this care plan, the nursing diagnosis "pain" is included under the diagnostic label of altered comfort.

c. **low back pain** related to:
1. decreased activity
2. abnormal posture and walking pattern and spasm associated with cerebellar and corticospinal tract lesions.

□ ▬▬▬▬▬▬▬▬▬▬▬▬▬▬▬▬▬▬▬▬

DESIRED OUTCOMES	**NURSING ACTIONS AND *SELECTED RATIONALES***

4. The client will experience diminished discomfort as evidenced by:
   a. verbalization of same
   b. relaxed facial expression and body positioning
   c. stable vital signs.

4.a. Determine how client usually responds to pain.
   b. Assess for nonverbal signs of discomfort (e.g. wrinkled brow; rubbing cheek, extremities, or lower back; clenched fists; reluctance to move; restlessness; diaphoresis; facial pallor or flushing; change in B/P; tachycardia).
   c. Assess verbal complaints of discomfort. Ask client to be specific about location, severity, and type of discomfort.
   d. Assess for factors that seem to aggravate and alleviate discomfort.
   e. Implement measures *to reduce discomfort*:
      1. perform actions *to reduce fear and anxiety about the discomfort* (e.g. assure client that actions will be taken to diminish discomfort, support hope that the discomfort will diminish following the period of disease exacerbation)
      2. perform actions *to reduce low back pain*:
         a. provide a firm mattress or place a bed board under mattress for added support
         b. instruct and assist client to maintain spine in proper alignment
         c. implement measures *to keep client from bending, twisting, and turning* (e.g. keep personal articles within easy reach, assist him/her to put on shoes or slippers)
         d. consult physician regarding an order for diathermy, massage, or ultrasonic heat treatment
         e. increase activity as allowed and tolerated
      3. instruct client to keep head and neck in good alignment *(forward flexion of the head can elicit Lhermitte's sign that results in transient electric-like shocks down the body)*
      4. provide or assist with nonpharmacological measures for relief of pain (e.g. back rub, position change, transcutaneous electrical nerve stimulation, guided imagery, biofeedback, quiet conversation, restful environment, diversional activities)
      5. monitor for therapeutic and nontherapeutic effects of the following medications if administered:
         a. ACTH and/or corticosteroids *to control signs and symptoms associated with exacerbation or disease progression*
         b. carbamazepine or phenytoin *to reduce facial pain and, in some instances, paresthesias*
         c. antidepressants *to alter the client's sensation of discomfort*
         d. muscle relaxants (e.g. baclofen, dantrolene) *to reduce spasm of the back muscles.*
   f. Consult physician if above measures fail to provide adequate relief of discomfort.
   g. Prepare client for nerve block or rhizotomy as ordered if severe pain persists following period of disease exacerbation.

□ ▬▬▬▬▬▬▬▬▬▬▬▬▬▬▬▬▬▬▬▬

5. NURSING DIAGNOSIS

Sensory-perceptual alteration: visual related to existing optic nerve lesions and/or inflammation of the optic nerve associated with exacerbation.

□ ▬▬▬▬▬▬▬▬▬▬▬▬▬▬▬▬▬▬▬▬

DESIRED OUTCOMES	NURSING ACTIONS AND *SELECTED RATIONALES*

5. The client will not experience further progression of visual disturbances.	5.a. Assess for visual disturbances (e.g. diplopia, blurred vision, dimmed vision, ophthalmoplegia, visual field cut).
	b. Monitor for therapeutic and nontherapeutic effects of ACTH and/or corticosteroids if administered *to control signs and symptoms associated with exacerbation or disease progression.*
	c. If vision is impaired:
	  1. provide an eyepatch or frosted lens for client to wear *in order to reduce diplopia if present*
	  2. remind client to turn head and "scan" environment *in order to compensate for visual field cut if present*
	  3. implement measures to prevent falls and cuts (see Nursing Diagnosis 16, actions b and d)
	  4. avoid startling client (e.g. speak client's name and identify yourself when entering room and before any physical contact, describe activities and reasons for various noises in the room)
	  5. assist client with personal hygiene he/she is unable to perform independently
	  6. identify where items are placed on the plate or tray, cut food, open packages, or feed client if necessary
	  7. assist with activities that require reading (e.g. menu selection, mail, legal documents)
	  8. provide auditory rather than visual diversionary activities.
	d. Consult physician if visual impairments worsen.

6. NURSING DIAGNOSIS

Impaired verbal communication related to ataxia, tremors, and spasticity of the muscles of speech associated with cerebellar lesions.

DESIRED OUTCOMES	NURSING ACTIONS AND *SELECTED RATIONALES*

6. The client will communicate needs and desires effectively.	6.a. Assess for difficulties in verbal communication (e.g. slow, scanning speech pattern; difficulty with articulation).
	b. Monitor for therapeutic and nontherapeutic effects of ACTH and/or corticosteroids if administered *to control signs and symptoms associated with exacerbation or disease progression.*
	c. Implement measures *to facilitate communication:*
	  1. maintain a patient, calm approach; listen carefully, avoid interrupting client, and allow ample time for communication
	  2. maintain a quiet environment *so that client does not have to raise voice to be heard*
	  3. ask questions that require short answers or nod of head
	  4. provide materials necessary for communication (e.g. magic slate, pad and pencil, flash cards)
	  5. ensure that intravenous therapy does not interfere with the client's ability to write

6. answer call signal in person rather than using the intercommunication system
7. make frequent rounds *to ascertain client's needs*
8. if client is frustrated or fatigued, try to anticipate needs *in order to minimize the necessity of verbal communication*
9. consult speech pathologist regarding methods for dealing with speech impairments; reinforce exercises and techniques prescribed
10. monitor for therapeutic and nontherapeutic effects of muscle relaxants (e.g. baclofen, dantrolene) if administered *to reduce muscle spasm.*

d. Inform significant others and health care personnel of approaches being used to maximize client's ability to communicate.

e. Consult physician if client experiences increasing impairment of verbal communication.

7. NURSING DIAGNOSIS

Impaired skin integrity: irritation or breakdown related to:

a. prolonged or uneven pressure on tissues associated with decreased mobility and use of splints or braces;
b. frequent contact with irritants associated with urinary and bowel incontinence.

DESIRED OUTCOMES	NURSING ACTIONS AND *SELECTED RATIONALES*

7. The client will maintain skin integrity as evidenced by:
a. absence of redness and irritation
b. no skin breakdown.
	7.a. Inspect the skin (especially bone prominences, dependent areas, skin under braces or splints, and perineum) for pallor, redness, and breakdown.
	b. Refer to Care Plan on Immobility, Nursing Diagnosis 7, action b, for measures to prevent skin breakdown associated with decreased mobility.
	c. Implement measures *to decrease skin irritation and prevent breakdown resulting from incontinence:*
	  1. perform actions to reduce episodes of urinary and bowel incontinence (see Nursing Diagnoses 11, action b.2 and 13, action b)
	  2. assist client to thoroughly cleanse and dry perineal area after each episode of incontinence; apply a protective ointment or cream (e.g. Sween cream, Desitin, A & D ointment, Vaseline)
	  3. use soft tissue to cleanse perianal area
	  4. apply a perianal pouch if bowel incontinence is a persistent problem
	  5. avoid direct contact of skin with Chux (e.g. place turn sheet or bed pad over Chux).
	d. Implement measures *to prevent skin irritation and breakdown resulting from prolonged or uneven pressure from splints or braces:*
	  1. instruct and assist client to apply the braces or splints correctly
	  2. provide additional padding over bone prominences if indicated
	  3. keep skin under braces or splints clean and dry
	  4. consult physician or orthotist regarding readjustment of braces or splints if skin is reddened or client complains of discomfort.
	e. If skin breakdown occurs:
	  1. notify physician
	  2. continue with above measures to prevent further irritation and breakdown
	  3. perform decubitus care as ordered or per standard hospital policy
	  4. monitor client closely and report signs and symptoms of infection (e.g. elevated temperature; redness, warmth, and edema around area of breakdown; unusual drainage from site).

□ ▬▬▬▬▬▬▬▬▬▬▬▬▬▬▬▬▬▬▬▬

8. NURSING DIAGNOSIS

Fatigue related to:

a. increased energy expenditure associated with spasticity and tremors;
b. increased psychological stress associated with new and/or intensified signs and symptoms and anticipated effects of residual impairments on usual life style and roles;
c. altered neurotransmission associated with MS;
d. difficulty resting and sleeping associated with fear, anxiety, and discomfort.

□ ▬▬▬▬▬▬▬▬▬▬▬▬▬▬▬▬▬▬▬▬

DESIRED OUTCOMES	NURSING ACTIONS AND *SELECTED RATIONALES*

8. The client will experience a reduction in fatigue as evidenced by:
a. verbalization of feelings of increased energy
b. increased interest in surroundings and ability to concentrate
c. decreased emotional lability.
	8.a. Assess for signs and symptoms of fatigue (e.g. verbalization of continuous, overwhelming lack of energy; lack of interest in surroundings; decreased ability to concentrate; increased emotional lability).
	b. Implement measures *to reduce fatigue:*
	  1. perform actions *to promote rest:*
	    a. maintain activity restrictions as ordered
	    b. minimize environmental activity and noise
	    c. schedule nursing care and diagnostic procedures to allow periods of uninterrupted rest
	    d. limit the number of visitors and their length of stay
	    e. assist client with self-care activities as needed
	    f. keep supplies and personal articles within easy reach
	    g. implement measures to reduce fear and anxiety (see Nursing Diagnosis 1)
	    h. implement measures to promote sleep (see Care Plan on Immobility, Nursing Diagnosis 12, action c)
	    i. implement measures to facilitate client's psychological adjustment to the effects of MS (see Nursing Diagnoses 19; 20, action d; 21; and 22, action d)
	    j. implement measures to reduce spasticity and tremors (see Nursing Diagnosis 9, action a.2.h)
	  2. instruct client in energy-saving techniques (e.g. using shower chair when showering, sitting to brush teeth or comb hair)
	  3. keep room temperature below 75°F and instruct client to avoid using hot water for showers and baths *(increased body temperature increases metabolic rate and reduces transmission of impulses along affected nerves)*
	  4. perform actions to maintain an adequate nutritional status (see Nursing Diagnosis 2)
	  5. monitor for therapeutic and nontherapeutic effects of the following medications if administered:
	    a. ACTH and/or corticosteroids *to control symptoms associated with exacerbation or disease progression*
	    b. amantadine hydrochloride (Symmetrel), *which increases neurotransmission in the central nervous system and has been found to reduce fatigue in some clients with MS*
	  6. increase client's activity gradually as allowed and tolerated.
	c. Consult physician if signs and symptoms of fatigue persist or worsen.

□ ▉▉▉▉▉▉▉▉▉▉▉▉▉▉▉▉▉▉▉▉▉▉▉▉▉▉▉▉

9. NURSING DIAGNOSIS

Impaired physical mobility related to:

a. unsteady gait, tremors, weakness, spasticity, and impaired coordination associated with cerebellar and corticospinal tract lesions;
b. prescribed activity restrictions during the period of exacerbation;
c. fatigue and discomfort;
d. reluctance to move associated with fear of injury.

□ ▉▉▉▉▉▉▉▉▉▉▉▉▉▉▉▉▉▉▉▉▉▉▉▉▉▉▉▉

DESIRED OUTCOMES	NURSING ACTIONS AND *SELECTED RATIONALES*

9.a. The client will achieve maximum physical mobility within limitations imposed by the disease process and treatment plan.	9.a.1. Assess for factors that impair physical mobility (e.g. impaired coordination, unsteady gait, tremors, spasticity, fatigue, pain, reluctance to move because of fear of injury).
	2. Implement measures *to increase mobility:*
	  a. monitor for therapeutic and nontherapeutic effects of ACTH and/or corticosteroids if administered *to control signs and symptoms associated with exacerbation or disease progression*
	  b. perform actions to reduce discomfort (see Nursing Diagnosis 4, action e)
	  c. perform actions to reduce fatigue (see Nursing Diagnosis 8, action b)
	  d. perform actions to prevent falls (see Nursing Diagnosis 16, action b) *in order to decrease client's fear of injury*
	  e. reinforce instructions, activities, and exercise plan recommended by physical and/or occupational therapists
	  f. instruct client in and assist with correct use of mobility aids (e.g. cane, braces, splints, walker, crutches) if appropriate
	  g. instruct client in and assist with range of motion exercises at least 4 times/day
	  h. perform actions *to reduce or control spasticity and tremors:*
	    1. implement measures to reduce fear and anxiety (see Nursing Diagnosis 1) and promote client's psychological adjustment to the effects of MS (see Nursing Diagnoses 19; 20, action d; 21; and 22, action d) *in order to reduce stress (tremors have been noted to increase during periods of stress)*
	    2. provide or assist with nonpharmacological measures of reducing spasticity (e.g. massage, biofeedback, stretching exercises, water exercises if pool is available, warm bath or whirlpool)
	    3. encourage client to utilize patterning *(this technique of tracing and repeating basic movement patterns may help reduce tremors)*
	    4. apply braces and splints as ordered to immobilize joints *(this limits random movement, which in turn helps control tremors and spasms)*
	    5. assist client with the application of weights to feet and/or ankles or to walker or cane *(the weights increase stability, which in turn reduces tremor)*
	    6. place client in prone position as tolerated *to decrease flexor spasms*
	    7. monitor for therapeutic and nontherapeutic effects of skeletal muscle relaxants (e.g. baclofen, dantrolene) if administered
	    8. prepare client for:
	      a. neurectomy, rhizotomy, or cordotomy if indicated *to treat unmanageable spasticity*
	      b. thalamotomy if indicated *to treat unmanageable tremors.*
	3. Increase activity and participation in self-care activities as allowed and tolerated.

4. Provide praise and encouragement for all efforts to increase physical mobility when allowed.
5. Encourage the support of significant others. Allow them to assist with range of motion exercises, positioning, and activity if desired.

| 9.b. The client will not experience problems associated with immobility. | 9.b. Refer to Care Plan on Immobility for actions to prevent problems associated with immobility. |

☐ ████████████████████████████████████

10. NURSING DIAGNOSIS

Self-care deficit related to impaired physical mobility and visual impairments.

☐ ████████████████████████████████████

DESIRED OUTCOMES	NURSING ACTIONS AND *SELECTED RATIONALES*

10. The client will perform self-care activities within physical limitations imposed by the disease process and treatment plan.	10.a. Refer to Care Plan on Immobility, Nursing Diagnosis 9, for measures related to assessment of, planning for, and meeting the client's self-care needs.
	b. Implement additional measures *to facilitate the client's ability to perform self-care activities:*
	1. perform actions to increase mobility (see Nursing Diagnosis 9, action a.2)
	2. perform actions *to enable client to feed self:*
	  a. reinforce use of adaptive devices (e.g. broad-handled utensils, hand braces) if indicated
	  b. provide client with weighted eating utensils or apply weight to hands or wrists if tremors are present
	  c. open containers, butter bread, and cut meat for client if necessary
	3. if vision is impaired, identify where all needed objects are located.

☐ ████████████████████████████████████

11. NURSING DIAGNOSIS

Altered patterns of urinary elimination:

a. **retention** related to hypotonic bladder associated with interruption of afferent pathways from bladder;
b. **incontinence** related to poor sphincter control and reduced bladder capacity associated with spastic bladder (resulting from lesions of efferent pathways of the corticospinal tract);
c. **urgency and frequency** related to spastic bladder associated with lesions of efferent pathways of the corticospinal tract.

☐ ████████████████████████████████████

DESIRED OUTCOMES	NURSING ACTIONS AND *SELECTED RATIONALES*
11.a. The client will not experience urinary retention (see Care Plan on Immobility, Nursing Diagnosis 10, for outcome criteria).	11.a.1. Refer to Care Plan on Immobility, Nursing Diagnosis 10, for measures related to assessment, prevention, and management of urinary retention. 2. Assist with urodynamic studies (e.g. cystometrogram) if ordered. 3. Instruct and encourage client to perform urethral stimulation if indicated *in order to initiate voiding.*

11.b. The client will experience urinary continence.

11.b.1. Monitor for urinary incontinence.
    2. Implement measures *to maintain urinary continence:*
      a. offer bedpan or urinal or assist client to commode or bathroom every 2–3 hours
      b. allow client to assume a normal position for voiding unless contraindicated *in order to promote complete bladder emptying*
      c. instruct client to perform perineal exercises (e.g. stopping and starting stream during voiding; pressing buttocks together, then relaxing the muscles) *in order to improve urinary sphincter tone*
      d. limit oral fluid intake in the evening *to decrease possibility of nighttime incontinence*
      e. instruct client to avoid drinking caffeinated beverages such as colas, coffee, and tea *(caffeine is a mild diuretic and may make urinary control more difficult)*
      f. monitor for therapeutic and nontherapeutic effects of the following medications if administered:
        1. alpha-adrenergic agonists (e.g. ephedrine) *to increase urinary sphincter tone*
        2. antispasmodics (e.g. ditropan, propantheline bromide) *to reduce bladder spasm.*
    3. If urinary incontinence persists:
      a. consult physician about intermittent catheterization, insertion of indwelling catheter, or use of external catheter or penile clamp
      b. provide emotional support to client and significant others.

11.c. The client will experience decreased urgency and frequency as evidenced by:
1. statements of decreased urgency
2. decrease in the number of times he/she urinates.

11.c.1. Assess for signs and symptoms of urgency and frequency (e.g. statements of needing to urinate immediately, increase in number of times client urinates).
    2. If client is experiencing urgency and frequency:
      a. monitor for therapeutic and nontherapeutic effects of antispasmodics (e.g. ditropan, propantheline bromide) if administered *to reduce bladder spasm and resultant symptoms of urgency and frequency*
      b. have bedpan or commode readily available to client
      c. consult physician if signs and symptoms of urgency and frequency persist or worsen.

□ ▬▬▬▬▬▬▬▬▬▬▬▬▬▬▬▬▬▬▬▬

12. NURSING DIAGNOSIS

Constipation related to decreased activity and decreased intake of fluid and foods high in fiber associated with dysphagia, anorexia, and difficulty feeding self.

□ ▬▬▬▬▬▬▬▬▬▬▬▬▬▬▬▬▬▬▬▬

DESIRED OUTCOMES	NURSING ACTIONS AND *SELECTED RATIONALES*
12. The client will maintain usual bowel elimination pattern.	12. Refer to Care Plan on Immobility, Nursing Diagnosis 11, for measures related to assessment, prevention, and management of constipation.

□ ▬▬▬▬▬▬▬▬▬▬▬▬▬▬▬▬▬▬▬▬

13. NURSING DIAGNOSIS

Bowel incontinence related to loss of sphincter control associated with lesions of efferent pathways of the corticospinal tract.

□ ▬▬▬▬▬▬▬▬▬▬▬▬▬▬▬▬▬▬▬▬

UNIT VI

DESIRED OUTCOMES	NURSING ACTIONS AND *SELECTED RATIONALES*

13. The client will maintain bowel control as evidenced by absence of episodes of incontinence.

13.a. Monitor for bowel incontinence.
  b. Implement measures *to reduce the risk of bowel incontinence:*
    1. instruct client to perform perineal exercises (e.g. relaxing and tightening perineal and gluteal muscles) *in order to strengthen anal sphincter*
    2. have commode or bedpan readily available to client
    3. initiate a bowel training program if appropriate.
  c. If bowel incontinence occurs:
    1. provide client with disposable liners for underwear or disposable undergarments such as Attends
    2. review and revise bowel training program
    3. provide emotional support to client and significant others.

□ ▬▬▬▬▬▬▬▬▬▬▬▬▬▬▬▬▬▬▬▬▬▬▬▬▬▬▬▬▬▬

14. NURSING DIAGNOSIS

Altered thought processes: impaired memory, decreased ability to problem-solve, and inappropriate emotional responses related to cerebral lesions and fatigue.

□ ▬▬▬▬▬▬▬▬▬▬▬▬▬▬▬▬▬▬▬▬▬▬▬▬▬▬▬▬▬▬

DESIRED OUTCOMES	NURSING ACTIONS AND *SELECTED RATIONALES*

14. The client will adapt to temporary or permanent alterations in thought processes as evidenced by:
  a. utilization of techniques to aid memory
  b. usual or improved problem-solving abilities
  c. decrease in episodes of inappropriate responses.

14.a. Assess client for alterations in thought processes (e.g. impaired memory, decreased ability to problem-solve, emotional lability).
  b. Ascertain from significant others client's usual intellectual and emotional functioning.
  c. Implement measures *to reduce alterations in thought processes:*
    1. perform actions to reduce fatigue (see Nursing Diagnosis 8, action b)
    2. monitor for therapeutic and nontherapeutic effects of ACTH and/or corticosteroids if administered *to control symptoms associated with exacerbation or disease progression.*
  d. If client shows evidence of altered thought processes:
    1. implement measures *to assist client to adapt to impaired memory:*
      a. encourage client to write down questions or concerns he/she may have
      b. provide written or taped instructions/information whenever possible for client to review as often as necessary
    2. implement measures *to assist client to adapt to impaired reasoning ability:*
      a. keep environmental stimuli to a minimum during treatments, conversations, and teaching sessions
      b. allow adequate time for teaching sessions and clarification of information
      c. encourage client to validate decisions
      d. assist client to problem-solve as necessary
    3. implement measures *to stop inappropriate, spontaneous laughing or crying when it occurs:*
      a. if client is crying inappropriately, instruct him/her to hold mouth open
      b. provide distraction (e.g. clap hands, whistle loudly)
    4. maintain realistic expectations of client's ability to learn, comprehend, and remember information provided
    5. monitor for therapeutic and nontherapeutic effects of antidepressants and antipsychotic medications if administered *to assist in managing emotional lability and controlling behavior*

6. encourage significant others to be supportive of client; instruct them in methods of dealing with the alterations in thought processes
7. discuss physiological basis for alterations in thought processes with client and significant others; inform them that these changes may improve during treatment and following the period of disease exacerbation
8. consult physician if client demonstrates increased alterations in thought processes or is unable to adapt to existing ones.

15. NURSING DIAGNOSIS

Potential for infection:

a. **pneumonia** related to:
   1. aspiration associated with difficulty swallowing
   2. decreased resistance to infection during administration of ACTH and/or corticosteroids
   3. stasis of secretions in the lungs associated with poor cough effort and decreased mobility;
b. **urinary tract infection** related to urinary stasis, indwelling catheter if present, and decreased resistance to infection during administration of ACTH and/or corticosteroids.

DESIRED OUTCOMES	NURSING ACTIONS AND *SELECTED RATIONALES*
15.a. The client will not develop pneumonia (see Care Plan on Immobility, Nursing Diagnosis 13, outcome a, for outcome criteria).	15.a.1. Refer to Care Plan on Immobility, Nursing Diagnosis 13, action a, for measures related to assessment, prevention, and treatment of pneumonia. 2. Implement measures to prevent aspiration (see Nursing Diagnosis 17, action d) *in order to further reduce the risk of pneumonia.*
15.b. The client will remain free of urinary tract infection (see Care Plan on Immobility, Nursing Diagnosis 13, outcome b, for outcome criteria).	15.b. Refer to Care Plan on Immobility, Nursing Diagnosis 13, action b, for measures related to assessment, prevention, and treatment of urinary tract infection.

16. NURSING DIAGNOSIS

Potential for trauma related to:

a. falls associated with weakness; muscle spasms; unsteady gait; tremors; paresthesias; and impaired proprioception, coordination, and vision;
b. burns associated with paresthesias, impaired motor function and vision, and altered thought processes;
c. cuts associated with tremors, muscle spasms, and impaired coordination and vision.

DESIRED OUTCOMES	NURSING ACTIONS AND *SELECTED RATIONALES*

16. The client will not experience falls, burns, or cuts.

16.a. Determine whether conditions predisposing client to falls, burns, or cuts (e.g. weakness, gait disturbances, muscle spasms, tremors, visual disturbances, altered thought processes, paresthesias) exist.
  b. Implement measures *to prevent falls:*
    1. keep bed in low position with side rails up when client is in bed
    2. keep needed items within easy reach
    3. encourage client to request assistance whenever needed; have call signal within easy reach
    4. use lap belt when client is in chair if indicated
    5. instruct client to wear shoes with nonskid soles and low heels when ambulating
    6. avoid unnecessary clutter in room
    7. accompany client during ambulation utilizing a transfer safety belt
    8. instruct client to concentrate on body balance and movement when ambulating
    9. provide ambulatory aids (e.g. walker, cane) if the client is weak or unsteady on feet
    10. assist with application of braces and splints as ordered *to provide additional support to the extremities*
    11. reinforce instructions from physical therapist regarding correct transfer and ambulation techniques
    12. instruct client to ambulate in well-lit areas and to utilize handrails if needed
    13. do not rush client; allow adequate time for trips to the bathroom and ambulation in hallway
    14. if vision is impaired:
      a. orient to surroundings, room, and arrangement of furniture
      b. assist client with ambulation by walking a half step ahead of client and describing approaching objects or obstacles; instruct client to grasp back of nurse's arm during ambulation
    15. perform actions to reduce or control spasticity and tremors (see Nursing Diagnosis 9, action a.2.h)
    16. encourage client to rest before ambulation
    17. increase activity gradually.
  c. Implement measures *to prevent burns:*
    1. let hot foods or fluids cool slightly before serving *to reduce the risk of burns if spills occur*
    2. supervise client while smoking if indicated
    3. assess temperature of bath water and heating pad before and during use.
  d. Assist client with tasks that require fine motor skills (e.g. shaving) *in order to prevent cuts.*
  e. Include client and significant others in planning and implementing measures to prevent injury.
  f. If injury does occur, initiate appropriate first aid measures and notify physician.

17. NURSING DIAGNOSIS

Potential for aspiration related to impaired swallowing.

DESIRED OUTCOMES	NURSING ACTIONS AND *SELECTED RATIONALES*

17. The client will not aspirate secretions and foods/fluids as evidenced by:
   a. clear breath sounds
   b. resonant percussion note over lungs
   c. respiratory rate at 16–20/minute
   d. absence of dyspnea
   e. absence of cyanosis.

17.a. Assess for factors that indicate potential for aspiration (e.g. difficulty swallowing, choking on secretions and foods/fluids).
   b. Assess for signs and symptoms of aspiration of secretions or foods/fluids (e.g. rhonchi, dull percussion note over lungs, tachycardia, rapid respirations, dyspnea, cyanosis).
   c. Monitor chest x-ray results. Report findings of pulmonary infiltrate.
   d. Implement measures *to reduce the risk of aspiration:*
      1. position client in side-lying or semi- to high Fowler's position at all times
      2. have suction equipment readily available for use
      3. perform oropharyngeal suctioning, encourage client to use tonsil-tip suction, and provide oral care as often as needed *to remove oral secretions*
      4. withhold foods/fluids if client is experiencing severe dysphagia
      5. if oral intake is allowed:
         a. perform actions to improve ability to swallow (see Nursing Diagnosis 3, action b)
         b. decrease environmental stimuli during meals and snacks *so client can concentrate on chewing and swallowing*
         c. provide small, frequent meals rather than 3 large ones *to decrease risk of gastric distention and regurgitation*
         d. allow ample time for meals
         e. instruct client to avoid laughing or talking while eating and drinking
         f. maintain client in high Fowler's position during and for at least 30 minutes after meals and snacks
         g. assist client with oral hygiene after eating *to ensure that food particles do not remain in mouth.*
   e. If signs and symptoms of aspiration occur:
      1. perform tracheal suctioning
      2. notify physician
      3. prepare client for chest x-ray.

□ ▬▬▬▬▬▬▬▬▬▬▬▬▬▬▬▬▬▬▬▬▬▬▬▬▬

18. NURSING DIAGNOSIS

Sexual dysfunction:

a. **decreased libido** related to weakness; fatigue; fear of rejection by desired partner, urinary or bowel incontinence, and spasms of hips and legs; diminished sensation in genital area; and altered self-concept;
b. **impotence** related to lesions of the spinal cord.

□ ▬▬▬▬▬▬▬▬▬▬▬▬▬▬▬▬▬▬▬▬▬▬▬▬▬

DESIRED OUTCOMES	NURSING ACTIONS AND *SELECTED RATIONALES*

18. The client will demonstrate beginning acceptance of changes in sexual functioning as evidenced by:
   a. verbalization of a perception of self as sexually acceptable and adequate
   b. maintenance of relationships with significant others.

18.a. Refer to Care Plan on Immobility, Nursing Diagnosis 15, for measures related to assessment and management of sexual dysfunction.
   b. Implement additional measures *to promote optimal sexual functioning:*
      1. perform actions to improve self-concept (see Nursing Diagnosis 19)
      2. perform actions *to decrease the possibility of rejection by partner:*
         a. assist the partner to acknowledge both positive and negative feelings
         b. if appropriate, involve partner in care (e.g. bathing, dressing, exercising) *to facilitate adjustment to and integration of the change in client's body image*
      3. reinforce the importance of rest before and after sexual activity

3. reinforce the importance of rest before and after sexual activity
4. if incontinence of urine or stool is a problem:
    a. reinforce adherence to bowel and bladder training programs *to decrease risk of incontinence*
    b. encourage client to void and/or defecate just before intercourse or other sexual activity
5. reinforce the use of skeletal muscle relaxants routinely or before sexual activity if indicated *to control hip and leg spasms*
6. provide information about penile prosthesis if appropriate
7. discuss alternative methods of becoming a parent (e.g. adoption, artificial insemination) if of concern to client.

---

19. NURSING DIAGNOSIS

Disturbance in self-concept* related to motor and sensory deficits; incontinence; dependence on others to meet self-care needs; feeling of powerlessness; alterations in sexual functioning, life style, and roles; and altered thought processes.

---

* This diagnostic label includes the nursing diagnoses of body image disturbance and self-esteem disturbance.

DESIRED OUTCOMES	NURSING ACTIONS AND *SELECTED RATIONALES*

19. The client will demonstrate beginning adaptation to changes in physical and mental functioning, life style, roles, and level of independence (see Care Plan on Immobility, Nursing Diagnosis 16, for outcome criteria).	19.a. Refer to Care Plan on Immobility, Nursing Diagnosis 16, for measures related to assessment and promotion of a positive self-concept.
	 b. Implement additional measures *to assist client to adapt to changes in body functioning, level of independence, life style, and roles:*
	 1. reinforce actions to assist client to cope with effects of MS (see Nursing Diagnosis 20, action d)
	 2. reinforce actions to promote optimal sexual functioning (see Nursing Diagnosis 18)
	 3. discuss techniques the client can utilize *to adapt to alterations in thought processes:*
	   a. make lists, jot down messages, and refer to these notes rather than relying on his/her memory
	   b. place self in a calm environment when making decisions and problem-solving
	   c. validate decisions, clarify information, and seek assistance to problem-solve if indicated
	 4. perform actions to maintain continence of urine and stool (see Nursing Diagnoses 11, action b.2 and 13, action b)
	 5. reinforce the use of an external catheter, penile clamp, waterproof liners for underwear, or absorbent undergarments (e.g. Attends) if incontinence is not well controlled by prescribed measures
	 6. reinforce methods of adapting to visual impairments (e.g. scan environment, wear frosted lens or eyepatch)
	 7. reinforce use of mobility aids (e.g. walker, braces, cane) and adaptive devices (e.g. weighted eating utensils) *to increase independence.*

20. NURSING DIAGNOSIS

Ineffective individual coping related to:

a. fear, anxiety, discomfort, and fatigue;
b. lack of control over the disease process;
c. inability to predict pattern of disease progression;
d. changes in usual body functioning, thought processes, life style, and roles;
e. inadequate support system.

DESIRED OUTCOMES	NURSING ACTIONS AND *SELECTED RATIONALES*

20. The client will demonstrate the use of effective coping skills as evidenced by:
a. willingness to participate in treatment plan and self-care activities
b. verbalization of ability to cope with the effects of MS
c. identification of stressors
d. utilization of appropriate problem-solving techniques
e. recognition and utilization of available support systems.
	20.a. Assess effectiveness of client's coping strategies by observing behavior and noting strengths, weaknesses, ability to express feelings and concerns, and willingness to participate in the treatment plan.
	b. Assess for and report signs and symptoms that may indicate ineffective coping (e.g. sleep disturbances, increasing fatigue, increased difficulty concentrating, irritability, verbalization of inability to cope, inability to problem-solve).
	c. Allow time for client to adjust psychologically to the diagnosis and planned treatment, residual effects of MS, and anticipated life-style and role changes.
	d. Implement measures *to promote effective coping:*
	  1. perform actions to reduce fear and anxiety (see Nursing Diagnosis 1)
	  2. perform actions to reduce discomfort (see Nursing Diagnosis 4, action e)
	  3. perform actions to reduce fatigue (see Nursing Diagnosis 8, action b)
	  4. arrange for a visit with another who has successfully adjusted to diagnosis and effects of MS
	  5. teach client the rationale for treatments, encourage maximum participation in treatment regimen, and allow choices whenever possible *to enable him/her to maintain a sense of control over life;* stress that exacerbation or disease progression is not necessarily reflective of client's failure to adhere to treatment program
	  6. instruct client in effective problem-solving techniques (e.g. accurate identification of stressors, determination of various options to solve problem)
	  7. assist client through methods such as role playing to prepare for negative reactions from others because of neurological impairments
	  8. if client is incontinent, instruct in ways to minimize the problem *so that socialization with others is possible* (e.g. placing liners in underwear, wearing absorbent undergarments such as Attends)
	  9. assist client to maintain usual daily routines whenever possible
	  10. provide diversional activities according to client's interests and abilities
	  11. assist client as he/she starts to plan for necessary life-style and role changes; provide input on realistic prioritization of problems that need to be dealt with
	  12. set up a home evaluation appointment with occupational and physical therapists *so that changes in home environment (e.g. installation of ramps and handrails, widening doorways, altering kitchen facilities) can be completed before client's discharge*
	  13. assist the client and significant others to identify ways that personal and family goals can be adjusted rather than abandoned
	  14. inform client that he/she will have days when impairments worsen; assure client that this may be temporary and the result of physical and/or emotional stress or fatigue rather than an indication of deteriorating neurological status

15. assist client to identify and utilize available support systems; provide information regarding available community resources that can assist client and significant others in coping with effects of MS (e.g. Multiple Sclerosis Society; vocational rehabilitation; sexual, family, individual and/or financial counseling).

e. Encourage continued emotional support from significant others.

f. Encourage the client to share with significant others the kind of support that would be most beneficial (e.g. listening, inspiring hope, providing reassurance and accurate information).

g. Assess for and support behaviors suggesting positive adaptation to changes experienced (e.g. participation in treatment plan and self-care activities, communication of the ability to cope).

h. Consult physician about psychological or vocational rehabilitation counseling if appropriate. Initiate a referral if necessary.

21. NURSING DIAGNOSIS

Powerlessness related to:

a. physical limitations, impaired verbal communication, and sensory-perceptual impairments;
b. dependence on others to meet basic needs;
c. feeling of loss of control over life;
d. alterations in usual roles, relationships, and future plans associated with residual impairments.

DESIRED OUTCOMES	NURSING ACTIONS AND *SELECTED RATIONALES*
21. The client will demonstrate increasing feelings of control over his/her situation (see Care Plan on Immobility, Nursing Diagnosis 17, for outcome criteria).	21.a. Refer to Care Plan on Immobility, Nursing Diagnosis 17, for measures related to assessment of feelings of powerlessness and measures to promote client's feeling of control over his/her situation.

b. Implement additional measures *to reduce client's feeling of powerlessness:*
1. perform actions to facilitate communication (see Nursing Diagnosis 6, action c) *in order to enable client to interact meaningfully with others*
2. perform actions to promote effective coping (see Nursing Diagnosis 20, action d) *in order to promote an increased sense of control over his/her situation*
3. support realistic hope about the effects of medication therapy, physical and occupational therapy programs, and use of adaptive devices on future independence
4. discuss with significant others the client's need to maintain as much control over his/her life as possible; stress the necessity of their encouraging and allowing the client to actively participate in physical and occupational therapy program scheduling and discharge planning.

22. NURSING DIAGNOSIS

Grieving* related to existing and anticipated loss of physical and mental functioning.

---

* This diagnostic label includes anticipatory grieving and grieving following the actual losses/changes.

DESIRED OUTCOMES	**NURSING ACTIONS AND *SELECTED RATIONALES***

22. The client will demonstrate beginning progression through the grieving process as evidenced by:
   a. verbalization of feelings about the effects of MS on his/her life
   b. expression of grief
   c. participation in treatment plan and self-care activities
   d. utilization of available support systems
   e. verbalization of a plan for integrating prescribed follow-up care into life style.

22.a. Determine the client's perception of the impact of MS on his/her future.
   b. Determine how the client usually expresses grief.
   c. Observe for signs of grieving (e.g. changes in eating habits, insomnia, anger, noncompliance, denial).
   d. Implement measures *to facilitate the grieving process:*
      1. assist client to acknowledge losses and changes experienced *so grief work can begin*; assess for factors that may hinder or facilitate acknowledgment
      2. discuss the grieving process and assist client to accept the stages of grieving as an expected response to actual and/or anticipated changes or losses; support the realization that grief may recur *because of the relapsing, degenerative nature of the disease*
      3. allow time for client to progress through the stages of grieving (denial, anger, bargaining, depression, acceptance [Kübler-Ross, 1969]); be aware that not every stage is experienced or expressed by all individuals
      4. provide an atmosphere of care and concern (e.g. provide privacy, be available and nonjudgmental, display empathy and respect) *so that client will feel free to verbalize both positive and negative feelings and concerns*
      5. perform actions *to promote trust* (e.g. answer questions honestly, provide requested information)
      6. encourage the expression of anger and sadness about the losses and changes experienced
      7. encourage client to express his/her feelings in whatever ways are comfortable (e.g. writing, drawing, conversation)
      8. perform actions to facilitate effective coping (see Nursing Diagnosis 20, action d)
      9. perform actions *to support realistic hope:*
         a. if appropriate, reassure client that he/she may experience a lengthy period of disease remission
         b. focus on what the client is able to accomplish/perform independently with and without the use of adaptive devices
         c. state that although there is no known cure at this time, research is continuing.
   e. Assess for and support behaviors suggesting successful resolution of grief (e.g. verbalizing feelings about losses in mental and physical function, expressing sorrow, focusing on ways to adapt to losses).
   f. Explain the stages of the grieving process to significant others. Encourage their support and understanding.
   g. Provide information regarding counseling services and support groups that might be of assistance to client in working through grief.
   h. Arrange for visit from clergy if desired by client.
   i. Monitor for therapeutic and nontherapeutic effects of antidepressants if administered.
   j. Consult physician regarding referral for counseling if signs of dysfunctional grieving (e.g. persistent denial of losses or changes, excessive anger or sadness, hysteria, suicidal behaviors, phobias) occur.

23. NURSING DIAGNOSIS

Altered family processes related to change in family roles and structure associated with disability of family member and the inability to predict how long remissions will last and what deficits will remain after each exacerbation of MS.

DESIRED OUTCOMES	NURSING ACTIONS AND *SELECTED RATIONALES*

23. The family members* will demonstrate beginning adjustment to changes in family roles and structure as evidenced by:
    a. verbalization of ways to adapt to required role and life-style changes
    b. active participation in decision making and client's rehabilitation
    c. positive interactions with one another.

23.a. Identify components of the family and their patterns of communication and role expectations.
 b. Assess for signs and symptoms of alterations in family processes (e.g. statements of not being able to accept client's disabilities or diagnosis of MS or to make necessary role and life-style changes, inability to make decisions, inability or refusal to participate in client's rehabilitation, negative family interactions).
 c. Implement measures *to facilitate family members' adjustment to changes in family roles and structure:*
    1. encourage verbalization of feelings about client's disabilities and MS and the effect of these on the family structure
    2. reinforce physician's explanations of the disease and planned treatment and rehabilitation
    3. provide privacy *so that family members and client can share their feelings with one another;* stress the importance and facilitate the use of good communication techniques
    4. assist family members to progress through their own grieving process; explain that during this progression, they may encounter times when they need to focus on meeting their own rather than the client's needs
    5. emphasize the need for family members to obtain adequate rest and nutrition and to identify and utilize stress management techniques *so that they are better able to emotionally and physically deal with the changes and losses experienced*
    6. encourage and assist family members to identify coping strategies for dealing with the client's disabilities and disease process and its effects on the family
    7. include family members in decision making about client and his/her care; convey appreciation for their input and continued support of client
    8. encourage and allow family members to participate in client's care; provide necessary instruction and stress the importance of allowing the client to utilize adaptive devices and mobility aids *so that he/she can maintain as much independence as possible*
    9. assist family members to identify resources that could assist them in coping with their feelings and meeting their immediate and long-term needs (e.g. counseling and social services; pastoral care; service, church, and MS support groups); initiate a referral if indicated.
 d. Consult physician if family members continue to demonstrate difficulty adapting to changes in roles and family structure.

---

* The term "family members" is being used here to include client's significant others.

□ ▬▬▬▬▬▬▬▬▬▬▬▬▬▬

24. NURSING DIAGNOSIS

Knowledge deficit regarding follow-up care.

□ ▬▬▬▬▬▬▬▬▬▬▬▬▬▬

DESIRED OUTCOMES	NURSING ACTIONS AND *SELECTED RATIONALES*

24.a. The client will identify ways to maintain an optimal level of independence.

24.a.1. Instruct client in ways *to maintain an optimal level of independence:*
    a. encourage measures *to maintain or improve physical mobility:*
       1. use a walker or cane as needed
       2. wear braces or splints as ordered
       3. adhere to a planned exercise program

4. continue with measures to reduce or control spasticity and tremors (e.g. warm baths, massage, stretching exercises, swimming or water exercises, sleeping or resting in the prone position, taking muscle relaxants and antispasmodics as ordered)
   b. encourage use of adaptive devices (e.g. weighted eating utensils, wrist splints)
   c. reinforce use of techniques to assist client in adapting to alterations in thought processes (see Nursing Diagnosis 19, action b.3)
   d. reinforce use of methods that can help the client adapt to visual impairments (e.g. visual scanning, wearing frosted lens or eyepatch).
2. Allow time for questions, clarification, and return demonstration.

24.b. The client will identify ways to decrease the risk of disease exacerbation.	24.b.1. Instruct client in ways *to decrease risk of an exacerbation:* a. avoid or control emotional stress b. avoid extremes in temperature (e.g. hot baths, drafts, very cold or hot weather) c. eat a well-balanced diet d. maintain a balanced program of rest and exercise e. decrease the risk of infection by avoiding contact with persons who have respiratory tract infections and maintaining good personal hygiene f. avoid becoming pregnant *(the physical and emotional stress can cause an exacerbation);* emphasize need to notify health care provider immediately if pregnancy does occur and to adhere to prescribed prenatal care. 2. Assist client to identify ways he/she can make appropriate changes in life style to reduce risk of disease exacerbation. Provide information about stress management classes, physical fitness programs, Planned Parenthood, and nutritional counseling if indicated.
24.c. The client will identify ways to manage incontinence.	24.c.1. Encourage adherence to bowel and bladder training programs established with client. 2. Instruct client in the following if appropriate: a. Credé technique, urethral or rectal stimulation, and Valsalva maneuver b. perineal exercises c. use of underwear liners or disposable, absorbent undergarments such as Attends d. use of penile clamp and/or external catheter e. intermittent catheterization f. care of an indwelling catheter and collection devices. 3. Allow time for questions, clarification, and return demonstration.
24.d. The client will verbalize ways to manage and cope with fatigue.	24.d. Instruct client in ways *to manage and cope with fatigue:* 1. view fatigue as a protective mechanism and/or a manageable disease symptom rather than a problematic limitation 2. determine ways that activity can be modified *to conserve energy and prevent excessive fatigue* (e.g. alternate light and heavy tasks, take short rests during an activity, sit during an activity whenever possible) 3. determine if life demands are realistic in light of physical status and adjust short- and long-term goals accordingly 4. avoid situations that are particularly fatiguing such as those that are boring, frustrating, or require prolonged or strenuous physical activity 5. attempt to remain in environments where temperature is less than 75°F and avoid using hot water for baths and showers *(an increased body temperature promotes fatigue by increasing metabolic rate and reducing transmission of impulses along affected nerves)* 6. participate in a regular exercise program as prescribed *to reduce anxiety and stress and improve or maintain muscle tone and activity tolerance.*
24.e. The client will identify appropriate safety measures.	24.e.1. Instruct client to wear an MS Medic-Alert band. 2. Instruct client to inform all health care providers that he/she has MS. 3. Reinforce methods *to decrease risk of physical injury:* a. concentrate on body position, movement, and balance b. allow ample time for all activity c. wear alternating eyepatch or frosted lens and scan environment continually if appropriate

UNIT VI

d. use mobility aids if necessary
e. avoid contact with anything very hot or cold
f. keep environment well-lit and uncluttered
g. wear shoes or slippers with nonskid soles and flat heels.

24.f. The client will state signs and symptoms to report to the health care provider.

24.f. Instruct client to report:
1. increase in or development of:
   a. spasticity, tremors
   b. weakness, fatigue
   c. pain
   d. difficulty speaking and/or swallowing
   e. numbness, tingling, and/or burning sensations
   f. visual disturbances (e.g. dimmed, blurred, or double vision)
   g. severe mood swings
   h. constipation or loss of bowel control
   i. urinary retention, incontinence, urgency, or frequency
   j. forgetfulness, difficulty solving problems
2. inability to maintain recommended activity level
3. skin irritation or breakdown
4. cough productive of purulent, green, or rust-colored sputum
5. temperature elevation
6. cloudy, foul-smelling urine
7. increased restriction of any joint motion
8. cessation of menses and tender breasts *(could indicate pregnancy).*

24.g. The client will identify community resources that can assist with home management and adjustment to changes in life style, body functioning, and roles.

24.g.1. Provide information about community resources that can assist the client and significant others with home management and adjustment to changes in life style, body functioning, and roles (e.g. local chapters of the American Red Cross and Multiple Sclerosis Society, home health agencies, social services, Visiting Nurse Association, individual and family counselors).
2. Initiate a referral if indicated.

24.h. The client will verbalize an understanding of and a plan for adhering to recommended follow-up care including future appointments with health care provider and physical and occupational therapists and medications prescribed.

24.h.1. Reinforce the importance of keeping appointments with the health care provider and physical and occupational therapists.
2. Explain the rationale for, side effects of, and importance of taking prescribed medications (e.g. antispasmodics, antidepressants, muscle relaxants).
3. Implement measures *to improve client compliance:*
   a. include significant others in teaching sessions if possible
   b. encourage questions and allow time for reinforcement or clarification of information provided
   c. provide written instructions on future appointments with health care provider and physical and occupational therapists, medications prescribed, and signs and symptoms to report.

Reference

Kübler-Ross, E. On death and dying. New York: Macmillan, 1969.

Spinal Cord Injury

Spinal cord injury can result from a contusion, compression, or actual severance of the spinal cord and from alterations in blood supply to the cord. Factors responsible for these conditions include trauma, tumors, edema, hematoma, ruptured intervertebral disc, and degenerative or disease-related changes of the spinal column. The injuries can be classified by type (e.g. flexion, flexion-rotation, compression, extension), level (cervical, thoracic, lumbar, sacral), degree of cord involvement (complete, incomplete), and functional ability (e.g. paraplegic, quadriplegic). The impairments of motor and sensory function depend on the level of the spinal cord injury; the higher the level of the spinal cord injury, the greater the loss of body function.

This care plan focuses on the adult client hospitalized with transection of the spinal cord at the level of the fifth cervical vertebra (C5). Spinal cord transection at this level results in loss of most deep tendon reflexes and motor function below the clavicles; however, full neck, upper shoulder, and biceps muscle control and elbow flexion are retained. Sensory function is intact above the clavicles and in certain areas of the deltoids and forearms and may be present to some degree in areas below the level of the lesion. Immediately after the injury, spinal shock (complete loss of motor, sensory, autonomic, and reflex activity below the level of the lesion) occurs and may last hours to weeks. After extensive rehabilitation, the client who has sustained a C5 transection should be able to do things such as operate an electric wheelchair; feed self using adaptive devices; utilize reflex activity to achieve an erection and stimulate bowel and bladder elimination; turn in bed using arm slings; and operate a typewriter, computer, and telephone using adaptive devices.

Initially, goals of care are to sustain life and prevent further injury by stabilizing the vertebral column and controlling spinal cord edema. Subsequently, goals of care are to mobilize the client, assist him/her to regain as much independence as possible, and facilitate psychological adjustment to the effects of the injury.

DISCHARGE CRITERIA

Prior to discharge, the client will:

- identify ways to prevent complications associated with spinal cord injury and immobility
- demonstrate the ability to correctly use and care for adaptive devices
- identify ways to manage bowel and bladder dysfunction
- state signs and symptoms to report to the health care provider
- identify community resources that can assist with home management and adjustment to changes resulting from spinal cord injury
- share thoughts and feelings about the effects of spinal cord injury on self-concept, life style, and roles
- verbalize an understanding of and a plan for adhering to recommended follow-up care including future appointments with health care provider and occupational and physical therapists and medications prescribed.

Use in conjunction with the Care Plan on Immobility.

NURSING/COLLABORATIVE DIAGNOSES

1. Anxiety □ *271*
2. Altered systemic tissue perfusion □ *272*
3. Ineffective breathing patterns:
   a. hyperventilation
   b. hypoventilation □ *273*
4. Ineffective airway clearance □ *274*
5. Altered nutrition: less than body requirements □ *274*
6. Altered comfort:
   a. headache
   b. shoulder pain
   c. neck pain
   d. intermittent pain and paresthesias in areas below level of lesion □ *275*
7. Ineffective thermoregulation □ *276*
8. Sensory-perceptual alterations:
   a. visual: limited visual field
   b. tactile: loss of sensation below clavicles □ *277*
9. Impaired skin integrity: irritation or breakdown □ *277*
10. Impaired physical mobility □ *278*
11. Self-care deficit □ *279*
12. Altered patterns of urinary elimination:
    a. retention
    b. incontinence □ *280*
13. Constipation □ *281*
14. Bowel incontinence □ *282*
15. Sleep pattern disturbance □ *282*
16. Potential for infection:
    a. pneumonia
    b. urinary tract infection □ *283*
17. Potential for trauma □ *284*
18. Potential for aspiration □ *284*
19. Dysreflexia □ *285*
20. Potential complications:
    a. further injury to the spinal cord
    b. thromboembolism
    c. gastrointestinal (GI) bleeding
    d. contractures □ *286*
21. Sexual dysfunction:
    a. decreased libido
    b. decreased ability to control and maintain an erection □ *288*
22. Disturbance in self-concept □ *289*
23. Ineffective individual coping □ *290*
24. Powerlessness □ *291*
25. Grieving □ *292*
26. Social isolation □ *293*
27. Altered family processes □ *293*
28. Knowledge deficit regarding follow-up care □ *294*

1. NURSING DIAGNOSIS

Anxiety related to unfamiliar environment; lack of understanding of diagnostic tests, diagnosis, and treatment; loss of motor and sensory function; application of immobilization device to stabilize the cervical spine; and anticipated effect of the spinal cord injury on life style and roles.

DESIRED OUTCOMES	NURSING ACTIONS AND *SELECTED RATIONALES*

1. The client will experience a reduction in fear and anxiety as evidenced by:
   a. verbalization of feeling less anxious or fearful
   b. relaxed facial expression
   c. usual skin color
   d. verbalization of an understanding of hospital routines, diagnostic tests, diagnosis, and treatments.

1.a. Assess client for signs and symptoms of fear and anxiety (e.g. verbalization of fears and concerns; tenseness; irritability; diaphoresis; facial tension, pallor, or flushing; noncompliance with treatment plan).
   b. Ascertain effectiveness of current coping skills.
   c. Implement measures *to reduce fear and anxiety:*
      1. assure client that staff members are nearby; place client in a room close to the nurses' station until his/her anxiety decreases and a call signal can be adapted to the client's specific motor and sensory impairments
      2. explain necessity of frequent neurological checks and the importance of his/her cooperation during these checks
      3. offer physical and emotional support during insertion of skull tongs or application of a halo device:
         a. assure client that tongs penetrate only the outer table of the skull, not the brain
         b. assure client that very little pain is associated with the tong insertion, but that the procedure will be quite loud since bone is such a good sound conductor
         c. assure client that only a small amount of hair is clipped at each tong insertion site
      4. explain the purpose and safety features of the turning frame, circular electric bed, or kinetic bed if appropriate
      5. assure client that measures have been taken to keep him/her from falling off bed/frame (e.g. side rails up if in bed, safety straps on turning frames and circular electric bed)
      6. explain the sensations the client may experience when frame or circular electric bed is turned (e.g. closed-in feeling, momentary dizziness); assure him/her that these sensations disappear when turns are completed
      7. once emergency stabilization procedures have been done:
         a. orient to hospital environment, equipment, and routines
         b. explain all diagnostic tests (e.g. spine x-rays, dermatome and myotome mapping)
         c. introduce staff who will be participating in his/her care; if possible, maintain consistency in staff assigned to his/her care *to provide feelings of stability and comfort with the environment*
         d. maintain a calm, confident manner when interacting with client
         e. avoid startling client (e.g. speak client's name and identify yourself when entering room and before physical contact, place self in client's visual field whenever possible during care and conversation)
         f. encourage verbalization of fear and anxiety; provide feedback
         g. reinforce physician's explanations and clarify any misconceptions client may have about spinal cord injury, treatment plan, and prognosis
         h. explain treatments that may be done to reduce edema of and around injured area of spinal cord (e.g. hypothermia, myelotomy, hyperbaric oxygen therapy)
         i. explain that the flaccid paralysis and lack of reflexes following the injury result from spinal shock; emphasize that some reflex activity will return after spinal shock subsides
         j. provide a calm, restful environment

UNIT VI

     k. instruct in relaxation techniques and encourage participation in diversional activities

     l. perform actions to assist client to cope with effects of the injury and its implications (see Nursing Diagnosis 23, action d)

     m. encourage significant others to project a caring, concerned attitude without obvious anxiousness

     n. if comfortable for nurse and client, reinforce verbal messages of caring by touching areas where client has sensation (e.g. shoulders, head, neck, face); encourage significant others to do the same

     o. arrange for a visit from clergy if client desires

     p. monitor for therapeutic and nontherapeutic effects of antianxiety agents if administered.

  d. Include significant others in orientation and teaching sessions and encourage their continued support of the client.

  e. Provide information based on current needs of client and significant others at a level they can understand. Encourage questions and clarification of information provided.

  f. Consult physician if above actions fail to control fear and anxiety.

2. NURSING DIAGNOSIS

Altered systemic tissue perfusion related to:

a. decreased cardiac output associated with:
 1. bradycardia and hypotension resulting from the loss of sympathetic nervous system response (especially during period of spinal shock)
 2. hypovolemia resulting from positional diuresis and decreased oral fluid intake
 3. decreased venous return
 4. decreased diastolic filling time due to an increased heart rate resulting from an imbalance in autonomic nervous system activity occurring after period of spinal shock
 5. cardiac deconditioning resulting from prolonged immobility;
b. peripheral pooling of blood associated with loss of sympathetic nervous system control over peripheral vessels (especially during period of spinal shock) and decreased venous return resulting from a loss of muscle tone in extremities (occurs because of paralysis of extremities and decreased mobility).

DESIRED OUTCOMES	NURSING ACTIONS AND *SELECTED RATIONALES*
2. The client will maintain adequate systemic tissue perfusion as evidenced by: a. B/P and pulse within normal range for client and stable with position change b. unlabored respirations at 16–20/minute c. usual mental status d. skin warm and usual color e. palpable peripheral pulses f. capillary refill time less than 3 seconds g. urine output at least 30 cc/hour.	2.a. Assess for and report signs and symptoms of diminished systemic tissue perfusion: 1. significant decrease in B/P 2. resting pulse rate less than 60 or greater than 100 beats/minute 3. decline in systolic B/P of at least 15 mm Hg with a concurrent rise in pulse when client is changed from horizontal to sitting or vertical position 4. rapid or labored respirations 5. restlessness, slow responses, confusion 6. cool, pale, mottled, or cyanotic skin 7. diminished or absent peripheral pulses 8. capillary refill time greater than 3 seconds 9. urine output less than 30 cc/hour. b. Implement measures *to maintain adequate systemic tissue perfusion:* 1. avoid activities that cause increased vagal stimulation (e.g. suctioning) during period of spinal shock unless absolutely necessary *in order to prevent further reduction in pulse rate*

2. perform actions *to reduce cardiac workload:*
   a. instruct client to avoid activities that create a Valsalva response (e.g. holding breath when being turned)
   b. implement measures to reduce fear and anxiety (see Nursing Diagnosis 1, action c)
   c. implement measures to improve breathing pattern and promote effective airway clearance (see Nursing Diagnoses 3, actions a and c and 4) *in order to ensure adequate oxygenation*
   d. place client in a semi- to high Fowler's position when allowed and tolerated
   e. provide frequent, small meals rather than 3 large ones *(large meals require an increased blood supply to gastrointestinal tract for digestion)*
3. perform actions *to prevent peripheral pooling of blood and/or increase venous return:*
   a. perform passive range of motion of extremities at least every 2 hours while client is awake
   b. position lower extremities properly; do not put pillows under client's knees, use the knee gatch, or allow client to sit for long periods
   c. apply thigh-high elastic wraps or antiembolic hose as ordered; remove for 30–60 minutes each shift
   d. assist with intermittent venous compression using pneumatic cuffs or boots if ordered
   e. elevate foot of bed for 20-minute intervals several times a shift unless contraindicated
   f. apply an abdominal binder before placing client in an upright position *(the binder increases pressure on the aorta and limits the amount of blood that will be able to flow to and pool in extremities)*
   g. monitor for therapeutic and nontherapeutic effects of sympathomimetics (e.g. ephedrine) if administered before sitting or vertical positioning
4. monitor for therapeutic and nontherapeutic effects of fluid replacement therapy if administered
5. when oral intake is allowed, encourage a minimum fluid intake of at least 2500 cc/day unless contraindicated
6. change client's position slowly and gradually progress him/her to an upright position using a recliner, wheelchair, or tilt table when allowed and tolerated *to allow time for remaining autoregulatory mechanisms to adjust to position changes*
7. discourage smoking *(smoking decreases oxygen availability and causes vasoconstriction).*

c. Consult physician if signs and symptoms of decreased systemic tissue perfusion persist or worsen.

3. NURSING DIAGNOSIS

Ineffective breathing patterns:

a. **hyperventilation** related to fear and anxiety;
b. **hypoventilation** related to impaired chest expansion associated with weakness or paralysis of abdominal and intercostal muscles and diaphragm, recumbent positioning, and immobility.

DESIRED OUTCOMES	NURSING ACTIONS AND *SELECTED RATIONALES*
3. The client will maintain an effective breathing pattern	3.a. Refer to Care Plan on Immobility, Nursing Diagnosis 3, for measures related to assessment and improvement of breathing patterns.

(see Care Plan on Immobility, Nursing Diagnosis 3, for outcome criteria).

   b. Monitor for and report a significant decline in vital capacity measurements.
   c. Implement additional measures *to improve breathing pattern:*
     1. perform actions to reduce fear and anxiety (see Nursing Diagnosis 1, action c)
     2. instruct client to breathe slowly if he/she is hyperventilating
     3. place client in a rocking bed or chair if ordered *to promote gravitational movement of the diaphragm*
     4. encourage and assist client to perform exercises that can help strengthen the accessory muscles used in breathing (e.g. shoulder shrugs *to strengthen the trapezius muscles)* when allowed and tolerated.

4. NURSING DIAGNOSIS

Ineffective airway clearance related to stasis of secretions associated with immobility and poor cough effort resulting from paralysis of abdominal and intercostal muscles and weakened diaphragm.

DESIRED OUTCOMES	NURSING ACTIONS AND *SELECTED RATIONALES*

4. The client will maintain clear, open airways (see Care Plan on Immobility, Nursing Diagnosis 4, for outcome criteria).

   4.a. Refer to Care Plan on Immobility, Nursing Diagnosis 4, for measures related to assessment and promotion of effective airway clearance.
     b. Implement measures *to facilitate the client's cough efforts in order to further promote effective airway clearance:*
     1. place client in a horizontal position during cough efforts unless contraindicated (*promotes a more effective forced expiration by decreasing the effects of gravity on the diaphragm)*
     2. use the "quad" coughing method (place palm of hand under client's diaphragm and push up on abdominal muscles as he/she exhales).

5. NURSING DIAGNOSIS

Altered nutrition: less than body requirements related to decreased oral intake associated with:

a. anorexia resulting from:
   1. anxiety, depression, boredom, slowed metabolic rate (results from decreased activity), and constipation
   2. early satiety associated with decreased gastrointestinal motility (slowed motility is due to loss of autonomic nervous system function [especially during period of spinal shock], decreased activity, and the hypercalcemia that may occur with prolonged immobility);
b. fear of choking while in positions necessary for spine immobilization (e.g. horizontal, neck hyperextended);
c. inability to feed self as a result of loss of motor function.

DESIRED OUTCOMES	NURSING ACTIONS AND *SELECTED RATIONALES*

5. The client will maintain an adequate nutritional status (see Care Plan on Immobility, Nursing Diagnosis 6, for outcome criteria).

5.a. Refer to Care Plan on Immobility, Nursing Diagnosis 6, for measures related to assessment and maintenance of nutritional status.
   b. Implement additional measures *to improve oral intake and maintain an adequate nutritional status:*
   1. perform actions to reduce fear and anxiety (see Nursing Diagnosis 1, action c)
   2. facilitate client's psychological adjustment to effects of spinal cord injury (see Nursing Diagnoses 22; 23, action d; 24; and 25, action d)
   3. perform actions to prevent constipation (see Nursing Diagnosis 13, action e)
   4. feed client until he/she is able to feed self using adaptive devices
   5. perform actions to improve client's ability to swallow while spine is immobilized (see Nursing Diagnosis 18, action d.5) *in order to decrease risk of and subsequently his/her fear of choking.*

UNIT VI

□ ▮▮▮▮▮▮▮▮▮▮▮▮▮▮▮▮▮▮▮▮▮▮▮▮▮▮▮▮▮▮▮

6. NURSING DIAGNOSIS

Altered comfort:*

a. **headache** related to fear, anxiety, and increase in sound conduction associated with presence of skull tongs;
b. **shoulder pain** related to muscle strain associated with increasing use of upper arms and shoulders and/or development of contractures;
c. **neck pain** related to muscle stiffness while stabilization device is in place and muscle strain associated with increased use of neck muscles following removal of stabilization device;
d. **intermittent pain and paresthesias in areas below level of lesion** related to irritation of nerve roots (believed to be associated with instability at the site of injury and/or scar tissue formation).

---

* In this care plan, the nursing diagnosis "pain" is included under the diagnostic label of altered comfort.

□ ▮▮▮▮▮▮▮▮▮▮▮▮▮▮▮▮▮▮▮▮▮▮▮▮▮▮▮▮▮▮▮

DESIRED OUTCOMES	NURSING ACTIONS AND *SELECTED RATIONALES*

6. The client will experience diminished discomfort as evidenced by:
   a. verbalization of same
   b. relaxed facial expression
   c. increased participation in activities when allowed
   d. stable vital signs.

6.a. Determine how the client usually responds to pain.
   b. Assess for nonverbal signs of discomfort (e.g. grimacing or tense facial expression, wrinkled brow, reluctance to turn head or move shoulders when increased activity is allowed, restlessness, change in B/P, tachycardia).
   c. Assess verbal complaints of discomfort. Ask client to be specific about location, severity, and type of discomfort.
   d. Assess for factors that seem to aggravate and alleviate discomfort.
   e. Implement measures *to reduce discomfort:*
   1. perform actions *to relieve headache:*
      a. minimize environmental stimuli (e.g. provide a calm environment, restrict visitors, dim lights)
      b. implement measures to reduce fear and anxiety (see Nursing Diagnosis 1, action c)
      c. avoid letting any object come in contact with skull tongs
      d. cover tips of halo device with rubber corks *to diminish sounds if tips are inadvertently hit*
      e. apply cool cloth to forehead if client desires

2. perform actions *to reduce shoulder and/or neck pain:*
   a. implement measures to prevent contractures (see Collaborative Diagnosis 20, action d)
   b. when moving client, provide support to neck and utilize turn sheet rather than pushing or pulling on shoulders
   c. apply neck support (e.g. soft cervical collar) if ordered following removal of stabilization device
   d. massage client's shoulders, being careful to avoid area around or over cervical spine until fracture has stabilized
   e. consult physician about application of heat or cold to shoulders and neck
3. maintain immobilization of the cervical spine as ordered *to prevent further nerve root injury or irritation*
4. provide or assist with additional nonpharmacological measures for pain relief (e.g. position change if allowed, relaxation techniques, guided imagery, quiet conversation, diversional activities)
5. monitor for therapeutic and nontherapeutic effects of the following if administered:
   a. aspirin or acetaminophen *to reduce headache and muscle aches and pains* (avoid use of narcotic analgesics *to prevent further depression of respiratory function)*
   b. medications such as phenytoin or carbamazepine *to control pain and paresthesias below the level of the lesion (these medications inhibit neuromuscular transmission).*

f. Consult physician if above measures fail to provide adequate relief of discomfort.

☐ ▬▬▬▬▬▬▬▬▬▬▬▬▬▬▬▬▬▬▬▬▬▬▬

7. NURSING DIAGNOSIS

Ineffective thermoregulation related to autonomic nervous system dysfunction (results in an inability of the vessels below the level of the lesion to dilate further in response to heat or to constrict in response to cold).

☐ ▬▬▬▬▬▬▬▬▬▬▬▬▬▬▬▬▬▬▬▬▬▬▬

DESIRED OUTCOMES	NURSING ACTIONS AND *SELECTED RATIONALES*

7. The client will experience effective thermoregulation as evidenced by:
a. verbalization of comfortable body temperature above the level of the lesion
b. absence of excessively warm or cool skin
c. temperature between 36–38°C.
	7.a. Assess for signs and symptoms of ineffective thermoregulation (e.g. complaints of feeling too warm or too cold, excessively warm or cool skin).
	b. Monitor temperature. Report temperature less than 36°C or greater than 38°C.
	c. Implement measures *to maintain effective thermoregulation:*
	  1. perform actions *to prevent hypothermia:*
	    a. maintain room temperature at 70°F
	    b. provide extra clothing or bedding as necessary
	    c. protect client from drafts
	    d. apply warming blanket as ordered
	    e. provide warm liquids for client to drink
	  2. perform actions *to prevent hyperthermia:*
	    a. maintain room temperature at 70°F
	    b. avoid use of excessive clothing or bedding
	    c. use tepid rather than hot water when bathing client
	    d. apply cooling blanket as ordered.
	d. Consult physician if above measures fail to maintain effective thermoregulation.

8. NURSING DIAGNOSIS

Sensory-perceptual alterations:

a. **visual: limited visual field** related to decreased ability to move head associated with immobilization devices used to stabilize the cervical spine;
b. **tactile: loss of sensation below clavicles** related to loss of integrity of ascending spinal pathways.

DESIRED OUTCOMES	NURSING ACTIONS AND *SELECTED RATIONALES*
8.a. The client will experience adequate visual stimulation as evidenced by verbalization of same.	8.a.1. Assess for conditions that can limit the client's visual field (e.g. stabilization of spine with a halo device, use of turning frame or circular electric bed). 2. Implement measures *to provide visual stimulation:* a. provide prism glasses for use when client is supine b. position mirrors in strategic places *to provide increased visualization of surroundings* c. place self within client's visual field when talking with him/her; instruct others to do the same d. put posters, pictures, or cards on the ceiling or suspend objects such as mobiles from ceiling *so client can view objects when supine* e. if client is on a turning frame or circular electric bed, place objects of interest (e.g. posters, clock, flowers, cards, small TV, pictures) on the floor within client's visual field when he/she is in prone position.
8.b. The client will experience adequate tactile stimulation as evidenced by verbalization of same.	8.b.1. Ascertain areas of body where client can perceive tactile sensation (usually face, neck, shoulders, and upper chest). 2. Implement measures *to provide tactile stimulation:* a. touch client on shoulders, face, head, and neck; encourage significant others to do the same b. obtain materials of various textures (e.g. sandpaper, cotton, leather) to rub gently on areas of sensation c. consult occupational therapist for additional ways to provide tactile stimulation.

9. NURSING DIAGNOSIS

Impaired skin integrity: irritation or breakdown related to:

a. prolonged pressure on tissues associated with decreased mobility and presence of stabilization device;
b. increased fragility of the skin in lower extremities associated with edema resulting from venous stasis (occurs as a result of decreased muscle activity and poor vascular tone);
c. frequent contact with irritants associated with urinary and/or bowel incontinence.

DESIRED OUTCOMES	NURSING ACTIONS AND *SELECTED RATIONALES*

9. The client will maintain skin integrity as evidenced by:
   a. absence of redness and irritation
   b. no skin breakdown.

9.a. Inspect the skin (especially bone prominences, dependent areas, pin sites, perineum, areas under stabilization device, and areas of decreased sensation and/or edema) for pallor, redness, and breakdown.
b. Refer to Care Plan on Immobility, Nursing Diagnosis 7, action b, for measures to prevent skin breakdown associated with decreased mobility.
c. Implement measures *to prevent skin irritation and breakdown resulting from pressure of the stabilization device:*
   1. provide adequate padding (e.g. foam, silicone gel, water pads) on each side of turning frame or circular electric bed
   2. turn client every 2 hours as ordered
   3. if client is wearing a stabilization vest or jacket:
      a. ensure that skin beneath it is kept clean and dry
      b. if it is unlined, make sure client wears a clean, dry, wrinkle-free, cotton t-shirt underneath it
      c. if it is lined, ensure that lining is always clean and dry
      d. consult physician and orthotist if vest or jacket is creating excessive pressure on any skin area.
d. Implement measures *to decrease risk of skin breakdown in dependent areas:*
   1. perform actions to prevent peripheral pooling of blood and increase venous return (see Nursing Diagnosis 2, action b.3) *in order to prevent dependent edema*
   2. handle edematous areas carefully.
e. Implement measures *to prevent skin irritation and breakdown resulting from urinary and bowel incontinence:*
   1. perform actions to prevent urinary and bowel incontinence (see Nursing Diagnoses 12, actions b.2–4 and 14, actions b and c)
   2. thoroughly cleanse and dry perineal area after each bowel movement and episode of incontinence; apply a protective ointment or cream (e.g. Sween cream, Desitin, A & D ointment, Vaseline)
   3. use soft tissue to cleanse perineal area
   4. apply a perianal pouch if bowel incontinence is a persistent problem
   5. avoid direct contact of skin with Chux (e.g. place turn sheet or bed pad over Chux).
f. If skin breakdown occurs:
   1. notify physician
   2. continue with above measures to prevent further irritation and breakdown
   3. perform decubitus care as ordered or per standard hospital policy
   4. monitor client closely and report signs and symptoms of infection (e.g. elevated temperature; redness, warmth, and edema around area of breakdown; unusual drainage from site).

10. NURSING DIAGNOSIS

Impaired physical mobility related to quadriplegia, restrictions imposed by treatment plan to stabilize spine, and spasticity (occurs due to absence of central nervous system control and stimulation of reflex arcs following period of spinal shock).

DESIRED OUTCOMES	NURSING ACTIONS AND *SELECTED RATIONALES*

10.a. The client will achieve maximum physical mobility within limitations imposed

10.a.1. Assess for factors that impair physical mobility (e.g. loss of motor function below level of injury, restrictions imposed during spinal stabilization, spasticity following spinal shock).

by quadriplegia and the treatment plan.

2. Implement measures *to increase mobility:*
   a. instruct client in and assist with active and active-resistive exercises of neck, shoulders, and biceps when allowed by physician
   b. perform passive range of motion to areas client is not able to move
   c. when activity is allowed, instruct client in ways to move his/her body (e.g. hook arm over side rail to assist in turning self, trigger flexor spasm of knees to help swing legs over side of bed during transfer to and from wheelchair)
   d. instruct client in and assist with correct use of mobility aids (e.g. sliding board, electric wheelchair) as activity progresses
   e. reinforce instructions, activities, and exercise plan recommended by physical and occupational therapists
   f. perform actions *to reduce spasticity if spasms are excessive and interfere with attempts to properly position client and increase mobility:*
      1. avoid stimulating extremities or muscle groups (e.g. do not jar bed, do not touch easily stimulated areas unnecessarily)
      2. implement measures to prevent conditions such as urinary tract infection, muscle tightening from staying in one position too long, fatigue, and chills *(these conditions can cause a stimulatory response)*
      3. provide or assist with nonpharmacological measures for reducing spasticity (e.g. biofeedback, stretching exercises, warm bath or whirlpool, local application of heat or cold)
   g. provide adequate rest periods before activity sessions.
3. Provide praise and encouragement for all efforts to increase physical mobility.
4. Encourage the support of significant others. Allow them to assist with range of motion exercises, positioning, and activity if desired.
5. Consult physician if client is unable to achieve expected level of mobility or if range of motion becomes restricted.

10.b. The client will not experience problems associated with immobility.

10.b. Refer to Care Plan on Immobility for actions to prevent problems associated with immobility.

□ ▬▬▬▬▬▬▬▬▬▬▬▬▬▬▬

11. NURSING DIAGNOSIS

Self-care deficit related to discomfort and impaired physical mobility associated with quadriplegia, spasticity, and activity restrictions imposed by treatment plan.

□ ▬▬▬▬▬▬▬▬▬▬▬▬▬▬▬

DESIRED OUTCOMES	NURSING ACTIONS AND *SELECTED RATIONALES*

11. The client will demonstrate increased participation in self-care activities within the limitations imposed by the treatment plan and quadriplegia.

11.a. Assess for factors that interfere with client's ability to perform self-care (e.g. discomfort, motor deficits, activity restrictions associated with treatment plan).
   b. With client, develop a realistic plan for meeting daily physical needs. Inform client that with rehabilitation and use of adaptive devices, he/she should be able to:
      1. feed self once meal has been set up
      2. wash face and chest
      3. comb front and sides of hair, brush teeth, shave self with an electric razor
      4. participate in dressing upper body.
   c. When condition stabilizes and physician allows, implement measures *to facilitate client's ability to perform self-care activities:*

UNIT VI

1. perform actions to increase mobility (see Nursing Diagnosis 10, action a.2)
2. perform actions to reduce discomfort (see Nursing Diagnosis 6, action e)
3. consult occupational therapist regarding adaptive devices available; reinforce use of these devices, which may include:
   a. rocker feeder, overhead sling, plate guard, sandwich holder, and broad-handled and/or swivel utensils for feeding self
   b. flexor-hinge splint or universal cuff to aid in brushing teeth, combing hair, and shaving self with electric razor
   c. bath mitt for bathing
   d. Velcro fasteners *to facilitate dressing*
4. schedule care at a time when client is most likely to be able to participate (e.g. when analgesics are at peak action, after rest periods, not immediately after treatments or meals)
5. keep needed objects within easy reach
6. allow adequate time for accomplishment of self-care activities.

d. Provide positive feedback for all efforts and accomplishments of self-care.

e. Assist client with those activities he/she is unable to perform using adaptive devices.

f. Inform significant others of client's abilities to participate in own care. Explain the importance of encouraging and allowing client to maintain an optimal level of independence.

□ ■■

12. NURSING DIAGNOSIS

Altered patterns of urinary elimination:

a. **retention** related to:
   1. atony of bladder wall and contraction of external urinary sphincter during period of spinal shock
   2. incomplete bladder emptying associated with spasticity of external urinary sphincter following period of spinal shock
   3. pooling of urine in kidney and bladder associated with prolonged horizontal positioning;
b. **incontinence** related to spasticity of the bladder following period of spinal shock (with upper motor neuron involvement, the reflex arcs remain intact but are uninhibited; this results in involuntary voiding).

□ ■■

DESIRED OUTCOMES	NURSING ACTIONS AND *SELECTED RATIONALES*

12.a. The client will not experience urinary retention as evidenced by:
1. absence of suprapubic distention
2. balanced intake and output.
	12.a.1. Assess for and report signs and symptoms of urinary retention (e.g. suprapubic distention, intake greater than output).
	2. Catheterize client if ordered *to determine amount of residual urine.*
	3. Assist with urodynamic studies (e.g. cystometrogram) if ordered.
	4. Implement measures *to prevent urinary retention during period of spinal shock:*
	  a. perform intermittent catheterization or insert indwelling urinary catheter as ordered
	  b. perform actions to maintain patency of urinary catheter if present (e.g. keep tubing free of kinks).
	5. Implement measures *to promote complete bladder emptying after period of spinal shock:*
	  a. stimulate trigger zones of the reflex sacral arc (e.g. tap suprapubic area, stroke or massage abdomen, stroke inner thigh, perform anal sphincter stretching, pull pubic hair); repeat stimulus as necessary (the

goal is to have a residual urine of less than 100 cc); if stimulation of the trigger zones is not effective, continue to provide the stimulation periodically *(it may take up to 9 months for strong reflex sacral arc activity to return)*
  b. place client in a sitting position for voiding unless contraindicated
  c. perform the Credé technique unless contraindicated *to facilitate emptying of the bladder*
  d. monitor for therapeutic and nontherapeutic effects of antispasmodics (e.g. propantheline, oxybutynin) if administered *to decrease spasticity of the external urinary sphincter.*
6. If signs and symptoms of urinary retention persist after the period of spinal shock despite implementation of above actions:
  a. perform intermittent catheterizations as ordered
  b. prepare client for insertion of an indwelling catheter (urethral or suprapubic) if indicated
  c. provide emotional support to client and significant others.

<table>
<tr><td>12.b. The client will experience urinary continence.</td><td>12.b.1. Monitor for urinary incontinence.
2. Implement measures *to prevent urinary incontinence:*
  a. space fluid intake evenly throughout the day *in order to prevent overdistention of the bladder at any one time (overdistention can cause increased bladder spasm and subsequent incontinence)*
  b. limit oral fluid intake in the evening *to decrease risk of nighttime incontinence*
  c. instruct client to avoid drinking caffeinated beverages such as colas, coffee, and tea *(caffeine is a mild diuretic and the increased urine production can cause overdistention of bladder and bladder spasm with subsequent incontinence)*
  d. allow client to assume a sitting position for voiding unless contraindicated *to promote complete bladder emptying*
  e. instruct client and others to avoid stimulating trigger zones at times other than during bladder care
  f. monitor for therapeutic and nontherapeutic effects of antispasmodics (e.g. oxybutynin, propantheline) if administered *to decrease spasticity of the bladder.*
3. If incontinence persists, carefully review bladder training program and revise as needed.
4. If reflex voiding cannot be controlled, consult physician regarding use of an external catheter or, if absolutely necessary, insertion of an indwelling urinary catheter.</td></tr>
</table>

□ ▬▬▬▬▬▬▬▬▬▬▬▬▬▬▬▬▬

13. NURSING DIAGNOSIS

Constipation related to:

a. decreased gastrointestinal motility associated with decreased activity and loss of abdominal muscle tone;
b. lack of awareness of stool in rectum.

□ ▬▬▬▬▬▬▬▬▬▬▬▬▬▬▬▬▬

DESIRED OUTCOMES	NURSING ACTIONS AND *SELECTED RATIONALES*

13. The client will evacuate soft, formed stool every 2–3 days or per his/her usual routine.	13.a. Ascertain client's usual bowel habits.
	  b. Monitor and record bowel movements including frequency, consistency, and shape.
	  c. Assess for signs and symptoms that may accompany constipation (e.g. headache, anorexia, nausea, abdominal distention).

d. Assess bowel sounds. Report a pattern of decreasing bowel sounds.
e. Implement measures *to prevent constipation* (the following are usually included in a bowel training program):
    1. assist client to select foods high in fiber (e.g. nuts, bran, whole grains, raw fruits and vegetables, dried fruits)
    2. encourage client to maintain a minimum fluid intake of 2500 cc/day unless contraindicated
    3. encourage client to drink warm liquids *in order to stimulate peristalsis*
    4. establish a routine time for defecation; try to schedule it 20 or 30 minutes after a meal *to take advantage of gastrocolic reflex*
    5. increase activity as allowed and tolerated
    6. perform digital stimulation and/or insert rectal suppository *to stimulate reflex peristalsis and emptying of rectum*
    7. place client in high Fowler's position or on commode once spine is stabilized and client is able to tolerate position changes
    8. allow ample time for bowel evacuation (may take up to an hour after rectal stimulation)
    9. monitor for therapeutic and nontherapeutic effects of stool softeners and laxatives if administered.
f. Check for impaction if client has not had a bowel movement in 3 days, he/she is passing liquid stool, or if other signs and symptoms of constipation are present. Administer oil retention and/or cleansing enemas as ordered followed by digital removal of stool if necessary.
g. Carefully review bowel training program and revise it as needed.

□ ▬▬▬▬▬▬▬▬▬▬▬▬▬▬▬▬▬▬▬▬▬▬▬▬

14. NURSING DIAGNOSIS

Bowel incontinence related to lack of voluntary control over anal sphincter and lack of awareness of stool in rectum.

□ ▬▬▬▬▬▬▬▬▬▬▬▬▬▬▬▬▬▬▬▬▬▬▬▬

DESIRED OUTCOMES	NURSING ACTIONS AND *SELECTED RATIONALES*
14. The client will not experience bowel incontinence.	14.a. Monitor episodes of bowel incontinence. b. Establish and adhere to a bowel training program *in order to evacuate the rectum at regularly scheduled intervals and reduce the risk of incontinence.* (Bowel training program is outlined in Nursing Diagnosis 13, action e.) c. If bowel incontinence occurs despite implementation of above, carefully review bowel training program and revise it as needed.

□ ▬▬▬▬▬▬▬▬▬▬▬▬▬▬▬▬▬▬▬▬▬▬▬▬

15. NURSING DIAGNOSIS

Sleep pattern disturbance related to:

a. inability to assume usual sleep position associated with loss of motor function and use of devices to immobilize the spine (e.g. halo device, turning frame, circular bed);
b. frequent assessments and treatments;
c. fear and anxiety;
d. unfamiliar environment;
e. decreased physical activity.

□ ▬▬▬▬▬▬▬▬▬▬▬▬▬▬▬▬▬▬▬▬▬▬▬▬

DESIRED OUTCOMES	NURSING ACTIONS AND *SELECTED RATIONALES*
15. The client will attain necessary amounts of sleep within the parameters of the treatment regimen (see Care Plan on Immobility, Nursing Diagnosis 12, for outcome criteria).	15.a. Refer to Care Plan on Immobility, Nursing Diagnosis 12, for measures related to assessment and promotion of sleep. b. Implement additional measures *to promote sleep:* 1. assist client to assume a comfortable sleep position within limits of treatment plan (e.g. if client is more comfortable prone than supine, it may be possible to alter turning schedule to allow prone position for 3 rather than 2 hours during the night) 2. perform actions to decrease fear and anxiety (see Nursing Diagnosis 1, action c) 3. progress activity as allowed and tolerated.

□ ▬▬▬▬▬▬▬▬▬▬▬▬▬▬▬▬▬▬▬▬▬▬▬▬

16. NURSING DIAGNOSIS

Potential for infection:

a. **pneumonia** related to:
   1. stasis of secretions in the lungs associated with decreased mobility and poor cough effort resulting from paralysis of abdominal and intercostal muscles and weakened diaphragm;
   2. aspiration associated with difficulty swallowing while in positions necessary for spine immobilization (e.g. flat, supine; neck hyperextended);
b. **urinary tract infection** related to urinary stasis, alkaline urine associated with hypercalciuria, tears in the bladder mucosa resulting from distention, and intermittent catheterizations or indwelling catheter if present.

□ ▬▬▬▬▬▬▬▬▬▬▬▬▬▬▬▬▬▬▬▬▬▬▬▬

DESIRED OUTCOMES	NURSING ACTIONS AND *SELECTED RATIONALES*
16.a. The client will not develop pneumonia (see Care Plan on Immobility, Nursing Diagnosis 13, outcome a, for outcome criteria).	16.a.1. Refer to Care Plan on Immobility, Nursing Diagnosis 13, action a, for measures related to assessment, prevention, and treatment of pneumonia. 2. Implement additional measures *to prevent pneumonia:* a. perform actions to improve breathing pattern and promote effective airway clearance (see Nursing Diagnoses 3, actions a and c and 4) b. perform actions to reduce the risk of aspiration (see Nursing Diagnosis 18, action d).
16.b. The client will remain free of urinary tract infection as evidenced by: 1. clear urine 2. no unusual odor to urine 3. absence of chills and fever 4. absence of WBCs, bacteria, and/or nitrites in urine 5. negative urine culture.	16.b.1. Assess for and report signs and symptoms of urinary tract infection (e.g. cloudy, foul-smelling urine; elevated temperature; chills). 2. Monitor urinalysis and report presence of WBCs, bacteria, and/or nitrites. 3. Obtain a urine specimen for culture and sensitivity if ordered. Report abnormal results. 4. Refer to Care Plan on Immobility, Nursing Diagnosis 13, actions b.4 and 5, for measures related to prevention and treatment of urinary tract infection. 5. Implement measures to prevent urinary retention (see Nursing Diagnosis 12, actions a.4–6) *in order to further reduce the risk of urinary tract infection.*

UNIT
VI

17. NURSING DIAGNOSIS

Potential for trauma related to:

a. falls associated with loss of motor function, use of turning frame or circular electric bed, and spasticity;
b. burns associated with loss of motor and sensory function.

DESIRED OUTCOMES	NURSING ACTIONS AND *SELECTED RATIONALES*
17. The client will not experience falls or burns.	17.a. Determine whether conditions predisposing the client to falls and burns (e.g. loss of motor and sensory function, placement on turning frame or circular electric bed, spasticity) exist. b. Implement measures *to prevent falls:* 1. if client is in a standard hospital bed, keep bed in low position with side rails up 2. keep safety belts securely fastened when client is on a turning frame, in a circular electric bed, or in a chair *(severe and/or unexpected spasms can propel client onto the floor)* 3. obtain adequate assistance when turning client or transferring him/her from bed to stretcher or chair; utilize instructions from physical therapist on correct transfer techniques 4. encourage client to request assistance whenever needed; have pressure-sensitive call signal or whistle readily available to client 5. do not rush client; allow adequate time for him/her to assist with transfer and position changes 6. perform actions to decrease spasticity (see Nursing Diagnosis 10, action a.2.f). c. Implement measures *to prevent burns:* 1. let hot foods or fluids cool slightly before serving *in order to reduce risk of burns if spills occur* 2. supervise client while smoking 3. assess temperature of bath water and heating pad before and during use 4. when client is up in a wheelchair, instruct him/her to avoid placing self next to heaters or stoves. d. Include client and significant others in planning and implementing measures to prevent injury. e. If injury does occur, initiate appropriate first aid and notify physician.

18. NURSING DIAGNOSIS

Potential for aspiration related to difficulty swallowing associated with inability to flex neck when stabilization device is in place.

DESIRED OUTCOMES	NURSING ACTIONS AND *SELECTED RATIONALES*
18. The client will not aspirate secretions and foods/fluids as evidenced by:	18.a. Assess for factors that indicate potential for aspiration (e.g. inability to flex neck, choking on secretions and foods/fluids). b. Assess for signs and symptoms of aspiration of secretions or foods/fluids

a. clear breath sounds
b. resonant percussion note over lungs
c. respiratory rate at 16–20/minute
d. absence of dyspnea
e. absence of cyanosis.

(e.g. rhonchi, dull percussion note over lungs, tachycardia, rapid respirations, dyspnea, cyanosis).
c. Monitor chest x-ray results. Report findings of pulmonary infiltrate.
d. Implement measures *to reduce the risk of aspiration during the time that client is unable to flex neck due to the presence of stabilization device:*
   1. position client in side-lying, semi- to high Fowler's, or prone position as often as allowed
   2. have suction equipment readily available for use
   3. perform oropharyngeal suctioning and provide oral care as often as needed *to remove oral secretions*
   4. withhold oral foods/fluids if client is experiencing severe dysphagia
   5. when oral intake is allowed, perform actions *to improve swallowing and reduce the risk of choking:*
      a. maintain client in the following position during and for 30 minutes after meals and snacks:
         1. prone position if on turning frame
         2. prone position or, if allowed and tolerated, vertical position if on circular electric bed
         3. high Fowler's position if in halo device
      b. decrease external stimuli when client is eating and drinking *so he/she can concentrate on swallowing*
      c. encourage client to use a straw for all liquids and to take small sips and sip slowly when drinking
      d. provide small, frequent meals rather than 3 large ones *to decrease risk of gastric distention and regurgitation*
      e. cut food in bite-size pieces and remind client to chew food thoroughly
      f. allow ample time for meals
      g. instruct client to avoid laughing or talking while eating and drinking
      h. assist client with oral hygiene after eating *to ensure that food particles do not remain in mouth.*
e. If signs and symptoms of aspiration occur:
   1. perform tracheal suctioning
   2. notify physician
   3. prepare client for chest x-ray.

19. NURSING DIAGNOSIS

Dysreflexia related to uninhibited response of the sympathetic nervous system to noxious stimuli below the level of the cord injury after the period of spinal shock.

DESIRED OUTCOMES	NURSING ACTIONS AND *SELECTED RATIONALES*

19. The client will not experience dysreflexia as evidenced by:
    a. vital signs within normal range for client
    b. skin dry and usual color above the level of the injury
    c. no complaints of headache, nasal congestion, or blurred vision.

19.a. Assess for signs and symptoms of dysreflexia:
   1. sudden rise in B/P (may go as high as 300/140 mm Hg)
   2. bradycardia (a parasympathetic nervous system response to the increased B/P)
   3. flushing and profuse diaphoresis above level of injury
   4. severe, pounding headache
   5. nasal congestion
   6. blurred vision.
b. Implement measures *to prevent stimulation of the sympathetic nervous system in order to prevent dysreflexia:*
   1. perform actions to prevent overdistention of the bladder and bowel (see Nursing Diagnoses 12, actions a.4–6 and 13, actions e–g)
   2. perform actions *to prevent pressure on any area of the client's body below the level of the cord injury:*

UNIT VI

   a. change his/her position frequently
   b. ensure that overbed tray is not resting on client
   c. ensure that clothing is not constrictive and shoes are not too tight
   3. perform good nail care *(ingrown nails can cause sympathetic stimulation)*
   4. perform actions to prevent and treat urinary tract infection and urinary calculi (see Nursing Diagnosis 16, actions b.4 and 5 and Care Plan on Immobility, Collaborative Diagnosis 14, actions c.4 and 5)
   5. apply a topical anesthetic agent to any existing pressure sores
   6. apply a local anesthetic (e.g. Nupercainal ointment) or administer a ganglionic blocking agent (e.g. Inversine) if ordered before performing actions that may result in an exaggerated sympathetic response (e.g. urinary catheterization, removal of a fecal impaction, administration of an enema, bladder irrigation, care of any wound below the level of the injury).
 c. If signs and symptoms of dysreflexia occur:
   1. immediately raise head of bed and lower client's legs unless contraindicated *(this will usually decrease B/P significantly)*
   2. monitor B/P and pulse frequently
   3. assess for and, if possible, alleviate the condition causing sympathetic stimulation
   4. notify physician immediately if signs and symptoms persist or if complications resulting from severe hypertension (e.g. seizures, intraocular hemorrhage, cerebrovascular accident) occur
   5. monitor for therapeutic and nontherapeutic effects of intravenous antihypertensives (e.g. diazoxide, hydralazine, nitroprusside) if administered
   6. notify all staff of client's episode of dysreflexia *since such episodes can recur*
   7. prepare client for pelvic or pudendal nerve sectioning or posterior rhizotomy if indicated (these procedures may be necessary if client continues to have frequent episodes of dysreflexia)
   8. provide emotional support to client and significant others.

□ ▋▋▋▋▋▋▋▋▋▋▋▋▋▋▋▋▋▋▋▋▋▋▋▋

20. COLLABORATIVE DIAGNOSIS

Potential complications:

a. **further injury to the spinal cord** related to ascending inflammation and/or ischemia, compression of cord by hematoma or bone fragments, and/or ineffective stabilization of the injured area;

b. **thromboembolism** related to venous stasis associated with immobility and decreased vasomotor tone;

c. **gastrointestinal (GI) bleeding** related to:
   1. development of a stress ulcer (continued stress causes vagal stimulation that results in gastric hyperacidity and multiple diffuse erosions of the gastric and duodenal mucosa)
   2. irritation of the gastric mucosa associated with side effects of certain medications (e.g. corticosteroids, carbamazepine, phenytoin, some muscle relaxants);

d. **contractures** related to prolonged immobility of joints and severe spasticity.

□ ▋▋▋▋▋▋▋▋▋▋▋▋▋▋▋▋▋▋▋▋▋▋▋▋

DESIRED OUTCOMES	NURSING ACTIONS AND *SELECTED RATIONALES*
20.a. The client will not experience spinal cord injury above the level of C5	20.a.1. Assess for and report signs and symptoms of ascending spinal cord injury: a. respiratory failure (e.g. rapid, shallow respirations; dusky or cyanotic skin color; drowsiness; confusion)

as evidenced by:
1. stable respiratory status
2. stable B/P and pulse
3. stable or improved motor and sensory function.

b. significant decrease in pulse, significant change in B/P
c. further loss of motor and sensory function.
2. Implement measures *to prevent further injury to the spinal cord:*
    a. perform actions *to maintain stabilization of the cervical spine:*
        1. do not release skeletal traction or readjust halo device unless ordered
        2. if skeletal traction is present, keep traction rope and weights hanging freely
        3. always use turn sheet and adequate assistance when repositioning client; never use the bars of the halo device as handles
        4. check pin sites of halo or traction device every shift; notify physician if pins are loose
        5. if stabilization device fails (e.g. pins fall out, traction weights drop, rods on halo device disconnect):
            a. stabilize client's head, neck, and shoulders with hands and/or sandbags
            b. notify physician immediately
    b. remind staff to utilize the jaw thrust method rather than hyperextending client's neck if respiratory distress occurs
    c. monitor for therapeutic and nontherapeutic effects of corticosteroids if administered *to reduce inflammation of and around injured area of spinal cord.*
3. If signs and symptoms of ascending spinal cord injury occur:
    a. continue with above actions
    b. assist with intubation or tracheotomy and mechanical ventilation
    c. prepare client for surgical removal of the hematoma or bone fragments that may be compressing the cord or for laminectomy and fusion to stabilize a fracture if indicated
    d. provide emotional support to client and significant others.

20.b. The client will not develop a venous thrombus or pulmonary embolism (see Care Plan on Immobility, Collaborative Diagnosis 14, outcomes a.1 and 2, for outcome criteria).

20.b.1. Refer to Care Plan on Immobility, Collaborative Diagnosis 14, actions a.1 and 2, for measures related to assessment, prevention, and treatment of a venous thrombus and pulmonary embolism.
2. Implement additional measures *to prevent venous thrombus:*
    a. position firm pillow between client's legs if spasms tend to cause legs to cross
    b. instruct client to notify staff if legs cross *so that they can be repositioned properly.*

20.c. The client will not experience GI bleeding as evidenced by:
1. no complaints of shoulder pain
2. absence of occult or frank blood in stool and gastric contents
3. B/P and pulse within normal range for client
4. RBC, Hct., and Hgb. levels within normal range.

20.c.1. Assess for and report signs and symptoms of GI bleeding (e.g. complaints of shoulder pain [this is a referred pain], frank or occult blood in stool or gastric contents, decreased B/P, increased pulse).
2. Monitor RBC, Hct., and Hgb. levels. Report declining values.
3. Implement measures *to prevent ulceration of the gastric or duodenal mucosa:*
    a. perform actions to decrease fear and anxiety (see Nursing Diagnosis 1, action c)
    b. encourage client to reduce intake of foods/fluids that are acidic, spicy, or high in caffeine (e.g. chocolate, colas, coffee, tea)
    c. administer ulcerogenic medications (e.g. corticosteroids, phenytoin, carbamazepine, some muscle relaxants) with meals or snacks *to decrease gastric irritation*
    d. monitor for therapeutic and nontherapeutic effects of histamine$_2$ receptor antagonists (e.g. cimetidine, ranitidine, famotidine), antacids, and mucosal barrier fortifiers (e.g. sucralfate) if administered.
4. If signs and symptoms of GI bleeding occur:
    a. insert nasogastric tube and maintain suction as ordered
    b. assist with iced water or saline gastric lavage, transendoscopic electrocoagulation, selective arterial embolization, endoscopic laser photocoagulation, and/or intra-arterial administration of vasopressors (e.g. vasopressin) if ordered
    c. monitor for therapeutic and nontherapeutic effects of blood products and/or volume expanders if administered
    d. prepare client for surgery (e.g. ligation of bleeding vessels, partial gastrectomy) if indicated
    e. provide emotional support to client and significant others
    f. refer to Care Plan on Peptic Ulcer for additional care measures.

UNIT VI

20.d. The client will maintain normal range of motion.

20.d.1. Refer to Care Plan on Immobility, Collaborative Diagnosis 14, action d, for measures related to assessment and prevention of contractures.
2. Implement measures to reduce spasticity (see Nursing Diagnosis 10, action a.2.f) *in order to further reduce risk of contractures.*

☐ ▬▬▬▬▬▬▬▬▬▬▬▬▬▬▬▬▬▬▬▬▬▬▬▬▬▬

21. NURSING DIAGNOSIS

Sexual dysfunction:

a. **decreased libido** related to:
1. loss of sensory and motor function below the level of spinal cord injury
2. presence of a urinary catheter and/or fear of urinary and bowel incontinence
3. alteration in self-concept
4. fear of rejection by desired partner
5. fear of dysreflexia (genital stimulation may cause dysreflexia);
b. **decreased ability to control and maintain an erection** related to loss of ability to have a psychogenic erection (only reflexogenic erection is possible).

☐ ▬▬▬▬▬▬▬▬▬▬▬▬▬▬▬▬▬▬▬▬▬▬▬▬▬▬

DESIRED OUTCOMES	NURSING ACTIONS AND *SELECTED RATIONALES*

21. The client will demonstrate beginning acceptance of changes in sexual functioning as evidenced by:
   a. verbalization of a perception of self as sexually acceptable and adequate
   b. maintenance of relationships with significant others.

21.a. Assess for signs and symptoms of sexual dysfunction (e.g. verbalization of sexual concerns, failure to maintain relationships with significant others, limitations imposed by loss of motor and sensory function).
b. Determine attitudes, knowledge, and concerns about the effects of the spinal cord injury on sexual functioning.
c. Communicate interest, understanding, and respect for the values of the client and his/her partner.
d. Provide accurate information about effects of spinal cord injury on sexual functioning. Encourage questions and clarify misconceptions.
e. Facilitate communication between the client and his/her partner. Assist them to identify issues that may affect their sexual relationship.
f. Implement measures *to decrease the possibility of rejection by partner:*
   1. assist the partner to acknowledge both positive and negative feelings
   2. if appropriate, involve partner in care (e.g. bathing, dressing, transfer activities, bowel and bladder care) *to facilitate adjustment to and integration of the change in client's body image.*
g. Arrange for uninterrupted privacy during hospital stay if desired by the couple.
h. Implement measures to improve self-concept (see Nursing Diagnosis 22).
i. If appropriate, suggest alternative methods of sexual gratification and use of adaptive aids. Encourage partner to explore erogenous areas on the client's lips, neck, and ears.
j. Discuss ways to be creative in expressing sexuality (e.g. verbalizing fantasies, cuddling).
k. Inform male client and his partner of techniques for eliciting and maintaining reflexogenic erection (e.g. direct stimulation of genitalia, stroke inner thigh, stimulate the rectum, manipulate the urinary catheter).
l. If client experiences episodes of dysreflexia, instruct him/her to consult physician about ways to prevent it during sexual activity (e.g. take a ganglionic blocking agent before sexual activity, have partner apply a local anesthetic to area being stimulated).
m. If client has difficulty maintaining an erection, encourage him to discuss the possibility of a penile prosthesis with physician if desired.
n. Discuss alternative methods of parenting (e.g. adoption, artificial insemination) if of concern to client.
o. Inform female client that vaginal lubrication can occur by local stimulation or can be enhanced by using a water-soluble lubricant.

p. If client has an indwelling urethral catheter, instruct him/her on ways to fold and secure the catheter tubing.
q. If incontinence of urine or stool is a problem, instruct client to:
    1. have bowel care performed several hours before sexual activity
    2. limit fluid intake 2 hours before sexual activity
    3. have bladder emptied immediately before sexual activity.
r. Instruct client to establish a relaxed, unhurried atmosphere for sexual activity.
s. Provide explicit films and literature if desired by client and/or partner.
t. Include partner in above discussions and encourage his/her continued support of the client.
u. Consult physician when client is ready for sexual counseling and/or sexual counseling appears indicated.

---

22. NURSING DIAGNOSIS

Disturbance in self-concept* related to:

a. dependence on others to meet self-care needs;
b. feeling of powerlessness;
c. change in appearance associated with temporary presence of devices to immobilize the spine, necessity of wheelchair use, spasticity following period of spinal shock, and muscle atrophy (especially in lower extremities);
d. infertility (in males only) associated with:
    1. possible loss of ability to ejaculate
    2. possibility of retrograde ejaculation (can result from impaired innervation of the bladder neck)
    3. decreased sperm formation and viability resulting from testicular atrophy and impaired temperature regulation in the testes (occurs as a result of decreased scrotal reflexes);
e. changes in body functioning, life style, and roles.

---

* This diagnostic label includes the nursing diagnoses of body image disturbance and self-esteem disturbance.

DESIRED OUTCOMES	NURSING ACTIONS AND *SELECTED RATIONALES*

22. The client will demonstrate beginning adaptation to changes in body functioning, appearance, life style, roles, and level of independence (see Care Plan on Immobility, Nursing Diagnosis 16, for outcome criteria).	22.a. Refer to Care Plan on Immobility, Nursing Diagnosis 16, for measures related to assessment and promotion of a positive self-concept.
	    b. Implement additional measures *to promote a positive self-concept:*
	      1. reinforce actions to assist client to cope with effects of the spinal cord injury (see Nursing Diagnosis 23, action d)
	      2. perform actions to prevent urinary and bowel incontinence (see Nursing Diagnoses 12, actions b.2–4 and 14, actions b and c)
	      3. perform actions to reduce client's feelings of powerlessness (see Nursing Diagnosis 24)
	      4. perform actions to facilitate the grieving process (see Nursing Diagnosis 25, action d)
	      5. assure client that tongs and halo device are temporary and will be removed as soon as internal stabilization of the spine occurs; if brace or collar is needed after removal of the cranial pins, assist client to select clothing that makes the spinal support less obvious (e.g. high-collared shirts, loose-fitting shirts, capes rather than jackets)
	      6. demonstrate acceptance of client using techniques such as therapeutic touch and frequent visits

7. encourage client contact with others *so that he/she can test and establish a new self-image*
8. reinforce measures that may assist client to adjust to alterations in sexual functioning (see Nursing Diagnosis 21, actions c–t)
9. perform actions to increase the client's ability to perform self-care (see Nursing Diagnosis 11, action c) *in order to increase client's sense of independence*
10. provide privacy during client's attempts at self-care *in order to minimize embarrassment that he/she may feel because of deficits and clumsiness*
11. use terms such as disabled or handicapped rather than cripple or invalid; avoid use of slang (e.g. quad, gimp).

☐ ▄▄▄▄▄▄▄▄▄▄▄▄▄▄▄▄▄▄▄▄▄▄▄▄▄▄▄▄▄▄▄▄▄▄

23. NURSING DIAGNOSIS

Ineffective individual coping related to:

a. fear and anxiety;
b. changes in body functioning, life style, and roles;
c. need for lengthy rehabilitation;
d. inadequate support system.

☐ ▄▄▄▄▄▄▄▄▄▄▄▄▄▄▄▄▄▄▄▄▄▄▄▄▄▄▄▄▄▄▄▄▄▄

DESIRED OUTCOMES	NURSING ACTIONS AND *SELECTED RATIONALES*

23. The client will demonstrate the use of effective coping skills as evidenced by:
a. willingness to participate in treatment plan and self-care activities
b. verbalization of ability to cope with the effects of the spinal cord injury
c. identification of stressors
d. utilization of appropriate problem-solving techniques
e. recognition and utilization of available support systems.
	23.a. Assess effectiveness of client's coping strategies by observing behavior and noting strengths, weaknesses, ability to express feelings and concerns, and willingness to participate in the treatment plan.
	b. Assess for and report signs and symptoms that may indicate ineffective coping (e.g. sleep disturbances, increasing fatigue, difficulty concentrating, irritability, verbalization of inability to cope, inability to problem-solve).
	c. Allow time for client to adjust psychologically to the diagnosis and planned treatment, residual effects of the spinal cord injury, and anticipated life-style and role changes.
	d. Implement measures *to promote effective coping:*
	  1. arrange for a visit from another who has successfully adjusted to a similar injury
	  2. perform actions to decrease fear and anxiety (see Nursing Diagnosis 1, action c)
	  3. assist client to maintain usual daily routines whenever possible
	  4. include the client in planning of care, encourage maximum participation in treatment plan, and allow choices whenever possible *to enable him/her to maintain a sense of control over life*
	  5. instruct client in effective problem-solving techniques (e.g. accurate identification of stressors, determination of various options to solve problem)
	  6. if client is experiencing severe spasticity:
	    a. reinforce measures to reduce severity of the spasms (see Nursing Diagnosis 10, action a.2.f)
	    b. reinforce ways that spasms can be beneficial (e.g. help swing legs from bed to wheelchair, initiate arm movements, maintain an erection, evacuate bowels)
	    c. inform client that spasticity will stabilize in 1–2 years
	  7. inform client that there will be times when spasticity is worse, bowel and bladder programs are less effective, and efforts at self-care are less successful; assure him/her that these are temporary results of physical

and/or emotional stress or fatigue rather than an indication of deteriorating neurological status

8. provide diversional activities according to client's interests and abilities
9. assist client as he/she starts to plan for necessary life-style and role changes; provide input on realistic prioritization of problems that need to be dealt with
10. assist the client and significant others to identify ways that personal and family goals can be adjusted rather than abandoned
11. assist client to prepare for negative reactions from others because of his/her quadriplegia
12. set up a home evaluation appointment with occupational and physical therapists *so that the home environment will be wheelchair accessible before client's discharge*
13. assist client to identify and utilize available support systems; provide information regarding available community resources that can assist client and significant others in coping with effects of the injury (e.g. spinal cord injury groups).

   e. Encourage continued emotional support from significant others.
   f. Encourage the client to share with significant others the kind of support that would be most beneficial (e.g. listening, inspiring hope, providing reassurance and accurate information).
   g. Assess for and support behaviors suggesting positive adaptation to changes experienced (e.g. verbalization of ability to cope, recognition and utilization of available support systems).
   h. Consult physician about psychological or vocational rehabilitation counseling if appropriate. Initiate a referral if necessary.

□ ▬▬▬▬▬▬▬▬▬▬▬▬▬▬▬▬▬▬▬▬▬▬▬▬▬▬

24. NURSING DIAGNOSIS

Powerlessness related to:

a. quadriplegia;
b. dependence on others to meet basic needs;
c. feeling of loss of control over life;
d. alterations in usual roles, relationships, and future plans associated with effects of the injury and need for extensive and lengthy rehabilitation.

□ ▬▬▬▬▬▬▬▬▬▬▬▬▬▬▬▬▬▬▬▬▬▬▬▬▬▬

DESIRED OUTCOMES	NURSING ACTIONS AND *SELECTED RATIONALES*

24. The client will demonstrate increasing feelings of control over his/her situation (see Care Plan on Immobility, Nursing Diagnosis 17, for outcome criteria).	24.a. Refer to Care Plan on Immobility, Nursing Diagnosis 17, for measures related to assessment of feelings of powerlessness and measures to promote client's feelings of control over his/her situation.
	  b. Implement additional measures *to reduce client's feelings of powerlessness:*
	    1. perform actions to promote effective coping (see Nursing Diagnosis 23, action d) *in order to promote an increased sense of control over his/her situation*
	    2. support realistic hope about effects of rehabilitation on future independence
	    3. discuss with significant others client's need to maintain as much control over his/her life as possible; stress the necessity of their encouraging and allowing the client to actively participate in rehabilitation program scheduling and discharge planning.

UNIT VI

25. NURSING DIAGNOSIS

Grieving* related to loss of motor and sensory function and the effects of this loss on future life style and roles.

_____

* This diagnostic label includes anticipatory grieving and grieving following the actual losses/changes.

DESIRED OUTCOMES	NURSING ACTIONS AND *SELECTED RATIONALES*

25. The client will demonstrate beginning progression through the grieving process as evidenced by:
  a. verbalization of feelings about the loss of motor and sensory function and its effects on his/her life
  b. expression of grief
  c. participation in treatment plan and self-care activities
  d. utilization of available support systems
  e. verbalization of a plan for integrating prescribed follow-up care into life style.

25.a. Determine the client's perception of the impact of the spinal cord injury on his/her future.

b. Determine how the client usually expresses grief.

c. Observe for signs of grieving (e.g. changes in eating habits, insomnia, anger, noncompliance, denial).

d. Implement measures *to facilitate the grieving process:*
  1. assist client to acknowledge the losses and changes experienced *so grief work can begin;* assess for factors that may hinder or facilitate acknowledgment
  2. discuss the grieving process and assist client to accept the stages of grieving as an expected response to the actual and anticipated losses/changes; support the realization that grief may recur *because of the lengthy rehabilitation process and extensiveness of the losses/changes*
  3. allow time for client to progress through the stages of grieving (denial, anger, bargaining, depression, acceptance [Kübler-Ross, 1969]); be aware that not every stage is experienced or expressed by all individuals
  4. provide an atmosphere of care and concern (e.g. provide privacy, be available and nonjudgmental, display empathy and respect) *so that client will feel free to verbalize both positive and negative feelings and concerns*
  5. perform actions *to promote trust* (e.g. answer questions honestly, provide requested information)
  6. encourage the expression of anger and sadness about the losses and changes experienced; recognize displacement of anger and assist client to see actual cause of angry feelings and resentment; establish limits on abusive behavior
  7. encourage client to express his/her feelings in whatever ways are comfortable (e.g. conversation)
  8. perform actions to facilitate effective coping (see Nursing Diagnosis 23, action d)
  9. support realistic hope about effects of rehabilitation on future independence.

e. Assess for and support behaviors suggesting successful resolution of grief (e.g. verbalizing feelings about losses, expressing sorrow, focusing on ways to adapt to changes and losses).

f. Explain the stages of the grieving process to significant others. Encourage their support and understanding.

g. Provide information about counseling services and support groups that might assist client in working through grief.

h. Arrange for visit from clergy if desired by client.

i. Monitor for therapeutic and nontherapeutic effects of antidepressants if administered.

j. Consult physician about referral for counseling if signs of dysfunctional grieving (e.g. persistent denial of losses or changes, excessive anger or sadness, hysteria, suicidal behaviors, phobias) occur.

26. NURSING DIAGNOSIS

Social isolation related to:

a. immobility associated with quadriplegia and treatment plan for spine stabilization;
b. prolonged hospitalization;
c. depression associated with quadriplegia and its effect on future life style.

DESIRED OUTCOMES	NURSING ACTIONS AND *SELECTED RATIONALES*

26. The client will experience a decreased sense of isolation as evidenced by:
a. maintenance of relationships with significant others and casual acquaintances
b. verbalization of decreasing loneliness and feelings of rejection.
	26.a. Ascertain client's usual degree of social interaction.
	b. Assess for and report behaviors indicative of social isolation (e.g. decreased interaction with significant others and staff; expression of feelings of rejection, abandonment, or being different from others; hostility; sad affect).
	c. Encourage client to express feelings of rejection and aloneness. Provide feedback and support.
	d. Implement measures *to decrease social isolation:*
	  1. provide client with an effective method for contacting nurses' station (e.g. whistle, pressure-sensitive pad under shoulder or upper arm)
	  2. perform actions to reduce depression by implementing measures to facilitate client's psychological adjustment to effects of spinal cord injury (see Nursing Diagnoses 22; 23, action d; 24; and 25, action d)
	  3. encourage and assist client to use the telephone
	  4. set up a schedule of visiting times so that client will not go for long periods of time without visitors
	  5. schedule time each day to sit and talk with client
	  6. when client is allowed up in wheelchair, routinely move him/her to a more stimulating environment (e.g. hall, lounge, occupational therapy unit, garden)
	  7. assist client to identify a few persons he/she feels comfortable with and encourage interactions with them
	  8. change room assignments as feasible *to provide client with roommate with similar interests*
	  9. support any appropriate movement away from social isolation.
	e. Consult physician if signs and symptoms of social isolation persist or worsen.

27. NURSING DIAGNOSIS

Altered family processes related to change in family roles and structure associated with disability of family member and need for extensive rehabilitation.

DESIRED OUTCOMES	NURSING ACTIONS AND *SELECTED RATIONALES*
27. The family members* will demonstrate beginning	27.a. Identify components of the family and their patterns of communication and role expectations.

* The term "family member" is being used here to include client's significant others.

adjustment to changes in family roles and structure as evidenced by:
a. verbalization of ways to adapt to required role and life-style changes
b. active participation in decision making and client's rehabilitation
c. positive interactions with one another.

b. Assess for signs and symptoms of alterations in family processes (e.g. statements of not being able to accept client's quadriplegia or to make necessary role and life-style changes, inability to make decisions, inability or refusal to participate in client's rehabilitation, negative family interactions).

c. Implement measures *to facilitate family members' adjustment to changes in family roles and structure:*
1. encourage verbalization of feelings about client's quadriplegia and the effect of this on the family structure
2. reinforce physician's explanations of the injury and planned treatment and rehabilitation
3. provide privacy *so that family members and client can share their feelings with one another;* stress the importance and facilitate the use of good communication techniques
4. assist family members to progress through their own grieving process; explain that during this progression, they may encounter times when they need to focus on meeting their own rather than the client's needs
5. emphasize the need for family members to obtain adequate rest and nutrition and to identify and utilize stress management techniques *so that they are better able to emotionally and physically deal with the changes and losses experienced*
6. encourage and assist family members to identify coping strategies for dealing with the client's quadriplegia and its effects on the family
7. include family members in decision making about client and his/her care; convey appreciation for their input and continued support of client
8. encourage and allow family members to participate in client's care; provide necessary instruction and stress the importance of allowing the client to utilize adaptive devices and mobility aids *so that he/she can progress toward independence in whatever activities possible*
9. assist family members to identify resources that could assist them in coping with their feelings and meeting their immediate and long-term needs (e.g. counseling and social services; pastoral care; service, church, and spinal cord injury groups); initiate a referral if indicated.

d. Consult physician if family members continue to demonstrate difficulty adapting to changes in roles and family structure.

□ ▬▬▬▬▬▬▬▬▬▬▬▬▬▬▬▬▬

28. NURSING DIAGNOSIS

Knowledge deficit regarding follow-up care.*

---

* Although the client may not be able to perform many of the actions mentioned because of physical deficits, he/she must be aware of the appropriate actions in order to provide proper instruction to significant others and/or attendant and maintain an active role in rehabilitation.

□ ▬▬▬▬▬▬▬▬▬▬▬▬▬▬▬▬▬

DESIRED OUTCOMES	NURSING ACTIONS AND *SELECTED RATIONALES*

28.a. The client will identify ways to prevent complications associated with spinal cord injury and immobility.	28.a.1. Refer to Care Plan on Immobility, Nursing Diagnosis 19, action a, for instructions related to ways to prevent complications associated with immobility.
	2. Instruct client in additional ways *to prevent complications associated with spinal cord injury:*
	  a. position firm pillow between legs if spasms tend to cause legs to cross *(helps to prevent thrombophlebitis and adduction contractures)*
	  b. wear an abdominal binder when changing from reclining to a sitting position and take vasoconstrictor drugs as ordered *to prevent dizziness and fainting*

   c. implement measures to reduce severe spasticity (e.g. avoid fatigue and chills, change position at least every 2 hours, take muscle relaxants as prescribed) *in order to increase mobility and prevent contractures*

   d. use full-length and long-handled mirrors to examine all skin surfaces daily

   e. place adequate padding (e.g. foam, silicone gel, water pads) on chairs and bed *to prevent skin breakdown*

   f. implement measures *to prevent hyperthermia* (e.g. use tepid rather than hot bath water, keep environmental temperature in a comfortable range, avoid excessive clothing or blankets)

   g. implement measures *to prevent hypothermia* (e.g. wear adequate amounts of clothing, keep environmental temperature in a comfortable range, drink warm liquids)

   h. implement measures *to prevent falls* (e.g. always use safety belt during transfers and when in chair, be certain to have adequate assistance for transfer activity)

   i. implement measures *to prevent burns:*
     1. always check temperature of shower or bath water before use (can use bath water thermometer or have attendant check water temperature)
     2. never smoke when alone
     3. let hot foods/fluids cool slightly before attempting to feed self *to decrease risk of burns resulting from spills*
     4. never sit in a chair that is next to a stove, heater, or major source of heat

   j. implement measures *to prevent dysreflexia:*
     1. prevent bladder or bowel distention
     2. change position frequently
     3. seek medical attention at first sign of infection, persistent pressure area, ingrown toenail, or urinary calculi
     4. apply a topical anesthetic to area being stimulated or take a ganglionic blocking agent as ordered (routinely or before activities known to precipitate dysreflexia).

3. Demonstrate the following procedures to client, significant others, and care givers:
   a. "quad" coughing technique
   b. skin care
   c. proper positioning
   d. transfer techniques
   e. active and passive range of motion exercises
   f. application of antiembolic hose, abdominal binder, and heel and elbow protectors
   g. emergency treatment of dysreflexia (e.g. elevate head of bed and lower client's legs, alleviate causative factor, administer ganglionic blocking agent).

4. Allow time for questions, clarification, and return demonstration.

28.b. The client will demonstrate the ability to correctly use and care for adaptive devices.	**28.b.1.** Reinforce instructions of physical and occupational therapists on use of adaptive devices. Allow time for questions, clarification, and return demonstration.
	2. Instruct client in proper care of adaptive devices (e.g. replace worn parts, clean wheel hubs and crossbars of wheelchairs per manufacturer's instruction, keep wheelchair tires properly inflated).
28.c. The client will identify ways to manage bowel and bladder dysfunction.	**28.c.1.** Reinforce bladder and bowel training programs. (General guidelines are included in Nursing Diagnoses 12, actions a.5 and b.2 and 13, action e, but the exact program will vary with each client.)
	2. Demonstrate bowel care (e.g. digital stimulation, insertion of suppositories, administration of enemas) and bladder care (e.g. stimulation techniques, application of external catheter, intermittent catheterization, emptying of urinary collection bag). Allow time for questions, clarification, and return demonstration.

28.d. The client will state signs and symptoms to report to the health care provider.	**28.d.** Instruct the client to report the following:
	   1. cloudy, foul-smelling urine
	   2. nausea and vomiting

3. cough productive of purulent, green, or rust-colored sputum
4. difficulty breathing or increased shortness of breath with activity
5. persistent shoulder pain
6. fever, chills
7. uncontrollable diaphoresis
8. unsuccessful bowel and/or bladder training programs
9. swelling or redness of lower extremities
10. increased restriction of any joint motion
11. signs and symptoms of dysreflexia (e.g. severe, pounding headache; ringing in ears; slow pulse; flushing and diaphoresis above level of injury; nasal congestion) that do not subside once the stimulus is removed
12. any area of persistent skin irritation or breakdown
13. indications of pregnancy (stress that appropriate prenatal care should be initiated as soon as possible).

28.e. The client will identify community resources that can assist with home management and adjustment to changes resulting from spinal cord injury.

28.e.1. Inform client and significant others of community resources that can assist with home management and adjustment to changes resulting from spinal cord injury (e.g. spinal cord injury support and social groups; Visiting Nurse Association; community health agencies; local service groups; financial, individual, family, and vocational rehabilitation counselors).
2. Initiate a referral if indicated.

28.f. The client will verbalize an understanding of and a plan for adhering to recommended follow-up care including future appointments with health care provider and occupational and physical therapists and medications prescribed.

28.f.1. Reinforce the importance of keeping scheduled follow-up visits with health care provider and occupational and physical therapists.
2. Explain the rationale for, side effects of, and importance of taking prescribed medications (e.g. ganglionic blocking agents, antispasmodics, muscle relaxants, antidepressants).
3. Implement measures designed *to improve client compliance:*
   a. include significant others and caregivers in teaching sessions
   b. encourage questions and allow time for reinforcement or clarification of information provided
   c. provide written instructions on scheduled appointments with health care provider and occupational and physical therapists, medications prescribed, and signs and symptoms to report.

☐ ▬▬▬▬▬▬▬▬▬▬▬▬▬▬▬▬▬▬▬▬▬▬▬

Reference

Kübler-Ross. On death and dying. New York: Macmillan, 1969.

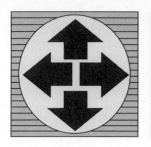
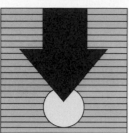
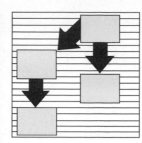
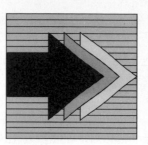
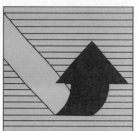

Unit VII

Nursing Care of the Client with Disturbances of Cardiovascular Function

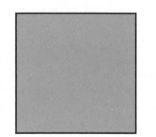

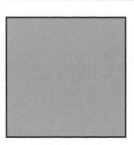

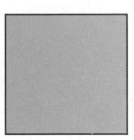

Angina Pectoris

Angina pectoris is a syndrome characterized by transient episodes of substernal or precordial chest pain that are due to a coronary blood supply that is insufficient to meet myocardial oxygen needs. Angina attacks are usually associated with atherosclerosis of a major coronary artery. The atherosclerotic vessels are unable to dilate and therefore cannot supply sufficient blood to the myocardium at times when the myocardial oxygen needs are increased. Other conditions that can compromise coronary blood flow are spasm and/or thrombosis of a coronary artery, generalized vasoconstriction, hypotension, hypovolemia, and aortic stenosis. Factors that reduce oxygen availability (e.g. anemia, smoking, oxyhemoglobin disorders) or increase cardiac workload (e.g. physical or emotional stress, smoking, exposure to cold, heavy meals, mitral regurgitation) may precipitate or increase the frequency of angina attacks by widening the gap between oxygen needs and availability.

There are several types of angina pectoris. The most common type is chronic stable angina that is usually precipitated by physical exertion or emotional stress, lasts 3–5 minutes, and is relieved by rest and nitroglycerin. Other types include unstable or crescendo angina, variant or Prinzmetal's angina, nocturnal angina, angina decubitus, and intractable or refractory angina. These various types differ in relation to severity of the attack, refractoriness of the pain, and typical precipitants of the attack. In all types of angina, the pain usually occurs in the substernal or precordial area; may or may not radiate; and is described as a heavy, gripping, squeezing, burning, or aching pain.

This care plan focuses on the adult client hospitalized during an attack of chest pain suspected to be angina. The goals of care are to relieve pain, prevent complications, and educate the client regarding follow-up care.

DISCHARGE CRITERIA

Prior to discharge, the client will:

- verbalize a basic understanding of angina pectoris
- identify factors that may precipitate angina attacks and ways to control these factors
- identify modifiable cardiovascular risk factors and ways to reduce these factors
- verbalize an understanding of the rationale for and constituents of the prescribed diet
- demonstrate accuracy in counting pulse
- verbalize an understanding of medication therapy including rationale for, side effects of, schedule for taking, and importance of taking as prescribed
- state signs and symptoms to report to the health care provider
- identify community resources that can assist in making necessary life-style changes and adjusting to the effects of angina pectoris
- verbalize an understanding of and a plan for adhering to recommended follow-up care including future appointments with health care provider.

NURSING/COLLABORATIVE DIAGNOSES

1. Anxiety □ *299*
2. Pain: radiating or nonradiating substernal or precordial chest pain □ *300*
3. Potential complications:
   a. arrhythmias
   b. myocardial infarction □ *301*
4. Knowledge deficit regarding follow-up care □ *302*

1. NURSING DIAGNOSIS

Anxiety related to unfamiliar environment; severe pain; sense of impending death; lack of understanding of diagnostic tests, diagnosis, and treatment plan; and implications of angina pectoris on future life style and roles.

DESIRED OUTCOMES	NURSING ACTIONS AND *SELECTED RATIONALES*

1. The client will experience a reduction in fear and anxiety as evidenced by:
   a. verbalization of feeling less anxious or fearful
   b. relaxed facial expression and body movements
   c. stable vital signs
   d. usual skin color
   e. verbalization of an understanding of hospital routines, diagnostic procedures, diagnosis, and treatments.

1.a. Assess client for signs and symptoms of fear and anxiety (e.g. verbalization of fears and concerns; tenseness; tremors; irritability; restlessness; diaphoresis; tachypnea; tachycardia; elevated blood pressure; facial tension, pallor, or flushing; noncompliance with treatment plan).
   b. Ascertain effectiveness of current coping skills.
   c. Implement measures *to reduce fear and anxiety:*
      1. provide care in a calm, confident manner
      2. if client is having severe pain:
         a. do not leave him/her alone during period of acute distress
         b. perform actions to relieve pain (see Nursing Diagnosis 2, action e)
      3. once period of acute distress has subsided:
         a. orient to hospital environment, equipment, and routines; include an explanation of cardiac monitoring equipment
         b. keep cardiac monitor out of client's view and the sound turned as low as possible
         c. introduce staff who will be participating in his/her care; if possible, maintain consistency in staff assigned to his/her care *to provide feelings of stability and comfort with the environment*
         d. assure client that staff members are nearby; respond to call signal as soon as possible
         e. encourage verbalization of fear and anxiety; provide feedback
         f. explain all diagnostic tests:
            1. serum cardiac enzyme levels, EKG, nuclear imaging, and vectorcardiography *to rule out myocardial infarction*
            2. serum triglyceride and cholesterol levels and lipoprotein profile *to determine the presence and type of hyperlipidemia*
            3. upper gastrointestinal series and cholecystogram *to rule out gastrointestinal disorders*
            4. exercise stress test and nuclear imaging *to determine if angina pectoris is stress induced*
            5. angiography and nuclear imaging *to determine need for percutaneous transluminal coronary angioplasty or coronary artery bypass grafting*
         g. reinforce physician's explanations and clarify any misconceptions client may have about angina pectoris, the treatment plan, and prognosis; stress to client that he/she has not had a "heart attack"
         h. reinforce physician's explanation of percutaneous transluminal coronary angioplasty (PTCA) if planned
         i. initiate preoperative teaching if heart surgery is planned
         j. instruct in relaxation techniques and encourage participation in diversional activities
         k. assist client to identify specific stressors and ways to cope with them
         l. allow client to discuss concerns about future life style and roles; focus on the need for alteration in rather than elimination of activities
         m. encourage significant others to project a caring, concerned attitude without obvious anxiousness
         n. monitor for therapeutic and nontherapeutic effects of antianxiety agents if administered.
   d. Include significant others in orientation and teaching sessions and encourage their continued support of the client.

UNIT VII

e. Provide information based on current needs of client and significant others at a level they can understand. Encourage questions and clarification of information provided.
f. Consult physician if above actions fail to control fear and anxiety.

□ ▬▬

2. NURSING DIAGNOSIS

Pain: radiating or nonradiating substernal or precordial chest pain related to decreased myocardial oxygenation (an insufficient oxygen supply forces the myocardium to convert to anaerobic metabolism resulting in lactic acid release; lactic acid acts as an irritant to myocardial neural receptors).

□ ▬▬

DESIRED OUTCOMES	NURSING ACTIONS AND *SELECTED RATIONALES*

2. The client will experience diminished chest, arm, neck, and jaw pain as evidenced by:
a. verbalization of pain relief
b. relaxed facial expression and body positioning
c. increased participation in activities
d. stable vital signs.
	2.a. Determine how the client usually responds to pain.
	b. Assess for nonverbal signs of pain (e.g. wrinkled brow; clenched fists; rubbing of neck, jaw, or arm; reluctance to move; clutching chest; restlessness; shallow, guarded respirations; diaphoresis; facial pallor or flushing; change in B/P; tachycardia).
	c. Assess verbal complaints of pain. Ask client to be specific about onset, location, type, severity, and duration of pain.
	d. Assess for factors that seem to aggravate and alleviate pain.
	e. Implement measures *to relieve pain:*
	  1. monitor for therapeutic and nontherapeutic effects of nitrates (e.g. nitroglycerin, isosorbide dinitrate) and nitrites (e.g. amyl nitrite) if administered *(the vasodilatory effect of these medications reduces preload and afterload, which decreases cardiac workload and myocardial oxygen consumption)*
	  2. perform additional actions *to improve myocardial oxygenation:*
	    a. maintain oxygen therapy as ordered
	    b. maintain client on bedrest in a semi- to high Fowler's position
	    c. implement measures to reduce fear and anxiety (see Nursing Diagnosis 1, action c)
	  3. consult physician about administration of a narcotic analgesic if pain is unrelieved by above measures within 15–20 minutes (these medications are usually administered intravenously *because injections are poorly absorbed if tissue perfusion is decreased; intramuscular injections also elevate serum enzyme levels, which may alter assessment of myocardial damage)*
	  4. provide or assist with nonpharmacological measures for pain relief (e.g. back rub, position change, relaxation techniques, quiet conversation, restful environment, diversional activities).
	f. Consult physician if pain persists or worsens.
	g. Implement measures *to prevent recurrent angina attacks:*
	  1. perform actions *to reduce cardiac workload and myocardial oxygen requirements:*
	    a. place client in a semi- to high Fowler's position
	    b. instruct client to avoid activities that create a Valsalva response (e.g. straining to have a bowel movement, bending at the waist, holding breath while moving)
	    c. promote physical and emotional rest
	    d. provide frequent, small meals rather than 3 large ones *(large meals require an increase in blood supply to gastrointestinal tract for digestion)*
	    e. discourage intake of foods/fluids high in caffeine such as coffee, tea,

chocolate, and colas *(caffeine is a myocardial stimulant and increases myocardial oxygen consumption)*
  f. discourage smoking *(smoking has a cardiostimulatory effect, causes vasoconstriction, and reduces oxygen availability)*
  g. increase activity gradually
  h. monitor for therapeutic and nontherapeutic effects of the following medications if administered:
    1. beta-adrenergic blocking agents (e.g. propranolol, pindolol, atenolol, nadolol, timolol, metoprolol) *to decrease myocardial contractility and heart rate, thereby reducing myocardial oxygen consumption*
    2. calcium-channel blockers (e.g. nifedipine, verapamil, diltiazem) *to produce peripheral and coronary artery dilation and decrease the force of myocardial contractility*
  2. perform actions as ordered to treat anemia, hypertension, hypotension, hyperthyroidism, or chronic obstructive pulmonary disease *(these conditions reduce oxygen availability and/or increase cardiac workload).*

□ ▆▆▆▆▆▆▆▆▆▆▆▆▆▆▆▆▆▆▆▆▆▆▆▆▆▆▆▆▆▆▆▆▆▆

3. COLLABORATIVE DIAGNOSIS

Potential complications:

a. **arrhythmias** related to cellular irritability associated with myocardial hypoxia;
b. **myocardial infarction** related to severe, prolonged, myocardial ischemia.

□ ▆▆▆▆▆▆▆▆▆▆▆▆▆▆▆▆▆▆▆▆▆▆▆▆▆▆▆▆▆▆▆▆▆▆

DESIRED OUTCOMES	NURSING ACTIONS AND *SELECTED RATIONALES*

3.a. The client will not experience cardiac arrhythmias as evidenced by:
  1. regular apical pulse at 60–100 beats/minute
  2. equal apical and radial pulses
  3. absence of syncope and palpitations
  4. EKG reading showing normal sinus rhythm.

3.a.1. Assess for and report signs and symptoms of arrhythmias (e.g. irregular apical pulse; pulse rate below 60 or above 100 beats/minute; apical-radial pulse deficit; syncope; palpitations; abnormal rate, rhythm, or configurations on EKG).
  2. Implement measures *to improve myocardial oxygenation in order to prevent arrhythmias:*
    a. monitor for therapeutic and nontherapeutic effects of nitrates (e.g. nitroglycerin, isosorbide dinitrate) and nitrites (e.g. amyl nitrite) if administered *to reduce preload and afterload, which decreases cardiac workload and myocardial oxygen consumption*
    b. maintain oxygen therapy as ordered
    c. perform actions to reduce cardiac workload and myocardial oxygen requirements (see Nursing Diagnosis 2, action g.1).
  3. If arrhythmias occur:
    a. initiate cardiac monitoring if not already being done
    b. monitor for therapeutic and nontherapeutic effects of the following medications if administered:
      1. Class I antiarrhythmics (e.g. phenytoin, tocainide, lidocaine, flecainide, procainamide, disopyramide, quinidine) *to interfere directly with depolarization*
      2. Class II antiarrhythmics (e.g. propranolol) *to block beta-adrenergic stimulation*
      3. Class III antiarrhythmics (e.g. bretylium, amiodarone) *to prolong the duration of the action potential*
      4. Class IV antiarrhythmics (e.g. verapamil, diltiazem) *to block the slow inward depolarizing current*
      5. anticholinergic agents (e.g. atropine) or sympathomimetics (e.g. ephedrine, isoproterenol) *to increase heart rate*
      6. cardiac glycosides (e.g. digitalis) *to decrease heart rate*

c. restrict client's activity based on his/her tolerance and severity of the arrhythmia

d. maintain oxygen therapy as ordered

e. assist with cardioversion if performed

f. assess cardiovascular status closely and report signs and symptoms of inadequate tissue perfusion (e.g. decline in B/P; cool, clammy, mottled skin; cyanosis; diminished peripheral pulses; declining urine output; increased restlessness and agitation; shortness of breath)

g. have emergency cart readily available for cardiopulmonary resuscitation.

3.b. The client will not experience a myocardial infarction as evidenced by:
1. resolution of chest pain within 15–20 minutes
2. stable vital signs
3. no elevation or only slight elevation of cardiac enzymes
4. absence of ST segment elevation, T wave changes, and pathological Q wave on EKG reading.

3.b.1. Assess for and report signs and symptoms of a myocardial infarction (e.g. chest pain that lasts longer than 20 minutes and is not relieved by a short-acting nitrate or nitrite; increase in pulse rate; decline in B/P; labored respirations; marked elevation of cardiac enzymes [CPK-MB is the first to increase]; ST segment elevation, T wave changes, and/or pathological Q wave on EKG [ST segment elevation can also occur in Prinzmetal's angina]).

2. Implement measures to improve myocardial oxygenation (see action a.2 in this diagnosis).

3. If signs and symptoms of a myocardial infarction occur:
a. initiate cardiac monitoring if not already being done
b. maintain client on strict bedrest in a semi- to high Fowler's position
c. maintain oxygen therapy as ordered
d. monitor for therapeutic and nontherapeutic effects of the following medications if administered:
1. morphine sulfate *to reduce pain and anxiety and decrease cardiac workload*
2. vasodilators *to reduce preload and/or afterload*
3. positive inotropic agents *to improve cardiac output*
4. beta-adrenergic blocking agents *to reduce sympathetic stimulation of the heart*
e. initiate cardiopulmonary resuscitation if indicated
f. provide emotional support to client and significant others
g. refer to Care Plan on Myocardial Infarction for additional care measures.

4. NURSING DIAGNOSIS

Knowledge deficit regarding follow-up care.

DESIRED OUTCOMES	NURSING ACTIONS AND *SELECTED RATIONALES*
4.a. The client will verbalize a basic understanding of angina pectoris.	4.a. Explain angina pectoris in terms the client can understand. Utilize teaching aids (e.g. pamphlets, diagrams) whenever possible.
4.b. The client will identify factors that may precipitate angina attacks and ways to control these factors.	4.b.1. Inform the client of factors that may precipitate angina pectoris (e.g. strenuous or isometric exercises, change in usual sexual habits and/or partner, straining to have a bowel movement, consumption of a large meal, exposure to extreme cold, strong emotions, smoking). 2. Provide the following instructions regarding ways *to reduce risk of precipitating an angina attack:* a. take sublingual nitroglycerin 5–10 minutes before strenuous activity or sexual intercourse and during times of high emotional stress b. adhere to a planned and regular isotonic exercise program (e.g. walking, biking, swimming) c. avoid isometric exercise (e.g. weight lifting, muscle tightening or setting)

d. stop any activity that causes chest pain, shortness of breath, palpitations, dizziness, or extreme fatigue and weakness

e. begin a cardiovascular fitness program when approved by physician

f. adhere to the following precautions regarding sexual activity:

  1. avoid intercourse for 2–3 hours after a heavy meal or alcohol consumption

  2. assume usual positions and experiment with ones that may reduce exertion (e.g. side-lying, partner on top)

  3. rest before and after intercourse

  4. avoid anal intercourse *(may initiate a vasovagal response)*

  5. maintain consistency in sexual partners.

4.c. The client will identify modifiable cardiovascular risk factors and ways to reduce these factors.

4.c.1. Inform client that the following modifiable factors have been shown to contribute to heart disease:

  a. obesity

  b. diet high in saturated fat and cholesterol

  c. sedentary life style

  d. smoking

  e. heavy alcohol intake (more than 2 ounces of ethanol/day on a regular basis)

  f. hypertension

  g. stressful life style.

2. Assist client to identify ways he/she can make appropriate changes in life style to reduce above factors.

3. Instruct client to take antihyperlipidemic medications (e.g. clofibrate, nicotinic acid, cholestyramine, probucol) and antiplatelet agents (e.g. sulfinpyrazone, aspirin, dipyridamole) as prescribed.

4.d. The client will verbalize an understanding of the rationale for and constituents of the prescribed diet.

4.d.1. Explain the rationale for a diet low in saturated fat and cholesterol.

2. Instruct client to reduce intake of foods high in saturated (animal) fat and cholesterol (e.g. butter, cheese, ice cream, egg yolks, shrimp, cashew nuts, organ meats).

3. If physician has recommended a diet high in fiber, explain that soluble fiber is believed by some to control progression of atherosclerosis. Provide a list of foods high in soluble fiber (e.g. oat bran, most fruits and vegetables, dried peas and beans).

4.e. The client will demonstrate accuracy in counting pulse.

4.e.1. Teach client to count his/her pulse, being alert to the regularity of the rhythm.

2. Allow time for return demonstration and accuracy check.

4.f. The client will verbalize an understanding of medication therapy including rationale for, side effects of, schedule for taking, and importance of taking as prescribed.

4.f.1. Explain the rationale for, side effects of, and importance of taking the medications prescribed.

2. If client is discharged on nitroglycerin, instruct to:

  a. avoid alcohol when using nitroglycerin *(both cause vasodilation and may precipitate severe hypotension when used concurrently)*

  b. have tablets readily available at all times

  c. take a tablet before strenuous activity or in emotionally stressful situations

  d. take one tablet when chest pain occurs and another every 5 minutes up to a total of 3 times if necessary; notify physician if pain persists

  e. place tablets under tongue and allow them to dissolve thoroughly before swallowing

  f. store tablets in a cool place in a light-resistant, airtight bottle or stainless steel container and replace tablets every 6 months; when opening bottle for initial use, remove cotton plug and do not replace it

  g. avoid rising to a standing position quickly after taking nitroglycerin *in order to reduce dizziness associated with its vasodilatory effect*

  h. recognize that dizziness, flushing, and mild headache may occur after taking nitroglycerin; instruct client to notify physician if severe headache or fainting occurs

  i. if nitroglycerin skin patches are prescribed:

    1. provide instructions about correct application, skin care, need to rotate sites, and frequency of change

    2. caution client that activities that increase blood flow to the skin

(e.g. exercise, hot bath, sauna) can cause a sudden reduction in blood pressure.

3. If client is discharged on a beta-adrenergic blocking agent (e.g. propranolol, metoprolol, atenolol, nadolol, timolol, pindolol), instruct to:
   a. take the medication on a regular basis and consistently either before or after meals *to minimize variations in absorption*
   b. check pulse before taking medication; consult physician if pulse rate is more irregular or below 60 beats/minute
   c. avoid skipping doses, trying to make up for missed doses, altering the prescribed dose, or discontinuing medication without physician's permission
   d. change from a lying to a sitting or standing position slowly *in order to prevent dizziness*
   e. avoid prolonged standing *to reduce pooling of blood in legs*
   f. avoid alcohol intake or drink moderately (less than 2 ounces of ethanol/day).
4. If client is discharged on a calcium-channel blocker (e.g. nifedipine, verapamil, diltiazem), instruct to:
   a. avoid skipping doses, altering the prescribed dose, or discontinuing medication without physician's permission
   b. change from a lying to a sitting or standing position slowly *in order to prevent dizziness*
   c. keep a record of the need for nitroglycerin while on calcium-channel blocker; report an increasing need for nitroglycerin
   d. keep medication in a cool place in an airtight, light-resistant container.
5. Instruct client to consult physician before taking other prescription and nonprescription medications.
6. Instruct client to inform all health care providers of medications being taken.

4.g. The client will state signs and symptoms to report to the health care provider.

4.g. Stress the importance of reporting the following signs and symptoms:
1. chest pain unrelieved by rest and/or nitroglycerin taken every 5 minutes for 15 minutes
2. shortness of breath
3. irregular pulse or a resting pulse less than 60 or greater than 100 beats/minute
4. fainting spells
5. diminished activity tolerance
6. increase in severity or frequency of angina attacks.

4.h. The client will identify community resources that can assist in making necessary life-style changes and adjusting to the effects of angina pectoris.

4.h.1. Provide information about community resources that can assist client in making life-style changes and adjusting to effects of angina pectoris (e.g. weight loss, stop smoking, and stress management programs; American Heart Association; YMCA; counseling services).
2. Initiate a referral if indicated.

4.i. The client will verbalize an understanding of and a plan for adhering to recommended follow-up care including future appointments with health care provider.

4.i.1. Reinforce the importance of keeping follow-up appointments with health care provider.
2. Implement measures *to improve client compliance:*
   a. include significant others in teaching sessions if possible
   b. encourage questions and allow time for reinforcement or clarification of information provided
   c. provide written instructions regarding future appointments with health care provider, dietary modifications, activity level, medications prescribed, and signs and symptoms to report.

Congestive Heart Failure

Congestive heart failure (CHF) is a syndrome characterized by vascular congestion and an inability of the heart to pump sufficient amounts of blood to meet the body's metabolic needs. Congestive heart failure can result from conditions that impair normal cardiac function (e.g. coronary artery disease, inflammatory heart conditions, cardiomyopathy, myocardial infarction, arrhythmias, constrictive pericarditis, valvular defects) or cause a prolonged increase in cardiac workload (e.g. hypertension, obesity, severe infection, thyrotoxicosis, fluid overload, pulmonary hypertension, prolonged physical or emotional stress, anemia).

Congestive heart failure is a chronic condition resulting from dysfunction of one or both ventricles. Signs and symptoms are dependent on which side of the heart is failing as well as whether there is forward or backward failure. Symptoms of forward failure are due to low cardiac output and symptoms of backward failure are associated with blood flow backup. Left-sided heart failure is the result of left ventricular damage (particularly common after a myocardial infarction) or hypertrophy resulting from the ventricle having to pump blood against increased resistance. In left-sided failure there is reduced emptying of the left ventricle, which results in decreased systemic tissue perfusion as well as blood flow backup in the left atrium and pulmonary vasculature. Pulmonary vascular congestion leads to pulmonary edema with symptoms such as dyspnea, cyanosis, and adventitious breath sounds. Right-sided heart failure is a result of right ventricular damage or hypertrophy due to the right ventricle having to pump blood against increased resistance in the pulmonary vessels. The effect of this is reduced emptying of the right ventricle. This leads to decreased pulmonary blood flow as well as backup of blood in the right atrium and peripheral venous congestion, which is manifested by peripheral edema and signs of major organ enlargement and dysfunction.

As long as the body's compensatory mechanisms (sympathetic nervous system activation, renin-angiotensin-aldosterone release, antidiuretic hormone release, cardiac dilation and hypertrophy) are able to maintain adequate tissue perfusion, a state of compensated heart failure is maintained. If the myocardium is severely damaged and intrinsic compensatory mechanisms fail to maintain adequate cardiac output and tissue perfusion, a state of decompensated heart failure exists. If therapeutic measures fail to reverse this state, cardiogenic shock ensues, resulting in tissue anoxia and death.

This care plan focuses on the adult client with signs and symptoms of decompensated right- and left-sided heart failure hospitalized for diagnosis, identification of causative factors, and treatment. The goals of care are to reduce cardiac workload, improve cardiac output, prevent complications, and educate the client regarding follow-up care.

UNIT VII

DISCHARGE CRITERIA

Prior to discharge, the client will:

- identify modifiable cardiovascular risk factors and ways to reduce these factors
- verbalize an understanding of the rationale for and constituents of a diet low in sodium, saturated fat, and cholesterol
- demonstrate accuracy in counting pulse
- verbalize an understanding of medication therapy including rationale for, side effects of, schedule for taking, and importance of taking as prescribed
- state signs and symptoms to report to the health care provider
- identify community resources that can assist with home management and adjustment to changes resulting from congestive heart failure
- share feelings and concerns about changes in body functioning and usual roles and life style
- verbalize an understanding of and a plan for adhering to recommended follow-up care including future appointments with health care provider and activity limitations.

Use in conjunction with the Care Plan on Immobility.

NURSING/COLLABORATIVE DIAGNOSES

1. Anxiety □ *306*
2. Decreased cardiac output □ *307*
3. Altered respiratory function:
   a. ineffective breathing patterns
   b. ineffective airway clearance
   c. impaired gas exchange □ *309*
4. Altered fluid balance:
   a. fluid volume excess
   b. third-spacing of fluid □ *310*
5. Altered nutrition: less than body requirements □ *312*
6. Altered comfort: nausea and vomiting □ *313*
7. Impaired skin integrity: irritation and breakdown □ *313*
8. Altered oral mucous membrane: dryness □ *314*
9. Activity intolerance □ *315*
10. Self-care deficit □ *315*
11. Constipation □ *316*
12. Altered thought processes: slowed verbal responses, shortened attention span, impaired memory, and confusion □ *316*
13. Sleep pattern disturbance □ *317*
14. Potential for trauma □ *317*
15. Potential complications:
    a. impaired renal function
    b. impaired liver function
    c. thromboembolism
    d. cardiogenic shock □ *318*
16. Disturbance in self-concept □ *320*
17. Grieving □ *321*
18. Noncompliance □ *322*
19. Knowledge deficit regarding follow-up care □ *323*

1. NURSING DIAGNOSIS

Anxiety related to unfamiliar environment; difficulty breathing; and lack of understanding of diagnostic tests, the diagnosis, treatments, and prognosis.

DESIRED OUTCOMES	NURSING ACTIONS AND *SELECTED RATIONALES*
1. The client will experience a reduction in fear and anxiety as evidenced by: a. verbalization of feeling less anxious or fearful b. relaxed facial expression and body movements c. stable vital signs	1.a. Assess client for signs and symptoms of fear and anxiety (e.g. verbalization of fears and concerns; tenseness; tremors; irritability; restlessness; increased dyspnea; diaphoresis; tachycardia; elevated blood pressure; facial tension, pallor, or flushing; noncompliance with treatment plan). Validate perceptions carefully, remembering that some behaviors may result from tissue hypoxia or fluid imbalance. b. Ascertain effectiveness of current coping skills. c. Implement measures *to reduce fear and anxiety:*

d. usual skin color
e. verbalization of an understanding of hospital routines, diagnostic procedures, diagnosis, treatments, and prognosis.

1. maintain a calm, confident manner when interacting with client
2. if client is in acute respiratory distress:
   a. do not leave him/her alone during this period
   b. perform actions to improve respiratory status (see Nursing Diagnosis 3, action e)
   c. perform actions *to reduce feeling of suffocation:*
      1. open curtains and doors
      2. approach client from the side rather than face-on *(close face-on contact may make client feel closed in)*
      3. limit the number of visitors in room at any one time
      4. remove unnecessary equipment from room
      5. administer oxygen via nasal cannula rather than mask if possible
3. encourage significant others to project a caring, concerned attitude without obvious anxiousness
4. once the period of acute respiratory distress has subsided:
   a. orient to hospital environment, equipment, and routines
   b. introduce staff who will be participating in his/her care; if possible, maintain consistency in staff assigned to his/her care *to provide feelings of stability and comfort with the environment*
   c. assure client that staff members are nearby; respond to call signal as soon as possible
   d. provide a calm, restful environment
   e. keep cardiac monitor out of client's view and the sound turned as low as possible
   f. encourage verbalization of fear and anxiety; provide feedback
   g. explain all diagnostic tests (e.g. blood studies, chest x-ray, EKG, nuclear imaging, echocardiography, carotid and/or jugular pulse tracing, pulmonary artery catheterization and pressure measurements)
   h. reinforce physician's explanations and clarify any misconceptions the client may have about CHF, the treatment plan, and prognosis
   i. reinforce physician's explanation of invasive measures or surgery that may be performed to improve cardiovascular status (e.g. intra-aortic balloon pump [IABP], artificial heart or ventricular assist device implant, heart transplant)
   j. instruct in relaxation techniques and encourage participation in diversional activities
   k. assist client to identify specific stressors and ways to cope with them
   l. monitor for therapeutic and nontherapeutic effects of antianxiety agents if administered.
d. Include significant others in orientation and teaching sessions and encourage their continued support of the client.
e. Provide information based on current needs of client and significant others at a level they can understand. Encourage questions and clarification of information provided.
f. Consult physician if above actions fail to control fear and anxiety.

☐ ▬▬▬▬▬▬▬▬▬▬▬▬▬▬▬▬▬▬▬▬▬▬▬▬▬

2. NURSING DIAGNOSIS

Decreased cardiac output related to an inability of the heart to pump effectively associated with myocardial damage or hypertrophy.

☐ ▬▬▬▬▬▬▬▬▬▬▬▬▬▬▬▬▬▬▬▬▬▬▬▬▬

DESIRED OUTCOMES	NURSING ACTIONS AND *SELECTED RATIONALES*

2. The client will have improved cardiac output as evidenced by:
  a. B/P within normal range for client
	2.a. Assess for signs and symptoms of decreased cardiac output:
	  1. drop of 20 mm Hg in systolic B/P, a systolic pressure below 80 mm Hg, or a continual drop of 5–10 mm Hg in systolic pressure with each reading
	  2. irregular pulse

b. apical pulse audible, regular, and between 60–100 beats/minute
c. resolution of gallop rhythms
d. B/P and pulse stable with position change
e. unlabored respirations at 16–20/minute
f. improved breath sounds
g. usual mental status
h. absence of lightheadedness or syncope
i. palpable peripheral pulses
j. stronger amplitude of carotid pulse
k. improved skin color and temperature
l. capillary refill time less than 3 seconds
m. urine output at least 30 cc/hour
n. decrease in peripheral edema, neck vein distention, ascites
o. decline in weight toward client's normal
p. hemodynamic measurements such as pulmonary artery pressure (PAP), pulmonary capillary wedge pressure (PCWP), cardiac output (CO), and central venous pressure (CVP) returning toward normal range
q. BUN and serum creatinine and alkaline phosphatase levels returning toward normal range.

3. pulse rate less than 60 or greater than 100 beats/minute
4. muffled heart sounds or softening of a pre-existing murmur
5. presence of an S_3 and/or S_4 gallop rhythm
6. decline in systolic B/P of at least 15 mm Hg with a concurrent rise in pulse when client sits up
7. rapid, labored, or irregular respirations
8. crackles and diminished or absent breath sounds
9. restlessness, confusion
10. lightheadedness, syncope
11. diminished or absent peripheral pulses
12. decreased amplitude of carotid pulse
13. cool, pale, mottled, or cyanotic skin
14. capillary refill time greater than 3 seconds
15. urine output less than 30 cc/hour
16. peripheral edema, distended neck veins, ascites
17. persistent or marked weight gain
18. decreased CO; increased PAP, PCWP, and CVP (use internal jugular vein pulsation method to estimate CVP if monitoring device not present)
19. elevated BUN and serum creatinine and alkaline phosphatase levels.

b. Monitor EKG readings and report arrhythmias.
c. Monitor chest x-ray results. Report findings of cardiomegaly, pleural effusion, or pulmonary edema.
d. Implement measures *to improve cardiac output:*
  1. perform actions *to reduce cardiac workload:*
    a. place client in a semi- to high Fowler's position
    b. instruct client to avoid activities that create a Valsalva response (e.g. straining to have a bowel movement, bending at the waist, holding breath while moving)
    c. implement measures to promote physical and emotional rest
    d. implement measures to improve respiratory status (see Nursing Diagnosis 3, action e) *in order to improve alveolar gas exchange and promote adequate tissue oxygenation*
    e. discourage smoking *(smoking has a cardiostimulatory effect, causes vasoconstriction, and reduces oxygen availability)*
    f. provide frequent, small meals rather than 3 large ones *(large meals require an increase in blood supply to gastrointestinal tract for digestion)*
    g. discourage intake of foods/fluids high in caffeine such as coffee, tea, chocolate, and colas *(caffeine is a myocardial stimulant and increases myocardial oxygen consumption)*
    h. increase activity gradually
    i. implement measures to prevent and treat fluid volume excess (see Nursing Diagnosis 4, action d.1)
    j. apply rotating tourniquets according to hospital policy if ordered *to reduce vascular congestion*
    k. implement measures as ordered to treat anemia, hypertension, hyperthyroidism, and chronic obstructive pulmonary disease *(these conditions increase cardiac workload)*
  2. monitor for therapeutic and nontherapeutic effects of the following medications if administered:
    a. positive inotropic agents (e.g. digitalis preparations, dobutamine, dopamine, amrinone) *to improve myocardial contractility*
    b. arterial dilators (e.g. hydralazine, minoxidil) *to decrease afterload*
    c. nitrates (e.g. nitroglycerin) and balanced vasodilators (e.g. prazosin, nitroprusside) *to decrease preload and afterload*
    d. calcium-channel blocking agents (e.g. nifedipine) *to decrease afterload*
    e. angiotensin-converting enzyme inhibitors (e.g. captopril, enalapril) *to decrease peripheral vascular resistance and suppress aldosterone output*
  3. prepare client for insertion of intra-aortic balloon pump (IABP) or surgery (e.g. artificial heart or ventricular assist device implant, heart transplant) if indicated.
e. Consult physician if signs and symptoms of decreased cardiac output persist or worsen.

3. NURSING DIAGNOSIS

Altered respiratory function:*

a. **ineffective breathing patterns** related to:
   1. fear and anxiety
   2. loss of alveolar elasticity associated with vascular engorgement
   3. restricted lung expansion resulting from pleural effusion and pressure on the diaphragm as a result of peritoneal fluid accumulation
   4. respiratory depressant and/or stimulant effects of hypoxia, hypercapnea, and diminished cerebral blood flow;
b. **ineffective airway clearance** related to fluid accumulation in the alveoli and bronchioles associated with pulmonary edema and poor cough effort associated with weakness and fatigue;
c. **impaired gas exchange** related to:
   1. ineffective breathing patterns and airway clearance
   2. thickened alveolar-capillary membrane associated with pulmonary edema
   3. decreased systemic tissue perfusion associated with decreased cardiac output.

* This diagnostic label includes the following nursing diagnoses: ineffective breathing pattern, ineffective airway clearance, and impaired gas exchange (Carpenito, 1989).

DESIRED OUTCOMES	NURSING ACTIONS AND *SELECTED RATIONALES*

3. The client will experience adequate respiratory function as evidenced by:
   a. normal rate, rhythm, and depth of respirations
   b. decreased dyspnea
   c. usual or improved breath sounds
   d. usual mental status
   e. usual skin color
   f. blood gases within normal range.

3.a. Assess for signs and symptoms of altered respiratory function:
   1. rapid, shallow, slow, or irregular respirations
   2. dyspnea, orthopnea
   3. use of accessory muscles when breathing
   4. adventitious breath sounds (e.g. rhonchi, crackles)
   5. diminished or absent breath sounds
   6. persistent cough productive of frothy or blood-tinged sputum
   7. restlessness, irritability
   8. confusion, somnolence
   9. dusky or cyanotic skin color.
   b. Monitor blood gas values. Report abnormal results.
   c. Monitor for and report significant changes in ear oximetry and capnograph results.
   d. Monitor chest x-ray results and report abnormalities.
   e. Implement measures *to improve respiratory status:*
      1. perform actions to improve cardiac output (see Nursing Diagnosis 2, action d) *in order to improve tissue perfusion and reduce fluid accumulation in the lungs*
      2. perform actions to reduce fear and anxiety (see Nursing Diagnosis 1, action c)
      3. instruct client to breathe slowly if he/she is hyperventilating
      4. place client in a semi- to high Fowler's position; position overbed table so client can lean forward on it if desired
      5. if client is on bedrest, assist him/her to turn at least every 2 hours
      6. instruct client to deep breathe or use inspiratory exerciser at least every 2 hours
      7. perform actions *to facilitate removal of pulmonary secretions:*
         a. instruct and assist client to cough every 1–2 hours
         b. implement measures *to liquefy tenacious secretions:*
            1. humidify inspired air as ordered

2. assist with administration of mucolytic agents via nebulizer or IPPB (IPPB may not be utilized *because it increases intrathoracic pressure, which causes impairment of venous blood flow to the right atrium*)
3. maintain the maximum fluid intake allowed

c. assist with or perform postural drainage, percussion, and vibration if ordered

d. perform tracheal suctioning if needed

e. monitor for therapeutic and nontherapeutic effects of expectorants if administered

8. maintain oxygen therapy as ordered (initially, high concentrations may be used *to overcome the pressure barrier caused by alveolar fluid accumulation*)

9. instruct client to avoid intake of gas-forming foods/fluids (e.g. beans, cauliflower, cabbage, onions, carbonated beverages) and large meals *in order to prevent gastric distention and a further increase in pressure on the diaphragm*

10. discourage smoking *(smoking irritates the respiratory tract, causes an increase in mucus production, impairs ciliary function, and decreases oxygen availability)*

11. increase activity as allowed and tolerated

12. administer central nervous system depressants (e.g. narcotic analgesics, sedatives) judiciously; hold medication and consult physician if respiratory rate is less than 12/minute

13. monitor for therapeutic and nontherapeutic effects of the following if administered:

a. medications to improve cardiac output (see Nursing Diagnosis 2, action d.2)

b. diuretics *to decrease pulmonary fluid accumulation*

c. morphine sulfate *to decrease pulmonary vascular congestion (its vasodilatory action reduces cardiac workload and eventually improves left ventricular emptying, which results in increased blood return from the pulmonary veins); morphine also reduces the apprehension associated with dyspnea*

d. theophylline *to dilate the bronchioles and reduce pulmonary vascular congestion by increasing cardiac output and promoting diuresis*

14. assist with thoracentesis and/or paracentesis if performed *to allow increased lung expansion.*

f. Consult physician if signs and symptoms of impaired respiratory function persist or worsen.

4. NURSING/COLLABORATIVE DIAGNOSIS

Altered fluid balance:

a. **fluid volume excess** related to high levels of aldosterone and antidiuretic hormone (ADH) associated with decreased renal blood flow (inadequate renal blood flow results in increased secretion of aldosterone and ADH);

b. **third-spacing of fluid** related to:
1. increased intravascular pressure associated with fluid volume excess
2. low plasma colloid osmotic pressure if serum albumin is decreased due to malnutrition or impaired liver function (results from hepatic venous congestion).

DESIRED OUTCOMES

NURSING ACTIONS AND *SELECTED RATIONALES*

4. The client will experience resolution of fluid imbalance as evidenced by:
   a. decline in weight toward client's normal
   b. B/P and pulse within normal range for client and stable with position change
   c. resolution of gallop rhythms
   d. balanced intake and output
   e. resolution of peripheral edema, ascites, neck vein distention
   f. Hct. returning toward normal range
   g. CVP within normal range
   h. less labored respirations
   i. improved breath sounds
   j. usual mental status.

4.a. Assess for signs and symptoms of the following:
   1. fluid volume excess:
      a. history of significant weight gain (greater than 0.5 kg/day)
      b. elevated B/P and pulse (B/P may not be elevated if fluid has shifted out of vascular space)
      c. development or worsening of S_3 and/or S_4 gallop rhythm
      d. intake greater than output
      e. low Hct. (may be normal or even increased if fluid has shifted out of the vascular space)
      f. distended neck veins
      g. elevated CVP (use internal jugular vein pulsation method to estimate CVP if monitoring device not present)
   2. third-spacing:
      a. peripheral edema
      b. ascites as evidenced by:
         1. increase in abdominal girth (abdominal girth should be measured daily at the same time and in same location on abdomen with client in same position)
         2. dull percussion note over abdomen with finding of shifting dullness
         3. presence of abdominal fluid wave
         4. bulging flanks and protruding umbilicus
      c. dyspnea, orthopnea
      d. crackles and diminished or absent breath sounds
      e. change in mental status
      f. decline in systolic B/P of at least 15 mm Hg with a concurrent rise in pulse when client changes from lying to sitting position.
   b. Monitor chest x-ray results. Report findings of vascular congestion, pleural effusion, or pulmonary edema.
   c. Monitor serum albumin levels. Report below-normal levels *(albumin maintains plasma colloid osmotic pressure)*.
   d. Implement measures *to restore fluid balance:*
      1. perform actions *to reduce fluid volume excess:*
         a. maintain fluid restrictions as ordered
         b. restrict sodium intake as ordered (sodium is usually restricted to 2–3 gm/day)
         c. monitor for therapeutic and nontherapeutic effects of the following medications if administered:
            1. diuretics *to increase excretion of water*
            2. positive inotropic agents and arterial vasodilators *to increase cardiac output and subsequently improve renal blood flow*
         d. assist with phlebotomy if performed *to reduce blood volume*
      2. perform actions *to prevent third-spacing and promote mobilization of fluid back into the vascular space:*
         a. implement measures to reduce fluid volume excess (see action d.1 in this diagnosis)
         b. encourage client to lie flat periodically as tolerated *(lying flat promotes reshifting of fluid into the vascular space)*
         c. implement measures *to increase colloid osmotic pressure:*
            1. provide a diet high in protein and still within the prescribed sodium restriction (e.g. poultry, fish, protein supplements) *to increase serum protein levels*
            2. monitor for therapeutic and nontherapeutic effects of salt-poor albumin infusions if administered
            3. assist with intravenous administration of ascitic fluid if indicated (the fluid is obtained by paracentesis using an ultra-filtration device and then administered intravenously *to replace the albumin that is lost; it is given in conjunction with diuretics to mobilize fluid into the vascular space for diuresis)*.
   e. Consult physician if signs and symptoms of fluid imbalance persist or worsen.

5. NURSING DIAGNOSIS

Altered nutrition: less than body requirements related to:

a. decreased oral intake associated with anorexia, nausea, weakness, fatigue, dyspnea, and dislike of the prescribed diet;
b. loss of nutrients associated with vomiting;
c. impaired absorption and transport of nutrients associated with poor tissue perfusion.

DESIRED OUTCOMES	NURSING ACTIONS AND *SELECTED RATIONALES*

5. The client will maintain an adequate nutritional status as evidenced by:
a. dry weight within normal range for client's age, height, and build (dry weight is achieved after fluid volume excess has been resolved)
b. normal BUN and serum albumin, protein, Hct., Hgb., cholesterol, and lymphocyte levels
c. triceps skinfold measurements within normal range
d. improved strength and activity tolerance
e. healthy oral mucous membrane.
	5.a. Assess the client for signs and symptoms of malnutrition:
	  1. dry weight below normal for client's age, height, and build
	  2. abnormal BUN and low serum albumin, protein, Hct., Hgb., cholesterol, and lymphocyte levels
	  3. triceps skinfold measurements less than normal for build
	  4. weakness and fatigue
	  5. stomatitis.
	b. Reassess nutritional status on a regular basis and report decline.
	c. Monitor percentage of meals eaten.
	d. Assess the client to determine causes of inadequate intake (e.g. nausea, dislike of diet, fatigue, dyspnea, anorexia).
	e. Implement measures *to improve nutritional status:*
	  1. perform actions *to improve oral intake:*
	    a. implement measures to relieve nausea and vomiting (see Nursing Diagnosis 6, action b)
	    b. provide oral care before meals
	    c. serve small portions of nutritious foods/fluids that are appealing to the client
	    d. obtain a dietary consult if necessary to assist client in selecting foods/fluids that meet nutritional needs, dietary restrictions, and preferences
	    e. instruct client to use herbs, spices, and salt substitutes if approved by physician *in order to make low-sodium diet more palatable*
	    f. place client in a high Fowler's position for meals *to help relieve dyspnea*
	    g. encourage a rest period before meals *to minimize fatigue*
	    h. provide a clean, relaxed, pleasant atmosphere
	    i. allow adequate time for meals; reheat food if necessary
	    j. increase activity as allowed and tolerated *(activity stimulates appetite)*
	  2. perform actions to improve cardiac output (see Nursing Diagnosis 2, action d) *in order to increase tissue perfusion and the absorption and transport of nutrients*
	  3. ensure that meals are well balanced and high in essential nutrients
	  4. monitor for therapeutic and nontherapeutic effects of vitamins and minerals if administered.
	f. Perform a 72-hour calorie count if nutritional status declines or fails to improve.
	g. Consult physician regarding alternative methods of providing nutrition (e.g. parenteral nutrition, tube feedings) if client does not consume enough food or fluids to meet nutritional needs.

6. NURSING DIAGNOSIS

Altered comfort: nausea and vomiting related to stimulation of the vomiting center associated with:

a. vagal and/or sympathetic stimulation resulting from vascular congestion in the heart and gastrointestinal tract;
b. cortical stimulation resulting from stress;
c. chemoreceptor trigger zone stimulation by certain medications (e.g. digitalis preparations, morphine sulfate).

DESIRED OUTCOMES	NURSING ACTIONS AND *SELECTED RATIONALES*

6. The client will experience relief of nausea and vomiting as evidenced by:
a. verbalization of relief of nausea
b. absence of vomiting.
	6.a. Assess client to determine factors that contribute to nausea and vomiting (e.g. receiving morphine sulfate, activity, eating, fear, anxiety, elevated digoxin level).
	b. Implement measures *to prevent nausea and vomiting:*
	  1. perform actions to improve cardiac output (see Nursing Diagnosis 2, action d) *in order to reduce vascular congestion in the heart and gastrointestinal tract*
	  2. monitor serum digoxin levels and report elevated values (be alert to a low serum potassium level *because it may precipitate digitalis toxicity*)
	  3. perform actions to reduce fear and anxiety (see Nursing Diagnosis 1, action c)
	  4. eliminate noxious sights and smells from the environment *(noxious stimuli cause cortical stimulation of the vomiting center)*
	  5. encourage client to take deep, slow breaths when nauseated
	  6. encourage client to change positions slowly *(movement stimulates chemoreceptor trigger zone)*
	  7. provide oral hygiene after each emesis and before meals
	  8. instruct client to ingest foods and fluids slowly
	  9. instruct client to avoid foods/fluids that irritate gastric mucosa (e.g. spicy foods; citrus fruits or juices; caffeine-containing items such as chocolate, coffee, tea, and colas)
	  10. instruct client to eat dry foods (e.g. toast, crackers) and avoid drinking liquids with meals if nauseated
	  11. instruct client to rest after eating with head of bed elevated
	  12. monitor for therapeutic and nontherapeutic effects of antiemetics if administered.
	c. Consult physician if above measures fail to control nausea and vomiting.

7. NURSING DIAGNOSIS

Impaired skin integrity: irritation and breakdown related to:

a. prolonged pressure on tissues associated with decreased mobility;
b. increased fragility of the skin associated with edema, poor tissue perfusion, and malnutrition.

DESIRED OUTCOMES	NURSING ACTIONS AND *SELECTED RATIONALES*

7. The client will maintain skin integrity as evidenced by:
a. absence of redness and irritation
b. no skin breakdown.
	7.a. Inspect the skin, especially bone prominences and dependent and edematous areas, for pallor, redness, and breakdown.
	b. Refer to Care Plan on Immobility, Nursing Diagnosis 7, action b, for measures to prevent skin breakdown associated with decreased mobility.
	c. Implement additional measures *to prevent skin breakdown:*
	  1. perform actions *to improve tissue perfusion and reduce edema:*
	    a. implement measures to increase cardiac output (see Nursing Diagnosis 2, action d)
	    b. implement measures to restore fluid balance (see Nursing Diagnosis 4, action d)
	    c. implement measures *to reduce fluid accumulation in dependent areas:*
	      1. assist with range of motion exercises
	      2. turn client at least every 2 hours
	      3. elevate lower extremities
	      4. apply elastic wraps or hose to lower extremities as ordered
	      5. apply a scrotal support if scrotal edema is present
	  2. handle edematous areas carefully
	  3. maintain an optimal nutritional status (see Nursing Diagnosis 5, action e).
	d. If skin breakdown occurs:
	  1. notify physician
	  2. continue with above measures to prevent further irritation and breakdown
	  3. perform decubitus care as ordered or per standard hospital policy
	  4. monitor client closely and report signs and symptoms of infection (e.g. elevated temperature; redness, warmth, and edema around area of breakdown; unusual drainage from site).

8. NURSING DIAGNOSIS

Altered oral mucous membrane: dryness related to prolonged oxygen therapy (oxygen is a dry gas and will dehydrate the respiratory mucous membranes if exposure is prolonged).

DESIRED OUTCOMES	NURSING ACTIONS AND *SELECTED RATIONALES*

8. The client will maintain a moist, intact oral mucous membrane.	8.a. Assess client every shift for dryness of the oral mucosa.
	b. Implement measures *to decrease dryness of oral mucous membrane:*
	  1. instruct and assist client to perform good oral hygiene as often as needed; avoid products such as lemon-glycerin swabs and commercial mouthwashes containing alcohol *(these have a drying or irritating effect on oral mucous membrane)*
	  2. encourage client to rinse mouth frequently with water
	  3. lubricate client's lips with Vaseline, K-Y jelly, ChapStick, Blistex, or mineral oil when oral care is given
	  4. encourage client to breathe through nose if possible
	  5. encourage client not to smoke *(smoking further irritates and dries the mucosa)*
	  6. encourage the maximum fluid intake allowed
	  7. encourage client to use artificial saliva (e.g. Moi-stir, Salivart) *to lubricate the mucous membrane.*
	c. If oral mucosa is irritated or cracked, implement measures *to relieve discomfort and promote healing:*
	  1. assist client to select soft, bland, and nonacidic foods
	  2. instruct client to avoid foods/fluids that are extremely hot or cold

3. use a soft bristle brush or low-pressure power spray for oral care
4. monitor for therapeutic and nontherapeutic effects of topical anesthetics, oral protective pastes, and topical and systemic analgesics if administered.

d. Consult physician if dryness, irritation, and discomfort persist.

□ ▬▬▬▬▬▬▬▬▬▬▬▬▬▬▬▬▬▬▬▬▬

9. NURSING DIAGNOSIS

Activity intolerance related to:

a. tissue hypoxia associated with impaired alveolar gas exchange and decreased tissue perfusion (a result of decreased cardiac output);
b. inadequate nutritional status;
c. difficulty resting and sleeping due to dyspnea, frequent assessments and treatments, fear, and anxiety.

□ ▬▬▬▬▬▬▬▬▬▬▬▬▬▬▬▬▬▬▬▬▬

DESIRED OUTCOMES	NURSING ACTIONS AND *SELECTED RATIONALES*
9. The client will demonstrate an increased tolerance for activity (see Care Plan on Immobility, Nursing Diagnosis 8, for outcome criteria).	9.a. Refer to Care Plan on Immobility, Nursing Diagnosis 8, for measures related to assessment and improvement of activity tolerance. b. Implement additional measures *to promote rest and improve activity tolerance:* 1. maintain activity restrictions as ordered 2. perform actions to reduce fear and anxiety (see Nursing Diagnosis 1, action c) 3. perform actions to promote sleep (see Nursing Diagnosis 13) 4. perform actions to improve respiratory status (see Nursing Diagnosis 3, action e) *in order to relieve dyspnea and improve tissue oxygenation* 5. perform actions to increase cardiac output (see Nursing Diagnosis 2, action d) 6. perform actions to improve nutritional status (see Nursing Diagnosis 5, action e) 7. increase client's activity gradually as allowed and tolerated; explain that activity is increased gradually *to prevent a sudden increase in cardiac workload.*

□ ▬▬▬▬▬▬▬▬▬▬▬▬▬▬▬▬▬▬▬▬▬

10. NURSING DIAGNOSIS

Self-care deficit related to weakness, fatigue, dyspnea, altered thought processes, and activity restrictions imposed by the treatment plan.

□ ▬▬▬▬▬▬▬▬▬▬▬▬▬▬▬▬▬▬▬▬▬

DESIRED OUTCOMES	NURSING ACTIONS AND *SELECTED RATIONALES*
10. The client will demonstrate increased participation in self-care activities within limitations imposed by the	10.a. Refer to Care Plan on Immobility, Nursing Diagnosis 9, for measures related to assessment of, planning for, and meeting client's self-care needs. b. Implement additional measures *to facilitate client's ability to perform self-care activities:*

disease process and
treatment plan.

1. perform actions to increase strength and activity tolerance (see Nursing Diagnosis 9)
2. perform actions to improve respiratory status and relieve dyspnea (see Nursing Diagnosis 3, action e)
3. perform actions to improve cardiac output (see Nursing Diagnosis 2, action d) *in order to improve activity tolerance and increase cerebral blood flow and thereby improve thought processes.*

11. NURSING DIAGNOSIS

Constipation related to decreased mobility, anxiety, vascular congestion in the bowel, and decreased intake of fluid and foods high in fiber.

DESIRED OUTCOMES	NURSING ACTIONS AND *SELECTED RATIONALES*

11. The client will maintain usual bowel elimination pattern.

11.a. Ascertain client's usual bowel elimination habits.
b. Monitor and record bowel movements including frequency, consistency, and shape.
c. Assess for signs and symptoms that may accompany constipation such as headache, anorexia, nausea, abdominal distention and cramping, and feeling of fullness or pressure in abdomen or rectum.
d. Assess bowel sounds. Report a pattern of decreasing bowel sounds.
e. Implement measures *to prevent constipation:*
  1. perform actions to improve cardiac output (see Nursing Diagnosis 2, action d) *in order to reduce vascular congestion in the bowel*
  2. encourage client to defecate whenever the urge is felt
  3. allow client to use commode for bowel movements if possible *(using a bedpan may actually require more energy than getting up to the commode)*; provide privacy and adequate ventilation
  4. encourage client to relax during attempts to defecate *in order to promote relaxation of the levator ani muscle and external anal sphincter*
  5. instruct client to select foods high in fiber and within dietary restrictions of sodium and saturated fat (e.g. bran, whole grains, raw fruits and vegetables, dried fruits)
  6. maintain the maximum fluid intake allowed
  7. encourage client to drink warm liquids *in order to stimulate peristalsis*
  8. increase activity as allowed and tolerated
  9. monitor for therapeutic and nontherapeutic effects of stool softeners and/or laxatives if administered.
f. Avoid enemas and manual removal of stool if possible *(both cause vagal stimulation).*
g. Consult physician if signs and symptoms of constipation persist.

12. NURSING DIAGNOSIS

Altered thought processes: slowed verbal responses, shortened attention span, impaired memory, and confusion related to cerebral hypoxia associated with impaired alveolar gas exchange and inadequate cerebral tissue perfusion due to decreased cardiac output.

DESIRED OUTCOMES	NURSING ACTIONS AND *SELECTED RATIONALES*

12. The client will regain usual thought processes as evidenced by:
    a. improved verbal response time
    b. longer attention span
    c. improved memory
    d. improved level of orientation.

12.a. Assess client for alterations in thought processes (e.g. slowed verbal responses, shortened attention span, impaired memory, confusion).
   b. Ascertain from significant others client's usual level of intellectual functioning.
   c. Implement measures to improve cardiac output and respiratory status (see Nursing Diagnoses 2, action d and 3, action e) *in order to increase cerebral oxygenation and improve thought processes.*
   d. If client shows evidence of altered thought processes:
      1. allow adequate time for communication and performance of activities
      2. repeat instructions as necessary using clear, simple language
      3. reorient client to person, place, and time as necessary
      4. write out a schedule of daily activities for client to refer to if desired
      5. encourage significant others to be supportive of client; instruct them to reorient client as necessary
      6. assure client and significant others that usual thought processes will usually be regained once acute heart failure has been resolved
      7. consult physician if alterations in thought processes worsen.

☐ ▬▬▬▬▬▬▬▬▬▬▬▬▬▬▬▬▬▬▬▬

UNIT VII

13. NURSING DIAGNOSIS

Sleep pattern disturbance related to unfamiliar environment, frequent assessments and treatments, decreased physical activity, fear, anxiety, and inability to assume usual sleep position due to orthopnea.

☐ ▬▬▬▬▬▬▬▬▬▬▬▬▬▬▬▬▬▬▬▬

DESIRED OUTCOMES	NURSING ACTIONS AND *SELECTED RATIONALES*

13. The client will attain optimal amounts of sleep within the parameters of the treatment regimen (see Care Plan on Immobility, Nursing Diagnosis 12, for outcome criteria).

13.a. Refer to Care Plan on Immobility, Nursing Diagnosis 12, for measures related to assessment and promotion of sleep.
   b. Implement additional measures *to promote sleep:*
      1. perform actions to improve respiratory status (see Nursing Diagnosis 3, action e) *in order to relieve dyspnea*
      2. assist client to assume a comfortable sleep position (e.g. bed in reverse Trendelenburg position with client in usual recumbent position, head of bed elevated with arms supported on pillows, resting forward on overbed table with good pillow support, sitting in chair)
      3. maintain oxygen therapy during sleep if indicated
      4. ensure good room ventilation *to reduce feeling of suffocation*
      5. increase activity as allowed and tolerated
      6. perform actions to reduce fear and anxiety (see Nursing Diagnosis 1, action c).

☐ ▬▬▬▬▬▬▬▬▬▬▬▬▬▬▬▬▬▬▬▬

14. NURSING DIAGNOSIS

Potential for trauma related to falls associated with dizziness, syncope, weakness, and altered thought processes resulting from inadequate tissue oxygenation due to impaired alveolar gas exchange and decreased tissue perfusion (a result of decreased cardiac output).

☐ ▬▬▬▬▬▬▬▬▬▬▬▬▬▬▬▬▬▬▬▬

DESIRED OUTCOMES	NURSING ACTIONS AND *SELECTED RATIONALES*

14. The client will not experience falls.

14.a. Determine whether conditions predisposing client to falls (e.g. weakness, fatigue, dizziness, confusion) exist.

   b. Implement measures *to prevent falls:*
1. keep bed in low position with side rails up when client is in bed
2. keep needed items within easy reach
3. encourage client to request assistance whenever needed; have call signal within easy reach
4. use lap belt when client is in chair if indicated
5. instruct client to wear shoes with nonskid soles and low heels when ambulating
6. avoid unnecessary clutter in room
7. accompany client during ambulation utilizing a transfer safety belt if he/she is weak or dizzy
8. provide ambulatory aids (e.g. walker, cane) if client is weak or unsteady on feet
9. instruct client to ambulate in well-lit areas and to utilize handrails if needed
10. do not rush client; allow adequate time for trips to the bathroom and ambulation in hallway
11. instruct and assist client to change positions slowly *to reduce dizziness associated with an orthostatic drop in B/P*
12. perform actions to improve cardiac output (see Nursing Diagnosis 2, action d) *in order to improve cerebral blood flow and reduce dizziness, syncope, and alterations in thought processes*
13. perform actions to increase strength and activity tolerance (see Nursing Diagnosis 9).

   c. If client is confused or irrational, implement additional measures *to reduce risk of falls:*
1. reorient frequently to surroundings and necessity of adhering to safety precautions
2. provide constant supervision (e.g. staff member, significant other) if indicated
3. use jacket or wrist restraints or safety alarm device if necessary *to reduce the risk of client's getting out of bed or chair unattended*
4. monitor for therapeutic and nontherapeutic effects of antianxiety and antipsychotic medications if administered.

   d. Include client and significant others in planning and implementing measures to prevent falls.

   e. If falls occur, initiate appropriate first aid measures and notify physician.

☐ ▉▉▉▉▉▉▉▉▉▉▉▉▉▉▉▉▉▉▉▉▉▉▉▉▉▉

15. COLLABORATIVE DIAGNOSIS

Potential complications:

a. **impaired renal function** related to inadequate renal blood flow associated with low cardiac output, volume depletion (a result of third-spacing), and venous congestion;

b. **impaired liver function** related to hepatic venous congestion;

c. **thromboembolism** related to venous stasis associated with decreased cardiac output and decreased mobility;

d. **cardiogenic shock** related to inability of heart, intrinsic compensatory mechanisms, and treatments to maintain adequate tissue perfusion to vital organs.

☐ ▉▉▉▉▉▉▉▉▉▉▉▉▉▉▉▉▉▉▉▉▉▉▉▉▉▉

DESIRED OUTCOMES	NURSING ACTIONS AND *SELECTED RATIONALES*

15.a. The client will maintain adequate renal function as evidenced by:
1. urine output at least 30 cc/hour
2. urine specific gravity between 1.010–1.030
3. BUN and serum creatinine levels within normal range.

15.a.1. Assess for and report signs and symptoms of impaired renal function (e.g. urine output less than 30 cc/hour, urine specific gravity fixed at or less than 1.010, elevated BUN and serum creatinine levels).
   2. Collect a 24-hour urine specimen if ordered. Report decreased creatinine clearance.
   3. Implement measures *to maintain adequate renal blood flow:*
     a. perform actions to improve cardiac output (see Nursing Diagnosis 2, action d)
     b. perform actions to restore fluid balance (see Nursing Diagnosis 4, action d) *in order to reduce venous congestion and prevent hypovolemia resulting from third-spacing.*
   4. If signs and symptoms of impaired renal function occur:
     a. continue with above actions
     b. administer diuretics as ordered
     c. consult physician about possible need to reduce the digitalis dosage *(digitalis is excreted by the kidney and will quickly reach toxic levels when renal function is impaired)*
     d. assess for and report signs of acute renal failure (e.g. oliguria or anuria; further weight gain; increasing edema; elevated B/P; lethargy and confusion; increasing BUN and serum creatinine, phosphorus, and potassium levels)
     e. prepare client for dialysis if indicated
     f. refer to Care Plan on Renal Failure for additional care measures.

15.b. The client will maintain adequate liver function as evidenced by:
1. no unusual bleeding
2. stable or improved mental status
3. absence of jaundice, asterixis, fetor hepaticus
4. serum bilirubin, GGT, ALT (SGPT), alkaline phosphatase (ALP), prothrombin, albumin, and ammonia levels within normal range.

15.b.1. Assess for and report signs and symptoms of impaired liver function:
     a. unusual bleeding (e.g. petechiae; frank or occult blood in stools, urine, or vomitus; bleeding gums; epistaxis)
     b. jaundice
     c. elevated serum bilirubin, GGT, ALT (SGPT), alkaline phosphatase (ALP), and ammonia levels
     d. decreasing serum albumin
     e. increased prothrombin time.
   2. Implement measures to improve cardiac output (see Nursing Diagnosis 2, action d) *in order to reduce hepatic venous congestion.*
   3. If signs and symptoms of impaired liver function occur:
     a. institute bleeding precautions (e.g. prevent trauma, use electric rather than straight-edge razor, brush teeth gently)
     b. consult physician before administering known or potential hepatotoxins (e.g. isoniazid, methyldopa, acetaminophen, sulfonamides)
     c. if client is taking a potassium-depleting diuretic (e.g. thiazide, furosemide), assess for and report signs and symptoms of hypokalemia (e.g. muscle weakness and cramping, arrhythmias, hypoactive or absent bowel sounds, low serum potassium), *which may precipitate hepatic coma*
     d. assess for and report signs and symptoms of hepatic encephalopathy (e.g. decline in mental status and motor skills, slurred speech, asterixis, fetor hepaticus)
     e. refer to Care Plan on Cirrhosis for additional care measures.

15.c. The client will not develop a venous thrombus or pulmonary embolism (see Care Plan on Immobility, Collaborative Diagnosis 14, outcomes a.1 and 2, for outcome criteria).

15.c.1. Refer to Care Plan on Immobility, Collaborative Diagnosis 14, actions a.1 and 2, for measures related to assessment, prevention, and treatment of a venous thrombus and pulmonary embolism.
   2. Implement measures to improve cardiac output (see Nursing Diagnosis 2, action d) *in order to decrease venous stasis and further reduce risk of thrombus development.*

15.d. The client will not develop cardiogenic shock as evidenced by:
1. stable or improved mental status

15.d.1. Assess for and immediately report signs and symptoms of cardiogenic shock:
     a. increased restlessness, lethargy, or confusion
     b. decrease in systolic B/P of 30 mm Hg or a systolic pressure below 80 mm Hg

UNIT VII

2. stable vital signs
3. palpable peripheral pulses
4. stable or stronger carotid pulse amplitude
5. stable or improved skin color and temperature
6. urine output at least 20 cc/hour
7. CVP and PCWP within normal range.

c. pulse rate greater than 100 beats/minute
d. diminished or absent peripheral pulses
e. further decrease in amplitude of carotid pulse
f. increased coolness and duskiness or cyanosis of skin
g. urine output less than 20 cc/hour
h. elevated CVP and PCWP.

2. Implement measures to improve cardiac output (see Nursing Diagnosis 2, action d) *in order to prevent cardiogenic shock.*

3. If signs and symptoms of cardiogenic shock occur:
   a. continue with above actions to improve cardiac output
   b. implement additional measures *to increase the myocardial oxygen supply:*
      1. maintain oxygen therapy as ordered
      2. assist with hyperbaric oxygenation and extracorporeal membrane oxygenation (ECMO) if indicated
   c. implement additional measures *to decrease oxygen utilization:*
      1. maintain client on strict bedrest
      2. assist with measures to induce hypothermia if ordered
   d. monitor for therapeutic and nontherapeutic effects of the following if administered:
      1. sympathomimetics (e.g. dopamine, dobutamine, isoproterenol, norepinephrine) *to increase cardiac output and maintain arterial pressure*
      2. antiarrhythmic agents *to increase cardiac output*
      3. vasodilators (e.g. nitroprusside, nitroglycerin) *to decrease cardiac workload* (sympathomimetics are given in conjunction with vasodilators *to maintain mean arterial pressure*)
      4. cardiac glycosides *to improve cardiac output*
      5. intravenous infusions of insulin, potassium, and hypertonic glucose *to provide an energy source for the cells*
      6. intravenous sodium bicarbonate *to correct acidosis* (reserved for treatment of severe acidosis when pH is less than 7.1)
   e. assist with insertion of hemodynamic monitoring device (e.g. Swan-Ganz catheter) and intra-aortic balloon pump (IABP) if indicated
   f. provide emotional support to client and significant others.

□ ▬▬▬▬▬▬▬▬▬▬▬▬▬▬▬▬▬▬

16. NURSING DIAGNOSIS

Disturbance in self-concept* related to:

a. dependence on others to meet self-care needs;
b. change in appearance (e.g. ascites, generalized edema);
c. altered thought processes;
d. possible alterations in usual sexual activities associated with weakness, fatigue, and prescribed activity limitations;
e. stigma of having a chronic illness;
f. possible changes in life style and roles.

---

* This diagnostic label includes the nursing diagnoses of body image disturbance and self-esteem disturbance.

□ ▬▬▬▬▬▬▬▬▬▬▬▬▬▬▬▬▬▬

DESIRED OUTCOMES	NURSING ACTIONS AND *SELECTED RATIONALES*
16. The client will demonstrate beginning adaptation to changes in appearance, body	16.a. Refer to Care Plan on Immobility, Nursing Diagnosis 16, for measures related to assessment and promotion of a positive self-concept. b. Implement additional measures *to promote a positive self-concept:*

functioning, life style, and roles (see Care Plan on Immobility, Nursing Diagnosis 16, for outcome criteria).

1. assist the client *to attain and maintain optimal independence:*
   a. perform actions to increase client's strength and activity tolerance (see Nursing Diagnosis 9)
   b. consult social services and occupational therapist about a home visit before discharge *in order to identify appropriate energy-saving techniques based on client's current living situation*
   c. reinforce the benefits of utilizing portable oxygen if prescribed
2. encourage significant others to allow client to do what he/she is able *so that independence can be re-established and/or self-esteem redeveloped*
3. teach client the rationale for treatments and encourage maximum participation in treatment regimen *to enable him/her to maintain a sense of control over life*
4. provide information about and encourage utilization of community agencies or support groups (e.g. vocational rehabilitation; sexual, family, and/or individual counseling; "coronary clubs").
c. Ensure that client and significant others have similar expectations and understanding of future life style.
d. Assist the client and significant others to identify ways that personal and family goals can be adjusted rather than abandoned.
e. Assure client that generalized swelling and altered thought processes are usually temporary.

17. NURSING DIAGNOSIS

Grieving* related to loss of normal function of the heart, possible changes in life style, and uncertainty of prognosis.

---

* This diagnostic label includes anticipatory grieving and grieving following the actual losses/changes.

DESIRED OUTCOMES	NURSING ACTIONS AND *SELECTED RATIONALES*

17. The client will demonstrate beginning progression through the grieving process as evidenced by:
   a. verbalization of feelings about CHF
   b. expression of grief
   c. participation in treatment plan and self-care activities
   d. utilization of available support systems
   e. verbalization of a plan for integrating prescribed follow-up care into life style.

17.a. Determine the client's perception of the impact of CHF on his/her future.
   b. Determine how client usually expresses grief.
   c. Observe for signs of grieving (e.g. changes in eating habits, insomnia, anger, noncompliance, denial).
   d. Implement measures *to facilitate the grieving process:*
   1. assist the client to acknowledge the loss of normal heart function and the need to alter usual life style *so grief work can begin*; assess for factors that may hinder or facilitate acknowledgment
   2. discuss the grieving process and assist client to accept the stages of grieving as an expected response to the changes experienced
   3. allow time for client to progress through the stages of grieving (denial, anger, bargaining, depression, acceptance [Kübler-Ross, 1969]; be aware that not every stage is experienced or expressed by all individuals
   4. assist client to identify personal strengths that have helped him/her to cope in previous situations of loss or change
   5. perform actions *to promote trust* (e.g. answer questions honestly, provide requested information)
   6. provide an atmosphere of care and concern (e.g. provide privacy, be available and nonjudgmental, display empathy and respect) *so that client will feel free to verbalize both positive and negative feelings and concerns*
   7. encourage the expression of anger and sadness about having CHF
   8. encourage client to express his/her feelings in whatever ways are comfortable (e.g. writing, drawing, conversation)
   9. support realistic hope regarding the prognosis.

UNIT VII

e. Assess for and support behaviors suggesting successful resolution of grief (e.g. verbalizing feelings about changes, expressing sorrow, focusing on ways to adapt to changes).
f. Explain the stages of the grieving process to significant others. Encourage their support and understanding.
g. Provide information regarding counseling services and support groups that might assist client in working through grief.
h. Arrange for a visit from clergy if desired by client.
i. Monitor for therapeutic and nontherapeutic effects of antidepressants if administered.
j. Consult physician regarding referral for counseling if signs of dysfunctional grieving (e.g. persistent denial of losses or changes, excessive anger or sadness, hysteria, suicidal behaviors, phobias) occur.

☐ ▬▬▬▬▬▬▬▬▬▬▬▬▬▬▬▬▬▬▬▬▬▬

18. NURSING DIAGNOSIS

Noncompliance* related to:

a. lack of understanding of the implications of not following the prescribed treatment plan;
b. difficulty modifying personal habits (e.g. smoking, alcohol intake, diet);
c. insufficient financial resources;
d. dysfunctional grieving.

* This diagnostic label includes both an informed decision by client not to comply and an inability to comply due to circumstances beyond client's control.

☐ ▬▬▬▬▬▬▬▬▬▬▬▬▬▬▬▬▬▬▬▬▬▬

DESIRED OUTCOMES	NURSING ACTIONS AND *SELECTED RATIONALES*

18. The client will demonstrate the probability of future compliance with the prescribed treatment plan as evidenced by:
   a. willingness to learn about and participate in treatments and care
   b. statements reflecting ways to modify personal habits and integrate treatments into life style
   c. statements reflecting an understanding of the implications of not following the prescribed treatment plan.

18.a. Assess for indications that the client may be unwilling or unable to comply with the prescribed treatment plan:
   1. statements reflecting that he/she was unable to manage care at home
   2. failure to adhere to treatment plan while in hospital (e.g. not adhering to dietary modifications and fluid restrictions, refusing medications)
   3. statements reflecting a lack of understanding of factors that may cause further progression of heart failure
   4. statements reflecting an unwillingness or inability to modify personal habits and integrate necessary treatments into life style
   5. statements reflecting the view that heart failure resolves completely or is hopeless and that efforts to comply with the treatment plan are useless.
   b. Implement measures *to improve client compliance:*
   1. explain CHF in terms the client can understand; stress the fact that CHF is a chronic disease and that adherence to the treatment program is necessary *in order to delay and/or prevent complications*
   2. encourage questions and clarify any misconceptions the client has regarding CHF and its effects
   3. encourage client to participate in treatment plan
   4. provide instructions on measuring intake and output, weighing self, counting pulse, and calculating dietary sodium content; allow time for return demonstration; determine areas of difficulty and misunderstanding and reinforce teaching as necessary
   5. provide client with written instructions about medications, signs and symptoms to report, measuring intake and output, weighing self, counting pulse, and calculating diet

6. assist client to identify ways he/she can incorporate treatments into life style; focus on modifications of life style rather than complete change
7. encourage the client to discuss his/her concerns regarding the cost of hospitalization, medications, and lifelong follow-up care; obtain a social service consult to assist the client with financial planning and to obtain financial aid if indicated
8. perform actions to facilitate the grieving process (see Nursing Diagnosis 17, action d)
9. initiate and reinforce discharge teaching outlined in Nursing Diagnosis 19 *in order to promote a sense of control and self-reliance*
10. provide information about and encourage utilization of community resources that can assist client to make necessary life-style changes (e.g. cardiovascular fitness, weight loss, and stop smoking programs).

c. Assess for and reinforce behaviors suggesting future compliance with changes in personal habits and prescribed treatments (e.g. statements reflecting ways to modify personal habits, active interest and participation in treatment plan).
d. Include significant others in explanations and teaching sessions and encourage their support.
e. Reinforce need for client to assume responsibility for managing as much of care as possible.
f. Consult physician regarding referrals to community health agencies if continued instruction, support, or supervision is needed.

☐ ▬▬▬▬▬▬▬▬▬▬▬▬▬▬▬▬▬▬▬

19. NURSING DIAGNOSIS

Knowledge deficit regarding follow-up care.

☐ ▬▬▬▬▬▬▬▬▬▬▬▬▬▬▬▬▬▬▬

DESIRED OUTCOMES	NURSING ACTIONS AND *SELECTED RATIONALES*
19.a. The client will identify modifiable cardiovascular risk factors and ways to reduce these factors.	19.a.1. Inform client that the following modifiable factors have been shown to contribute to heart disease: a. obesity b. diet high in saturated fat and cholesterol c. sedentary life style d. smoking e. heavy alcohol intake (more than 2 ounces of ethanol/day on a regular basis) f. hypertension g. stressful life style. 2. Assist client to identify ways he/she can make appropriate changes in life style to reduce the above factors. Provide information about weight reduction plans; stress management classes; and cardiovascular fitness, stop smoking, and alcohol rehabilitation programs if appropriate. Initiate a referral if indicated.
19.b. The client will verbalize an understanding of the rationale for and constituents of a diet low in sodium, saturated fat, and cholesterol.	19.b.1. Explain the rationale for a diet low in sodium, saturated fat, and cholesterol. 2. Provide the following information *about decreasing sodium intake* (recommended restriction is usually 2 gm sodium [5 gm salt]/day): a. be aware that the terms salt and sodium are often used interchangeably but are not synonymous; there is 40% sodium in table salt b. read food labels and calculate sodium content of items (often expressed in milligrams [2 gm is 2000 mg])

      c. do not add salt when cooking foods or to prepared foods
      d. avoid foods/fluids and additives high in sodium (e.g. baking soda, tomato juice, bouillon, meat tenderizer, processed meats, sauerkraut, catsup, canned soups and vegetables, salty snacks)
      e. reduce sodium content in vegetables and meats by boiling, discarding the water, adding fresh water, and reboiling.
   3. Provide the following instructions on ways *to reduce intake of saturated fat and cholesterol:*
      a. decrease intake of foods high in saturated fat and cholesterol (e.g. butter, cheese, ice cream, egg yolks, shrimp, cashew nuts, organ meats)
      b. avoid fried foods
      c. trim fat off meats and remove all poultry skin.
   4. Obtain a dietary consult to assist client in planning meals that will meet prescribed dietary modifications.

19.c. The client will demonstrate accuracy in counting pulse.

19.c.1. Teach the client how to count his/her pulse, being alert to the regularity of the rhythm.
   2. Allow time for return demonstration and accuracy check.

19.d. The client will verbalize an understanding of medication therapy including rationale for, side effects of, schedule for taking, and importance of taking as prescribed.

19.d.1. Explain the rationale for, side effects of, and importance of taking the medications prescribed.
   2. If client is discharged on a digitalis preparation, instruct to:
      a. take pulse before taking digitalis (should be a resting pulse rate taken at least 5 minutes after any activity); consult physician before taking medication if pulse rate is more irregular than usual or below 60 or above 120 beats/minute
      b. avoid altering dosage or trying to make up for missed doses
      c. promptly report a loss of usual appetite, nausea, vomiting, headache, diarrhea, muscle weakness, and visual disturbances.
   3. If client is discharged on a diuretic, instruct to:
      a. take once-daily doses or the larger dose in the morning *to minimize nighttime urination*
      b. weigh self daily and keep a record of daily weights
      c. avoid alcohol intake *(the combined vasodilating effect of alcohol and volume-depleting effect of a diuretic greatly increase the tendency toward orthostatic hypotension)*
      d. change from a lying to standing position slowly if experiencing dizziness or lightheadedness with position change
      e. increase intake of foods/fluids high in potassium (e.g. oranges, bananas, figs, dates, tomatoes, potatoes, raisins, apricots, Gatorade, fruit juices) if taking a potassium-depleting diuretic
      f. notify physician if unable to tolerate food or fluids *(dehydration can develop rapidly if intake is poor and client continues to take diuretic)*
      g. avoid salt substitutes with a high potassium content if discharged on a potassium-sparing diuretic (e.g. triamterene, spironolactone)
      h. report the following signs and symptoms:
         1. weight gain of 1 pound a day for 3 days
         2. swelling of ankles, feet, or abdomen
         3. weight loss of more than 5 pounds a week
         4. excessive thirst
         5. severe dizziness or episodes of fainting
         6. muscle weakness or cramping, nausea, vomiting, irregular pulse, or increased pulse rate.
   4. Instruct client to consult physician before taking other prescription and nonprescription medication.
   5. Instruct client to inform all health care providers of medications being taken.

19.e. The client will state signs and symptoms to report to the health care provider.

19.e. Instruct client to report:
   1. weight gain of more than 1 pound a day for 3 days
   2. swelling of ankles, feet, or abdomen
   3. persistent cough
   4. increasing shortness of breath
   5. chest pain
   6. significant change in pulse

7. increased weakness and fatigue
8. frequent nighttime urination
9. signs and symptoms of digitalis toxicity (see action d.2.c in this diagnosis)
10. side effects of diuretic therapy (see actions d.3.h.3–6 in this diagnosis).

19.f. The client will identify community resources that can assist with home management and adjustment to changes resulting from CHF.

19.f.1. Provide information regarding community resources that can assist with home management and adjustment to changes resulting from CHF (e.g. Visiting Nurse Association, Meals on Wheels, home health agencies, transportation services, American Heart Association, counseling services).
2. Initiate a referral if indicated.

19.g. The client will verbalize an understanding of and a plan for adhering to recommended follow-up care including future appointments with health care provider and activity limitations.

19.g.1. Reinforce the importance of keeping follow-up appointments with health care provider.
2. Provide the following instructions regarding activity:
   a. progress activity gradually and only as tolerated
   b. stop any activity that causes shortness of breath, chest pain, dizziness, or significant fatigue
   c. plan and adhere to rest periods during the day
   d. adhere to physician's recommendations about activities that should be avoided
   e. notify physician if activity tolerance declines
   f. reduce dyspnea and fatigue during sexual activity by:
      1. avoiding sexual activity when unusually fatigued
      2. resting before and after sexual activities
      3. waiting 2–3 hours after a heavy meal before engaging in sexual activity
      4. identifying and using positions that minimize energy expenditure (e.g. side-lying, partner on top)
      5. using portable oxygen during sexual activities.
3. Refer to Nursing Diagnosis 18, action b, for measures to improve client compliance.

☐ ▬▬▬▬▬▬▬▬▬▬▬▬▬▬▬▬▬▬▬▬▬▬▬▬▬▬▬

References

Carpenito, LJ. Handbook of nursing diagnosis (3rd ed.). Philadelphia: J.B. Lippincott Company, 1989.
Kübler-Ross, E. On death and dying. New York: Macmillan, 1989.

Heart Surgery: Coronary Artery Bypass Grafting (CABG) or Valve Replacement

Heart surgery is performed for a variety of reasons including myocardial revascularization; valve repair or replacement; repositioning of vessels; heart transplant; and repair of septal defects, aneurysms, and coarctation of the aorta. Two common heart surgeries are coronary artery bypass grafting (CABG), which is done to treat severe coronary artery disease, and heart valve replacement. CABG involves removing a segment of the saphenous vein and grafting it to the aorta at a point on the coronary artery distal to the obstruction and/or grafting the internal mammary artery directly to the diseased coronary artery. Heart valve replacement involves replacing the stenotic or regurgitant valve with a mechanical prosthesis (e.g. Starr-Edwards valve, Bjork-Shiley valve) or a biological (e.g. porcine) valve.

Both CABG and valve replacement surgeries are performed through a midline sternotomy or anterolateral thoracotomy. Cardiopulmonary bypass (extracorporeal circulation) is maintained during surgery by a heart-lung machine that performs vital gas exchange functions; maintains the desired body temperature; filters the blood for thrombi, emboli, or impurities; and recirculates the blood into the arterial system. Cold cardioplegia (infusing a cold solution containing potassium into the aortic

root and pericardium) is often performed to cool the myocardium and reduce its oxygen requirements. Prior to closing the chest, epicardial pacer wires are often placed on the atria and/or ventricles and connected to an external demand pacemaker. A chest tube is inserted to drain blood from the mediastinum, and if the pleura was opened, an additional chest tube is placed in the pleural cavity to evacuate air and blood and promote lung re-expansion.

This care plan focuses on the adult client hospitalized for either coronary artery bypass grafting (CABG) or valve replacement surgery. Preoperatively, a major goal of care is to reduce fear and anxiety. Goals of postoperative care are to maintain comfort, prevent complications, and educate the client regarding follow-up care.

DISCHARGE CRITERIA

Prior to discharge, the client will:

- identify modifiable cardiovascular risk factors and ways to reduce these factors
- verbalize an understanding of the rationale for and constituents of a diet low in sodium, saturated fat, and cholesterol
- verbalize an understanding of activity restrictions and the rate of activity progression
- verbalize an understanding of medication therapy including rationale for, side effects of, schedule for taking, and importance of taking as prescribed
- state signs and symptoms to report to the health care provider
- identify community resources that can assist with cardiac rehabilitation and adjustment to having had heart surgery
- verbalize an understanding of and a plan for adhering to recommended follow-up care including future appointments with health care provider, wound care, and pain management.

NURSING/COLLABORATIVE DIAGNOSES

Preoperative
  1. Anxiety □ *327*
Postoperative
  1. Decreased cardiac output □ *328*
  2. Altered systemic tissue perfusion □ *330*
  3. Ineffective breathing patterns:
      a. hypoventilation
      b. hyperventilation □ *330*
  4. Altered fluid and electrolyte balance:
      a. fluid volume excess or water intoxication
      b. fluid volume deficit, hypokalemia, hyponatremia, hypochloremia, and metabolic alkalosis
      c. hyperkalemia
      d. hypocalcemia
      e. metabolic acidosis □ *331*
  5. Pain:
      a. chest pain
      b. leg pain □ *333*

6. Activity intolerance □ *333*
7. Altered thought processes: cardiac psychosis (agitation, impaired memory and judgment, paranoia, confusion, hallucinations, combativeness) □ *334*
8. Potential for infection: pneumonia □ *335*
9A. Potential cardiac complications:
   1. myocardial infarction (MI)
   2. arrhythmias
   3. congestive heart failure (CHF)
   4. pericarditis or postpericardiotomy syndrome
   5. cardiac tamponade
   6. graft embolization, graft site separation, or paravalvular leaks
   7. cardiogenic shock □ *335*
9B. Potential extracardiac complications:
   1. bleeding
   2. thromboembolism
   3. cerebral ischemia
   4. impaired renal function
   5. atelectasis
   6. hemopneumothorax □ *339*
10. Knowledge deficit regarding follow-up care □ *343*

Preoperative

Use in conjunction with the Standardized Preoperative Care Plan.

1. NURSING DIAGNOSIS

Anxiety related to:

a. unfamiliar environment;
b. lack of understanding of diagnostic tests, planned surgery, and postoperative course;
c. effects of anesthesia and anticipated postoperative discomfort and disfigurement;
d. economic factors associated with surgery and hospitalization;
e. possible alterations in life style and roles;
f. possibility of death.

DESIRED OUTCOMES	NURSING ACTIONS AND *SELECTED RATIONALES*
1. The client will experience a reduction in fear and anxiety (see Standardized Preoperative	1.a. Refer to Standardized Preoperative Care Plan, Nursing Diagnosis 1, for measures related to assessment and reduction of fear and anxiety. b. Implement additional measures *to reduce fear and anxiety:*

Care Plan, Nursing Diagnosis 1, for outcome criteria).

1. explain all diagnostic tests that may be performed to determine cardiac status (e.g. EKG, phonocardiogram, echocardiogram, nuclear imaging, cardiac catheterization)
2. arrange for a visit from an intensive care nurse or a visit to the intensive care unit; assure client and significant others that transfer to intensive care after heart surgery is routine
3. explain the rationale for cardiac monitoring equipment, respirator, chest tubes, arterial and venous lines, nasogastric tube, and urinary catheter
4. if bypass grafting is planned, inform client that he/she may have leg incisions as well as a chest incision
5. inform client that the clicking sound that may be present after replacement of some valves is normal
6. explain to client that a very cold feeling will persist for several hours after surgery if the body temperature has been lowered during surgery
7. with client, establish an alternative method of communicating (e.g. magic slate, word board, flash cards, signals) to be used while he/she is on the respirator
8. encourage client to discuss fear of disfigurement, disability, and death; clarify any misconceptions the client may have
9. focus on postoperative care (this promotes a feeling in client that he/she will survive surgery)
10. arrange for a visit with a person who has had successful heart surgery.

☐ ▬▬▬▬▬▬▬▬▬▬▬▬▬▬▬▬▬▬▬▬▬▬▬▬▬▬▬▬

Postoperative

Use in conjunction with the Standardized Postoperative Care Plan.

☐ ▬▬▬▬▬▬▬▬▬▬▬▬▬▬▬▬▬▬▬▬▬▬▬▬▬▬▬▬

1. NURSING DIAGNOSIS

Decreased cardiac output related to:

a. pre-existing compromise in cardiac function;
b. trauma to the heart during surgery;
c. hypovolemia associated with surgical blood loss and persistent bleeding post-operatively; excessive loss of fluids resulting from nasogastric tube drainage, vomiting, and diuretic therapy; and decreased fluid intake;
d. hypotension associated with medication therapy (e.g. anesthetics, narcotics), hypovolemia, rapid body warming following surgery, decreased mobility, and development of cardiac complications.

☐ ▬▬▬▬▬▬▬▬▬▬▬▬▬▬▬▬▬▬▬▬▬▬▬▬▬▬▬▬

DESIRED OUTCOMES	NURSING ACTIONS AND *SELECTED RATIONALES*
1. The client will maintain adequate cardiac output as evidenced by: a. B/P within range of 120–90/80–70 b. apical pulse audible, regular, and between 60–100 beats/minute	1.a. Assess for and report signs and symptoms of: 1. hypovolemia (e.g. low B/P; resting pulse rate greater than 100 beats/minute; decline in B/P of at least 15 mm Hg with a concurrent rise in pulse when client sits up; cool, pale, or cyanotic skin; diminished or absent peripheral pulses; urine output less than 30 cc/hour; low central venous, left atrial, and pulmonary pressures) 2. hypotension (systolic B/P persistently below 100 mm Hg) 3. decreased cardiac output:

c. equal apical and radial pulses
d. absence of or no increase in intensity of gallop rhythms
e. B/P and pulse stable with position change
f. unlabored respirations at 16–20/minute
g. normal breath sounds
h. usual mental status
i. absence of lightheadedness or syncope
j. palpable peripheral pulses
k. normal amplitude of carotid pulse
l. skin warm and usual color
m. capillary refill time less than 3 seconds
n. urine output at least 30 cc/hour
o. hemodynamic measurements such as pulmonary artery pressure (PAP), pulmonary capillary wedge pressure (PCWP), left atrial pressure (LAP), cardiac output (CO), and central venous pressure (CVP) within normal limits
p. BUN and serum creatinine and alkaline phosphatase levels within normal range.

a. drop of 20 mm Hg in systolic B/P, a systolic pressure below 90 mm Hg, or a continual drop of 5–10 mm Hg in systolic pressure with each reading
b. irregular pulse
c. pulse rate less than 60 or greater than 100 beats/minute
d. apical-radial pulse deficit
e. muffled heart sounds
f. presence of an S_3 and/or S_4 gallop rhythm
g. decline in systolic B/P of at least 15 mm Hg with a concurrent rise in pulse when client sits up
h. rapid, labored, or irregular respirations
i. crackles and diminished or absent breath sounds
j. restlessness, confusion
k. lightheadedness, syncope
l. diminished or absent peripheral pulses
m. decreased amplitude of carotid pulse
n. cool, pale, mottled, or cyanotic skin
o. capillary refill time greater than 3 seconds
p. urine output less than 30 cc/hour
q. decreased CO; increased PAP, PCWP, LAP, and CVP (use internal jugular vein pulsation method to estimate CVP if monitoring device not present)
r. elevated BUN and serum creatinine and alkaline phosphatase levels.

b. Implement measures *to maintain adequate cardiac output:*
  1. perform actions *to reduce cardiac workload:*
     a. place client in a semi- to high Fowler's position
     b. instruct client to avoid activities that create a Valsalva response (e.g. straining to have a bowel movement, bending at the waist, holding breath while moving)
     c. implement measures to promote rest (see Standardized Postoperative Care Plan, Nursing Diagnosis 10, action b.1)
     d. maintain oxygen therapy as ordered
     e. discourage smoking (*smoking has a cardiostimulatory effect, causes vasoconstriction, and reduces oxygen availability*)
     f. provide frequent, small meals rather than 3 large ones (*large meals require an increase in blood supply to gastrointestinal tract for digestion*)
     g. discourage intake of foods/fluids high in caffeine such as coffee, tea, chocolate, and colas (*caffeine is a myocardial stimulant and increases myocardial oxygen consumption*)
     h. implement measures to prevent or treat fluid volume excess (see Postoperative Nursing Diagnosis 4, action a)
     i. increase activity gradually
  2. monitor for therapeutic and nontherapeutic effects of positive inotropic agents (e.g. digitalis preparations, dopamine) if administered *to increase myocardial contractility*
  3. perform actions *to prevent and treat hypovolemia:*
     a. administer blood and/or volume expanders as ordered
     b. maintain a minimum fluid intake of 1000 cc/day unless ordered otherwise
     c. implement measures to prevent and control bleeding (see Postoperative Collaborative Diagnosis 9.B, actions 1.d and e)
  4. perform actions *to prevent hypotension:*
     a. monitor B/P closely before and after administering negative inotropic agents (e.g. propranolol), vasodilators, and narcotic analgesics
     b. consult physician before giving negative inotropic and vasodilating agents if B/P is below 110/70 mm Hg
     c. administer narcotic analgesics judiciously, being alert to the synergistic effect of the narcotic ordered and the anesthetic that was used during surgery
     d. implement measures to prevent and treat hypovolemia (see action b.3 in this diagnosis)
     e. increase activity gradually
     f. monitor for therapeutic and nontherapeutic effects of sympathomimetics (e.g. norepinephrine, dopamine) if administered
  5. perform actions to prevent and treat postoperative cardiac complications

UNIT VII

(see Postoperative Collaborative Diagnosis 9.A, actions 1.c; 2.b and c; 3.c and d; 4.b; 5.b and c; 6.b and c; and 7.b and c).

    c. Consult physician if signs and symptoms of decreased cardiac output persist or worsen.

2. NURSING DIAGNOSIS

Altered systemic tissue perfusion related to:

a. hypovolemia associated with fluid loss and decreased fluid intake;
b. peripheral pooling of blood associated with decreased venous return resulting from a loss of vasomotor tone associated with anesthesia, some medications (e.g. narcotic analgesics), and decreased activity;
c. vasoconstriction associated with hypothermia (hypothermia may be utilized to lower the metabolic rate during surgery or may result from cool operating and recovery room temperatures);
d. decreased cardiac output.

DESIRED OUTCOMES	NURSING ACTIONS AND *SELECTED RATIONALES*
2. The client will maintain adequate systemic tissue perfusion (see Standardized Postoperative Care Plan, Nursing Diagnosis 2, for outcome criteria).	2.a. Refer to Standardized Postoperative Care Plan, Nursing Diagnosis 2, for measures related to assessment and maintenance of adequate systemic tissue perfusion. b. Implement measures to maintain adequate cardiac output (see Postoperative Nursing Diagnosis 1, action b) *in order to improve systemic tissue perfusion.*

3. NURSING DIAGNOSIS

Ineffective breathing patterns:

a. **hypoventilation** related to depressant effects of anesthesia and some medications (e.g. narcotic analgesics, muscle relaxants), weakness, reluctance to breathe deeply due to chest incision pain and fear of dislodging chest tube, and pressure on the diaphragm due to abdominal distention;
b. **hyperventilation** related to:
    1. fear and anxiety
    2. excessive ventilatory assistance
    3. compensation for metabolic or respiratory acidosis and decreased tissue oxygenation.

DESIRED OUTCOMES	NURSING ACTIONS AND *SELECTED RATIONALES*
3. The client will maintain an effective breathing pattern (see Standardized	3.a. Refer to Standardized Postoperative Care Plan, Nursing Diagnosis 3, for measures related to assessment and management of ineffective breathing patterns.

Postoperative Care Plan, Nursing Diagnosis 3, for outcome criteria).

b. Implement additional measures *to improve breathing pattern:*
  1. assure client that the chest tube is sutured in place and that deep breathing will not dislodge the tube
  2. perform actions to prevent or treat metabolic acidosis (see Postoperative Nursing Diagnosis 4, action e.2)
  3. perform actions to maintain adequate systemic tissue perfusion (see Postoperative Nursing Diagnosis 2) *in order to improve tissue oxygenation*
  4. monitor mechanical ventilation carefully *to ensure that ventilatory rate and pressures are correct.*

c. Consult physician if:
  1. ineffective breathing patterns continue
  2. signs and symptoms of impaired gas exchange (e.g. confusion, restlessness, irritability, cyanosis, decreased PaO_2 and increased $PaCO_2$ levels) are present
  3. signs and symptoms of respiratory acidosis (e.g. change in mental status, rapid pulse, dizziness, headache, feeling of fullness in head, muscle twitching, seizures, elevated $PaCO_2$ and low pH) occur
  4. signs and symptoms of respiratory alkalosis (e.g. inability to concentrate, lightheadedness, palpitations, circumoral paresthesias, numbness and tingling of extremities, diaphoresis, tinnitus, blurred vision, low $PaCO_2$ and elevated pH) occur.

4. NURSING/COLLABORATIVE DIAGNOSIS

Altered fluid and electrolyte balance:

a. **fluid volume excess or water intoxication** related to:
  1. the hemodilution technique used to prime the heart-lung machine
  2. vigorous fluid and blood replacement therapy during and immediately after surgery
  3. increased production of antidiuretic hormone (ADH) and aldosterone post-operatively (output of these hormones is stimulated by trauma, pain, anesthetic agents, and narcotic analgesics)
  4. reabsorption of third-space fluid approximately 3 days after surgery
  5. renal or cardiac insufficiency;

b. **fluid volume deficit, hypokalemia, hyponatremia, hypochloremia, and metabolic alkalosis** related to excessive loss of fluid and electrolytes associated with vomiting, nasogastric tube drainage, and diuretic therapy (the hemodilution technique used to prime the heart-lung machine further contributes to the hypokalemia, hyponatremia, and hypochloremia);

c. **hyperkalemia** related to metabolic acidosis (high serum hydrogen levels cause cellular potassium to shift into vascular space), red cell hemolysis while on heart-lung machine, and renal insufficiency;

d. **hypocalcemia** related to alkalosis (reduces the level of available calcium) and multiple blood transfusions during surgery (the citrate in stored blood binds calcium);

e. **metabolic acidosis** related to hyperkalemia (high serum potassium levels cause cellular hydrogen to shift into the vascular space) and lactic acid release associated with tissue hypoxia.

DESIRED OUTCOMES	NURSING ACTIONS AND *SELECTED RATIONALES*
4.a. The client will not experience fluid volume excess or water intoxication	4.a.1. Refer to Standardized Postoperative Care Plan, Nursing Diagnosis 5, action b, for measures related to assessment, prevention, and management of fluid volume excess and water intoxication.

(see Standardized Postoperative Care Plan, Nursing Diagnosis 5, outcome b, for outcome criteria).

2. Implement additional measures *to prevent or treat fluid volume excess and water intoxication:*
   a. perform actions to maintain adequate renal blood flow (see Postoperative Collaborative Diagnosis 9.B, action 4.c)
   b. perform actions to maintain an adequate cardiac output (see Postoperative Nursing Diagnosis 1, action b)
   c. maintain fluid and sodium restrictions as ordered (2500 cc fluid and 3–4 gm sodium restrictions are common).

4.b. The client will not experience fluid volume deficit, hypokalemia, hyponatremia, hypochloremia, and metabolic alkalosis (see Standardized Postoperative Care Plan, Nursing Diagnosis 5, outcome a, for outcome criteria).

4.b. Refer to Standardized Postoperative Care Plan, Nursing Diagnosis 5, action a, for measures related to assessment, prevention, and treatment of fluid volume deficit, hypokalemia, hyponatremia, hypochloremia, and metabolic alkalosis.

4.c. The client will maintain a safe serum potassium level as evidenced by:
1. regular pulse at 60–100 beats/minute
2. usual muscle tone and strength
3. normal bowel sounds
4. serum potassium within normal range.

4.c.1. Assess for and report signs and symptoms of hyperkalemia (e.g. slow or irregular pulse; paresthesias; muscle weakness and flaccidity; hyperactive bowel sounds with diarrhea and intestinal colic; EKG reading showing peaked T wave, prolonged PR interval, and/or widened QRS; elevated serum potassium level).
2. Implement measures *to prevent or treat hyperkalemia:*
   a. maintain dietary restrictions of potassium if ordered
   b. perform actions to prevent or treat metabolic acidosis (see action e.2 in this diagnosis) *in order to decrease cellular release of potassium*
   c. perform actions to maintain adequate renal blood flow (see Postoperative Collaborative Diagnosis 9.B, action 4.c) *in order to promote normal excretion of potassium*
   d. if signs and symptoms of hyperkalemia are present, consult physician before administering prescribed potassium supplements
   e. request fresh blood if transfusions are necessary (*the potassium content of stored blood is higher than that of fresh blood*)
   f. monitor for therapeutic and nontherapeutic effects of the following if administered:
      1. loop diuretics (e.g. ethacrynic acid, furosemide) *to increase renal excretion of potassium*
      2. cation-exchange resins (e.g. Kayexalate) *to increase potassium excretion via the intestines (act by exchanging sodium for potassium)*
      3. intravenous insulin and hypertonic glucose solutions *to enhance transport of potassium back into cells.*
3. Consult physician if signs and symptoms of hyperkalemia persist or worsen.

4.d. The client will maintain a safe serum calcium level as evidenced by:
1. usual mental status
2. regular pulse at 60–100 beats/minute
3. negative Chvostek's and Trousseau's signs
4. absence of paresthesias, muscle cramps, tetany, seizure activity
5. serum calcium within normal range.

4.d.1. Assess for and report signs and symptoms of hypocalcemia (e.g. change in mental status; cardiac arrhythmias; positive Chvostek's and Trousseau's signs; numbness and tingling of fingers, toes, and circumoral area; muscle cramps; tetany; seizures; low serum calcium level).
2. Implement measures *to prevent or treat hypocalcemia:*
   a. perform actions *to prevent binding of ionized calcium:*
      1. implement measures to prevent metabolic alkalosis (see Standardized Postoperative Care Plan, Nursing Diagnosis 5, action a.3)
      2. implement measures to improve breathing pattern (see Postoperative Nursing Diagnosis 3, actions a and b) *in order to prevent respiratory alkalosis*
   b. request fresh blood if additional transfusions are necessary (*the citrate in stored blood binds calcium*)
   c. provide sources of calcium and vitamin D (e.g. dairy products) in diet
   d. administer activated vitamin D and calcium supplements as ordered.
3. If signs and symptoms of hypocalcemia occur:
   a. institute seizure precautions
   b. have intravenous calcium preparation readily available.

4.e. The client will maintain acid-base balance as evidenced by:
1. usual mental status
2. unlabored respirations at 16–20/minute
3. absence of headache, nausea, and vomiting
4. blood gases within normal range
5. anion gap less than 16 mEq/liter.

4.e.1. Assess for and report signs and symptoms of metabolic acidosis (e.g. drowsiness; disorientation; stupor; rapid, deep respirations; headache; nausea and vomiting; low pH and CO_2 content and negative base excess; anion gap greater than 16 mEq/liter).
2. Implement measures *to prevent or treat metabolic acidosis:*
   a. perform actions to maintain adequate systemic tissue perfusion (see Postoperative Nursing Diagnosis 2) *in order to reduce tissue hypoxia and the resultant lactic acid release*
   b. perform actions to prevent or treat hyperkalemia (see action c.2 in this diagnosis) *in order to decrease cellular release of hydrogen*
   c. monitor for therapeutic and nontherapeutic effects of sodium bicarbonate if administered (reserved for use in severe acidosis when pH is less than 7.1).
3. Consult physician if signs and symptoms of acidosis persist or worsen.

5. NURSING DIAGNOSIS

Pain:

a. **chest pain** related to tissue trauma associated with the surgery and tissue irritation associated with the presence of chest tube(s);
b. **leg pain** related to tissue trauma associated with excision of the saphenous vein for graft use.

DESIRED OUTCOMES	NURSING ACTIONS AND *SELECTED RATIONALES*
5. The client will experience diminished pain (see Standardized Postoperative Care Plan, Nursing Diagnosis 7.A, for outcome criteria).	5.a. Refer to Standardized Postoperative Care Plan, Nursing Diagnosis 7.A, for measures related to assessment and management of postoperative pain. b. Securely anchor chest tube(s) *to decrease discomfort resulting from movement of tube(s).*

6. NURSING DIAGNOSIS

Activity intolerance related to:

a. tissue hypoxia associated with diminished systemic tissue perfusion and anemia resulting from blood loss and red cell hemolysis (red cells are traumatized by heart-lung machine);
b. difficulty resting and sleeping due to frequent assessments and treatments, discomfort, fear, and anxiety.

DESIRED OUTCOMES	NURSING ACTIONS AND *SELECTED RATIONALES*
6. The client will demonstrate an increased tolerance for activity (see Standardized	6.a. Refer to Standardized Postoperative Care Plan, Nursing Diagnosis 10, for measures related to assessment and improvement of activity tolerance. b. Implement additional measures *to improve activity tolerance:*

Postoperative Care Plan,
Nursing Diagnosis 10, for
outcome criteria).

1. perform actions to maintain adequate systemic tissue perfusion (see
   Postoperative Nursing Diagnosis 2)
2. perform actions to improve breathing pattern (see Postoperative Nursing
   Diagnosis 3, actions a and b) and promote effective airway clearance (see
   Standardized Postoperative Care Plan, Nursing Diagnosis 4, action b) *in
   order to maintain adequate alveolar gas exchange*
3. encourage client to increase intake of foods high in iron (e.g. organ
   meats, apricots, figs, green leafy vegetables, whole-grain and enriched
   breads and cereals) *to help resolve anemia*
4. monitor for therapeutic and nontherapeutic effects of whole blood or
   packed red cells if administered
5. increase client's activity gradually as allowed and tolerated; explain to
   client that a progressive and gradual increase in activity is necessary *in
   order to strengthen the myocardium without causing a sudden increase
   in cardiac workload.*

7. NURSING DIAGNOSIS

**Altered thought processes: cardiac psychosis (agitation, impaired memory and
judgment, paranoia, confusion, hallucinations, combativeness)** related to
prolonged time on heart-lung machine; prolonged deep anesthesia; and sleep deprivation and sensory overload associated with fear, anxiety, pain, frequent assessments and treatments, and noise from monitoring devices.

DESIRED OUTCOMES	NURSING ACTIONS AND *SELECTED RATIONALES*

7. The client will regain usual
   thought processes as
   evidenced by:
   a. usual memory and
      judgment
   b. absence of agitation,
      paranoia, hallucinations,
      confusion, combativeness.

7.a. Assess client for signs and symptoms of cardiac psychosis (e.g. impaired
     memory and judgment, agitation, paranoia, confusion, hallucinations,
     combativeness).
   b. Ascertain from significant others client's usual personality and level of
      intellectual functioning.
   c. Implement measures *to prevent cardiac psychosis:*
      1. perform actions *to reduce fear and anxiety* (e.g. explain treatments; keep
         monitor out of client's view; be readily available to client; project a calm,
         confident manner)
      2. perform actions to promote sleep (see Standardized Postoperative Care
         Plan, Nursing Diagnosis 15, action c)
      3. perform actions to reduce pain (see Postoperative Nursing Diagnosis 5)
      4. perform actions *to minimize environmental stimuli:*
         a. plan assessments, treatments, and care activities to allow periods of
            uninterrupted rest
         b. dim lights in room
         c. keep auditory level on monitors as low as possible
         d. avoid unnecessary conversations in or directly outside of client's room
         e. restrict the number of visitors and their length of stay.
   d. If client shows evidence of cardiac psychosis:
      1. initiate appropriate safety precautions (e.g. side rails up, accompany
         when out of bed)
      2. reorient client to person, place, and time as necessary
      3. allow adequate time for communication and performance of activities
      4. repeat instructions as necessary using clear, simple language
      5. perform actions *to reduce paranoia:*
         a. explain treatments and care activities thoroughly
         b. follow through with actions/activities you have told client you will
            perform

6. encourage significant others to be supportive of client; instruct them to reorient client as necessary
7. assure client and significant others that symptoms client is experiencing are not unusual and should gradually subside
8. monitor for therapeutic and nontherapeutic effects of antianxiety and antipsychotic agents if administered
9. consult physician if signs of cardiac psychosis persist or worsen.

8. NURSING DIAGNOSIS

Potential for infection: pneumonia related to stasis of pulmonary secretions and aspiration.

DESIRED OUTCOMES	NURSING ACTIONS AND *SELECTED RATIONALES*
8. The client will not develop pneumonia (see Standardized Postoperative Care Plan, Nursing Diagnosis 16, outcome a, for outcome criteria).	8.a. Refer to Standardized Postoperative Care Plan, Nursing Diagnosis 16, action a, for measures related to assessment, prevention, and treatment of pneumonia. b. Assure client that chest tube is sutured in place and that coughing and deep breathing will not dislodge the tube or disrupt the suture line.

9.A. COLLABORATIVE DIAGNOSIS

Potential cardiac complications:

1. **myocardial infarction (MI)** related to insufficient coronary blood flow intraoperatively or postoperatively;
2. **arrhythmias** related to altered myocardial conductivity associated with trauma to the heart during surgery, electrolyte imbalance (particularly potassium and calcium), pericarditis, acid-base imbalances, and hypoxia;
3. **congestive heart failure (CHF)** related to preoperative myocardial hypertrophy and further damage to the myocardium during surgery;
4. **pericarditis or postpericardiotomy syndrome** related to:
   a. an inflammatory response that occurs with the surgery, an infarction, or an infection
   b. residual blood left in the pericardial sac;
5. **cardiac tamponade** related to blood or fluid accumulation in the pericardial sac and/or mediastinum;
6. **graft embolization, graft site separation, or paravalvular leaks** related to surgical trauma, loss of integrity of suture line, and/or postoperative hypertension (there is an increased risk of separation and leakage if hypertension occurs; hypertension is of greatest risk the first 24 hours postoperatively due to high catecholamine output and fluid loading during surgery as well as vasoconstriction induced by hypothermia);
7. **cardiogenic shock** related to:
   a. rupture of any cardiac structure
   b. inability of the damaged heart, intrinsic compensatory mechanisms, and treatment measures to maintain adequate tissue perfusion to vital organs.

DESIRED OUTCOMES	NURSING ACTIONS AND *SELECTED RATIONALES*

9.A.1. The client will not experience an MI as evidenced by:
    a. no episodes of sudden, severe, and persistent chest pain
    b. stable vital signs
    c. cardiac enzyme levels declining toward normal range
    d. absence of ST segment elevation, T wave changes, and pathological Q wave on EKG reading.

9.A.1.a. Assess for and report signs and symptoms of a myocardial infarction (e.g. sudden, severe, and persistent chest pain; dyspnea; fall in mean arterial pressure in presence of normal CVP; further increase in cardiac enzymes; significant ST segment elevation, T wave changes, and/or pathological Q wave on EKG reading).
    b. Implement measures to maintain adequate cardiac output (see Postoperative Nursing Diagnosis 1, action b) *in order to improve myocardial blood supply and reduce the risk of myocardial infarction.*
    c. If signs and symptoms of a myocardial infarction occur:
      1. initiate cardiac monitoring if not already being done
      2. maintain client on strict bedrest in a semi- to high Fowler's position
      3. maintain oxygen therapy as ordered
      4. monitor for therapeutic and nontherapeutic effects of the following medications if administered:
        a. morphine sulfate *to reduce pain and anxiety and decrease cardiac workload*
        b. vasodilators *to reduce preload and/or afterload*
        c. positive inotropic agents *to improve cardiac output*
        d. beta-adrenergic blocking agents *to reduce sympathetic stimulation of the heart*
      5. initiate cardiopulmonary resuscitation if indicated
      6. provide emotional support to client and significant others
      7. refer to Care Plan on Myocardial Infarction for additional care measures.

9.A.2. The client will not experience cardiac arrhythmias as evidenced by:
    a. regular apical pulse at 60–100 beats/minute
    b. equal apical and radial pulses
    c. absence of syncope and palpitations
    d. EKG reading showing normal sinus rhythm.

9.A.2.a. Assess for and report signs and symptoms of arrhythmias (e.g. irregular apical pulse; pulse rate below 60 or above 100 beats/minute; apical-radial pulse deficit; syncope; palpitations; abnormal rate, rhythm, or configurations on EKG).
    b. Implement measures *to prevent arrhythmias:*
      1. perform actions to maintain adequate cardiac output and myocardial blood flow (see Postoperative Nursing Diagnosis 1, action b)
      2. maintain oxygen therapy as ordered
      3. perform actions to maintain electrolyte and acid-base balance (see Postoperative Nursing Diagnosis 4, actions b, c.2, d.2, and e.2)
      4. perform actions to improve breathing pattern (see Postoperative Nursing Diagnosis 3, actions a and b) and promote effective airway clearance (see Standardized Postoperative Care Plan, Nursing Diagnosis 4, action b) *in order to improve tissue oxygenation and prevent respiratory acidosis or alkalosis (myocardial conductivity is altered by hypoxia and acid-base imbalance).*
    c. If arrhythmias occur:
      1. initiate cardiac monitoring if not already being done
      2. monitor for therapeutic and nontherapeutic effects of the following medications if administered:
        a. Class I antiarrhythmics (e.g. phenytoin, tocainide, lidocaine, flecainide, procainamide, disopyramide, quinidine) *to interfere directly with depolarization*
        b. Class II antiarrhythmics (e.g. propranolol) *to block beta-adrenergic stimulation*
        c. Class III antiarrhythmics (e.g. bretylium, amiodarone) *to prolong the duration of the action potential*
        d. Class IV antiarrhythmics (e.g. verapamil, diltiazem) *to block the slow inward depolarizing current*
        e. anticholinergic agents (e.g. atropine) or sympathomimetics (e.g. ephedrine, isoproterenol) *to increase heart rate*
        f. cardiac glycosides (e.g. digitalis) *to decrease the heart rate*
      3. restrict client's activity based on his/her tolerance and severity of arrhythmia
      4. maintain oxygen therapy as ordered
      5. have emergency cart readily available for defibrillation, cardioversion, or cardiopulmonary resuscitation
      6. maintain temporary pacemaker function as ordered.

9.A.3. The client will not develop CHF as evidenced by:
   a. stable vital signs
   b. audible heart sounds without an S₃ or S₄ or softening of pre-existing murmurs
   c. normal breath sounds
   d. absence of or no increase in dyspnea and orthopnea
   e. palpable peripheral pulses and stronger carotid pulse amplitude
   f. balanced intake and output
   g. stable weight
   h. CVP within normal range
   i. absence of peripheral edema; distended neck veins; enlarged, tender liver
   j. BUN and serum creatinine and alkaline phosphatase levels within normal range.

9.A.3.a Assess for and report signs and symptoms of CHF:
   1. significant increase in pulse rate
   2. softened or muffled heart sounds
   3. development of or intensified S₃ and/or S₄ gallop rhythm
   4. crackles and diminished or absent breath sounds
   5. dyspnea, orthopnea
   6. displaced apical impulse
   7. diminished or absent peripheral pulses
   8. decreased amplitude of carotid pulse
   9. intake greater than output
   10. weight gain
   11. elevated CVP
   12. peripheral edema
   13. distended neck veins
   14. enlarged, tender liver
   15. elevated BUN and serum creatinine and alkaline phosphatase levels.
   b. Monitor chest x-ray results. Report findings of cardiomegaly, pleural effusion, or pulmonary edema.
   c. Implement measures *to prevent CHF:*
      1. perform actions to maintain adequate cardiac output (see Postoperative Nursing Diagnosis 1, action b)
      2. monitor for therapeutic and nontherapeutic effects of positive inotropic agents (e.g. digitalis preparations, dopamine) if administered *to increase myocardial contractility.*
   d. If signs and symptoms of CHF occur:
      1. continue with above actions
      2. monitor for therapeutic and nontherapeutic effects of medications that may be administered *to reduce vascular congestion and/or cardiac workload* (e.g. diuretics, cardiotonics, vasodilators, morphine sulfate)
      3. apply rotating tourniquets according to hospital policy if ordered *to reduce pulmonary vascular congestion*
      4. refer to Care Plan on Congestive Heart Failure for additional care measures.

9.A.4. The client will experience resolution of pericarditis or postpericardiotomy syndrome if it occurs as evidenced by:
   a. fewer complaints of substernal or precordial pain
   b. absence of pericardial friction rub
   c. unlabored respirations at 16–20/minute
   d. temperature declining toward normal
   e. WBC count and sedimentation rate declining toward normal range.

9.A.4.a. Assess for and report signs and symptoms of pericarditis and postpericardiotomy syndrome:
   1. substernal or precordial pain that frequently radiates to left shoulder, neck, and arm; is intensified during deep inspiration; and usually is relieved by sitting up
   2. pericardial friction rub (may be transient)
   3. dyspnea, tachypnea
   4. persistent temperature elevation
   5. further increase in WBC count and sedimentation rate (both will be elevated as a result of the surgery)
   6. chest x-ray and echocardiography results showing cardiomegaly and pericardial effusion.
   b. If signs and symptoms of pericarditis or postpericardiotomy syndrome occur:
      1. allay client's anxiety (client may believe that symptoms indicate a "heart attack")
      2. monitor for therapeutic and nontherapeutic effects of medications that may be administered *to reduce inflammation* (e.g. aspirin, indomethacin, ibuprofen, corticosteroids)
      3. assess for and immediately report signs of cardiac tamponade (see action 5.a.2 in this diagnosis for list of signs)
      4. prepare client for and assist with pericardiocentesis if indicated.

9.A.5. The client will not experience cardiac tamponade as evidenced by:
   a. stable vital signs
   b. audible heart sounds
   c. absence of neck vein

9.A.5.a. Assess for and immediately report:
   1. a sudden cessation of chest tube drainage or a sudden increase in bleeding from the midline incision *(may indicate accumulation of fluid in the mediastinum or pericardium, which can lead to cardiac tamponade)*
   2. signs and symptoms of cardiac tamponade (e.g. rapid and continual decline in B/P; narrowed pulse pressure; pulsus paradoxus; weak,

distention on inspiration
d. normal amplitude of waves on EKG
e. CVP and pulmonary pressures within normal limits.

rapid pulse; distant or muffled heart sounds; neck vein distention on inspiration; decreased amplitude of waves on EKG; increased CVP and pulmonary pressures).
b. Implement measures *to reduce the risk of cardiac tamponade:*
 1. administer medications to treat pericarditis or postpericardiotomy syndrome (see action 4.b.2 in this diagnosis) *in order to reduce inflammation and fluid accumulation in the pericardial sac*
 2. perform actions *to maintain patency and integrity of chest drainage system:*
  a. maintain water seal and suction levels as ordered
  b. maintain air occlusive dressing over chest tube insertion site
  c. tape all connections securely
  d. milk or strip mediastinal tube(s) every 1–2 hours if ordered (milking or stripping of mediastinal tube[s] is thought to be unnecessary and of little value by some clinicians)
  e. always keep drainage system below client's chest level
  f. keep chest drainage and suction tubing free of kinks
 3. if mediastinal tube(s) becomes obstructed:
  a. assist with clearing of the tube(s) using a Fogarty catheter
  b. prepare client for surgical intervention (e.g. removal of clots, insertion of another chest tube) if indicated.
c. If signs and symptoms of cardiac tamponade occur, prepare client for pericardiocentesis or further surgery as indicated.

9.A.6. The client will not experience graft embolization, graft site separation, or paravalvular leakage as evidenced by signs and symptoms of adequate cardiac output (see Postoperative Nursing Diagnosis 1 for outcome criteria).

9.A.6.a. Assess for and report signs and symptoms of graft embolization, graft site separation, and paravalvular leakage (manifested by signs and symptoms of decreased cardiac output [see Postoperative Nursing Diagnosis 1, action a.3]).
b. Implement measures *to minimize the risk of graft embolization, graft site separation, and paravalvular leakage:*
 1. monitor for therapeutic and nontherapeutic effects of low-dose heparin and antiplatelet agents (e.g. aspirin, dipyridamole) if administered *to reduce the risk of graft embolization*
 2. perform actions *to prevent and control hypertension* (the goal is to maintain systolic pressure close to 110 mm Hg) *in order to decrease the risk of suture line separation and paravalvular leakage:*
  a. implement measures to promote rest (see Standardized Postoperative Care Plan, Nursing Diagnosis 10, action b.1)
  b. implement measures *to reduce fear and anxiety* (e.g. explain treatments; keep monitor out of client's view; be readily available to client; project a calm, confident manner)
  c. monitor for therapeutic and nontherapeutic effects of vasodilators (e.g. captopril, nitroprusside) if administered.
c. If signs and symptoms of graft embolization, graft separation, or paravalvular leakage occur, prepare the client for further surgery if indicated.

9.A.7. The client will not develop cardiogenic shock as evidenced by:
a. stable or improved mental status
b. stable vital signs
c. palpable peripheral pulses
d. stable or improved skin color and temperature
e. urine output at least 20 cc/hour
f. stable or stronger carotid pulse amplitude
g. CVP, PCWP, and LAP within normal range.

9.A.7.a. Assess for and immediately report signs and symptoms of cardiogenic shock:
 1. increased restlessness, lethargy, or confusion
 2. decrease in systolic B/P of 30 mm Hg or a systolic pressure below 80 mm Hg
 3. pulse rate greater than 100 beats/minute
 4. diminished or absent peripheral pulses
 5. increased coolness and duskiness or cyanosis of skin
 6. urine output less than 20 cc/hour
 7. further decrease in amplitude of carotid pulse
 8. elevated CVP, PCWP, and LAP.
b. Implement measures *to prevent cardiogenic shock:*
 1. perform actions to maintain adequate cardiac output (see Postoperative Nursing Diagnosis 1, action b)
 2. perform actions to prevent and control hypertension (see action 6.b.2 in this diagnosis) *to decrease the risk of rupture of any cardiac structure.*
c. If signs and symptoms of cardiogenic shock occur:
 1. continue with actions to improve cardiac output

2. implement additional measures *to increase myocardial oxygen supply:*
   a. maintain oxygen therapy as ordered
   b. assist with hyperbaric oxygenation and extracorporeal membrane oxygenation (ECMO) if indicated
3. implement additional measures *to reduce oxygen utilization:*
   a. maintain client on strict bedrest
   b. assist with measures to induce hypothermia if ordered
4. monitor for therapeutic and nontherapeutic effects of the following if administered:
   a. sympathomimetics (e.g. dopamine, dobutamine, isoproterenol, norepinephrine) *to increase cardiac output and maintain arterial pressure*
   b. antiarrhythmic agents *to increase cardiac output*
   c. vasodilators (e.g. nitroprusside, nitroglycerin) *to decrease cardiac workload* (sympathomimetics are given in conjunction with vasodilators *to maintain arterial pressure*)
   d. intravenous infusions of insulin, potassium, and hypertonic glucose *to provide an energy source for the cells*
   e. intravenous sodium bicarbonate *to correct acidosis* (reserved for use in severe acidosis when pH is less than 7.1)
5. prepare client for insertion of intra-aortic balloon pump (IABP) or further surgery (e.g. repair of ruptured cardiac structure, ventricular assist device implant) if indicated
6. provide emotional support to client and significant others.

9.B. COLLABORATIVE DIAGNOSIS

Potential extracardiac complications:

1. **bleeding** related to:
   a. alteration in platelet function and destruction of clotting factors associated with utilization of heart-lung machine during surgery
   b. incomplete neutralization of the heparin used to prime the heart-lung machine
   c. anticoagulant therapy (relevant primarily for clients who have had valve replacement);
2. **thromboembolism** related to:
   a. trauma to the coronary arteries and donor vessels during grafting procedure
   b. mural thrombi formation at the prosthetic valve site
   c. incomplete filtration of air by heart-lung machine
   d. formation of microemboli associated with incomplete emptying of cardiac chambers if atrial fibrillation occurs
   e. venous stasis associated with diminished cardiac output and decreased mobility;
3. **cerebral ischemia** related to low cardiac output or an embolus;
4. **impaired renal function** related to deposit of hemolyzed red blood cells in renal tubules or inadequate renal blood flow associated with low cardiac output, hypovolemia, an embolus, or vasoconstriction during cardiopulmonary bypass;
5. **atelectasis** related to:
   a. hypoventilation associated with depressant effects of anesthesia and some medications, weakness, chest incision pain, fear of dislodging chest tube(s), and abdominal distention
   b. obstruction of the bronchioles with retained secretions;
6. **hemopneumothorax** related to the accumulation of air and blood in the pleural space if the pleura was opened during surgery.

DESIRED OUTCOMES	NURSING ACTIONS AND *SELECTED RATIONALES*

9.B.1. The client will not experience unusual bleeding as evidenced by:
  a. gradual decline in amount of bloody drainage from chest tube(s)
  b. skin and mucous membranes free of bleeding, petechiae, and ecchymosis
  c. absence of unusual joint pain or swelling
  d. no increase in abdominal girth
  e. absence of frank or occult blood in stool, urine, and vomitus
  f. usual menstrual flow
  g. vital signs within normal range for client
  h. stable or improved Hct. and Hgb.
  i. usual mental status.

9.B.1.a. Assess client for and report signs and symptoms of unusual bleeding:
  1. excessive amount of bloody drainage from chest tubes (200 cc/hour is maximum amount expected in first 4–6 hours; drainage should then markedly decline) and/or change in color of drainage from dark red to a bright red
  2. continuous oozing of blood from incisions
  3. petechiae
  4. multiple ecchymotic areas
  5. bleeding gums
  6. frequent or uncontrollable episodes of epistaxis
  7. unusual oozing from injection sites
  8. unusual joint pain or swelling
  9. increase in abdominal girth
  10. hematemesis, melena, red or smoke-colored urine
  11. hypermenorrhea
  12. significant drop in B/P accompanied by an increased pulse rate
  13. decline in Hct. and Hgb. levels
  14. restlessness, confusion.
  b. Monitor coagulation test results (e.g. prothrombin time, activated partial thromboplastin time, platelet count, bleeding time). Report abnormal values.
  c. If coagulation test results are abnormal or Hct. and Hgb. levels decline, test all stools, urine, and vomitus for occult blood. Report positive results.
  d. Implement measures *to prevent bleeding:*
    1. use the smallest gauge needle possible when giving injections and performing venous or arterial punctures
    2. apply gentle, prolonged pressure after injections and venous or arterial punctures
    3. take B/P only when necessary and avoid overinflating the cuff
    4. caution client to avoid activities that increase potential for trauma (e.g. shaving with a straight-edge razor, cutting nails, using stiff bristle toothbrush or dental floss)
    5. pad side rails if client is confused or restless
    6. remove hazardous objects from pathway *to prevent bumps or falls*
    7. instruct client to avoid blowing nose forcefully or straining to have a bowel movement; consult physician regarding order for decongestants, stool softeners, and/or laxatives if indicated
    8. monitor for therapeutic and nontherapeutic effects of the following medications and blood products if administered:
      a. vitamin K (e.g. phytonadione, menadione)
      b. protamine sulfate
      c. platelets
      d. plasma or whole blood.
  e. If bleeding occurs and does not subside spontaneously:
    1. apply firm, prolonged pressure to bleeding area if possible
    2. if epistaxis occurs, place client in a high Fowler's position and apply pressure and ice packs to nasal area
    3. maintain oxygen therapy as ordered
    4. perform iced water or saline lavage as ordered *to control gastric bleeding*
    5. administer vitamin K (e.g. phytonadione) and blood products (e.g. fresh frozen plasma, whole blood, platelets) as ordered
    6. prepare client for return to surgery if indicated
    7. provide emotional support to client and significant others.

9.B.2. The client will not develop a thromboembolism as evidenced by:
  a. palpable peripheral pulses

9.B.2.a. Assess for and report signs and symptoms of:
  1. venous thrombus (e.g. pain, swelling, unusual warmth or redness, and/or positive Homan's sign in extremity)
  2. arterial thrombus or embolus (e.g. diminished or absent peripheral pulses; pallor, cyanosis, coolness, numbness, and/or pain in extremity)

b. usual skin temperature and color of extremities

c. absence of pain in extremities

d. absence of sudden chest pain, cough, hemoptysis

e. usual mental status

f. usual sensory and motor function.

3. cerebral ischemia (see action 3.a in this diagnosis for a list of signs and symptoms)

4. pulmonary embolism (e.g. sudden, severe chest pain; cough; hemoptysis; dyspnea; cyanosis; increased restlessness; transient weakness or faintness).

b. Implement measures to prevent and treat a venous thrombus and pulmonary embolism (see Standardized Postoperative Care Plan, Collaborative Diagnosis 19, actions c.1.b and c and c.2.b and c).

c. Implement measures *to prevent development of mural thrombi and microemboli:*

1. perform actions to prevent and treat arrhythmias (see Postoperative Collaborative Diagnosis 9.A, actions 2.b and c) *in order to reduce stasis of blood in cardiac chambers*

2. monitor for therapeutic and nontherapeutic effects of anticoagulants (e.g. heparin, warfarin) or antiplatelet agents (e.g. aspirin, dipyridamole) if administered prophylactically.

d. If signs and symptoms of an arterial thromboembolism occur:

1. maintain client on strict bedrest with lower extremities in a level or slightly dependent position *to improve arterial blood flow*

2. prepare client for diagnostic studies (e.g. Doppler ultrasound, plethysmography, oscillometry)

3. implement measures *to promote vasodilation in the obstructed extremity:*
   a. administer peripheral vasodilating agents (e.g. papaverine, cyclandelate) as ordered
   b. keep lower extremities warm
   c. assist with a lumbar sympathetic block if performed *to decrease vasoconstrictor tone*

4. monitor for therapeutic and nontherapeutic effects of heparin and thrombolytic agents (e.g. streptokinase, tissue plasminogen activator [tPA], urokinase) if administered

5. refer to action 3.c in this diagnosis for additional care measures if signs and symptoms of cerebral ischemia occur

6. prepare client for surgical intervention (e.g. thromboembolectomy, revascularization) if indicated

7. provide emotional support to client and significant others.

9.B.3. The client will maintain adequate cerebral blood flow as evidenced by:

a. absence of dizziness, syncope, visual disturbances

b. mentally alert and oriented

c. pupils equal and normally reactive to light

d. normal motor and sensory function.

9.B.3.a. Assess for and report signs and symptoms of cerebral ischemia:

1. dizziness, syncope

2. blurred or dimmed vision, diplopia, change in visual field

3. decreased level of consciousness

4. unequal pupils or a sluggish or absent pupillary reaction to light (be aware that pupils may be dilated if CO_2 level is high and constricted if client is receiving sympathomimetics)

5. paresthesias, motor weakness, paralysis

6. seizures.

b. Implement measures *to promote adequate cerebral blood flow:*

1. keep head of bed flat until B/P is stabilized at a satisfactory level (at least 100 mm Hg systolic)

2. keep head and neck in proper alignment

3. perform actions to maintain adequate cardiac output (see Postoperative Nursing Diagnosis 1, action b)

4. perform actions to prevent development of mural thrombi and microemboli (see action 2.c in this diagnosis).

c. If signs and symptoms of cerebral ischemia occur:

1. continue with above measures

2. maintain client on bedrest with head of bed flat unless contraindicated

3. monitor for and report progression of signs and symptoms

4. initiate appropriate safety measures (e.g. side rails up, seizure precautions)

5. monitor for therapeutic and nontherapeutic effects of peripheral vasodilators (e.g. cyclandelate, papaverine, isoxsuprine) if administered *to improve cerebral blood flow*

6. provide emotional support to client and significant others

UNIT VII

7. refer to Care Plan on Cerebrovascular Accident for additional care measures if signs and symptoms persist.

9.B.4. The client will maintain adequate renal function as evidenced by:
   a. urine output at least 30 cc/hour
   b. urine specific gravity between 1.010–1.030
   c. BUN and serum creatinine levels within normal range.

9.B.4.a. Assess for and report signs and symptoms of impaired renal function (e.g. urine output less than 30 cc/hour, urine specific gravity fixed at or less than 1.010, elevated BUN and serum creatinine levels).
   b. Collect 24-hour urine specimen if ordered. Report decreased creatinine clearance.
   c. Implement measures *to maintain adequate renal blood flow:*
      1. maintain a minimum fluid intake of 1000 cc/day unless ordered otherwise
      2. perform actions to maintain adequate cardiac output (see Postoperative Nursing Diagnosis 1, action b)
      3. perform actions to prevent mural thrombi and microemboli (see action 2.c in this diagnosis).
   d. If signs and symptoms of impaired renal function occur:
      1. continue with above actions
      2. administer diuretics as ordered
      3. assess for and report signs of acute renal failure (e.g. oliguria or anuria; weight gain; edema; elevated B/P; lethargy and confusion; increasing BUN and serum creatinine, phosphorus, and potassium levels)
      4. prepare client for dialysis if indicated
      5. refer to Care Plan on Renal Failure for additional care measures.

9.B.5. The client will not develop atelectasis (see Standardized Postoperative Care Plan, Collaborative Diagnosis 19, outcome b, for outcome criteria).

9.B.5.a. Refer to Standardized Postoperative Care Plan, Collaborative Diagnosis 19, action b, for measures related to assessment, prevention, and treatment of atelectasis.
   b. Assure client that chest tube is sutured in place and that coughing and deep breathing will not dislodge the tube or disrupt the incision.

9.B.6. The client will experience normal lung re-expansion postoperatively as evidenced by:
   a. normal breath sounds and percussion note by 3rd–4th postoperative day
   b. unlabored respirations at 16–20/minute
   c. blood gases returning toward normal
   d. chest x-ray showing lung re-expansion.

9.B.6.a. Assess for and immediately report signs and symptoms of:
      1. malfunction of chest drainage system (e.g. respiratory distress, sudden cessation of drainage, excessive bubbling in water seal chamber, significant increase in subcutaneous emphysema)
      2. extended pneumothorax (e.g. extended area of absent breath sounds and hyperresonant percussion note; further increase in pulse rate; respiratory distress; sudden, sharp chest pain; cyanosis; restlessness; confusion)
      3. hemothorax (e.g. diminished or absent breath sounds with dull percussion note over affected area, further increase in pulse rate, dyspnea, cyanosis).
   b. Monitor blood gases. Report values that have worsened.
   c. Monitor chest x-ray results. Report findings of delayed lung re-expansion.
   d. Implement measures *to promote lung re-expansion and prevent further lung collapse:*
      1. perform actions *to maintain patency and integrity of chest drainage system:*
         a. maintain water seal and suction levels as ordered
         b. maintain air occlusive dressing over chest tube insertion site
         c. tape all connections securely
         d. milk or strip tubes if ordered
         e. keep chest drainage and suction tubing free of kinks
         f. keep drainage system below client's chest level at all times
      2. perform actions to improve breathing pattern (see Postoperative Nursing Diagnosis 3, actions a and b) and promote effective airway clearance (see Standardized Postoperative Care Plan, Nursing Diagnosis 4, action b).
   e. If signs and symptoms of extended pneumothorax or hemothorax occur:
      1. maintain client on bedrest in a semi- to high Fowler's position
      2. maintain oxygen therapy as ordered
      3. assess for and immediately report signs and symptoms of mediastinal shift (e.g. severe dyspnea, increased restlessness and agitation, rapid and/or irregular pulse rate, cyanosis, shift in point of apical impulse and trachea toward unaffected side)

4. assist with clearing of existing chest tube and/or insertion of a new tube
5. prepare client for surgery to ligate bleeding vessels if indicated
6. provide emotional support to client and significant others.

□ ▬▬▬▬▬▬▬▬▬▬▬▬▬▬▬

10. NURSING DIAGNOSIS

Knowledge deficit regarding follow-up.

□ ▬▬▬▬▬▬▬▬▬▬▬▬▬▬▬

DESIRED OUTCOMES	NURSING ACTIONS AND *SELECTED RATIONALES*

10.a. The client will identify modifiable cardiovascular risk factors and ways to reduce these factors.

10.a.1. Inform client that the following modifiable factors have been shown to contribute to cardiovascular disease:
  a. obesity
  b. diet high in saturated fat and cholesterol
  c. sedentary life style
  d. smoking
  e. heavy alcohol intake (more than 2 ounces of ethanol/day on a regular basis)
  f. stressful life style
  g. hypertension.
2. Assist the client to identify ways he/she can make appropriate changes in life style to reduce above factors. Provide information about stress management classes and weight loss, cardiovascular fitness, stop smoking, and alcohol rehabilitation programs. Initiate a referral if indicated.

10.b. The client will verbalize an understanding of the rationale for and constituents of a diet low in sodium, saturated fat, and cholesterol.

10.b.1. Explain the rationale for a diet low in sodium, saturated fat, and cholesterol.
2. Provide the following information *about decreasing sodium intake:*
  a. be aware that the terms salt and sodium are often used interchangeably but are not synonymous; there is 40% sodium in table salt
  b. read food labels and calculate sodium content of items (often expressed in milligrams [1 gm is 1000 mg])
  c. do not add salt when cooking foods or to prepared foods
  d. avoid foods/fluids and additives high in sodium (e.g. baking soda, tomato juice, bouillon, meat tenderizer, processed meats, sauerkraut, catsup, canned soups and vegetables, salty snacks)
  e. reduce sodium content in vegetables and meats by boiling, discarding the water, adding fresh water, and reboiling.
3. Provide the following instructions on ways *to reduce intake of saturated fat and cholesterol:*
  a. decrease intake of foods high in saturated fat and cholesterol (e.g. butter, cheese, ice cream, egg yolks, shrimp, cashew nuts, organ meats)
  b. avoid fried foods
  c. trim fat off meats and remove all poultry skin.
4. If physician has recommended a diet high in fiber, explain that soluble fiber is believed by some to reduce the progression of atherosclerosis. Provide a list of foods high in soluble fiber (e.g. oat bran, most fruits and vegetables, dried peas and beans).
5. Obtain a dietary consult to assist client in planning meals that will meet the prescribed limitations of sodium, saturated fat, and cholesterol.

10.c. The client will verbalize an understanding of activity restrictions and the rate of activity progression.

10.c.1. Reinforce physician's instructions regarding activity progression.
2. Inform client that activity progression will depend on extent of surgery and his/her activity tolerance.
3. Instruct client to avoid lifting heavy objects *in order to allow the incision to heal and prevent a sudden increase in cardiac workload.*
4. Instruct client to begin a cardiovascular fitness program when allowed by physician.

10.d. The client will verbalize an understanding of medication therapy including rationale for, side effects of, schedule for taking, and importance of taking as prescribed.

10.d.1. Explain the rationale for, side effects of, and importance of taking medications prescribed.
2. If client has had a valve replacement and is discharged on a coumarin derivative (e.g. dicumarol, warfarin, phenprocoumon), instruct to:
   a. keep scheduled appointments for periodic blood studies to monitor coagulation times
   b. take medication at the same time each day *in order to maintain a therapeutic blood level*
   c. avoid regular and/or excessive intake of alcohol *(may alter responsiveness to coumarins)*
   d. avoid taking over-the-counter products containing aspirin or other salicylates *(these products enhance the action of coumarins)*
   e. take the following precautions *to minimize risk of bleeding:*
      1. avoid taking aspirin, aspirin-containing products, and ibuprofen
      2. use an electric rather than a straight-edge razor
      3. floss and brush teeth gently
      4. cut nails carefully
      5. avoid situations that could result in injury (e.g. contact sports)
      6. avoid blowing nose forcefully
      7. avoid straining to have a bowel movement
   f. report prolonged or excessive bleeding from skin, nose, or mouth; blood in urine, vomitus, or stools; prolonged or excessive menses; excessive bruising; severe headache; or sudden abdominal or back pain
   g. apply firm, prolonged pressure to any bleeding area if possible
   h. wear a Medic-Alert band identifying self as being on anticoagulant therapy.
3. Instruct client to inform physician before taking other prescription and nonprescription medications.
4. Instruct client to inform all health care providers of medications being taken.

10.e. The client will state signs and symptoms to report to the health care provider.

10.e.1. Refer to Standardized Postoperative Care Plan, Nursing Diagnosis 20, action c, for signs and symptoms to report to the health care provider.
2. Instruct client to report these additional signs and symptoms:
   a. chest pain that seems unrelated to incisional discomfort
   b. development of or increased shortness of breath
   c. dizziness, fainting
   d. increased fatigue and weakness
   e. weight gain greater than 3 pounds a week
   f. swelling of extremities, face, or abdomen
   g. persistent cough especially if productive of yellow, green, rust-colored, or frothy sputum
   h. significant change in pulse rate or rhythm (check with physician about client's need to monitor pulse at home).

10.f. The client will identify community resources that can assist with cardiac rehabilitation and adjustment to having had heart surgery.

10.f.1. Provide information about community resources that can assist client with cardiac rehabilitation and adjustment to having had heart surgery (e.g. American Heart Association, YMCA, counseling services).
2. Initiate a referral if indicated.

10.g. The client will verbalize an understanding of and a plan for adhering to recommended follow-up care including future

10.g.1. Refer to Standardized Postoperative Care Plan, Nursing Diagnosis 20, for routine postoperative instructions and measures to improve client compliance.
2. If client had a saphenous vein graft, inform him/her that it takes approximately 6 weeks for circulation in leg to return to normal and that

appointments with health care provider, wound care, and pain management.

he/she should wear antiembolic hose during waking hours and keep operative leg on a footstool when sitting until all swelling has subsided.
3. If client had a valve replacement, instruct him/her not to have dental work for 6 months and to inform health care providers of valve surgery so prophylactic anti-infectives may be started before any dental work, invasive diagnostic procedures, or surgery.

Hypertension

Hypertension is defined as a sustained elevation of arterial blood pressure at a level of 140/90 or higher. Isolated systolic hypertension refers to a systolic pressure over 160 mm Hg with a diastolic pressure less than 90 mm Hg. Hypertension is classified as primary (essential or idiopathic) or secondary. Primary hypertension, which constitutes approximately 90% of the cases, has an unknown etiology. Secondary hypertension occurs as a result of hormone therapy and other pathological conditions such as Cushing's syndrome, increased intracranial pressure, renal disease, pheochromocytoma, and coarctation of the aorta. Hypertension is classified according to the degree of severity, ranging from Class I (mild hypertension with a diastolic pressure between 90–104 mm Hg) to Class III (severe hypertension with a diastolic pressure above 115 mm Hg). Accelerated or malignant hypertension is characterized by a sudden and rapid rise of diastolic pressure above 120 mm Hg and concurrent Grade III–IV retinopathy. When the pressure elevation causes an immediate threat to the client's life, hypertensive crisis exists.

The basic pathophysiological mechanism causing hypertension is an increase in peripheral vascular resistance. The increased resistance can be due to increased intravascular fluid volume (associated with chronic sodium and water retention) and/or narrowing of the vessels (due to loss of vascular elasticity or excessive vasoconstriction resulting from excessive or prolonged sympathetic nervous system stimulation or altered renin-angiotensin levels). In order to maintain adequate tissue perfusion when the peripheral vascular resistance is increased, the heart must pump harder. A prolonged increase in cardiac workload eventually leads to ventricular hypertrophy and heart failure. The prolonged increase in vascular pressure causes widespread pathological changes in the large and small blood vessels and eventually results in atherosclerosis, thrombosis, and aneurysm formation. The end result of all the changes in the cardiovascular system is a decreased blood supply to the tissues with end-organ damage occurring most often in the eyes, kidneys, brain, and heart.

Initial treatment of hypertension is usually nonpharmacological and consists of dietary modification as well as weight reduction, stress management, and control of other risk factors as indicated. If a conservative approach does not achieve the desired control of blood pressure, pharmacological therapy is initiated, utilizing a stepped-care approach. This 1–4 stepped-care approach progresses from use of a diuretic or beta-adrenergic blocking agent to use of combinations of drugs until the desired control of blood pressure is achieved with a minimum of side effects.

This care plan focuses on the adult client with severe hypertension hospitalized during an accelerated or malignant phase or in hypertensive crisis. The goals of care are to lower the blood pressure to a safe level, reduce fear and anxiety, prevent complications, and educate the client regarding follow-up care.

DISCHARGE CRITERIA

Prior to discharge, the client will:

- verbalize a basic understanding of hypertension and its effects on the body
- identify modifiable cardiovascular risk factors and ways to reduce these factors
- verbalize an understanding of medication therapy including rationale for, side effects of, schedule for taking, and importance of taking as prescribed
- verbalize an understanding of the rationale for and constituents of the recommended diet

- demonstrate accuracy in taking, reading, and recording blood pressure
- state signs and symptoms to report to the health care provider
- identify community resources that can assist in making life-style changes necessary for effective control of hypertension
- share feelings and concerns about hypertension and its effects on life style
- verbalize an understanding of and a plan for adhering to recommended follow-up care including future appointments with health care provider and activity level.

NURSING/COLLABORATIVE DIAGNOSES

1. Anxiety ☐ *346*
2. Altered systemic tissue perfusion ☐ *347*
3A. Altered comfort: headache ☐ *348*
3B. Altered comfort: nausea and vomiting ☐ *349*
4. Activity intolerance ☐ *350*
5. Self-care deficit ☐ *350*
6. Potential complications:
   a. hypertensive encephalopathy and/or cerebral ischemia
   b. ischemic heart disease (angina and/or myocardial infarction)
   c. arterial thromboembolism
   d. impaired renal function
   e. congestive heart failure (CHF)
   f. retinopathy
   g. hypovolemic shock ☐ *351*
7. Ineffective individual coping ☐ *355*
8. Noncompliance ☐ *356*
9. Knowledge deficit regarding follow-up care ☐ *357*

---

1. NURSING DIAGNOSIS

Anxiety related to unfamiliar environment; necessity for urgent treatment; existing symptoms; possibility of severe disability or sudden death; and lack of understanding of diagnostic tests, diagnosis, and treatment plan.

DESIRED OUTCOMES	NURSING ACTIONS AND *SELECTED RATIONALES*

1. The client will experience a reduction in fear and anxiety as evidenced by:
  a. verbalization of feeling less anxious or fearful
  b. relaxed facial expression and body movements
  c. vital signs returning to normal range for client
	1.a. Assess client for signs and symptoms of fear and anxiety (e.g. verbalization of fears and concerns; tenseness; tremors; irritability; restlessness; diaphoresis; tachypnea; tachycardia; further elevation of blood pressure; facial tension, pallor, or flushing; noncompliance with treatment plan). Validate perceptions carefully, remembering that some behaviors may result from decreased tissue perfusion and neurological changes.
	  b. Ascertain effectiveness of current coping skills.
	  c. Implement measures *to reduce fear and anxiety:*
	    1. orient to hospital environment, equipment, and routines

d. usual skin color
e. verbalization of an understanding of hospital routines, diagnostic tests, diagnosis, and treatments.

2. provide a calm, restful environment
3. introduce staff who will be participating in his/her care; if possible, maintain consistency in staff assigned to his/her care *to provide feelings of stability and comfort with the environment*
4. assure client that staff members are nearby; respond to call signal as soon as possible
5. maintain a calm, confident manner when interacting with client
6. encourage verbalization of fear and anxiety; provide feedback
7. inform client that many of current symptoms such as headache, vomiting, and visual disturbances will resolve when B/P is well controlled
8. explain all diagnostic tests that may be performed to determine the cause and residual effects of hypertension:
   a. blood studies (e.g. triglyceride, cholesterol, catecholamine, cortisol, urea nitrogen, creatinine, and renin levels; lipoprotein profile)
   b. urine studies (e.g. catecholamine, cortisol, and protein levels)
   c. EKG, chest x-ray
   d. intravenous pyelogram, isotope renography
   e. angiography
9. reinforce physician's explanations and clarify any misconceptions the client may have about hypertension, the treatment plan, and prognosis
10. perform actions to reduce discomfort (see Nursing Diagnoses 3.A, action 5 and 3.B, action 2)
11. instruct in relaxation techniques and encourage participation in diversional activities
12. perform actions to assist client to cope with the diagnosis and its implications (see Nursing Diagnosis 7, action d)
13. encourage significant others to project a caring, concerned attitude without obvious anxiousness
14. monitor for therapeutic and nontherapeutic effects of antianxiety agents if administered.
d. Include significant others in orientation and teaching sessions and encourage their continued support of client.
e. Provide information based on current needs of client and significant others at a level they can understand. Encourage questions and clarification of information provided.
f. Consult physician if above actions fail to control fear and anxiety.

□ ▬▬▬▬▬▬▬▬▬▬▬▬▬▬▬▬▬▬▬▬▬▬

2. NURSING DIAGNOSIS

Altered systemic tissue perfusion related to increased peripheral vascular resistance.

□ ▬▬▬▬▬▬▬▬▬▬▬▬▬▬▬▬▬▬▬▬▬▬

DESIRED OUTCOMES	NURSING ACTIONS AND *SELECTED RATIONALES*
2. The client will maintain adequate systemic tissue perfusion as evidenced by: a. B/P and pulse declining toward normal range b. unlabored respirations at 16–20/minute c. usual mental status d. skin warm and usual color e. palpable peripheral pulses f. capillary refill time less than 3 seconds	2.a. Assess for and report signs and symptoms of diminished systemic tissue perfusion: 1. further increase in B/P and pulse (may indicate the body's attempt to compensate for diminished tissue perfusion) 2. rapid or labored respirations 3. restlessness, slow responses, confusion 4. cool, pale, mottled, or cyanotic skin 5. diminished or absent peripheral pulses 6. capillary refill time greater than 3 seconds 7. urine output less than 30 cc/hour. b. Implement measures *to reduce vascular resistance and control hypertension in order to improve systemic tissue perfusion*:

g. urine output at least 30 cc/
hour.

1. monitor for therapeutic and nontherapeutic effects of the following
   medications if administered *to reduce B/P:*
   a. diuretics *(decrease peripheral vascular resistance by reducing
      intravascular fluid volume;* some thiazide and related sulfonamide
      diuretics *also decrease peripheral vascular resistance)*
   b. adrenergic inhibiting agents:
      1. central-acting adrenergic inhibitors (e.g. clonidine, methyldopa,
         guanabenz)
      2. alpha-adrenergic blockers (e.g. prazosin, phentolamine)
      3. peripheral-acting adrenergic inhibitors (e.g. reserpine,
         guanethidine)
      4. beta-adrenergic blockers (e.g. propranolol, metoprolol, atenolol,
         nadolol, timolol)
      5. combined alpha- and beta-adrenergic blockers (e.g. labetalol)
   c. vasodilators (e.g. minoxidil, hydralazine, nitroprusside, diazoxide,
      trimethaphan); this group of medications is most often used when
      immediate reduction of B/P is necessary
   d. angiotensin-converting enzyme inhibitors (e.g. captopril, enalapril)
   e. calcium-channel blocking agents (e.g. nifedipine, verapamil, diltiazem)
2. perform actions *to reduce sympathetic nervous system stimulation:*
   a. implement measures to reduce fear and anxiety (see Nursing Diagnosis
      1, action c)
   b. implement measures to reduce discomfort (see Nursing Diagnoses 3.A,
      action 5 and 3.B, action 2)
   c. implement measures to promote rest (see Nursing Diagnosis 4, action
      b.1)
   d. discourage intake of foods/fluids high in caffeine such as coffee, tea,
      chocolate, and colas *(caffeine stimulates the sympathetic nervous
      system)*
3. discourage smoking *(smoking causes vasoconstriction; it also contributes
   to decreased tissue oxygenation by reducing oxygen availability)*
4. maintain fluid and dietary sodium restrictions as ordered *to reduce fluid
   retention*
5. instruct and assist client to avoid selecting foods high in saturated fat
   and cholesterol (e.g. butter, ice cream, egg yolks, shrimp, cashew nuts,
   organ meats) *in order to prevent further progression of atherogenesis*
6. monitor for therapeutic and nontherapeutic effects of antihyperlipidemic
   agents (e.g. clofibrate, nicotinic acid, cholestyramine, probucol) if
   administered *to prevent further atherogenesis of vessels.*

c. Consult physician if signs and symptoms of diminished systemic tissue
   perfusion persist or worsen.

☐ ▬▬▬▬▬▬▬▬▬▬▬▬▬▬▬▬▬▬▬▬▬

3.A. NURSING DIAGNOSIS

Altered comfort:* headache related to increased cerebral vascular pressure resulting from severe hypertension.

_____

* In this care plan, the nursing diagnosis of "pain" is included under the diagnostic label of altered
comfort.

☐ ▬▬▬▬▬▬▬▬▬▬▬▬▬▬▬▬▬▬▬▬▬

DESIRED OUTCOMES	NURSING ACTIONS AND *SELECTED RATIONALES*
3.A. The client will obtain relief of headache as evidenced by: 1. verbalization of headache relief	3.A.1. Determine how the client usually responds to pain. 2. Assess for nonverbal signs of headache (e.g. reluctance to move head, rubbing head, avoidance of bright lights and noises, wrinkled brow, clenched fists). 3. Assess verbal complaints of discomfort. Ask client to be specific about

2. relaxed facial expression and body positioning
3. increased participation in activities.

type, location, and severity of headache. (The headache is usually occipital, present upon waking, and subsides once the client is up and moving around.)
4. Assess for factors that seem to aggravate and alleviate the headache.
5. Implement measures *to relieve headache:*
   a. perform actions to reduce vascular resistance and control hypertension (see Nursing Diagnosis 2, action b)
   b. perform actions *to minimize environmental stimuli* (e.g. provide a calm environment, restrict visitors, dim lights)
   c. avoid jarring bed or startling client *to minimize risk of sudden movements*
   d. provide or assist with nonpharmacological measures for headache relief (e.g. cool cloth to forehead, back and neck rubs, elevation of head, relaxation techniques, guided imagery, diversional activities)
   e. monitor for therapeutic and nontherapeutic effects of analgesics if administered.
6. Consult physician if above actions fail to relieve headache.

□ ▬▬▬▬▬▬▬▬▬▬▬▬▬▬▬▬▬▬▬▬

3.B. NURSING DIAGNOSIS

Altered comfort: nausea and vomiting related to stimulation of the vomiting center associated with cortical stimulation due to pain, stress, and an increase in intra-cranial pressure.

□ ▬▬▬▬▬▬▬▬▬▬▬▬▬▬▬▬▬▬▬▬

DESIRED OUTCOMES	NURSING ACTIONS AND *SELECTED RATIONALES*

3.B. The client will experience relief of nausea and vomiting as evidenced by:
1. verbalization of relief of nausea
2. absence of vomiting.

3.B.1. Assess the client to determine factors that contribute to nausea and vomiting (e.g. headache, elevation of B/P, movement, anxiety).
2. Implement measures *to reduce nausea and vomiting:*
   a. perform actions to reduce vascular resistance and control hypertension (see Nursing Diagnosis 2, action b)
   b. perform actions to relieve headache (see Nursing Diagnosis 3.A, action 5)
   c. perform actions to reduce fear and anxiety (see Nursing Diagnosis 1, action c)
   d. eliminate noxious sights and smells from the environment *(noxious stimuli cause cortical stimulation of the vomiting center)*
   e. encourage client to change positions slowly *(movement stimulates chemoreceptor trigger zone)*
   f. encourage client to take deep, slow breaths when nauseated
   g. provide oral hygiene after each emesis and before meals
   h. provide small, frequent meals rather than 3 large ones
   i. instruct client to ingest foods and fluids slowly
   j. instruct client to avoid foods/fluids that irritate the gastric mucosa (e.g. spicy foods; citrus fruits or juices; caffeine-containing items such as chocolate, coffee, tea, and colas)
   k. provide carbonated beverages for client to sip if nauseated
   l. instruct client to eat dry foods (e.g. toast, crackers) and avoid drinking liquids with meals if nauseated
   m. instruct client to rest after eating with head of bed elevated
   n. monitor for therapeutic and nontherapeutic effects of antiemetics if administered.
3. Consult physician if above measures fail to control nausea and vomiting.

UNIT VII

4. NURSING DIAGNOSIS

Activity intolerance related to:

a. decreased tissue oxygenation associated with inadequate tissue perfusion;
b. difficulty resting and sleeping associated with fear, anxiety, frequent assessments, and discomfort.

DESIRED OUTCOMES	NURSING ACTIONS AND *SELECTED RATIONALES*

4. The client will demonstrate an increased tolerance for activity as evidenced by:
  a. verbalization of feeling less fatigued and weak
  b. ability to perform activities of daily living without exertional dyspnea, chest pain, diaphoresis, dizziness, or a significant change in vital signs.
	4.a. Assess for signs and symptoms of activity intolerance:
	  1. statements of fatigue and weakness
	  2. exertional dyspnea, chest pain, diaphoresis, or dizziness
	  3. decrease in pulse rate or an increase in rate of 20 beats/minute above resting rate
	  4. pulse rate not returning to preactivity level within 5 minutes after stopping activity
	  5. decreased blood pressure or an increase in diastolic pressure of 15 mm Hg with activity.
	  b. Implement measures *to improve activity tolerance:*
	    1. perform actions *to promote rest:*
	      a. maintain activity restrictions
	      b. minimize environmental activity and noise
	      c. schedule nursing care and diagnostic procedures to allow periods of uninterrupted rest
	      d. limit the number of visitors and their length of stay
	      e. assist client with self-care activities as needed
	      f. keep supplies and personal articles within easy reach
	      g. implement measures to reduce fear and anxiety (see Nursing Diagnosis 1, action c)
	      h. implement measures to reduce discomfort (see Nursing Diagnoses 3.A, action 5 and 3.B, action 2)
	    2. perform actions to reduce vascular resistance and improve systemic tissue perfusion (see Nursing Diagnosis 2, action b)
	    3. instruct client in energy-saving techniques (e.g. using shower chair when showering, sitting to brush teeth or comb hair)
	    4. maintain an optimal nutritional status
	    5. increase client's activity gradually as allowed and tolerated.
	  c. Instruct client to:
	    1. report a decreased tolerance for activity
	    2. stop any activity that causes chest pain, shortness of breath, dizziness, or extreme fatigue or weakness.
	  d. Consult physician if signs and symptoms of activity intolerance persist or worsen.

5. NURSING DIAGNOSIS

Self-care deficit related to activity intolerance, discomfort, and prescribed activity restrictions.

DESIRED OUTCOMES	NURSING ACTIONS AND *SELECTED RATIONALES*

5. The client will demonstrate increased participation in self-care activities within physical limitations and/or prescribed activity restrictions.

5.a. Assess for factors that interfere with the client's ability to perform self-care (e.g. weakness, fatigue, headache).
 b. With client, develop a realistic plan for meeting daily physical needs.
 c. Encourage maximum independence within limitations imposed by activity tolerance, prescribed activity restrictions, and discomfort.
 d. Implement measures *to facilitate client's ability to perform self-care activities:*
   1. perform actions to increase activity tolerance (see Nursing Diagnosis 4, action b)
   2. schedule care at a time when client is most likely to be able to participate (e.g. when analgesics are at peak action, after rest periods, not immediately after meals or treatments)
   3. keep needed objects within easy reach
   4. allow adequate time for accomplishment of self-care activities.
 e. Provide positive feedback for all efforts and accomplishments of self-care.
 f. Assist client with those activities he/she is unable to perform independently.
 g. Inform significant others of client's abilities to perform own care. Explain the importance of encouraging and allowing client to maintain an optimal level of independence within prescribed activity restrictions and his/her activity tolerance level.

□ ▬▬▬▬▬▬▬▬▬▬▬▬▬▬▬▬▬▬▬▬▬▬▬▬▬

6. COLLABORATIVE DIAGNOSIS

Potential complications:

 a. **hypertensive encephalopathy and/or cerebral ischemia** related to impaired cerebral blood flow associated with spasms of cerebral vessels, cerebral edema, an arterial thrombus or embolus, and intracerebral hemorrhage (can occur as a result of increased vascular pressure);
 b. **ischemic heart disease (angina and/or myocardial infarction)** related to:
   1. myocardial oxygen deficiency associated with increased myocardial oxygen utilization as a result of the increased cardiac workload created by hypertension
   2. decreased coronary blood flow associated with atherosclerosis (a long-term result of hypertension and accelerated by further increases in vascular pressure);
 c. **arterial thromboembolism** related to damage to the intima of the blood vessels associated with prolonged or excessive arterial vascular pressure;
 d. **impaired renal function** related to vascular changes in the kidneys associated with effects of prolonged or severe hypertension;
 e. **congestive heart failure (CHF)** related to the prolonged increase in cardiac workload that results from having to pump against increased peripheral vascular resistance;
 f. **retinopathy** related to progressive deterioration and focal spasms of the retinal arterioles associated with prolonged and/or excessive arterial vascular pressure;
 g. **hypovolemic shock** related to blood loss associated with rupture of an abdominal aneurysm as a result of excessive intravascular pressure (aneurysms result from thinning of the arterial wall due to a prolonged increase in pressure).

□ ▬▬▬▬▬▬▬▬▬▬▬▬▬▬▬▬▬▬▬▬▬▬▬▬▬

DESIRED OUTCOMES	NURSING ACTIONS AND *SELECTED RATIONALES*

6.a. The client will maintain adequate cerebral blood

6.a.1. Assess for and report signs and symptoms of cerebral edema and cerebral ischemia:

flow without signs and symptoms of cerebral edema as evidenced by:
1. absence of dizziness, syncope, visual disturbances
2. absence or resolution of headache
3. reduction in nausea and vomiting
4. mentally alert and oriented
5. pupils equal and normally reactive to light
6. normal motor and sensory function.

a. dizziness, syncope
b. blurred or dimmed vision, diplopia, scotoma or any other change in visual field
c. persistent or increasing headache
d. nausea and vomiting
e. decreased level of consciousness
f. unequal pupils or a sluggish or absent pupillary reaction to light
g. paresthesias, motor weakness, paralysis
h. seizures.
2. Observe and document progression of symptoms (this information may aid in differentiating hypertensive encephalopathy from a cerebrovascular accident).
3. Implement measures to promote adequate cerebral blood flow:
   a. perform actions to reduce vascular resistance and improve systemic tissue perfusion (see Nursing Diagnosis 2, action b)
   b. perform actions to prevent an increase in intracranial pressure:
      1. implement measures to relieve nausea and vomiting (see Nursing Diagnosis 3.B, action 2)
      2. implement measures to prevent constipation in order to reduce straining during bowel movements:
         a. provide a diet high in fiber (e.g. bran, whole grains, fresh fruits and vegetables, dried fruits)
         b. encourage the maximum fluid intake allowed
         c. consult physician regarding order for stool softeners and laxatives
      3. encourage client to keep head and neck in proper alignment to promote adequate venous return
   c. monitor for therapeutic and nontherapeutic effects of peripheral vasodilators (e.g. cyclandelate, papaverine, isoxsuprine) if administered.
4. If signs and symptoms of cerebral edema or cerebral ischemia occur:
   a. continue with above measures
   b. maintain client on bedrest with head of bed elevated 20–30°
   c. monitor for and report progression of signs and symptoms
   d. initiate appropriate safety measures (e.g. side rails up, seizure precautions)
   e. monitor for therapeutic and nontherapeutic effects of osmotic diuretics (e.g. mannitol) and corticosteroids (e.g. dexamethasone, methylprednisolone) if administered to decrease cerebral edema
   f. provide emotional support to client and significant others
   g. refer to Care Plan on Cerebrovascular Accident for additional care measures if signs and symptoms persist.

6.b. The client will not experience episodes of myocardial ischemia as evidenced by:
1. absence of chest pain
2. unlabored respirations at 16–20/minute
3. normal cardiac enzymes
4. normal EKG readings.

6.b.1. Assess for signs and symptoms of myocardial ischemia (e.g. sudden chest pain, dyspnea).
2. Implement measures to prevent myocardial ischemia:
   a. perform actions to reduce vascular resistance and control hypertension (see Nursing Diagnosis 2, action b)
   b. perform additional actions to reduce cardiac workload:
      1. maintain oxygen therapy as ordered
      2. place client in a semi- to high Fowler's position
      3. provide small, frequent meals (large meals require an increased blood supply to the gastrointestinal tract for digestion)
      4. instruct client to avoid activities that create a Valsalva response (e.g. straining to have a bowel movement, bending at the waist, holding breath while moving)
      5. increase activity gradually as allowed and tolerated.
3. If signs and symptoms of myocardial ischemia occur:
   a. obtain blood specimens for cardiac enzyme levels and have EKG done as ordered; report significant elevation of cardiac enzymes and a significant ST segment elevation, T wave changes, or pathological Q wave on EKG reading (indicative of myocardial infarction)
   b. maintain client on strict bedrest in a semi- to high Fowler's position
   c. maintain oxygen therapy as ordered
   d. monitor for therapeutic and nontherapeutic effects of nitrates if administered to promote peripheral vasodilation and reduce cardiac workload
   e. if chest pain is unrelieved by nitrates, prepare to administer

medications that may be utilized to treat myocardial infarction (e.g. morphine sulfate, vasodilators, positive inotropic agents)
f. initiate cardiopulmonary resuscitation if indicated
g. provide emotional support to client and significant others
h. refer to Care Plans on Angina Pectoris and Myocardial Infarction for additional care measures.

6.c. The client will not develop an arterial thrombus or embolus as evidenced by: 1. palpable peripheral pulses 2. usual skin temperature and color in extremities 3. absence of pain in extremities 4. usual sensory and motor function 5. absence of dizziness, syncope, visual disturbances 6. mentally alert and oriented 7. pupils equal and normally reactive to light.	6.c.1. Assess for and report signs and symptoms of: a. arterial thrombus or embolus (e.g. diminished or absent peripheral pulses; pallor, cyanosis, coolness, numbness, and/or pain in extremity) b. cerebral ischemia (see action a.1 in this diagnosis for a list of signs and symptoms). 2. Implement measures to reduce vascular resistance and control hypertension (see Nursing Diagnosis 2, action b) *in order to reduce risk of arterial thrombus development.* 3. If signs and symptoms of an arterial thromboembolism occur: a. maintain client on strict bedrest with lower extremities in a level or slightly dependent position *to improve arterial blood flow* b. prepare client for diagnostic studies (e.g. Doppler ultrasound, plethysmography, oscillometry) c. implement measures *to promote vasodilation in the obstructed extremity:* 1. administer peripheral vasodilators (e.g. papaverine, cyclandelate) as ordered 2. keep lower extremities warm 3. assist with a lumbar sympathetic block if performed *to decrease vasoconstrictor tone* d. monitor for therapeutic and nontherapeutic effects of heparin and thrombolytic agents (e.g. streptokinase, tissue plasminogen activator [tPA], urokinase) if administered e. refer to action a.4 in this diagnosis for additional care measures if signs and symptoms of cerebral ischemia occur f. prepare client for surgical intervention (e.g. thromboembolectomy, revascularization) if indicated g. provide emotional support to client and significant others.
6.d. The client will maintain adequate renal function as evidenced by: 1. urine output at least 30 cc/hour 2. urine specific gravity between 1.010–1.030 3. BUN and serum creatinine levels within normal range.	6.d.1. Assess for and report signs and symptoms of impaired renal function (e.g. urine output less than 30 cc/hour, urine specific gravity fixed at or less than 1.010, elevated BUN and serum creatinine levels). 2. Collect a 24-hour urine specimen if ordered. Report decreased creatinine clearance. 3. Implement measures *to maintain adequate renal blood flow:* a. perform actions to reduce vascular resistance and improve systemic tissue perfusion (see Nursing Diagnosis 2, action b) b. maintain an adequate fluid intake (if client is on a fluid restriction, maintain the maximum fluid intake allowed) *to reduce risk of dehydration.* 4. If signs and symptoms of impaired renal function occur: a. continue with above actions b. administer diuretics as ordered c. assess for and report signs of acute renal failure (e.g. oliguria or anuria; weight gain; edema; increasing B/P; lethargy and confusion; increasing BUN and serum creatinine, phosphorus, and potassium levels) d. prepare client for dialysis if indicated e. refer to Care Plan on Renal Failure for additional care measures.
6.e. The client will not develop CHF as evidenced by: 1. vital signs returning toward normal range for client 2. audible heart sounds 3. no increase in the intensity of S_3 or S_4 or	6.e.1. Assess for and report signs and symptoms of CHF: a. tachycardia b. softened or muffled heart sounds c. development of or intensified S_3 and/or S_4 gallop rhythm d. crackles and diminished or absent breath sounds e. dyspnea, orthopnea f. displaced apical impulse g. diminished or absent peripheral pulses

softening of pre-existing murmurs
4. normal breath sounds
5. absence of or no increase in dyspnea and orthopnea
6. palpable peripheral pulses and normal carotid pulse amplitude
7. balanced intake and output
8. stable weight
9. CVP within normal range
10. absence of peripheral edema; distended neck veins; enlarged, tender liver
11. BUN and serum creatinine and alkaline phosphatase levels within normal range.

h. decline in amplitude of carotid pulse (hypertension may cause an increased carotid pulse amplitude because the left ventricle has to pump harder; low-output failure may eventually ensue with a decline in the carotid pulse amplitude)
i. intake greater than output
j. weight gain
k. elevated CVP
l. peripheral edema
m. distended neck veins
n. enlarged, tender liver
o. elevated BUN and serum creatinine and alkaline phosphatase levels.
2. Monitor chest x-ray results. Report findings of cardiomegaly, pleural effusion, or pulmonary edema.
3. Implement measures *to prevent CHF:*
   a. perform actions to reduce vascular resistance and control hypertension (see Nursing Diagnosis 2, action b)
   b. perform additional actions to reduce cardiac workload (see action b.2.b in this diagnosis)
4. If signs and symptoms of CHF occur:
   a. continue with above actions
   b. monitor for therapeutic and nontherapeutic effects of medications that may be administered *to reduce vascular congestion and/or cardiac workload* (e.g. diuretics, cardiotonics, vasodilators, morphine sulfate)
   c. assist with phlebotomy if performed *to reduce blood volume*
   d. apply rotating tourniquets according to hospital policy if ordered *to reduce pulmonary vascular congestion*
   e. provide emotional support to client and significant others
   f. refer to Care Plan on Congestive Heart Failure for additional care measures.

6.f. The client will not experience progression of retinopathy.

6.f.1. Determine client's baseline retinal vascular and visual status by:
a. examining the fundus of the eye for indications of mild retinal vascular damage (e.g. increased light reflex; arteriolar tortuosity, narrowing, and irregularity; arteriovenous nicking) to more severe retinal vascular damage (e.g. small retinal hemorrhages, soft exudates, papilledema)
b. assessing for symptoms of blurred vision, scotoma, and partial or total blindness.
2. Implement measures to reduce vascular resistance and control hypertension (see Nursing Diagnosis 2, action b) *in order to prevent progression of retinal vascular damage.*
3. If vision is impaired:
   a. implement measures *to prevent injury:*
      1. orient client to surroundings, room, and arrangement of furniture
      2. keep side rails up and call signal within reach
      3. place desired personal articles within reach and assist client to identify their location
      4. instruct client to request assistance as needed
      5. assist client with ambulation by walking a half step ahead of client and describing approaching objects or obstacles; instruct client to grasp back of nurse's arm during ambulation
      6. avoid unnecessary clutter in room
      7. provide adequate lighting in room
   b. avoid startling client (e.g. speak client's name and identify yourself when entering room and before any physical contact, describe activities and reasons for various noises in the room)
   c. assist client with personal hygiene he/she is unable to perform independently
   d. identify where items are placed on the plate or tray, cut food, open packages, or feed client if necessary
   e. assist with activities that require reading (e.g. menu selection, mail, legal documents).
4. Reassess retinal vascular and visual status regularly and consult physician if signs and symptoms of retinopathy worsen.

6.g. The client will not develop hypovolemic shock as

6.g.1. Assess for and report signs and symptoms of:
a. abdominal aneurysm (e.g. abnormal abdominal pulsations; bruits over

evidenced by:
1. usual mental status
2. stable vital signs
3. skin warm and usual color
4. palpable peripheral pulses
5. capillary refill time less than 3 seconds
6. urine output at least 30 cc/hour.

major abdominal vessels; recent onset of constant abdominal, lumbar, or pelvic pain)
    b. leaking aneurysm (e.g. increasing abdominal girth; hematoma of scrotum, perineum, or penis; diminishing peripheral pulses; new or increased complaints of lumbar, pelvic, abdominal, or groin pain; declining Hct. and Hgb. levels)
    c. hypovolemic shock:
       1. restlessness, agitation, confusion
       2. significant decrease in B/P
       3. decline in B/P of at least 15 mm Hg with concurrent rise in pulse when client changes from lying to sitting or standing position
       4. resting pulse rate greater than 100 beats/minute
       5. rapid or labored respirations
       6. cool, pale, or cyanotic skin
       7. diminished or absent peripheral pulses
       8. capillary refill time greater than 3 seconds
       9. urine output less than 30 cc/hour.
2. Implement measures *to prevent rupture of an existing aneurysm:*
    a. perform actions to reduce vascular resistance and control hypertension (see Nursing Diagnosis 2, action b)
    b. instruct client to avoid activities that create a Valsalva response (e.g. straining to have a bowel movement, bending at the waist, holding breath while moving).
3. If signs and symptoms of hypovolemic shock occur:
    a. place client flat in bed unless contraindicated
    b. monitor vital signs frequently
    c. administer oxygen as ordered
    d. monitor for therapeutic and nontherapeutic effects of blood products and/or volume expanders if administered
    e. prepare client for surgical repair of ruptured aneurysm if planned
    f. provide emotional support to client and significant others.

7. NURSING DIAGNOSIS

Ineffective individual coping related to fear, anxiety, need to alter life style, knowledge that condition is chronic and will require lifelong medical supervision and medication therapy, uncomfortable side effects of some antihypertensive agents, and inadequate support system.

DESIRED OUTCOMES	NURSING ACTIONS AND *SELECTED RATIONALES*

7. The client will demonstrate the use of effective coping skills as evidenced by:
 a. willingness to participate in treatment plan and self-care activities
 b. verbalization of ability to cope with hypertension and its management
 c. identification of stressors
 d. utilization of appropriate problem-solving techniques
 e. recognition and
	7.a. Assess effectiveness of client's coping strategies by observing behavior and noting strengths, weaknesses, ability to express feelings and concerns, and willingness to participate in the treatment plan.
	 b. Assess for and report signs and symptoms that may indicate ineffective coping (e.g. sleep disturbances, increasing fatigue, difficulty concentrating, irritability, decreased tolerance of headache, verbalization of inability to cope, inability to problem-solve).
	 c. Allow time for client to adjust psychologically to diagnosis, planned treatment, and anticipated life-style and role changes.
	 d. Implement measures *to promote effective coping:*
	   1. arrange for a visit with another who has successfully adjusted to hypertension
	   2. perform actions to reduce fear and anxiety (see Nursing Diagnosis 1, action c)

UNIT VII

utilization of available support systems.

3. include client in planning of care, encourage maximum participation in treatment plan, and allow choices when possible *to enable him/her to maintain a sense of control*
4. assist client to maintain usual daily routines whenever possible
5. instruct client in effective problem-solving techniques (e.g. identification of stressors, determination of various options to solve problem)
6. assist client as he/she starts to plan for necessary life-style and role changes after discharge; provide input on realistic prioritization of problems that need to be dealt with
7. assist the client and significant others to identify ways that personal and family goals can be adjusted rather than abandoned
8. assist client to identify and utilize available support systems; provide information regarding available community resources that can assist client in coping with effects of hypertension (e.g. counseling services, stress management classes, local support groups)
9. monitor for therapeutic and nontherapeutic effects of antidepressants if administered.
   e. Encourage continued emotional support from significant others.
   f. Assess for and support behaviors suggesting positive adaptation to changes experienced (e.g. active participation in the treatment plan, verbalization of plans for altering life style).
   g. Consult physician about psychological or vocational rehabilitation counseling if appropriate. Initiate a referral if necessary.

---

8. NURSING DIAGNOSIS

Noncompliance* related to:

a. lack of understanding of the implications of not following the prescribed treatment plan;
b. difficulty modifying personal habits (e.g. smoking, alcohol intake, dietary preferences) and uncomfortable side effects of some antihypertensive agents;
c. insufficient financial resources.

---

* This diagnostic label includes both an informed decision by client not to comply and an inability to comply due to circumstances beyond the client's control.

DESIRED OUTCOMES	NURSING ACTIONS AND *SELECTED RATIONALES*
8. The client will demonstrate the probability of future compliance with the prescribed treatment plan as evidenced by: a. willingness to learn about and participate in treatments and care b. statements reflecting ways to modify personal habits and integrate treatments into life style c. statements reflecting an understanding of the implications of not following the prescribed treatment plan.	8.a. Assess for indications that the client may be unwilling or unable to comply with the prescribed treatment plan: 1. statements reflecting that he/she was unable to manage care at home 2. failure to adhere to treatment plan while in hospital (e.g. not adhering to dietary modifications and fluid restrictions, refusing medications) 3. statements reflecting a lack of understanding of factors that may cause progression of hypertension 4. statements reflecting an unwillingness or inability to modify personal habits and integrate necessary treatments into life style 5. statements reflecting view that hypertension will reverse itself or that the situation is hopeless and efforts to comply with treatments are useless 6. statements reflecting that the side effects of medications are too uncomfortable and that he/she feels better when not taking medication. b. Implement measures *to improve client compliance:* 1. explain hypertension in terms the client can understand; stress the fact

that hypertension is a chronic condition and that adherence to the treatment plan is necessary *in order to delay and/or prevent complications*

2. encourage questions and clarify any misconceptions client has about hypertension and its effects
3. perform actions to assist client to cope with diagnosis and its effects (see Nursing Diagnosis 7, action d)
4. provide instructions on and encourage client to participate in the treatment plan (e.g. calculating sodium and fat intake, measuring fluid intake, monitoring blood pressure); determine areas of misunderstanding and reinforce teaching as necessary
5. provide client with written instructions about dietary modifications, signs and symptoms to report, medication therapy, blood pressure monitoring, and exercise regimen
6. assist client to identify ways he/she can incorporate treatments into life style; focus on modifications of life style rather than complete change
7. initiate and reinforce discharge teaching outlined in Nursing Diagnosis 9 *in order to promote a sense of control and self-reliance*
8. provide information about and encourage utilization of community resources that can assist client to make necessary life-style changes (e.g. cardiovascular fitness, weight loss, and stop smoking programs)
9. encourage client to discuss his/her concerns regarding the cost of medications and visits with health care provider; obtain a social service consult to assist the client with financial planning and to obtain financial aid if indicated
10. encourage client to attend follow-up educational classes.

c. Assess for and reinforce behaviors suggesting future compliance with prescribed treatments (e.g. statements reflecting plans for integrating treatments into life style, statements reflecting an understanding of hypertension and its long-term effects).
d. Include significant others in explanations and teaching sessions and encourage their support.
e. Reinforce the need for the client to assume responsibility for managing as much of care as possible.
f. Consult physician regarding referrals to community health agencies if continued instruction or supervision is needed.

9. NURSING DIAGNOSIS

Knowledge deficit regarding follow-up care.

DESIRED OUTCOMES	NURSING ACTIONS AND *SELECTED RATIONALES*
9.a. The client will verbalize a basic understanding of hypertension and its effects on the body.	9.a. Explain hypertension and its effects in terms client can understand. Utilize available teaching aids (e.g. pictures, videotapes).
9.b. The client will identify modifiable cardiovascular risk factors and ways to reduce these factors.	9.b.1. Inform client that the following modifiable factors have been shown to contribute to vascular disease and hypertension: a. obesity b. diet high in salt, saturated fat, and cholesterol c. sedentary life style d. smoking e. heavy alcohol intake (more than 2 ounces of ethanol/day on a regular basis) f. stressful life style.

2. Assist the client to identify ways he/she can make appropriate changes in life style to reduce the modifiable cardiovascular risk factors. Provide information about weight reduction plans; stress management classes; and cardiovascular fitness, stop smoking, and alcohol rehabilitation programs. Initiate a referral if indicated.

3. Instruct client to take antihyperlipidemic medications (e.g. clofibrate, nicotinic acid, cholestyramine, probucol) and antiplatelet agents (e.g. sulfinpyrazone, aspirin, dipyridamole) as prescribed.

9.c. The client will verbalize an understanding of medication therapy including rationale for, side effects of, schedule for taking, and importance of taking as prescribed.

9.c.1. Explain the rationale for, side effects of, and importance of taking medications prescribed.

2. If client is discharged on a diuretic, instruct to:
   a. take once-daily dose or the larger dose in the morning *to minimize nighttime urination*
   b. weigh self daily and keep a record of daily weights
   c. avoid alcohol intake *(the combined vasodilating effect of alcohol and volume-depleting effect of a diuretic greatly increase the tendency toward orthostatic hypotension)*
   d. change from a lying to a standing position slowly if experiencing dizziness or lightheadedness with position change
   e. increase intake of foods/fluids high in potassium (e.g. oranges, bananas, figs, dates, tomatoes, potatoes, raisins, apricots, Gatorade, fruit juices) if taking a potassium-depleting diuretic
   f. notify physician if unable to tolerate food or fluids *(dehydration can develop rapidly if intake is poor and client continues to take a diuretic)*
   g. avoid salt substitutes with a high potassium content if discharged on a potassium-sparing diuretic (e.g. triamterene, spironolactone)
   h. report the following signs and symptoms:
      1. weight gain of 1 pound a day for 3 days
      2. swelling of ankles, feet, or abdomen
      3. weight loss of more than 5 pounds a week
      4. excessive thirst
      5. severe dizziness or episodes of fainting
      6. muscle weakness or cramping, nausea, vomiting, irregular pulse, or increased pulse rate.

3. If client is discharged on another antihypertensive such as an adrenergic inhibiting agent, vasodilator, or angiotensin-converting enzyme inhibitor, instruct to:
   a. take medication on a regular schedule
   b. avoid skipping doses, altering prescribed dose, making up for missed doses, or discontinuing medication without permission of health care provider
   c. be alert to expected side effects such as mood changes, impotence, weight gain, and dry mouth; these side effects often subside with time but should be reported if they interfere with life style
   d. implement measures *to reduce severity of orthostatic hypotension:*
      1. rise from a lying to standing position by sitting up slowly, sitting for a few minutes, then standing slowly
      2. sleep with head slightly elevated
      3. perform actions *to decrease peripheral venous pooling:*
         a. avoid prolonged standing
         b. do leg exercises when lying down
         c. wear support stockings when up
   e. implement measures *to prevent unnecessary vasodilation:*
      1. avoid hot baths, steam rooms, and saunas
      2. avoid drinking alcoholic beverages.

4. Instruct the client to consult health care provider before taking other prescription and nonprescription medications.

9.d. The client will verbalize an understanding of the rationale for and constituents of the recommended diet.

9.d.1. Explain the rationale for the recommended dietary modifications (usually a diet low in sodium, saturated fat, and cholesterol is recommended; additional recommendations may include increasing foods high in calcium and increasing soluble dietary fiber [e.g. oat bran] intake).

2. Depending on the physician's recommendations:

a. provide the following information *about decreasing sodium intake* (recommended restriction is usually 2 gm sodium [5 gm salt]/day):
   1. be aware that the terms salt and sodium are often used interchangeably but are not synonymous; there is 40% sodium in table salt
   2. read food labels and calculate sodium content of items (often expressed in milligrams [2 gm is 2000 mg])
   3. do not add salt when cooking foods or to prepared foods
   4. avoid foods/fluids and additives high in sodium (e.g. baking soda, tomato juice, bouillon, meat tenderizer, processed meats, sauerkraut, catsup, canned soups and vegetables, salty snacks)
   5. reduce sodium content in vegetables and meats by boiling, discarding the water, adding fresh water, and reboiling
   6. do not restrict milk and cheese intake to lower sodium *(there is some evidence that increasing calcium intake lowers blood pressure)*
b. provide the following instructions on ways *to reduce intake of saturated fat and cholesterol:*
   1. decrease intake of foods high in saturated fat and cholesterol (e.g. butter, ice cream, egg yolks, shrimp, cashew nuts, organ meats)
   2. avoid fried foods
   3. trim fat off meats and remove all poultry skin.
3. If the client is taking an MAO inhibitor, instruct him/her to avoid foods/fluids containing tyramine (e.g. cheese, fava or broad bean pods, cured meats, figs, beer, red wine, pickled foods, yeast extract), caffeine-containing items (e.g. coffee, tea, chocolate, colas), and tyramine-containing medications (e.g. many cold medicines and nasal decongestants) *in order to reduce the risk of precipitating hypertensive crisis.*

9.e. The client will demonstrate accuracy in taking, reading, and recording blood pressure.

9.e.1. Teach client to take, read, and record blood pressure.
2. Allow time for return demonstration and accuracy check.
3. Instruct client to monitor and record blood pressure weekly (or more often if directed by physician) and bring record of pressures to visits with health care provider.

9.f. The client will state signs and symptoms to report to the health care provider.

9.f. Instruct the client to report:
1. headache present upon awakening
2. sudden and continued increase of B/P (if B/P is monitored at home)
3. chest pain
4. shortness of breath
5. significant weight gain or swelling of the extremities
6. changes in vision
7. frequent or uncontrollable nosebleeds
8. severe depression or emotional lability
9. side effects of diuretic therapy (see actions c.2.h.3–6 in this diagnosis)
10. side effects of antihypertensives (see action c.3.c in this diagnosis).

9.g. The client will identify community resources that can assist in making life-style changes necessary for effective control of hypertension.

9.g.1. Provide information regarding community resources and support groups that can assist client in making life-style changes that are necessary for effective control of hypertension (e.g. American Heart Association; "coronary clubs"; stop smoking, alcohol rehabilitation, and weight loss programs; stress management classes; counseling services).
2. Initiate a referral if indicated.

9.h. The client will verbalize an understanding of and a plan for adhering to recommended follow-up care including future appointments with health care provider and activity level.

9.h.1. Reinforce the importance of keeping follow-up appointments with health care provider and continuing lifelong medical supervision.
2. Reinforce the physician's instructions regarding activity level.
3. Refer to Nursing Diagnosis 8, action b, for measures to improve client compliance.

Myocardial Infarction

A myocardial infarction (MI) occurs as a result of severe ischemia of the heart muscle, which is caused by a sudden and prolonged interruption of coronary blood flow. The coronary artery occlusion can result from atherosclerosis, a thrombus, or arterial spasm. Sustained ischemia causes irreversible cellular damage and tissue necrosis, which result in many biochemical and morphological changes in the necrotic or infarcted area. Major manifestations of these changes include intense, crushing chest pain unrelieved by nitroglycerin; release of cardiac enzymes; and functional alterations caused by reduced contractility and altered electrical properties of the heart. The location of the infarct depends on which coronary vessel is occluded. Most infarctions occur in the left ventricle. An infarction may involve only a partial thickness (subendocardial infarction) or the entire thickness (transmural infarction) of the myocardium. Prognosis is largely influenced by the size and location of the infarct, concurrent cardiovascular status, effectiveness of compensatory mechanisms, and the promptness and effectiveness of treatment.

This care plan focuses on the adult client hospitalized during an attack of crushing chest pain and severe dyspnea for definitive diagnosis and management of a myocardial infarction. The goals of care are to prevent extension of the infarction, reduce fear and anxiety, relieve pain, improve cardiac output, prevent complications, and educate the client regarding follow-up care.

DISCHARGE CRITERIA

Prior to discharge, the client will:

- verbalize a basic understanding of a myocardial infarction
- demonstrate accuracy in counting pulse
- identify modifiable cardiovascular risk factors and ways to reduce these factors
- verbalize an understanding of the rationale for and constituents of a diet low in sodium, saturated fat, and cholesterol
- verbalize an understanding of medication therapy including rationale for, side effects of, schedule for taking, and importance of taking as prescribed
- verbalize an understanding of activity restrictions and the rate at which activity can be progressed
- state signs and symptoms to report to the health care provider
- identify community resources that can assist with cardiac rehabilitation and adjustment to the effects of a myocardial infarction
- share feelings and concerns about changes in body functioning and usual roles and life style
- verbalize an understanding of and a plan for adhering to recommended follow-up care including future appointments with health care provider.

Use in conjunction with the Care Plan on Immobility.

NURSING/COLLABORATIVE DIAGNOSES

1. Anxiety ☐ *361*
2. Decreased cardiac output ☐ *362*
3. Ineffective breathing patterns ☐ *364*

   4. Impaired gas exchange □ *365*
   5. Altered electrolyte balance:
      a. metabolic acidosis
      b. hyperkalemia
      c. hypokalemia □ *365*
  6A. Altered comfort: chest pain that may radiate to arm, neck, jaw, or back □ *366*
  6B. Altered comfort: nausea and vomiting □ *367*
   7. Activity intolerance □ *368*
   8. Impaired physical mobility □ *368*
   9. Self-care deficit □ *369*
  10. Constipation □ *369*
  11. Sleep pattern disturbance □ *370*
  12. Potential complications:
      a. arrhythmias
      b. congestive heart failure (CHF) and pulmonary edema
      c. thromboembolism
      d. rupture of the heart wall, papillary muscle, septum, or an aneurysm
      e. pericarditis
      f. recurrent MI
      g. cardiogenic shock □ *371*
  13. Sexual dysfunction: decreased libido and/or impotence □ *375*
  14. Disturbance in self-concept □ *375*
  15. Grieving □ *376*
  16. Knowledge deficit regarding follow-up care □ *377*

□ ▬▬▬▬▬▬▬▬▬▬▬▬▬▬▬▬▬▬▬▬▬▬▬▬▬▬▬▬▬▬▬▬▬▬

1. NURSING DIAGNOSIS

Anxiety related to unfamiliar environment; severe pain; difficulty breathing; feeling of suffocation; possibility of severe disability or impending death; and lack of understanding of diagnostic tests, the diagnosis, and treatment plan.

□ ▬▬▬▬▬▬▬▬▬▬▬▬▬▬▬▬▬▬▬▬▬▬▬▬▬▬▬▬▬▬▬▬▬▬

DESIRED OUTCOMES	NURSING ACTIONS AND *SELECTED RATIONALES*

1. The client will experience a reduction in fear and anxiety as evidenced by:
a. verbalization of feeling less anxious or fearful
b. relaxed facial expression and body movements
c. stable vital signs
d. usual skin color
e. verbalization of an understanding of hospital routines, diagnostic procedures, the diagnosis, and treatments.
	1.a. Assess client for signs and symptoms of fear and anxiety (e.g. verbalization of fears and concerns; tenseness; tremors; irritability; restlessness; increased dyspnea; diaphoresis; tachycardia; facial tension, pallor, or flushing; noncompliance with treatment plan). Validate perceptions carefully, remembering that some behaviors may result from hypoxia or fluid and electrolyte imbalances.
	   b. Ascertain effectiveness of current coping skills.
	   c. Implement measures *to reduce fear and anxiety:*
	     1. provide care in a calm, confident manner
	     2. if client is having severe pain and/or dyspnea:
	       a. do not leave alone during period of acute distress
	       b. perform actions to improve breathing pattern (see Nursing Diagnosis 3, action d)
	       c. perform actions to reduce pain (see Nursing Diagnosis 6.A, action 5)

    d. perform actions *to reduce feeling of suffocation:*
      1. open curtains and doors
      2. approach client from the side rather than face-on *(close face-on contact may make the client feel closed in)*
      3. limit the number of persons in room at any one time
      4. remove unnecessary equipment from room
      5. administer oxygen via nasal cannula rather than mask if possible
  3. encourage significant others to project a caring, concerned attitude without obvious anxiousness
  4. once the period of acute distress has subsided:
    a. orient to hospital environment, equipment, and routines; include an explanation of cardiac monitoring devices
    b. introduce staff who will be participating in his/her care; if possible, maintain consistency in staff assigned to his/her care *to provide feelings of stability and comfort with the environment*
    c. assure client that staff members are nearby; respond to call signal as soon as possible
    d. keep cardiac monitor out of client's view and the sound turned as low as possible
    e. encourage verbalization of fear and anxiety; provide feedback
    f. reinforce physician's explanation of invasive measures that may be performed to improve coronary blood flow (e.g. intra-aortic balloon pump [IABP]; streptokinase, urokinase, or tissue plasminogen activator [tPA] infusion; percutaneous transluminal coronary angioplasty [PTCA]) if planned
    g. explain all diagnostic tests (e.g. serum cardiac enzyme levels, chest x-ray, EKG, nuclear imaging, vectorcardiography, echocardiography, coronary angiography, exercise stress test)
    h. reinforce physician's explanations and clarify any misconceptions client may have about an MI, the treatment plan, and prognosis
    i. instruct in relaxation techniques and encourage participation in diversional activities
    j. assist client to identify specific stressors and ways to cope with them
  5. monitor for therapeutic and nontherapeutic effects of antianxiety agents if administered.
  d. Include significant others in orientation and teaching sessions and encourage their continued support of the client.
  e. Provide information based on current needs of client and significant others at a level they can understand. Encourage questions and clarification of information provided.
  f. Consult physician if above actions fail to control fear and anxiety.

□ ▬▬▬▬▬▬▬▬▬▬▬▬▬▬▬▬▬▬▬▬▬▬▬▬▬

2. NURSING DIAGNOSIS

Decreased cardiac output related to altered conductivity and contractility of the heart associated with myocardial damage.

□ ▬▬▬▬▬▬▬▬▬▬▬▬▬▬▬▬▬▬▬▬▬▬▬▬▬

DESIRED OUTCOMES	NURSING ACTIONS AND *SELECTED RATIONALES*

2. The client will have improved cardiac output as evidenced by:
  a. B/P within normal range for client
	2.a. Assess for and report signs and symptoms of an MI:
	  1. sudden, severe, and persistent chest pain (be aware that 15–20% of MIs may be painless, especially in the elderly)
	  2. dyspnea
	  3. elevated CPK (CK)-MB

b. apical pulse audible, regular, and between 60–100 beats/minute
c. absence of gallop rhythms
d. B/P and pulse stable with position change
e. unlabored respirations at 16–20/minute
f. normal breath sounds
g. usual mental status
h. absence of lightheadedness or syncope
i. palpable peripheral pulses
j. stronger amplitude of carotid pulse
k. improved skin color and temperature
l. capillary refill time less than 3 seconds
m. urine output at least 30 cc/hour
n. hemodynamic measurements such as pulmonary artery pressure (PAP), pulmonary capillary wedge pressure (PCWP), cardiac output (CO), and central venous pressure (CVP) returning toward normal range.

4. elevated LDH_1 and LDH_2 (an LDH_1 level that is higher than the LDH_2 is a reliable indicator of acute MI)
5. elevated WBC count and/or AST (SGOT); these tests are not specific for myocardial injury but support the diagnosis when CPK-MB, LDH_1, and LDH_2 are elevated
6. temperature elevation *(reflects tissue destruction and resulting inflammation)*
7. EKG readings showing ST segment elevation, T wave changes, and/or the presence of pathological Q waves.

b. Assess for and report signs and symptoms of decreased cardiac output:
1. drop of 20 mm Hg in systolic B/P, a systolic pressure below 80 mm Hg, or a continual drop of 5–10 mm Hg in systolic pressure with each reading
2. irregular pulse
3. pulse rate less than 60 or greater than 100 beats/minute
4. muffled heart sounds
5. presence of S_3 and/or S_4 gallop rhythm
6. decline in systolic B/P of at least 15 mm Hg with a concurrent rise in pulse when the client sits up
7. rapid, labored, or irregular respirations
8. crackles and diminished or absent breath sounds
9. restlessness, confusion
10. lightheadedness, syncope
11. diminished or absent peripheral pulses
12. decreased amplitude of carotid pulse
13. cool, pale, mottled, or cyanotic skin
14. capillary refill time greater than 3 seconds
15. urine output less than 30 cc/hour
16. decreased CO; increased PAP, PCWP, and CVP (use internal jugular vein pulsation method to estimate CVP if monitoring device not present).

c. Implement measures *to improve cardiac output:*
1. perform actions *to reduce cardiac workload:*
   a. place client in a semi- to high Fowler's position
   b. instruct client to avoid activities that create a Valsalva response (e.g. straining to have a bowel movement, bending at the waist, holding breath while moving)
   c. promote physical and emotional rest
   d. implement measures to improve gas exchange (see Nursing Diagnosis 4, action d) *in order to promote adequate tissue oxygenation*
   e. discourage smoking *(smoking has a cardiostimulatory effect, causes vasoconstriction, and reduces oxygen availability)*
   f. provide frequent, small meals rather than 3 large ones *(large meals require an increase in blood supply to gastrointestinal tract for digestion)*
   g. discourage intake of foods/fluids high in caffeine such as coffee, tea, chocolate, and colas *(caffeine is a myocardial stimulant and increases myocardial oxygen consumption)*
   h. implement measures *to prevent fluid volume excess:*
      1. maintain fluid restriction as ordered
      2. restrict sodium intake as ordered (2–3 gm sodium restriction is common)
      3. monitor for therapeutic and nontherapeutic effects of diuretics if administered
   i. increase activity gradually
   j. implement measures as ordered to treat anemia, hypotension, hypertension, hyperthyroidism, and chronic obstructive pulmonary disease *(these conditions reduce myocardial oxygen availability and/or increase cardiac workload)*
2. monitor for therapeutic and nontherapeutic effects of the following if administered:
   a. positive inotropic agents (e.g. digitalis preparations, dobutamine, dopamine, amrinone) *to improve myocardial contractility* (the use of these agents is controversial *because they can increase myocardial oxygen requirements; it has also been shown that digitalis preparations increase myocardial irritability in the first 48 hours after an MI)*

    b. nitrates (e.g. nitroglycerin) *to reduce cardiac workload by decreasing preload and afterload*

    c. beta-adrenergic blocking agents (e.g. timolol, propranolol, metoprolol, atenolol, nadolol, pindolol) *to reduce cardiac workload by blocking sympathetic stimulation of the heart* (these agents are contraindicated if signs and symptoms of congestive heart failure develop)

    d. calcium-channel blocking agents (e.g. nifedipine, verapamil, diltiazem) *to increase coronary blood flow and reduce cardiac workload by decreasing afterload*

    e. antiarrhythmics (e.g. quinidine, procainamide) if arrhythmias exist *to improve cardiac output by increasing diastolic filling time*

    f. intravenous infusions of insulin, potassium, and hypertonic glucose *to provide a source of energy for the damaged myocardium*

    3. prepare client for invasive measures that may be used *to improve coronary blood flow* (e.g. streptokinase, urokinase, or tissue plasminogen activator [tPA] infusion; intra-aortic balloon pump [IABP]; percutaneous transluminal coronary angioplasty [PTCA]) if planned.

  d. Consult physician if signs and symptoms of decreased cardiac output persist or worsen.

☐ ▬▬▬▬▬▬▬▬▬▬▬▬▬▬▬▬▬▬▬▬▬▬▬▬▬▬▬▬▬▬▬▬

3. NURSING DIAGNOSIS

Ineffective breathing patterns related to pain, fear, anxiety, depressant effects of some medications (e.g. narcotics, sedatives), and respiratory depressant and/or stimulant effects of hypoxia and diminished cerebral blood flow.

☐ ▬▬▬▬▬▬▬▬▬▬▬▬▬▬▬▬▬▬▬▬▬▬▬▬▬▬▬▬▬▬▬▬

DESIRED OUTCOMES	NURSING ACTIONS AND *SELECTED RATIONALES*

3. The client will maintain an effective breathing pattern as evidenced by:
a. normal rate, rhythm, and depth of respirations
b. decreased dyspnea
c. blood gases within normal range.
	3.a. Assess for signs and symptoms of ineffective breathing patterns (e.g. shallow, guarded respirations; dyspnea; use of accessory muscles for breathing; respiratory rate less than 16 or greater than 20/minute).
	b. Monitor blood gases. Report abnormal results.
	c. Monitor for and report significant changes in ear oximetry and capnograph results.
	d. Implement measures *to improve breathing pattern:*
	  1. perform actions to decrease pain (see Nursing Diagnosis 6.A, action 5)
	  2. perform actions to improve cardiac output (see Nursing Diagnosis 2, action c) *in order to promote adequate tissue perfusion*
	  3. perform actions to improve gas exchange (see Nursing Diagnosis 4, action d) *in order to promote adequate tissue oxygenation*
	  4. perform actions to decrease fear and anxiety (see Nursing Diagnosis 1, action c)
	  5. place client in a semi- to high Fowler's position unless contraindicated
	  6. while client is on bedrest, assist him/her to turn at least every 2 hours
	  7. instruct client to deep breathe or use inspiratory exerciser at least every 2 hours
	  8. increase activity as allowed and tolerated
	  9. administer central nervous system depressants (e.g. narcotic analgesics, sedatives) judiciously; hold medication and consult physician if respiratory rate is less than 12/minute.
	e. Consult physician if ineffective breathing patterns persist or worsen.

□

4. NURSING DIAGNOSIS

Impaired gas exchange related to:

a. ineffective breathing patterns;
b. decreased systemic tissue perfusion associated with decreased cardiac output.

□

DESIRED OUTCOMES	NURSING ACTIONS AND *SELECTED RATIONALES*

4. The client will experience adequate O_2/CO_2 exchange as evidenced by:
a. usual mental status
b. usual skin color
c. decreased dyspnea
d. blood gases within normal range.
	4.a. Assess for and report signs and symptoms of impaired gas exchange:
	   1. restlessness or irritability
	   2. confusion, somnolence
	   3. dusky or cyanotic skin
	   4. dyspnea.
	  b. Monitor blood gas values. Report abnormal results.
	  c. Monitor for and report significant changes in ear oximetry and capnograph results.
	  d. Implement measures *to improve gas exchange:*
	   1. perform actions to improve breathing pattern (**see** Nursing Diagnosis 3, action d)
	   2. perform actions to improve cardiac output (see Nursing Diagnosis 2, action c) *in order to promote adequate systemic tissue perfusion*
	   3. maintain oxygen therapy as ordered
	   4. discourage smoking *(smoking decreases oxygen availability and causes vasoconstriction).*
	  e. Consult physician if signs and symptoms of impaired gas exchange persist or worsen.

□

5. COLLABORATIVE DIAGNOSIS

Altered electrolyte balance:

a. **metabolic acidosis** related to excessive lactic acid production associated with anaerobic metabolism (due to tissue hypoxia resulting from inadequate cardiac output);
b. **hyperkalemia** related to metabolic acidosis and myocardial tissue destruction (both conditions result in cellular release of potassium);
c. **hypokalemia** related to loss of potassium associated with vomiting, diuretic therapy, and excessive excretion of potassium if renal function is adequate while serum potassium level is increased.

□

DESIRED OUTCOMES	NURSING ACTIONS AND *SELECTED RATIONALES*
5.a. The client will maintain acid-base balance as evidenced by: 1. usual mental status	5.a.1. Assess for and report signs and symptoms of metabolic acidosis (e.g. drowsiness; disorientation; stupor; rapid, deep respirations; headache; nausea and vomiting; low pH and CO_2 content and negative base excess; anion gap greater than 16 mEq/liter).

UNIT VII

2. unlabored respirations at 16–20/minute
3. absence of headache, nausea, and vomiting
4. blood gases within normal range
5. anion gap less than 16 mEq/liter.

2. Implement measures *to prevent or treat metabolic acidosis:*
   a. perform actions to improve cardiac output (see Nursing Diagnosis 2, action c) *in order to promote adequate tissue perfusion and oxygenation and prevent excessive lactic acid production*
   b. monitor for therapeutic and nontherapeutic effects of sodium bicarbonate if administered (reserved for use in severe acidosis when the pH is less than 7.1).
3. Consult physician if signs and symptoms of metabolic acidosis persist or worsen.

5.b. The client will maintain a safe serum potassium level as evidenced by:
   1. regular pulse at 60–100 beats/minute
   2. usual muscle tone and strength
   3. normal bowel sounds
   4. serum potassium within normal range.

5.b.1. Assess for and report signs and symptoms of:
   a. hyperkalemia (e.g. slow or irregular pulse; paresthesias; muscle weakness and flaccidity; hyperactive bowel sounds with diarrhea and intestinal colic; EKG reading showing peaked T wave, prolonged PR interval, and/or widened QRS; elevated serum potassium level)
   b. hypokalemia (e.g. irregular pulse; muscle weakness and cramping; paresthesias; nausea and vomiting; hypoactive or absent bowel sounds; drowsiness; EKG reading showing ST segment depression, T wave inversion or flattening, and presence of U waves; low serum potassium level).
2. Implement measures *to prevent or treat hyperkalemia:*
   a. perform actions to prevent or treat metabolic acidosis (see action a.2 in this diagnosis) *in order to decrease cellular release of potassium*
   b. maintain dietary restrictions of potassium as ordered
   c. if signs and symptoms of hyperkalemia are present, consult physician before administering prescribed potassium supplements
   d. monitor for therapeutic and nontherapeutic effects of the following if administered:
      1. loop diuretics (e.g. ethacrynic acid, furosemide) *to increase renal excretion of potassium*
      2. cation-exchange resins (e.g. Kayexalate) *to increase potassium excretion via the intestines (act by exchanging sodium for potassium)*
      3. intravenous insulin and hypertonic glucose solutions *to enhance transport of potassium back into cells.*
3. Implement measures *to prevent or treat hypokalemia:*
   a. perform actions to reduce nausea and vomiting (see Nursing Diagnosis 6.B, action 2)
   b. maintain intravenous and oral potassium replacements as ordered (monitor serum potassium and urine output closely when giving supplemental potassium and consult physician if potassium level increases above normal and/or urine output is less than 30 cc/hour)
   c. if client is taking a potassium-depleting diuretic or if signs and symptoms of hypokalemia are present, encourage intake of foods/fluids high in potassium (e.g. bananas, oranges, potatoes, raisins, figs, apricots, dates, tomatoes, Gatorade, fruit juices) when oral intake is allowed.
4. Consult physician if signs and symptoms of potassium imbalance persist or worsen.

□ ▬▬▬▬▬▬▬▬▬▬▬▬▬▬▬▬▬▬▬▬▬▬▬

6.A. NURSING DIAGNOSIS

Altered comfort:* chest pain that may radiate to arm, neck, jaw, or back related to reduced coronary blood flow (a decreased oxygen supply forces the myocardium to convert to anaerobic metabolism resulting in lactic acid release; lactic acid acts as an irritant to myocardial neural receptors).

---

* In this care plan, the nursing diagnosis "pain" is included under the diagnostic label of altered comfort.

□ ▬▬▬▬▬▬▬▬▬▬▬▬▬▬▬▬▬▬▬▬▬▬▬

DESIRED OUTCOMES	NURSING ACTIONS AND *SELECTED RATIONALES*

6.A. The client will experience diminished chest, arm, neck, jaw, and back pain as evidenced by:
1. verbalization of pain relief
2. relaxed facial expression and body positioning
3. increased participation in activities
4. stable vital signs.
	6.A.1. Determine how the client usually responds to pain.
	2. Assess for nonverbal signs of pain (e.g. wrinkled brow; rubbing neck, jaw, or arm; clenched fists; reluctance to move; clutching chest; restlessness; shallow, guarded respirations; diaphoresis; facial pallor or flushing; change in B/P; tachycardia).
	3. Assess verbal complaints of pain. Ask client to be specific about onset, location, type, severity, and duration of pain.
	4. Assess for factors that seem to aggravate and alleviate pain.
	5. Implement measures *to reduce pain:*
	  a. maintain oxygen therapy as ordered *to increase the myocardial oxygen supply*
	  b. monitor for therapeutic and nontherapeutic effects of the following medications if administered:
	    1. narcotic analgesics (an intravenous rather than an intramuscular route should be used *because injections will be poorly absorbed if tissue perfusion is decreased; intramuscular injections also elevate serum enzyme levels which may interfere with assessment of myocardial damage);* consult physician before giving morphine sulfate if client has bradycardia or hypotension
	    2. nitrates (e.g. nitroglycerin)
	  c. perform actions to reduce cardiac workload (see Nursing Diagnosis 2, action c.1) *in order to decrease myocardial oxygen consumption*
	  d. provide or assist with nonpharmacological measures for pain relief (e.g. neck and shoulder massage, back rub, position change, relaxation techniques, quiet conversation, restful environment, diversional activities).
	6. Consult physician if above measures fail to provide adequate pain relief.

□ ▬▬▬▬▬▬▬▬▬▬▬▬▬▬▬▬▬▬▬▬▬▬▬▬▬▬

6.B. NURSING DIAGNOSIS

Altered comfort: nausea and vomiting related to stimulation of the vomiting center associated with:

1. vagal and/or sympathetic stimulation resulting from inflammation of visceral receptors in the heart;
2. cortical stimulation due to pain and stress.

□ ▬▬▬▬▬▬▬▬▬▬▬▬▬▬▬▬▬▬▬▬▬▬▬▬▬▬

DESIRED OUTCOMES	NURSING ACTIONS AND *SELECTED RATIONALES*

6.B. The client will experience relief of nausea and vomiting as evidenced by:
1. verbalization of relief of nausea
2. absence of vomiting.
	6.B.1. Assess client to determine factors that contribute to nausea and vomiting (e.g. pain, fear, anxiety).
	2. Implement measures *to reduce nausea and vomiting:*
	  a. perform actions to reduce pain (see Nursing Diagnosis 6.A, action 5)
	  b. eliminate noxious sights and smells from the environment (*noxious stimuli cause cortical stimulation of the vomiting center*)
	  c. encourage client to change positions slowly (*movement stimulates the chemoreceptor trigger zone*)
	  d. provide oral hygiene after each emesis and before meals
	  e. provide small, frequent meals rather than 3 large ones
	  f. instruct client to ingest foods and fluids slowly
	  g. instruct client to avoid foods/fluids that irritate the gastric mucosa (e.g. spicy foods; citrus fruits or juices; caffeine-containing items such as chocolate, coffee, tea, and colas)

UNIT
VII

   h. instruct client to eat dry foods (e.g. toast, crackers) and avoid drinking liquids with meals if nauseated
   i. provide carbonated beverages for client to sip if nauseated
   j. encourage client to take deep, slow breaths if nauseated
   k. instruct client to rest after eating with head of bed elevated
   l. perform actions to reduce fear and anxiety (see Nursing Diagnosis 1, action c)
   m. monitor for therapeutic and nontherapeutic effects of antiemetics if administered.
   3. Consult physician if above measures fail to control nausea and vomiting.

☐ ▬▬▬▬▬▬▬▬▬▬▬▬▬▬▬▬▬▬▬▬▬▬

7. NURSING DIAGNOSIS

Activity intolerance related to:

a. tissue hypoxia associated with impaired alveolar gas exchange and decreased tissue perfusion (a result of decreased cardiac output);
b. difficulty resting and sleeping associated with discomfort, dyspnea, frequent assessments and treatments, fear, and anxiety.

☐ ▬▬▬▬▬▬▬▬▬▬▬▬▬▬▬▬▬▬▬▬▬▬

DESIRED OUTCOMES	NURSING ACTIONS AND *SELECTED RATIONALES*
7. The client will demonstrate an increased tolerance for activity (see Care Plan on Immobility, Nursing Diagnosis 8, for outcome criteria).	7.a. Refer to Care Plan on Immobility, Nursing Diagnosis 8, for measures related to assessment and improvement of activity tolerance. b. Implement additional measures *to promote rest and improve activity tolerance:* 1. maintain activity restrictions as ordered 2. perform actions to reduce fear and anxiety (see Nursing Diagnosis 1, action c) 3. perform actions to promote sleep (see Nursing Diagnosis 11) 4. perform actions to improve breathing pattern and gas exchange (see Nursing Diagnoses 3, action d and 4, action d) *in order to relieve dyspnea and improve tissue oxygenation* 5. perform actions to reduce discomfort (see Nursing Diagnoses 6.A, action 5 and 6.B, action 2) 6. perform actions to increase cardiac output (see Nursing Diagnosis 2, action c) 7. increase client's activity gradually as allowed and tolerated (desired activity level by time of discharge is moderate-energy activities of 3–5 metabolic equivalents [METS]).

☐ ▬▬▬▬▬▬▬▬▬▬▬▬▬▬▬▬▬▬▬▬▬▬

8. NURSING DIAGNOSIS

Impaired physical mobility related to weakness and fatigue, fear that movement will precipitate chest pain and another "heart attack," and activity restrictions imposed by the treatment plan.

☐ ▬▬▬▬▬▬▬▬▬▬▬▬▬▬▬▬▬▬▬▬▬▬

DESIRED OUTCOMES	NURSING ACTIONS AND *SELECTED RATIONALES*

8.a. The client will maintain an optimal level of physical mobility within physical limitations and prescribed activity restrictions.	8.a.1. Assess for factors that impair physical mobility (e.g. weakness, fatigue, reluctance to move because of fear of precipitating pain and another "heart attack," restrictions imposed by treatment plan).
	2. Implement measures *to increase mobility:*
	  a. perform actions to control pain (see Nursing Diagnosis 6.A, action 5)
	  b. perform actions to improve strength and activity tolerance (see Nursing Diagnosis 7)
	  c. reassure the client that gradual progression of activity is designed to strengthen the heart and is not likely to cause another MI.
	3. Increase activity and participation in self-care activities as allowed and tolerated.
	4. Provide praise and encouragement for all efforts to increase physical mobility.

8.b. The client will not experience problems associated with immobility.	8.b. Refer to Care Plan on Immobility for actions to prevent problems associated with immobility if client is to remain on bedrest for longer than 48 hours.

9. NURSING DIAGNOSIS

Self-care deficit related to dyspnea and impaired physical mobility associated with weakness, fatigue, fear of precipitating chest pain and another "heart attack," and prescribed activity restrictions.

DESIRED OUTCOMES	NURSING ACTIONS AND *SELECTED RATIONALES*

9. The client will demonstrate increased participation in self-care activities within physical limitations and prescribed activity restrictions.	9.a. Refer to Care Plan on Immobility, Nursing Diagnosis 9, for measures related to assessment of, planning for, and meeting client's self-care needs.
	  b. Implement additional measures *to facilitate client's ability to perform self-care activities:*
	    1. perform actions to improve gas exchange (see Nursing Diagnosis 4, action d) *in order to relieve dyspnea*
	    2. perform actions to increase mobility (see Nursing Diagnosis 8, action a.2).

10. NURSING DIAGNOSIS

Constipation related to decreased mobility, anxiety, use of narcotics, and fear that straining will precipitate another "heart attack."

DESIRED OUTCOMES	NURSING ACTIONS AND *SELECTED RATIONALES*

10. The client will maintain usual bowel elimination pattern.	10.a. Ascertain client's usual bowel elimination habits.
	   b. Monitor and record bowel movements including frequency, consistency, and shape.
	   c. Assess for signs and symptoms that may accompany constipation such as headache, anorexia, nausea, abdominal distention and cramping, and feeling of fullness or pressure in abdomen or rectum.
	   d. Assess bowel sounds. Report a pattern of decreasing bowel sounds.
	   e. Implement measures *to prevent constipation:*
	      1. encourage client to defecate whenever the urge is felt
	      2. allow client to use a commode rather than a bedpan for bowel movements *(use of a bedpan may actually require more energy than getting up to the commode);* provide privacy and adequate ventilation
	      3. encourage client to relax during attempts to defecate *in order to promote relaxation of the levator ani muscle and the external anal sphincter*
	      4. maintain the maximum fluid intake allowed
	      5. instruct client to select foods high in fiber and within dietary restrictions of sodium and saturated fat (e.g. bran, whole grains, raw fruits and vegetables, dried fruits)
	      6. encourage client to drink warm liquids *to stimulate peristalsis*
	      7. increase activity as allowed and tolerated
	      8. monitor for therapeutic and nontherapeutic effects of stool softeners and/or laxatives if administered.
	   f. Avoid enemas and manual removal of stool if possible *(both cause vagal stimulation).*
	   g. Consult physician if signs and symptoms of constipation persist.

11. NURSING DIAGNOSIS

Sleep pattern disturbance related to frequent assessments and treatments, decreased physical activity, fear, anxiety, discomfort, and inability to assume usual sleep position due to orthopnea.

DESIRED OUTCOMES	NURSING ACTIONS AND *SELECTED RATIONALES*

11. The client will attain optimal amounts of sleep within the parameters of the treatment regimen (see Care Plan on Immobility, Nursing Diagnosis 12, for outcome criteria).	11.a. Refer to Care Plan on Immobility, Nursing Diagnosis 12, for measures related to assessment and promotion of sleep.
	   b. Implement additional measures *to promote sleep:*
	      1. perform actions to reduce discomfort (see Nursing Diagnoses 6.A, action 5 and 6.B, action 2)
	      2. perform actions to improve gas exchange (see Nursing Diagnosis 4, action d) *in order to reduce orthopnea*
	      3. assist client to assume a comfortable sleep position (e.g. bed in reverse Trendelenburg position with client in usual recumbent sleep position, head of bed elevated with arms supported on pillows, resting forward on overbed table with good pillow support)
	      4. maintain oxygen therapy during sleep if indicated
	      5. ensure good room ventilation
	      6. perform actions to reduce fear and anxiety (see Nursing Diagnosis 1, action c).

12. COLLABORATIVE DIAGNOSIS

Potential complications:

a. **arrhythmias** related to altered myocardial conductivity associated with digitalis therapy, hypoxia, electrolyte and acid-base imbalances, or damage to conduction pathways and/or excessive sympathetic and/or parasympathetic stimulation during the infarction;

b. **congestive heart failure (CHF) and pulmonary edema** related to pump failure and the resultant vascular congestion;

c. **thromboembolism** related to:
 1. formation of mural thrombi on the infarcted endocardium
 2. formation of microemboli associated with incomplete emptying of cardiac chambers if atrial fibrillation or CHF occurs
 3. venous stasis associated with diminished cardiac output and decreased mobility;

d. **rupture of the heart wall, papillary muscle, septum, or an aneurysm** related to necrosis and/or thinning of areas of the myocardium;

e. **pericarditis** related to extension of the infarction to the pericardial surface (usually develops 2–3 days after the infarction) or an autoimmune response known as Dressler's syndrome (post-MI syndrome), which can occur 1–4 weeks after the MI;

f. **recurrent MI** related to continued or increased stress on the heart;

g. **cardiogenic shock** related to:
 1. rupture of any cardiac structure
 2. inability of the damaged heart, intrinsic compensatory mechanisms, and treatment measures to maintain adequate tissue perfusion to vital organs (the release of myocardial depressant factor as a result of inadequate splanchnic circulation further complicates this process).

DESIRED OUTCOMES	NURSING ACTIONS AND *SELECTED RATIONALES*

12.a. The client will not experience cardiac arrhythmias as evidenced by:
1. regular apical pulse at 60–100 beats/minute
2. equal apical and radial pulses
3. absence of syncope and palpitations
4. EKG reading showing normal sinus rhythm.
	12.a.1. Assess for and report signs and symptoms of arrhythmias (e.g. irregular apical pulse; pulse rate below 60 or above 100 beats/minute; apical-radial pulse deficit; syncope; palpitations; abnormal rate, rhythm, or configurations on EKG). Monitor closely for arrhythmias if client is taking a digitalis preparation *(digitalis seems to increase the tendency for arrhythmias when given within the first 48 hours after MI)*.
	  2. Implement measures *to prevent arrhythmias:*
	    a. perform actions to improve cardiac output (see Nursing Diagnosis 2, action c) *in order to promote adequate myocardial tissue perfusion and oxygenation*
	    b. perform actions to prevent and treat metabolic acidosis (see Collaborative Diagnosis 5, action a.2)
	    c. perform actions to maintain serum potassium within a safe range (see Collaborative Diagnosis 5, actions b.2 and 3).
	  3. If arrhythmias occur:
	    a. initiate cardiac monitoring if not already being done
	    b. monitor for therapeutic and nontherapeutic effects of the following medications if administered:
	      1. Class I antiarrhythmics (e.g. phenytoin, tocainide, lidocaine, flecainide, procainamide, disopyramide, quinidine) *to interfere directly with depolarization*
	      2. Class II antiarrhythmics (e.g. propranolol) *to block beta-adrenergic stimulation*
	      3. Class III antiarrhythmics (e.g. bretylium, amiodarone) *to prolong the duration of the action potential*

4. Class IV antiarrhythmics (e.g. verapamil, diltiazem) *to block the slow inward depolarizing current*
5. anticholinergic agents (e.g. atropine) or sympathomimetics (e.g. ephedrine, isoproterenol) *to increase heart rate*
6. cardiac glycosides (e.g. digitalis) *to decrease the heart rate*
   c. restrict client's activity based on his/her tolerance and severity of arrhythmia
   d. maintain oxygen therapy as ordered
   e. assist with cardioversion if performed
   f. assess cardiovascular status closely and report signs and symptoms of inadequate tissue perfusion (e.g. decline in B/P; cool, clammy, mottled skin; cyanosis; diminished peripheral pulses; declining urine output; increased restlessness and agitation; increased shortness of breath)
   g. prepare client for insertion of pacemaker if planned
   h. have emergency cart readily available for cardiopulmonary resuscitation.

12.b. The client will not develop CHF and pulmonary edema as evidenced by:
1. vital signs within normal range for client
2. audible heart sounds without an S₃ or S₄ or softening of pre-existing murmurs
3. normal breath sounds
4. absence of or no increase in dyspnea and orthopnea
5. palpable peripheral pulses and stronger carotid pulse amplitude
6. balanced intake and output
7. stable weight
8. CVP within normal range
9. absence of peripheral edema; distended neck veins; enlarged, tender liver
10. BUN and serum creatinine and alkaline phosphatase levels within normal range.

12.b.1. Assess for and report signs and symptoms of CHF (clients taking beta-adrenergic blocking agents are more susceptible to CHF *because these medications decrease myocardial contractility*):
   a. tachycardia
   b. softened or muffled heart sounds
   c. development of or intensified S₃ and/or S₄ gallop rhythm
   d. crackles and diminished or absent breath sounds
   e. increased shortness of breath
   f. displaced apical impulse
   g. diminished or absent peripheral pulses
   h. decreased amplitude of carotid pulse
   i. intake greater than output
   j. weight gain
   k. elevated CVP
   l. peripheral edema
   m. distended neck veins
   n. enlarged, tender liver
   o. elevated BUN and serum creatinine and alkaline phosphatase levels.
2. Monitor chest x-ray results. Report findings of cardiomegaly, pleural effusion, or pulmonary edema.
3. Implement measures *to prevent CHF*:
   a. perform actions to improve cardiac output (see Nursing Diagnosis 2, action c)
   b. perform actions as ordered to treat arrhythmias and hypertension if present *(these conditions increase cardiac workload and contribute to development of CHF)*.
4. If signs and symptoms of CHF occur:
   a. continue with above actions
   b. monitor for therapeutic and nontherapeutic effects of medications that may be administered *to reduce vascular congestion and/or cardiac workload* (e.g. diuretics, cardiotonics, vasodilators, morphine sulfate)
   c. assist with phlebotomy if performed *to reduce blood volume*
   d. apply rotating tourniquets according to hospital policy if ordered *to reduce pulmonary vascular congestion*
   e. refer to Care Plan on Congestive Heart Failure for additional care measures.

12.c. The client will not develop a thromboembolism as evidenced by:
1. palpable peripheral pulses
2. usual skin temperature and color of extremities
3. absence of pain in extremities
4. absence of sudden chest pain, cough, hemoptysis

12.c.1. Assess for and report signs and symptoms of:
   a. venous thrombus (e.g. pain, swelling, unusual warmth or redness, and/or positive Homan's sign in extremity)
   b. arterial thrombus or embolus (e.g. diminished or absent peripheral pulses; pallor, cyanosis, coolness, numbness, and/or pain in extremity)
   c. cerebral ischemia (e.g. decreased level of consciousness, alteration in usual sensory and motor function, seizures)
   d. pulmonary embolism (e.g. sudden, severe chest pain; cough; hemoptysis; increased dyspnea; cyanosis; increased restlessness).
2. Implement measures *to prevent the development of mural thrombi and microemboli*:

5. usual mental status
6. usual sensory and motor function.

    a. perform actions to prevent and treat arrhythmias and CHF (see actions a.2 and 3 and b.3 and 4 in this diagnosis) *in order to reduce stasis of blood in the cardiac chambers*
    b. monitor for therapeutic and nontherapeutic effects of anticoagulants (e.g. heparin, warfarin) or antiplatelet agents (e.g. aspirin, dipyridamole) if administered prophylactically.
3. Implement measures to prevent and treat a venous thrombus and pulmonary embolism (see Care Plan on Immobility, Collaborative Diagnosis 14, actions a.1.b and c and a.2.b and c).
4. If signs and symptoms of an arterial thromboembolism occur:
    a. maintain client on strict bedrest with lower extremities in a level or slightly dependent position *to improve arterial blood flow*
    b. prepare client for diagnostic studies (e.g. Doppler ultrasound, plethysmography, oscillometry)
    c. implement measures *to promote vasodilation in the obstructed extremity:*
       1. administer peripheral vasodilating agents (e.g. papaverine, cyclandelate) as ordered
       2. keep lower extremities warm
       3. assist with a lumbar sympathetic block if performed *to decrease vasoconstrictor tone*
    d. monitor for therapeutic and nontherapeutic effects of heparin and thrombolytic agents (e.g. streptokinase, tissue plasminogen activator [tPA], urokinase) if administered
    e. prepare client for surgical intervention (e.g. thromboembolectomy, revascularization) if indicated
    f. provide emotional support to client and significant others.
5. If signs and symptoms of cerebral ischemia occur:
    a. maintain client on bedrest with head of bed flat unless contraindicated
    b. initiate appropriate safety precautions (e.g. side rails up, seizure precautions)
    c. monitor for and report progression of symptoms
    d. provide emotional support to client and significant others
    e. refer to Care Plan on Cerebrovascular Accident for additional care measures if signs and symptoms persist.

12.d. The client will not experience rupture of any cardiac structure as evidenced by absence of signs of acute heart failure and/or cardiogenic shock (see outcomes b and g in this diagnosis for outcome criteria).

12.d.1. Assess for signs and symptoms of the following:
    a. ventricular aneurysm (e.g. bulges seen on cardiac x-rays, persistent ST segment elevation on EKG readings, arrhythmias, identification of aneurysm on angiography reports)
    b. papillary muscle rupture leading to mitral regurgitation (e.g. holosystolic murmur at apex, apical thrills, severe dyspnea, chest pain, syncope)
    c. ventricular septal defect (e.g. systolic murmur at left sternal border; loud, widely split S_2; identification of defect on cardiac catheterization reports)
    d. heart wall rupture leading to cardiac tamponade (e.g. rapid and continual decrease in B/P, narrowing pulse pressure, pulsus paradoxus, distant or muffled heart sounds, neck vein distention on inspiration) and electromechanical dissociation.
2. Assess for and immediately report signs and symptoms of acute heart failure and/or cardiogenic shock (see actions b.1 and 2 and g.1 in this diagnosis), which may occur as a result of rupture of an aneurysm or cardiac structure.
3. Implement measures to reduce cardiac workload (see Nursing Diagnosis 2, action c.1) *in order to reduce risk of rupture of an aneurysm or other cardiac structure.*
4. If signs and symptoms of rupture occur:
    a. maintain client on bedrest
    b. assist with pericardiocentesis if performed
    c. assist with measures to treat cardiogenic shock (see action g.3 in this diagnosis)
    d. prepare client for surgical intervention (e.g. valve replacement, repair of ventricular septal defect, aneurysmectomy) if planned
    e. provide emotional support to client and significant others.

UNIT VII

12.e. The client will experience resolution of pericarditis if it develops as evidenced by:
1. fewer complaints of substernal or precordial pain
2. absence of pericardial friction rub
3. unlabored respirations at 16–20/minute
4. temperature declining toward normal
5. WBC count and sedimentation rate declining toward normal range.

12.e.1. Assess for and report signs and symptoms of pericarditis:
   a. substernal or precordial pain that frequently radiates to left shoulder, neck, and arm; is intensified during deep inspiration; and usually is relieved by sitting up
   b. pericardial friction rub (may be transient)
   c. increased dyspnea, tachypnea
   d. persistent temperature elevation
   e. further increase in WBC count and sedimentation rate (both will be elevated as a result of the infarction)
   f. chest x-ray and echocardiography results showing cardiomegaly and pericardial effusion.
2. If signs and symptoms of pericarditis occur:
   a. allay client's anxiety (client may believe that symptoms indicate recurrent MI)
   b. monitor for therapeutic and nontherapeutic effects of medications that may be administered *to reduce inflammation* (e.g. aspirin, indomethacin, ibuprofen, corticosteroids)
   c. assess for and immediately report signs of cardiac tamponade (e.g. rapid and continual decline in B/P; narrowed pulse pressure; pulsus paradoxus; weak, rapid pulse; distant or muffled heart sounds; neck vein distention on inspiration; decreased amplitude of waves on EKG; increased CVP and pulmonary pressures)
   d. prepare client for and assist with pericardiocentesis if indicated.

12.f. The client will not experience a recurrent MI as evidenced by:
1. no further episodes of persistent chest pain
2. stable vital signs
3. cardiac enzyme levels declining toward normal range
4. improved EKG readings.

12.f.1. Assess for and report signs and symptoms of a recurrent MI (e.g. recurrent episode of sudden, severe, and persistent chest pain; increased dyspnea; significant change in vital signs; recurrent increase in cardiac enzymes; increased ST segment elevation, pathological Q waves, and/or T wave changes on EKG reading).
2. Implement measures to improve cardiac output (see Nursing Diagnosis 2, action c) *in order to reduce risk of a recurrent MI.*
3. If signs and symptoms of myocardial infarction recur, continue with measures identified in this care plan.

12.g. The client will not develop cardiogenic shock as evidenced by:
1. stable or improved mental status
2. stable vital signs
3. palpable peripheral pulses
4. stable or improved skin color and temperature
5. urine output at least 20 cc/hour
6. stable or stronger carotid pulse amplitude
7. CVP and PCWP within normal range.

12.g.1. Assess for and immediately report signs and symptoms of cardiogenic shock:
   a. increased restlessness, lethargy, or confusion
   b. decrease in systolic B/P of 30 mm Hg or a systolic pressure below 80 mm Hg
   c. pulse rate greater than 100 beats/minute
   d. diminished or absent peripheral pulses
   e. increased coolness and duskiness or cyanosis of skin
   f. urine output less than 20 cc/hour
   g. further decrease in amplitude of carotid pulse
   h. elevated CVP and PCWP.
2. Implement measures to improve cardiac output (see Nursing Diagnosis 2, action c) *in order to prevent cardiogenic shock.*
3. If signs and symptoms of cardiogenic shock occur:
   a. continue with above actions to improve cardiac output
   b. implement additional measures *to increase myocardial oxygen supply:*
      1. maintain oxygen therapy as ordered
      2. assist with hyperbaric oxygenation and extracorporeal membrane oxygenation (ECMO) if indicated
   c. implement additional measures *to reduce oxygen utilization:*
      1. maintain client on strict bedrest
      2. assist with measures to induce hypothermia if ordered
   d. monitor for therapeutic and nontherapeutic effects of the following if administered:
      1. sympathomimetics (e.g. dopamine, dobutamine, isoproterenol, norepinephrine) *to increase cardiac output and maintain arterial pressure*
      2. antiarrhythmic agents *to increase cardiac output*
      3. vasodilators (e.g. nitroprusside, nitroglycerin) *to decrease cardiac workload* (sympathomimetics are given in conjunction with vasodilators *to maintain arterial pressure*)

4. intravenous infusions of insulin, potassium, and hypertonic glucose *to provide an energy source for the cells*
5. intravenous sodium bicarbonate *to correct acidosis* (reserved for use in severe acidosis when the pH is less than 7.1)

e. assist with insertion of hemodynamic monitoring device (e.g. Swan-Ganz catheter) and intra-aortic balloon pump (IABP) if indicated

f. provide emotional support to client and significant others.

---

13. NURSING DIAGNOSIS

Sexual dysfunction: decreased libido and/or impotence related to an altered self-concept, fear of sexual inadequacy and/or death during coitus, and the effects of some medications (e.g. beta-adrenergic blocking agents).

DESIRED OUTCOMES	NURSING ACTIONS AND *SELECTED RATIONALES*
13. The client will perceive self as sexually adequate and acceptable (see Care Plan on Immobility, Nursing Diagnosis 15, for outcome criteria).	13.a. Refer to Care Plan on Immobility, Nursing Diagnosis 15, for measures related to assessment and management of sexual dysfunction. b. Implement additional measures *to promote optimal sexual functioning:* 1. provide accurate information about effects of sexual activity on cardiac function; encourage questions and clarify any misconceptions 2. perform actions to promote a positive self-concept (see Nursing Diagnosis 14) 3. inform client that anxiety, fatigue, and certain medications (e.g. beta blockers) can cause impotence; encourage client to discuss persistent impotence with physician and assure him that impotence is usually reversible.

---

14. NURSING DIAGNOSIS

Disturbance in self-concept* related to:

a. dependence on others to meet self-care needs;
b. need to alter usual sexual activities to comply with treatment plan;
c. perceived loss of normal body functioning;
d. possible changes in life style, vocation, and roles.

---

* This diagnostic label includes the nursing diagnoses of body image disturbance and self-esteem disturbance.

DESIRED OUTCOMES	NURSING ACTIONS AND *SELECTED RATIONALES*
14. The client will demonstrate beginning adaptation to changes in body functioning, life style, and roles (see Care	14.a. Refer to Care Plan on Immobility, Nursing Diagnosis 16, for measures related to assessment and promotion of a positive self-concept. b. Implement additional measures *to promote a positive self-concept:* 1. clarify misconceptions about future limitations on activity; inform client

Plan on Immobility, Nursing
Diagnosis 16, for outcome
criteria).

that the majority of persons are able to return to gainful employment
after an MI

2. perform actions to promote optimal sexual functioning (see Nursing
Diagnosis 13)

3. increase activity and participation in self-care activities as allowed and
tolerated *to reduce feelings of dependency*

4. encourage significant others to allow client to do what he/she is able *so
that independence can be re-established and self-esteem redeveloped*

5. teach client the rationale for treatments and encourage maximum
participation in the treatment regimen *to enable him/her to have a
sense of control over life*

6. provide information about and encourage utilization of community
agencies or support groups (e.g. vocational rehabilitation, "coronary
clubs," counseling services).

c. Ensure that client and significant others have similar expectations and
understanding of future life style.

d. Assist the client and significant others to identify ways that personal and
family goals can be adjusted rather than abandoned.

15. NURSING DIAGNOSIS

Grieving* related to loss of normal function of the heart, possible changes in life
style and roles, and uncertainty of prognosis.

---

* This diagnostic label includes anticipatory grieving and grieving following the actual losses/changes.

DESIRED OUTCOMES	NURSING ACTIONS AND *SELECTED RATIONALES*

15. The client will demonstrate
beginning progression
through the grieving process
as evidenced by:
   a. verbalization of feelings
   about having had an MI
   b. expression of grief
   c. participation in treatment
   plan and self-care
   activities
   d. utilization of available
   support systems
   e. verbalization of a plan for
   integrating prescribed
   follow-up care into life
   style.

15.a. Determine the client's perception of impact of having had an MI on his/her
future.

b. Determine how the client usually expresses grief.

c. Observe for signs of grieving (e.g. changes in eating habits, insomnia,
anger, noncompliance, denial).

d. Implement measures *to facilitate the grieving process:*

1. assist the client to acknowledge the loss of normal heart function and
the need to alter usual life style *so grief work can begin;* assess for
factors that may hinder or facilitate acknowledgment

2. discuss the grieving process and assist client to accept the stages of
grieving as an expected response to the changes experienced

3. allow time for client to progress through the stages of grieving (denial,
anger, bargaining, depression, acceptance [Kübler-Ross, 1969]); be
aware that not every stage is experienced or expressed by all individuals

4. assist client to identify personal strengths that have helped him/her to
cope in previous situations of loss or change

5. perform actions *to promote trust* (e.g. answer questions honestly,
provide requested information)

6. provide an atmosphere of care and concern (e.g. provide privacy, be
available and nonjudgmental, display empathy and respect) *so that
client will feel free to verbalize both positive and negative feelings and
concerns*

7. encourage the expression of anger and sadness about having had an MI

8. encourage client to express his/her feelings in whatever ways are
comfortable (e.g. writing, drawing, conversation)

9. support realistic hope regarding the prognosis.

e. Assess for and support behaviors suggesting successful resolution of grief (e.g. verbalizing feelings about changes, expressing sorrow, focusing on ways to adapt to changes).

f. Explain the stages of the grieving process to significant others. Encourage their support and understanding.

g. Provide information regarding counseling services and support groups that might assist client in working through grief.

h. Arrange for a visit from clergy if desired by client.

i. Monitor for therapeutic and nontherapeutic effects of antidepressants if administered.

j. Consult physician regarding referral for counseling if signs of dysfunctional grieving (e.g. persistent denial of losses or changes, excessive anger or sadness, hysteria, suicidal behaviors, phobias) occur.

---

16. NURSING DIAGNOSIS

Knowledge deficit regarding follow-up care.

DESIRED OUTCOMES	NURSING ACTIONS AND *SELECTED RATIONALES*
16.a. The client will verbalize a basic understanding of a myocardial infarction.	16.a. Explain a myocardial infarction in terms the client can understand. Utilize appropriate teaching aids (e.g. pictures, videotapes, heart models). Inform client that it takes approximately 6–8 weeks for the heart to heal after a myocardial infarction.
16.b. The client will demonstrate accuracy in counting pulse.	16.b.1. Teach client how to count his/her pulse, being alert to the regularity of the rhythm. 2. Allow time for return demonstration and accuracy check.
16.c. The client will identify modifiable cardiovascular risk factors and ways to reduce these factors.	16.c.1. Inform client that the following modifiable factors have been shown to contribute to heart disease: a. obesity b. diet high in saturated fat and cholesterol c. sedentary life style d. smoking e. heavy alcohol intake (more than 2 ounces of ethanol/day on a regular basis) f. hypertension g. stressful life style. 2. Assist the client to identify ways he/she can make appropriate changes in life style to reduce the above factors. Provide information about weight reduction plans; stress management classes; and cardiovascular fitness, stop smoking, and alcohol rehabilitation programs. Initiate a referral if indicated. 3. Instruct client to take antihyperlipidemic medications (e.g. clofibrate, nicotinic acid, cholestyramine, probucol) and antiplatelet agents (e.g. sulfinpyrazone, aspirin, dipyridamole) as prescribed.
16.d. The client will verbalize an understanding of the rationale for and constituents of a diet low in sodium, saturated fat, and cholesterol.	16.d.1. Explain the rationale for a diet low in sodium, saturated fat, and cholesterol. 2. Provide the following information *about decreasing sodium intake* (recommended restriction is usually 2 gm sodium [5 gm salt]/day): a. be aware that the terms salt and sodium are often used interchangeably but are not synonymous; there is 40% sodium in table salt b. read food labels and calculate sodium content of items (often expressed in milligrams [2 gm is 2000 mg])

      c. do not add salt when cooking foods or to prepared foods

      d. avoid foods/fluids and additives high in sodium (e.g. baking soda, tomato juice, bouillon, meat tenderizer, processed meats and cheeses, sauerkraut, catsup, canned soups and vegetables, salty snacks)

      e. reduce sodium content in vegetables and meats by boiling, discarding the water, adding fresh water, and reboiling.

   3. Provide the following instructions on ways *to reduce intake of saturated fat and cholesterol:*

      a. decrease intake of foods high in saturated fat and cholesterol (e.g. butter, cheese, ice cream, egg yolks, shrimp, cashew nuts, organ meats)

      b. avoid fried foods

      c. trim fat off meats and remove all poultry skin.

   4. If physician has recommended a diet high in fiber, explain that soluble fiber is believed by some to reduce the progression of atherosclerosis. Provide a list of foods high in soluble fiber (e.g. oat bran, most fruits and vegetables, dried peas and beans).

   5. Obtain a dietary consult to assist client in planning meals that will meet the prescribed limitations of sodium, saturated fat, and cholesterol.

16.e. The client will verbalize an understanding of medication therapy including rationale for, side effects of, schedule for taking, and importance of taking as prescribed.

16.e.1. Explain the rationale for, side effects of, and importance of taking the medications prescribed.

   2. If client is discharged on nitroglycerin, instruct to:

      a. avoid alcohol when using nitroglycerin (*both cause vasodilation and may precipitate severe hypotension when used concurrently*)

      b. have tablets readily available at all times

      c. take a tablet before strenuous activity and in emotionally stressful situations

      d. take one tablet when chest pain occurs and another every 5 minutes up to a total of 3 times if necessary; notify physician if pain persists

      e. place tablets under tongue and allow them to dissolve thoroughly before swallowing

      f. store tablets in a cool place in a light-resistant, airtight bottle or stainless steel container and replace tablets every 6 months; when opening bottle for initial use, remove cotton plug and do not replace it

      g. avoid rising to a standing position quickly after taking nitroglycerin *in order to reduce dizziness associated with its vasodilatory effect*

      h. recognize that dizziness, flushing, and mild headache may occur after taking nitroglycerin; instruct client to notify physician if severe headache or fainting occurs

      i. if nitroglycerin skin patches are prescribed:

        1. provide instructions about correct application, skin care, need to rotate sites, and frequency of change

        2. caution client that activities that increase blood flow to the skin (e.g. exercise, hot bath, sauna) can cause a sudden reduction in blood pressure.

   3. If client is discharged on a digitalis preparation, instruct to:

      a. take pulse before taking digitalis (should be a resting pulse rate taken at least 5 minutes after any activity); consult physician before taking medication if pulse rate is more irregular than usual or below 60 or above 120 beats/minute

      b. avoid altering dosage or trying to make up for missed doses

      c. promptly report a loss of usual appetite, nausea, vomiting, headache, diarrhea, muscle weakness, and visual disturbances.

   4. If client is discharged on a beta-adrenergic blocking agent (e.g. propranolol, metoprolol, timolol, atenolol, nadolol, pindolol) instruct to:

      a. take the medication on a regular basis and consistently either before or after meals *to minimize variations in absorption*

      b. check pulse before taking medication; consult physician before taking medication if pulse rate is more irregular or below 60 beats/minute

      c. avoid skipping doses, altering the prescribed dose, trying to make up for missed doses, and discontinuing medication without physician's permission

      d. change from a lying to a sitting or standing position slowly *in order to prevent dizziness*

    e. avoid prolonged standing *to reduce pooling of blood in legs*

    f. avoid alcohol intake or drink moderately (less than 2 ounces of ethanol/day).

5. If client is discharged on a calcium-channel blocker (e.g. nifedipine, verapamil, diltiazem), instruct to:

    a. avoid skipping doses, altering the prescribed dose, or discontinuing medication without physician's permission

    b. change from a lying to a sitting or standing position slowly *in order to prevent dizziness*

    c. keep a record of the need for nitroglycerin while on calcium-channel blocker; report an increasing need for nitroglycerin

    d. keep medication in a cool place in an airtight, light-resistant container.

6. Instruct the client to consult physician before taking other prescription and nonprescription medications.

7. Instruct client to inform all health care providers of medications being taken.

16.f. The client will verbalize an understanding of activity restrictions and the rate at which activity can be progressed.	16.f.1. Reinforce physician's instructions about activity limitations. Instruct client to:

    a. gradually rebuild activity tolerance by adhering to the planned exercise program (often begins with a walking program)

    b. take frequent rest periods for about 4–8 weeks after discharge

    c. avoid physical conditioning programs such as jogging and aerobic dancing until advised by physician

    d. avoid static or isometric exercises such as weight lifting or hand gripping

    e. stop any activity that causes chest pain, shortness of breath, palpitations, dizziness, or extreme fatigue or weakness

    f. keep appointment for stress testing if planned

    g. begin cardiovascular fitness program when approved by physician.

2. Reinforce instructions regarding sexual activity:

    a. sexual activity with usual partner can be resumed after the prescribed length of time (many physicians consider a client ready to resume sexual activity when he/she is able to climb 2 flights of stairs briskly without dyspnea or angina)

    b. assume usual position for intercourse and experiment with ones that may reduce exertion (e.g. side-lying, partner on top)

    c. a new sexual relationship can be started but may result in greater energy expenditure until it becomes a more familiar or usual experience

    d. take nitroglycerin before sexual activity *in order to prevent angina*

    e. rest before and after sexual activity

    f. wait 2–3 hours after a heavy meal or alcohol consumption before engaging in sexual activity

    g. avoid sexual activity when fatigued or stressed

    h. avoid anal intercourse *(may cause a vasovagal response)*

    i. engage in foreplay before intercourse *because it causes a gradual increase in heart rate.*

16.g. The client will state signs and symptoms to report to the health care provider.	16.g. Instruct the client to report:

1. chest pain unrelieved by nitroglycerin
2. shortness of breath
3. significant weight gain or swelling of extremities
4. irregular pulse or a significant unexpected change in the pulse rate
5. persistent impotence or decreased libido
6. signs and symptoms of digitalis toxicity (see action e.3.c in this diagnosis).

16.h. The client will identify community resources that can assist with cardiac rehabilitation and adjustment to the effects of a myocardial infarction.	16.h.1. Provide information on community resources and support groups that can assist client with cardiac rehabilitation and adjustment to the effects of MI (e.g. American Heart Association, YMCA, "coronary clubs," counseling services).

2. Initiate a referral if indicated.

UNIT VII

16.i. The client will verbalize an understanding of and a plan for adhering to recommended follow-up care including future appointments with health care provider.

16.i.1. Reinforce the importance of keeping follow-up appointments with health care provider.
2. Implement measures *to improve client compliance:*
   a. include significant others in teaching sessions if possible
   b. encourage questions and allow time for reinforcement or clarification of information provided
   c. provide written instructions on future appointments with health care provider, dietary modifications, activity progression, medications prescribed, and signs and symptoms to report.

Reference

Kübler-Ross, E. On death and dying. New York: Macmillan, 1969.

Pacemaker Insertion

A pacemaker is an electrical device used to stimulate the heart to beat regularly when a person has symptomatic SA-AV node conduction disturbances. Pacemakers are implanted to treat bradyarrhythmias, particularly complete heart block, and certain tachyarrhythmias that have been refractory to medical therapy and are resulting in diminished cardiac output.

Pacemakers are either temporary or permanent. Temporary pacemakers are used in emergency situations to regulate the heart rate. They are implanted via a transvenous or transthoracic approach and regulated by an external pacemaker device.

Permanent pacemakers are utilized for long-term management of certain arrhythmias. There are a number of permanent programmable pacemakers available. They are described by a 3-letter-code nomenclature system sanctioned by the Intersociety Commission for Heart Disease (ICHD). The code specifies the chamber being paced, the chamber being sensed, and the pacemaker response to the stimulus. Insertion of a permanent pacemaker is most commonly performed under local anesthesia using a transvenous approach. The electrodes are usually placed in the right ventricle but can also be placed in the right atrium or in both locations. The pulse generator is then implanted in a subcutaneous pouch in the chest or abdomen. There are two basic modes of pacing, demand and asynchronous or fixed rate. The majority of pacemakers implanted today are demand pacemakers that are triggered only when the client's heart rate drops below a preset level. Most pacemakers inserted at this time have lithium batteries that last 6–10 years. Recent advances in pacemaker technology, however, have resulted in the development of pacemakers that can be reprogrammed and recharged externally and nuclear-powered ones that have a life span of 15–20 years.

This care plan focuses on the adult client hospitalized for a transvenous insertion of a permanent demand pacemaker under local anesthesia. Preoperative goals of care are to maintain adequate cardiac output and assist the client to adjust psychologically to the idea of having a permanent pacemaker. Postoperatively, the goals of care are to maintain comfort, prevent complications, and educate the client regarding follow-up care.

DISCHARGE CRITERIA

Prior to discharge, the client will:

- verbalize a basic understanding of the rationale for and function of a permanent pacemaker
- demonstrate accuracy in counting pulse

- demonstrate the ability to correctly perform range of motion exercises of arm and shoulder on the side of pacemaker insertion
- identify appropriate safety precautions associated with having a permanent pacemaker
- state signs and symptoms to report to the health care provider
- verbalize an understanding of and a plan for adhering to recommended follow-up care including future appointments with health care provider, medications prescribed, wound care, and activity restrictions.

NURSING/COLLABORATIVE DIAGNOSES

Preoperative
1. Anxiety □ *381*
2. Decreased cardiac output □ *382*

Postoperative
1. Potential complications:
   a. pacemaker malfunction (e.g. failure to capture, fire, or sense; runaway pacer)
   b. frozen shoulder syndrome □ *383*
2. Knowledge deficit regarding follow-up care □ *385*

Preoperative

Use in conjunction with the Standardized Preoperative Care Plan.

---

1. NURSING DIAGNOSIS

Anxiety related to unfamiliar environment, lack of understanding of surgical procedure, anticipated postoperative discomfort, possibility of pacemaker malfunction, and possible changes in life style as a result of having a pacemaker.

DESIRED OUTCOMES	NURSING ACTIONS AND *SELECTED RATIONALES*
1. The client will experience a reduction in fear and anxiety as evidenced by:	1.a. Refer to Standardized Preoperative Care Plan, Nursing Diagnosis 1, for measures related to assessment and reduction of fear and anxiety. b. Implement additional measures *to reduce fear and anxiety:*

a. verbalization of feeling less anxious or fearful
b. relaxed facial expression and body movements
c. stable vital signs
d. usual skin color
e. verbalization of an understanding of the planned surgical procedure
f. verbalization of an understanding that pacemakers are safe and that postoperative activity restrictions will be minimal.

1. explain rationale for and basic function of a pacemaker
2. inform client that pacemakers are electrically safe and will not be harmed by usual daily activities except contact sports
3. inform client of the expected life span of the particular pacemaker he/she is to have implanted; depending on the kind to be implanted, explain that only the generator will need to be replaced when the battery gets weak or that it can be recharged externally
4. discuss the client's concerns regarding whether his/her occupation and/or hobbies can be done safely with a pacemaker in place; if the occupation or interests involve contact with high-voltage electrical equipment, electrical cautery, diathermy, running automobile engines, or radar equipment, instruct him/her to consult physician about the safety of continuing these activities.

2. NURSING DIAGNOSIS

Decreased cardiac output related to the existing arrhythmia.

DESIRED OUTCOMES	NURSING ACTIONS AND *SELECTED RATIONALES*

2. The client will maintain adequate cardiac output as evidenced by:
   a. systolic B/P of at least 80 mm Hg
   b. palpable peripheral pulses
   c. no increase in number or duration of syncopal episodes
   d. usual mental status
   e. absence of cyanosis
   f. urine output at least 30 cc/hour.

2.a. Assess client upon admission for baseline data regarding status of cardiac output. Expect that many of the following signs and symptoms of low cardiac output will be present:
   1. B/P less than 110/70 or below normal for client
   2. irregular pulse
   3. pulse rate less than 60 or greater than 100 beats/minute
   4. muffled heart sounds
   5. presence of an S_3 and/or S_4 gallop rhythm
   6. decline in systolic B/P of at least 15 mm Hg with a concurrent rise in pulse when client sits up
   7. rapid, labored, or irregular respirations
   8. crackles and diminished or absent breath sounds
   9. restlessness, confusion
   10. lightheadedness, syncope
   11. diminished peripheral pulses
   12. decreased amplitude of carotid pulse
   13. cool, pale, or mottled skin
   14. capillary refill time greater than 3 seconds
   15. increased CVP (use internal jugular vein pulsation method to estimate CVP)
   16. increased BUN and serum creatinine and alkaline phosphatase levels
   17. chest x-ray findings of cardiomegaly, pleural effusion, or pulmonary edema.
b. Monitor EKG readings and report worsening of or additional arrhythmias.
c. Reassess cardiac status frequently and report the following signs and symptoms that may indicate the need for emergency pacemaker insertion:
   1. systolic B/P below 80 mm Hg
   2. absent peripheral pulses
   3. prolonged or increased frequency of syncopal episodes
   4. persistent decline in mental status
   5. cyanosis
   6. urine output less than 30 cc/hour.

d. Implement measures *to maintain an adequate cardiac output before surgery:*
1. perform actions *to reduce cardiac workload:*
   a. maintain activity restrictions as ordered
   b. place client in a semi- to high Fowler's position
   c. instruct client to avoid activities that create a Valsalva response (e.g. straining to have a bowel movement, bending at the waist, holding breath while moving)
   d. promote physical and emotional rest
   e. maintain oxygen therapy as ordered
   f. discourage smoking *(smoking has a cardiostimulatory effect, causes vasoconstriction, and reduces oxygen availability)*
   g. provide frequent, small meals rather than 3 large ones *(large meals require an increased blood supply to the gastrointestinal tract for digestion)*
   h. discourage intake of foods/fluids high in caffeine such as coffee, tea, chocolate, and colas *(caffeine is a myocardial stimulant and increases myocardial oxygen consumption)*
2. monitor for therapeutic and nontherapeutic effects of the following medications if administered:
   a. antiarrhythmics (e.g. propranolol, procainamide, disopyramide, quinidine, phenytoin, lidocaine, bretylium) *to treat tachyarrhythmias*
   b. anticholinergic agents (e.g. atropine) or sympathomimetics (e.g. ephedrine, isoproterenol) *to increase heart rate*
3. notify physician if serum potassium level is abnormal *(abnormal potassium levels affect myocardial conductivity)*
4. if client is in heart block, consult physician before giving any prescribed digitalis preparations *(digitalis preparations delay AV node conductivity).*

UNIT VII

Postoperative

Use in conjunction with the Standardized Postoperative Care Plan.

---

1. COLLABORATIVE DIAGNOSIS

Potential complications:

a. **pacemaker malfunction (e.g. failure to capture, fire, or sense; runaway pacer)** related to:
   1. faulty equipment or contact with electrical hazards
   2. displacement or breakage of the pacemaker catheter associated with improper or excessive movement;
b. **frozen shoulder syndrome** related to restricted arm movement on the operative side.

DESIRED OUTCOMES	NURSING ACTIONS AND *SELECTED RATIONALES*

1.a. The client will experience normal pacemaker function as evidenced by:
1. regular pulse at a rate within 2–3 beats of the preset level
2. stable B/P
3. absence of fatigue, lightheadedness, dizziness, syncope, confusion, dyspnea
4. EKG readings showing pacer spikes before the QRS complex when the pulse rate falls below the preset rate.

1.a.1. Ascertain the method of pacing being used and the rate set by the physician in surgery. Use this information when assessing pacemaker function.
2. Assess for and report signs and symptoms of:
   a. pacemaker malfunction:
      1. discrepancy of more than 5 beats/minute between apical pulse rate and preset pacemaker rate
      2. significant decline in B/P
      3. unexplained fatigue
      4. lightheadedness, dizziness, syncope, confusion
      5. dyspnea
      6. EKG readings showing any of the following:
         a. absence of pacer spikes when heart rate falls below the preset level
         b. pacer spikes following normal QRS complexes at a rate higher than the preset pacemaker rate
         c. absence of QRS complex following a pacer spike
         d. presence of premature beats
   b. pacemaker catheter dislodgment or breakage:
      1. hiccups and/or contractions of the intercostal muscles (occur as a result of perforation of the ventricle and resultant pacemaker stimulation of the diaphragm and/or intercostal muscles)
      2. rapid and continual decline in B/P, narrowed pulse pressure, pulsus paradoxus, distant or muffled heart sounds, neck vein distention on inspiration, and decreased amplitude of waves on EKG (indicative of cardiac tamponade, which can result from ventricular perforation).
3. Implement measures *to prevent pacemaker malfunction:*
   a. perform actions *to provide an electrically safe environment:*
      1. do not use any equipment with a frayed cord or in any other state of disrepair
      2. make sure all electrical equipment in client's vicinity is properly grounded (e.g. use cords with three-prong plugs); note: if client has a temporary rather than permanent pacemaker, cover any metal part on the output terminal or the pacer wire with nonconductive tape and wear rubber gloves when handling exposed pacer wires
      3. do not attach client to two or more pieces of electrical equipment simultaneously unless they are on common ground
   b. perform actions *to prevent catheter dislodgment and breakage:*
      1. maintain activity restrictions as ordered *to allow fibrosis to begin to form around the electrode*
      2. instruct client to limit movement of the arm and shoulder on the side of pacemaker insertion for the first 72 hours after surgery
      3. instruct client to avoid coughing and report any nausea; consult physician about order for antitussive and antiemetic *to prevent coughing and vomiting (both activities may dislodge the electrode).*
4. If signs and symptoms of pacemaker malfunction or dislodgment occur:
   a. turn client onto left side *(helps achieve placement of the electrode against the ventricle wall)*
   b. follow manufacturer's suggestions for problem-solving (e.g. place a magnet over the pacemaker site to convert a demand pacer to a fixed rate, then recheck the pulse rate and EKG reading); report results. Note: if client has a temporary rather than a permanent pacemaker, check and adjust sensitivity dial, EKG lead position, external pacemaker connections, and battery function as indicated
   c. prepare client for surgical repair or replacement of pacemaker if indicated
   d. provide emotional support to client and significant others.

1.b. The client will not develop a frozen shoulder as evidenced by the ability to

1.b.1. Instruct and assist client with gentle, full range of motion exercises of arm and shoulder on operative side as soon as allowed (usually by 3rd postoperative day).

move arm and shoulder on the operative side through full range of motion within 72 hours after surgery.

2. Notify physician if client is unable to move arm and shoulder on operative side through full range of motion.

2. NURSING DIAGNOSIS

Knowledge deficit regarding follow-up care.

DESIRED OUTCOMES	NURSING ACTIONS AND *SELECTED RATIONALES*
2.a. The client will verbalize a basic understanding of the rationale for and function of a permanent pacemaker.	2.a.1. Reinforce preoperative teaching regarding the rationale for and basic function of a permanent pacemaker. 2. Review manufacturer's instruction manual with client and provide him/her with a copy to keep.
2.b. The client will demonstrate accuracy in counting pulse.	2.b.1. Teach the client how to count his/her pulse, being alert to the regularity of the rhythm. 2. Allow time for return demonstration and accuracy check.
2.c. The client will demonstrate the ability to correctly perform range of motion exercises of arm and shoulder on the side of pacemaker insertion.	2.c.1. Teach client range of motion exercises for arm and shoulder on the side of pacemaker insertion. Instruct client to perform range of motion exercises at least 4 times/day and to do the exercises slowly and gently *in order to prevent dislodgment of the pacemaker catheter.* 2. Allow adequate time for questions, clarification, and return demonstration.
2.d. The client will identify appropriate safety precautions associated with having a permanent pacemaker.	2.d. Instruct the client to adhere to the following safety precautions: 1. avoid participation in contact sports 2. avoid pressure on the insertion site and pulse generator (e.g. do not wear constrictive clothing or purse strap over the shoulder on operative side) 3. avoid close proximity with high-voltage electrical equipment, electrical cautery, diathermy, television or radio transmitters, radar equipment, older model microwave ovens, radiation, and magnetic force machines 4. move away from any electrical device if dizziness, lightheadedness, or decline in pulse rate occurs; caution client that some store antitheft devices may also affect pacemaker function 5. if planning to travel, obtain name of a physician and/or pacemaker clinic at point(s) of destination 6. alert airport personnel to pacemaker (the pacemaker will set off the security alarm) and request a seat away from the galley *since most meals are heated in a microwave oven* 7. always wear a Medic-Alert tag and carry a pacemaker identification card; identification card should have insertion date, model and serial number of pacemaker, type of lead placement, and rate setting 8. check pulse daily *to monitor for pacemaker malfunction* 9. have pulse generator monitored regularly as instructed at end of expected lifespan of pacemaker battery or if there is any indication that the pacemaker is not functioning properly; inform client that monitoring may be done at the physician's office, at a pacemaker clinic, or by a telephone monitoring device.

2.e. The client will state signs and symptoms to report to the health care provider.

2.e.1. Refer to Standardized Postoperative Care Plan, Nursing Diagnosis 20, action c, for signs and symptoms to report to the health care provider.
2. Instruct client to report these additional signs and symptoms:
   a. irregular pulse
   b. pulse rate increase or decrease of more than 5 beats from the preset rate
   c. unexplained fatigue
   d. lightheadedness, dizziness, fainting spell
   e. shortness of breath
   f. swelling of extremities
   g. persistent and unexplained weight gain
   h. chest pain.

2.f. The client will verbalize an understanding of and a plan for adhering to recommended follow-up care including future appointments with health care provider, medications prescribed, wound care, and activity restrictions.

2.f.1. Refer to Standardized Postoperative Care Plan, Nursing Diagnosis 20, for routine postoperative instructions and measures to improve client compliance.
2. Instruct client to progress activity as tolerated.
3. Instruct client to limit vigorous movement and stress on arms and shoulders for first 6 weeks after surgery.
4. Instruct client to inform health care providers of pacemaker insertion so prophylactic anti-infectives may be started before any dental work, invasive diagnostic procedures, or surgery.

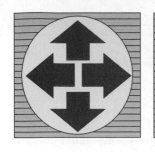
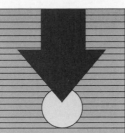
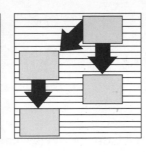
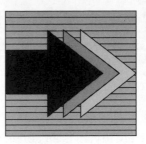
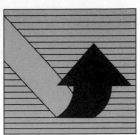

Unit VIII

Nursing Care of the Client with Disturbances of Peripheral Vascular Function

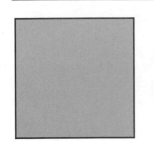

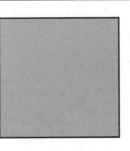
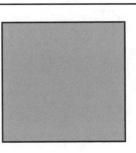
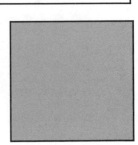

Abdominal Aortic Aneurysm Repair

An abdominal aortic aneurysm is an abnormal dilation of the arterial wall and is usually located between the renal arteries and iliac branches of the aorta. Aneurysms can be classified according to gross appearance (i.e. fusiform, saccular), etiology (e.g. mycotic, hypertensive), and location (e.g. femoral, abdominal aortic). Aneurysm formation is most often associated with atherosclerosis and hypertension but may also result from trauma, congenital vascular disease, cystic medionecrosis, syphilis, and infection. Surgical resection of the dilated area and replacement with a prosthetic graft is the most effective treatment of an aneurysm that is 5–6 cm or larger or is symptomatic.

This care plan focuses on the adult client hospitalized for elective surgical repair of an abdominal aortic aneurysm. Preoperatively, goals of care are to reduce fear and anxiety and decrease the risk of aneurysm rupture. The goals of postoperative care are to maintain comfort, prevent complications, and educate the client regarding follow-up care.

DISCHARGE CRITERIA

Prior to discharge, the client will:

- identify modifiable cardiovascular risk factors and ways to reduce these factors
- state signs and symptoms of complications to report to the health care provider
- verbalize an understanding of and a plan for adhering to recommended follow-up care including future appointments with health care provider, medications prescribed, activity level, and wound care.

NURSING/COLLABORATIVE DIAGNOSES

Preoperative
1. Anxiety □ 389
2. Potential complications:
   a. hypovolemic shock
   b. distal embolization □ 389
Postoperative
1. Altered fluid and electrolyte balance:
   a. third-spacing of fluid
   b. fluid volume excess or water intoxication
   c. fluid volume deficit, hyponatremia, hypokalemia, hypochloremia, and metabolic alkalosis □ 391
2. Potential complications:
   a. hypovolemic shock
   b. lower extremity embolization
   c. bowel ischemia
   d. impaired renal function and spinal cord ischemia □ 392
3. Sexual dysfunction:
   a. decreased libido
   b. impotence □ 394
4. Knowledge deficit regarding follow-up care □ 395

Preoperative

Use in conjunction with the Standardized Preoperative Care Plan.

1. NURSING DIAGNOSIS

Anxiety related to unfamiliar environment; lack of understanding of diagnosis, diagnostic tests, and preoperative and postoperative procedures; effects of anesthesia; anticipated postoperative discomfort; possible loss of sexual functioning; and risk of death.

DESIRED OUTCOMES	NURSING ACTIONS AND *SELECTED RATIONALES*

1. The client will experience a reduction in fear and anxiety (see Standardized Preoperative Care Plan, Nursing Diagnosis 1, for outcome criteria).	1.a. Refer to Standardized Preoperative Care Plan, Nursing Diagnosis 1, for measures related to the assessment and reduction of fear and anxiety.
	b. Implement additional measures *to reduce preoperative fear and anxiety:*
	  1. explain all diagnostic tests (e.g. chest and abdominal x-rays, blood tests, ultrasonography, angiography, computed tomography)
	  2. orient to intensive care unit if appropriate
	  3. describe and explain the rationale for equipment such as cardiac monitor, respirator, intravenous and intra-arterial lines, Doppler flowmeter, nasogastric tube, and urinary catheter
	  4. explain that B/P may be taken in both arms and thighs *in order to better evaluate systemic circulatory status*
	  5. establish an alternative method of communicating with client (e.g. paper and pencil, magic slate) if he/she is expected to be on a respirator postoperatively
	  6. reinforce physician's explanations and clarify misconceptions client may have about effects of the surgery on sexual functioning (e.g. impotence).

2. COLLABORATIVE DIAGNOSIS

Potential complications:

a. **hypovolemic shock** related to excessive blood loss associated with rupture of the aneurysm;

b. **distal embolization** related to mobilization of a thrombus from the affected artery.

DESIRED OUTCOMES	NURSING ACTIONS AND *SELECTED RATIONALES*
2.a. The client will not develop hypovolemic shock as evidenced by:	2.a.1. Assess for and immediately report signs and symptoms of conditions that indicate impending aneurysm rupture: a. leaking aneurysm:

UNIT
VIII

1. usual mental status
2. stable vital signs
3. skin warm and usual color
4. palpable peripheral pulses
5. capillary refill time less than 3 seconds
6. urine output at least 30 cc/hour.

1. increasing abdominal girth
2. hematoma of scrotum, perineum, or penis
3. frank or occult gastrointestinal bleeding
4. declining RBC, Hct., and Hgb. levels
5. new or increased complaints of lumbar, pelvic, or groin pain *(accumulation of blood causes irritation of and pressure on the tissues and nerves)*
6. diminishing peripheral pulses
7. further decline in thigh B/P as compared with B/P in arm (in clients with abdominal aortic aneurysms, thigh B/P is usually slightly lower than B/P in arms)

  b. expanding aneurysm:
1. new or increased complaints of lumbar, flank, or groin pain *(results from pressure on lumbar nerves)*
2. increased size of pulsating mass in abdomen
3. increasing sense of fullness, nausea, or vomiting *(results from pressure on duodenum or mesenteric nerve root)*
4. decreasing motor and sensory function of lower extremities *(results from pressure on lumbar, sacral, or femoral nerves).*

2. Assess for and report signs and symptoms of hypovolemic shock:
  a. restlessness, agitation, confusion
  b. significant decrease in B/P
  c. decline in B/P of at least 15 mm Hg with concurrent rise in pulse when client changes from lying to sitting or standing position
  d. resting pulse rate greater than 100 beats/minute
  e. rapid or labored respirations
  f. cool, pale, or cyanotic skin
  g. diminished or absent peripheral pulses
  h. capillary refill time greater than 3 seconds
  i. urine output less than 30 cc/hour.

3. Implement measures *to decrease risk of aneurysm rupture:*
  a. instruct client to avoid elevating legs when in bed, using knee gatch, sitting for prolonged periods, and crossing legs *in order to prevent restriction of peripheral blood flow and increased pressure on aneurysm site*
  b. perform actions *to prevent a generalized increase in blood pressure:*
    1. limit client's activity as ordered
    2. instruct client to avoid activities that create a Valsalva response (e.g. straining to have a bowel movement, bending at the waist, holding breath while moving, lifting heavy objects)
    3. implement measures to reduce fear and anxiety (see Preoperative Nursing Diagnosis 1)
  c. monitor for therapeutic and nontherapeutic effects of diuretics and antihypertensives if administered *to reduce blood volume and/or vascular pressure in the dilated vessel.*

4. If signs and symptoms of hypovolemic shock occur:
  a. place client flat in bed unless contraindicated
  b. monitor vital signs frequently
  c. administer oxygen as ordered
  d. monitor for therapeutic and nontherapeutic effects of the following if administered:
    1. blood products and/or volume expanders (these need to be used with caution *since increased vascular pressure can extend a tear at site of rupture)*
    2. vasopressors (may be administered for a short time *to maintain arterial pressure)*
  e. assist with insertion of Swan-Ganz catheter, intra-aortic balloon pump, and central venous catheter if indicated
  f. prepare client for emergency surgical repair of aneurysm if indicated
  g. provide emotional support to client and significant others.

2.b. The client will not experience distal embolization as evidenced by:

2.b.1. Assess for and report signs and symptoms of distal embolization (e.g. diminished or absent peripheral pulses; cool, pale, or mottled extremities; colicky or diffuse abdominal pain; new or increased lumbar, groin, or leg pain).

1. palpable peripheral pulses
2. usual warmth and color of extremities
3. absence of or no increase in abdominal, lumbar, groin, or leg pain.

2. Implement measures to decrease B/P (see actions a.3.b and c in this diagnosis) *in order to reduce risk of embolization.*
3. If signs and symptoms of distal embolization occur:
   a. continue with above measures to decrease B/P
   b. maintain client on strict bedrest
   c. prepare client for embolectomy if indicated
   d. provide emotional support to client and significant others.

Postoperative

Use in conjunction with the Standardized Postoperative Care Plan.

1. NURSING/COLLABORATIVE DIAGNOSIS

Altered fluid and electrolyte balance:

a. **third-spacing of fluid** related to increased permeability of the inflamed mesenteric and peritoneal vessels with major abdominal surgery (occurs during first 24–36 hours after surgery);
b. **fluid volume excess or water intoxication** related to:
   1. vigorous fluid replacement
   2. increased production of antidiuretic hormone (ADH) and aldosterone (output of these hormones is stimulated by trauma, pain, anesthetic agents, and narcotic analgesics)
   3. reabsorption of third-space fluid (occurs about the 3rd postoperative day)
   4. fluid retention associated with renal insufficiency due to inadequate blood flow to the kidneys during surgery;
c. **fluid volume deficit, hyponatremia, hypokalemia, hypochloremia, and metabolic alkalosis** related to excessive loss of fluid and electrolytes associated with vomiting and nasogastric tube drainage.

DESIRED OUTCOMES	NURSING ACTIONS AND *SELECTED RATIONALES*
1.a. The client will experience resolution of third-spacing within expected time postoperatively as evidenced by: 1. absence of peripheral edema and ascites 2. unlabored respirations between 16–20/minute 3. normal breath sounds 4. usual mental status 5. B/P and pulse within normal range for client and stable with position change.	1.a.1. Assess for and report signs and symptoms of third-spacing: a. peripheral edema b. ascites c. dyspnea, orthopnea d. crackles and diminished or absent breath sounds e. change in mental status f. decline in systolic B/P of at least 15 mm Hg with a concurrent rise in pulse when client changes from lying to sitting position. 2. Monitor for therapeutic and nontherapeutic effects of salt-poor albumin infusions if administered *to promote mobilization of fluid back into the vascular space and reduce further third-spacing by increasing colloid osmotic pressure.* 3. Consult physician if signs and symptoms of third-spacing worsen or fail to resolve within expected length of time (reabsorption usually begins on 3rd postoperative day).

UNIT
VIII

1.b. The client will not experience fluid volume excess or water intoxication (see Standardized Postoperative Care Plan, Nursing Diagnosis 5, outcome b, for outcome criteria).

1.b. Refer to Standardized Postoperative Care Plan, Nursing Diagnosis 5, action b, for measures related to assessment, prevention, and treatment of fluid volume excess and water intoxication.

1.c. The client will maintain fluid and electrolyte balance (see Standardized Postoperative Care Plan, Nursing Diagnosis 5, outcome a, for outcome criteria).

1.c. Refer to Standardized Postoperative Care Plan, Nursing Diagnosis 5, action a, for measures related to assessment, prevention, and treatment of fluid and electrolyte imbalance.

☐ ▬▬▬▬▬▬▬▬▬▬▬▬▬▬▬▬▬▬▬▬▬▬▬▬

2. COLLABORATIVE DIAGNOSIS

Potential complications:

a. **hypovolemic shock** related to blood loss during surgery, third-space fluid shift, vomiting, nasogastric tube drainage, inadequate fluid replacement, and hemorrhage associated with graft separation;
b. **lower extremity embolization** related to dislodgment of necrotic debris or clot from surgical site;
c. **bowel ischemia** related to diminished blood supply to bowel associated with ligation of the mesenteric and hypogastric arteries during surgery, hypovolemia, and embolization;
d. **impaired renal function and spinal cord ischemia** related to insufficient blood flow to these areas associated with hypovolemia, prolonged aortic clamp time, and embolization.

☐ ▬▬▬▬▬▬▬▬▬▬▬▬▬▬▬▬▬▬▬▬▬▬▬▬

DESIRED OUTCOMES	NURSING ACTIONS AND *SELECTED RATIONALES*

2.a. The client will not develop hypovolemic shock (see Standardized Postoperative Care Plan, Collaborative Diagnosis 19, outcome a, for outcome criteria).

2.a.1. Assess for and report signs and symptoms of leakage at graft site:
 a. new or expanding hematoma of incision site, scrotum, perineum, or penis
 b. increased abdominal girth
 c. new or increased complaints of lumbar, pelvic, or groin pain
 d. increasing feeling of abdominal or gastric fullness unrelated to oral intake
 e. diminishing or absent peripheral pulses
 f. decreased motor and sensory function in lower extremities
 g. declining B/P, increasing pulse
 h. decreasing RBC, Hct., and Hgb. values.
 2. Assess for and report signs and symptoms of hypovolemic shock (see Standardized Postoperative Care Plan, Collaborative Diagnosis 19, action a.3).
 3. Implement measures *to prevent hypovolemic shock:*
 a. perform actions *to prevent and treat hypovolemia:*
 1. implement measures to prevent vomiting (see Standardized Postoperative Care Plan, Nursing Diagnosis 7.C, action 2)
 2. provide maximum fluid intake allowed (a fluid restriction is often

ordered *to prevent fluid overload and reduce pressure in the surgical area)*
3. administer blood and/or volume expanders as ordered
4. monitor for therapeutic and nontherapeutic effects of salt-poor albumin infusions if administered *to promote mobilization of fluid back into the vascular space and reduce further third-spacing by increasing colloid osmotic pressure*

b. perform actions *to reduce stress on graft site in order to prevent graft separation:*
1. instruct client to avoid positions that compromise peripheral blood flow (e.g. elevating legs when in bed, use of knee gatch, sitting for prolonged periods, crossing legs)
2. implement measures to reduce accumulation of gastrointestinal gas and fluid, prevent nausea and vomiting, and prevent or control hiccoughs (see Standardized Postoperative Care Plan, Nursing Diagnoses 7.B, action 3; 7.C, action 2; and 7.D)
3. implement measures to prevent fluid volume excess and water intoxication (see Standardized Postoperative Care Plan, Nursing Diagnosis 5, action b.3)
4. instruct client to avoid activities that create a Valsalva response (e.g. straining to have a bowel movement, bending at the waist, holding breath while moving)
5. instruct client to avoid vigorous coughing; consult physician about an order for an antitussive if indicated
6. monitor for therapeutic and nontherapeutic effects of diuretics and antihypertensives if administered *to reduce blood volume and/or vascular resistance.*

4. If signs and symptoms of hypovolemic shock occur:
a. place client flat in bed unless contraindicated
b. monitor vital signs frequently
c. administer oxygen as ordered
d. monitor for therapeutic and nontherapeutic effects of blood products and/or volume expanders if administered (these need to be used with caution if graft separation is suspected)
e. prepare client for surgical repair of the graft if indicated
f. provide emotional support to client and significant others.

2.b. The client will not experience lower extremity embolization as evidenced by: 1. palpable peripheral pulses 2. usual warmth and color of extremities.	**2.b.1.** Assess for and report signs and symptoms of lower extremity embolization: a. diminishing or absent femoral, popliteal, posterior tibial, or dorsalis pedis pulses (there may be a brief absence of pulses after surgery *due to vasospasm or hypothermia)* b. cool, pale, or mottled extremities. 2. Implement measures *to reduce risk of lower extremity embolization:* a. limit client's activity as ordered b. instruct client to avoid activities that create a Valsalva response (e.g. straining to have a bowel movement, bending at the waist, holding breath while moving) *in order to prevent dislodgment of clot.* 3. If signs and symptoms of lower extremity embolization occur, prepare client for embolectomy if indicated.
2.c. The client will not develop bowel ischemia as evidenced by: 1. absence of blood in stools 2. absence of diarrhea 3. absence of colicky or diffuse abdominal pain 4. soft, nontender abdomen.	**2.c.1.** Assess bowel sounds. Report bowel sounds that fail to return to normal within expected length of time. 2. Assess for and report signs and symptoms of bowel ischemia (e.g. blood in stools, diarrhea, complaints of colicky or diffuse abdominal pain, distended abdomen). 3. Monitor WBC count. Report values of 20,000 to 30,000/mm³ *(this could indicate bowel necrosis or gangrene).* 4. Implement measures to prevent hypovolemic shock (see action a.3 in this diagnosis) *in order to maintain adequate blood supply to the bowel.* 5. If signs and symptoms of bowel ischemia occur: a. monitor for therapeutic and nontherapeutic effects of anti-infectives if administered b. prepare client for bowel resection with anastomosis or colostomy if extensive bowel tissue necrosis or gangrenous patches are present c. provide emotional support to client and significant others.

UNIT
VIII

2.d. The client will maintain adequate renal function as evidenced by:
1. urine output at least 30 cc/hour
2. urine specific gravity between 1.010–1.030
3. BUN and serum creatinine levels within normal range.

2.d.1. Assess for and report signs and symptoms of impaired renal function (e.g. urine output less than 30 cc/hour, urine specific gravity fixed at or less than 1.010, elevated BUN and serum creatinine levels).
2. Collect a 24-hour urine specimen if ordered. Report decreased creatinine clearance.
3. Implement measures to prevent hypovolemic shock (see action a.3 in this diagnosis) *in order to maintain adequate renal blood flow.*
4. If signs and symptoms of impaired renal function occur:
    a. assess for and report signs of acute renal failure (e.g. oliguria or anuria; weight gain; edema; elevated B/P; lethargy and confusion; increasing BUN and serum creatinine, phosphorus, and potassium levels)
    b. prepare client for embolectomy and/or dialysis if indicated
    c. refer to Care Plan on Renal Failure for additional care measures.

2.e. The client will not develop spinal cord ischemia as evidenced by:
1. normal motor and sensory function of lower extremities
2. usual bowel and bladder function.

2.e.1. Assess for and report signs and symptoms of spinal cord ischemia (e.g. decreased motor and sensory function of lower extremities, urinary retention or incontinence, bowel incontinence).
2. Implement measures to prevent hypovolemic shock (see action a.3 in this diagnosis) *in order to maintain adequate blood supply to the spinal cord.*
3. If signs and symptoms of spinal cord ischemia occur:
    a. implement measures *to protect lower extremities from injury* (e.g. avoid use of heating pad on areas of decreased sensation)
    b. implement measures *to maintain optimal mobility* (e.g. assist client with range of motion exercises, position extremities in functional alignment)
    c. initiate and maintain bowel and bladder training programs if indicated
    d. prepare client for embolectomy if indicated
    e. provide emotional support to client and significant others
    f. refer to Care Plan on Spinal Cord Injury for additional care measures if decreased motor and sensory function persist.

□ ▐▬▬▬▬▬▬▬▬▬▬▬▬▬▬▬▬▬▬▬▬▬▬

3. NURSING DIAGNOSIS

Sexual dysfunction:

a. **decreased libido** related to operative site discomfort and fear of graft site bleeding;
b. **impotence** related to:
    1. diminished blood flow in the internal iliac arteries associated with prolonged aortic clamp time during surgery, hypovolemia, embolization, and graft occlusion
    2. damage to the inferior mesenteric plexus during surgery.

□ ▐▬▬▬▬▬▬▬▬▬▬▬▬▬▬▬▬▬▬▬▬▬▬

DESIRED OUTCOMES	NURSING ACTIONS AND *SELECTED RATIONALES*

3. The client will demonstrate beginning acceptance of changes in sexual functioning as evidenced by:
a. verbalization of a perception of self as sexually acceptable and adequate

3.a. Assess for signs and symptoms of sexual dysfunction (e.g. verbalization of sexual concerns, failure to maintain relationships with significant others).
b. Determine client's attitudes, knowledge, and concerns about possible effects of the surgery on sexual functioning and activities.
c. Communicate interest, understanding, and respect for the values of client and his/her partner.
d. Provide accurate information about effects of the surgery on sexual functioning. Encourage questions and clarify misconceptions.

b. maintenance of relationships with significant others.

e. Facilitate communication between the client and his/her partner. Assist them to identify issues that may affect their sexual relationship.

f. Arrange for uninterrupted privacy during hospital stay if desired by the couple.

g. If client is concerned that operative site discomfort will interfere with usual sexual activity:
   1. assure him/her that the discomfort is temporary and will diminish as incision heals
   2. encourage alternatives to intercourse or use of positions that decrease pressure on the surgical site (e.g. side-lying).

h. Reinforce the physician's instructions regarding when client can resume sexual activity. Assure him/her that the suture lines and graft site will be secure.

i. If impotence is a problem:
   1. encourage client to discuss it with physician *(impotence may be due to reversible factors such as antihypertensive medications [especially beta blockers] or poorly controlled secondary health problems rather than a permanent consequence of the surgery)*
   2. suggest alternative methods of sexual gratification and use of assistive devices if appropriate
   3. discuss ways to be creative in expressing sexuality (e.g. massage, fantasies, cuddling)
   4. provide information regarding penile prosthesis if appropriate
   5. discuss alternative methods of becoming a parent (e.g. artificial insemination, adoption) if appropriate.

j. Include partner in above discussions and encourage his/her continued support of the client.

k. Consult physician if counseling appears indicated.

4. NURSING DIAGNOSIS

Knowledge deficit regarding follow-up care.

DESIRED OUTCOMES	NURSING ACTIONS AND *SELECTED RATIONALES*
4.a. The client will identify modifiable cardiovascular risk factors and ways to reduce these factors.	4.a.1. Inform the client of modifiable factors that have been shown to contribute to vascular disease: a. obesity b. diet high in saturated fat and cholesterol c. sedentary life style d. smoking e. heavy alcohol intake (more than 2 ounces of ethanol/day on a regular basis) f. stressful life style. 2. Assist the client to identify ways he/she can make appropriate changes in life style. Provide information about stress management classes and weight loss, stop smoking, cardiovascular fitness, and alcohol rehabilitation programs if appropriate. Initiate a referral if indicated.
4.b. The client will state signs and symptoms of complications to report to the health care provider.	4.b.1. Refer to Standardized Postoperative Care Plan, Nursing Diagnosis 20, action c, for signs and symptoms to report to the health care provider. 2. Instruct client to report these additional signs and symptoms: a. sudden or gradual increase in lower back, flank, groin, or operative site pain b. increased coolness or pallor of lower extremities c. increased weakness and fatigue

d. decreased movement and/or sensation in lower extremities
e. decreased urine output
f. dark brown, bloody, or persistent diarrhea
g. swelling of extremities
h. increased bruising of incision site, perineum, scrotum, or penis
i. impotence.

4.c. The client will verbalize an understanding of and a plan for adhering to recommended follow-up care including future appointments with health care provider, medications prescribed, activity level, and wound care.	4.c.1. Refer to Standardized Postoperative Care Plan, Nursing Diagnosis 20, for routine postoperative instructions and measures to improve client compliance. 2. Reinforce the physician's instructions regarding: a. need to avoid lifting objects over 10 pounds b. need to avoid participating in strenuous exercise c. importance of scheduling adequate rest periods d. need to avoid sitting for prolonged periods.

Carotid Endarterectomy

Carotid endarterectomy is the surgical removal of atherosclerotic plaque from the intima of the carotid artery. The most common site of plaque formation in the carotid artery is at the bifurcation. Access to this extracranial area is gained through an incision along the anterior sternocleidomastoid muscle. Surgery is performed to restore adequate cerebral circulation and to reduce the risk of cerebral embolization and stroke.

This care plan focuses on the adult client hospitalized for a carotid endarterectomy. Preoperatively, the goals of care are to reduce fear and anxiety and maintain adequate cerebral tissue perfusion. Postoperative goals of care are to maintain comfort, prevent complications, and educate the client regarding follow-up care.

DISCHARGE CRITERIA

Prior to discharge, the client will:

• identify ways to prevent or slow the progression of atherosclerosis
• identify ways to manage symptoms resulting from cranial nerve damage if it has occurred
• state signs and symptoms to report to the health care provider
• verbalize an understanding of and a plan for adhering to recommended follow-up care including future appointments with health care provider, medications prescribed, activity level, and wound care.

NURSING/COLLABORATIVE DIAGNOSES

Preoperative
1. Altered cerebral tissue perfusion □ 397
Postoperative
1. Potential complications:

a. cerebral ischemia
b. respiratory distress
c. cranial nerve injury (particularly the facial, hypoglossal, glosso-pharyngeal, vagus, and/or accessory nerves) □ *398*
2. Knowledge deficit regarding follow-up care □ *400*

Preoperative

Use in conjunction with the Standardized Preoperative Care Plan.

1. NURSING DIAGNOSIS

Altered cerebral tissue perfusion related to an interruption in cerebral blood flow associated with partial or complete occlusion of the carotid artery by atherosclerotic plaque or a thrombus.

DESIRED OUTCOMES	NURSING ACTIONS AND *SELECTED RATIONALES*
1. The client will maintain adequate cerebral tissue perfusion as evidenced by: a. mentally alert and oriented b. absence of dizziness, syncope, visual disturbances c. pupils equal and normally reactive to light d. normal motor and sensory function.	1.a. Assess client upon admission for baseline data regarding status of cerebral tissue perfusion. Include: 1. level of consciousness 2. presence of syncope or complaints of dizziness 3. presence of visual disturbances (e.g. blurred or dimmed vision, diplopia, hemianopsia) 4. pupillary size and reactivity 5. motor and sensory function. b. Implement measures *to maintain adequate cerebral tissue perfusion:* 1. monitor for therapeutic and nontherapeutic effects of peripheral vasodilators (e.g. cyclandelate, papaverine, isoxsuprine) if administered 2. perform actions *to reduce risk of a cerebral embolism:* a. implement measures to reduce fear and anxiety (see Standardized Preoperative Care Plan, Nursing Diagnosis 1, action d) *in order to prevent hypertension resulting from stress* b. monitor for therapeutic and nontherapeutic effects of the following medications if administered: 1. antihypertensives (these medications are usually discontinued at least 48 hours before surgery *in order to reduce risk of a critical drop in B/P during surgery*) 2. anticoagulants (e.g. warfarin, heparin) or antiplatelet agents (e.g. aspirin, dipyridamole); these medications are usually discontinued at least 48 hours before surgery *in order to reduce risk of intraoperative and postoperative hemorrhage.* c. Reassess neurological status frequently and report changes that could indicate decreasing cerebral tissue perfusion and necessitate postponement or cancellation of planned surgery (e.g. increasing agitation or lethargy,

confusion, increased episodes of syncope, blurred vision, diplopia, change in visual field, numbness and tingling of face and/or extremities, aphasia, hemiparesis, hemiplegia, seizures).

Postoperative

Use in conjunction with the Standardized Postoperative Care Plan.

1. COLLABORATIVE DIAGNOSIS

Potential complications:

a. **cerebral ischemia** related to:
   1. prolonged carotid artery clamp time during surgery and/or vasospasm from clamping and manipulation of cerebral vessels
   2. hypovolemia associated with intraoperative and/or postoperative blood loss
   3. compression of cerebral vessels due to a hematoma or edema
   4. embolization during or after surgery;
b. **respiratory distress** related to airway obstruction associated with tracheal compression (due to a hematoma and/or edema in the surgical area) and aspiration (especially if there is laryngeal or hypoglossal nerve injury);
c. **cranial nerve injury (particularly the facial, hypoglossal, glossopharyngeal, vagus, and/or accessory nerves)** related to trauma to the nerves as a result of surgery or blood accumulation and edema in the surgical area.

DESIRED OUTCOMES	NURSING ACTIONS AND *SELECTED RATIONALES*

1.a. The client will maintain adequate cerebral blood flow as evidenced by:
1. absence of dizziness, syncope, visual disturbances
2. mentally alert and oriented
3. pupils equal and normally reactive to light
4. normal motor and sensory function.
	1.a.1. Assess for and report signs and symptoms of:
	a. excessive operative site bleeding (e.g. large hematoma formation; continued bright red bleeding from incision or drain [a drain is sometimes left in for about 24 hours after surgery]; decreasing RBC, Hct., and Hgb. levels)
	b. hypovolemic shock (see Standardized Postoperative Care Plan, Collaborative Diagnosis 19, action a.3)
	c. cerebral ischemia:
	  1. dizziness, syncope
	  2. blurred or dimmed vision, diplopia, change in visual field
	  3. decreased level of consciousness
	  4. unequal pupils or a sluggish or absent pupillary reaction to light
	  5. paresthesias, motor weakness, paralysis
	  6. seizures.
	2. Implement measures *to promote adequate cerebral blood flow:*
	a. perform actions to prevent or treat hypovolemic shock (see Standardized Postoperative Care Plan, Collaborative Diagnosis 19, actions a.4 and 5)
	b. perform actions *to reduce pressure on carotid vessels:*
	  1. maintain patency of drain (e.g. keep tubing free of kinks, empty collection device as often as necessary) if present *in order to prevent hematoma formation*

   2. monitor for therapeutic and nontherapeutic effects of corticosteroids if administered *to reduce surgical site edema*
   3. instruct client to support head and neck with hands during position changes and avoid turning head abruptly or hyperextending neck *in order to reduce stress on the suture line and decrease risk of operative site bleeding*

c. keep head and neck in proper alignment
d. perform actions *to control hypertension* (e.g. maintain fluid and activity restrictions, administer antihypertensive medications) as ordered *to reduce risk of operative site bleeding and dislodgment of any existing thrombi*
e. monitor for therapeutic and nontherapeutic effects of peripheral vasodilators (e.g. cyclandelate, papaverine, isoxsuprine) if administered.

3. If signs and symptoms of cerebral ischemia occur:
   a. continue with above measures
   b. maintain client on bedrest with head of bed flat unless contraindicated
   c. monitor for and report progression of signs and symptoms
   d. initiate appropriate safety measures (e.g. side rails up, seizure precautions)
   e. provide emotional support to client and significant others
   f. refer to Care Plan on Cerebrovascular Accident for additional care measures if signs and symptoms persist.

1.b. The client will not experience respiratory distress as evidenced by:
   1. unlabored respirations at 16–20/minute
   2. absence of stridor and sternocleidomastoid muscle retraction
   3. usual skin color
   4. usual mental status
   5. blood gases within normal range.

1.b.1. Assess for and immediately report:
   a. increased edema or expanding hematoma in surgical area
   b. deviation of trachea from midline
   c. persistent or increased difficulty swallowing
   d. signs and symptoms of respiratory distress (e.g. rapid and/or labored respirations, stridor, sternocleidomastoid muscle retraction, cyanosis, restlessness, agitation)
   e. abnormal blood gases
   f. significant changes in ear oximetry and capnograph results.

2. Have tracheostomy and suction equipment readily available.
3. Implement measures *to prevent respiratory distress:*
   a. perform actions *to prevent compression of trachea:*
      1. instruct client to support head and neck with hands during position changes and avoid turning head abruptly or hyperextending neck *in order to reduce stress on the suture line and decrease risk of operative site bleeding*
      2. maintain patency of drain (e.g. keep tubing free of kinks, empty collection device as often as necessary) if present *in order to prevent hematoma formation*
      3. perform actions *to minimize edema of surgical site:*
         a. keep head of bed elevated 30° unless contraindicated
         b. apply ice bag to incisional area as ordered
      4. monitor for therapeutic and nontherapeutic effects of the following medications if administered:
         a. corticosteroids *to reduce operative site edema*
         b. antihypertensive medications *(increased B/P can cause strain on the suture line and result in bleeding and hematoma formation)*
   b. perform actions *to reduce risk of aspiration if client is having difficulty swallowing:*
      1. perform oral, pharyngeal, or tracheal suctioning if needed
      2. withhold food and fluids if gag reflex is absent or if dysphagia is severe
      3. place client in high Fowler's position during and for 30 minutes after meals and snacks unless contraindicated
      4. assist client to select foods that are easy to swallow (e.g. custards, applesauce, pureed food)
      5. reinforce techniques *to improve swallowing* (e.g. flex neck slightly, stroke throat)
      6. provide good oral care after eating *to ensure that no food particles are left in mouth.*

4. If signs and symptoms of respiratory distress occur:
   a. place client in a high Fowler's position unless contraindicated
   b. loosen neck dressing if it appears tight

    c. administer oxygen as ordered

    d. assist with bronchoscopy (may be performed if aspiration has occurred), intubation, or emergency tracheostomy if indicated

    e. prepare client for evacuation of hematoma or surgical repair of the bleeding vessel if indicated

    f. provide emotional support to client and significant others.

1.c. The client will experience beginning resolution of cranial nerve damage if it occurs as evidenced by:
1. gradual return of usual facial muscle tone, movements, and sensation
2. increased ability to chew and swallow
3. improved speech
4. return of usual shoulder movements.

1.c.1. Assess for signs and symptoms of the following:
    a. facial nerve damage (e.g. facial ptosis, loss of blink reflex on affected side, impaired sense of taste)
    b. vagus and glossopharyngeal nerve damage (e.g. difficulty swallowing, hoarseness, loss of gag reflex, inability to speak clearly, asymmetrical movement of vocal cords and soft palate when saying "ah")
    c. accessory nerve damage (e.g. unilateral shoulder sag, difficulty raising arm to horizontal position and raising shoulder against resistance)
    d. hypoglossal nerve damage (e.g. tongue biting when chewing, tongue deviation toward affected side, difficulty swallowing and speaking).

2. Monitor for therapeutic and nontherapeutic effects of corticosteroids if administered *to reduce edema in surgical area*.

3. If signs and symptoms of cranial nerve damage occur:
    a. if there is damage to the facial, hypoglossal, vagus, and/or glossopharyngeal nerves:
        1. withhold oral foods/fluids until gag reflex returns and client is better able to chew and swallow
        2. provide parenteral nutrition or tube feedings if necessary until oral intake is allowed and tolerated
        3. consult speech pathologist regarding techniques to improve swallowing and speech
        4. instruct client to add extra sweeteners or seasonings to foods if desired *in order to compensate for altered sense of taste*
        5. obtain a dietary consult to assist client to select foods/fluids that he/she likes, meet nutritional needs, and are easy to chew and swallow
        6. implement measures *to facilitate swallowing* (e.g. place client in high Fowler's position with head erect and chin tilted forward when he/she is eating or drinking, gently stroke client's throat when he/she is swallowing)
        7. implement measures *to facilitate communication* (e.g. maintain quiet environment; provide pen and pencil, magic slate, or flash cards; listen carefully when client speaks)
        8. implement measures *to prevent corneal irritation if blink reflex is decreased or absent* (e.g. instill isotonic eyedrops routinely, tape eyelid shut)
    b. if there is damage to the accessory nerve, instruct client in and assist with exercises *to prevent atrophy of trapezius and sternocleidomastoid muscles* (e.g. shoulder flexion, abduction, and external rotation; wall climbing with fingers; shoulder shrugs)
    c. provide emotional support to client and significant others; assure them that the nerve damage is usually not permanent, but caution them that the symptoms may take months to resolve.

□ ▬▬▬▬▬▬▬▬▬▬▬▬▬▬▬▬▬

2. NURSING DIAGNOSIS

Knowledge deficit regarding follow-up care.

□ ▬▬▬▬▬▬▬▬▬▬▬▬▬▬▬▬▬

DESIRED OUTCOMES	NURSING ACTIONS AND *SELECTED RATIONALES*

2.a. The client will identify ways to prevent or slow the

2.a.1. Inform the client that the following conditions contribute to atherosclerosis:

progression of
atherosclerosis.

a. obesity
b. diet high in saturated fat and cholesterol
c. sedentary life style
d. smoking
e. heavy alcohol intake (more than 2 ounces of ethanol/day on a regular basis)
f. hypertension
g. stressful life style.

2. Assist client to identify ways he/she can make appropriate changes in life style to reduce above factors. Provide information about stress management classes and cardiovascular fitness, weight loss, stop smoking, and alcohol rehabilitation programs if appropriate. Initiate a referral if indicated.

3. Provide instruction regarding diet low in saturated fat and cholesterol if indicated. Additional recommended dietary modifications may include increasing intake of foods high in soluble fiber (e.g. oat bran, most fruits and vegetables, dried peas and beans).

4. Instruct client to take antihyperlipidemic medications (e.g. clofibrate, nicotinic acid, cholestyramine, probucol) and antiplatelet agents (e.g. aspirin, sulfinpyrazone, dipyridamole) as prescribed.

2.b. The client will identify ways to manage symptoms resulting from cranial nerve damage if it has occurred.

2.b.1. If symptoms of hypoglossal, facial, vagus, and/or glossopharyngeal nerve damage are present:
a. reinforce exercises and techniques to improve swallowing and speaking ability
b. assist client in identifying foods that are both nutritious and easy to chew and swallow; obtain a dietary consult if needed
c. instruct client to increase the amount of sweeteners and seasonings he/she usually uses and/or to try different seasonings in foods or beverages if sense of taste is altered
d. stress the need to rest voice if hoarseness is present
e. demonstrate appropriate eye care (e.g. instilling isotonic eyedrops, taping eyelid shut) if blink reflex is diminished or absent.

2. If signs and symptoms of accessory nerve damage are present, reinforce exercises that should be performed to prevent shoulder muscle atrophy.

3. Allow time for questions, clarification, and return demonstration.

2.c. The client will state signs and symptoms to report to the health care provider.

2.c.1. Refer to Standardized Postoperative Care Plan, Nursing Diagnosis 20, action c, for signs and symptoms to report to the health care provider.

2. Instruct client to report these additional signs and symptoms:
a. increased swelling or purple discoloration at wound site
b. new or increased difficulty chewing and swallowing
c. double vision, blurred vision, "blind spots"
d. increased hoarseness or slurred speech
e. dizziness
f. numbness, tingling, or muscle weakness
g. increasing lethargy
h. tremors, seizures
i. failure of cranial nerve damage to resolve as expected.

2.d. The client will verbalize an understanding of and a plan for adhering to recommended follow-up care including future appointments with health care provider, medications prescribed, activity level, and wound care.

2.d. Refer to Standardized Postoperative Care Plan, Nursing Diagnosis 20, for routine postoperative instructions and measures to improve client compliance.

Femoropopliteal Bypass

Lower extremity arterial bypass is performed to treat peripheral artery insufficiency that has not responded well to conservative management. The impaired blood flow can occur as a result of acute conditions (e.g. trauma, embolization) but most often is due to atherosclerotic changes in the vessels. The femoropopliteal arterial segment is the most common site of occlusion in persons with lower extremity arterial disease, although significant narrowing of the aortoiliac, popliteal-tibial, and peroneal segments may also occur. The diseased arterial segment can be removed and replaced with a synthetic graft but the most common procedure is to bypass the segment using a synthetic or autologous graft. The saphenous vein is the preferred graft for femoropopliteal bypass because it is thick walled and has an adequate lumen diameter. Prior to grafting the saphenous vein proximal and distal to the occluded femoropopliteal arterial segment, reversal of the vein or division of its valve cusps is done to allow unimpeded arterial blood flow. Surgical intervention is indicated when intermittent claudication becomes disabling, foot pain is present at rest, or lower extremity ischemic ulcers or gangrene is present.

This care plan focuses on the adult client with atherosclerotic occlusion of the femoropopliteal arterial segment who has been hospitalized for a femoropopliteal bypass. Preoperatively, goals of care are to reduce fear and anxiety, relieve discomfort in the affected lower extremity, and reduce the risk of embolization. The goals of postoperative care are to maintain comfort, prevent complications, and educate the client regarding follow-up care.

DISCHARGE CRITERIA

Prior to discharge, the client will:

- identify ways to prevent or slow the progression of atherosclerosis
- identify ways to promote blood flow in the operative extremity
- state signs and symptoms of complications to report to the health care provider
- verbalize an understanding of and a plan for adhering to recommended follow-up care including future appointments with health care provider, medications prescribed, activity level, and wound care.

NURSING/COLLABORATIVE DIAGNOSES

Preoperative
1. Altered peripheral tissue perfusion □ *403*
2. Altered comfort:
   a. intermittent claudication and rest pain
   b. paresthesias (burning, numbness, tingling) □ *403*
3. Potential complication: distal arterial embolization □ *404*
Postoperative
1. Altered peripheral tissue perfusion □ *405*
2. Potential complications:
   a. hypovolemic shock
   b. graft occlusion
   c. compartment syndrome
   d. saphenous nerve damage □ *406*
3. Knowledge deficit regarding follow-up care □ *408*

Preoperative

Use in conjunction with the Standardized Preoperative Care Plan.

1. NURSING DIAGNOSIS

Altered peripheral tissue perfusion related to diminished blood flow in the affected lower extremity associated with atherosclerotic changes in the femoral and popliteal arteries.

DESIRED OUTCOMES	NURSING ACTIONS AND *SELECTED RATIONALES*

1. The client will not experience further reduction in blood flow in the affected lower extremity as evidenced by:
a. no increase in lower extremity discomfort
b. no further decrease in or absence of peripheral pulses
c. no increase in capillary refill time
d. usual temperature and color of extremity.
	1.a. Assess for signs and symptoms of a further reduction in blood flow in the affected lower extremity:
	  1. intermittent claudication occurring with increased intensity and/or with less activity than previously
	  2. development of or increase in intensity of rest pain (the foot and toe pain that occurs when the client is resting in a horizontal position results from decreased blood flow to the skin and subcutaneous tissue; because it occurs in the absence of lower extremity muscle activity, it reflects a severe reduction in the femoropopliteal arterial blood flow)
	  3. diminishing peripheral pulses
	  4. increase in usual capillary refill time
	  5. increased coolness and cyanosis of foot and lower leg.
	b. Implement measures *to prevent further reduction in and/or improve blood flow in the affected lower extremity:*
	  1. discourage positions that compromise blood flow in lower extremities (e.g. crossing legs, pillows under knees, use of knee gatch, elevating legs when in bed, sitting for long periods)
	  2. discourage smoking *(smoking causes vasoconstriction)*
	  3. maintain a comfortable room temperature and provide client with adequate clothing, warm socks, and blankets *(exposure to cold causes generalized vasoconstriction)*
	  4. place a bed cradle over lower extremities *to minimize pressure from bed linens*
	  5. encourage short walks and Buerger-Allen exercises as tolerated
	  6. monitor for therapeutic and nontherapeutic effects of pentoxifylline (Trental) if administered *to improve capillary blood flow.*
	c. Consult physician if signs and symptoms of further reduction in lower extremity tissue perfusion occur.

2. NURSING DIAGNOSIS

Altered comfort:*

a. **intermittent claudication and rest pain** related to diminished arterial blood flow in the affected lower extremity (ischemia results in release of anaerobic metab-

---

* In this care plan, the nursing diagnosis "pain" is included under the diagnostic label of altered comfort.

olites such as lactic acid, which irritate the muscle, skin, and subcutaneous tissue of the affected lower extremity);

b. **paresthesias (burning, numbness, tingling)** related to peripheral neuropathies (ischemia results in release of anaerobic metabolites such as lactic acid, which irritate the nerve endings of the affected lower extremity).

☐ ▬▬▬▬▬▬▬▬▬▬▬▬▬▬▬▬▬▬▬▬▬

DESIRED OUTCOMES	NURSING ACTIONS AND *SELECTED RATIONALES*

2. The client will experience diminished lower extremity discomfort as evidenced by verbalization of reduced cramping, burning, aching, numbness, and tingling of the affected lower leg, foot, and toes.	2.a. Determine how the client usually responds to discomfort.
	b. Assess for signs and symptoms of discomfort in the affected lower extremity:
	  1. intermittent claudication (e.g. complaints of cramping [usually in the calf muscle] during ambulation)
	  2. rest pain (e.g. awakening at night with complaints of severe burning or aching in foot or toes)
	  3. peripheral neuropathies (e.g. complaints of burning, numbness, and/or tingling of the lower leg or foot).
	c. Assess for factors that aggravate and alleviate discomfort.
	d. Implement measures *to reduce discomfort in the affected extremity:*
	  1. perform actions to prevent further reduction in and/or improve blood flow in the affected lower extremity (see Preoperative Nursing Diagnosis 1, action b)
	  2. perform actions *to reduce the number of episodes of intermittent claudication:*
	    a. encourage client to stop activity minutes before he/she usually experiences muscle cramping (intermittent claudication is predictable and the client is often aware of how far or how long he/she can ambulate before the discomfort begins or intensifies)
	    b. maintain client on bedrest if he/she is experiencing severe intermittent claudication *(limiting activity decreases muscle contractions in and subsequent ischemia of the affected lower extremity)*
	  3. if client is experiencing rest pain in the affected extremity, perform actions *to facilitate gravity flow of arterial blood to the ischemic area:*
	    a. allow client to sleep in a recliner with legs in a dependent position or, if in bed, to hang affected lower leg over the side of the bed
	    b. instruct client to avoid horizontal positioning and elevation of affected extremity for prolonged periods
	  4. provide or assist with nonpharmacological measures for relief of discomfort (e.g. relaxation techniques, guided imagery, quiet conversation, diversional activity)
	  5. monitor for therapeutic and nontherapeutic effects of analgesics if administered.
	e. Consult physician if above measures fail to provide adequate relief of discomfort.

☐ ▬▬▬▬▬▬▬▬▬▬▬▬▬▬▬▬▬▬▬▬▬

3. COLLABORATIVE DIAGNOSIS

Potential complication: distal arterial embolization related to mobilization of a thrombus (if present) from the atherosclerotic femoral and/or popliteal arteries.

☐ ▬▬▬▬▬▬▬▬▬▬▬▬▬▬▬▬▬▬▬▬▬

DESIRED OUTCOMES	NURSING ACTIONS AND *SELECTED RATIONALES*

3. The client will not experience distal arterial embolization of the affected extremity as evidenced by:
   a. no complaints of sudden, severe toe or foot pain
   b. no further decrease in or absence of peripheral pulses
   c. usual temperature, color, and sensation of foot.

3.a. Assess for and report signs and symptoms of distal arterial embolization of the affected extremity (e.g. sudden, severe pain in toes or foot; further decrease in or absence of peripheral pulses; cold, cyanotic, numb foot).
   b. Implement measures *to prevent mobilization of a thrombus if present:*
      1. limit activity as ordered
      2. perform actions *to prevent a generalized increase in blood pressure:*
         a. implement measures to reduce fear and anxiety (see Standardized Preoperative Care Plan, Nursing Diagnosis 1, action d)
         b. monitor for therapeutic and nontherapeutic effects of antihypertensives if administered
      3. do not massage affected lower extremity
      4. protect affected leg from trauma (e.g. pad side rails if client is restless).
   c. If signs and symptoms of distal arterial embolization occur:
      1. maintain client on strict bedrest with lower extremities in a level or slightly dependent position *to improve arterial blood flow*
      2. prepare client for diagnostic studies (e.g. Doppler ultrasound, oscillometry)
      3. implement measures *to promote vasodilation in the obstructed extremity:*
         a. administer peripheral vasodilators (e.g. papaverine, cyclandelate) as ordered
         b. keep lower extremities warm
         c. assist with a lumbar sympathetic block if performed *to decrease vasoconstrictor tone*
      4. monitor for therapeutic and nontherapeutic effects of heparin and thrombolytic agents (e.g. streptokinase, tissue plasminogen activator [tPA], urokinase) if administered
      5. prepare client for embolectomy if indicated
      6. provide emotional support to client and significant others.

Postoperative

Use in conjunction with the Standardized Postoperative Care Plan.

1. NURSING DIAGNOSIS

Altered peripheral tissue perfusion related to diminished blood flow in the operative extremity associated with:

a. trauma to the surrounding vessels during surgery;
b. inflammation of the femoral and popliteal arteries at the sites of graft anastomosis;
c. edema resulting from decreased venous return and dissection around the perivascular lymphatics;
d. venous stasis resulting from decreased mobility and insufficient venous return if the saphenous vein was used for the bypass graft (can result in impaired venous return until collateral venous circulation improves).

UNIT
VIII

DESIRED OUTCOMES	NURSING ACTIONS AND *SELECTED RATIONALES*

1. The client will maintain adequate blood flow in the operative extremity as evidenced by:
   a. gradual resolution of leg pain
   b. palpable peripheral pulses
   c. adequate Doppler flow readings in operative extremity
   d. absence of coolness and cyanosis in foot and lower leg
   e. gradual resolution of edema in operative extremity
   f. capillary refill time less than 3 seconds.

1.a. Assess for and report signs and symptoms of inadequate blood flow in the operative extremity:
   1. pain unrelieved by prescribed analgesics
   2. diminished or absent pulses (the pulses may be difficult to palpate *because of edema in the operative extremity*)
   3. diminished or absent Doppler flow readings over operative extremity
   4. extreme coolness or cyanosis of foot and lower leg
   5. increase in edema in the operative extremity
   6. capillary refill time greater than 3 seconds.
  b. Implement measures *to promote adequate blood flow in operative extremity:*
   1. avoid 90° flexion of the hip as much as possible (e.g. place client in high Fowler's position for meals only, limit length of time that client is in straight-back chair, provide recliner for client's use when sitting up)
   2. limit length of time that operative leg is in dependent position (e.g. allow client to sit up for meals only; encourage short, frequent walks rather than long walks)
   3. avoid hyperextension and extreme flexion of the knee (e.g. maintain knee in a neutral or slightly flexed position)
   4. if lower extremity edema is present:
      a. apply elastic wraps or antiembolic hose and remove and reapply as ordered
      b. assist with intermittent venous compression using pneumatic cuffs or boots if ordered
      c. elevate foot of bed 15° as ordered *to promote venous return without compromising arterial flow*
   5. place a bed cradle over lower extremities *to minimize pressure from bed linens*
   6. instruct client to perform active foot and leg exercises for 5–10 minutes every 1–2 hours while awake
   7. maintain a minimum fluid intake of 2500 cc/day unless contraindicated *to prevent fluid volume deficit and the resultant increased blood viscosity*
   8. discourage smoking *(smoking causes vasoconstriction)*
   9. maintain a comfortable room temperature and provide client with adequate clothing, warm socks, and blankets *(exposure to cold causes generalized vasoconstriction).*

□ ▬▬▬▬▬▬▬▬▬▬▬▬▬▬▬▬▬▬▬▬▬▬

2. COLLABORATIVE DIAGNOSIS

Potential complications:

a. **hypovolemic shock** related to hemorrhage associated with graft separation and fluid volume deficit associated with excessive fluid loss and inadequate fluid replacement;
b. **graft occlusion** related to kinking of graft and inadequate vessel diameter at sites of anastomosis;
c. **compartment syndrome** related to leg edema associated with inflammation resulting from surgical trauma, reperfusion of the ischemic muscles, and dissection around the perivascular lymphatics;
d. **saphenous nerve damage** related to surgical trauma or actual nerve dissection during surgery.

□ ▬▬▬▬▬▬▬▬▬▬▬▬▬▬▬▬▬▬▬▬▬▬

DESIRED OUTCOMES	**NURSING ACTIONS AND *SELECTED RATIONALES***

2.a. The client will not develop hypovolemic shock (see Standardized Postoperative Care Plan, Collaborative Diagnosis 19, outcome a, for outcome criteria).

2.a.1. Assess for and report signs and symptoms of bleeding at the sites of graft anastomosis:
    a. swelling and/or discoloration of incisional areas
    b. diminished or absent peripheral pulses
    c. decreased motor and sensory function in operative extremity.
  2. Refer to Standardized Postoperative Care Plan, Collaborative Diagnosis 19, action a, for measures related to assessment, prevention, and treatment of hypovolemic shock.
  3. Implement measures *to prevent graft separation in order to further reduce the risk of hypovolemic shock:*
    a. perform actions *to reduce pressure at the sites of graft anastomosis:*
      1. implement measures to prevent and treat fluid volume excess (see Standardized Postoperative Care Plan, Nursing Diagnosis 5, action b.3)
      2. monitor for therapeutic and nontherapeutic effects of antihypertensives if administered (must be used with caution *to avoid inadequate perfusion of the graft*)
    b. perform actions *to prevent trauma to sites of graft anastomosis* (e.g. avoid prolonged sitting; ensure that antiembolic hose, elastic wraps, or pneumatic cuffs or boots are not too tight).

2.b. The client will not experience graft occlusion in the operative extremity as evidenced by:
  1. no complaints of sudden, severe toe or foot pain
  2. palpable peripheral pulses
  3. improved capillary refill time
  4. absence of cyanosis, increasing coolness, and diminishing sensation in the foot.

2.b.1. Assess for and report signs and symptoms of graft occlusion in the operative extremity (e.g. sudden, severe pain in toes or foot; diminishing or absent peripheral pulses; increasing capillary refill time; cyanosis, increasing coolness, and diminished sensation in the foot).
  2. Avoid prolonged flexion of the knee (e.g. limit sitting as ordered, do not place pillows under knees when in bed) *in order to reduce the risk of graft occlusion.*
  3. If signs and symptoms of graft occlusion occur:
    a. maintain client on bedrest with operative leg in horizontal position
    b. prepare client for surgical intervention (e.g. straightening of graft, widening of lumen at site[s] of anastomosis) if indicated
    c. provide emotional support to client and significant others.

2.c. The client will not experience compartment syndrome in the operative extremity as evidenced by:
  1. no complaints of increasing foot and lower leg pain
  2. no statements of feelings of new or increasing numbness and tingling in foot and lower leg or tightness and tenseness of calf muscle
  3. no decrease in or absence of peripheral pulses
  4. absence of cyanosis and coldness of lower leg and foot.

2.c.1. Assess for and report signs and symptoms of compartment syndrome in the operative extremity:
    a. complaints of increasing foot and lower leg pain
    b. statements of feelings of new or increasing numbness and tingling in foot and lower leg or tightness and tenseness of calf muscle
    c. diminishing or absent peripheral pulses
    d. cyanotic, cold foot and lower leg.
  2. Implement measures *to prevent increased tissue edema in operative leg in order to reduce the risk of development of compartment syndrome:*
    a. limit length of time that operative leg is in a dependent position (e.g. limit sitting and walking as ordered)
    b. elevate operative extremity 15° if ordered.
  3. If signs and symptoms of compartment syndrome occur:
    a. maintain client on bedrest
    b. assess for and report brown discoloration of urine *(could indicate myoglobinuria resulting from the release of myoglobin from the damaged muscle cells; if there is an excessive amount of myoglobin released, it can get trapped in the renal tubules and cause renal failure)*
    c. prepare client for a fasciotomy as ordered
    d. provide emotional support to client and significant others.

2.d. The client will have resolution of or adapt to operative extremity

2.d.1. Assess for and report signs and symptoms of saphenous nerve damage (e.g. numbness, tingling, and hypersensitivity of the operative extremity).
  2. If signs and symptoms of saphenous nerve damage are present:

UNIT VIII

saphenous nerve damage if it has occurred.

a. adhere to and instruct client in the following safety precautions:
   1. wear shoes or slippers whenever out of bed
   2. do not apply heat or cold to the affected extremity
   3. test temperature of bath water before use
   4. protect operative extremity from trauma
b. reinforce information from physician regarding permanence of numbness, tingling, and hypersensitivity (these symptoms are permanent if the nerve was severed intentionally or inadvertently during surgery; if the nerve was just traumatized, the symptoms are temporary and expected to resolve within 1 year)
c. consult physician if signs and symptoms increase in severity.

☐ ▬▬▬▬▬▬▬▬▬▬▬▬▬▬▬▬▬▬▬▬▬▬▬▬▬

3. NURSING DIAGNOSIS

Knowledge deficit regarding follow-up care.

☐ ▬▬▬▬▬▬▬▬▬▬▬▬▬▬▬▬▬▬▬▬▬▬▬▬▬

DESIRED OUTCOMES	NURSING ACTIONS AND *SELECTED RATIONALES*

3.a. The client will identify ways to prevent or slow the progression of atherosclerosis.	3.a.1. Inform the client that the following conditions contribute to atherosclerosis:
	  a. obesity
	  b. diet high in saturated fat and cholesterol
	  c. sedentary life style
	  d. smoking
	  e. heavy alcohol intake (more than 2 ounces of ethanol/day on a regular basis)
	  f. hypertension
	  g. stressful life style.
	2. Assist client to identify ways he/she can make appropriate changes in life style to reduce above factors. Provide information about stress management classes and cardiovascular fitness, weight loss, stop smoking, and alcohol rehabilitation programs if appropriate. Initiate a referral if indicated.
	3. Provide dietary instruction for a diet low in saturated fat and cholesterol if indicated. Additional recommended dietary modifications may include increasing intake of foods high in soluble fiber (e.g. oat bran, most fruits and vegetables, dried peas and beans).
	4. Instruct client to take antihyperlipidemic medications (e.g. clofibrate, nicotinic acid, cholestyramine, probucol) as prescribed.

3.b. The client will identify ways to promote blood flow in the operative extremity.	3.b. Provide the following instructions about ways *to promote blood flow in the operative extremity:* 1. avoid wearing constrictive clothing (e.g. garters, girdles, knee-high stockings) 2. avoid positions that compromise blood flow (e.g. pillows under knees, crossing legs, sitting or standing for prolonged periods) 3. wear antiembolic or support hose while awake; put on before arising 4. do active foot and leg exercises for 5 minutes every hour while awake 5. maintain a regular exercise program (walking and swimming are recommended) 6. stop smoking 7. drink at least 10 glasses of liquid/day 8. avoid chronic constipation (*causes decreased venous return as a result of straining and increased intra-abdominal pressure*).

3.c. The client will state signs and symptoms of complications to report to the health care provider.

3.c.1. Refer to Standardized Postoperative Care Plan, Nursing Diagnosis 20, action c, for signs and symptoms to report to the health care provider.
2. Instruct client to report these additional signs and symptoms:
   a. sudden or gradual increase in operative leg or foot pain
   b. increased swelling or purple discoloration at incision sites
   c. pallor, coldness, or bluish color of the operative extremity
   d. diminishing or sudden absence of peripheral pulses (client may be instructed to monitor his/her peripheral pulses)
   e. significant increase in swelling of operative extremity (edema is expected to resolve gradually in 1–6 weeks)
   f. increasing numbness and/or tingling sensation of lower leg or foot.

3.d. The client will verbalize an understanding of and a plan for adhering to recommended follow-up care including future appointments with health care provider, medications prescribed, activity level, and wound care.

3.d.1. Refer to Standardized Postoperative Care Plan, Nursing Diagnosis 20, for routine postoperative instructions and measures to improve client compliance.
2. Reinforce the physician's instructions regarding:
   a. importance of scheduling adequate rest periods
   b. need to avoid sitting or standing for prolonged periods.

Thrombophlebitis

Thrombophlebitis is a condition in which a clot (thrombus) and inflammation of the vein wall are present. Factors that may contribute to inflammation and thrombus formation in a vein are trauma to the endothelium of a vessel, venous stasis, and hypercoagulability. Both superficial and deep veins may be affected. Signs and symptoms experienced by the client are a result of venous obstruction.

This care plan focuses on the adult client hospitalized for treatment of deep vein thrombophlebitis in a lower extremity. The goals of care are to reduce discomfort, promote adequate peripheral circulation, prevent complications, and educate the client regarding follow-up care.

DISCHARGE CRITERIA

Prior to discharge, the client will:

- identify ways to promote venous blood flow and reduce the risk of recurrent thrombus formation
- verbalize an understanding of medication therapy including rationale for, side effects of, schedule for taking, importance of taking as prescribed, and method of administration
- identify precautions necessary to prevent bleeding associated with anticoagulant therapy
- state signs and symptoms to report to the health care provider
- verbalize an understanding of and a plan for adhering to recommended follow-up care including future appointments with health care provider and activity level.

☐ ▄▄▄▄▄▄▄▄▄▄▄▄▄▄▄▄▄▄▄▄▄▄▄▄▄▄▄▄▄▄

Use in Conjunction with the Care Plan on Immobility.

☐ ▄▄▄▄▄▄▄▄▄▄▄▄▄▄▄▄▄▄▄▄▄▄▄▄▄▄▄▄▄▄

NURSING/COLLABORATIVE DIAGNOSES

1. Anxiety ☐ *410*
2. Altered peripheral tissue perfusion ☐ *411*
3. Pain: affected extremity ☐ *411*
4. Impaired skin integrity: breakdown ☐ *412*
5. Impaired physical mobility ☐ *413*
6. Self-care deficit ☐ *413*
7. Potential complications:
   a. pulmonary embolism
   b. chronic venous insufficiency (postphlebitic syndrome)
   c. phlegmasia alba or cerulea dolens (sudden massive swelling and pallor progressing to cyanosis of extremity)
   d. bleeding ☐ *414*
8. Knowledge deficit regarding follow-up care ☐ *415*

☐ ▄▄▄▄▄▄▄▄▄▄▄▄▄▄▄▄▄▄▄▄▄▄▄▄▄▄▄▄▄▄

1. NURSING DIAGNOSIS

Anxiety related to unfamiliar environment; pain; lack of understanding of diagnostic tests, diagnosis, and treatment plan; and fear of dislodging thrombus.

☐ ▄▄▄▄▄▄▄▄▄▄▄▄▄▄▄▄▄▄▄▄▄▄▄▄▄▄▄▄▄▄

DESIRED OUTCOMES	NURSING ACTIONS AND *SELECTED RATIONALES*

1. The client will experience a reduction in fear and anxiety (see Care Plan on Immobility, Nursing Diagnosis 1, for outcome criteria).	1.a. Refer to Care Plan on Immobility, Nursing Diagnosis 1, for measures related to assessment and reduction of fear and anxiety.
	b. Implement additional measures *to reduce fear and anxiety:*
	  1. explain all diagnostic tests (e.g. venography or phlebography, isotope studies, Doppler ultrasound, impedance plethysmography)
	  2. reassure client that strict adherence to the treatment plan greatly reduces risk of thrombus dislodgment
	  3. perform actions to reduce pain (see Nursing Diagnosis 3, action e)
	  4. if surgical intervention is planned, begin preoperative teaching.

2. NURSING DIAGNOSIS

Altered peripheral tissue perfusion related to diminished venous blood flow in affected extremity associated with venous obstruction resulting from thrombophlebitis and venous stasis resulting from decreased mobility.

DESIRED OUTCOMES	NURSING ACTIONS AND *SELECTED RATIONALES*

2. The client will have improved venous blood flow in the affected extremity as evidenced by:
   a. diminished pain in extremity
   b. improved skin color of extremity
   c. diminished edema in extremity
   d. increased Doppler flow reading over vessels in extremity.

2.a. Assess for signs and symptoms of thrombophlebitis and impaired venous blood flow in the affected extremity:
   1. tenderness and pain in extremity
   2. warmth and redness in affected area
   3. edema of extremity (assess by measuring and comparing circumference of affected and unaffected calf or thigh)
   4. positive Homan's sign in extremity (not always a reliable indicator)
   5. diminished or absent Doppler flow reading over vessels in extremity.
   b. In the acute phase, implement measures *to improve venous blood flow:*
   1. maintain activity restrictions as ordered (client is usually on complete bedrest for 4–7 days)
   2. elevate legs above heart level
   3. discourage positions that compromise venous blood flow (e.g. crossing legs, pillows under knees, use of knee gatch, sitting for long periods)
   4. discourage smoking *(smoking causes vasoconstriction)*
   5. maintain a minimum fluid intake of 2500 cc/day unless contraindicated *to prevent dehydration and increased blood viscosity, which leads to hypercoagulability*
   6. consult physician about application of heat to affected extremity (some physicians do not prescribe heat *because they believe vasodilation increases the likelihood of mobilizing the thrombus)*
   7. place a bed cradle over lower extremities *to relieve pressure from bed linens*
   8. monitor for therapeutic and nontherapeutic effects of anticoagulants (e.g. heparin, warfarin) if administered
   9. prepare client for surgical intervention (e.g. thrombectomy, insertion of an intracaval filtering device) or injection of a thrombolytic agent (e.g. urokinase, tissue plasminogen activator [tPA], streptokinase) if indicated.
   c. After the period of high risk for an embolus (usually 4–7 days), implement additional measures *to promote venous blood flow:*
   1. instruct client to perform active foot and leg exercises for 5–10 minutes every 1–2 hours while awake
   2. begin progressive ambulation
   3. consult physician about applying antiembolic hose or elastic wraps to legs before ambulation
   4. remind client to avoid prolonged sitting and standing.
   d. Consult physician if signs and symptoms of thrombophlebitis and impaired venous blood flow in affected extremity persist or worsen.

3. NURSING DIAGNOSIS

Pain: affected extremity related to vein inflammation, obstructed blood flow, and swelling.

DESIRED OUTCOMES	NURSING ACTIONS AND *SELECTED RATIONALES*

3. The client will experience diminished pain in the affected extremity as evidenced by:
a. verbalization of pain relief
b. relaxed facial expression and body positioning
c. increased participation in activities when allowed
d. stable vital signs.
	3.a. Determine how the client usually responds to pain.
	b. Assess for nonverbal signs of pain (e.g. rubbing of affected area, wrinkled brow, clenched fists, reluctance to move, restlessness, diaphoresis, facial pallor or flushing, change in B/P, tachycardia).
	c. Assess verbal complaints of pain. Ask client to be specific about location, severity, and type of pain.
	d. Assess for factors that seem to aggravate and alleviate pain.
	e. Implement measures *to reduce pain:*
	  1. perform actions to improve venous blood flow (see Nursing Diagnosis 2, actions b and c)
	  2. apply heat to affected area as ordered (use caution when applying heat *because sensation may be diminished in the affected area due to decreased circulation; this increases risk of burns*)
	  3. perform actions *to protect the affected extremity from trauma, pressure, or excessive movement:*
	    a. avoid jarring the bed
	    b. use a bed cradle or footboard *to relieve pressure from bed linens*
	    c. support extremity with a pillow during position changes
	    d. maintain activity restrictions as ordered
	    e. instruct client to move affected extremity slowly and cautiously
	  4. provide or assist with nonpharmacological measures for pain relief (e.g. position change, relaxation techniques, guided imagery, quiet conversation, restful environment, diversional activities)
	  5. monitor for therapeutic and nontherapeutic effects of analgesics and anti-inflammatory agents if administered.
	f. Explain to client and significant others that the painful extremity should not be rubbed to relieve pain (*rubbing could dislodge the thrombus*).
	g. Consult physician if above measures fail to provide adequate pain relief.

□ ▬▬▬▬▬▬▬▬▬▬▬▬▬▬▬▬▬▬▬▬▬▬

4. NURSING DIAGNOSIS

Impaired skin integrity: breakdown related to:

a. prolonged pressure on tissues associated with decreased mobility;
b. development of stasis ulcers in the affected extremity associated with venous insufficiency;
c. increased skin fragility associated with edema in the affected extremity.

□ ▬▬▬▬▬▬▬▬▬▬▬▬▬▬▬▬▬▬▬▬▬▬

DESIRED OUTCOMES	NURSING ACTIONS AND *SELECTED RATIONALES*

4. The client will maintain skin integrity as evidenced by:
a. absence of redness and irritation
b. no skin breakdown.
	4.a. Inspect the skin (especially bone prominences, dependent areas, and affected extremity) for pallor, redness, and breakdown.
	b. Refer to Care Plan on Immobility, Nursing Diagnosis 7, action b, for measures to prevent skin breakdown associated with decreased mobility.
	c. Implement measures *to prevent skin breakdown in involved extremity:*
	  1. perform actions to improve venous blood flow (see Nursing Diagnosis 2, actions b and c)
	  2. perform actions *to protect affected extremity from trauma and excessive pressure:*
	    a. use a bed cradle or footboard *to relieve pressure from bed linens*
	    b. keep heel off bed by elevating extremity on pillows, placing water-filled glove under heel, or using heel protector
	    c. instruct and assist client to move affected extremity cautiously

    d. remove antiembolic hose or elastic wraps once/shift for 30–60 minutes
    e. apply heat cautiously.
d. If skin breakdown occurs:
    1. notify physician
    2. continue with above measures to prevent further irritation and breakdown
    3. perform decubitus care as ordered or per standard hospital policy
    4. implement measures to treat stasis ulcers (e.g. anti-infective or debriding ointments, Unna's paste boot, wet to dry dressings)
    5. monitor client closely and report signs and symptoms of infection (e.g. elevated temperature; redness, warmth, and edema around area of breakdown; unusual drainage from site).

5. NURSING DIAGNOSIS

Impaired physical mobility related to activity restrictions imposed by the treatment plan and reluctance to move because of pain and fear of dislodging the thrombus.

DESIRED OUTCOMES	NURSING ACTIONS AND *SELECTED RATIONALES*

5.a. The client will maintain an optimal level of physical mobility within the restrictions imposed by the treatment plan.	5.a.1. Assess for factors that impair physical mobility (e.g. reluctance to move because of pain or fear of dislodging the thrombus, activity restrictions imposed by treatment plan).
	     2. Implement measures *to increase mobility:*
	       a. perform actions to reduce pain (see Nursing Diagnosis 3, action e)
	       b. reassure client that a certain amount of movement is desirable and will not dislodge the thrombus
	       c. assist client with range of motion exercises to unaffected extremities at least 4 times/day.
	     3. Increase activity and participation in self-care activities as allowed.
	     4. Encourage the support of significant others. Allow them to assist with positioning and physical care if desired.

5.b. The client will not experience problems associated with immobility.	5.b. Refer to Care Plan on Immobility for actions to prevent problems associated with immobility if client is to remain on bedrest for longer than 48 hours.

6. NURSING DIAGNOSIS

Self-care deficit related to impaired mobility associated with pain, fear, and activity restrictions.

DESIRED OUTCOMES	NURSING ACTIONS AND *SELECTED RATIONALES*
6. The client will perform self-care activities within physical limitations and prescribed activity restrictions.	6.a. Refer to Care Plan on Immobility, Nursing Diagnosis 9, for measures related to assessment of, planning for, and meeting the client's self-care needs. b. Implement measures to increase mobility (see Nursing Diagnosis 5, action a.2) *in order to further facilitate client's ability to perform self-care activities.*

□ ▬▬▬▬▬▬▬▬▬▬▬▬▬▬▬▬▬▬▬▬▬▬▬▬▬▬▬▬

7. COLLABORATIVE DIAGNOSIS

Potential complications:

a. **pulmonary embolism** related to dislodgment of thrombus;
b. **chronic venous insufficiency (postphlebitic syndrome)** related to residual vein damage from thrombophlebitis;
c. **phlegmasia alba or cerulea dolens (sudden massive swelling and pallor progressing to cyanosis of extremity)** related to thrombosis of the ileofemoral and femoral veins;
d. **bleeding** related to prolonged coagulation time associated with anticoagulant therapy.

□ ▬▬▬▬▬▬▬▬▬▬▬▬▬▬▬▬▬▬▬▬▬▬▬▬▬▬▬▬

DESIRED OUTCOMES	NURSING ACTIONS AND *SELECTED RATIONALES*

7.a. The client will not experience a pulmonary embolism as evidenced by:
1. absence of sudden chest pain, cough, hemoptysis
2. unlabored respirations
3. stable vital signs
4. usual skin color
5. usual mental status
6. blood gases within normal range.
	7.a.1. Assess for and report signs and symptoms of a pulmonary embolism:
	  a. sudden chest pain
	  b. cough and/or hemoptysis
	  c. dyspnea, tachypnea
	  d. tachycardia, hypotension
	  e. pallor, cyanosis
	  f. restlessness, agitation
	  g. low PaO_2.
	2. Implement measures *to prevent a pulmonary embolism:*
	  a. perform actions *to prevent dislodgment of thrombus:*
	    1. maintain client on complete bedrest as ordered
	    2. do not exercise affected extremity during acute phase of thrombophlebitis
	    3. never massage affected extremity
	    4. caution client to avoid activities that create a Valsalva response (e.g. straining to have a bowel movement, bending at the waist, holding breath while moving)
	  b. monitor for therapeutic and nontherapeutic effects of anticoagulants (e.g. heparin, warfarin) if administered.
	3. If signs and symptoms of a pulmonary embolism occur:
	  a. maintain client on strict bedrest in a semi- to high Fowler's position
	  b. maintain oxygen therapy as ordered
	  c. prepare client for diagnostic tests (e.g. blood gases, lung scan, venography, pulmonary angiography)
	  d. monitor for therapeutic and nontherapeutic effects of the following medications if administered:
	    1. heparin
	    2. thrombolytic agents (e.g. streptokinase, tissue plasminogen activator [tPA], urokinase)
	    3. vasoconstrictors (may be necessary *to maintain mean arterial pressure if shock occurs*)
	  e. prepare client for surgical intervention (e.g. embolectomy) if indicated
	  f. provide emotional support to client and significant others
	  g. refer to Care Plan on Pulmonary Embolism for additional care measures.

7.b. The client will not experience chronic venous insufficiency in the affected extremity as evidenced by: 1. absence of skin ulcerations 2. resolution of edema 3. return of usual skin color	7.b.1. Assess for and report signs and symptoms of chronic venous insufficiency in the affected extremity (e.g. skin ulcerations, usually over the medial malleolus; persistent edema; unusual skin pigmentation; cyanosis of foot when in dependent position). 2. Implement measures to promote venous blood flow (see Nursing Diagnosis 2, actions b and c). 3. If signs and symptoms of chronic venous insufficiency occur: a. continue with above actions to promote venous blood flow

as thrombophlebitis resolves.

7.c. The client will have resolution of phlegmasia alba or cerulea dolens if it occurs as evidenced by:
1. resolution of edema in affected extremity
2. return of usual skin color in affected extremity as thrombophlebitis resolves.

7.d. The client will not experience unusual bleeding as evidenced by:
1. skin and mucous membranes free of bleeding, petechiae, and ecchymosis
2. absence of unusual joint pain or swelling
3. no increase in abdominal girth
4. absence of frank or occult blood in stool, urine, and vomitus
5. usual menstrual flow
6. vital signs within normal range for client
7. stable Hct. and Hgb.
8. usual mental status.

b. implement measures to prevent and treat skin breakdown in affected extremity (see Nursing Diagnosis 4, actions c and d).

7.c.1. Assess for and report signs and symptoms of phlegmasia alba or cerulea dolens (e.g. sudden massive swelling of extremity, pallor or cyanosis of extremity, marked distention of veins in extremity).
2. If signs and symptoms of phlegmasia alba or cerulea dolens occur:
a. implement measures to improve venous blood flow (see Nursing Diagnosis 2, actions b and c)
b. prepare client for surgical intervention (e.g. thrombectomy, inferior vena cava plication, insertion of intracaval filtering device) if indicated
c. provide emotional support to client and significant others.

7.d.1. Assess client for and report signs and symptoms of unusual bleeding:
a. petechiae
b. multiple ecchymotic areas
c. bleeding gums
d. frequent or uncontrollable episodes of epistaxis
e. unusual oozing from injection sites
f. unusual joint pain or swelling
g. increase in abdominal girth
h. hematemesis, melena, red or smoke-colored urine
i. hypermenorrhea
j. significant drop in B/P accompanied by an increased pulse rate
k. decline in Hct. and Hgb. levels
l. restlessness and confusion.
2. Monitor coagulation test results (e.g. prothrombin time, activated partial thromboplastin time, partial thromboplastin time). Report values that are greater than 2½ times the control time.
3. If coagulation test results are abnormal or Hct. and Hgb. levels decline, test all stool, urine, and vomitus for occult blood. Report positive results.
4. Implement measures *to prevent bleeding:*
a. use smallest gauge needle possible when giving injections and performing venous or arterial punctures
b. apply gentle, prolonged pressure after injections and venous or arterial punctures
c. take B/P only when necessary and avoid overinflating the cuff
d. caution client to avoid activities that increase the potential for trauma (e.g. shaving with a straight-edge razor, cutting nails, using stiff bristle toothbrush or dental floss)
e. pad side rails if client is confused or restless
f. remove hazardous objects from pathway *to prevent bumps or falls*
g. instruct client to avoid blowing nose forcefully or straining to have a bowel movement; consult physician about an order for decongestants, stool softeners, and/or laxatives if indicated.
5. If bleeding occurs and does not subside spontaneously:
a. apply firm, prolonged pressure to bleeding area if possible
b. if epistaxis occurs, place client in a high Fowler's position and apply pressure and ice packs to nasal area
c. maintain oxygen therapy as ordered
d. perform iced water or saline lavage as ordered *to control gastric bleeding*
e. administer protamine sulfate (antidote for heparin) and vitamin K (e.g. phytonadione) as ordered
f. prepare client for surgical repair of bleeding vessels if indicated
g. provide emotional support to client and significant others.

8. NURSING DIAGNOSIS

Knowledge deficit regarding follow-up care.

DESIRED OUTCOMES	NURSING ACTIONS AND *SELECTED RATIONALES*

8.a. The client will identify ways to promote venous blood flow and reduce the risk of recurrent thrombus formation.

8.a. Provide the following instructions on ways *to promote venous blood flow and reduce risk of recurrent thrombus development:*
1. avoid wearing constrictive clothing (e.g. garters, girdles, knee-high stockings)
2. avoid positions that compromise blood flow (e.g. pillows under knees, crossing legs, prolonged sitting or standing)
3. wear antiembolic or support hose if daily activities involve prolonged standing
4. do active foot and leg exercises for 5 minutes every hour while awake
5. maintain a regular exercise program (walking and swimming are recommended)
6. elevate lower extremities when lying down
7. avoid exposure to extreme cold and stop smoking *(both cause vasoconstriction)*
8. avoid trauma to the affected extremity
9. avoid use of oral contraceptives and estrogen preparations *(these have been shown to increase risk of thrombus development)*
10. drink at least 10 glasses of liquid/day
11. maintain an ideal body weight for age, height, and build
12. eat a diet low in saturated fat *(saturated fat contributes to atherogenesis, which narrows the vessels)*
13. avoid chronic constipation *(causes decreased venous return as a result of straining and increased intra-abdominal pressure)*
14. take anticoagulant or antiplatelet agents as prescribed.

8.b. The client will verbalize an understanding of medication therapy including rationale for, side effects of, schedule for taking, importance of taking as prescribed, and method of administration.

8.b.1. Explain the rationale for, side effects of, and importance of taking medications prescribed.
2. If client is discharged on a coumarin derivative (e.g. dicumarol, warfarin, phenprocoumon) or heparin, instruct to:
   a. keep scheduled appointments for periodic blood studies to monitor coagulation times
   b. take or administer medication at the same time each day *in order to maintain a therapeutic blood level*
   c. avoid taking over-the-counter products containing aspirin or other salicylates *(these enhance the action of coumarins)*
   d. avoid regular and/or excessive intake of alcohol *(may alter responsiveness to coumarins and heparin)*
   e. report prolonged or excessive bleeding from skin, nose, or mouth; blood in urine, vomitus, sputum, or stool; prolonged or excessive menses; excessive bruising; severe headache; or sudden abdominal or back pain
   f. wear a Medic-Alert band identifying self as being on anticoagulant therapy.
3. If client is to administer own subcutaneous heparin, instruct in proper injection technique and appropriate sites to use. Allow time for practice and return demonstration.
4. Instruct client to inform physician of any other prescription and nonprescription medications he/she is taking.
5. Instruct client to inform all health care providers of medications being taken.

8.c. The client will identify precautions necessary to prevent bleeding associated with anticoagulant therapy.

8.c.1. Instruct client about ways *to minimize risk of bleeding:*
   a. avoid taking aspirin, aspirin-containing products, and ibuprofen
   b. use an electric rather than straight-edge razor
   c. floss and brush teeth gently
   d. cut nails carefully
   e. avoid situations that could result in injury (e.g. contact sports)
   f. avoid blowing nose forcefully
   g. avoid straining to have a bowel movement.
2. Instruct client to control any bleeding by applying firm, prolonged pressure to the area if possible.

8.d. The client will state signs and symptoms to report to the health care provider.

8.d. Instruct client to report:
1. recurrent redness, swelling, or pain in extremity
2. bluish color of the affected extremity
3. sudden chest pain accompanied by shortness of breath
4. unusual bleeding (see action b.2.e in this diagnosis)
5. skin breakdown on affected extremity.

8.e. The client will verbalize an understanding of and a plan for adhering to recommended follow-up care including future appointments with health care provider and activity level.

8.e.1. Reinforce importance of keeping follow-up appointments with health care provider.
2. Reinforce physician's instructions regarding activity limitations.
3. Implement measures *to improve client compliance:*
   a. include significant others in teaching sessions if possible
   b. encourage questions and allow time for reinforcement and clarification of information provided
   c. provide written instructions regarding future appointments with health care provider, medications prescribed, activity restrictions, signs and symptoms to report, and future laboratory studies.

□□

UNIT VIII

Vein Ligation

Vein ligation is the surgical treatment for severe varicose veins, which are dilated, tortuous vessels most often found in the lower extremities. The venous dilation may be due to a primary intrinsic weakness in the vessel wall or conditions that contribute to venous stasis in the lower extremities (e.g. thrombophlebitis, prolonged standing, ascites, obesity, pregnancy, an abdominal tumor). Prolonged venous dilation causes pressure on the valves of the involved vessels and eventually leads to valvular incompetence, which results in further vessel dilation.

Surgical intervention for varicose veins is indicated if the client is experiencing chronic venous insufficiency, recurrent thrombophlebitis, or cosmetic disfigurement. The surgery involves ligation of the affected vessel(s) above the varicosities followed by removal of the affected portion of the vein and its incompetent tributaries. This usually requires multiple incisions in the affected extremity.

This care plan focuses on the adult client hospitalized for a saphenous vein ligation. Preoperatively, the goals of care are to reduce fear and anxiety and relieve discomfort in the affected extremity. The goals of care postoperatively are to maintain comfort, prevent complications, and educate the client regarding follow-up care.

DISCHARGE CRITERIA

Prior to discharge, the client will:

- identify ways to promote venous blood flow and prevent the development of varicosities in other vessels
- identify appropriate safety precautions if paresthesias are present
- state signs and symptoms to report to the health care provider
- verbalize an understanding of and a plan for adhering to recommended follow-up care including future appointments with health care provider, medications prescribed, wound care, and activity restrictions.

NURSING/COLLABORATIVE DIAGNOSES

Preoperative
1. Pain: leg aches and cramps □ *418*
Postoperative
1. Altered peripheral tissue perfusion □ *419*
2. Potential complication: saphenous nerve damage □ *419*
3. Knowledge deficit regarding follow-up care □ *420*

Preoperative

Use in conjunction with the Standardized Preoperative Care Plan.

---

1. NURSING DIAGNOSIS

Pain: leg aches and cramps related to venous obstruction.

DESIRED OUTCOMES	NURSING ACTIONS AND *SELECTED RATIONALES*

1. The client will experience diminished leg aches and cramps as evidenced by:
a. verbalization of same
b. relaxed facial expression and body positioning
c. increased participation in activities.
	1.a. Determine how the client usually responds to pain.
	b. Assess for nonverbal signs of pain (e.g. wrinkled brow, clenched fists, frequent position changes, restlessness, rubbing legs).
	c. Assess verbal complaints of pain. Ask client to be specific about location, severity, and type of pain.
	d. Assess for factors that seem to aggravate and alleviate pain.
	e. Implement measures *to reduce leg aches and cramps:*
	  1. perform actions *to improve venous return:*
	    a. encourage client to ambulate frequently
	    b. instruct client to avoid prolonged standing or sitting, crossing legs, or use of knee gatch or pillows under knees
	    c. elevate foot of bed whenever client is in bed
	  2. provide or assist with nonpharmacological measures for pain relief (e.g. position change, relaxation techniques, range of motion of affected extremity, quiet conversation, restful environment, diversional activities)
	  3. monitor for therapeutic and nontherapeutic effects of analgesics if administered.
	f. Explain to client that the painful extremity should not be rubbed to relieve discomfort *(rubbing could dislodge a formed thrombus).*
	g. Consult physician if above measures fail to provide adequate relief of pain.

Postoperative

Use in conjunction with the Standardized Postoperative Care Plan.

1. NURSING DIAGNOSIS

Altered peripheral tissue perfusion related to diminished blood flow in the operative extremity associated with surgical excision of the saphenous vein and its tributaries, trauma to surrounding vessels during surgery, and venous stasis associated with decreased mobility.

DESIRED OUTCOMES	NURSING ACTIONS AND *SELECTED RATIONALES*

1. The client will maintain adequate blood flow in the operative extremity as evidenced by:
   a. gradual resolution of postoperative leg pain
   b. palpable peripheral pulses
   c. adequate Doppler flow readings in operative extremity
   d. extremity warm and usual color
   e. gradual resolution of edema in operative extremity
   f. capillary refill time in toes less than 3 seconds.

1.a. Assess for and report signs and symptoms of inadequate blood flow in the operative extremity:
   1. pain unrelieved by prescribed analgesics and elevation of extremity
   2. diminished or absent pulses (the pulses may be difficult to palpate *because of edema in the operative extremity)*
   3. diminished or absent Doppler flow readings in operative extremity
   4. extreme coolness or cyanosis of toes
   5. increase in edema in the operative extremity
   6. capillary refill time in toes greater than 3 seconds.
  b. Implement measures *to promote adequate blood flow in operative extremity:*
   1. keep foot of bed elevated 15–20° *in order to promote venous return without compromising arterial flow*
   2. apply elastic wraps or antiembolic hose and remove and reapply as ordered (some physicians may want them removed only for dressing changes)
   3. place a bed cradle over lower extremities *to minimize pressure from bed linens*
   4. instruct client to perform active foot and leg exercises for 5–10 minutes every 1–2 hours while awake
   5. discourage positions that compromise blood flow to and from the lower extremities (e.g. crossing legs, pillows under knees, use of knee gatch)
   6. maintain a minimum fluid intake of 2500 cc/day unless contraindicated *to prevent dehydration and the resultant increased blood viscosity*
   7. discourage smoking *(smoking causes vasoconstriction)*
   8. when ambulation is allowed (usually 24–48 hours after surgery):
     a. encourage client to ambulate for 5 minutes at regular intervals
     b. instruct client not to sit or stand still *(these activities cause venous stasis).*
  c. Consult physician if signs and symptoms of inadequate blood flow in operative extremity persist or worsen.

2. COLLABORATIVE DIAGNOSIS

Potential complication: saphenous nerve damage related to surgical trauma.

DESIRED OUTCOMES	NURSING ACTIONS AND *SELECTED RATIONALES*

2. The client will experience resolution of saphenous nerve damage if it occurs as evidenced by: diminished numbness, tingling, and hypersensitivity of the operative extremity.	2.a. Assess for and report signs and symptoms of saphenous nerve damage (e.g. numbness, tingling, and hypersensitivity of the operative extremity).
	b. If signs and symptoms of saphenous nerve damage occur:
	  1. adhere to and instruct client *on the following safety precautions:*
	    a. wear shoes or slippers whenever out of bed
	    b. do not apply heat or cold to the affected extremity
	    c. test temperature of bath water before use
	    d. protect operative extremity from trauma
	  2. reinforce information from physician regarding permanence of numbness, tingling, and hypersensitivity (these symptoms are usually temporary but may take months to resolve)
	  3. consult physician if signs and symptoms increase in severity.

□ ▬▬▬▬▬▬▬▬▬▬▬▬▬▬▬▬▬▬▬▬

3. NURSING DIAGNOSIS

Knowledge deficit regarding follow-up care.

□ ▬▬▬▬▬▬▬▬▬▬▬▬▬▬▬▬▬▬▬▬

DESIRED OUTCOMES	NURSING ACTIONS AND *SELECTED RATIONALES*

3.a. The client will identify ways to promote venous blood flow and prevent the development of varicosities in other vessels.	3.a. Provide the following instructions about ways *to promote venous blood flow and prevent development of varicosities in other vessels:*
	  1. avoid wearing constrictive clothing (e.g. garters, girdles, knee-high stockings)
	  2. avoid positions that compromise blood flow (e.g. pillows under knees, crossing legs, sitting or standing for prolonged periods)
	  3. wear antiembolic or support hose while awake; put on before arising
	  4. elevate legs for 2–3 minutes every few hours and, if possible, sleep with legs elevated
	  5. do active foot and leg exercises for 5 minutes every hour while awake
	  6. maintain a regular exercise program (walking and swimming are recommended)
	  7. stop smoking
	  8. drink at least 10 glasses of liquid/day
	  9. maintain an ideal weight for age, height, and build; obtain a dietary consult or refer client to a weight loss program if appropriate
	  10. avoid chronic constipation *(causes decreased venous return as a result of straining and increased intra-abdominal pressure).*

3.b. The client will identify appropriate safety precautions if paresthesias are present.	3.b. Reinforce instructions regarding safety precautions to prevent injury to the operative extremity if paresthesias are present (see Postoperative Collaborative Diagnosis 2, action b.1).

3.c. The client will state signs and symptoms to report to the health care provider.	3.c.1. Refer to Standardized Postoperative Care Plan, Nursing Diagnosis 20, action c, for signs and symptoms to report to the health care provider.
	  2. Instruct client to report these additional signs and symptoms:
	    a. diminished sensation in operative extremity
	    b. coldness or bluish color in operative extremity
	    c. significant increase in swelling of operative extremity that does not resolve with elevation of the extremity
	    d. pain in calf of operative extremity when walking
	    e. sudden chest pain accompanied by shortness of breath
	    f. recurrence of dilated, tortuous vessels in extremities.

3.d. The client will verbalize an understanding of and a plan for adhering to recommended follow-up care including future appointments with health care provider, medications prescribed, wound care, and activity restrictions.

3.d.1. Refer to Standardized Postoperative Care Plan, Nursing Diagnosis 20, for routine postoperative instructions and measures to improve client compliance.
2. Reinforce physician's instructions regarding restrictions on standing and sitting.
3. Reinforce physician's instructions regarding wearing antiembolic or support hose.

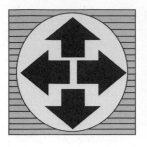
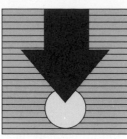
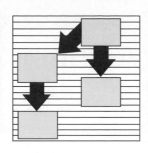
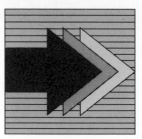
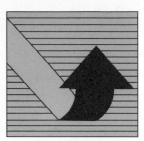

Unit IX

Nursing Care of the Client with Disturbances of Respiratory Function

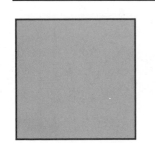
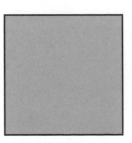
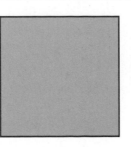
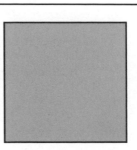
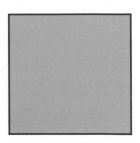

Asthma

Asthma is the term used to describe recurrent, usually reversible, diffuse obstructive airway disease associated with hyperreactivity of the airways. The syndrome is characterized by episodes of dyspnea, wheezing, and coughing that result from constriction of bronchial smooth muscle, excess mucus production, and mucosal edema. The basic pathologic process involves a hypersensitive response of the mast cells, sensory and motor neurons of the vagal reflex arc, bronchial smooth muscles, and mucous glands.

Asthma is classified according to the factor that causes the hypersensitive response. It can be extrinsic (atopic, allergic, exogenous, noninfectious), intrinsic (nonatropic, nonallergic, endogenous, infectious), or most often a mixture of the two. The extrinsic type usually begins in childhood and is the result of an antigen-antibody reaction stimulated by environmental allergens. The onset of the intrinsic type of asthma usually occurs about age 35 and is commonly associated with a history of recurrent respiratory tract infections. Symptoms can range from mild with diffuse wheezes and no evidence of impaired air exchange to severe with significant wheezing and marked respiratory distress. Asthma attacks can last for a few minutes to several hours with the frequency of occurrence varying from person to person. Between attacks, most asthmatics are asymptomatic, but some may experience a degree of chronic bronchospasm.

This care plan focuses on the adult client hospitalized during an acute asthma attack. The goals of care are to relieve respiratory distress, provide emotional support, and educate the client regarding follow-up care.

DISCHARGE CRITERIA

Prior to discharge, the client will:

- identify ways to decrease the risk of an asthma attack
- verbalize an understanding of medication therapy including rationale for, side effects of, methods of administering, and importance of taking as prescribed
- state signs and symptoms to report to the health care provider
- share thoughts and feelings about the effects of asthma on life style and self-concept
- identify community resources that can assist in making necessary life-style changes and coping with the effects of asthma
- verbalize an understanding of and a plan for adhering to recommended follow-up care including chest physiotherapy and future appointments with health care provider.

NURSING/COLLABORATIVE DIAGNOSES

1. Anxiety ☐ 425
2. Ineffective airway clearance ☐ 426
3. Ineffective breathing patterns:
   a. hyperventilation
   b. hypoventilation ☐ 427
4. Fluid volume deficit ☐ 428
5. Pain: chest ☐ 429
6. Activity intolerance ☐ 429
7. Sleep pattern disturbance ☐ 430
8. Potential complications:
   a. atelectasis
   b. status asthmaticus
   c. respiratory failure ☐ 431
9. Ineffective individual coping ☐ 432
10. Knowledge deficit regarding follow-up care ☐ 433

1. NURSING DIAGNOSIS

Anxiety related to:

a. unfamiliar environment;
b. lack of understanding of diagnosis, diagnostic tests, and treatments;
c. difficulty breathing and feeling of suffocation associated with respiratory distress during the acute attack;
d. possibility of recurrent asthma attacks.

DESIRED OUTCOMES	NURSING ACTIONS AND *SELECTED RATIONALES*

1. The client will experience a reduction in fear and anxiety as evidenced by:
  a. verbalization of feeling less anxious or fearful
  b. relaxed facial expression and body movements
  c. stable vital signs
  d. usual skin color
  e. verbalization of an understanding of hospital routines, diagnosis, diagnostic tests, and treatments.
	1.a. Assess client for signs and symptoms of fear and anxiety (e.g. verbalization of fears and concerns; tenseness; tremors; irritability; restlessness; increased dyspnea; diaphoresis; elevated blood pressure; tachycardia; facial tension, pallor, or flushing; noncompliance with treatment plan).
	  b. Ascertain effectiveness of current coping skills.
	  c. Implement measures *to reduce fear and anxiety:*
	    1. maintain a calm, confident manner when interacting with client
	    2. do not leave client alone during period of acute respiratory distress
	    3. perform actions to improve respiratory status (see Nursing Diagnoses 2, action b and 3, action e) *in order to relieve dyspnea*
	    4. perform actions *to decrease client's feeling of suffocation:*
	      a. open curtains and doors
	      b. approach client from the side rather than face-on *(close face-on contact may make client feel closed in)*
	      c. limit number of visitors in room at any one time
	      d. remove unnecessary equipment from room
	      e. administer oxygen via nasal cannula rather than mask if possible
	    5. reassure client that asthma attacks are usually controlled by medication therapy
	    6. encourage significant others to project a caring, concerned attitude without obvious anxiousness
	    7. assure client that increased cough and expectoration of copious amounts of thick, tenacious sputum do not indicate another asthma attack but rather are characteristic of the end of the attack
	    8. when acute respiratory distress has subsided:
	      a. orient to hospital environment, equipment, and routines
	      b. introduce staff who will be participating in his/her care; if possible, maintain consistency in staff assigned to his/her care *to provide feelings of stability and comfort with the environment*
	      c. assure client that staff members are nearby; respond to call signal as soon as possible
	      d. provide a calm, restful environment
	      e. encourage verbalization of fear and anxiety; provide feedback
	      f. reinforce physician's explanations and clarify any misconceptions client may have about asthma, the treatment plan, and prognosis
	      g. assist client to identify factors that may have precipitated the asthma attack; discuss methods of alleviating or controlling these factors
	      h. explain all diagnostic tests (e.g. chest x-ray, pulmonary function studies, sputum cultures, blood gas analysis, WBC count, serum immunoglobulin levels)
	      i. instruct in relaxation techniques and encourage participation in diversional activities
	      j. perform actions to assist client to cope with the diagnosis and its implications (see Nursing Diagnosis 9, action e)
	      k. monitor for therapeutic and nontherapeutic effects of antianxiety agents if administered.

UNIT
IX

d. Include significant others in orientation and teaching sessions and encourage their continued support of client.
e. Provide information based on current needs of client and significant others at a level they can understand. Encourage questions and clarification of information provided.
f. Consult physician if above actions fail to control fear and anxiety.

☐ ▬▬▬▬▬▬▬▬▬▬▬▬▬▬▬▬▬▬▬▬▬▬▬▬

2. NURSING DIAGNOSIS

Ineffective airway clearance related to:

a. bronchospasm associated with release of chemical mediators (e.g. leukotrienes, histamine) from the mast cells of bronchial tissues and acetylcholine (a result of parasympathetic nervous system stimulation) in response to mechanical and chemical irritation of the airways;
b. bronchial mucosal wall edema associated with increased capillary permeability resulting from the release of chemical mediators (e.g. leukotrienes, histamine) from mast cells;
c. increased production of mucus associated with stimulation of the goblet mucus-producing cells;
d. tenacious sputum associated with fluid volume deficit resulting from mouth breathing, hyperventilation, increased production of mucus, and decreased oral intake during attack and subsequent period of fatigue;
e. decreased cough effort following the asthma attack associated with fatigue.

☐ ▬▬▬▬▬▬▬▬▬▬▬▬▬▬▬▬▬▬▬▬▬▬▬▬

DESIRED OUTCOMES	NURSING ACTIONS AND *SELECTED RATIONALES*

2. The client will attain clear, open airways as evidenced by:
   a. improved breath sounds
   b. normal rate and depth of respirations
   c. absence of dyspnea
   d. absence of cyanosis.

2.a. Assess for signs and symptoms of ineffective airway clearance (e.g. adventitious breath sounds; rapid, shallow respirations; dyspnea; cyanosis).
  b. Implement measures *to promote effective airway clearance:*
    1. monitor for therapeutic and nontherapeutic effects of the following medications if administered *to open the client's airways during the acute attack:*
      a. methylxanthine-derivative bronchodilators (e.g. theophylline), sympathomimetic bronchodilators (e.g. terbutaline, epinephrine, metaproterenol, albuterol), and/or anticholinergics (e.g. atropine, ipratropium) *to relieve bronchial smooth muscle spasm*
      b. corticosteroids *to reduce inflammation*
    2. perform actions *to promote effective airway clearance after the acute attack:*
      a. instruct and assist client to turn, cough, and deep breathe every 1–2 hours
      b. reinforce correct use of inspiratory exerciser at least every 2 hours
      c. increase activity as allowed and tolerated
      d. implement measures *to facilitate removal of pulmonary secretions:*
        1. assist client to a sitting position during cough efforts *in order to most efficiently utilize accessory muscles*
        2. augment cough efforts by placing hands on client's upper abdomen and exerting upward pressure during exhalation
        3. perform actions *to liquefy pulmonary secretions:*
          a. maintain a fluid intake of at least 3000 cc/day unless contraindicated (intravenous therapy is usually needed to supplement oral intake during acute attack and subsequent period of fatigue)
          b. humidify inspired air
          c. assist with administration of mucolytic agents via nebulizer treatment

4. perform tracheal suctioning if needed
5. assist with or perform postural drainage, percussion, and vibration if ordered
6. monitor for therapeutic and nontherapeutic effects of expectorants if administered

e. continue to administer bronchodilators and corticosteroids as ordered
f. implement measures *to prevent recurrent bronchospasm or bronchoconstriction:*
1. instruct client to avoid drinking cold liquids (*these can cause bronchospasm*)
2. avoid exposure to irritating substances such as smoke, powder, flowers, and perfume
3. obtain dietary consult if indicated to assist client in selecting foods/fluids that he/she is not allergic to (allergies are often to eggs, chocolate, wheat, or foods/fluids containing yellow dye No. 5)
4. consult physician about administration of antihistamines or decongestants if client is experiencing nasal stuffiness and postnasal drip (*postnasal drip can stimulate the cholinergic reflex mechanism and cause bronchospasm*); use these medications cautiously *because they can cause drying of respiratory mucosa, which makes mucus more tenacious*
5. consult physician before administering any medications such as propranolol, timolol, and nadolol that have a nonselective beta-adrenergic blocking effect (*these medications have a bronchoconstricting effect*)
6. monitor for therapeutic and nontherapeutic effects of cromolyn sodium if administered *to inhibit the release of chemical mediators (e.g. histamine) from the mast cells.*

c. Consult physician if:
1. signs and symptoms of ineffective airway clearance persist
2. signs and symptoms of impaired gas exchange (e.g. confusion, restlessness, irritability, cyanosis, decreased PaO_2 and increased $PaCO_2$ levels) are present.

3. NURSING DIAGNOSIS

Ineffective breathing patterns:

a. **hyperventilation** related to fear and anxiety;
b. **hypoventilation** related to weakness, fatigue, and reluctance to breathe deeply due to chest pain (results from muscle strain associated with use of accessory muscles for breathing and excessive coughing during and immediately after the asthma attack).

DESIRED OUTCOMES	NURSING ACTIONS AND *SELECTED RATIONALES*
3. The client will resume an effective breathing pattern as evidenced by: a. normal rate, rhythm, and depth of respirations b. absence of dyspnea c. blood gases within normal range.	3.a. Assess for signs and symptoms of ineffective breathing patterns (e.g. shallow, rapid respirations; dyspnea; use of accessory muscles for breathing). b. Monitor blood gases. Report abnormal results. c. Monitor for and report significant changes in ear oximetry and capnograph results. d. Assist with pulmonary function studies if done *to evaluate respiratory status and/or effectiveness of treatment measures.* e. Implement measures *to improve breathing pattern:* 1. perform actions to decrease fear and anxiety (see Nursing Diagnosis 1, action c)

2. perform actions to reduce chest pain (see Nursing Diagnosis 5, action e)
3. place client in semi- to high Fowler's position
4. perform actions to increase strength and activity tolerance (see Nursing Diagnosis 6, action b)
5. instruct client to deep breathe or use inspiratory exerciser at least every 2 hours
6. administer or assist with IPPB treatments if ordered following the asthma attack
7. instruct and assist client with diaphragmatic and pursed-lip breathing techniques at least every 2 hours if appropriate
8. assist client to turn at least every 2 hours while in bed
9. increase activity as allowed and tolerated
10. avoid administering central nervous system depressants (e.g. narcotic analgesics, sedatives, muscle relaxants) unless absolutely necessary *(these can further depress respiratory status).*

f. Consult physician if:
1. ineffective breathing patterns persist
2. signs and symptoms of impaired gas exchange (e.g. confusion, restlessness, irritability, cyanosis, decreased PaO_2 and increased $PaCO_2$ levels) are present.

4. NURSING DIAGNOSIS

Fluid volume deficit related to:

a. excessive fluid loss during the asthma attack associated with hyperventilation, increased production of pulmonary secretions, and mouth breathing;
b. decreased oral fluid intake associated with dyspnea and fatigue.

DESIRED OUTCOMES	NURSING ACTIONS AND *SELECTED RATIONALES*

4. The client will not experience fluid volume deficit as evidenced by:
   a. normal skin turgor
   b. moist mucous membranes
   c. weight loss no greater than 0.5 kg/day
   d. B/P and pulse within normal range for client and stable with position change
   e. Hct. within normal range
   f. balanced intake and output
   g. urine specific gravity between 1.010–1.030.

4.a. Assess for and report signs and symptoms of fluid volume deficit:
   1. decreased skin turgor
   2. dry mucous membranes, thirst
   3. weight loss greater than 0.5 kg/day
   4. low B/P and/or decline in systolic B/P of at least 15 mm Hg with concurrent rise in pulse when client sits up
   5. weak, rapid pulse
   6. elevated Hct.
   7. output less than intake with urine specific gravity higher than 1.030 (reflects an actual rather than potential water loss).
 b. Implement measures *to prevent or treat fluid volume deficit:*
   1. perform actions to control asthma attack and prevent recurrence (see Nursing Diagnosis 2, actions b.1 and 2.e and f) *in order to reduce hyperventilation and production of pulmonary secretions*
   2. maintain a fluid intake of at least 3000 cc/day unless contraindicated
   3. maintain intravenous fluid therapy as ordered.
 c. Consult physician if signs and symptoms of fluid volume deficit persist or worsen.

5. NURSING DIAGNOSIS

Pain: chest related to muscle strain associated with use of accessory muscles for breathing and excessive coughing during and immediately following the asthma attack.

DESIRED OUTCOMES	NURSING ACTIONS AND *SELECTED RATIONALES*

5. The client will experience diminished chest pain as evidenced by:
a. verbalization of pain relief
b. relaxed facial expression and body positioning
c. increased participation in activities
d. usual depth and rate of respirations
e. stable vital signs.
	5.a. Determine how the client usually responds to pain.
	b. Assess for nonverbal signs of pain (e.g. wrinkled brow; clenched fists; rubbing of chest; reluctance to move; restlessness; shallow, guarded respirations; diaphoresis; facial pallor or flushing; change in B/P; tachycardia).
	c. Assess verbal complaints of pain. Ask client to be specific about location, type, and severity of pain.
	d. Assess for factors that seem to aggravate and alleviate pain.
	e. Implement measures *to reduce chest pain:*
	  1. provide or assist with nonpharmacological measures for pain relief (e.g. back rub, position change, relaxation techniques, quiet conversation, restful environment, diversional activities)
	  2. consult physician regarding application of heat to painful area
	  3. monitor for therapeutic and nontherapeutic effects of mild analgesics if administered (narcotic analgesics are contraindicated *because of their respiratory depressant effects*).
	f. Consult physician if above measures fail to reduce pain.

6. NURSING DIAGNOSIS

Activity intolerance related to:

a. decreased tissue oxygenation if it occurs as a result of ineffective airway clearance and breathing patterns;

b. difficulty resting and sleeping associated with dyspnea, persistent coughing, frequent assessments and treatments, fear, anxiety, side effects of medication therapy (e.g. some bronchodilators), and chest pain;

c. increased energy expenditure associated with strenuous breathing efforts and persistent coughing.

DESIRED OUTCOMES	NURSING ACTIONS AND *SELECTED RATIONALES*

6. The client will demonstrate an increased tolerance for activity as evidenced by:
a. verbalization of feeling less fatigued and weak
b. ability to perform activities of daily living without
	6.a. Assess for signs and symptoms of activity intolerance:
	  1. statements of fatigue and weakness
	  2. increased dyspnea and chest pain, diaphoresis, or dizziness
	  3. decrease in pulse rate or an increase in rate of 20 beats/minute above resting rate
	  4. pulse rate not returning to preactivity level within 5 minutes after stopping activity

UNIT IX

increased dyspnea and chest pain, diaphoresis, dizziness, or a significant change in vital signs.

5. decreased blood pressure or an increase in diastolic pressure of 15 mm Hg with activity.
    b. Implement measures *to improve activity tolerance:*
       1. perform actions *to promote rest:*
          a. maintain activity restrictions if ordered
          b. minimize environmental activity and noise
          c. schedule nursing care and diagnostic procedures to allow periods of uninterrupted rest
          d. limit the number of visitors and their length of stay
          e. assist client with self-care activities
          f. keep supplies and personal articles within easy reach
          g. implement measures to reduce fear and anxiety (see Nursing Diagnosis 1, action c)
          h. implement measures to improve respiratory status (see Nursing Diagnoses 2, action b and 3, action e) *in order to relieve dyspnea*
          i. implement measures to promote sleep (see Nursing Diagnosis 7, action c)
          j. implement measures to reduce chest pain (see Nursing Diagnosis 5, action e)
       2. instruct client in energy-saving techniques (e.g. using shower chair when showering, sitting to brush teeth or comb hair)
       3. perform actions to improve respiratory status (see Nursing Diagnoses 2, action b and 3, action e)
       4. encourage use of bronchodilators before activity if ordered
       5. reinforce the use of controlled breathing patterns (e.g. inhaling through nose and exhaling slowly through pursed lips) during activity if indicated
       6. encourage client to use oxygen as needed during self-care activities and ambulation; keep portable oxygen equipment readily available for client's use
       7. increase client's activity gradually as allowed and tolerated.
    c. Instruct client to:
       1. report a decreased tolerance for activity
       2. stop any activity that causes increased chest pain or shortness of breath, dizziness, or extreme fatigue or weakness.
    d. Consult physician if signs and symptoms of activity intolerance persist or worsen.

□ ▰▰▰▰▰▰▰▰▰▰▰▰▰▰▰▰▰▰▰▰▰▰▰▰

7. NURSING DIAGNOSIS

Sleep pattern disturbance related to fear, anxiety, dyspnea, persistent coughing, chest pain, frequent assessments and treatments, and side effects of some medications (e.g. some bronchodilators).

□ ▰▰▰▰▰▰▰▰▰▰▰▰▰▰▰▰▰▰▰▰▰▰▰▰

DESIRED OUTCOMES	NURSING ACTIONS AND *SELECTED RATIONALES*
7. The client will attain optimal amounts of sleep within the parameters of the treatment regimen as evidenced by: a. statements of feeling well rested b. usual behavior c. absence of frequent yawning, thick speech, dark circles under eyes.	7.a. Assess for signs and symptoms of a sleep pattern disturbance: 1. verbal complaints of difficulty falling asleep, not feeling well rested, sleep interruptions, or awakening earlier or later than desired 2. behavior changes (e.g. irritability, disorganization, lethargy) 3. frequent yawning, thick speech, dark circles under eyes, slight hand tremors. b. Determine the client's usual sleep habits. c. Implement measures *to promote sleep:* 1. perform actions to decrease fear and anxiety (see Nursing Diagnosis 1, action c)

2. perform actions to improve respiratory status (see Nursing Diagnoses 2, action b and 3, action e) *in order to relieve dyspnea*
3. perform actions to reduce chest pain (see Nursing Diagnosis 5, action e)
4. assist client to assume a comfortable sleep position (e.g. bed in reverse Trendelenburg position with client in usual recumbent sleep position, head of bed elevated with arms supported on pillows, resting forward on overbed table with good pillow support, sitting in chair)
5. maintain oxygen therapy during sleep if indicated
6. ensure good room ventilation
7. allow client to continue usual sleep practices (e.g. position, time, bedtime rituals) if possible
8. determine measures that have been helpful to client in the past (e.g. milk, warm drinks, warm bath) and incorporate in plan of care
9. encourage participation in relaxing diversional activities in early evening hours
10. provide a quiet, restful atmosphere
11. discourage intake of foods and fluids high in caffeine (e.g. chocolate, coffee, tea, colas), especially in the evening
12. satisfy basic needs such as hunger, comfort, and warmth before sleep
13. have client empty bladder just before bedtime
14. utilize relaxation techniques (e.g. progressive relaxation exercises, back massage, meditation, soft music) before sleep
15. perform actions *to provide for periods of uninterrupted sleep (90- to 120-minute periods of uninterrupted sleep are considered essential):*
    a. restrict visitors during rest periods
    b. group care (e.g. medications, treatments, physical care, assessments) whenever possible
16. monitor for therapeutic and nontherapeutic effects of sedatives and hypnotics if administered.
d. Consult physician if signs of sleep deprivation persist or worsen.

8. COLLABORATIVE DIAGNOSIS

Potential complications:

a. **atelectasis** related to hypoventilation and obstruction of the bronchioles with mucus;
b. **status asthmaticus** related to severe unresolved bronchospasm or bronchoconstriction;
c. **respiratory failure** related to hypoxemia associated with ineffective breathing patterns and airway obstruction.

DESIRED OUTCOMES	NURSING ACTIONS AND *SELECTED RATIONALES*
8.a. The client will not develop atelectasis following the asthma attack as evidenced by: 1. normal breath sounds 2. resonant percussion note over lungs 3. pulse and respiratory rates within normal limits for client	8.a.1. Assess for and report signs and symptoms of atelectasis following the asthma attack (e.g. diminished or absent breath sounds, dull percussion note over a particular area, increased pulse and respiratory rates, elevated temperature). 2. Monitor chest x-ray results. Report findings of atelectasis. 3. Implement measures *to prevent atelectasis:* a. perform actions to promote effective airway clearance (see Nursing Diagnosis 2, action b) b. perform actions to improve breathing pattern (see Nursing Diagnosis 3, action e).

4. afebrile status.

4. If signs and symptoms of atelectasis occur:
   a. increase frequency of turning, coughing, deep breathing, and use of inspiratory exerciser
   b. consult physician if signs and symptoms of atelectasis persist or worsen.

8.b. The client will not experience status asthmaticus as evidenced by cessation of the asthma attack within expected time.

8.b.1. Assess for and report signs and symptoms of an asthma attack that worsen or do not subside within the expected length of time (usually 1 hour).
2. Implement measures to control the asthma attack (see Nursing Diagnosis 2, action b.1).
3. If signs and symptoms of status asthmaticus occur:
   a. assess for and report signs and symptoms of respiratory failure (see action c.1 in this diagnosis)
   b. assess for and report signs and symptoms of heart failure (e.g. tachycardia, cyanosis, peripheral edema, softened or muffled heart sounds, distended neck veins)
   c. monitor for therapeutic and nontherapeutic effects of neuromuscular blocking agents (e.g. curare) if administered *to produce respiratory paralysis* (the client receiving neuromuscular blocking agents will need mechanical ventilation)
   d. provide emotional support to client and significant others.

8.c. The client will not experience respiratory failure as evidenced by:
1. respiratory rate above 8 and below 30/minute
2. usual skin color
3. usual mental status
4. PaO$_2$ above 50 mm Hg and PaCO$_2$ below 50 mm Hg.

8.c.1. Assess for and report signs and symptoms of severe respiratory distress (e.g. rapid, shallow respirations; sternocleidomastoid muscle retraction; dusky or cyanotic skin color; drowsiness; confusion).
2. Monitor blood gas values. Report abnormal values or values that have worsened.
3. Monitor for and report worsening of ear oximetry and capnograph results.
4. Implement measures *to prevent respiratory failure:*
   a. perform actions to improve respiratory status (see Nursing Diagnoses 2, action b and 3, action e)
   b. assess for and report conditions that might further compromise respiratory status (e.g. cardiac arrhythmias, low B/P, atelectasis, severe stress).
5. If signs and symptoms of respiratory failure occur:
   a. continue with above actions
   b. assist with intubation, mechanical ventilation, and transfer to intensive care unit if indicated
   c. provide emotional support to client and significant others.

□ ▬▬▬▬▬▬▬▬▬▬▬▬▬▬▬▬▬▬▬▬▬▬▬▬▬▬▬

9. NURSING DIAGNOSIS

Ineffective individual coping related to unpredictable and variable nature of asthma attacks, fear of precipitating another asthma attack, necessity of altering life style to avoid recurrent attacks, and inadequate support system.

□ ▬▬▬▬▬▬▬▬▬▬▬▬▬▬▬▬▬▬▬▬▬▬▬▬▬▬▬

DESIRED OUTCOMES	NURSING ACTIONS AND *SELECTED RATIONALES*

9. The client will demonstrate the use of effective coping skills as evidenced by:
   a. willingness to participate in treatment plan and self-care activities
   b. verbalization of ability to cope with asthma

9.a. Assess effectiveness of client's coping strategies by observing behavior and noting strengths, weaknesses, ability to express feelings and concerns, and willingness to participate in and adhere to the treatment plan.
b. Assess for and report signs and symptoms that may indicate ineffective coping (e.g. lack of participation in treatment plan, sleep disturbances, increasing fatigue, tendency to overuse inhalants, reluctance to be discharged, increase in number of asthma attacks, verbalization of inability to cope, inability to problem-solve).

c. identification of stressors
d. utilization of appropriate problem-solving techniques
e. recognition and utilization of available support systems.

c. Allow time for client to adjust psychologically to the fact that he/she had an asthma attack and that additional medication therapy and life-style changes may be necessary to prevent future attacks.
d. Inform client that it may take many alterations in medication therapy (e.g. type, dose) to arrive at an effective balance between control of symptoms and tolerable side effects.
e. Implement measures *to promote effective coping:*
   1. if indicated, arrange for a visit with an asthmatic who has successfully adjusted to the disease
   2. perform actions to decrease fear and anxiety (see Nursing Diagnosis 1, action c)
   3. include client in the planning of care, encourage maximum participation in treatment plan, and allow choices when possible *to enable client to maintain a sense of control*
   4. instruct client in effective problem-solving techniques (e.g. accurate identification of stressors, determination of various options to solve problem)
   5. assist client to maintain usual daily routines whenever possible
   6. discuss ways client can realistically gain some control over factors that can precipitate an asthma attack (e.g. avoidance of irritating substances, stress reduction, maintenance of optimal physical and psychological health); focus on alterations in rather than elimination of usual activities
   7. encourage client to continue involvement in social activities and previous hobbies; if previous interests are contraindicated, encourage development of new ones
   8. assist client to identify and utilize available support systems; provide information on available community resources that can assist client and significant others to cope with effects of the disease (e.g. local chapter of American Lung Association, support groups, counseling services).
f. Encourage continued emotional support from significant others.
g. Assess for and support behaviors suggesting positive adaptation to changes experienced (e.g. active participation in treatment plan and self-care, improved sleep pattern, verbalization of ability to cope, utilization of effective problem-solving strategies).
h. Consult physician about psychological or vocational rehabilitation counseling if appropriate. Initiate a referral if necessary.

UNIT
IX

10. NURSING DIAGNOSIS

Knowledge deficit regarding follow-up care.

DESIRED OUTCOMES	NURSING ACTIONS AND *SELECTED RATIONALES*
10.a. The client will identify ways to decrease the risk of an asthma attack.	10.a.1. Instruct client in ways *to decrease risk of an asthma attack:* a. remain indoors as much as possible when pollution levels are high b. avoid irritants such as tobacco smoke, perfumes, aerosol cleaners, paint fumes, and solvents whenever possible c. wear a mask or scarf over nose and mouth when exposed to high levels of irritants such as smoke, fumes, pollen, and mold spores d. implement dust control measures (e.g. place a plastic cover around mattress, vacuum and dust living area thoroughly once a week, remove items such as shag carpets and overstuffed chairs when possible) e. maintain a balanced program of exercise and rest f. avoid contact with persons who have respiratory tract infections

g. if medication therapy includes the use of inhalants, clean and replace home inhalation therapy equipment as instructed *to reduce the risk of respiratory tract infections*

h. control or eliminate stress factors

i. avoid substances (e.g. medications, foods, fabrics) that have caused allergic reactions in the past

j. use a properly cleaned and maintained room humidifier as needed *to moisturize dry indoor air*

k. avoid exposure to cold air and drafts

l. stop smoking

m. receive immunizations against influenza and pneumococcal pneumonia

n. continue with program of desensitization (immunotherapy) if prescribed to treat existing allergies

o. take medications (e.g. cromolyn sodium, bronchodilators, corticosteroids) as prescribed.

2. Reinforce importance of early recognition of signs and symptoms of an impending asthma attack (e.g. tightness in chest, increased wheezing or coughing, increased requirement for inhalant, decreased activity tolerance, difficulty breathing when lying down).

3. Instruct client to perform the following actions if signs and symptoms of an impending asthma attack occur:

a. take medications (e.g. bronchodilators, corticosteroids) as prescribed

b. practice relaxation techniques

c. take a hot shower (unless it makes symptoms worse), sit near a vaporizer, and continue to drink plenty of fluids

d. eliminate precipitating or aggravating factors.

4. Caution client to consult physician about anticipated value of costly investments such as air purifiers or dramatic life-style changes (e.g. moving, changing jobs) if being done solely as a method of controlling asthma condition.

10.b. The client will verbalize an understanding of medication therapy including rationale for, side effects of, methods of administering, and importance of taking as prescribed.

10.b.1. Provide instructions regarding medications prescribed:

a. clarify which medications should be taken routinely (e.g. cromolyn sodium, theophylline, corticosteroids) and which are to be used in an acute attack (e.g. epinephrine, terbutaline, metaproterenol)

b. reinforce correct method of administering drugs; if client is to administer own subcutaneous injections and/or use inhalers or nebulizers, demonstrate procedures; allow time for questions, clarification, and return demonstration

c. reinforce protocols for the adjustment of medication therapy (e.g. some clients are instructed to monitor their peak expiratory flow rate [PEFR] using a peak flowmeter and to increase the dose of their bronchodilator if the PEFR decreases)

d. caution client that the overuse of medications may trigger asthma attacks

e. if client is discharged on theophylline, instruct him/her to:

1. take the medication with food *to minimize nausea, vomiting, and epigastric pain*

2. report signs and symptoms of overdose (persistent nausea and vomiting, headache, exaggerated reflexes, fine muscle tremors, rapid pulse, seizures)

3. take medication on a regular basis *to maintain therapeutic blood levels*

4. have blood theophylline levels evaluated periodically.

2. Instruct client to consult health care provider before taking additional prescription and nonprescription medications.

10.c. The client will state signs and symptoms to report to the health care provider.

10.c. Instruct client to report:

1. increasing agitation (this could be a side effect of medication therapy and health care provider may be able to alter type, dose, or scheduling of medication)

2. asthma attack that is not controlled by usual methods

3. increased need for medications to prevent or treat asthma attacks

4. increasing frequency of asthma attacks
5. decreasing activity tolerance and increased shortness of breath
6. temperature elevation lasting longer than 3 days
7. cough productive of green, purulent, or rust-colored sputum
8. signs and symptoms of theophylline overdose (see action b.1.e.2 in this diagnosis).

10.d. The client will identify community resources that can assist in making necessary life-style changes and coping with the effects of asthma.	10.d.1. Provide information on community resources that can assist client to make necessary life-style changes and cope with the effects of asthma (e.g. American Lung Association, stop smoking programs, stress management classes, counseling services, vocational rehabilitation agencies). 2. Initiate a referral if indicated.

10.e. The client will verbalize an understanding of and a plan for adhering to recommended follow-up care including chest physiotherapy and future appointments with health care provider.	10.e.1. Reinforce the importance of keeping future appointments with health care provider and having periodic laboratory studies as prescribed.
	 2. Reinforce instructions regarding chest physiotherapy (e.g. oxygen administration, postural drainage, chest percussion and vibration, breathing exercises) if indicated. Allow time for questions, clarification, and return demonstration.
	 3. Implement measures *to improve client compliance:*
	   a. include significant others in teaching sessions if possible
	   b. encourage questions and allow time for reinforcement and clarification of information provided
	   c. provide written instructions on scheduled appointments with health care provider, medications prescribed, signs and symptoms to report, and future laboratory and pulmonary function studies.

UNIT
IX

Cancer of the Lung

Cancer of the lung, a malignant neoplasm involving lung tissue, is the leading cause of cancer-related deaths in the United States today. The rising incidence of cancer of the lung in both men and women is related to several factors, the chief of which is smoking. Other factors include environmental pollution and occupational exposure to carcinogens such as asbestos, radioactive substances, arsenic, nickel, iron oxide, and chromium.

Cancer of the lung may occur as a primary tumor or as a metastasis from a primary site elsewhere in the body. The World Health Organization has identified 14 categories of primary lung neoplasms. Over 90% of these arise from the bronchial epithelium and can be grouped into small cell lung cancer (SCLC) or one of the three non–small cell types of lung cancer (NSCLC), which include epidermoid or squamous cell, adenocarcinoma, and large cell. The four histological types of bronchogenic carcinoma vary in relation to where they arise in the lung, responsiveness to the major modes of treatment, pattern of spread, clinical course, and prognosis. Epidermoid and adenocarcinoma are the most common types. Epidermoid is almost always associated with smoking, usually occurs as a central tumor, and produces early symptoms of local disease because of bronchial obstruction. It generally spreads by direct extension to surrounding tissue and has the best 5-year survival rate. Adenocarcinoma occurs most frequently in the periphery of the lungs, has a slow growth rate, tends not to produce symptoms until late in the course of the disease, and occurs more frequently in women and nonsmokers. Large cell tumors are similar to the epidermoid type, although they tend to arise in the peripheral area of the lung. Small cell lung carcinoma tends to occur in the hilar or perihilar area, is a systemic disease at the time of diagnosis, and has a very poor prognosis. It is the type most frequently associated with paraneoplastic syndromes, which may predate x-ray evidence of the lung tumor by many months. The regional lymph nodes, bones, brain, liver, and adrenal glands are common sites of metastasis of lung cancer.

The treatment selected depends on the type of tumor and whether or not metastasis has occurred. The treatment of choice for NSCLC is surgical resection of the tumor if feasible. Radiation therapy may be used adjunctively to surgery or alone for cure or palliation. Clients who present with metastasis at diagnosis are candidates for chemotherapy, although the results in clinical trials have been disappointing. Immunotherapy has also been used with limited success. Aggressive combination chemotherapy is the treatment of choice for SCLC because of the systemic nature of the disease at diagnosis. Response of the client primarily depends on the extensiveness of the disease.

This care plan focuses on the adult client hospitalized for staging and initiation of treatment for cancer of the lung. The goals of care are to reduce fear and anxiety, provide emotional support, relieve symptoms associated with the disease process and its treatment, and educate the client regarding follow-up care. If surgery is planned, this care plan should be used in conjunction with the Care Plan on Lung Surgery.

DISCHARGE CRITERIA

Prior to discharge, the client will:

- identify ways to improve oxygenation status and maximize pulmonary health
- demonstrate proper chest physiotherapy techniques
- identify ways to minimize the risk of infection
- verbalize ways to improve appetite and maintain an adequate nutritional status
- verbalize ways to manage chronic syndrome of inappropriate antidiuretic hormone (SIADH)
- identify ways to prevent injury associated with weakness, fatigue, and/or neuromuscular deficits if they are present
- state signs and symptoms to report to the health care provider
- share thoughts and feelings about the diagnosis of lung cancer, the prognosis, and the effects of the disease process and its treatment on self-concept, life style, and roles
- identify community resources that can assist with home management and adjustment to changes resulting from the diagnosis and the effects of treatment
- verbalize an understanding of and a plan for adhering to recommended follow-up care including future appointments with health care provider, medications prescribed, activity level, and plans for subsequent treatment.

Use in conjunction with the Care Plans on Chemotherapy, External Radiation Therapy, and Immobility if appropriate.

NURSING/COLLABORATIVE DIAGNOSES

1. Anxiety □ *437*
2. Altered respiratory function:
   a. ineffective breathing patterns
   b. ineffective airway clearance
   c. impaired gas exchange □ *438*
3. Altered fluid and electrolyte balance:
   a. hypercalcemia
   b. fluid volume deficit, hyponatremia, hypokalemia, and hypochloremia
   c. metabolic acidosis
   d. metabolic alkalosis □ *440*

UNIT
IX

1. NURSING DIAGNOSIS

Anxiety related to unfamiliar environment; current signs and symptoms; lack of understanding of the diagnosis, staging procedures, and treatment plan; anticipated effects of cancer and its treatment on body functioning and usual life style and roles; and probability of premature death.

DESIRED OUTCOMES	NURSING ACTIONS AND *SELECTED RATIONALES*
1. The client will experience a reduction in fear and anxiety as evidenced by:	1.a. Assess client on admission for: 1. fears, misconceptions, and level of understanding about lung cancer, tests to stage the disease, and possible treatment modes

a. verbalization of feeling less anxious or fearful
b. relaxed facial expression and body movements
c. stable vital signs
d. usual skin color
e. verbalization of an understanding of hospital routines, diagnosis, staging procedures, treatment plan and its effects, and prognosis.

2. perception of anticipated results of diagnostic tests and planned treatment
3. significance of the diagnosis of lung cancer
4. availability of an adequate support system
5. past experiences with cancer and its treatment
6. signs and symptoms of fear and anxiety (e.g. verbalization of fears and concerns; tenseness; tremors; irritability; restlessness; diaphoresis; tachycardia; tachypnea; elevated blood pressure; facial tension, pallor, or flushing; noncompliance with treatment plan).

b. Ascertain effectiveness of current coping skills.
c. Refer to Care Plan on Immobility, Nursing Diagnosis 1, action c, for measures to reduce fear and anxiety.
d. Implement additional measures to reduce fear and anxiety:
  1. explain all diagnostic tests performed to stage lung cancer (tests will vary according to the histological type of tumor and client's symptoms):
     a. chest x-ray and lung scan or tomogram
     b. serial sputum specimens for cytology
     c. bronchoscopy, mediastinoscopy
     d. laser photoradiation
     e. biopsies (may include peripheral nodular lesions; lymph nodes such as scalene, mediastinal, or supraclavicular; pleura; bone marrow [if unexplained anemia present])
     f. barium swallow if esophageal symptoms present
     g. thoracentesis
     h. arterial blood gases
     i. pulmonary function studies
     j. liver, bone, and/or brain scans
     k. blood chemistry
     l. pulmonary angiogram
  2. refer to Nursing Diagnosis 1, action c, in Care Plans on Chemotherapy and External Radiation for measures to reduce fear and anxiety associated with planned treatment
  3. perform actions to reduce pain (see Nursing Diagnosis 6)
  4. perform actions to relieve dyspnea:
     a. perform actions to improve respiratory status (see Nursing Diagnosis 2, action e)
     b. assist client to identify and avoid particular activities that precipitate or increase dyspnea
     c. instruct client in and assist with strategies such as position changes, relaxation exercises, and diversional activities
  5. inform client that the amount of blood in sputum does not necessarily correlate with severity of the disease; provide an opaque, covered container for sputum expectoration and collection to reduce fear associated with hemoptysis
  6. perform actions to assist client to cope with the diagnosis and its implications (see Nursing Diagnosis 17).
e. Include significant others in orientation and teaching sessions and encourage their continued support of client.
f. Provide information based on current needs of client and significant others at a level they can understand. Encourage questions and clarification of information provided.
g. Consult physician if above actions fail to control fear and anxiety.

□ ▬▬▬▬▬▬▬▬▬▬▬▬▬▬▬▬

2. NURSING DIAGNOSIS

Altered respiratory function:*

a. **ineffective breathing patterns** related to:
  1. fear, anxiety, pain
  2. depressant effects of narcotic analgesics

---

* This diagnostic label includes the following nursing diagnoses: ineffective breathing pattern, ineffective airway clearance, and impaired gas exchange (Carpenito, 1989).

3. restricted lung expansion associated with:
   a. paralysis of hemidiaphragm if the tumor involves the phrenic nerve
   b. pleural effusion (may result from obstruction of blood and lymph flow by tumor and/or inflammation in the area surrounding tumor)
   c. weakness
   d. compression of lung tissue by tumor;
b. **ineffective airway clearance** related to:
   1. excessive mucus production associated with inflammation of lung tissue resulting from the disease process
   2. stasis of secretions associated with poor cough effort, airway obstruction due to the presence of tumor, and decreased activity;
c. **impaired gas exchange** related to:
   1. decrease in effective lung surface associated with compression and/or replacement of lung tissue by neoplastic cells
   2. ineffective breathing patterns and airway clearance.

☐ ███

DESIRED OUTCOMES	NURSING ACTIONS AND *SELECTED RATIONALES*

2. The client will experience adequate respiratory function as evidenced by:
   a. normal rate, rhythm, and depth of respirations
   b. decreased dyspnea
   c. usual or improved breath sounds
   d. usual mental status
   e. usual skin color
   f. blood gases within normal range.

2.a. Assess for and report signs and symptoms of altered respiratory function:
   1. rapid, shallow, slow, or irregular respirations
   2. dyspnea, orthopnea
   3. use of accessory muscles when breathing
   4. adventitious breath sounds (e.g. crackles, wheezes)
   5. diminished or absent breath sounds
   6. restlessness, irritability
   7. confusion, somnolence
   8. dusky or cyanotic skin color.
 b. Monitor blood gases. Report abnormal results.
 c. Monitor for and report significant changes in ear oximetry and capnograph results.
 d. Monitor chest x-ray results and report abnormalities.
 e. Implement measures *to improve respiratory status:*
   1. place client in a semi- to high Fowler's position; position overbed table so client can lean on it if desired
   2. perform actions to reduce fear and anxiety (see Nursing Diagnosis 1, actions c and d)
   3. perform actions to reduce pain (see Nursing Diagnosis 6)
   4. instruct client to breathe slowly if he/she is hyperventilating
   5. maintain oxygen therapy as ordered
   6. instruct and assist client to turn every 2 hours if mobility is impaired
   7. instruct client to deep breathe and use inspiratory exerciser at least every 2 hours
   8. perform actions *to facilitate removal of pulmonary secretions:*
      a. instruct and assist client to cough every 1–2 hours; splint chest *to increase comfort and effectiveness*
      b. implement measures *to liquefy tenacious secretions:*
         1. maintain a fluid intake of 2500 cc/day unless contraindicated
         2. humidify inspired air as ordered
         3. assist with administration of mucolytic agents via nebulizer or IPPB treatments
      c. assist with or perform postural drainage, percussion, and vibration if ordered
      d. perform tracheal suctioning if needed
      e. monitor for therapeutic and nontherapeutic effects of expectorants if administered
   9. instruct client to avoid gas-forming foods/fluids (e.g. beans, cauliflower, cabbage, onions, carbonated beverages) and large meals *in order to prevent abdominal distention and increased pressure on the diaphragm*
   10. discourage smoking *(smoking irritates the respiratory tract, causes an increase in mucus production, impairs ciliary function, and decreases oxygen availability)*

UNIT IX

11. protect client from exposure to irritating substances (e.g. smoke, flowers, perfume)
12. increase activity as tolerated
13. administer central nervous system depressants (e.g. narcotics, sedatives) judiciously; hold medications and consult physician if respiratory rate is less than 12/minute
14. monitor for therapeutic and nontherapeutic effects of the following medications if administered:
    a. corticosteroids *to decrease inflammation*
    b. bronchodilators
    c. chemotherapeutic agents *to reduce tumor mass*
15. assist with thoracentesis if performed *to remove excessive pleural fluid and improve lung expansion*
16. prepare client for laser treatment if planned *to remove bronchial obstruction.*

f. Consult physician if signs and symptoms of impaired respiratory function persist or worsen.

3. NURSING/COLLABORATIVE DIAGNOSIS

Altered fluid and electrolyte balance:

a. **hypercalcemia** related to:
   1. demineralization of the bone associated with decreased activity and metastasis to the bone if it has occurred
   2. ectopic production of parathyroid hormone or other osteolytic substance by tumor cells;
b. **fluid volume deficit, hyponatremia, hypokalemia, and hypochloremia** related to:
   1. decreased oral intake associated with:
      a. anorexia
      b. dysphagia and oral, pharyngeal, and esophageal pain resulting from mucositis due to chemotherapy
      c. nausea
   2. excessive loss of fluid and electrolytes associated with:
      a. persistent vomiting resulting from side effects of radiation therapy and/or chemotherapy
      b. diarrhea resulting from side effects of chemotherapy;
c. **metabolic acidosis** related to hyponatremia and persistent diarrhea associated with side effects of chemotherapy;
d. **metabolic alkalosis** related to hypokalemia, hypochloremia, and persistent vomiting associated with side effects of radiation therapy and/or chemotherapy.

DESIRED OUTCOMES	NURSING ACTIONS AND *SELECTED RATIONALES*
3.a. The client will maintain a safe serum calcium level (see Care Plan on Immobility, Collaborative Diagnosis 5, for outcome criteria).	3.a. Refer to Care Plan on Immobility, Collaborative Diagnosis 5, for measures related to assessment, prevention, and treatment of hypercalcemia.
3.b. The client will maintain fluid, electrolyte, and acid-base balance (see Care Plan on External Radiation, Nursing Diagnosis 2, outcomes a and b, for outcome criteria).	3.b. Refer to Care Plan on External Radiation, Nursing Diagnosis 2, actions a and b, for measures related to assessment and management of fluid, electrolyte, and acid-base balance.

4. NURSING DIAGNOSIS

Altered nutrition: less than body requirements related to:*

a. decreased oral intake associated with:
   1. anorexia resulting from:
      a. depression, fear, and anxiety
      b. fatigue and discomfort
      c. taste alteration associated with:
         1. change in the sense of smell and the threshold for bitter, sweet, sour, and salt taste (particularly red meat, coffee, tea, tomatoes, and chocolate) related to the release of tumor byproducts into the bloodstream
         2. zinc, copper, nickel, niacin, and vitamin A deficiency and increased serum levels of calcium and lactate related to the disease process
      d. alteration in the metabolism of proteins, fats, and carbohydrates
      e. early satiety associated with direct stimulation of the satiety center by an-orexigenic factors (e.g. peptides) secreted by tumor cells
      f. increased concentration of neurotransmitters in the brain and/or derange-ments in the serotoninergic system associated with the disease process
   2. pharyngeal and esophageal pain resulting from mucositis associated with side effects of radiation therapy to upper chest and/or cytotoxic drugs
   3. dysphagia and nausea
   4. oral pain resulting from stomatitis associated with side effects of cytotoxic drugs;
b. loss of nutrients associated with persistent vomiting;
c. elevated metabolic rate associated with an increased and continuous energy uti-lization by rapidly proliferating malignant cells;
d. utilization of available nutrients by the malignant cells rather than the host;
e. failure of feeding center to induce a sufficient increase in the intake of food to match increase in metabolic needs;
f. inefficient and accelerated metabolism of proteins, fats, and carbohydrates as-sociated with the disease process.

---

* Some of the etiologic factors presented here are currently under investigation.

DESIRED OUTCOMES	NURSING ACTIONS AND *SELECTED RATIONALES*
4. The client will maintain an adequate nutritional status (see Care Plan on External Radiation, Nursing Diagnosis 3, for outcome criteria).	4. Refer to Care Plan on External Radiation, Nursing Diagnosis 3, for measures related to assessment and promotion of an optimal nutritional status.

5. NURSING DIAGNOSIS

Impaired swallowing related to:

a. esophageal invasion or compression by tumor;
b. oral, pharyngeal, and esophageal pain;
c. dry mouth and viscous oral secretions associated with changes in the quantity and quality of saliva resulting from stomatitis and decreased oral intake.

UNIT
IX

DESIRED OUTCOMES	NURSING ACTIONS AND *SELECTED RATIONALES*
5. The client will experience an improvement in swallowing (see Care Plan on External Radiation, Nursing Diagnosis 4, for outcome criteria).	5. Refer to Care Plan on External Radiation, Nursing Diagnosis 4, for measures related to assessment and improvement of impaired swallowing.

□ ▬▬▬▬▬▬▬▬▬▬▬▬▬▬▬▬▬▬▬▬▬▬▬

6. NURSING DIAGNOSIS

Pain:

a. **tissue and skeletal pain** related to pressure from tumor and enlarged lymph nodes, nerve involvement, excessive coughing episodes, and metastasis to the bone (particularly the ribs, spine, and pelvis) or other organs if it has occurred;

b. **pleuritic pain** related to inflammation and tumor involvement of the parietal pleura;

c. **pain within the irradiated area** related to a cumulative dose of 3200–3600 rads and exposed nerve endings associated with moist desquamation if it occurs;

d. **pharyngeal and esophageal pain** related to inflammation and/or ulceration of the mucosa associated with radiation to upper chest and/or side effects of cytotoxic drugs;

e. **oral pain** related to stomatitis associated with the side effects of cytotoxic drugs.

□ ▬▬▬▬▬▬▬▬▬▬▬▬▬▬▬▬▬▬▬▬▬▬▬

DESIRED OUTCOMES	NURSING ACTIONS AND *SELECTED RATIONALES*

6. The client will experience diminished pain (see Care Plan on External Radiation, Nursing Diagnosis 5.A, for outcome criteria).	6.a. Refer to Care Plan on External Radiation, Nursing Diagnosis 5.A, for measures related to assessment and management of pain.
	b. Implement additional measures *to reduce pain:*
	  1. perform actions *to reduce bone pain:*
	    a. move client carefully; obtain adequate assistance when needed
	    b. when turning client, log roll and support all extremities
	    c. utilize smooth motions when moving client; avoid pushing or pulling on body parts
	    d. caution client to avoid sudden twisting or turning
	    e. provide a firm mattress or place a bed board under mattress for added support
	    f. utilize a bed cradle *to protect affected extremities from excessive weight of bed linens*
	    g. monitor for therapeutic and nontherapeutic effects of anti-inflammatory agents if administered
	  2. perform actions *to reduce pleuritic pain:*
	    a. instruct and assist client to splint chest with hands or pillow when deep breathing, coughing, and changing position
	    b. position on affected side for 2-hour periods *to reduce stretching of the inflamed pleura*
	    c. assist with an intercostal nerve block if performed *for intractable pain*
	  3. perform actions to control coughing (see Nursing Diagnosis 11, action b.4).

7. NURSING DIAGNOSIS

Impaired verbal communication related to:

a. mucositis of the pharynx associated with chemotherapy and/or radiation therapy to tumor site;
b. hoarseness associated with involvement of the recurrent laryngeal nerve by tumor extension into the mediastinum.

DESIRED OUTCOMES	NURSING ACTIONS AND *SELECTED RATIONALES*
7. The client will communicate needs and desires effectively.	7. Refer to Care Plan on External Radiation, Nursing Diagnosis 6, for measures related to assessment and management of impaired verbal communication.

8. NURSING DIAGNOSIS

Fatigue related to:

a. accumulation of cellular waste products associated with rapid lysis of cancerous and normal cells exposed to cytotoxic drugs and/or radiation;
b. inability to rest and sleep;
c. anxiety and depression associated with the diagnosis, the treatment regimen and its effects, the need to alter usual activities, and the inability to fulfill usual roles;
d. increased energy expenditure associated with dyspnea and an increase in the basal metabolic rate resulting from continuous, active tumor growth.

DESIRED OUTCOMES	NURSING ACTIONS AND *SELECTED RATIONALES*

8. The client will experience a reduction in fatigue (see Care Plan on External Radiation, Nursing Diagnosis 9, for outcome criteria).	8.a. Refer to Care Plan on External Radiation, Nursing Diagnosis 9, for measures related to assessment, prevention, and management of fatigue.
	b. Implement additional measures *to promote rest and reduce fatigue:*
	  1. perform actions to reduce pain (see Nursing Diagnosis 6)
	  2. perform actions to relieve dyspnea (see Nursing Diagnosis 1, action d.4)
	  3. perform actions to promote sleep (see Nursing Diagnosis 11).

9. NURSING DIAGNOSIS

Activity intolerance related to:

a. tissue hypoxia associated with impaired alveolar gas exchange and anemia (caused by chemotherapy-induced bone marrow suppression and nutritional deficits);
b. malnutrition;
c. inability to rest and sleep.

UNIT
IX

DESIRED OUTCOMES	NURSING ACTIONS AND *SELECTED RATIONALES*

9. The client will demonstrate an increased tolerance for activity (see Care Plan on External Radiation, Nursing Diagnosis 10, for outcome criteria).	9.a. Refer to Care Plan on External Radiation, Nursing Diagnosis 10, for measures related to assessment and improvement of activity tolerance.
	b. Implement additional measures *to promote rest and improve activity tolerance:*
	  1. perform actions to reduce pain (see Nursing Diagnosis 6)
	  2. perform actions to relieve dyspnea (see Nursing Diagnosis 1, action d.4)
	  3. perform actions to promote sleep (see Nursing Diagnosis 11)
	  4. perform actions to improve respiratory status (see Nursing Diagnosis 2, action e) *in order to improve tissue oxygenation*
	  5. if oxygen therapy is necessary during activity, keep portable oxygen equipment readily available for client's use.

10. NURSING DIAGNOSIS

Self-care deficit related to activity intolerance, fatigue, and discomfort associated with the disease process, diagnostic tests, and/or the side effects of radiation therapy or treatment with cytotoxic drugs.

DESIRED OUTCOMES	NURSING ACTIONS AND *SELECTED RATIONALES*

10. The client will demonstrate increased participation in self-care activities within limitations imposed by the disease process and treatment plan.	10.a. Refer to Care Plan on External Radiation, Nursing Diagnosis 11, for measures related to assessment of, planning for, and meeting client's self-care needs.
	b. Implement additional measures *to further facilitate client's ability to perform self-care:*
	  1. perform actions to reduce fatigue and improve activity tolerance (see Nursing Diagnoses 8 and 9)
	  2. perform actions to reduce pain (see Nursing Diagnosis 6).

11. NURSING DIAGNOSIS

Sleep pattern disturbance related to fear, anxiety, unfamiliar environment, decreased activity, persistent cough, frequent assessments and treatments, inability to assume usual sleep position due to orthopnea, and discomfort associated with the disease process and side effects of treatment.

DESIRED OUTCOMES	NURSING ACTIONS AND *SELECTED RATIONALES*
11. The client will attain optimal amounts of sleep within the parameters of the treatment	11.a. Refer to Care Plan on Immobility, Nursing Diagnosis 12, for measures related to assessment and promotion of sleep. b. Implement additional measures *to promote sleep:*

regimen (see Care Plan on Immobility, Nursing Diagnosis 12, for outcome criteria).

1. perform actions to reduce fear and anxiety (see Nursing Diagnosis 1, actions c and d)
2. perform actions to improve respiratory status (see Nursing Diagnosis 2, action e) *in order to relieve orthopnea*
3. perform actions to reduce pain (see Nursing Diagnosis 6)
4. perform actions *to control coughing:*
   a. instruct client to avoid intake of very hot or cold foods/fluids *(these can stimulate cough)*
   b. protect client from irritants (e.g. flowers, smoke, powder)
   c. encourage client not to smoke *(smoking irritates the respiratory tract)*
   d. humidify inspired air as ordered
   e. monitor for therapeutic and nontherapeutic effects of antitussives if administered
5. assist client to assume a comfortable sleep position (e.g. bed in reverse Trendelenburg position with client in usual recumbent sleep position, head of bed elevated with arms supported on pillows, resting forward on overbed table with good pillow support, sitting in chair)
6. ensure good room ventilation
7. maintain oxygen therapy during sleep if indicated.

12. NURSING DIAGNOSIS

Altered thought processes: slowed verbal responses, impaired memory, irritability, shortened attention span, and/or confusion related to:

a. cerebral hypoxia associated with decreased oxygen-carrying capacity of the blood due to anemia and impaired alveolar gas exchange;
b. depressant effects of hypercalcemia on the central nervous system.

UNIT IX

DESIRED OUTCOMES	NURSING ACTIONS AND *SELECTED RATIONALES*
12. The client will experience an improvement in thought processes as evidenced by: a. improved verbal response time b. improved memory c. longer attention span d. absence of irritability and confusion.	12.a. Assess client for alterations in thought processes (e.g. slowed verbal responses, impaired memory, shortened attention span, irritability, confusion). b. Ascertain from significant others client's usual level of intellectual functioning. c. Implement measures *to maintain optimal thought processes:* 1. perform actions to improve respiratory status (see Nursing Diagnosis 2, action e) 2. perform actions to prevent and treat hypercalcemia (see Care Plan on Immobility, Collaborative Diagnosis 5, action b). d. If client shows evidence of altered thought processes: 1. allow adequate time for communication and performance of activities 2. repeat instructions as necessary using clear, simple language 3. reorient client to person, place, and time as necessary 4. write out a schedule of activities for client to refer to if desired 5. encourage significant others to be supportive of client; instruct them to reorient client as necessary 6. inform client and significant others that intellectual and emotional functioning usually improve once serum calcium levels have returned to normal and oxygenation has improved 7. consult physician if alterations in thought processes persist or worsen.

☐ ▬▬▬▬▬▬▬▬▬▬▬▬▬▬▬▬▬▬▬▬▬▬▬

13. NURSING DIAGNOSIS

Potential for infection related to:

a. stasis of pulmonary secretions associated with airway obstruction, poor cough effort, and decreased activity;
b. decreased resistance to infection associated with malnutrition, general debilitation, and immunosuppressive side effects of cytotoxic drugs;
c. break in skin integrity associated with radiation-induced desquamation.

☐ ▬▬▬▬▬▬▬▬▬▬▬▬▬▬▬▬▬▬▬▬▬▬▬

DESIRED OUTCOMES	NURSING ACTIONS AND *SELECTED RATIONALES*
13. The client will not develop infection (see Care Plan on External Radiation, Nursing Diagnosis 14, for outcome criteria).	13.a. Refer to Care Plan on External Radiation, Nursing Diagnosis 14, for measures related to assessment, prevention, and treatment of infection. b. Implement measures to facilitate removal of pulmonary secretions (see Nursing Diagnosis 2, action e.8) *in order to prevent pneumonia.*

☐ ▬▬▬▬▬▬▬▬▬▬▬▬▬▬▬▬▬▬▬▬▬▬▬

14. NURSING DIAGNOSIS

Potential for trauma related to falls associated with:

a. confusion and lethargy resulting from impaired gas exchange and hypercalcemia;
b. weakness resulting from nutritional and sleep deficits, anemia, impaired alveolar gas exchange, fluid and electrolyte imbalances, and side effects of radiation therapy and/or chemotherapy.

☐ ▬▬▬▬▬▬▬▬▬▬▬▬▬▬▬▬▬▬▬▬▬▬▬

DESIRED OUTCOMES	NURSING ACTIONS AND *SELECTED RATIONALES*

14. The client will not experience falls.	14.a. Determine whether conditions predisposing client to falls (e.g. weakness, lethargy, confusion) exist.
	b. Refer to Care Plan on External Radiation, Nursing Diagnosis 15, action b, for measures related to prevention of falls.
	c. Implement additional measures *to reduce risk of falls:*
	  1. perform actions to prevent or treat hypercalcemia (see Care Plan on Immobility, Collaborative Diagnosis 5, action b) *in order to help maintain mental alertness and normal neuromuscular function*
	  2. perform actions to improve respiratory status (see Nursing Diagnosis 2, action e) *in order to facilitate gas exchange and reduce cerebral hypoxia*
	  3. perform actions to reduce fatigue and improve activity tolerance (see Nursing Diagnoses 8 and 9)
	  4. if client is confused or irrational:
	    a. reorient frequently to surroundings and necessity of adhering to safety precautions
	    b. provide constant supervision (e.g. staff member, significant other) if indicated
	    c. use jacket or wrist restraints or safety alarm device if necessary *to reduce risk of client's getting out of bed or chair unattended*
	    d. monitor for therapeutic and nontherapeutic effects of antianxiety and antipsychotic medications if administered.

    d. Include client and significant others in planning and implementing
       measures to prevent falls.
    e. If falls occur, initiate appropriate first aid and notify physician.

15.A. COLLABORATIVE DIAGNOSIS

Potential pulmonary complications:

1. **atelectasis** related to bronchial obstruction by secretions or tumor and restricted lung expansion associated with presence of tumor, enlarged lymph nodes, or pleural effusion;
2. **lung abscess** related to stasis of secretions and necrosis of tissue within and around tumor.

DESIRED OUTCOMES	NURSING ACTIONS AND *SELECTED RATIONALES*
15.A.1. The client will not develop atelectasis (refer to Care Plan on Immobility, Collaborative Diagnosis 14, outcome b, for outcome criteria).	15.A.1.a. Refer to Care Plan on Immobility, Collaborative Diagnosis 14, action b, for measures related to assessment, prevention, and treatment of atelectasis. b. Implement measures to improve respiratory status (see Nursing Diagnosis 2, action e) *in order to further reduce risk of atelectasis.*

15.A.2. The client will not develop a lung abscess as evidenced by:
a. absence of chills and fever
b. vital signs within normal range for client
c. usual breath sounds for client
d. resonant percussion note over lungs
e. cough productive of clear mucus only
f. no increase in chest pain.
	15.A.2.a. Assess for and report signs and symptoms of a lung abscess (e.g. chills; fever; tachycardia; tachypnea; diminished or absent breath sounds; dull percussion note over a particular lung area; cough productive of purulent, foul-smelling sputum; increased chest pain).
	b. Monitor chest x-ray and lung scan results. Report findings of lung abscess.
	c. Implement measures *to prevent pooling of pulmonary secretions:*
	  1. instruct and assist client to turn every 2 hours if mobility is impaired
	  2. perform actions to facilitate removal of pulmonary secretions (see Nursing Diagnosis 2, action e.8).
	d. If signs and symptoms of a lung abscess occur:
	  1. implement measures to improve respiratory status (see Nursing Diagnosis 2, action e)
	  2. prepare client for surgical drainage of abscess if indicated
	  3. monitor for therapeutic and nontherapeutic effects of anti-infectives if administered
	  4. provide emotional support to client and significant others.

15.B. COLLABORATIVE DIAGNOSIS

Potential metastatic extrapulmonary manifestations of cancer of the lung:

1. **Pancoast's syndrome** related to invasion of adjacent structures such as the brachial plexus, ribs, spine, and sympathetic nerve trunks by a superior sulcus (thoracic inlet) tumor (occurs most frequently with squamous cell carcinoma);
2. **superior vena cava syndrome (SVCS)** related to obstruction of the superior vena cava associated with extrinsic pressure by tumor or enlarged lymph nodes, intraluminal thrombosis, or invasion of venous wall by tumor cells (occurs most frequently with a superior mediastinal or hilar mass);

3. **pathologic fractures** related to demineralization of the bone associated with bone metastasis if it has occurred and complicated further by disuse osteoporosis resulting from decreased activity.

DESIRED OUTCOMES	NURSING ACTIONS AND *SELECTED RATIONALES*

15.B.1. The client will experience optimal relief of symptoms associated with Pancoast's syndrome as evidenced by:
  a. reduced pain in shoulder, scapular area, upper chest, arm, neck, and axilla
  b. reduction of signs and symptoms of Horner's syndrome.

15.B.1.a. Assess for and report signs and symptoms of Pancoast's syndrome:
  1. pain in shoulder, scapular area, upper chest, arm, neck, or axilla
  2. ipsilateral miosis, partial ptosis, enophthalmos, and flushing with inability to sweat (these signs and symptoms are indicative of Horner's syndrome, which is part of Pancoast's syndrome and occurs when tumor spreads into inferior cervical sympathetic ganglion).
  b. If signs and symptoms of Pancoast's syndrome occur:
    1. prepare client for percutaneous needle biopsy of tumor
    2. administer analgesics as ordered
    3. prepare client for external radiation therapy and en bloc resection of the tumor if indicated
    4. provide emotional support to client and significant others.

15.B.2. The client will experience optimal relief of symptoms associated with SVCS as evidenced by:
  a. decreased dyspnea
  b. absence of edema of face, arms, and hands
  c. absence of plethora
  d. absence of hoarseness, increased chest pain, headache, vertigo, blurred vision
  e. usual mental status.

15.B.2.a. Assess for and report signs and symptoms of SVCS (e.g. increased dyspnea; swelling of the face, arms, or hands; erythema of face, neck, or upper trunk [plethora]; prominent superficial veins over upper body; hoarseness; increased chest pain; headache; vertigo; blurred vision; confusion; lethargy; seizures). Symptoms may become more pronounced if client bends forward or lies flat for an extended period.
  b. If signs and symptoms of SVCS occur:
    1. prepare client for the following diagnostic tests if planned:
      a. chest x-ray, computed tomography
      b. invasive studies such as bronchoscopy, lymph node and bone marrow biopsies, thoracentesis, mediastinoscopy, or limited thoracotomy *to determine histological diagnosis and appropriate treatment* (controversy exists regarding the use of invasive procedures and the need to establish a tissue diagnosis prior to initiation of treatment)
    2. implement measures to improve respiratory status (see Nursing Diagnosis 2, action e) *in order to decrease dyspnea*
    3. elevate arms on pillows *to reduce edema*
    4. prepare client for the following if planned (intervention selected depends on etiology, type of obstruction, and severity of symptoms):
      a. external radiation therapy (treatment of choice for NSCLC with a reduction of symptoms usually occurring within 3–7 days after initiation of treatment)
      b. combination chemotherapy if histological diagnosis is SCLC (drugs are usually administered via lower extremity vein *because of impaired blood flow in arms*)
      c. surgery such as superior vena cava bypass or radical excision of SVC with grafting if SVCS is due to thrombosis or if client is experiencing severe symptoms such as airway obstruction or cerebral compromise (symptom relief is usually attained within 48 hours)
    5. monitor for therapeutic and nontherapeutic effects of the following medications if administered:
      a. anticonvulsants *to control seizures resulting from cerebral edema*
      b. corticosteroids *to decrease inflammation and edema at site of obstruction of superior vena cava*
      c. diuretics *to reduce edema* particularly if client is experiencing respiratory distress (provide only temporary relief and are used cautiously *because they can further decrease venous return*)
      d. thrombolytic agents (e.g. urokinase, tissue plasminogen activator [tPA], streptokinase) if etiology is intraluminal thrombosis

e. anticoagulants (e.g. heparin, warfarin) *to prevent thrombus formation as a result of venous stasis*
6. initiate appropriate emergency care if respiratory arrest, tracheal obstruction, and/or seizures occur
7. provide emotional support to client and significant others.

15.B.3. The client will not experience pathologic fractures (see Care Plan on Immobility, Collaborative Diagnosis 14, outcome e, for outcome criteria).

15.B.3. Refer to Care Plan on Immobility, Collaborative Diagnosis 14, action e, for measures related to assessment, prevention, and treatment of pathologic fractures.

15.C. COLLABORATIVE DIAGNOSIS

Potential nonmetastatic extrapulmonary manifestations of lung cancer:

1. **syndrome of inappropriate antidiuretic hormone (SIADH)** related to the unregulated synthesis and secretion of antidiuretic hormone (ADH) by tumor cells (occurs particularly with SCLC) and accentuated by the increased levels of ADH resulting from pain and stress;
2. **neuromuscular syndromes** (e.g. peripheral neuropathy, Eaton-Lambert syndrome, corticocerebellar degeneration) of unknown etiology (most are associated with SCLC);
3. **hypertrophic pulmonary osteoarthropathy** (may include clubbing of digits; inflammation of joints; and edema of feet, hands, or legs) of unknown etiology and primarily associated with epidermoid or adenocarcinoma of the lung;
4. **atypical Cushing's syndrome** related to bilateral adrenocortical hyperplasia associated with ectopic adrenocorticotropic hormone (ACTH) production.

DESIRED OUTCOMES	NURSING ACTIONS AND *SELECTED RATIONALES*

15.C.1. The client will experience a reduction in symptoms of SIADH if it develops as evidenced by:
  a. decline in weight toward normal
  b. balanced intake and output
  c. usual mental status
  d. absence of headache, muscle weakness, cellular edema, abdominal cramping, nausea, vomiting, seizure activity
  e. serum and urine sodium and osmolality levels within normal limits.

15.C.1.a. Assess for and report signs and symptoms of SIADH:
  1. sudden weight gain
  2. intake greater than output
  3. lethargy, confusion
  4. complaints of persistent headache
  5. muscle weakness
  6. fingerprint edema over sternum (indicative of cellular edema)
  7. abdominal cramping, nausea, vomiting
  8. seizures
  9. urine specific gravity greater than 1.012
  10. elevated urine sodium and osmolality levels
  11. low serum sodium and osmolality levels.
  b. Implement measures *to prevent accentuation of SIADH if it occurs:*
    1. perform actions to reduce pain (see Nursing Diagnosis 6)
    2. perform actions to reduce fear and anxiety (see Nursing Diagnosis 1, actions c and d).
  c. If signs and symptoms of SIADH occur:
    1. maintain fluid restrictions if ordered (usually 500–1000 cc/day) *to prevent further fluid retention*
    2. encourage intake of foods/fluids high in sodium (e.g. cured meats, processed cheese, soups, catsup, pickles, salty snacks, tomato juice, canned vegetables, bouillon)

3. initiate routine seizure precautions until serum sodium levels return to normal
4. monitor for therapeutic and nontherapeutic effects of the following if administered:
   a. diuretics (usually furosemide) *to aid in water excretion*
   b. infusions of normal or hypertonic saline solutions *to treat hyponatremia*
   c. lithium carbonate and demeclocycline *to promote water excretion (inhibit action of ADH at the renal tubular level)*
   d. urea *to promote osmotic diuresis*
5. prepare client for treatment of the underlying malignancy if planned
6. provide emotional support to client and significant others.

15.C.2. The client will attain optimal neuromuscular function as evidenced by:
  a. improved sensory and motor function
  b. improved mental status.

15.C.2.a. Assess for and report signs and symptoms of neuromuscular manifestations of lung cancer:
   1. weakness of proximal muscle groups particularly the pelvic girdle and thigh, usually manifested by difficulty in rising from a chair (indicative of Eaton-Lambert syndrome)
   2. paresthesias, loss of motor function of extremities
   3. vertigo, ataxia, dysarthria, dementia.
  b. If signs and symptoms of neuromuscular deficits occur:
   1. implement measures *to protect client from injury:*
      a. perform actions to prevent falls (see Nursing Diagnosis 14, actions b and c)
      b. perform actions *to prevent burns if paresthesias are present:*
         1. let hot foods or fluids cool slightly before serving *to reduce risk of burns if spills occur*
         2. supervise client while smoking if indicated
         3. assess temperature of bath water and heating pad before and during use
   2. implement measures to assist client to meet self-care needs (see Nursing Diagnosis 10)
   3. assist with range of motion and repetitive exercises of involved muscle groups *in order to improve muscle strength in client with Eaton-Lambert syndrome*
   4. monitor for therapeutic and nontherapeutic effects of guanidine hydrochloride if administered to client with Eaton-Lambert syndrome
   5. prepare client for treatment of underlying malignancy *(may result in regression of some symptoms)*
   6. provide emotional support to client and significant others.

15.C.3. The client will experience a reduction in symptoms associated with hypertrophic pulmonary osteoarthropathy if it develops as evidenced by:
  a. diminished joint swelling and pain
  b. ability to move joints freely
  c. reduced edema of feet, lower legs, and/or hands.

15.C.3.a. Assess for and report signs and symptoms of hypertrophic pulmonary osteoarthropathy (e.g. clubbing of digits; painful inflammation of joints; limitation of joint movement; edema of feet, lower legs, and/or hands).
  b. If signs and symptoms of hypertrophic pulmonary osteoarthropathy occur:
   1. implement measures to prevent falls (see Nursing Diagnosis 14, actions b and c)
   2. assist client with activities of daily living as necessary
   3. monitor for therapeutic and nontherapeutic effects of anti-inflammatory agents if administered
   4. prepare client for treatment of underlying malignancy if indicated *(reduction of tumor will result in a rapid regression of symptoms).*

15.C.4. The client will experience relief of symptoms associated with atypical Cushing's syndrome if it occurs as evidenced by:
  a. body weight returning toward normal
  b. increased muscle strength

15.C.4.a. Assess for and report signs and symptoms of atypical Cushing's syndrome (e.g. significant weight loss, muscle weakness, facial edema, mild hypertension, hyperglycemia, increased serum sodium, decreased serum potassium, increased pH and CO_2 content, increase in skin pigmentation).
  b. If signs and symptoms of atypical Cushing's syndrome occur:
   1. monitor for therapeutic and nontherapeutic effects of metyrapone or aminoglutethimide if administered *to inhibit adrenal steroid synthesis*

c. resolution of facial edema
d. B/P within normal range for client
e. serum glucose, sodium, and potassium within normal range
f. blood gases within normal range for client.

2. prepare client for treatment of the underlying malignancy if planned
3. provide emotional support to client and significant others.

---

16. NURSING DIAGNOSIS

Disturbance in self-concept* related to:

a. loss of normal body function;
b. change in appearance (e.g. excessive weight loss, hair loss associated with che-motherapy, skin changes associated with radiation therapy, gynecomastia asso-ciated with ectopic hormone production by tumor cells);
c. sterility associated with gonadal dysfunction resulting from cytotoxic drug therapy;
d. changes in sexual functioning associated with weakness, fatigue, dyspnea, pain, and anxiety;
e. dependence on others to meet self-care needs;
f. stigma associated with the diagnosis of cancer;
g. anticipated changes in life style and roles associated with effects of the disease process and its treatment.

---

* This diagnostic label includes the nursing diagnoses of body image disturbance and self-esteem dis-turbance.

DESIRED OUTCOMES	NURSING ACTIONS AND *SELECTED RATIONALES*
16. The client will demonstrate beginning adaptation to changes in appearance, body functioning, life style, and roles (see Care Plan on External Radiation, Nursing Diagnosis 18, for outcome criteria).	16. Refer to Care Plan on External Radiation, Nursing Diagnosis 18, for measures related to assessment and promotion of a positive self-concept.

---

17. NURSING DIAGNOSIS

Ineffective individual coping related to:

a. persistent discomfort associated with the disease process and the side effects of chemotherapy and/or external radiation therapy;
b. guilt associated with the diagnosis of lung cancer if a personal habit such as smok-ing was the major cause;
c. fear, anxiety, and depression associated with the diagnosis of lung cancer, effects of treatment, and poor prognosis;
d. inadequate support system.

DESIRED OUTCOMES	NURSING ACTIONS AND *SELECTED RATIONALES*
17. The client will demonstrate the use of effective coping skills (see Care Plan on External Radiation, Nursing Diagnosis 19, for outcome criteria).	17.a. Refer to Care Plan on External Radiation, Nursing Diagnosis 19, for measures related to assessment and management of ineffective coping. b. Assist the client to work through feelings of guilt about his/her smoking history.

□ ▬▬▬▬▬▬▬▬▬▬▬▬▬▬▬▬

18. NURSING DIAGNOSIS

Grieving* related to:

a. loss of normal function of the lung;
b. changes in body image associated with extrapulmonary manifestations of the disease and side effects of radiation therapy and/or chemotherapy;
c. alteration in usual life style and roles resulting from the disease process and its treatment;
d. diagnosis of cancer with probability of premature death.

───────────

* This diagnostic label includes anticipatory grieving and grieving following the actual losses/changes.

□ ▬▬▬▬▬▬▬▬▬▬▬▬▬▬▬▬

DESIRED OUTCOMES	NURSING ACTIONS AND *SELECTED RATIONALES*
18. The client will demonstrate beginning progression through the grieving process (see Care Plan on External Radiation, Nursing Diagnosis 20, for outcome criteria).	18. Refer to Care Plan on External Radiation, Nursing Diagnosis 20, for measures related to assessment and facilitation of grieving.

□ ▬▬▬▬▬▬▬▬▬▬▬▬▬▬▬▬

19. NURSING DIAGNOSIS

Knowledge deficit regarding follow-up care.

□ ▬▬▬▬▬▬▬▬▬▬▬▬▬▬▬▬

DESIRED OUTCOMES	NURSING ACTIONS AND *SELECTED RATIONALES*

19.a. The client will identify ways to improve oxygenation status and maximize pulmonary health.	19.a. Instruct client in ways *to improve oxygenation status and maximize pulmonary health:*
	1. schedule adequate rest periods
	2. avoid exposure to respiratory irritants:
	  a. stop smoking
	  b. avoid tobacco smoke, perfume, aerosol cleaners, paint fumes, and solvents whenever possible
	  c. avoid extremely hot and cold temperatures
	3. wear a mask or scarf over nose and mouth if exposure to high levels of irritants such as smoke, fumes, and dust is unavoidable

4. minimize risk of respiratory tract infections:
   a. avoid contact with persons with respiratory tract infections
   b. avoid crowds and poorly ventilated areas
   c. maintain good oral hygiene
   d. adhere to prescribed chest physiotherapy (e.g. postural drainage, vibration, percussion, breathing exercises)
   e. take medications such as bronchodilators, anti-infectives, and mucolytics as prescribed
   f. cleanse all respiratory care equipment properly
   g. drink at least 10 glasses of liquid/day.

19.b. The client will demonstrate proper chest physiotherapy techniques.

19.b.1. Reinforce instructions about chest physiotherapy including:
   a. use of equipment such as oxygen, IPPB machine, inspiratory exerciser, and humidifier
   b. postural drainage, percussion, and vibration techniques.
2. Allow time for questions, clarification, and return demonstration.

19.c. The client will identify ways to minimize the risk of infection.

19.c. Refer to Care Plan on External Radiation, Nursing Diagnosis 21, action g, for instructions related to preventing infection.

19.d. The client will verbalize ways to improve appetite and maintain an adequate nutritional status.

19.d. Refer to Care Plan on External Radiation, Nursing Diagnosis 21, action c, for instructions related to improving appetite and maintaining an adequate nutritional status.

19.e. The client will verbalize ways to manage chronic SIADH.

19.e. Provide the following instructions related to home management of chronic SIADH:
1. continue fluid restriction (usually 1 quart/day) if recommended by physician
2. take medications (e.g. urea, diuretics, demeclocycline) as prescribed
3. increase intake of foods/fluids high in sodium (e.g. cured meats, processed cheese, soups, catsup, pickles, salty snacks, bouillon)
4. increase intake of foods/fluids high in potassium (e.g. bananas, oranges, potatoes, raisins, figs, apricots, dates, tomatoes, Gatorade, most fruit juices) if discharged on a potassium-depleting diuretic
5. report an increase in signs and symptoms of SIADH (e.g. sudden weight gain, intake persistently greater than output, drowsiness, confusion, weakness, headache, nausea, abdominal cramping, seizures).

19.f. The client will identify ways to prevent injury associated with weakness, fatigue, and/or neuromuscular deficits if they are present.

19.f. Provide the following instructions on ways *to prevent injury if weakness, fatigue, and/or neuromuscular deficits are present:*
1. obtain assistance or utilize a cane or walker when ambulating
2. avoid use of ice packs on areas of decreased sensation
3. wear shoes or slippers with nonskid soles and low heels *to prevent falls*
4. reduce risk of burns by:
   a. letting hot foods and fluids cool slightly before eating
   b. testing bath water with a thermometer before use
   c. avoiding use of heating pads and hot water bottles on areas of decreased sensation
5. do not hurry; allow ample time for all activities.

19.g. The client will state signs and symptoms to report to the health care provider.

19.g.1. Instruct client to report the following:
   a. drainage from and/or persistent redness of biopsy site(s)
   b. signs and symptoms of hypercalcemia (e.g nausea, vomiting, increased thirst and urination, muscle weakness, confusion)
   c. persistent fever
   d. difficulty swallowing
   e. excessive weight loss
   f. increasing fatigue, weakness, and shortness of breath
   g. pain in shoulder, arm, or neck
   h. swollen, painful joints
   i. swelling of upper body
   j. persistent headache
   k. increasing cough productive of purulent, foul-smelling, or blood-tinged sputum

UNIT
IX

l. irritability, drowsiness, confusion

m. signs and symptoms of SIADH (see action e.5 in this diagnosis)

n. excessive depression or difficulty coping with the diagnosis.

2. If appropriate, refer to the Care Plan on Chemotherapy, Nursing Diagnosis 24, action l and/or the Care Plan on External Radiation, Nursing Diagnosis 21, action j, for additional signs and symptoms client should report if he/she is receiving chemotherapy and/or radiation therapy.

19.h. The client will identify community resources that can assist with home management and adjustment to changes resulting from the diagnosis and the effects of treatment.

19.h.1. Provide information about and encourage utilization of community resources that can assist client and significant others with home management and adjustment to the diagnosis of lung cancer and effects of prescribed treatment (e.g. American Cancer Society, Visiting Nurse Association, counselors, social service agencies, I Can Cope, Meals on Wheels, local support groups, Hospice).

2. Initiate a referral if indicated.

19.i. The client will verbalize an understanding of and a plan for adhering to recommended follow-up care including future appointments with health care provider, medications prescribed, activity level, and plans for subsequent treatment.

19.i.1. Reinforce physician's explanation of planned radiation therapy and/or chemotherapy schedule if appropriate. Stress importance of strictly following the prescribed protocol for radiation therapy and/or chemotherapy and keeping all appointments for follow-up supervision and laboratory work.

2. Explain rationale for, side effects of, and importance of taking medications prescribed.

3. Emphasize need for planned rest periods and for gauging activity according to tolerance.

4. Implement measures *to improve client compliance:*
   a. include significant others in teaching sessions if possible
   b. encourage questions and allow time for reinforcement and clarification of information provided
   c. provide written instructions regarding scheduled appointments with health care provider and for chemotherapy, radiation therapy, and laboratory work; medications prescribed; and signs and symptoms to report.

Reference

Carpenito LJ. Handbook of nursing diagnosis (3rd ed.). Philadelphia: J.B. Lippincott Company, 1989.

Chronic Obstructive Pulmonary Disease

Chronic obstructive pulmonary disease (COPD) is a term used to describe a group of diseases characterized by an increased resistance to airflow. The two diseases that are most often termed COPD are chronic bronchitis and emphysema.* Although one may be predominant,

* Bronchial asthma is included in the group only if it has resulted in irreversible lung damage and has merged into chronic bronchitis and emphysema.

both conditions are often present in the same person. Chronic bronchitis is defined clinically as a disease characterized by an excessive production of mucus in the bronchi accompanied by a cough that persists at least 3 months of the year for 2 consecutive years. Chronic inflammation of the bronchioles, hypertrophy and hyperplasia of the mucous glands, and thick mucus that cannot be mobilized because of the decreased ciliary activity are factors contributing to narrowing of the bronchioles and diminished airflow. In contrast, emphysema is characterized by dyspnea and only a mild cough. The impaired airflow is related to the loss of lung elasticity, hyperinflation of the alveoli, destruction of alveolar walls, and narrowed airways.

Causative factors of COPD include chronic irritation of the lungs by cigarette smoke, exposure to air pollution and chemical irritants, and recurrent respiratory tract infections. In some cases of emphysema, there is a destruction of lung tissue by proteolytic enzymes as a result of a genetic deficiency of alpha$_1$-antitrypsin. The normal process of aging also contributes to the development of COPD by causing diminished lung function due to loss of elastase with resultant dilation of the alveoli.

Diagnosis and treatment of COPD is usually done on an outpatient basis unless there is an exacerbation of symptoms that necessitates hospitalization. This care plan focuses on care of the adult client with COPD who is hospitalized during an acute exacerbation. Goals of care are to improve respiratory function, prevent complications, and educate the client regarding ways to manage existing symptoms and slow further progression of the disease process.

DISCHARGE CRITERIA

Prior to discharge, the client will:

- identify ways to prevent or minimize further pulmonary damage
- demonstrate proper breathing techniques and chest physiotherapy
- verbalize an understanding of medication therapy including rationale for, side effects of, method of administering, and importance of taking as prescribed
- identify appropriate safety measures related to COPD and its treatment
- state signs and symptoms to report to the health care provider
- share feelings and thoughts about the effects of COPD on life style and roles
- identify community resources that can assist with home management and adjustment to changes resulting from COPD
- verbalize an understanding of and a plan for adhering to recommended follow-up care including future appointments with health care provider and graded exercise program.

UNIT IX

Use in conjunction with the Care Plan on Immobility.

NURSING/COLLABORATIVE DIAGNOSES

1. Anxiety ☐ *456*
2. Altered respiratory function:
   a. ineffective breathing patterns
   b. ineffective airway clearance
   c. impaired gas exchange ☐ *457*
3. Fluid volume deficit ☐ *459*
4. Altered nutrition: less than body requirements ☐ *459*

5. Altered comfort: nausea and vomiting □ *460*
6. Impaired skin integrity: irritation and breakdown □ *461*
7. Altered oral mucous membrane: dryness □ *461*
8. Activity intolerance □ *462*
9. Self-care deficit □ *463*
10. Sleep pattern disturbance □ *463*
11. Potential for infection: pneumonia □ *464*
12. Potential for trauma □ *464*
13. Potential complications:
    a. thromboembolism
    b. gastrointestinal (GI) bleeding
    c. spontaneous pneumothorax
    d. right-sided heart failure
    e. respiratory failure □ *465*
14. Sexual dysfunction:
    a. decreased libido
    b. impotence □ *467*
15. Disturbance in self-concept □ *468*
16. Grieving □ *469*
17. Noncompliance □ *470*
18. Knowledge deficit regarding follow-up care □ *471*

1. NURSING DIAGNOSIS

Anxiety related to unfamiliar environment; dyspnea and feeling of suffocation; lack of understanding of diagnosis, diagnostic tests, treatment plan, and prognosis; and feeling of lack of control over progression of the disease.

DESIRED OUTCOMES	NURSING ACTIONS AND *SELECTED RATIONALES*

1. The client will experience a reduction in fear and anxiety as evidenced by:
   a. verbalization of feeling less anxious or fearful
   b. relaxed facial expression and body movements
   c. stable vital signs
   d. usual skin color
   e. verbalization of an understanding of hospital routines, diagnosis, diagnostic tests, treatments, and prognosis.

1.a. Assess client for signs and symptoms of fear and anxiety (e.g. verbalization of fears and concerns; tenseness; tremors; irritability; restlessness; diaphoresis; elevated blood pressure; increased respiratory rate; tachycardia; facial tension, pallor, or flushing; noncompliance with treatment plan). Validate perceptions carefully, remembering that some behavior may result from tissue hypoxia.
   b. Ascertain effectiveness of current coping skills.
   c. Implement measures *to reduce fear and anxiety:*
      1. maintain a calm, confident manner when interacting with client
      2. do not leave client alone during period of acute respiratory distress
      3. perform actions to improve respiratory status and relieve dyspnea (see Nursing Diagnosis 2, action f)
      4. perform actions *to decrease client's feeling of suffocation:*
         a. open curtains and doors
         b. approach client from the side rather than face-on (*close face-on contact may make client feel closed in*)
         c. limit number of visitors in room at any one time
         d. remove unnecessary equipment from room
         e. administer oxygen via nasal cannula rather than mask if possible

5. encourage significant others to project a caring, concerned attitude without obvious anxiousness
6. once the period of acute respiratory distress has subsided:
   a. introduce staff who will be participating in his/her care; if possible, maintain consistency in staff assigned to his/her care *to provide feelings of stability and comfort with the environment*
   b. orient to hospital environment, equipment, and routines
   c. assure client that staff members are nearby; respond to call signal as soon as possible
   d. provide a calm, restful environment
   e. encourage verbalization of fear and anxiety; provide feedback
   f. reinforce physician's explanations and clarify any misconceptions client may have about COPD, treatment plan, and prognosis
   g. explain all diagnostic tests (e.g. pulmonary function studies, sputum cultures, blood studies, chest x-ray)
   h. instruct in relaxation techniques and encourage participation in diversional activities
   i. assist client to identify factors that have precipitated the exacerbation and discuss methods of controlling these in the future
   j. monitor for therapeutic and nontherapeutic effects of antianxiety agents if administered.
d. Include significant others in orientation and teaching sessions and encourage their continued support of client.
e. Provide information based on current needs of client and significant others at a level they can understand. Encourage questions and clarification of information provided.
f. Consult physician if above actions fail to control fear and anxiety.

2. NURSING DIAGNOSIS

Altered respiratory function:*

a. **ineffective breathing patterns** related to fear, anxiety, and presence of a flattened diaphragm associated with prolonged hyperinflation of the lungs;
b. **ineffective airway clearance** related to:
   1. excessive mucus production and narrowing of the bronchioles associated with inflammation and hyperplasia of the bronchial walls (especially with bronchitis)
   2. narrowing or collapse of bronchioles associated with destruction of lung tissue by proteolytic enzymes (occurs primarily with emphysema)
   3. stasis of secretions associated with impaired ciliary function and poor cough effort;
c. **impaired gas exchange** related to:
   1. ineffective breathing patterns and airway clearance
   2. decrease in effective lung surface associated with destruction and fibrosis of alveolar walls.

---

* This diagnostic label includes the following nursing diagnoses: ineffective breathing pattern, ineffective airway clearance, and impaired gas exchange (Carpenito, 1989).

DESIRED OUTCOMES	NURSING ACTIONS AND *SELECTED RATIONALES*
2. The client will experience adequate respiratory function as evidenced by:	2.a. Assess for signs and symptoms of altered respiratory function: 1. shallow, rapid respirations 2. dyspnea, orthopnea

a. usual rate, rhythm, and depth of respirations
b. decreased dyspnea
c. usual or improved breath sounds
d. usual mental status
e. usual skin color
f. blood gases within normal range for client.

3. use of accessory muscles when breathing
4. adventitious breath sounds (e.g. rhonchi)
5. diminished or absent breath sounds
6. restlessness, irritability
7. confusion, somnolence
8. dusky or cyanotic skin color.

b. Monitor blood gases. Report abnormal results.

c. Monitor for and report significant changes in ear oximetry and capnograph results.

d. Monitor chest x-ray results and report abnormalities.

e. Assist with pulmonary function studies if done *to evaluate respiratory status and/or effectiveness of treatment measures.*

f. Implement measures *to improve respiratory status:*
1. place client in a semi- to high Fowler's position; position overbed table so client can lean on it if desired
2. perform actions to reduce fear and anxiety (see Nursing Diagnosis 1, action c)
3. maintain oxygen therapy as ordered (question any order for high oxygen concentration *since many persons with COPD are dependent on hypoxemia as the stimulus to breathe)*
4. instruct and assist client to turn every 2 hours if mobility is impaired
5. instruct client in and assist with diaphragmatic and pursed-lip breathing techniques
6. instruct client to deep breathe and use inspiratory exerciser at least every 2 hours
7. perform actions *to facilitate removal of pulmonary secretions:*
   a. instruct and assist client to cough every 1–2 hours
   b. implement measures *to liquefy tenacious secretions:*
      1. maintain a fluid intake of at least 2500 cc/day unless contraindicated
      2. humidify inspired air as ordered
      3. assist with administration of mucolytic agents via nebulizer
   c. assist with or perform postural drainage, percussion, and vibration if ordered
   d. perform tracheal suctioning if needed
   e. monitor for therapeutic and nontherapeutic effects of expectorants if administered
8. assist client to apply an elastic abdominal support if indicated *(the support forces the flattened diaphragm higher into thorax)*
9. instruct client to avoid large meals and gas-forming foods/fluids (e.g. beans, cauliflower, cabbage, onions, carbonated beverages) *in order to prevent gastric distention and increased pressure on the diaphragm*
10. discourage smoking *(smoking decreases oxygen availability, increases mucus production, and impairs ciliary function)*
11. protect client from exposure to irritating substances (e.g. smoke, flowers, perfume)
12. increase activity as allowed and tolerated
13. avoid use of central nervous system depressants such as narcotics, sedatives, and muscle relaxants *(these further depress respiratory status)*
14. monitor for therapeutic and nontherapeutic effects of the following medications if administered:
    a. bronchodilators
    b. corticosteroids *to decrease inflammation.*

g. Consult physician if:
1. signs and symptoms of altered respiratory function persist or worsen
2. signs and symptoms of respiratory acidosis (e.g. change in mental status, increased pulse, dizziness, headache, feeling of fullness in head, muscle twitching, seizures, increase in usual $PaCO_2$ and decline in pH) are present.

3. NURSING DIAGNOSIS

Fluid volume deficit related to:

a. increased fluid loss associated with vomiting and hyperventilation (can occur with fear, anxiety, and respiratory acidosis);
b. decreased oral fluid intake associated with anorexia, dyspnea, nausea, weakness, and fatigue.

DESIRED OUTCOMES	NURSING ACTIONS AND *SELECTED RATIONALES*

3. The client will not experience a fluid volume deficit as evidenced by:
   a. normal skin turgor
   b. moist mucous membranes
   c. weight loss no greater than 0.5 kg/day
   d. B/P and pulse within normal range for client and stable with position change
   e. Hct. within normal range for client
   f. balanced intake and output
   g. urine specific gravity between 1.010 and 1.030.

3.a. Assess for and report signs and symptoms of fluid volume deficit:
   1. decreased skin turgor
   2. dry mucous membranes, thirst
   3. weight loss greater than 0.5 kg/day
   4. low B/P and/or decline in systolic B/P of at least 15 mm Hg with concurrent rise in pulse when client sits up
   5. weak, rapid pulse
   6. increase in Hct. level (Hct. may normally be elevated in clients with COPD in an effort to compensate for chronic hypoxemia)
   7. output less than intake with urine specific gravity higher than 1.030 (reflects an actual rather than potential water deficit).
 b. Implement measures *to prevent or treat fluid volume deficit:*
   1. perform actions to prevent vomiting (see Nursing Diagnosis 5, action b)
   2. perform actions *to prevent hyperventilation:*
      a. implement measures to reduce fear and anxiety (see Nursing Diagnosis 1, action c)
      b. implement measures to improve respiratory status (see Nursing Diagnosis 2, action f) *in order to prevent respiratory acidosis, which causes hyperventilation*
   3. encourage a fluid intake of at least 2500 cc/day unless contraindicated
   4. maintain intravenous fluid therapy as ordered.
 c. Consult physician if signs and symptoms of fluid volume deficit persist or worsen.

4. NURSING DIAGNOSIS

Altered nutrition: less than body requirements related to:

a. decreased oral intake associated with:
   1. anorexia resulting from early satiety (can occur due to compression of stomach by flattened diaphragm), constipation, and depression
   2. nausea, dyspnea, weakness, and fatigue;
b. loss of nutrients associated with vomiting;
c. increased metabolic needs associated with increased energy expenditure resulting from strenuous breathing efforts and persistent coughing.

DESIRED OUTCOMES	NURSING ACTIONS AND *SELECTED RATIONALES*

4. The client will maintain an adequate nutritional status as evidenced by:
   a. weight within normal range for client's age, height, and build
   b. normal BUN and serum albumin, protein, cholesterol, and lymphocyte levels
   c. triceps skinfold measurements within normal range
   d. usual strength and activity tolerance
   e. healthy oral mucous membrane.

4.a. Assess client for signs and symptoms of malnutrition:
   1. weight below normal for client's age, height, and build
   2. abnormal BUN and low serum albumin, protein, cholesterol, and lymphocyte levels
   3. triceps skinfold measurement less than normal for build
   4. weakness and fatigue
   5. stomatitis.
 b. Reassess nutritional status on a regular basis and report decline.
 c. Monitor percentage of meals eaten.
 d. Assess client to determine causes of inadequate intake (e.g. nausea, dyspnea, anorexia, weakness, fatigue).
 e. Refer to Care Plan on Immobility, Nursing Diagnosis 6, actions e and g, for measures to maintain an adequate nutritional status.
 f. Implement additional measures *to improve oral intake:*
   1. perform actions to improve respiratory status (see Nursing Diagnosis 2, action f) *in order to relieve dyspnea and reduce fatigue*
   2. perform actions to prevent nausea and vomiting (see Nursing Diagnosis 5, action b)
   3. perform actions to improve self-concept and facilitate grieving (see Nursing Diagnoses 15 and 16, action d) *in order to reduce depression*
   4. place client in a high Fowler's position for meals *to help relieve dyspnea.*
 g. Perform a 72-hour calorie count if nutritional status declines or fails to improve.

---

5. NURSING DIAGNOSIS

Altered comfort: nausea and vomiting related to cortical stimulation of the vomiting center associated with fear, anxiety, and the taste and/or odor of sputum and some aerosol treatments.

DESIRED OUTCOMES	NURSING ACTIONS AND *SELECTED RATIONALES*

5. The client will experience relief of nausea and vomiting as evidenced by:
   a. verbalization of decreased nausea
   b. no episodes of vomiting.

5.a. Assess client to determine factors that contribute to nausea and vomiting (e.g. anxiety, copious sputum production, aerosol treatments).
 b. Implement measures *to prevent nausea and vomiting:*
   1. perform actions to reduce fear and anxiety (see Nursing Diagnosis 1, action c)
   2. eliminate noxious sights and smells from the environment; provide client with an opaque, covered container for expectorated sputum; empty container frequently and remove it from the table during mealtime if it is not needed *(noxious stimuli cause cortical stimulation of the vomiting center)*
   3. encourage client to take deep, slow breaths when nauseated
   4. encourage client to change positions slowly *(movement stimulates the chemoreceptor trigger zone)*
   5. provide oral hygiene after chest physiotherapy, aerosol treatments, and each emesis and before meals
   6. schedule treatments that assist in mobilizing the mucus (e.g. aerosol treatments, postural drainage, percussion, vibration) at least 1 hour before or after meals
   7. provide small, frequent meals rather than 3 large ones
   8. instruct client to ingest foods and fluids slowly

9. instruct client to avoid foods/fluids that irritate the gastric mucosa (e.g. spicy foods; citrus fruits or juices; caffeine-containing items such as chocolate, coffee, tea, and colas)
10. instruct client to rest after eating with head of bed elevated
11. encourage client to eat dry foods (e.g. toast, crackers) and avoid drinking liquids with meals if nauseated
12. monitor for therapeutic and nontherapeutic effects of antiemetics if administered.

c. Consult physician if above measures fail to prevent nausea and vomiting.

6. NURSING DIAGNOSIS

Impaired skin integrity: irritation and breakdown related to:

a. prolonged pressure on tissues associated with decreased mobility;
b. increased fragility of the skin associated with tissue hypoxia and malnutrition.

DESIRED OUTCOMES	NURSING ACTIONS AND *SELECTED RATIONALES*

6. The client will maintain skin integrity as evidenced by:
a. absence of redness and irritation
b. no skin breakdown.
	6.a. Inspect the skin, especially bone prominences, for pallor, redness, and breakdown.
	b. Refer to Care Plan on Immobility, Nursing Diagnosis 7, action b, for measures to prevent skin breakdown associated with decreased mobility.
	c. Implement additional measures *to prevent skin irritation and breakdown:*
	  1. perform actions to improve respiratory status (see Nursing Diagnosis 2, action f) *in order to improve tissue oxygenation*
	  2. perform actions to improve nutritional status (see Nursing Diagnosis 4, actions e and f).
	d. If skin breakdown occurs:
	  1. notify physician
	  2. continue with above measures to prevent further irritation and breakdown
	  3. perform decubitus care as ordered or per standard hospital policy
	  4. monitor client closely and report signs and symptoms of infection (e.g. elevated temperature; redness, warmth, and edema around area of breakdown; unusual drainage from site).

7. NURSING DIAGNOSIS

Altered oral mucous membrane: dryness related to prolonged oxygen therapy (oxygen is a dry gas and will dehydrate the respiratory mucous membranes if exposure is prolonged).

DESIRED OUTCOMES	NURSING ACTIONS AND *SELECTED RATIONALES*
7. The client will maintain a moist, intact oral mucous membrane.	7.a. Assess client every shift for dryness of the oral mucosa. b. Implement measures *to decrease dryness of the oral mucous membrane:* 1. instruct and assist client to perform good oral hygiene as often as

needed; avoid products such as lemon-glycerin swabs and commercial mouthwashes containing alcohol *(these products have a drying or irritating effect on the oral mucous membrane)*
2. encourage client to rinse mouth frequently with water
3. lubricate client's lips with Vaseline, K-Y jelly, ChapStick, Blistex, or mineral oil when oral care is given
4. encourage client to breathe through nose if possible
5. encourage client not to smoke *(smoking further irritates and dries the mucosa)*
6. encourage a fluid intake of at least 2500 cc/day unless contraindicated
7. encourage client to use artificial saliva (e.g. Moi-stir, Salivart, Xero-Lube) *to lubricate the mucous membrane.*
   c. If oral mucosa is irritated or cracked, implement measures *to relieve discomfort and promote healing:*
   1. assist client to select soft, bland, and nonacidic foods
   2. instruct client to avoid foods/fluids that are extremely hot or cold
   3. use a soft bristle brush or low-pressure power spray for oral care
   4. monitor for therapeutic and nontherapeutic effects of topical anesthetics, oral protective pastes, and topical and systemic analgesics if administered.
   d. Consult physician if dryness, irritation, and discomfort persist.

8. NURSING DIAGNOSIS

Activity intolerance related to:

a. tissue hypoxia associated with impaired gas exchange;
b. inadequate nutritional status;
c. difficulty resting and sleeping associated with dyspnea, excessive coughing (occurs with chronic bronchitis), fear, anxiety, frequent assessments and treatments, and side effects of medication therapy (e.g. some bronchodilators);
d. increased energy expenditure associated with strenuous breathing efforts and persistent coughing.

DESIRED OUTCOMES	NURSING ACTIONS AND *SELECTED RATIONALES*

8. The client will demonstrate an increased tolerance for activity (see Care Plan on Immobility, Nursing Diagnosis 8, for outcome criteria).	8.a. Refer to Care Plan on Immobility, Nursing Diagnosis 8, for measures related to assessment and improvement of activity tolerance.
	b. Implement additional measures *to promote rest and improve activity tolerance:*
	1. maintain activity restrictions if ordered
	2. perform actions to reduce fear and anxiety (see Nursing Diagnosis 1, action c)
	3. perform actions to promote sleep (see Nursing Diagnosis 10, actions a and b)
	4. perform actions *to control cough:*
	  a. instruct client to avoid intake of very hot or cold foods/fluids *(these can stimulate cough)*
	  b. protect client from irritants (e.g. flowers, smoke, powder)
	  c. monitor for therapeutic and nontherapeutic effects of antitussives if administered *to suppress cough during periods of rest and sleep*
	5. perform actions to improve respiratory status (see Nursing Diagnosis 2, action f) *in order to improve tissue oxygenation and relieve dyspnea*
	6. perform actions to improve nutritional status (see Nursing Diagnosis 4, actions e and f)

7. reinforce use of controlled breathing techniques (e.g. inhaling through nose and exhaling slowly through pursed lips) during activity
8. if oxygen therapy is necessary during activity, keep portable oxygen equipment readily available for client's use
9. increase client's activity gradually as allowed and tolerated; assist with graded exercises and physical conditioning program (e.g. measured level walks, treadmill, stationary bicycling) as ordered.

☐ ▰▰▰▰▰▰▰▰▰▰▰▰▰▰▰▰▰▰▰▰▰▰▰

9. NURSING DIAGNOSIS

Self-care deficit related to weakness, fatigue, and dyspnea.

☐ ▰▰▰▰▰▰▰▰▰▰▰▰▰▰▰▰▰▰▰▰▰▰▰

DESIRED OUTCOMES	NURSING ACTIONS AND *SELECTED RATIONALES*

9. The client will demonstrate increased participation in self-care activities within physical limitations and prescribed activity restrictions.	9.a. Assess for factors that interfere with client's ability to perform self-care (e.g. dyspnea, fatigue, weakness).
	b. With client, develop a realistic plan for meeting daily physical needs.
	c. Encourage maximum independence within limitations imposed by dyspnea, weakness, and fatigue.
	d. Implement measures *to facilitate client's ability to perform self-care activities:*
	  1. schedule care at a time when client is most likely to be able to participate:
	    a. a couple of hours after arising *(bronchial secretions and edema are greater immediately upon awakening because of client's inactivity through the night)*
	    b. after scheduled rest periods
	    c. not directly after meals or treatments when already fatigued
	  2. keep needed objects within easy reach
	  3. perform actions to increase strength and improve activity tolerance (see Nursing Diagnosis 8)
	  4. consult occupational therapist about adaptive devices available (e.g. long-handled hairbrush and shoehorn); reinforce use of these devices if indicated
	  5. allow adequate time for accomplishment of self-care activities.
	e. Provide positive feedback for all efforts and accomplishments of self-care.
	f. Assist client with those activities he/she is unable to perform independently.
	g. Inform significant others of client's abilities to perform own care. Explain the importance of encouraging and allowing client to maintain optimal level of independence within prescribed activity restrictions and his/her activity tolerance level.

☐ ▰▰▰▰▰▰▰▰▰▰▰▰▰▰▰▰▰▰▰▰▰▰▰

10. NURSING DIAGNOSIS

Sleep pattern disturbance related to fear, anxiety, unfamiliar environment, excessive coughing, inability to assume usual sleep position due to orthopnea, frequent assessments and treatments, and decreased activity.

☐ ▰▰▰▰▰▰▰▰▰▰▰▰▰▰▰▰▰▰▰▰▰▰▰

DESIRED OUTCOMES	NURSING ACTIONS AND *SELECTED RATIONALES*

10. The client will attain optimal amounts of sleep within the parameters of the treatment regimen (see Care Plan on Immobility, Nursing Diagnosis 12, for outcome criteria).	10.a. Refer to Care Plan on Immobility, Nursing Diagnosis 12, for measures related to assessment and promotion of sleep.
	b. Implement additional measures *to promote sleep:*
	  1. perform actions to reduce fear and anxiety (see Nursing Diagnosis 1, action c)
	  2. perform actions to improve respiratory status (see Nursing Diagnosis 2, action f) *in order to relieve orthopnea*
	  3. assist client to assume a comfortable sleep position (e.g. bed in reverse Trendelenburg position with client in usual recumbent sleep position, head of bed elevated with arms supported on pillows, resting forward on overbed table with good pillow support, sitting in chair)
	  4. ensure good room ventilation
	  5. maintain oxygen therapy during sleep if indicated
	  6. perform actions to control cough (see Nursing Diagnosis 8, action b.4).
	c. Reinforce need to avoid medications such as sedatives and hypnotics *(these medications further depress respiratory status).*

11. NURSING DIAGNOSIS

Potential for infection: pneumonia related to excessive mucus production (with chronic bronchitis) and stasis of secretions in the lungs.

DESIRED OUTCOMES	NURSING ACTIONS AND *SELECTED RATIONALES*
11. The client will not develop pneumonia (see Care Plan on Immobility, Nursing Diagnosis 13, outcome a, for outcome criteria).	11.a. Refer to Care Plan on Immobility, Nursing Diagnosis 13, action a, for measures related to the assessment, prevention, and treatment of pneumonia. b. Implement measures to improve respiratory status (see Nursing Diagnosis 2, action f) *in order to further decrease risk of pneumonia.*

12. NURSING DIAGNOSIS

Potential for trauma related to falls associated with:

a. confusion and lethargy resulting from cerebral hypoxia (may occur as a result of impaired gas exchange);
b. weakness and fatigue resulting from tissue hypoxia, malnutrition, and interruption in usual sleep pattern.

DESIRED OUTCOMES	NURSING ACTIONS AND *SELECTED RATIONALES*
12. The client will not experience falls.	12.a. Determine whether conditions predisposing client to falls (e.g. lethargy, confusion, weakness, fatigue) exist.

b. Implement measures *to prevent falls:*
   1. keep bed in low position with side rails up when client is in bed
   2. keep needed items within easy reach
   3. encourage client to request assistance whenever needed; have call signal within easy reach
   4. use lap belt when client is in chair if indicated
   5. instruct client to wear shoes with nonskid soles and low heels when ambulating
   6. avoid unnecessary clutter in room
   7. accompany client during ambulation utilizing a transfer safety belt if indicated
   8. provide ambulatory aids (e.g. walker, cane) if client is weak or unsteady on feet
   9. instruct client to ambulate in well-lit areas and to utilize handrails if needed
   10. do not rush client; allow adequate time for trips to the bathroom and ambulation in hallway
   11. perform actions to increase strength and improve activity tolerance (see Nursing Diagnosis 8).
c. If client is confused or irrational, implement additional measures *to reduce risk of falls:*
   1. reorient frequently to surroundings and necessity of adhering to safety precautions
   2. provide constant supervision (e.g. staff member, significant other) if indicated
   3. use jacket or wrist restraints or safety alarm device if necessary *to reduce the risk of client's getting out of bed or chair unattended*
   4. monitor for therapeutic and nontherapeutic effects of antianxiety and antipsychotic medications if administered.
d. Include client and significant others in planning and implementing measures to prevent falls.
e. If falls occur, initiate appropriate first aid measures and notify physician.

□ ▅▅▅▅▅▅▅▅▅▅▅▅▅▅▅▅▅▅▅▅▅

13. COLLABORATIVE DIAGNOSIS

Potential complications:

a. **thromboembolism** related to:
   1. venous stasis associated with decreased activity and increased blood viscosity
   2. hypercoagulability associated with increased blood viscosity due to fluid volume deficit and polycythemia (the body increases erythrocyte production in an effort to compensate for decreased circulating oxygen levels);
b. **gastrointestinal (GI) bleeding** related to development of a peptic ulcer associated with:
   1. increased gastric secretions resulting from stress
   2. increased back diffusion of hydrogen ions resulting from decreased gastric tissue oxygenation (occurs with hypoxemia)
   3. irritation of gastric mucosa by ulcerogenic medications (e.g. theophylline, corticosteroids);
c. **spontaneous pneumothorax** related to overdistention of alveoli and rupture of pleural blebs into the pleural cavity;
d. **right-sided heart failure** related to cor pulmonale associated with pulmonary hypertension (results from increased pulmonary vascular resistance to blood flow and a compensatory increase in cardiac output);
e. **respiratory failure** related to hypoxemia.

□ ▅▅▅▅▅▅▅▅▅▅▅▅▅▅▅▅▅▅▅▅▅

DESIRED OUTCOMES	NURSING ACTIONS AND *SELECTED RATIONALES*

13.a. The client will not develop a venous thrombus or pulmonary embolism (see Care Plan on Immobility, Collaborative Diagnosis 14, outcomes a.1 and 2, for outcome criteria).

13.a. Refer to Care Plan on Immobility, Collaborative Diagnosis 14, actions a.1 and 2, for measures related to assessment, prevention, and treatment of a venous thrombus and pulmonary embolism.

13.b. The client will not experience GI bleeding as evidenced by:
1. no complaints of epigastric discomfort and fullness
2. absence of occult or frank blood in stool and gastric contents
3. B/P and pulse within normal range for client
4. stable RBC, Hct., and Hgb. levels.

13.b.1. Assess for and report signs and symptoms of GI bleeding (e.g. complaints of epigastric discomfort or fullness, frank or occult blood in stool or gastric contents, decreased B/P, increased pulse).
  2. Monitor RBC, Hct., and Hgb. levels. Report declining values.
  3. Implement measures *to prevent ulceration of the gastric or duodenal mucosa:*
    a. perform actions to decrease fear and anxiety (see Nursing Diagnosis 1, action c)
    b. perform actions to improve respiratory status (see Nursing Diagnosis 2, action f) *in order to improve tissue oxygenation and prevent respiratory acidosis*
    c. instruct client to avoid foods/fluids that irritate gastric mucosa (e.g. spicy foods; citrus fruits or juices; caffeine-containing items such as chocolate, coffee, tea, and colas)
    d. administer ulcerogenic medications (e.g. corticosteroids, theophylline) with meals or snacks *to decrease gastric irritation*
    e. monitor for therapeutic and nontherapeutic effects of histamine$_2$ receptor antagonists (e.g. cimetidine, ranitidine, famotidine), antacids, and mucosal barrier fortifiers (e.g. sucralfate) if administered.
  4. If signs and symptoms of GI bleeding occur:
    a. insert nasogastric tube and maintain suction as ordered
    b. assist with iced water or saline gastric lavage, transendoscopic electrocoagulation, selective arterial embolization, endoscopic laser photocoagulation, and/or intra-arterial administration of vasopressors (e.g. vasopressin) if ordered
    c. monitor for therapeutic and nontherapeutic effects of blood products and/or volume expanders if administered
    d. prepare client for surgery if indicated
    e. provide emotional support to client and significant others
    f. refer to Care Plan on Peptic Ulcer for additional care measures.

13.c. The client will not experience spontaneous pneumothorax as evidenced by:
1. usual or improved breath sounds
2. usual respiratory rate and pattern
3. absence of chest pain and cyanosis
4. usual mental status
5. blood gases within normal range for client.

13.c.1. Assess for and immediately report signs and symptoms of pneumothorax (e.g. absent breath sounds with hyperresonant percussion note over involved area, increased dyspnea, tachycardia, chest pain, cyanosis, increased restlessness, confusion).
  2. Monitor blood gases. Report values that have worsened.
  3. Implement measures to improve respiratory status (see Nursing Diagnosis 2, action f) *in order to decrease further damage to alveoli and reduce the risk of pneumothorax.*
  4. If signs and symptoms of pneumothorax occur:
    a. maintain client on bedrest in a semi- to high Fowler's position
    b. maintain oxygen therapy as ordered
    c. assess for and immediately report signs and symptoms of mediastinal shift (e.g. severe dyspnea, increased restlessness and agitation, rapid and/or irregular heart rate, shift in point of apical impulse and trachea toward the unaffected side)
    d. prepare client for insertion of chest tube(s) if indicated
    e. provide emotional support to client and significant others.

13.d. The client will not develop right-sided heart failure as evidenced by:

13.d.1. Assess for and report signs and symptoms of right-sided heart failure:
    a. increase in pulse rate

1. vital signs within normal range for client
2. no increase in intensity of S_2 or development of a gallop or murmur over the pulmonic valve area
3. balanced intake and output
4. stable weight
5. CVP within normal range
6. absence of peripheral edema; distended neck veins; enlarged, tender liver
7. BUN and serum creatinine and alkaline phosphatase levels within normal range.

b. development of loud S_2 and/or gallop or murmur over the pulmonic valve area
c. intake greater than output
d. weight gain
e. elevated CVP
f. peripheral edema
g. distended neck veins
h. enlarged, tender liver
i. elevated BUN and serum creatinine and alkaline phosphatase levels.

2. Monitor chest x-ray results. Report findings of cardiomegaly.
3. Implement measures to improve respiratory status (see Nursing Diagnosis 2, action f) *in order to reduce cardiac workload and prevent right-sided heart failure.*
4. If signs and symptoms of right-sided heart failure occur:
   a. maintain oxygen therapy as ordered
   b. maintain fluid and sodium restrictions as ordered
   c. maintain client on strict bedrest in a semi- to high Fowler's position
   d. monitor for therapeutic and nontherapeutic effects of medications that may be administered *to reduce vascular congestion and/or cardiac workload* (e.g. diuretics, cardiotonics, vasodilators, morphine sulfate)
   e. assist with insertion of Swan-Ganz catheter if indicated
   f. refer to Care Plan on Congestive Heart Failure for additional care measures.

13.e. The client will not experience respiratory failure as evidenced by:
1. respiratory rate above 8 and below 30/minute
2. usual skin color
3. usual mental status
4. PaO_2 above 50 mm Hg and $PaCO_2$ below 50 mm Hg.

13.e.1. Assess for and report signs and symptoms of severe respiratory distress (e.g. increased rate and decreased depth of respirations, increased sternocleidomastoid muscle retraction, dusky or cyanotic skin color, drowsiness, confusion).
2. Monitor blood gases. Report values that have worsened.
3. Monitor for and report worsening of ear oximetry and capnograph results.
4. Implement measures *to prevent respiratory failure:*
   a. perform actions to improve respiratory status (see Nursing Diagnosis 2, action f)
   b. assess for and report conditions that might further compromise respiratory status (e.g. cardiac arrhythmias, respiratory acidosis, low B/P, pneumonia, pneumothorax, right-sided heart failure).
5. If signs and symptoms of respiratory failure occur:
   a. continue with above actions
   b. assist with intubation, mechanical ventilation, and transfer to intensive care unit if indicated
   c. continue with comfort measures such as keeping upper airways free of mucus and wiping face with cool cloth if aggressive life-saving techniques are not indicated; refer to Care Plan on Terminal Care if appropriate
   d. provide emotional support to client and significant others.

UNIT IX

14. NURSING DIAGNOSIS

Sexual dysfunction:

a. **decreased libido** related to depression, dyspnea, persistent cough, weakness, and fatigue;
b. **impotence** related to depression, fear, anxiety, disturbance in self-concept, and side effects of some medications.

DESIRED OUTCOMES	NURSING ACTIONS AND *SELECTED RATIONALES*

14. The client will perceive self as sexually adequate and acceptable (see Care Plan on Immobility, Nursing Diagnosis 15, for outcome criteria).	14.a. Refer to Care Plan on Immobility, Nursing Diagnosis 15, for measures related to assessment and management of sexual dysfunction.
	b. Implement additional measures *to promote optimal sexual functioning:*
	  1. perform actions to reduce fear and anxiety (see Nursing Diagnosis 1, action c)
	  2. perform actions to increase strength and improve activity tolerance (see Nursing Diagnosis 8)
	  3. perform actions to improve self-concept (see Nursing Diagnosis 15)
	  4. instruct client to take an antitussive before sexual activity if prescribed *to control cough*
	  5. instruct client in ways to reduce dyspnea during sexual activity (e.g. obtain adequate rest and use inhaled bronchodilators before sexual activity, use oxygen before and during sexual activity, assume positions such as side-lying that reduce energy expenditure).

☐ ▬▬▬▬▬▬▬▬▬▬▬▬▬▬▬▬▬▬▬▬

15. NURSING DIAGNOSIS

Disturbance in self-concept* related to:

a. change in appearance (e.g. "barrel" chest, clubbing of fingers, retraction of tissues around the neck and supraclavicular spaces);
b. dependence on others to meet self-care needs;
c. possible alterations in sexual functioning;
d. stigma of having a chronic illness;
e. possible changes in life style and roles.

---

* This diagnostic label includes the nursing diagnoses of body image disturbance and self-esteem disturbance.

☐ ▬▬▬▬▬▬▬▬▬▬▬▬▬▬▬▬▬▬▬▬

DESIRED OUTCOMES	NURSING ACTIONS AND *SELECTED RATIONALES*

15. The client will demonstrate beginning adaptation to changes in appearance, body functioning, level of independence, life style, and roles (see Care Plan on Immobility, Nursing Diagnosis 16, for outcome criteria).	15.a. Refer to Care Plan on Immobility, Nursing Diagnosis 16, for measures related to assessment and promotion of a positive self-concept.
	b. Implement additional measures *to assist client to adapt to changes in body functioning, level of independence, life style, and roles:*
	  1. if client is self-conscious about appearance, suggest clothing styles that make physical changes less apparent
	  2. perform actions to assist client to promote optimal sexual functioning (see Nursing Diagnosis 14)
	  3. assist client to attain and maintain optimal independence:
	    a. perform actions to increase strength and improve activity tolerance (see Nursing Diagnosis 8)
	    b. consult social services and occupational therapist about a home visit before discharge *to identify appropriate energy-saving techniques based on client's current living situation*
	    c. reinforce benefits of utilizing portable oxygen if prescribed
	  4. encourage significant others to allow client to do what he/she is able *so that independence can be re-established and/or self-esteem redeveloped*
	  5. teach client the rationale for treatments and encourage maximum participation in treatment regimen *to enable him/her to maintain a sense of control over life*
	  6. ensure that client and significant others have similar expectations and understanding of future life style

7. assist client and significant others to identify ways that personal and family goals can be adjusted rather than abandoned
8. provide information about and encourage utilization of community resources or support groups that can assist in adaptation to life-style and role changes (e.g. counselors, vocational rehabilitation services, American Lung Association, self-help groups, emphysema clubs).

16. NURSING DIAGNOSIS

Grieving* related to continued loss of lung function and changes in life style and roles.

* This diagnostic label includes anticipatory grieving and grieving following the actual losses/changes.

DESIRED OUTCOMES	NURSING ACTIONS AND *SELECTED RATIONALES*

16. The client will demonstrate beginning progression through the grieving process as evidenced by:
    a. verbalization of feelings about COPD
    b. expression of grief
    c. participation in treatment plan and self-care activities
    d. utilization of available support systems
    e. verbalization of a plan for integrating prescribed follow-up care into life style.

16.a. Determine the client's perception of the impact of COPD on his/her future.
   b. Determine how client usually expresses grief.
   c. Observe for signs of grieving (e.g. changes in eating habits, insomnia, anger, noncompliance, denial).
   d. Implement measures *to facilitate the grieving process:*
   1. assist client to acknowledge the loss of lung function *so grief work can begin*; assess for factors that may hinder or facilitate acknowledgment
   2. discuss the grieving process and assist client to accept the stages of grieving as an expected response to the actual and/or anticipated changes; support the realization that grief may recur *because of the chronic nature of the disease*
   3. allow time for client to progress through the stages of grieving (denial, anger, bargaining, depression, acceptance, [Kübler-Ross, 1969]); be aware that not every stage is experienced or expressed by all individuals
   4. provide an atmosphere of care and concern (e.g. provide privacy, be available and nonjudgmental, display empathy and respect) *so that client will feel free to verbalize both positive and negative feelings and concerns*
   5. perform actions *to promote trust* (e.g. answer questions honestly, provide requested information)
   6. encourage the expression of anger and sadness about the changes experienced
   7. encourage client to express his/her feelings in whatever ways are comfortable (e.g. writing, drawing, conversation)
   8. assist client to identify personal strengths that have helped him/her to cope in previous situations of loss and change
   9. support realistic hope about the success of treatment on the disease progression.
   e. Assess for and support behaviors suggesting successful resolution of grief (e.g. verbalizing feelings about changes, expressing sorrow, focusing on ways to adapt to changes that have occurred).
   f. Explain the stages of the grieving process to significant others. Encourage their support and understanding.
   g. Provide information regarding counseling services and support groups that might assist client in working through grief.
   h. Arrange for visit from clergy if desired by client.
   i. Monitor for therapeutic and nontherapeutic effects of antidepressants if administered.
   j. Consult physician regarding referral for counseling if signs of dysfunctional grieving (e.g. persistent denial of losses or changes, excessive anger or sadness, hysteria, suicidal behaviors, phobias) occur.

UNIT
IX

☐ ▬▬▬▬▬▬▬▬▬▬▬▬▬▬▬▬

17. NURSING DIAGNOSIS

Noncompliance*related to:

a. lack of understanding of the implications of not following the prescribed treatment plan;
b. difficulty modifying personal habits and integrating necessary treatments into life style;
c. insufficient financial resources;
d. dysfunctional grieving.

---

* This diagnostic label includes both an informed decision by client not to comply and an inability to comply due to circumstances beyond the client's control.

☐ ▬▬▬▬▬▬▬▬▬▬▬▬▬▬▬▬

DESIRED OUTCOMES	NURSING ACTIONS AND *SELECTED RATIONALES*

17. The client will demonstrate the probability of future compliance with the prescribed treatment plan as evidenced by:
    a. willingness to learn about and participate in treatments and care
    b. statements reflecting ways to modify personal habits and integrate treatments into life style
    c. statements reflecting an understanding of the implications of not following the prescribed treatment plan.

17.a. Assess for indications that the client may be unwilling or unable to comply with the prescribed treatment plan:
  1. statements reflecting that he/she was unable to manage care at home
  2. failure to adhere to treatment plan while in hospital (e.g. refusing to use proper breathing techniques, refusing medications)
  3. statements reflecting a lack of understanding of factors that may cause further progression of COPD
  4. statements reflecting an unwillingness or inability to modify personal habits and integrate necessary treatments into life style
  5. statements reflecting view that COPD is curable or that treatment will not affect the disease progression.

  b. Implement measures *to improve client compliance:*
  1. explain COPD in terms client can understand; stress the fact that COPD is a chronic disease and that adherence to the treatment program is necessary *in order to delay and/or prevent complications*
  2. encourage questions and clarify any misconceptions client has about COPD and its effects
  3. encourage client to participate in treatment plan (e.g. chest physiotherapy, breathing exercises)
  4. have client demonstrate breathing techniques and chest physiotherapy; determine areas of difficulty and misunderstanding and reinforce teaching as necessary
  5. initiate and reinforce the discharge teaching outlined in Nursing Diagnosis 18 *in order to promote a sense of control over disease progression*
  6. provide client with written instructions about breathing techniques, chest physiotherapy, ways to prevent further pulmonary damage, prescribed medications, signs and symptoms to report, and future appointments with health care provider
  7. assist client to identify ways he/she can incorporate treatments into life style; focus on modifications of life style rather than complete change
  8. encourage client to discuss his/her financial concerns regarding cost of hospitalization, medications, oxygen equipment, and lifelong follow-up care; obtain a social service consult to assist with financial planning and to obtain financial aid if indicated
  9. provide information about and encourage utilization of community resources that can assist client to make necessary life-style changes (e.g. American Lung Association; emphysema clubs; counseling, vocational, and social services; stop smoking programs).

  c. Assess for and reinforce behaviors suggesting future compliance with prescribed treatments (e.g. statements reflecting plans for integrating treatments into life style, active participation in treatment plan, changes in personal habits).

d. Include significant others in explanations and teaching sessions and encourage their support.
e. Reinforce the need for client to assume responsibility for managing as much of care as possible.
f. Consult physician about referrals to community health agencies if continued instruction, support, or supervision is needed.

18. NURSING DIAGNOSIS

Knowledge deficit regarding follow-up care.

DESIRED OUTCOMES	NURSING ACTIONS AND *SELECTED RATIONALES*

18.a. The client will identify ways to prevent or minimize further pulmonary damage.	18.a.1. Instruct client in ways *to prevent or minimize further pulmonary damage:*
	a. maintain overall general good health:
	  1. eat a well-balanced diet
	  2. schedule adequate rest periods *to avoid undue fatigue*
	  3. adhere to prescribed graded exercise program
	  4. control or eliminate factors that cause stress
	b. stop smoking
	c. avoid exposure to respiratory irritants such as tobacco smoke, perfumes, aerosol cleaners, paint fumes, and solvents
	d. remain indoors when air pollution levels are high and/or outdoor temperatures are extremely hot or cold
	e. wear a mask or scarf over nose and mouth if exposure to high levels of irritants such as smoke, fumes, and dust is unavoidable
	f. decrease the risk of respiratory tract infections:
	  1. avoid contact with persons who have respiratory tract infections
	  2. avoid crowds and poorly ventilated areas
	  3. receive immunizations against influenza and pneumococcal pneumonia
	  4. take anti-infective therapy as prescribed (many physicians instruct clients to begin anti-infective therapy if sputum color becomes yellow or green)
	  5. adhere to chest physiotherapy (e.g. postural drainage, vibration, percussion, breathing exercises) as ordered
	  6. take medications such as bronchodilators and mucolytics as prescribed
	  7. cleanse all respiratory care equipment properly
	  8. drink at least 10 glasses of liquid/day.
	2. Assist client in identifying ways he/she can make appropriate changes in personal habits and life style to reduce risk factors.

18.b. The client will demonstrate proper breathing techniques and chest physiotherapy.	18.b.1. Instruct client in proper breathing techniques and chest physiotherapy. Include: a. diaphragmatic breathing b. pursed-lip breathing c. use of equipment such as oxygen, inspiratory exerciser, and humidifier d. postural drainage, percussion, and vibration. 2. Allow time for questions, clarification, and return demonstration.
18.c. The client will verbalize an understanding of medication therapy including rationale for, side	18.c.1. Explain the rationale for, side effects of, and importance of taking medications prescribed. 2. Instruct in proper use of nebulizers and inhalants if prescribed. Allow time for client to practice the techniques.

UNIT IX

effects of, method of administering, and importance of taking as prescribed.

3. If client is discharged on theophylline, instruct to:
   a. take it with food *to minimize nausea, vomiting, and epigastric pain*
   b. take it on a regular basis as ordered *to maintain therapeutic blood levels*
   c. report signs and symptoms of overdose (e.g. persistent nausea and vomiting, headache, exaggerated reflexes, muscle tremors, seizures, rapid pulse)
   d. have blood theophylline levels evaluated periodically.
4. Reinforce the need to consult health care provider before taking additional prescription and nonprescription medications.

18.d. The client will identify appropriate safety measures related to COPD and its treatment.

18.d. Instruct client regarding the following safety measures:
1. do not smoke when using oxygen therapy
2. do not set oxygen flow rate at a level higher than prescribed by physician
3. always wear a Medic-Alert tag *to ensure that proper medications and appropriate oxygen flow rate are administered in emergency situations*
4. notify health care providers of the disease condition and current therapy.

18.e. The client will state signs and symptoms to report to the health care provider.

18.e. Instruct client to report:
1. change in sputum characteristics
2. sputum that does not return to usual color after 3 days of anti-infective therapy
3. cough that becomes worse
4. increased fatigue, weakness, and shortness of breath
5. increased need for medications and/or oxygen therapy
6. elevated temperature
7. increased restlessness, irritability, drowsiness, or confusion
8. increasing feeling of "tightness" of chest
9. chest pain with accompanying shortness of breath
10. persistent weight loss or sudden weight gain
11. swelling in ankles and/or feet
12. bright red or dark blood in stool or vomitus
13. epigastric pain
14. signs and symptoms of theophylline overdose (see action c.3.c in this diagnosis).

18.f. The client will identify community resources that can assist with home management and adjustment to changes resulting from COPD.

18.f.1. Provide information regarding community resources that can assist client and significant others with home management and adjustment to changes resulting from COPD (e.g. American Lung Association; emphysema clubs; counseling, vocational, and social services; Meals on Wheels; transportation services; home health agencies).
2. Initiate a referral if indicated.

18.g. The client will verbalize an understanding of and a plan for adhering to recommended follow-up care including future appointments with health care provider and graded exercise program.

18.g.1. Reinforce importance of lifelong follow-up care.
2. Reinforce physician's instructions about a graded exercise program.
3. Implement measures to improve client compliance (see Nursing Diagnosis 17, action b).

References

Carpenito, LJ. Handbook of nursing diagnosis (3rd ed.). Philadelphia: J.B. Lippincott Company, 1989.

Kübler-Ross, E. On death and dying. New York: Macmillan, 1969.

Lung Surgery

Lung surgery may consist of a pneumonectomy (removal of the entire lung), a lobectomy (removal of a lobe), or a segmental or wedge resection of a portion of a lung. A pneumonectomy is most commonly performed for treatment of cancer and extensive tuberculosis or bronchiectasis or for lung abscesses. A lobectomy or a segmental resection is indicated when the disease process is confined to a limited area of the lung. Either may be performed to remove benign or malignant tumors, small areas of bronchiectasis, and blebs or bullae. A wedge resection of a small portion of a lung is performed to biopsy lung tissue or to excise a small, well-defined lesion or nodule.

This care plan focuses on the adult client hospitalized for removal of a portion or all of a lung. Preoperative goals of care are to reduce fear and anxiety and assist the client to attain an optimal physical condition. The goals of postoperative care are to prevent and detect complications, maintain comfort, and educate the client regarding follow-up care. The care plan will need to be individualized according to the client's diagnosis, prognosis, and plans for subsequent treatment.

DISCHARGE CRITERIA

Prior to discharge, the client will:

- demonstrate the ability to perform prescribed arm and shoulder exercises
- state signs and symptoms of complications to report to the health care provider
- identify community resources that can assist with home management and adjustment to the diagnosis, effects of surgery, and adjunctive treatment if planned
- verbalize an understanding of and a plan for adhering to recommended follow-up care including future appointments with health care provider, medications prescribed, activity level, pain management, wound care, and subsequent treatment of the underlying disorder.

NURSING/COLLABORATIVE DIAGNOSES

Preoperative
1. Anxiety ☐ 474
2. Ineffective airway clearance ☐ 474
3. Impaired gas exchange ☐ 475
Postoperative
1. Altered respiratory function:
    a. ineffective breathing patterns:
        1. hypoventilation
        2. hyperventilation
    b. ineffective airway clearance
    c. impaired gas exchange ☐ 476
2. Pain:
    a. chest pain
    b. shoulder pain ☐ 477
3. Potential complications:
    a. extended pneumothorax
    b. hemothorax
    c. mediastinal shift
    d. acute pulmonary edema
    e. restricted arm and shoulder movement ☐ 477
4. Grieving ☐ 480
5. Knowledge deficit regarding follow-up care ☐ 481

Preoperative

Use in conjunction with the Standardized Preoperative Care Plan.

1. NURSING DIAGNOSIS

Anxiety related to unfamiliar environment; diagnosis; lack of understanding of diagnostic tests, surgical procedure, and postoperative management; effects of anesthesia; and anticipated postoperative pain and effects of loss of all or part of a lung on future activity.

DESIRED OUTCOMES	NURSING ACTIONS AND *SELECTED RATIONALES*
1. The client will experience a reduction in fear and anxiety (see Standardized Preoperative Care Plan, Nursing Diagnosis 1, for outcome criteria).	1.a. Refer to Standardized Preoperative Care Plan, Nursing Diagnosis 1, for measures related to assessment and reduction of fear and anxiety. b. Implement additional measures *to reduce fear and anxiety:* 1. explain all diagnostic tests performed to evaluate status of disease process or effectiveness of lung function (e.g. chest x-ray, lung scan, pulmonary function studies, arterial blood gases, bronchoscopy) 2. reinforce physician's explanations about anticipated effect of loss of lung tissue on future activities (client may experience decreased lung function depending on extensiveness of surgery) 3. provide instruction about the purpose of chest drainage system that will be present after partial removal of a lung (chest tubes are usually not inserted during a pneumonectomy; if one is in place, it is clamped).

2. NURSING DIAGNOSIS

Ineffective airway clearance related to:

a. excessive or tenacious pulmonary secretions associated with the underlying disease process;
b. ineffective cough effort associated with weakness and pain (may occur as a result of underlying disease process).

DESIRED OUTCOMES	NURSING ACTIONS AND *SELECTED RATIONALES*
2. The client will maintain clear, open airways as evidenced by: a. usual breath sounds b. usual rate and depth of respirations c. absence of dyspnea	2.a. Assess for signs and symptoms of ineffective airway clearance (e.g. adventitious breath sounds; rapid, shallow respirations; dyspnea; cyanosis). b. Implement measures *to promote effective airway clearance:* 1. instruct and assist client to turn, cough, and deep breathe every 1–2 hours 2. reinforce correct use of inspiratory exerciser at least every 2 hours

d. absence of cyanosis.

3. perform actions *to facilitate removal of pulmonary secretions:*
   a. implement measures *to liquefy tenacious secretions:*
      1. maintain a fluid intake of at least 2500 cc/day unless contraindicated
      2. humidify inspired air as ordered
      3. assist with administration of mucolytic agents via nebulizer or IPPB treatment
   b. assist with or perform postural drainage, percussion, and vibration if ordered
   c. perform tracheal suctioning if needed
   d. monitor for therapeutic and nontherapeutic effects of expectorants if administered
4. increase activity as allowed and tolerated
5. discourage smoking *(smoking causes an increase in mucus production and impairs ciliary function).*
c. Consult physician if signs and symptoms of ineffective airway clearance persist or worsen.

☐ ▇▇▇▇▇▇▇▇▇▇▇▇▇▇▇▇▇▇▇▇▇▇▇▇▇▇▇▇▇▇▇▇▇

3. NURSING DIAGNOSIS

Impaired gas exchange related to ineffective airway clearance and loss of effective lung surface associated with the respiratory disease process.

☐ ▇▇▇▇▇▇▇▇▇▇▇▇▇▇▇▇▇▇▇▇▇▇▇▇▇▇▇▇▇▇▇▇▇

DESIRED OUTCOMES	NURSING ACTIONS AND *SELECTED RATIONALES*

3. The client will experience adequate O_2/CO_2 exchange as evidenced by:
   a. usual mental status
   b. usual skin color
   c. absence of dyspnea
   d. blood gases within normal range for client.

3.a. Assess for and report signs and symptoms of impaired gas exchange:
   1. restlessness or irritability
   2. confusion, somnolence
   3. dusky or cyanotic skin color
   4. dyspnea.
b. Monitor blood gas values. Report abnormal results.
c. Monitor for and report significant changes in ear oximetry and capnograph results.
d. Implement measures *to improve gas exchange:*
   1. perform actions to promote effective airway clearance (see Preoperative Nursing Diagnosis 2, action b)
   2. place client in a semi- to high Fowler's position; position overbed table so client can rest on it if desired
   3. maintain oxygen therapy as ordered
   4. discourage smoking *(smoking decreases oxygen availability)*
   5. administer central nervous system depressants (e.g. narcotics, sedatives) judiciously; hold medication and consult physician if respiratory rate is less than 12/minute.
e. Consult physician if signs and symptoms of impaired gas exchange persist or worsen.

☐ ▬▬▬▬▬▬▬▬▬▬▬▬▬▬▬▬▬▬▬▬

Postoperative

Use in conjunction with the Standardized Postoperative Care Plan.

☐ ▬▬▬▬▬▬▬▬▬▬▬▬▬▬▬▬▬▬▬▬

1. NURSING DIAGNOSIS

Altered respiratory function:*

a. **ineffective breathing patterns:**
   1. **hypoventilation** related to depressant effects of anesthesia and some medications (e.g. narcotic analgesics), reluctance to breathe deeply due to incisional pain and fear of dislodging chest tube(s) if in place, restricted expansion of remaining lung due to positioning, weakness, and pressure on the diaphragm resulting from abdominal distention
   2. **hyperventilation** related to fear, anxiety, and discomfort;
b. **ineffective airway clearance** related to:
   1. stasis of secretions associated with decreased activity and poor cough effort resulting from depressant effects of anesthesia and some medications (e.g. narcotic analgesics), pain, and fatigue
   2. increased secretions associated with irritation of the respiratory tract (can result from inhalation anesthetics and endotracheal intubation)
   3. tenacious secretions associated with fluid loss and decreased fluid intake;
c. **impaired gas exchange** related to:
   1. ineffective breathing patterns and airway clearance
   2. inability of pulmonary system to compensate fully for the decrease in alveolar surface associated with the surgical removal of lung tissue.

---

 * This diagnostic label includes the following nursing diagnoses: ineffective breathing pattern, ineffective airway clearance, and impaired gas exchange (Carpenito, 1989).

☐ ▬▬▬▬▬▬▬▬▬▬▬▬▬▬▬▬▬▬▬▬

DESIRED OUTCOMES	NURSING ACTIONS AND *SELECTED RATIONALES*
1. The client will experience adequate respiratory function as evidenced by: a. improved rate, rhythm, and depth of respirations b. decreased dyspnea c. improved breath sounds d. usual mental status e. usual skin color f. blood gases returning toward normal range.	1.a. Assess for and report signs and symptoms of altered respiratory function: 1. rapid, shallow, slow, or irregular respirations 2. dyspnea, orthopnea 3. use of accessory muscles when breathing 4. adventitious breath sounds (e.g. crackles, rhonchi) 5. diminished or absent breath sounds over remaining lung tissue 6. restlessness, irritability 7. confusion, somnolence 8. dusky or cyanotic skin color. b. Monitor blood gases. Report values that have worsened. c. Monitor for and report significant changes in ear oximetry and capnograph results. d. Monitor chest x-ray results and report significant changes. e. Implement measures *to improve respiratory status:* 1. perform actions to improve breathing pattern and promote effective airway clearance (see Standardized Postoperative Care Plan, Nursing Diagnoses 3, action d and 4, action b) 2. perform actions to reduce pain (see Postoperative Nursing Diagnosis 2) 3. if chest tube(s) present, assure client that deep breathing and coughing will not dislodge the tube(s)

4. position client as ordered (e.g. on back or slightly tilted on operative side after pneumonectomy, on back or unoperative side following segmental or wedge resection) *to allow full expansion of remaining lung tissue*
5. maintain oxygen therapy as ordered
6. discourage smoking *(smoking depresses ciliary function, increases mucus production, and decreases oxygen availability)*
7. allow frequent rest periods *to compensate for the decreased respiratory capacity resulting from loss of lung tissue*
8. monitor for therapeutic and nontherapeutic effects of bronchodilators if administered.

f. Consult physician if signs and symptoms of impaired respiratory function persist or worsen.

□ ▬▬▬▬▬▬▬▬▬▬▬▬▬▬▬▬▬▬▬▬▬

2. NURSING DIAGNOSIS

Pain:

a. **chest pain** related to tissue trauma, irritation of intercostal nerves, and tissue irritation associated with surgical procedure and/or presence of chest tube(s);
b. **shoulder pain** related to inflammation of incised muscles.

□ ▬▬▬▬▬▬▬▬▬▬▬▬▬▬▬▬▬▬▬▬▬

DESIRED OUTCOMES	NURSING ACTIONS AND *SELECTED RATIONALES*

2. The client will experience diminished pain (see Standardized Postoperative Care Plan, Nursing Diagnosis 7.A, for outcome criteria).	2.a. Refer to Standardized Postoperative Care Plan, Nursing Diagnosis 7.A, for measures related to assessment and management of postoperative pain.
	b. Implement additional measures *to reduce pain:*
	  1. securely anchor or fasten chest tube(s) *to decrease discomfort resulting from movement of tube(s)*
	  2. provide adequate support (e.g. pillows, sling) to arm and shoulder on operative side.

□ ▬▬▬▬▬▬▬▬▬▬▬▬▬▬▬▬▬▬▬▬▬

3. COLLABORATIVE DIAGNOSIS

Potential complications:

a. **extended pneumothorax** related to surgical opening of pleura and chest tube malfunction;
b. **hemothorax** related to intraoperative or postoperative bleeding and/or chest tube malfunction;
c. **mediastinal shift** related to:
   1. increase in intrapleural pressure on the operative side following a lobectomy associated with an accumulation of fluid and air
   2. excessive negative pressure on operative side following pneumonectomy associated with inadequate serous fluid accumulation in the thoracic space (the position of the mediastinum is maintained by accumulation of serous fluid in the empty thoracic space)
   3. incorrect positioning following a pneumonectomy;
d. **acute pulmonary edema** related to:
   1. increased capillary permeability associated with hypoxia
   2. excessive hydrostatic pressure in the remaining pulmonary vessels associated

with removal of a large portion of the pulmonary vascular system if a pneumonectomy was performed;

e. **restricted arm and shoulder movement** related to decreased activity of the arm
and shoulder on the operative side and adhesion formation between incised muscles.

☐ ▮▮

DESIRED OUTCOMES	NURSING ACTIONS AND *SELECTED RATIONALES*

3.a. The client will experience normal lung re-expansion postoperatively as evidenced by:
1. normal breath sounds and percussion note over remaining lung tissue by 3rd–4th postoperative day
2. unlabored respirations at 16–20/minute
3. blood gases returning toward normal
4. chest x-ray showing lung re-expansion.
	3.a.1. Assess for and immediately report signs and symptoms of:
	  a. malfunction of chest drainage system (e.g. respiratory distress, sudden cessation of drainage, excessive bubbling in water seal chamber, significant increase in subcutaneous emphysema)
	  b. extended pneumothorax (e.g. extended area of absent breath sounds and hyperresonant percussion note; further increase in pulse rate; increased respiratory distress; sudden, sharp chest pain; cyanosis; restlessness; confusion).
	  2. Monitor blood gases. Report values that have worsened.
	  3. Monitor chest x-ray results. Report findings of delayed lung re-expansion.
	  4. Implement measures *to promote lung re-expansion and prevent extended pneumothorax:*
	    a. perform actions *to maintain patency and integrity of chest drainage system if present:*
	      1. maintain water seal and suction levels as ordered
	      2. maintain air occlusive dressing over chest tube insertion site
	      3. tape all connections securely
	      4. milk or strip tubes if ordered
	      5. keep chest drainage and suction tubing free of kinks
	      6. keep drainage system below client's chest level at all times
	    b. perform actions to improve respiratory status (see Postoperative Nursing Diagnosis 1, action e).
	  5. If signs and symptoms of extended pneumothorax occur:
	    a. maintain client on bedrest in a semi- to high Fowler's position
	    b. maintain oxygen therapy as ordered
	    c. assess for and immediately report signs and symptoms of mediastinal shift (see action c.1 in this diagnosis)
	    d. assist with clearing of existing chest tube and/or insertion of a new tube
	    e. provide emotional support to client and significant others.

3.b. The client will not develop hemothorax as evidenced by:
1. normal breath sounds and percussion note over remaining lung tissue by 3rd–4th postoperative day
2. unlabored respirations at 16–20/minute
3. usual skin color
4. blood gases returning toward normal range.
	3.b.1. Assess for and immediately report signs and symptoms of:
	  a. thoracic bleeding (e.g. unexpected bloody drainage from chest tubes, increase in bloody drainage on dressing, further decrease in Hct. and Hgb.)
	  b. hemothorax (e.g. diminished or absent breath sounds with dull percussion note over affected area, dyspnea, cyanosis).
	  2. Monitor blood gases. Report values that have worsened.
	  3. Implement measures to maintain patency and integrity of chest drainage system (see action a.4.a in this diagnosis) *in order to reduce risk of hemothorax.*
	  4. If signs and symptoms of hemothorax occur:
	    a. maintain client on bedrest in a semi- to high Fowler's position
	    b. maintain oxygen therapy as ordered
	    c. monitor for and report signs and symptoms of a mediastinal shift (see action c.1 in this diagnosis)
	    d. assess for and report signs and symptoms of shock (e.g. hypotension; increased pulse and respirations; urine output less than 30 cc/hour; cool, clammy skin; change in mental status)
	    e. monitor for therapeutic and nontherapeutic effects of blood products and/or volume expanders if administered
	    f. assist with clearing of existing chest tube(s), thoracentesis, or insertion of chest tube(s) if not already present

g. prepare client for surgical intervention to ligate bleeding vessels if indicated

h. provide emotional support to client and significant others.

3.c. The client will not develop mediastinal shift as evidenced by:
1. vital signs within normal range for client
2. usual skin color
3. point of apical impulse in 5th intercostal space near midclavicular line
4. trachea in midline position
5. blood gases returning toward normal range.

3.c.1. Assess for and immediately report signs and symptoms of mediastinal shift (e.g. severe dyspnea, restlessness and agitation, rapid and/or irregular pulse rate, cyanosis, shift in point of apical impulse, displacement of trachea away from midline).
2. Monitor blood gases and report values that have worsened.
3. Implement measures *to reduce risk of mediastinal shift:*
   a. keep chest tube clamped if one is in place after a pneumonectomy *(serous fluid accumulation is essential to maintain proper pressure gradient on operative side)*
   b. position client as ordered (e.g. on back or slightly tilted on operative side after pneumonectomy)
   c. perform actions to prevent and treat pneumothorax and hemothorax (see actions a.4 and 5 and b.3 and 4 in this diagnosis).
4. If signs and symptoms of mediastinal shift occur:
   a. maintain client on bedrest in a semi- to high Fowler's position
   b. maintain oxygen therapy as ordered
   c. if chest tube(s) malfunctioning or not present, assist with clearing of existing tube(s), thoracentesis, or insertion of new tube(s) if indicated
   d. assist with attempts to increase pressure in the empty thoracic space if shift occurs toward operative side following a pneumonectomy
   e. provide emotional support to client and significant others.

3.d. The client will not develop pulmonary edema as evidenced by:
1. vital signs within normal range for client
2. clear breath sounds and resonant percussion note over unoperative area
3. absence of productive, persistent cough
4. usual skin color
5. blood gases returning toward normal range.

3.d.1. Assess for and report signs and symptoms of pulmonary edema (e.g. severe dyspnea, tachycardia, dull percussion note over unoperative area, adventitious breath sounds, persistent cough productive of frothy and/or blood-tinged sputum, cyanosis).
2. Obtain blood gases as ordered. Report decline in PaO_2 and increase in $PaCO_2$.
3. Monitor for and report significant changes in ear oximetry and capnograph results.
4. Monitor chest x-ray results. Report findings of pulmonary edema.
5. Implement measures *to prevent hypoxia and reduce the risk of pulmonary edema:*
   a. perform actions to promote lung re-expansion (see action a.4 in this diagnosis)
   b. maintain oxygen therapy as ordered.
6. If signs and symptoms of pulmonary edema occur:
   a. continue with above measures to promote lung re-expansion and reduce hypoxia
   b. monitor for therapeutic and nontherapeutic effects of the following medications if administered:
      1. bronchodilators (e.g. theophylline) *to facilitate breathing*
      2. agents *to reduce pulmonary vascular congestion* (e.g. diuretics, morphine sulfate, cardiotonics)
   c. apply rotating tourniquets according to hospital policy if ordered *to reduce pulmonary vascular congestion.*

3.e. The client will maintain normal arm and shoulder function as evidenced by ability to move arm and shoulder on operative side through usual range of motion.

3.e.1. Assess for and report signs and symptoms of restricted arm and shoulder movement on operative side (e.g. inability to move arm and shoulder through usual range of motion, inability to use arm in activities of daily living).
2. Implement measures *to prevent restriction of arm and shoulder movement on operative side:*
   a. perform passive range of motion to arm and shoulder at least 2 times every 4–6 hours during first 24 hours postoperatively
   b. instruct client in and assist with active arm and shoulder exercises (e.g. shoulder shrugs, wall climbing with fingers) 10–20 times every 2 hours beginning the 1st or 2nd postoperative day
   c. perform actions to reduce pain (see Postoperative Nursing Diagnosis 2) *in order to increase client's ability and willingness to move arm and shoulder*

UNIT
IX

    d. encourage client to use arm on operative side in activities of daily living
    e. place frequently used articles and bedstand on operative side *so that client will be encouraged to reach with affected arm*
    f. anchor pull rope at foot of bed; encourage client to use arm on operative side to pull self to sitting position.
3. If signs and symptoms of restricted arm and shoulder movement occur:
    a. continue with above actions
    b. assist with planned physical therapy program
    c. provide emotional support to client and significant others.

---

4. NURSING DIAGNOSIS

Grieving* related to loss of all or part of a lung and anticipated changes in usual life style as a result of altered lung capacity.

---

* This diagnostic label includes anticipatory grieving and grieving following the actual losses/changes.

DESIRED OUTCOMES	NURSING ACTIONS AND *SELECTED RATIONALES*

4. The client will demonstrate beginning progression through the grieving process as evidenced by:
    a. verbalization of feelings about the loss of a lung and its effects on life style
    b. expression of grief
    c. participation in treatment plan and self-care activities
    d. utilization of available support systems
    e. verbalization of ways to modify current life style to compensate for altered lung capacity.

4.a. Determine client's perception of the impact of loss of all or part of a lung on his/her life style.
  b. Determine how client usually expresses grief.
  c. Observe for signs of grieving (e.g. changes in eating habits, insomnia, anger, noncompliance, denial).
  d. Implement measures *to facilitate the grieving process:*
    1. assist client to acknowledge the changes resulting from loss of lung function *so grief work can begin*; assess for factors that may hinder or facilitate acknowledgment
    2. discuss the grieving process and assist client to accept the stages of grieving as an expected response to his/her loss
    3. allow time for client to progress through the stages of grieving (denial, anger, bargaining, depression, acceptance [Kübler-Ross, 1969]); be aware that not every stage is experienced or expressed by all individuals
    4. provide an atmosphere of care and concern (e.g. provide privacy, be available and nonjudgmental, display empathy and respect) *so that client will feel free to verbalize both positive and negative feelings and concerns*
    5. perform actions *to promote trust* (e.g. answer questions honestly, provide requested information)
    6. encourage the expression of anger and sadness about the loss of the lung
    7. encourage client to express his/her feelings in whatever ways are comfortable (e.g. writing, drawing, conversation)
    8. assist client to identify personal strengths that have helped him/her to cope in previous situations of loss
    9. support realistic hope about the ability to resume his/her usual activities.
  e. Assess for and support behaviors suggesting successful resolution of grief (e.g. verbalizing feelings about the loss of a lung, expressing sorrow, focusing on ways to adapt to an altered lung capacity).
  f. Explain the stages of the grieving process to significant others. Encourage their support and understanding.
  g. Provide information regarding counseling services and support groups that might be of assistance to client in working through grief.
  h. Arrange for visit from clergy if desired by client.

i. Monitor for therapeutic and nontherapeutic effects of antidepressants if administered.

j. Consult physician regarding referral for counseling if signs of dysfunctional grieving (e.g. persistent denial of loss and necessary changes in life style, excessive anger or sadness, hysteria, suicidal behaviors, phobias) occur.

5. NURSING DIAGNOSIS

Knowledge deficit regarding follow-up care.

DESIRED OUTCOMES	NURSING ACTIONS AND *SELECTED RATIONALES*
5.a. The client will demonstrate the ability to perform prescribed arm and shoulder exercises.	5.a.1. Instruct client regarding importance of exercising the arm and shoulder on operative side. Emphasize that the exercises should be carried out at least 4 times/day for several weeks. 2. Demonstrate appropriate arm and shoulder exercises (e.g. shoulder shrugs, arm circles). 3. Allow time for questions, clarification, and return demonstration.

5.b. The client will state signs and symptoms of complications to report to the health care provider.	5.b.1. Refer to Standardized Postoperative Care Plan, Nursing Diagnosis 20, action c, for signs and symptoms to report to the health care provider.
	 2. Instruct the client to report these additional signs and symptoms:
	   a. increased discomfort in or decreased ability to move arm and shoulder on operative side
	   b. increased shortness of breath with activity.

5.c. The client will identify community resources that can assist with home management and adjustment to the diagnosis, effects of surgery, and adjunctive treatment if planned.	5.c.1. Provide information about community resources that can assist the client and significant others with home management and adjustment to the diagnosis, effects of surgery, and adjunctive treatment if planned (e.g. American Lung Association, American Cancer Society, Meals on Wheels, counselors, support groups, Visiting Nurse Association, home health agencies). 2. Initiate a referral if indicated.

5.d. The client will verbalize an understanding of and a plan for adhering to recommended follow-up care including future appointments with health care provider, medications prescribed, activity level, pain management, wound care, and subsequent treatment of the underlying disorder.	5.d.1. Refer to Standardized Postoperative Care Plan, Nursing Diagnosis 20, for routine postoperative instructions and measures to improve client compliance.
	 2. Reinforce physician's instructions about activity restrictions:
	   a. gauge activity according to tolerance and ensure adequate rest periods
	   b. stop any activity that causes excessive fatigue, dyspnea, or chest pain
	   c. avoid lifting heavy objects until complete healing of chest muscles has occurred (usually 3–6 months).
	 3. Inform client that numbness and discomfort in the operative area will persist for several weeks but is usually temporary. Explain that application of heat is sometimes helpful in relieving the discomfort.
	 4. Clarify plans for subsequent treatment of underlying disorder (e.g. chemotherapy, radiation therapy) if appropriate.

UNIT IX

References

Carpenito, LJ. Handbook of nursing diagnosis (3rd ed.). Philadelphia: J.B. Lippincott Company, 1989.

Kübler-Ross, E. On death and dying. New York: Macmillan, 1969.

Pneumonia

Pneumonia is an acute inflammation of lung tissue resulting from exposure to environmental irritants such as toxic chemicals, gases, and dust or pathogenic organisms such as bacteria, viruses, and fungi. Pneumonia can also result from aspiration of body secretions, food, fluid, and foreign objects.

Pneumonia is usually classified according to the causative organism or etiological factor. It may also be classified as community-acquired, hospital-acquired, atypical, or pneumonia in the immunocompromised host. The types differ in relation to the mechanism of lung invasion (e.g. inhalation, aspiration, vascular system), incubation period, signs and symptoms experienced by the client, complications that can result, and mortality rate. The most common type of pneumonia is community-acquired pneumococcal pneumonia. It occurs most often in winter and early spring, has an abrupt onset, and usually follows an upper respiratory infection.

This care plan focuses on the adult client hospitalized for treatment of pneumococcal pneumonia. Major goals of care are to improve respiratory function, relieve discomfort, prevent complications, and educate the client regarding follow-up care.

DISCHARGE CRITERIA

Prior to discharge, the client will:

- identify ways to maintain respiratory health
- state signs and symptoms to report to the health care provider
- verbalize an understanding of and a plan for adhering to recommended follow-up care including future appointments with health care provider, medications prescribed, and activity limitations.

Use in conjunction with the Care Plan on Immobility.

NURSING/COLLABORATIVE DIAGNOSES

1. Anxiety □ *483*
2. Altered respiratory function:
    a. ineffective breathing patterns:
        1. hypoventilation
        2. hyperventilation
    b. ineffective airway clearance
    c. impaired gas exchange □ *483*
3. Fluid volume deficit □ *485*
4. Altered nutrition: less than body requirements □ *485*
5A. Altered comfort: chills and excessive diaphoresis □ *486*
5B. Altered comfort: chest pain □ *486*
5C. Altered comfort: abdominal distention and gas pain □ *487*
5D. Altered comfort: nausea and vomiting □ *488*

□ ▬▬▬▬▬▬▬▬▬▬▬▬▬▬▬▬▬▬▬▬▬▬▬▬▬▬▬

1. NURSING DIAGNOSIS

Anxiety related to sudden onset of symptoms; unfamiliar environment; dyspnea; chest pain; and lack of understanding of diagnosis, diagnostic tests, and treatment plan.

□ ▬▬▬▬▬▬▬▬▬▬▬▬▬▬▬▬▬▬▬▬▬▬▬▬▬▬▬

DESIRED OUTCOMES	NURSING ACTIONS AND *SELECTED RATIONALES*

1. The client will experience a reduction in fear and anxiety (see Care Plan on Immobility, Nursing Diagnosis 1, for outcome criteria).	1.a. Refer to Care Plan on Immobility, Nursing Diagnosis 1, for measures related to assessment and reduction of fear and anxiety.
	b. Implement additional measures *to reduce fear and anxiety:*
	  1. explain all diagnostic tests (e.g. chest x-ray, serum and sputum studies, ear oximetry, capnography, pulmonary function studies, fiberoptic bronchoscopy, transtracheal aspiration of sputum)
	  2. perform actions to reduce chest pain (see Nursing Diagnosis 5.B, action 5)
	  3. perform actions to improve respiratory status (see Nursing Diagnosis 2, action f) *in order to reduce dyspnea.*

□ ▬▬▬▬▬▬▬▬▬▬▬▬▬▬▬▬▬▬▬▬▬▬▬▬▬▬▬

2. NURSING DIAGNOSIS

Altered respiratory function:*

a. **ineffective breathing patterns:**
   1. **hypoventilation** related to chest pain, pleural effusion, abdominal distention, weakness, and fatigue
   2. **hyperventilation** related to fear, anxiety, and infection;
b. **ineffective airway clearance** related to:
   1. copious, tenacious secretions associated with fluid volume deficit and increased mucus production resulting from the infectious process

---

* This diagnostic label includes the following nursing diagnoses: ineffective breathing pattern, ineffective airway clearance, and impaired gas exchange (Carpenito, 1989).

2. stasis of secretions associated with decreased activity, impaired ciliary function, and poor cough effort resulting from fatigue and chest pain;
c. **impaired gas exchange** related to ineffective breathing patterns and airway clearance and a decrease in effective lung surface associated with accumulation of secretions and consolidation of lung tissue.

DESIRED OUTCOMES	NURSING ACTIONS AND *SELECTED RATIONALES*

2. The client will experience adequate respiratory function as evidenced by:
   a. normal rate, rhythm, and depth of respirations
   b. decreasing dyspnea
   c. improved breath sounds
   d. usual mental status
   e. usual skin color
   f. blood gases within normal range.

2.a. Assess for and report signs and symptoms of altered respiratory function:
   1. rapid, shallow, or irregular respirations
   2. dyspnea, orthopnea
   3. use of accessory muscles when breathing
   4. diminished or absent breath sounds
   5. adventitious breath sounds (e.g. crackles, wheezes)
   6. restlessness, irritability
   7. confusion, somnolence
   8. dusky or cyanotic skin color.
   b. Monitor blood gases. Report abnormal results.
   c. Monitor for and report significant changes in ear oximetry and capnograph results.
   d. Monitor for and report an increasing amount of purulent or rust-colored sputum.
   e. Monitor chest x-ray results and report abnormalities.
   f. Implement measures *to improve respiratory status:*
      1. maintain client on bedrest as ordered during the acute phase *to reduce oxygen needs*
      2. place client in a semi- to high Fowler's position
      3. instruct and assist client to turn, cough, and deep breathe every 1–2 hours
      4. reinforce correct use of inspiratory exerciser at least every 2 hours
      5. perform actions *to facilitate removal of pulmonary secretions:*
         a. implement measures *to liquefy secretions:*
            1. maintain a fluid intake of at least 2500 cc/day unless contraindicated
            2. humidify inspired air as ordered
            3. assist with administration of mucolytic agents via nebulizer or IPPB treatment
         b. assist with or perform postural drainage, percussion, and vibration if ordered
         c. perform tracheal suctioning if needed
         d. monitor for therapeutic and nontherapeutic effects of expectorants if administered
      6. perform actions to reduce abdominal distention (see Nursing Diagnosis 5.C, action 3) *in order to prevent an increase in pressure on the diaphragm*
      7. perform actions to reduce fear and anxiety (see Nursing Diagnosis 1)
      8. perform actions to reduce chest pain (see Nursing Diagnosis 5.B, action 5)
      9. maintain oxygen therapy as ordered
      10. discourage smoking (*smoking depresses alveolar macrophage activity, impairs ciliary function, causes an increase in mucus production, and decreases oxygen availability*)
      11. increase activity as allowed and tolerated
      12. administer central nervous system depressants (e.g. narcotics, sedatives) judiciously; hold medication and consult physician if respiratory rate is less than 12/minute
      13. monitor for therapeutic and nontherapeutic effects of bronchodilators and anti-infectives if administered.
   g. Consult physician if signs and symptoms of impaired respiratory function persist or worsen.

3. NURSING DIAGNOSIS

Fluid volume deficit related to:

a. excessive fluid loss associated with vomiting, profuse diaphoresis, hyperventilation, and increased production of pulmonary secretions;
b. decreased oral fluid intake associated with anorexia, nausea, and dyspnea.

DESIRED OUTCOMES	NURSING ACTIONS AND *SELECTED RATIONALES*

3. The client will not experience a fluid volume deficit as evidenced by:
a. normal skin turgor
b. moist mucous membranes
c. weight loss no greater than 0.5 kg/day
d. B/P and pulse within normal range for client and stable with position change
e. Hct. within normal range
f. balanced intake and output
g. urine specific gravity between 1.010–1.030.
	3.a. Assess for and report signs and symptoms of fluid volume deficit:
	   1. decreased skin turgor
	   2. dry mucous membranes, thirst
	   3. weight loss greater than 0.5 kg/day
	   4. low B/P and/or decline in systolic B/P of at least 15 mm Hg with concurrent rise in pulse when client sits up
	   5. weak, rapid pulse
	   6. elevated Hct.
	   7. output less than intake with urine specific gravity higher than 1.030 (reflects an actual rather than potential water deficit).
	  b. Monitor client for profuse diaphoresis. Keep count of linen changes *to aid in estimating fluid loss.*
	  c. Implement measures *to prevent or treat fluid volume deficit:*
	   1. perform actions to reduce fever (see Nursing Diagnosis 6, action b) *in order to prevent profuse diaphoresis*
	   2. perform actions to improve oral intake (see Nursing Diagnosis 4)
	   3. perform actions to reduce nausea and vomiting (see Nursing Diagnosis 5.D, action 2)
	   4. perform actions to reduce fear and anxiety (see Nursing Diagnosis 1) *in order to decrease hyperventilation*
	   5. perform actions to resolve the infectious process (see Nursing Diagnosis 6, action b.1) *in order to reduce fever, decrease production of pulmonary secretions, and decrease hyperventilation*
	   6. maintain a fluid intake of at least 2500 cc/day unless contraindicated
	   7. maintain intravenous fluid therapy as ordered.
	  d. Consult physician if signs and symptoms of fluid volume deficit persist or worsen.

UNIT
IX

4. NURSING DIAGNOSIS

Altered nutrition: less than body requirements related to:

a. decreased oral intake associated with:
  1. anorexia resulting from discomfort, fatigue, and decreased activity
  2. nausea
  3. dyspnea;
b. loss of nutrients associated with vomiting;
c. increased metabolic rate associated with infection.

DESIRED OUTCOMES	NURSING ACTIONS AND *SELECTED RATIONALES*

4. The client will maintain an adequate nutritional status (see Care Plan on Immobility, Nursing Diagnosis 6, for outcome criteria).	4.a. Refer to Care Plan on Immobility, Nursing Diagnosis 6, for measures related to assessment and improvement of nutritional status.
	b. Implement additional measures *to improve oral intake and nutritional status:*
	  1. perform actions to relieve nausea and vomiting (see Nursing Diagnosis 5.D, action 2)
	  2. perform actions to reduce discomfort (see Nursing Diagnoses 5.A, actions 3 and 4; 5.B, action 5; and 5.C, action 3)
	  3. place client in a high Fowler's position for meals *to help relieve dyspnea.*

5.A. NURSING DIAGNOSIS

Altered comfort: chills and excessive diaphoresis related to persistent fever associated with the infectious process.

DESIRED OUTCOMES	NURSING ACTIONS AND *SELECTED RATIONALES*

5.A. The client will not experience discomfort associated with chills and diaphoresis as evidenced by:
1. verbalization of comfort
2. ability to rest.
	5.A.1. Assess client for chills and excessive diaphoresis.
	  2. Implement measures to reduce fever (see Nursing Diagnosis 6, action b).
	  3. Implement measures *to promote comfort if client is having chills:*
	    a. maintain a room temperature that is comfortable for client
	    b. protect client from drafts
	    c. provide extra blankets and clothing as needed
	    d. provide warm liquids to drink as tolerated.
	  4. Implement measures *to promote comfort if excessive diaphoresis is present:*
	    a. change linen and clothing whenever damp
	    b. bathe client and sponge his/her face as needed.
	  5. Consult physician if persistent temperature elevation leads to continued chills and excessive diaphoresis.

5.B. NURSING DIAGNOSIS

Altered comfort:* chest pain related to irritation of the parietal pleura associated with the inflammatory process and muscle strain associated with excessive coughing.

---

* In this care plan, the nursing diagnosis "pain" is included under the diagnostic label of altered comfort.

DESIRED OUTCOMES	NURSING ACTIONS AND *SELECTED RATIONALES*
5.B. The client will experience diminished chest pain as	5.B.1. Determine how the client usually responds to pain. 2. Assess for nonverbal signs of pain (e.g. wrinkled brow, clenched fists,

evidenced by:
1. verbalization of pain relief
2. relaxed facial expression and body positioning
3. increased participation in activities
4. improved breathing pattern.

reluctance to move, increased diaphoresis, tachycardia, guarding of affected side or areas of chest, shallow respirations).
3. Assess verbal complaints of pain. Ask client to be specific regarding location, severity, and type of pain.
4. Assess for factors that seem to aggravate and alleviate pain.
5. Implement measures *to reduce chest pain:*
   a. instruct and assist client to splint chest with hands or pillow when deep breathing, coughing, and changing position
   b. position on affected side for 2-hour periods *to reduce stretching of inflamed pleura*
   c. provide or assist with nonpharmacological measures for pain relief (e.g. back rub, position change, relaxation techniques, guided imagery, quiet conversation, restful environment, diversional activities)
   d. perform actions to decrease excessive coughing episodes (see Nursing Diagnosis 8, action b.1)
   e. monitor for therapeutic and nontherapeutic effects of analgesics if administered
   f. assist with intercostal nerve block if performed.
6. Consult physician if above actions fail to relieve chest pain.

□ ▮▮

5.C. NURSING DIAGNOSIS

Altered comfort: abdominal distention and gas pain related to persistent air swallowing during severe dyspneic episodes and decreased peristalsis associated with infection and decreased activity.

□ ▮▮

UNIT
IX

DESIRED OUTCOMES	NURSING ACTIONS AND *SELECTED RATIONALES*

5.C. The client will experience diminished abdominal distention and gas pain as evidenced by:
1. verbalization of decreased abdominal fullness and pain
2. relaxed facial expression and body positioning
3. decrease in abdominal distention.

5.C.1. Assess for nonverbal signs of abdominal distention and gas pain (e.g. clutching and guarding of abdomen, restlessness, reluctance to move, grimacing, increasing abdominal girth, increased dyspnea).
2. Assess for verbal complaints of abdominal fullness and gas pain.
3. Implement measures *to reduce accumulation of gastrointestinal gas and fluid:*
   a. encourage and assist client with frequent position changes and ambulation when allowed and tolerated *(activity stimulates peristalsis and expulsion of flatus)*
   b. instruct client to avoid activities such as chewing gum, sucking on hard candy, and smoking *in order to reduce air swallowing*
   c. encourage client to drink warm liquids *to stimulate peristalsis*
   d. instruct client to avoid gas-producing foods/fluids (e.g. carbonated beverages, cabbage, onions, popcorn, baked beans)
   e. apply heat to the abdomen for 20 minutes every 2–3 hours unless contraindicated
   f. consult physician regarding insertion of a rectal tube or administration of a return flow enema if indicated
   g. monitor for therapeutic and nontherapeutic effects of the following medications if administered:
      1. antiflatulents *to reduce gas accumulation*
      2. gastrointestinal stimulants (e.g. metoclopramide, bisacodyl) *to increase gastrointestinal motility.*
4. Consult physician if abdominal distention and gas pain persist or worsen.

☐ ▬▬▬▬▬▬▬▬▬▬▬▬▬▬▬▬▬▬▬▬

5.D. NURSING DIAGNOSIS

Altered comfort: nausea and vomiting related to stimulation of the vomiting center associated with:

1. vagal and/or sympathetic stimulation resulting from visceral irritation associated with abdominal distention;
2. cortical stimulation resulting from taste of some aerosol treatments, foul odor and taste of sputum, and stress.

☐ ▬▬▬▬▬▬▬▬▬▬▬▬▬▬▬▬▬▬▬▬

DESIRED OUTCOMES	NURSING ACTIONS AND *SELECTED RATIONALES*

5.D. The client will experience relief of nausea and vomiting as evidenced by:
1. verbalization of relief of nausea
2. absence of vomiting.
	5.D.1. Assess client to determine factors that contribute to nausea and vomiting (e.g. fear, anxiety, abdominal distention, copious sputum, aerosol treatments).
	  2. Implement measures *to prevent nausea and vomiting:*
	    a. perform actions to reduce fear and anxiety (see Nursing Diagnosis 1)
	    b. perform actions to decrease abdominal distention (see Nursing Diagnosis 5.C, action 3)
	    c. encourage client to take deep, slow breaths when nauseated
	    d. eliminate noxious sights and smells from the environment; provide client with an opaque, covered container for expectorated sputum; empty container frequently and remove it from the table during mealtime if it is not needed *(noxious stimuli cause cortical stimulation of the vomiting center)*
	    e. encourage client to change positions slowly *(movement stimulates the chemoreceptor trigger zone)*
	    f. provide oral hygiene after chest physiotherapy, aerosol treatments, and each emesis and before meals
	    g. schedule treatments that assist in mobilizing the mucus (e.g. aerosol treatments, postural drainage, percussion, vibration) at least 1 hour before or after meals
	    h. provide small, frequent meals rather than 3 large ones
	    i. instruct client to ingest foods and fluids slowly
	    j. instruct client to avoid foods/fluids that irritate the gastric mucosa (e.g. spicy foods; citrus fruits or juices; caffeine-containing items such as chocolate, coffee, tea, and colas)
	    k. encourage client to eat dry foods (e.g. toast, crackers) and avoid drinking liquids with meals if nauseated
	    l. instruct client to rest after eating with head of bed elevated
	    m. monitor for therapeutic and nontherapeutic effects of antiemetics if administered.
	  3. If above measures fail to control nausea and vomiting:
	    a. consult physician
	    b. be prepared to insert a nasogastric tube and maintain suction as ordered.

☐ ▬▬▬▬▬▬▬▬▬▬▬▬▬▬▬▬▬▬▬▬

6. NURSING DIAGNOSIS

Hyperthermia related to stimulation of the thermoregulatory center in the hypothalamus by endogenous pyrogens that are released in an infectious process.

☐ ▬▬▬▬▬▬▬▬▬▬▬▬▬▬▬▬▬▬▬▬

DESIRED OUTCOMES	**NURSING ACTIONS AND *SELECTED RATIONALES***

6. The client will experience resolution of hyperthermia as evidenced by:
a. skin usual color and temperature
b. pulse rate between 60–100 beats/minute
c. respirations 16–20/minute
d. normal body temperature.
	6.a. Assess for signs and symptoms of hyperthermia (e.g. warm, flushed skin; tachycardia; tachypnea; elevated temperature).
	b. Implement measures *to reduce fever:*
	  1. perform actions *to resolve the infectious process:*
	    a. implement measures to facilitate removal of pulmonary secretions (see Nursing Diagnosis 2, action f.5)
	    b. implement measures to promote rest (see Nursing Diagnosis 8)
	    c. implement measures to maintain an optimal nutritional status (see Nursing Diagnosis 4)
	    d. monitor for therapeutic and nontherapeutic effects of anti-infectives if administered
	  2. administer tepid sponge bath
	  3. apply cooling blanket as ordered
	  4. monitor for therapeutic and nontherapeutic effects of antipyretics if administered.
	c. Consult physician if temperature remains higher then 38°C.

---

7. NURSING DIAGNOSIS

Altered oral mucous membrane: dryness related to:

a. fluid volume deficit associated with increased fluid loss and decreased fluid intake;
b. oxygen therapy (oxygen is a dry gas and will dehydrate the respiratory mucous membranes if exposure is prolonged).

UNIT
IX

DESIRED OUTCOMES	**NURSING ACTIONS AND *SELECTED RATIONALES***

7. The client will maintain a moist, intact oral mucous membrane.	7.a. Assess client every shift for dryness of the oral mucosa.
	b. Implement measures *to decrease dryness of the oral mucous membrane:*
	  1. instruct and assist client to perform good oral hygiene as often as needed
	  2. encourage client to rinse mouth frequently with water
	  3. instruct client to avoid products such as lemon-glycerin swabs and commercial mouthwashes containing alcohol *(these products have a drying or irritating effect on the oral mucous membrane)*
	  4. lubricate client's lips with Vaseline, K-Y jelly, ChapStick, Blistex, or mineral oil when oral care is given
	  5. encourage client to breathe through nose if possible
	  6. encourage client not to smoke *(smoking further irritates and dries the mucosa)*
	  7. perform actions to prevent or treat fluid volume deficit (see Nursing Diagnosis 3, action c)
	  8. offer hot tea with lemon or warm lemonade at regular intervals unless contraindicated *to increase salivary flow*
	  9. encourage client to use artificial saliva (e.g. Moi-stir, Salivart, Xero-Lube) *to lubricate the mucous membrane.*
	c. If oral mucosa is irritated or cracked, implement measures *to relieve discomfort and promote healing:*
	  1. assist client to select soft, bland, and nonacidic foods
	  2. instruct client to avoid foods/fluids that are extremely hot or cold
	  3. use a soft bristle brush or low-pressure power spray for oral care
	  4. monitor for therapeutic and nontherapeutic effects of topical anesthetics, oral protective pastes, and topical and systemic analgesics if administered.
	d. Consult physician if dryness, irritation, and discomfort persist.

8. NURSING DIAGNOSIS

Activity intolerance related to:

a. tissue hypoxia associated with impaired gas exchange;
b. inability to rest and sleep associated with discomfort, excessive coughing, anxiety, dyspnea, and frequent assessments and treatments;
c. malnutrition.

DESIRED OUTCOMES	NURSING ACTIONS AND *SELECTED RATIONALES*

8. The client will demonstrate an increased tolerance for activity (see Care Plan on Immobility, Nursing Diagnosis 8, for outcome criteria).	8.a. Refer to Care Plan on Immobility, Nursing Diagnosis 8, for measures related to assessment and improvement of activity tolerance.
	b. Implement additional measures *to promote rest and improve activity tolerance:*
	  1. perform actions *to decrease excessive coughing episodes:*
	    a. protect client from irritants (e.g. flowers, smoke, powder)
	    b. instruct client to avoid intake of extremely hot or cold foods/fluids *(these can stimulate cough)*
	    c. monitor for therapeutic and nontherapeutic effects of antitussives if administered early in the acute phase when cough is usually nonproductive
	  2. perform actions to promote sleep (see Nursing Diagnosis 10)
	  3. perform actions to improve respiratory status (see Nursing Diagnosis 2, action f) *in order to improve tissue oxygenation and relieve dyspnea.*
	  4. perform actions to relieve discomfort (see Nursing Diagnoses 5.A, actions 3 and 4; 5.B, action 5; 5.C, action 3; and 5.D, action 2)
	  5. perform actions to improve nutritional status (see Nursing Diagnosis 4).

9. NURSING DIAGNOSIS

Self-care deficit related to decreased activity tolerance, reluctance to move associated with chest pain, and activity restrictions imposed by the treatment plan.

DESIRED OUTCOMES	NURSING ACTIONS AND *SELECTED RATIONALES*

9. The client will demonstrate increased participation in self-care activities within activity tolerance level and prescribed activity restrictions.	9.a. Refer to Care Plan on Immobility, Nursing Diagnosis 9, for measures related to assessment of, planning for, and meeting the client's self-care needs.
	b. Implement additional measures *to facilitate client's ability to perform self-care activities:*
	  1. perform actions to improve activity tolerance (see Nursing Diagnosis 8)
	  2. perform actions to reduce chest pain (see Nursing Diagnosis 5.B, action 5).

10. NURSING DIAGNOSIS

Sleep pattern disturbance related to fear, anxiety, unfamiliar environment, decreased activity, discomfort, excessive coughing, inability to assume usual sleep position due to dyspnea, and frequent assessments and treatments.

DESIRED OUTCOMES	NURSING ACTIONS AND *SELECTED RATIONALES*

10. The client will attain optimal amounts of sleep within the parameters of the treatment regimen (see Care Plan on Immobility, Nursing Diagnosis 12, for outcome criteria).	10.a. Refer to Care Plan on Immobility, Nursing Diagnosis 12, for measures related to assessment and promotion of sleep.
	   b. Implement additional measures *to promote sleep:*
	    1. perform actions to reduce fear and anxiety (see Nursing Diagnosis 1)
	    2. assist client to assume a comfortable sleep position (e.g. bed in reverse Trendelenburg position with client in usual recumbent sleep position, head of bed elevated with arms supported on pillows, resting forward on overbed table with good pillow support, sitting in chair)
	    3. maintain oxygen therapy during sleep if indicated
	    4. ensure good room ventilation
	    5. perform actions to reduce discomfort (see Nursing Diagnoses 5.A, actions 3 and 4; 5.B, action 5; 5.C, action 3; and 5.D, action 2)
	    6. perform actions to reduce excessive coughing episodes (see Nursing Diagnosis 8, action b.1)
	    7. perform actions to improve respiratory status (see Nursing Diagnosis 2, action f) *in order to relieve dyspnea.*

UNIT
IX

11. NURSING DIAGNOSIS

Potential for infection: superinfection (bacteremia, pericarditis, endocarditis, candidiasis, meningitis, septic arthritis) related to spread of a highly virulent organism via the bloodstream, resistance of organism to anti-infective agents, and elimination of natural bacterial flora by anti-infective agents.

DESIRED OUTCOMES	NURSING ACTIONS AND *SELECTED RATIONALES*

11. The client will not develop a superinfection as evidenced by:
a. gradual return of vital signs to normal
b. improved breath sounds
c. usual mental status
d. absence of joint pain and swelling
e. absence of unusual drainage from any body cavity
f. absence of unusual lesions
	11.a. Assess for and report signs and symptoms of a superinfection:
	    1. increase in temperature above previous levels
	    2. increase in dyspnea and pulse rate
	    3. cardiac arrhythmias
	    4. breath sounds that worsen or fail to improve
	    5. change in mental status
	    6. swollen, red, painful joints
	    7. unusual color, amount, and odor of vaginal drainage; perineal itching; white patches or ulcerated areas in the mouth or vagina *(fungal infections are common superinfections with anti-infective therapy)*
	    8. stiff neck, headache
	    9. increase in WBC count above previous levels and/or significant change in differential.

g. absence of stiff neck, headache
h. WBC and differential counts returning to normal
i. negative results of cultured specimens.

b. Obtain culture specimens (e.g. blood, urine, mouth, sputum, vaginal) as ordered. Report positive results.
c. Implement measures *to prevent a superinfection:*
   1. perform actions to resolve the infectious process (see Nursing Diagnosis 6, action b.1)
   2. use good handwashing technique and encourage client to do the same
   3. protect client from others with infection
   4. perform actions *to prevent urinary tract infection:*
      a. instruct and assist female client to wipe from front to back following urination and defecation
      b. keep perianal area clean
   5. reinforce importance of good oral care.
d. If signs and symptoms of a superinfection occur:
   1. continue with above measures
   2. implement appropriate comfort measures for symptoms experienced
   3. implement measures *to ensure client safety* (e.g. side rails up, assistance when up) if changes in mental status are present
   4. monitor for therapeutic and nontherapeutic effects of anti-infectives if administered.

12. COLLABORATIVE DIAGNOSIS

Potential complications:

a. **delayed resolution of pneumonia** related to infection by drug-resistant or highly virulent organisms and general debilitation;
b. **exudative pleural effusion** related to an increase in capillary permeability associated with the inflammatory process;
c. **atelectasis** related to ineffective breathing patterns, obstruction of bronchioles with mucus, and decreased surfactant production associated with reduced pulmonary blood flow if client is immobile (can result from decreased tissue perfusion);
d. **acute respiratory failure** related to a ventilation-perfusion imbalance associated with:
   1. ineffective breathing patterns and airway clearance
   2. decrease in effective lung surface resulting from atelectasis, accumulation of secretions, and consolidation of lung tissue.

DESIRED OUTCOMES	NURSING ACTIONS AND *SELECTED RATIONALES*
12.a. The client will experience resolution of pneumonia within the expected time.	12.a.1. Assess for and report signs and symptoms of delayed resolution of pneumonia: a. breath sounds that worsen or fail to improve b. persistent cyanosis, dyspnea, tachypnea c. persistent or recurrent temperature elevation and tachycardia d. failure of blood gases to return toward normal e. continued positive results of sputum cultures. 2. Implement measures to resolve the infectious process (see Nursing Diagnosis 6, action b.1). 3. Provide emotional support to client and significant others if pneumonia is slow to resolve and hospitalization is prolonged.
12.b. The client will experience resolution of pleural	12.b.1. Assess for and report signs and symptoms of pleural effusion: a. increase in or sudden absence of pleuritic pain

effusion if it occurs as evidenced by:
1. no increase in or sudden absence of pleuritic pain
2. unlabored respirations at 16–20/minute
3. usual chest excursion with respirations
4. resonant percussion note throughout lung fields
5. improved breath sounds.

    b. increased dyspnea
    c. bulging of intercostal spaces
    d. decreased chest movement on affected side
    e. dull percussion note, diminished or absent breath sounds, and decreased tactile fremitus over affected area.
2. Monitor chest x-ray and ultrasound results. Report findings of pleural effusion.
3. If signs and symptoms of pleural effusion occur:
    a. continue with actions to improve respiratory status (see Nursing Diagnosis 2, action f)
    b. implement measures to resolve the infectious process (see Nursing Diagnosis 6, action b.1)
    c. prepare client for a thoracentesis if indicated.

12.c. The client will not develop atelectasis (see Care Plan on Immobility, Collaborative Diagnosis 14, outcome b, for outcome criteria).

12.c.1. Refer to Care Plan on Immobility, Collaborative Diagnosis 14, action b, for measures related to assessment, prevention, and treatment of atelectasis.
2. Implement measures to improve respiratory status (see Nursing Diagnosis 2, action f) *in order to further reduce the risk of atelectasis.*

12.d. The client will not experience respiratory failure as evidenced by:
1. respiratory rate above 8 and below 30/minute
2. improved skin color
3. usual mental status
4. PaO$_2$ above 50 mm Hg and PaCO$_2$ below 50 mm Hg.

12.d.1. Assess for and report signs and symptoms of severe respiratory distress (e.g. rapid, shallow, and/or labored respirations; sternocleidomastoid muscle retraction; dusky or cyanotic skin color; drowsiness; restlessness; agitation; confusion).
2. Monitor blood gas values. Report values that worsen or fail to improve.
3. Monitor for and report significant changes in ear oximetry and capnograph results.
4. Implement measures *to prevent respiratory failure:*
    a. perform actions to improve respiratory status (see Nursing Diagnosis 2, action f)
    b. assess for and report conditions that might cause a further decline in respiratory status (e.g. cardiac arrhythmias, low B/P, fluid and electrolyte imbalances, atelectasis, superinfection, pleural effusion, severe abdominal distention).
5. If signs and symptoms of respiratory failure occur:
    a. continue with above actions to improve respiratory status
    b. assist with intubation, mechanical ventilation, and transfer to intensive care unit if indicated
    c. provide emotional support to client and significant others.

UNIT IX

13. NURSING DIAGNOSIS

Knowledge deficit regarding follow-up care.

DESIRED OUTCOMES	NURSING ACTIONS AND *SELECTED RATIONALES*

13.a. The client will identify ways to maintain respiratory health.

13.a. Instruct client in ways *to maintain respiratory health:*
1. consume a well-balanced diet
2. drink at least 10 glasses of liquid/day
3. maintain a balanced program of rest and exercise
4. avoid crowds during flu and cold season
5. avoid contact with persons who have respiratory infections
6. consult physician about vaccinations available if at high risk for recurrent pneumonia
7. continue cough and deep breathing exercises for at least 6–8 weeks after discharge and during any period of decreased physical activity or respiratory infection

8. maintain good oral hygiene by brushing teeth after eating and flossing at least twice a day *in order to reduce the number of organisms in the oropharynx*
9. avoid excessive alcohol intake and stop smoking *to prevent depression of pulmonary antimicrobial defenses*
10. avoid sudden changes in environmental temperature.

13.b. The client will state signs and symptoms to report to the health care provider.

13.b. Instruct client to report the following signs and symptoms:
1. persistent or recurrent temperature elevation
2. chills
3. increased difficulty breathing
4. increased restlessness, irritability, drowsiness, or confusion
5. chest pain
6. weight loss
7. persistent fatigue
8. persistent cough productive of purulent or rust-colored sputum
9. unusual color, amount, and odor of vaginal secretions
10. white patches or ulcerated areas in the mouth or vagina.

13.c. The client will verbalize an understanding of and a plan for adhering to recommended follow-up care including future appointments with health care provider, medications prescribed, and activity limitations.

13.c.1. Reinforce the importance of keeping follow-up appointments with health care provider.
2. Explain the rationale for, side effects of, and importance of taking medications prescribed (e.g. anti-infectives, expectorants, mucolytics).
3. Implement measures *to improve client compliance:*
   a. include significant others in all discharge teaching sessions if possible
   b. encourage questions and allow time for reinforcement and clarification of information provided
   c. provide written instructions regarding scheduled appointments with health care provider, medications prescribed, fluid requirements, respiratory care, and signs and symptoms to report.

Reference

Carpenito, LJ. Handbook of nursing diagnosis (3rd ed.). Philadelphia: J.B. Lippincott Company, 1989.

Pneumothorax

Pneumothorax is an accumulation of air in the pleural space that results in complete or partial collapse of the lung. If air enters the pleural space through an opening in the chest wall, the pneumothorax is usually classified as open; if there is no external wound, it is classified as closed. Both types can be further classified as traumatic, iatrogenic, or spontaneous depending on the etiology. In a traumatic pneumothorax, air enters the pleural space as a result of a penetrating or nonpenetrating chest injury. Pneumothorax that is surgically induced or occurs as a complication of a diagnostic or therapeutic measure (e.g. insertion of subclavian catheter, mechanical ventilation) is classified as iatrogenic. A spontaneous pneumothorax is one that occurs in the absence of accidental or intentional trauma. This type of pneumothorax may be further classified as primary if the cause is unknown or secondary if the pneumothorax is attributed to pre-existing lung disease such as emphysema, tuberculosis, or a malignancy.

Symptoms experienced by the client with a pneumothorax depend on the degree of lung collapse. In a small proportion of clients, no treatment is required. For the remainder, intervention is necessary to re-establish negative intrapleural pressure and re-expand the lung. Establishment of a chest drainage system is the treatment of choice. Resection of lung blebs and/or pleural scarification may also be indicated for the client who has experienced recurrent episodes of spontaneous pneumothorax.

This care plan focuses on the adult client hospitalized for diagnosis and treatment of a primary spontaneous pneumothorax. Goals of care are to maintain an adequate respiratory status, relieve discomfort, prevent complications, and educate the client regarding follow-up care.

DISCHARGE CRITERIA

Prior to discharge, the client will:

- demonstrate the ability to perform appropriate wound care
- identify ways to reduce the risk of recurrent spontaneous pneumothorax
- state signs and symptoms to report to the health care provider
- verbalize an understanding of and plan for adhering to recommended follow-up care including future appointments with health care provider, medications prescribed, and activity restrictions.

NURSING/COLLABORATIVE DIAGNOSES

1. Anxiety □ *495*
2. Ineffective breathing patterns □ *496*
3. Impaired gas exchange □ *497*
4. Pain:
   a. pleuritic pain
   b. discomfort at chest tube site □ *498*
5. Altered oral mucous membrane: dryness □ *498*
6. Sleep pattern disturbance □ *499*
7. Potential for infection: wound □ *500*
8. Potential complication: mediastinal shift □ *500*
9. Knowledge deficit regarding follow-up care □ *501*

1. NURSING DIAGNOSIS

Anxiety related to difficulty breathing; chest pain; unfamiliar environment; and lack of understanding of diagnostic tests, diagnosis, treatment measures, and prognosis.

DESIRED OUTCOMES	NURSING ACTIONS AND *SELECTED RATIONALES*
1. The client will experience a reduction in fear and anxiety as evidenced by:	1.a. Assess client for signs and symptoms of fear and anxiety (e.g. verbalization of fears and concerns; tenseness; tremors; irritability; restlessness; diaphoresis; tachypnea; tachycardia; elevated blood pressure; facial tension,

a. verbalization of feeling less anxious or fearful
b. relaxed facial expression and body movements
c. stable vital signs
d. usual skin color
e. verbalization of an understanding of hospital routines, diagnostic tests, diagnosis, treatment measures, and prognosis.

pallor, or flushing; noncompliance with treatment plan). Validate perceptions carefully, remembering that some behaviors may be due to tissue hypoxia and respiratory distress.

b. Ascertain effectiveness of current coping skills.

c. Implement measures *to reduce fear and anxiety:*
 1. orient to hospital environment, equipment, and routines
 2. introduce staff who will be participating in his/her care; if possible, maintain consistency in staff assigned to his/her care *to provide feelings of stability and comfort with the environment*
 3. assure client that staff members are nearby; respond to call signal as soon as possible
 4. maintain a calm, confident manner when interacting with client
 5. encourage verbalization of fear and anxiety; provide feedback
 6. reinforce the physician's explanations and clarify any misconceptions the client may have about the pneumothorax, treatment plan, and prognosis
 7. explain all diagnostic tests (e.g. blood gas analysis, capnography, ear oximetry, chest x-rays, thoracentesis)
 8. perform actions to reduce chest pain (see Nursing Diagnosis 4, action e)
 9. perform actions to improve gas exchange (see Nursing Diagnosis 3, action e) *in order to relieve respiratory distress*
 10. provide a calm, restful environment
 11. instruct in relaxation techniques and encourage participation in diversional activities once the period of acute pain and respiratory distress has subsided
 12. assist client to identify specific stressors and ways to cope with them
 13. encourage significant others to project a caring, concerned attitude without obvious anxiousness
 14. if surgical intervention is indicated, begin preoperative teaching
 15. monitor for therapeutic and nontherapeutic effects of antianxiety agents if administered.

d. Include significant others in orientation and teaching sessions and encourage their continued support of the client.

e. Provide information based on current needs of client and significant others at a level they can understand. Encourage questions and clarification of information provided.

f. Consult physician if above actions fail to control fear and anxiety.

☐ ▬▬▬▬▬▬▬▬▬▬▬▬▬▬▬▬▬▬▬▬

2. NURSING DIAGNOSIS

Ineffective breathing patterns related to chest pain, fear, and anxiety.

☐ ▬▬▬▬▬▬▬▬▬▬▬▬▬▬▬▬▬▬▬▬

DESIRED OUTCOMES	NURSING ACTIONS AND *SELECTED RATIONALES*

2. The client will maintain an effective breathing pattern as evidenced by:
a. normal rate, rhythm, and depth of respirations
b. decreased dyspnea
c. blood gases within normal range.
	2.a. Assess for signs and symptoms of ineffective breathing patterns (e.g. shallow respirations, hyperventilation, dyspnea, use of accessory muscles for breathing).
	b. Monitor blood gases. Report abnormal results.
	c. Monitor for and report significant changes in ear oximetry and capnograph results.
	d. Implement measures *to improve breathing pattern:*
	  1. perform actions to reduce chest pain (see Nursing Diagnosis 4, action e)
	  2. perform actions to reduce fear and anxiety (see Nursing Diagnosis 1, action c)
	  3. place client in a semi- to high Fowler's position unless contraindicated
	  4. if client is on bedrest, assist him/her to turn at least every 2 hours

5. instruct client to deep breathe or use inspiratory exerciser at least every 2 hours
6. instruct client to breathe slowly if he/she is hyperventilating
7. increase activity as allowed and tolerated
8. administer central nervous system depressants (e.g. narcotic analgesics, sedatives) judiciously; hold medication and consult physician if respiratory rate is less than 12/minute.
   e. Consult physician if ineffective breathing patterns persist or worsen.

□ ▬▬▬▬▬▬▬▬▬▬▬▬▬▬▬▬▬

3. NURSING DIAGNOSIS

Impaired gas exchange related to ineffective breathing patterns and a decrease in effective surface area of lung associated with lung collapse.

□ ▬▬▬▬▬▬▬▬▬▬▬▬▬▬▬▬▬

DESIRED OUTCOMES	NURSING ACTIONS AND *SELECTED RATIONALES*

3. The client will experience adequate O_2/CO_2 exchange as evidenced by:
   a. usual mental status
   b. usual skin color
   c. decreased dyspnea
   d. blood gases within normal range.

3.a. Assess for and report signs and symptoms of extended pneumothorax (e.g. decreased chest excursion on affected side; diminished or absent breath sounds with hyperresonant percussion note over affected area; rapid, shallow, and/or labored respirations; tachycardia; sudden, sharp chest pain; cyanosis; restlessness; confusion).
   b. Assess for and report signs and symptoms of impaired gas exchange:
   1. restlessness or irritability
   2. confusion, somnolence
   3. dusky or cyanotic skin color
   4. dyspnea.
   c. Monitor blood gas values. Report abnormal results.
   d. Monitor for and report significant changes in ear oximetry and capnograph results.
   e. Implement measures *to improve gas exchange:*
   1. perform actions *to promote lung re-expansion and prevent recurrent pneumothorax:*
      a. prepare client for and assist with needle aspiration of air or insertion of chest tube(s) if appropriate (chest tubes are usually inserted if the pneumothorax is greater than 15% of the hemithorax)
      b. if chest tube is inserted:
      1. perform actions *to maintain patency and integrity of chest drainage system:*
         a. maintain water seal and suction levels as ordered
         b. maintain air occlusive dressing over chest tube insertion site
         c. tape all connections securely
         d. milk or strip tube if ordered
         e. keep chest drainage and suction tubing free of kinks
         f. keep drainage system below client's chest level at all times
      2. assess for and report signs and symptoms that may indicate malfunction of chest drainage system (e.g. respiratory distress, sudden cessation of drainage, excessive bubbling in water seal chamber, subcutaneous emphysema)
      c. implement measures to improve breathing pattern (see Nursing Diagnosis 2, action d)
   2. maintain oxygen therapy as ordered
   3. discourage smoking *(smoking decreases oxygen availability)*
   4. maintain activity restrictions as ordered *to reduce oxygen demand.*
   f. Consult physician if signs and symptoms of impaired gas exchange persist or worsen.

UNIT IX

□ ▬▬▬▬▬▬▬▬▬▬▬▬▬▬▬

4. NURSING DIAGNOSIS

Pain:

a. **pleuritic pain** related to stretching of the parietal pleura as a result of air in the pleural space;
b. **discomfort at chest tube site** related to tissue irritation associated with presence and removal of chest tube(s).

□ ▬▬▬▬▬▬▬▬▬▬▬▬▬▬▬

DESIRED OUTCOMES	NURSING ACTIONS AND *SELECTED RATIONALES*

4. The client will experience diminished chest pain as evidenced by:
a. verbalization of pain relief
b. relaxed facial expression and body positioning
c. improved breathing pattern
d. increased participation in activities
e. stable vital signs.
	4.a. Determine how client usually responds to pain.
	b. Assess for nonverbal signs of pain (e.g. wrinkled brow, clenched fists, reluctance to move, diaphoresis, guarding of affected side of chest, shallow respirations, change in blood pressure, tachycardia).
	c. Assess verbal complaints of pain. Ask client to be specific regarding location, severity, and type of pain.
	d. Assess for factors that seem to aggravate and alleviate pain.
	e. Implement measures *to reduce chest pain:*
	  1. instruct and assist client to splint chest with hands or pillow when deep breathing, coughing, and changing position
	  2. provide or assist with nonpharmacological measures for pain relief (e.g. back rub, position change, relaxation techniques, guided imagery, quiet conversation, restful environment, diversional activities)
	  3. securely fasten or anchor chest tubes *to limit movement and resulting tissue irritation*
	  4. monitor for therapeutic and nontherapeutic effects of analgesics if administered
	  5. assist with intercostal nerve block if performed
	  6. administer analgesics as ordered prior to removal of chest tube(s).
	f. Consult physician if the above actions fail to provide adequate pain relief.

□ ▬▬▬▬▬▬▬▬▬▬▬▬▬▬▬

5. NURSING DIAGNOSIS

Altered oral mucous membrane: dryness related to mouth breathing and the prolonged administration of oxygen (oxygen is a dry gas and will dehydrate the respiratory mucous membranes if exposure is prolonged).

□ ▬▬▬▬▬▬▬▬▬▬▬▬▬▬▬

DESIRED OUTCOMES	NURSING ACTIONS AND *SELECTED RATIONALES*

5. The client will maintain a moist, intact oral mucous membrane.	5.a. Assess client every shift for dryness of the oral mucosa.
	b. Implement measures *to decrease dryness of the oral mucous membrane:*
	  1. instruct and assist client to perform good oral hygiene as often as needed
	  2. have client rinse mouth frequently with water
	  3. instruct client to avoid products such as lemon-glycerin swabs and commercial mouthwashes containing alcohol *(these products have a drying or irritating effect on the oral mucous membrane)*

4. lubricate client's lips with Vaseline, K-Y jelly, ChapStick, Blistex, or mineral oil when oral care is given
5. encourage client to breathe through nose if possible
6. encourage client not to smoke (*smoking further irritates and dries the mucosa*)
7. encourage a fluid intake of at least 2500 cc/day unless contraindicated
8. encourage client to use artificial saliva (e.g. Moi-stir, Salivart) *to lubricate the mucous membrane.*

c. If oral mucosa is irritated or cracked, implement measures *to relieve discomfort and promote healing:*
1. assist client to select soft, bland, and nonacidic foods
2. instruct client to avoid extremely hot or cold foods/fluids
3. use a soft bristle brush or low-pressure power spray for oral care
4. monitor for therapeutic and nontherapeutic effects of topical anesthetics, oral protective pastes, and topical and systemic analgesics if administered.

d. Consult physician if dryness, irritation, and discomfort persist.

6. NURSING DIAGNOSIS

Sleep pattern disturbance related to fear, anxiety, frequent assessments, chest pain, and inability to assume usual sleep position because of presence of chest tube(s) and dyspnea.

DESIRED OUTCOMES	NURSING ACTIONS AND *SELECTED RATIONALES*
6. The client will attain optimal amounts of sleep within the parameters of the treatment regimen as evidenced by: a. statements of feeling well rested b. usual behavior c. absence of frequent yawning, thick speech, dark circles under eyes.	6.a. Assess for signs and symptoms of a sleep pattern disturbance: 1. verbal complaints of difficulty falling asleep, not feeling well rested, sleep interruptions, or awakening earlier or later than desired 2. behavior changes (e.g. irritability, disorganization, lethargy) 3. frequent yawning, thick speech, dark circles under eyes, slight hand tremors). b. Determine the client's usual sleep habits. c. Implement measures *to promote sleep:* 1. perform actions to reduce fear and anxiety (see Nursing Diagnosis 1, action c) 2. perform actions to relieve chest pain (see Nursing Diagnosis 4, action e) 3. perform actions to improve gas exchange (see Nursing Diagnosis 3, action e) *in order to relieve dyspnea* 4. assist client to assume a comfortable sleep position (e.g. in semi- to high Fowler's position with arms supported on pillows, resting forward on overbed table with good pillow support) 5. maintain oxygen therapy during sleep if indicated 6. ensure good room ventilation 7. allow client to continue usual sleep practices (e.g. time, bedtime rituals) if possible 8. determine measures that have been helpful to the client in the past (e.g. milk, warm drinks) and incorporate in plan of care 9. discourage long periods of sleep during the day unless sleep deprivation exists or daytime sleep is usual for client 10. encourage participation in relaxing diversional activities in the early evening hours 11. provide a quiet, restful atmosphere 12. discourage intake of foods and fluids high in caffeine (e.g. chocolate, coffee, tea, colas), especially in the evening 13. satisfy basic needs such as hunger, comfort, and warmth before sleep

14. have client empty bladder just before bedtime
15. utilize relaxation techniques (e.g. progressive relaxation exercises, back massage, meditation, soft music) before sleep
16. perform actions *to provide for periods of uninterrupted sleep (90- to 120-minute periods of uninterrupted sleep are considered essential):*
    a. restrict visitors during rest periods
    b. group care (e.g. medications, treatments, physical care, assessments) whenever possible
17. monitor for therapeutic and nontherapeutic effects of sedatives and hypnotics if administered.
    d. Consult physician if signs of sleep deprivation persist or worsen.

7. NURSING DIAGNOSIS

Potential for infection: wound related to break in skin integrity associated with chest tube insertion.

DESIRED OUTCOMES	NURSING ACTIONS AND *SELECTED RATIONALES*
7. The client will remain free of wound infection as evidenced by: a. absence of chills and fever b. pulse within normal limits c. absence of redness, swelling, and unusual drainage around chest tube insertion site(s) d. absence of unusual drainage from chest tube(s) e. WBC count within normal range f. negative cultures of wound and chest tube drainage.	7.a. Assess for and report signs and symptoms of wound infection: 1. elevated temperature 2. chills 3. pattern of increased pulse or pulse rate greater than 100 beats/minute 4. redness, swelling, or unusual drainage around chest tube insertion site(s) 5. purulent drainage from chest tube(s) 6. elevated WBC count. b. Obtain culture specimens from wound site(s) and chest tube drainage as ordered. Report positive results. c. Implement measures *to prevent wound infection:* 1. maintain a fluid intake of at least 2500 cc/day unless contraindicated 2. use good handwashing technique and encourage client to do the same 3. maintain meticulous aseptic technique during chest tube insertion and removal and wound care 4. anchor chest tube(s) securely *in order to prevent irritation and breakdown of skin around insertion site(s) associated with excessive movement of tube(s)* 5. maintain an optimal nutritional status by encouraging a diet high in calories, protein, vitamins, and minerals. d. Monitor for therapeutic and nontherapeutic effects of anti-infectives if administered.

8. COLLABORATIVE DIAGNOSIS

Potential complication: mediastinal shift related to tension pneumothorax or hemothorax.

DESIRED OUTCOMES	NURSING ACTIONS AND *SELECTED RATIONALES*
8. The client will not develop mediastinal shift as evidenced by: a. vital signs within normal range for client b. usual skin color c. point of apical impulse in 5th intercostal space near midclavicular line d. trachea in midline position e. blood gases within normal range.	8.a. Assess for and immediately report signs and symptoms of mediastinal shift (e.g. severe dyspnea, increase in restlessness and agitation, rapid and/or irregular pulse, cyanosis, shift in point of apical impulse and trachea toward unaffected side) and/or hemothorax (e.g. further decrease in breath sounds with dull percussion note over affected area, increased dyspnea, cyanosis, increased pleuritic pain). b. Monitor blood gases and report values that have worsened. c. Implement measures to maintain patency and integrity of chest drainage system (see Nursing Diagnosis 3, action e.1.b.1) *in order to prevent pneumothorax and hemothorax and reduce the risk of mediastinal shift.* d. If signs and symptoms of mediastinal shift occur: 1. maintain client on bedrest in a semi- to high Fowler's position 2. maintain oxygen therapy as ordered 3. if chest tube(s) are malfunctioning or not present, assist with the insertion of new tube(s) or a thoracentesis if indicated 4. provide emotional support to client and significant others.

□ ▉▉▉▉▉▉▉▉▉ o ▉▉▉▉▉▉▉▉▉▉▉▉▉▉▉▉▉▉▉▉

9. NURSING DIAGNOSIS

Knowledge deficit regarding follow-up care.

□ ▉▉▉▉▉▉▉▉▉▉▉▉▉▉▉▉▉▉▉▉▉▉▉▉▉▉▉▉▉▉

DESIRED OUTCOMES	NURSING ACTIONS AND *SELECTED RATIONALES*
9.a. The client will demonstrate the ability to perform appropriate wound care.	9.a.1. Instruct client on care of chest tube insertion site (e.g. occlusive dressing). 2. Allow time for questions, clarification, and return demonstration.
9.b. The client will identify ways to reduce the risk of recurrent spontaneous pneumothorax.	9.b.1. Caution client to avoid situations and activities that would expose him/her to marked changes in atmospheric pressure (e.g. scuba diving). 2. Encourage client to stop smoking *(smoking increases the risk of recurrent pneumothorax).*
9.c. The client will state signs and symptoms to report to the health care provider.	9.c. Instruct client to report the following signs and symptoms: 1. difficulty breathing 2. chest pain 3. elevated temperature 4. chills 5. increased redness and warmth at wound site 6. purulent drainage from wound site.
9.d. The client will verbalize an understanding of and plan for adhering to recommended follow-up care including future appointments with health care provider, medications prescribed, and activity restrictions.	9.d.1. Reinforce importance of keeping follow-up appointments with health care provider. 2. Instruct client to avoid excessive physical exertion and lifting objects over 10 pounds until permitted by physician. 3. Reinforce physician's explanation about the possibility of recurrent spontaneous pneumothorax (occurs in approximately 50% of clients after initial episode). Assist client to develop plan for obtaining emergency assistance should spontaneous pneumothorax recur. 4. Explain the rationale for, side effects of, and importance of taking medications prescribed. 5. Implement measures *to improve client compliance:* a. include significant others in teaching sessions if possible

b. encourage questions and allow time for reinforcement and clarification of information provided
c. provide written instructions about wound care, signs and symptoms to report, future appointments with health care provider, medications prescribed, and activity restrictions.

□□

Pulmonary Embolism

Pulmonary embolism occurs when the pulmonary arteries or one of the branches is partially or completely occluded by an embolus. Most often the embolism originates as a thrombus in the deep veins of the legs or pelvis or, less frequently, the right atrium. The embolus may also be composed of air, fat (can occur as a result of a long bone fracture), amniotic fluid, or neoplastic cells that have entered the circulation. The classic signs and symptoms of a moderate-sized pulmonary embolism with some resultant pulmonary infarction include sudden dyspnea, tachypnea, tachycardia, restlessness, feel-ings of apprehension, chest pain, and hemoptysis. The severity of symptoms depends on the size and number of emboli, size of the blood vessel occluded, extent of vessel occlusion, and presence of pre-existing cardiopulmonary disease.

This care plan focuses on the adult client hospitalized for treatment of a pulmonary embolism resulting from a dislodged deep vein thrombus. The goals of care are to reduce fear and anxiety, maintain optimal respiratory function, prevent complications, and educate the client regarding follow-up care.

DISCHARGE CRITERIA

Prior to discharge, the client will:

- identify ways to prevent recurrent thrombus formation and pulmonary embolism
- verbalize an understanding of medication therapy including rationale for, side effects of, schedule for taking, importance of taking as prescribed, and method of administration
- identify precautions necessary to prevent bleeding associated with anticoagulant therapy
- state signs and symptoms to report to the health care provider
- verbalize an understanding of and a plan for adhering to recommended follow-up care including future appointments with health care provider and activity level.

□ ████████████████████████████████████

Use in conjunction with the Care Plan on Immobility.

□ ███████████████████████████████████████

NURSING/COLLABORATIVE DIAGNOSES

1. Anxiety □ *503*
2. Ineffective breathing patterns □ *504*
3. Impaired gas exchange □ *504*
4. Pain: chest □ *505*
5. Impaired physical mobility □ *506*
6. Self-care deficit □ *506*
7. Potential complications:
   a. right-sided heart failure
   b. extended or recurrent pulmonary embolism
   c. atelectasis
   d. bleeding □ *507*
8. Knowledge deficit regarding follow-up care □ *509*

□ ███████████████████████████████████████

1. NURSING DIAGNOSIS

Anxiety related to unfamiliar environment; dyspnea; chest pain; lack of understanding of diagnostic tests, diagnosis, and treatments; possibility of recurrent embolism; and threat of death.

□ ███████████████████████████████████████

DESIRED OUTCOMES	NURSING ACTIONS AND *SELECTED RATIONALES*

1. The client will experience a reduction in fear and anxiety as evidenced by:
   a. verbalization of feeling less anxious or fearful
   b. relaxed facial expression and body movements
   c. stable vital signs
   d. usual skin color
   e. verbalization of an understanding of hospital routines, diagnostic tests, diagnosis, and treatments.

1.a. Assess client for signs and symptoms of fear and anxiety (e.g. verbalization of fears and concerns; tenseness; tremors; irritability; restlessness; diaphoresis; tachypnea; tachycardia; elevated blood pressure; facial tension, pallor, or flushing; noncompliance with treatment plan). Validate perceptions carefully, remembering that some behavior may result from factors such as tissue hypoxia and pain.
   b. Ascertain effectiveness of current coping skills.
   c. Implement measures *to reduce fear and anxiety:*
      1. maintain a calm, confident manner when interacting with client
      2. do not leave client alone during period of acute respiratory distress
      3. perform actions to improve gas exchange (see Nursing Diagnosis 3, action d) *in order to relieve dyspnea*
      4. perform actions to reduce chest pain (see Nursing Diagnosis 4, action e)
      5. explain all diagnostic tests (e.g. perfusion lung scan, blood gases, venography, pulmonary angiography)
      6. reassure client that anxiety and "sense of doom" are common symptoms of pulmonary embolism and will diminish as condition stabilizes
      7. encourage significant others to project a caring, concerned attitude without obvious anxiousness
      8. when the acute respiratory distress and pain have subsided:
         a. orient to hospital environment, equipment, and routines
         b. introduce staff who will be participating in his/her care; if possible, maintain consistency in staff assigned to his/her care *to provide feelings of stability and comfort with the environment*
         c. assure client that staff members are nearby; respond to call signal as soon as possible

     d. provide a calm, restful environment
     e. encourage verbalization of fear and anxiety; provide feedback
     f. reinforce the physician's explanations and clarify any misconceptions the client may have about pulmonary embolism, the treatment plan, and prognosis
     g. instruct in relaxation techniques and encourage participation in diversional activities
     h. assist client to identify specific stressors and ways to cope with them
    9. monitor for therapeutic and nontherapeutic effects of antianxiety agents if administered.
  d. Include significant others in orientation and teaching sessions and encourage their continued support of client.
  e. Provide information based on current needs of client and significant others at a level they can understand. Encourage questions and clarification of information provided.
  f. Consult physician if above actions fail to control fear and anxiety.

☐ ▬▬▬▬▬▬▬▬▬▬▬▬▬▬▬▬▬▬▬▬

2. NURSING DIAGNOSIS

Ineffective breathing patterns related to fear, anxiety, chest pain, depressant effects of some medications (e.g. narcotic analgesics, sedatives), and stimulant effects of hypoxia.

☐ ▬▬▬▬▬▬▬▬▬▬▬▬▬▬▬▬▬▬▬▬

DESIRED OUTCOMES	NURSING ACTIONS AND *SELECTED RATIONALES*

2. The client will maintain an effective breathing pattern as evidenced by:
  a. normal rate, rhythm, and depth of respirations
  b. decreased dyspnea
  c. blood gases within normal range.
	2.a. Assess for signs and symptoms of ineffective breathing patterns (e.g. rapid, shallow respirations; dyspnea; use of accessory muscles for breathing).
	  b. Monitor blood gases. Report abnormal results.
	  c. Monitor for and report significant changes in ear oximetry and capnograph results.
	  d. Implement measures *to improve breathing pattern:*
	    1. perform actions to decrease pain (see Nursing Diagnosis 4, action e)
	    2. perform actions to decrease fear and anxiety (see Nursing Diagnosis 1, action c)
	    3. place client in a semi- to high Fowler's position unless contraindicated
	    4. if client is on bedrest, assist him/her to turn at least every 2 hours
	    5. instruct client to deep breathe or use inspiratory exerciser at least every 2 hours
	    6. administer central nervous system depressants (e.g. narcotic analgesics, sedatives) judiciously; hold medication and consult physician if respiratory rate is less than 12/minute
	    7. increase activity when allowed
	    8. perform actions to improve gas exchange (see Nursing Diagnosis 3, action d) *in order to reduce hypoxia.*
	  e. Consult physician if ineffective breathing patterns persist or worsen.

☐ ▬▬▬▬▬▬▬▬▬▬▬▬▬▬▬▬▬▬▬▬

3. NURSING DIAGNOSIS

Impaired gas exchange related to:

a. ineffective breathing patterns;
b. decreased pulmonary perfusion associated with partial or complete occlusion of

pulmonary arterial blood flow by the embolus and vasoconstriction resulting from the release of vasoactive substances from the clot;

c. reflex bronchoconstriction associated with the release of histamine, serotonin, and prostaglandins from the clot.

□ ▬▬▬▬▬▬▬▬▬▬▬▬▬▬▬▬▬▬▬▬▬▬▬

DESIRED OUTCOMES	NURSING ACTIONS AND *SELECTED RATIONALES*

3. The client will experience adequate O_2/CO_2 exchange as evidenced by:
   a. usual mental status
   b. usual skin color
   c. absence of dyspnea
   d. blood gases within normal range.

3.a. Assess for and report signs and symptoms of impaired gas exchange:
   1. restlessness or irritability
   2. confusion, somnolence
   3. dusky or cyanotic skin color
   4. dyspnea.
   b. Monitor blood gas values. Report abnormal results.
   c. Monitor for and report significant changes in ear oximetry and capnograph results.
   d. Implement measures *to improve gas exchange:*
      1. maintain client on bedrest *to reduce oxygen demand during acute respiratory distress*
      2. maintain oxygen therapy as ordered
      3. perform actions to improve breathing pattern (see Nursing Diagnosis 2, action d)
      4. discourage smoking *(smoking decreases oxygen availability)*
      5. monitor for therapeutic and nontherapeutic effects of the following medications if administered:
         a. anticoagulants (e.g. heparin, warfarin)
         b. thrombolytic agents (e.g. streptokinase, tissue plasminogen activator [tPA], urokinase) *to dissolve the embolus and improve pulmonary blood flow*
         c. methylxanthine-derivative bronchodilators (e.g. theophylline) and sympathomimetic bronchodilators (e.g. terbutaline, epinephrine, metaproterenol, isoproterenol).
   e. Consult physician if signs and symptoms of impaired gas exchange persist or worsen.

□ ▬▬▬▬▬▬▬▬▬▬▬▬▬▬▬▬▬▬▬▬▬▬▬

4. NURSING DIAGNOSIS

Pain: chest related to tissue hypoxia associated with decreased pulmonary tissue perfusion in the affected area.

□ ▬▬▬▬▬▬▬▬▬▬▬▬▬▬▬▬▬▬▬▬▬▬▬

DESIRED OUTCOMES	NURSING ACTIONS AND *SELECTED RATIONALES*

4. The client will experience diminished chest pain as evidenced by:
   a. verbalization of pain relief
   b. relaxed facial expression and body positioning
   c. increased participation in activities when allowed
   d. improved breathing pattern.

4.a. Determine how the client usually responds to pain.
   b. Assess for nonverbal signs of pain (e.g. rubbing chest, wrinkled brow, clenched fists, reluctance to move, diaphoresis, tachycardia, guarding of affected side of chest, shallow respirations).
   c. Assess verbal complaints of pain. Ask client to be specific regarding location, severity, and type of pain.
   d. Assess for factors that seem to aggravate and alleviate pain.
   e. Implement measures *to reduce pain:*
      1. perform actions to improve gas exchange (see Nursing Diagnosis 3, action d) *in order to reduce tissue hypoxia in the involved lung area*

UNIT IX

2. instruct and assist client to splint chest with hands or pillow when deep breathing, coughing, and changing position
3. provide or assist with nonpharmacological measures for pain relief (e.g. position change, back rub, relaxation techniques, restful environment, diversional activities)
4. monitor for therapeutic and nontherapeutic effects of analgesics if administered.

f. Consult physician if above actions fail to relieve pain.

5. NURSING DIAGNOSIS

Impaired physical mobility related to reluctance to move due to pain and fear of dislodging another thrombus and activity restrictions imposed by the treatment plan.

DESIRED OUTCOMES	NURSING ACTIONS AND *SELECTED RATIONALES*

5.a. The client will maintain an optimal level of physical mobility within the restrictions imposed by the treatment plan.	5.a.1. Assess for factors that impair physical mobility (e.g. reluctance to move because of pain or fear of dislodging another thrombus, activity restrictions imposed by treatment plan).
	2. Implement measures *to increase mobility:*
	  a. perform actions to reduce chest pain (see Nursing Diagnosis 4, action e)
	  b. reassure client that a certain degree of movement is necessary to prevent problems associated with decreased activity (e.g. stasis of secretions, muscle weakness, thrombus development) and should not dislodge a thrombus.
	3. Increase activity and participation in self-care activities as allowed.

5.b. The client will not experience problems associated with immobility.	5.b. Refer to Care Plan on Immobility for actions to prevent problems associated with decreased mobility if client is to remain on bedrest for longer than 48 hours.

6. NURSING DIAGNOSIS

Self-care deficit related to dyspnea and impaired mobility associated with pain, fear, and activity restrictions.

DESIRED OUTCOMES	NURSING ACTIONS AND *SELECTED RATIONALES*
6. The client will perform self-care activities within physical limitations and prescribed activity restrictions.	6.a. Assess for factors that interfere with the client's ability to perform self-care (e.g. reluctance to move because of pain or fear of recurrent embolism, dyspnea, activity restrictions imposed by treatment plan). b. Refer to Care Plan on Immobility, Nursing Diagnosis 9, for measures related to planning for and meeting client's self-care needs. c. Implement additional measures *to facilitate client's ability to perform self-care activities:*

1. perform actions to improve gas exchange and relieve dyspnea (see Nursing Diagnosis 3, action d)
2. perform actions to increase mobility (see Nursing Diagnosis 5, action a.2)
3. maintain oxygen therapy during self-care activities if indicated.

□ ▬▬▬▬▬▬▬▬▬▬▬▬▬▬▬▬▬▬▬▬▬▬▬▬▬▬▬▬▬▬

7. COLLABORATIVE DIAGNOSIS

Potential complications:

a. **right-sided heart failure** related to pulmonary hypertension associated with occlusion of a large pulmonary vessel by a massive embolus or occlusion of many smaller vessels by multiple diffuse emboli;

b. **extended or recurrent pulmonary embolism** related to ineffective treatment and/or continued presence of predisposing conditions;

c. **atelectasis** related to hypoventilation associated with chest pain and decreased surfactant production (can occur with reduced pulmonary blood flow resulting from the pulmonary embolism and decreased activity);

d. **bleeding** related to prolonged coagulation time associated with anticoagulant therapy.

□ ▬▬▬▬▬▬▬▬▬▬▬▬▬▬▬▬▬▬▬▬▬▬▬▬▬▬▬▬▬▬

DESIRED OUTCOMES	NURSING ACTIONS AND *SELECTED RATIONALES*

UNIT IX

7.a. The client will not develop right-sided heart failure as evidenced by:
1. vital signs within normal range for client
2. no increase in intensity of S_2 or development of a gallop or murmur over the pulmonic valve area
3. balanced intake and output
4. stable weight
5. CVP within normal range
6. absence of peripheral edema; distended neck veins; enlarged, tender liver
7. BUN and serum creatinine and alkaline phosphatase levels within normal range.

7.a.1. Assess for and report signs and symptoms of right-sided heart failure:
   a. tachycardia
   b. development of loud S_2 and/or gallop or murmur over the pulmonic valve area
   c. intake greater than output
   d. weight gain
   e. elevated CVP
   f. peripheral edema
   g. distended neck veins
   h. enlarged, tender liver
   i. elevated BUN and serum creatinine and alkaline phosphatase levels.
2. Monitor chest x-ray results. Report findings of cardiomegaly.
3. Monitor for therapeutic and nontherapeutic effects of medications administered *to treat the pulmonary embolism and thereby reduce pulmonary hypertension:*
   a. anticoagulant agents (e.g. heparin, warfarin)
   b. thrombolytic agents (e.g. urokinase, tissue plasminogen activator [tPA], streptokinase).
4. If signs and symptoms of right-sided heart failure occur:
   a. maintain oxygen therapy as ordered
   b. maintain client on strict bedrest in a semi- to high Fowler's position
   c. maintain fluid and sodium restrictions as ordered
   d. monitor for therapeutic and nontherapeutic effects of medications that may be administered *to reduce vascular congestion and/or cardiac workload* (e.g. diuretics, cardiotonics, vasodilators, morphine sulfate)
   e. assist with insertion of Swan-Ganz catheter if indicated
   f. refer to Care Plan on Congestive Heart Failure for additional care measures.

7.b. The client will not experience extension or recurrence of a pulmonary embolism as evidenced by:

7.b.1. Assess for and report signs and symptoms of extended or recurrent pulmonary embolism (e.g. development of, persistent, or increased chest pain, dyspnea, tachypnea, tachycardia, hypotension, pallor, cyanosis, restlessness, cough, or hemoptysis; declining PaO_2).

1. absence of or diminishing chest pain
2. unlabored respirations
3. stable vital signs
4. usual skin color
5. usual mental status
6. blood gases returning toward normal.

2. Monitor WBC count. Report levels that increase or fail to return to normal *(this may indicate tissue necrosis resulting from pulmonary infarction).*
3. Monitor for therapeutic and nontherapeutic effects of heparin and thrombolytic agents (e.g. urokinase, tissue plasminogen activator [tPA], streptokinase) if administered *to prevent extension of the embolism.*
4. Implement measures *to prevent recurrence of a pulmonary embolism:*
   a. perform actions to prevent and treat a venous thrombus (see Care Plan on Immobility, Collaborative Diagnosis 14, actions a.1.b and c)
   b. perform actions *to prevent dislodgment of thrombus:*
      1. maintain client on bedrest as ordered
      2. do not exercise or massage an extremity suspected of thrombosis
      3. caution client to avoid activities that create a Valsalva response (e.g. straining to have a bowel movement, bending at the waist, holding breath while moving).
5. If signs and symptoms of extended or recurrent pulmonary embolism occur:
   a. maintain client on strict bedrest in a semi- to high Fowler's position
   b. maintain oxygen therapy as ordered
   c. prepare client for diagnostic tests (e.g. perfusion lung scan, blood gases, venography, pulmonary angiography) if indicated
   d. monitor for therapeutic and nontherapeutic effects of the following medications if administered:
      1. thrombolytic agents (e.g. urokinase, tissue plasminogen activator [tPA], streptokinase)
      2. heparin
      3. vasoconstrictors (may be necessary *to maintain mean arterial pressure if shock occurs*)
   e. prepare client for surgical intervention (e.g. embolectomy) if indicated
   f. provide emotional support to client and significant others.

7.c. The client will not develop atelectasis (see Care Plan on Immobility, Collaborative Diagnosis 14, outcome b, for outcome criteria).

7.c.1. Refer to Care Plan on Immobility, Collaborative Diagnosis 14, action b, for measures related to assessment, prevention, and treatment of atelectasis.
2. Implement measures *to further reduce the risk of atelectasis:*
   a. perform actions to improve breathing pattern (see Nursing Diagnosis 2, action d)
   b. monitor for therapeutic and nontherapeutic effects of thrombolytic agents (e.g. streptokinase, tissue plasminogen activator [tPA], urokinase) *to dissolve the embolus and improve pulmonary blood flow.*

7.d. The client will not experience unusual bleeding as evidenced by:
1. skin and mucous membranes free of bleeding, petechiae, and ecchymosis
2. absence of unusual joint pain and swelling
3. no increase in abdominal girth
4. absence of frank or occult blood in stool, urine, and vomitus
5. usual menstrual flow
6. vital signs within normal range for client
7. stable Hct. and Hgb.
8. usual mental status.

7.d.1. Assess client for and report signs and symptoms of unusual bleeding:
   a. petechiae
   b. multiple ecchymotic areas
   c. bleeding gums
   d. frequent or uncontrollable episodes of epistaxis
   e. unusual oozing from injection sites
   f. unusual joint pain or swelling
   g. increase in abdominal girth
   h. hematemesis, melena, red or smoke-colored urine
   i. hypermenorrhea
   j. significant drop in B/P accompanied by an increased pulse rate
   k. decline in Hct. and Hgb. levels
   l. restlessness, confusion.
2. Monitor coagulation test results (e.g. prothrombin time, activated partial thromboplastin time, bleeding time). Report values that are greater than $2\frac{1}{2}$ times the control time.
3. If coagulation test results are abnormal or Hct. and Hgb. levels decline, test all stools, urine, and vomitus for occult blood. Report positive results.
4. Implement measures *to prevent bleeding:*
   a. use smallest gauge needle possible when giving injections and performing venous or arterial punctures
   b. apply gentle, prolonged pressure after injections and venous or arterial punctures
   c. take B/P only when necessary and avoid overinflating the cuff
   d. caution client to avoid activities that increase the potential for trauma (e.g. shaving with a straight-edge razor, cutting nails, using stiff bristle toothbrush or dental floss)

    e. pad side rails if client is confused or restless

    f. remove hazardous objects from pathway *to prevent bumps or falls*

    g. instruct client to avoid blowing nose forcefully or straining to have a bowel movement; consult physician about an order for decongestants, stool softeners, and/or laxatives if indicated.

5. If bleeding occurs and does not subside spontaneously:

    a. apply firm, prolonged pressure to bleeding area if possible

    b. if epistaxis occurs, place client in a high Fowler's position and apply pressure and ice packs to nasal area

    c. maintain oxygen therapy as ordered

    d. perform iced water or saline lavage as ordered *to control gastric bleeding*

    e. administer protamine sulfate (antidote for heparin) and vitamin K (e.g. phytonadione) as ordered

    f. prepare client for surgical repair of bleeding vessels if indicated

    g. provide emotional support to client and significant others.

8. NURSING DIAGNOSIS

Knowledge deficit regarding follow-up care.

DESIRED OUTCOMES	NURSING ACTIONS AND *SELECTED RATIONALES*

8.a. The client will identify ways to prevent recurrent thrombus formation and pulmonary embolism.	8.a.1. Provide the following instructions on ways *to promote venous blood flow and reduce risk of thrombus recurrence:*
	  a. avoid wearing constrictive clothing (e.g. garters, girdles, knee-high stockings)
	  b. avoid positions that compromise blood flow (e.g. pillows under knees, crossing legs, prolonged sitting or standing)
	  c. wear antiembolic or support hose if daily activities involve prolonged standing
	  d. do active foot and leg exercises for 5 minutes every hour while awake
	  e. maintain a regular exercise program (walking and swimming are recommended)
	  f. elevate lower extremities when lying down
	  g. avoid exposure to extreme cold and stop smoking *(both cause vasoconstriction)*
	  h. avoid use of oral contraceptives and estrogen preparations *(have been shown to increase the risk of thrombus development)*
	  i. drink at least 10 glasses of liquid/day
	  j. maintain an ideal body weight for age, height, and build
	  k. eat a diet low in saturated fat *(saturated fat contributes to atherogenesis, which narrows the vessels)*
	  l. avoid chronic constipation *(causes decreased venous return as a result of straining and increased intra-abdominal pressure)*
	  m. take anticoagulants and/or antiplatelet medications as prescribed.
	2. Instruct client to avoid trauma to or massage of any area of suspected thrombus formation *in order to decrease risk of pulmonary embolism.*
	3. Provide information regarding support groups that can assist the client to stop smoking, lose weight, and/or establish an exercise program if appropriate.

8.b. The client will verbalize an understanding of medication therapy including rationale for, side effects of, schedule	8.b.1. Explain the rationale for, side effects of, and importance of taking medications prescribed. 2. If client is discharged on a coumarin derivative (e.g. dicumarol, warfarin, phenprocoumon) or heparin, instruct to:

<table>
<tbody>
<tr>
<td>

for taking, importance of taking as prescribed, and method of administration.

</td>
<td>

   a. keep scheduled appointments for periodic blood studies to monitor coagulation times
   b. take or administer medication at same time each day
   c. avoid taking over-the-counter products containing aspirin or other salicylates *(these enhance the actions of coumarins)*
   d. avoid regular and/or excessive intake of alcohol *(may alter responsiveness to coumarins and heparin)*
   e. report prolonged or excessive bleeding from skin, nose, or mouth; blood in urine, vomitus, sputum, or stool; prolonged or excessive menses; excessive bruising; severe headache; and sudden abdominal or back pain
   f. wear a Medic-Alert band identifying self as being on anticoagulant therapy.
  3. If client is to administer own subcutaneous heparin, instruct in proper injection technique and appropriate sites.
  4. Instruct client to inform physician of any other prescription and nonprescription medications he/she is taking.
  5. Instruct client to inform all health care providers of medications being taken.

</td>
</tr>
</tbody>
</table>

8.c. The client will identify precautions necessary to prevent bleeding associated with anticoagulant therapy.

8.c.1. Instruct client about ways *to minimize the risk of bleeding while on anticoagulant therapy:*
   a. avoid taking aspirin, aspirin-containing products, and ibuprofen
   b. use an electric rather than straight-edge razor
   c. floss and brush teeth gently
   d. cut nails carefully
   e. avoid situations that could result in injury (e.g. contact sports)
   f. avoid blowing nose forcefully
   g. avoid straining to have a bowel movement.
  2. Instruct client to control any bleeding by applying firm, prolonged pressure to the area if possible.

8.d. The client will state signs and symptoms to report to the health care provider.

8.d. Stress the importance of reporting the following signs and symptoms:
  1. redness, swelling, or pain in extremity
  2. bluish color and/or persistent coolness of extremity
  3. sudden chest pain accompanied by shortness of breath
  4. unusual anxiousness or restlessness
  5. cough productive of blood-tinged sputum
  6. unusual bleeding (see action b.2.e in this diagnosis).

8.e. The client will verbalize an understanding of and a plan for adhering to recommended follow-up care including future appointments with health care provider and activity level.

8.e.1. Reinforce the importance of keeping follow-up appointments with health care provider.
  2. Reinforce the physician's instructions regarding activity limitations.
  3. Implement measures *to improve client compliance:*
   a. include significant others in teaching sessions if possible
   b. encourage questions and allow time for reinforcement and clarification of information provided
   c. provide written instructions regarding future appointments with health care provider, medications prescribed, activity restrictions, signs and symptoms to report, and future laboratory studies.

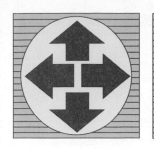

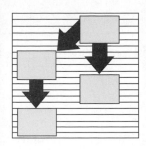
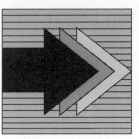
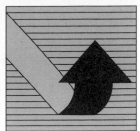

Unit X

Nursing Care of the Client with Disturbances of the Kidney and Urinary Tract

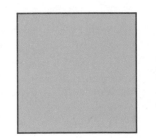

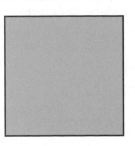
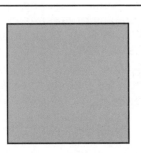
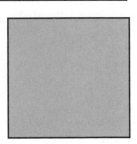

Cystectomy

Cystectomy is the removal of the bladder and is accompanied by a procedure to divert urinary flow. It may be performed to treat malignancy of the bladder, congenital bladder anomalies, neurogenic bladder, and strictures of or trauma to the urethra and/or ureters. It may also be performed to prevent further deterioration of renal function associated with chronic bladder infection. In men, a total cystectomy may include the removal of the prostate, bladder, urethra, and seminal vesicles. In women, it usually includes removal of the bladder and urethra. A pelvic lymph node dissection may also be done if the surgery is performed to treat a malignancy.

There are several ways to accomplish urinary diversion. The most common surgical method is the ileal or colon conduit. In this procedure, the ureters are implanted in the proximal end of an isolated piece of the terminal ileum or the colon and the distal end is then brought through the abdominal wall to create the stoma. Urinary flow can also be diverted to the rectum by means of a ureterosigmoidostomy. This type of diversion has the advantage of having no external stoma but is infrequently performed at the present time because it creates problems such as electrolyte imbalance, recurrent urinary tract infection, difficult daily management, and increased risk of colon malignancy in subsequent years. In clients who are not able to tolerate prolonged surgery, ureters can be implanted directly into the abdominal wall (cutaneous ureterostomy). There is a high rate of stomal stenosis with this procedure so it is usually reserved for clients whose life expectancy is very short. A newer method of urinary diversion is the Kock continent urostomy. In this procedure, a pouch is created from an isolated segment of the ileum and intussuscepting segments of the intestine are used to construct two nipple valves, which create a continent, nonrefluxing reservoir. The pouch initially has a small capacity (e.g. 150–200 cc), but eventually reaches 600 cc or more. It must be drained by means of a catheter 4–6 times a day. Although the client has a stoma, neither an external appliance nor nighttime drainage system is needed with this method of diversion.

This care plan focuses on the adult client hospitalized for a cystectomy and urinary diversion by means of an ileal conduit. The goals of preoperative care are to reduce fear and anxiety and prepare the client for the change in body image and function. Postoperatively, goals of care are to maintain peristomal skin integrity, prevent complications, facilitate psychological adjustment to the changes experienced, and educate the client regarding management of the urinary diversion and follow-up care.

DISCHARGE CRITERIA

Prior to discharge, the client will:

- verbalize a basic understanding of the anatomical changes that have occurred as a result of the surgery
- demonstrate ways to maintain stomal and peristomal skin integrity
- demonstrate proper technique for cleansing reusable ostomy equipment
- verbalize ways to prevent excessive skin growth over the stoma and peristomal area
- identify ways to control odor of ostomy drainage and pouch
- identify ways to prevent urinary tract infection
- state signs and symptoms to report to the health care provider
- share thoughts and feelings about altered urinary function and its effect on body image and life style
- identify appropriate community resources that can assist with home management and adjustment to changes resulting from the urinary diversion
- verbalize an understanding of and a plan for adhering to recommended follow-up care including future appointments with health care provider, wound care, activity level, and medications prescribed.

NURSING/COLLABORATIVE DIAGNOSES

Preoperative
1. Anxiety □ *513*
2. Knowledge deficit □ *514*

Postoperative
1. Impaired skin integrity:
   a. surgical incision
   b. impaired wound healing
   c. irritation or breakdown around suture lines and wound drains
   d. peristomal irritation or breakdown □ *515*
2. Potential for infection: urinary tract □ *518*
3. Potential complications:
   a. stomal changes
      1. prolapse
      2. excessive bleeding or irritation
      3. necrosis
   b. urinary obstruction
   c. peritonitis □ *518*
4. Sexual dysfunction:
   a. decreased libido
   b. impotence □ *520*
5. Disturbance in self-concept □ *522*
6. Ineffective individual coping □ *523*
7. Grieving □ *524*
8. Knowledge deficit regarding follow-up care □ *525*

UNIT
X

Preoperative

Use in conjunction with the Standardized Preoperative Care Plan.

1. NURSING DIAGNOSIS

Anxiety related to unfamiliar environment; lack of understanding of diagnostic tests and surgical procedure; effects of anesthesia; and anticipated postoperative discomfort, changes in body image and functioning, and effects of the urinary diversion on future life style and activities.

DESIRED OUTCOMES	NURSING ACTIONS AND *SELECTED RATIONALES*
1. The client will experience a reduction in fear and anxiety	1.a. Refer to Standardized Preoperative Care Plan, Nursing Diagnosis 1, for measures related to assessment and reduction of fear and anxiety.

(see Standardized Preoperative Care Plan, Nursing Diagnosis 1, for outcome criteria).

b. Implement additional measures *to reduce fear and anxiety:*
   1. explain diagnostic tests performed to evaluate effectiveness of urinary tract function and/or identify structural anomalies and presence of metastasis (e.g. cystoscopy, excretory urogram, cystogram, lymphangiogram, ultrasound of the bladder, bone scans, skeletal x-rays, pelvic scan, serum chemistry, urinalysis)
   2. show client and significant others a picture of a stoma *so that they will know what to expect*; explain that the stoma will shrink in size during the first 6 weeks postoperatively and that every attempt will be made to place the stoma in an area where the appliance will lie flat and be unobtrusive
   3. assure client that stoma has no pain receptors and will not be painful when touched
   4. explain that current ostomy collection devices are odorproof and available in sizes to fit various body contours
   5. explain that the stoma will begin to function immediately upon implantation of the ureters into the bowel segment and that a pouch, connected to a drainage system, will be applied in the operating room
   6. assure client that no dietary changes are necessary after the initial postoperative period
   7. if client will be in the intensive care unit for the first 48 hours after surgery, arrange for a visit to the unit or for a visit with an intensive care nurse; assure client and significant others that transfer to intensive care following a cystectomy is routine
   8. reinforce physician's explanation about the probability of impotence resulting from the surgical procedure; encourage client to verbalize feelings; provide feedback and support
   9. arrange for a visit with a person of similar age and same sex who has successfully adapted to a urinary diversion
   10. assure client that an ostomy need not alter life style (only contact sports are contraindicated).

☐ ▇▇▇▇▇▇▇▇▇▇▇▇▇▇▇▇▇▇▇▇▇▇▇▇▇▇▇▇▇

2. NURSING DIAGNOSIS

Knowledge deficit regarding hospital routines associated with surgery, physical preparation for the cystectomy and urinary diversion, and postoperative care and management of the ileal conduit.

☐ ▇▇▇▇▇▇▇▇▇▇▇▇▇▇▇▇▇▇▇▇▇▇▇▇▇▇▇▇▇

DESIRED OUTCOMES	NURSING ACTIONS AND *SELECTED RATIONALES*
2.a. The client will verbalize an understanding of usual preoperative and postoperative care and routines.	2.a.1. Refer to Standardized Preoperative Care Plan, Nursing Diagnosis 4, actions a.1–4, for information to include in preoperative teaching. 2. Explain measures utilized preoperatively to ensure that the bowel is adequately prepared (e.g. minimal-residue diet, enemas, cathartics, anti-infective therapy). 3. Inform client that a tentative stoma site will be mapped out preoperatively by the physician or enterostomal therapist. Explain that an optimal stoma site allows proper fit of an appliance, freedom of movement, and good visualization by client. 4. Explain that a urethral catheter will be in place (if the urethra has not been removed) *to drain excessive fluid from the space that had been occupied by the bladder.* 5. Inform client that a nasogastric tube will be in place for a few days postoperatively *to decompress the bowel and prevent excessive pressure on the intestinal anastomosis site.*

6. Explain that ureteral stents (small, firm catheters) will be inserted in surgery *to maintain patency of the ureters and protect the anastomoses between the ureters and the bowel segment.* The stents will extend from the stoma and are usually removed 7–10 days after surgery.
7. Allow time for questions and clarification of information provided.

2.b. The client will demonstrate the ability to perform techniques designed to prevent postoperative complications.

2.b. Refer to Standardized Preoperative Care Plan, Nursing Diagnosis 4, action b, for instructions on ways to prevent postoperative complications.

2.c. The client will verbalize an understanding of the postoperative function, appearance, and management of the ostomy.

2.c.1. Arrange for a visit with enterostomal therapist.
2. Reinforce basic information provided by physician and/or enterostomal therapist regarding:
   a. expected location of stoma
   b. expected appearance of stoma postoperatively (red, initially edematous)
   c. expected drainage (slight bleeding of stoma, mucus in urine [occurs *because the bowel mucosa normally secretes mucus*])
   d. management of the ostomy (e.g. skin care, odor control, use of various types of appliances)
   e. ostomy appliances that client will be using in the immediate postoperative period; provide visual aids and allow client to handle appliances if he/she desires; encourage client to try wearing an appliance partially filled with water *in order to experience how it feels.*

Postoperative

Use in conjunction with the Standardized Postoperative Care Plan.

UNIT X

1. NURSING DIAGNOSIS

Impaired skin integrity:

a. **surgical incision;**
b. **impaired wound healing** related to inadequate nutritional status, inadequate blood supply to wound area, stress on wound area, infection, preoperative radiation therapy (may have been done if the client's diagnosis was cancer of the bladder), and increased levels of glucocorticoids (levels usually rise with stress);
c. **irritation or breakdown around suture lines and wound drains** related to contact of the skin with wound drainage, pressure from drainage tubes, and use of tape;
d. **peristomal irritation or breakdown** related to:
   1. chemical irritation resulting from prolonged contact with urine (particularly alkaline urine), accumulation of urine crystals (alkaline encrustations), soap residue and perspiration under the appliance, and allergic reaction to substances used to secure the appliance
   2. mechanical irritation associated with frequent and/or improper removal of adhesives, skin cements, and tape; aggressive cleansing of peristomal area; pressure from appliance belt and plastic or metal drainage valves or clamps; and presence of urine crystals.

DESIRED OUTCOMES	NURSING ACTIONS AND *SELECTED RATIONALES*

1.a. The client will experience normal healing of surgical wounds (see Standardized Postoperative Care Plan, Nursing Diagnosis 9, outcome a, for outcome criteria).

1.a. Refer to Standardized Postoperative Care Plan, Nursing Diagnosis 9, action a, for measures related to assessment and promotion of normal wound healing.

1.b. The client will maintain skin integrity (see Standardized Postoperative Care Plan, Nursing Diagnosis 9, outcome b, for outcome criteria).

1.b.1. Inspect skin areas that are in contact with wound drainage, tape, and drainage tubings for signs of irritation and breakdown.
2. Assess for signs and symptoms of peristomal irritation and breakdown (e.g. redness, inflammation, and/or excoriation of peristomal skin; complaints of itching and burning under the appliance; inability to keep appliance on).
3. Refer to Standardized Postoperative Care Plan, Nursing Diagnosis 9, action b.2, for measures to prevent skin irritation and breakdown resulting from wound drainage, tape, and drainage tubings.
4. Implement measures *to prevent peristomal irritation and breakdown:*
    a. patch test all adhesives, sprays, solvents, and skin barriers before initial use; do not use products that cause redness, itching, burning, or inflammation
    b. change appliance only when necessary (e.g. as ordered, if appliance or seal is leaking, if client complains of burning or itching under seal); appliance should be able to remain in place for 3–5 days
    c. use a 2-piece appliance (barrier/flange and pouch) *so that collection bag can be changed without having to remove adhesive from the skin and easily applied over the stents* (a 1-piece appliance is commonly used once the stents are removed)
    d. perform actions *to reduce peristomal irritation during removal of appliance:*
        1. place drops of warm water or solvent at edge of flange or adhesive disc if necessary *to loosen adhesive* (allow time for adhesive to dissolve before pulling appliance off)
        2. remove appliance gently and in the direction of hair growth
        3. if solvent was used, wash and rinse the area completely after pouch is removed
    e. perform actions *to prevent urine from coming in contact with the skin when changing appliance:*
        1. change appliance when the ostomy is least active (in the morning before drinking liquids or when fluid intake has been reduced for a few hours)
        2. place a "wick" (rolled gauze pad), vaginal tampon, or tissue on the stoma opening when the appliance is off
    f. cleanse peristomal skin thoroughly with mild soap and water; rinse off all soap; use tepid rather than hot water *to prevent burns*
    g. apply skin sealants (e.g. United Skin Prep, Sween Prep, Hollister Skin Gel) or skin barriers composed of synthetic material (e.g. United Skin Barrier, Reliaseal, Stomahesive) before application of flange or stoma pouch; avoid the use of hydrophilic barriers (e.g. karaya) *because they attract and hold water and will dissolve when in contact with urine*
    h. perform actions *to prevent urine from contacting the skin when appliance is on:*
        1. utilize a skin barrier with an opening exactly the same size as the stoma *to prevent any contact of the peristomal skin with urine*
        2. measure diameter of stoma and select a pouch with an opening that is no more than 0.3 cm (⅛ inch) larger than stoma (it may be necessary to create a pattern to use for cutting pouch opening if stoma has an irregular shape and cannot be measured using appliance manufacturer's standard measuring guide)
        3. instruct and assist client to remeasure the stoma size frequently during first 6 weeks after surgery and to alter pouch opening as stomal edema decreases

    4. implement measures *to ensure an adequate seal:*
       a. avoid use of ointments or creams on peristomal skin *(these can interfere with adequate adhesive bonding)*
       b. follow manufacturer's instructions carefully when applying skin barrier or appliance
       c. use ostomy paste (e.g. Stomahesive paste, Premium paste) to fill in irregularities around stoma site (e.g. body folds, previous scars, retention sutures) before applying collection device
       d. apply firm pressure and remove all air pockets when applying flange or stoma pouch; place client in a supine position *to increase tautness of skin surface during application*
       e. use products with a flexible or convex backing or medical adhesive if needed
    5. empty pouch every 2–3 hours or when it is about ⅓ full *(the weight of pouch could cause it to separate from the skin)*
    6. position pouch so gravity flow facilitates drainage away from stoma and skin
    7. close valve or clamp tightly after emptying *to prevent leakage*
  i. if a belted appliance is used, fasten the belt so that 2 fingers can easily slip between belt and skin *in order to prevent excessive pressure on the skin*
  j. instruct and assist client to check appliance periodically to ensure that clamps or valves are not pressing on the skin
  k. perform actions *to prevent urine crystals from forming on peristomal skin:*
    1. implement measures *to maintain urine acidity:*
       a. assist client with active-resistive exercises *(muscle activity produces an acid end product)*
       b. encourage client to increase intake of foods/fluids that form an acid ash (e.g. cranberry and prune juice, meat, eggs, poultry, fish, grapes, whole grains)
       c. instruct client to decrease intake of milk, citrus fruits, and carbonated beverages *(these tend to alkalinize the urine)*
       d. administer medications as ordered *to acidify the urine* (e.g. ascorbic acid)
       e. refer to Postoperative Nursing Diagnosis 2, action d, for measures to prevent urinary tract infection *(urea-splitting organisms tend to alkalinize the urine)*
    2. replace equipment from which urine crystals cannot be completely removed
    3. be sure that stoma opening on pouch is only 0.3 cm (⅛ inch) larger than diameter of stoma
  l. if urine crystals are present on peristomal skin, remove flange or stoma pouch every 2–3 days and apply vinegar and water (1:1) compress to affected area for 30 minutes; remoisten compress frequently.
5. If signs and symptoms of peristomal skin irritation and breakdown occur:
  a. identify irritant
  b. cleanse area gently with warm water
  c. expose affected area to light or heat for 20–30 minutes when flange or stoma pouch is removed; keep heat source (e.g. hair dryer on lukewarm setting, heat lamp) about 30 cm (about 12 inches) away; cover stoma with a damp gauze pad *to prevent burns and to decrease risk of stomal swelling due to heat-induced increased blood flow*
  d. perform skin care according to physician's order or hospital protocol (usual care includes covering all irritated skin with a properly fitted, hypoallergenic, solid skin barrier and avoiding appliance changes unless there are signs of leakage)
  e. monitor for therapeutic and nontherapeutic effects of the following medications if applied:
    1. nystatin powder *to treat fungal infections*
    2. corticosteroids (e.g. triamcinolone) *to reduce inflammation associated with severe skin reactions*
  f. consult physician and/or enterostomal therapist if:
    1. condition of peristomal skin does not improve within 48 hours

2. signs and symptoms of infection (e.g. elevated temperature; redness, warmth, and edema around area of breakdown; unusual drainage or odor from site) are present.

☐ ▬▬▬▬▬▬▬▬▬▬▬▬▬▬▬▬▬▬▬▬

2. NURSING DIAGNOSIS

Potential for infection: urinary tract related to:

a. urinary stasis (the conduit always contains about 5 cc of residual urine);
b. bacterial invasion via the stoma or urethral catheter (if present);
c. reflux of urine associated with occlusion of the stoma, a refluxing ureteroileal anastomosis, and a full or improperly positioned collection pouch.

☐ ▬▬▬▬▬▬▬▬▬▬▬▬▬▬▬▬▬▬▬▬

DESIRED OUTCOMES	NURSING ACTIONS AND *SELECTED RATIONALES*

2. The client will remain free of urinary tract infection as evidenced by:
   a. no increase in cloudiness of and sediment in urine
   b. no unusual odor to urine
   c. absence of chills and fever
   d. absence of bacteria, nitrites, and WBCs in urine
   e. negative urine culture.

2.a. Assess for and report signs and symptoms of urinary tract infection (e.g. increased cloudiness of and sediment in urine, change in odor of urine, elevated temperature, chills).
b. Monitor urinalysis and report presence of WBCs, bacteria, and/or nitrites.
c. Obtain a urine specimen for culture and sensitivity if ordered. Report abnormal results.
d. Implement measures *to prevent urinary tract infection:*
   1. perform actions *to prevent urinary reflux and stasis:*
      a. implement measures to prevent urinary obstruction (see Postoperative Collaborative Diagnosis 3, action b.2)
      b. use a pouch with an antireflux valve whenever possible
      c. instruct and assist client to empty pouch when it is ⅓ full *in order to prevent reflux and reduce risk of bacterial growth resulting from stasis of urine in pouch*
      d. instruct and assist client to change to a bedside collection system before lying down for an extended period
      e. increase activity as tolerated
   2. ensure that any reusable pouch is cleansed thoroughly, rinsed, and allowed to dry completely between applications
   3. perform actions to maintain urine acidity (see Postoperative Nursing Diagnosis 1, action b.4.k.1)
   4. if a urethral catheter is in place, perform catheter care as often as needed *to prevent accumulation of mucus around the meatus.*
e. If signs and symptoms of urinary tract infection are present:
   1. continue with above actions
   2. monitor for therapeutic and nontherapeutic effects of anti-infectives if administered.

☐ ▬▬▬▬▬▬▬▬▬▬▬▬▬▬▬▬▬▬▬▬

3. COLLABORATIVE DIAGNOSIS

Potential complications:

a. **stomal changes:**
   1. **prolapse** related to pressure around the stoma and loss of integrity of suture line
   2. **excessive bleeding or irritation** related to aggressive cleansing techniques, poor appliance fit, and/or presence of urine crystals

    3. **necrosis** related to intraoperative and/or postoperative interruption of blood supply to the stoma;

  b. **urinary obstruction** related to:

    1. stenosis of the stoma associated with excessive edema, formation of scar tissue, or epithelial hyperplasia

    2. malfunctioning ureteral stents

    3. edema at the ureteroileal junction

    4. collection of mucus at stomal and/or ureteral openings;

  c. **peritonitis** related to:

    1. wound infection

    2. abscess formation

    3. leakage of urine and/or intestinal contents into the peritoneum associated with failure of the surgical anastomoses

    4. leakage of urine into and/or exposure of the peritoneum associated with retraction of peristomal skin (retraction can occur with slippage of the sutures or shrinkage of the supporting tissues).

DESIRED OUTCOMES	NURSING ACTIONS AND *SELECTED RATIONALES*

3.a. The client will maintain integrity of the stoma as evidenced by:
  1. dark pink or red coloring of stoma
  2. expected stomal height
  3. absence of excessive bleeding and increasing edema of the stoma.
	3.a.1. Assess for and report signs and symptoms of impaired stomal integrity (e.g. pale, dark red, blue-black, or magenta color of stoma; increased stomal height; increased stomal edema or bleeding). Use only clear appliances during immediate postoperative period *to allow easy visibility of stoma.*
	  2. Implement measures *to maintain integrity of stoma:*
	    a. perform actions to *maintain adequate stomal circulation:*
	      1. ensure that the openings of the skin barrier and pouch are the right size; be careful to center stoma in the opening *in order to prevent pressure on stoma*
	      2. use properly fitted flange and belt *to reduce peristomal pressure*
	    b. anchor flange and pouch securely *to prevent a shearing action across stoma*
	    c. cleanse stoma gently using a soft cloth, gauze, or tissue
	    d. perform actions to prevent or remove urine crystals (see Postoperative Nursing Diagnosis 1, actions b.4.k and l) *in order to prevent stomal irritation.*
	  3. If signs and symptoms of impaired stomal integrity occur:
	    a. perform wound care as ordered
	    b. prepare client for surgical revision of stoma if indicated
	    c. provide emotional support to client and significant others.

3.b. The client will not experience urinary obstruction as evidenced by:
  1. balanced intake and output beginning 48 hours postoperatively
  2. gradual resolution of abdominal tenderness and distention
  3. expected volume of drainage from abdominal wound.
	3.b.1. Assess for and report signs and symptoms of ureteral or stomal obstruction (e.g. sudden decrease in urinary output from stoma or ureteral stents, increasing abdominal tenderness and distention, increase in drainage from abdominal wound).
	  2. Implement measures *to prevent urinary obstruction:*
	    a. encourage a fluid intake of 2500 cc/day unless contraindicated *to flush conduit and prevent mucus from congealing*
	    b. irrigate ureteral stents as ordered *to maintain patency* (should be done with very little fluid and gently)
	    c. change pouch carefully *in order to avoid dislodgment of the ureteral stents that may be extending from stoma* (stents usually remain in place for 7–10 days postoperatively)
	    d. perform actions to maintain urine acidity (see Postoperative Nursing Diagnosis 1, action b.4.k.1) *in order to prevent inflammation and scarring of the stoma resulting from prolonged contact with alkaline urine.*
	  3. If signs and symptoms of urinary obstruction occur:

UNIT X

a. assess for signs and symptoms of hyperchloremic acidosis (e.g. fever, irregular pulse, lethargy, nausea, vomiting, diarrhea, muscle weakness) that may occur as a result of excessive absorption of chloride associated with prolonged stasis of urine in the conduit (may also be due to a lengthy conduit with poor peristalsis)

b. prepare client for dilation of the stoma, surgical revision of stoma or sites of anastomoses, and/or replacement of ureteral stents

c. provide emotional support to client and significant others.

3.c. The client will not develop peritonitis as evidenced by:
1. gradual resolution of abdominal pain
2. soft, nondistended abdomen
3. temperature declining toward normal
4. vital signs within normal range for client
5. gradual return of normal bowel sounds
6. WBC count declining toward normal.

3.c.1. Assess for and report signs and symptoms of peritonitis (e.g. increase in severity of abdominal pain; rebound tenderness; tense, rigid abdomen; temperature increase; tachycardia; tachypnea; hypotension; failure of bowel sounds to return to normal).

2. Monitor WBC counts. Report levels that increase or fail to decline toward normal.

3. Implement measures *to prevent peritonitis:*
a. perform actions to prevent and treat wound infection (see Standardized Postoperative Care Plan, Nursing Diagnosis 16, actions b.4 and 5)
b. perform actions *to maintain patency of wound drain(s) if present:*
   1. keep tubing free of kinks
   2. empty collection device as often as necessary
   3. maintain suction as ordered
c. perform actions *to prevent inadvertent removal of drain(s) if present:*
   1. use caution when changing dressings surrounding drain(s)
   2. provide extension tubing if necessary *to enable client to move without placing tension on the drain(s)*
   3. instruct client not to pull on drain(s) or drainage tubing
d. perform actions *to prevent urinary obstruction* (see action b.2 in this diagnosis) *in order to prevent resultant strain on and leakage from the suture line*
e. if peristomal skin is retracted, perform wound care as ordered *to facilitate the formation of granulation tissue in retracted area.*

4. If signs and symptoms of peritonitis occur:
a. withhold all food and fluid as ordered
b. place client on bedrest in a semi-Fowler's position *to assist in pooling or localizing gastrointestinal contents and urine in the pelvis rather than under the diaphragm*
c. insert a nasogastric tube and maintain suction as ordered
d. monitor for therapeutic and nontherapeutic effects of anti-infectives if administered
e. monitor for therapeutic and nontherapeutic effects of intravenous fluids and/or blood volume expanders if administered *to prevent or treat shock (shock can occur as a result of the escape of protein, fluid, and electrolytes into peritoneal cavity)*
f. prepare client for surgical intervention (e.g. repair of sites of anastomoses or retracted peristomal skin, drainage of abscess) if indicated
g. provide emotional support to client and significant others.

4. NURSING DIAGNOSIS

Sexual dysfunction:

a. **decreased libido** related to altered self-concept, fear of offensive odor or leakage of urine from the pouch, fear of rejection by desired partner, discomfort associated with the surgical incision, and grieving;
b. **impotence** related to damage to the sympathetic and parasympathetic nerve fibers that control erection (can occur with removal of bladder neck).

DESIRED OUTCOMES	NURSING ACTIONS AND *SELECTED RATIONALES*

4. The client will demonstrate beginning acceptance of changes in sexual functioning as evidenced by:
   a. verbalization of a perception of self as sexually acceptable and adequate
   b. maintenance of relationships with significant others
   c. statements reflecting beginning adjustment to the effects of the urinary diversion on sexuality.

4.a. Assess for signs and symptoms of sexual dysfunction (e.g. verbalization of sexual concerns, failure to maintain relationships with significant others, limitations imposed by nerve damage).
   b. Determine attitudes, knowledge, and concerns about the effects of the cystectomy and urinary diversion on sexual functioning.
   c. Communicate interest, understanding, and respect for the values of the client and his/her partner.
   d. Provide accurate information about effects of the cystectomy and urinary diversion on sexual functioning. Encourage questions and clarify misconceptions.
   e. Facilitate communication between the client and his/her partner. Assist them to identify issues that may affect their sexual relationship.
   f. Implement measures to facilitate psychological adjustment to the changes that have occurred (see Postoperative Nursing Diagnoses 5, actions d–s; 6, action d; and 7, action d).
   g. Instruct client in ways *to reduce risk of leakage of urine from the pouch during sexual activity:*
      1. empty appliance before sexual activity
      2. secure appliance seal with tape for added security.
   h. If client is concerned about odor, instruct him/her to:
      1. shower or bathe before sexual activity
      2. use an odorproof pouch or pouch deodorant
      3. use cologne or perfume if desired
      4. keep room well ventilated.
   i. Implement measures *to decrease possibility of rejection by partner:*
      1. provide support for the partner by helping him/her to acknowledge both positive and negative feelings about changes in the client
      2. if appropriate, involve partner in ostomy care *to facilitate adjustment to and integration of his/her partner's new body image.*
   j. If client is concerned about the presence of the stoma and appliance, discuss the possibility of:
      1. using opaque or patterned pouches or decorative pouch covers
      2. wearing underwear with the crotch removed (for females), boxer shorts (for males), or large elastic wraps around abdomen during sexual activity.
   k. Arrange for uninterrupted privacy during hospital stay if desired by the couple.
   l. If client is concerned that operative site discomfort will interfere with usual sexual activity:
      1. assure him/her that discomfort is temporary and will diminish as the incision heals
      2. encourage alternatives to intercourse or use of positions that decrease pressure on surgical site (e.g. side-lying).
   m. If impotence resulted from the surgical procedure:
      1. encourage client to discuss the possibility of a penile prosthesis with physician
      2. discuss ways to be creative in expressing sexuality (e.g. massage, fantasies, cuddling)
      3. suggest alternative methods of sexual gratification and use of assistive devices if appropriate
      4. discuss alternative methods of parenting (e.g. artificial insemination, adoption) if of concern to client.
   n. Inform client that written information regarding sexual activity when one has an ostomy is available from the United Ostomy Association and from manufacturers of ostomy appliances.
   o. Include partner in above discussions and encourage his/her continued support of the client.
   p. Consult physician and enterostomal therapist if counseling appears indicated.

UNIT X

5. NURSING DIAGNOSIS

Disturbance in self-concept* related to:

a. loss of bladder and ability to urinate normally;
b. temporary or permanent dependence on others to assist with ostomy management;
c. feeling of loss of control associated with altered urinary elimination;
d. change in appearance associated with the presence of a stoma;
e. changes in usual sexual functioning;
f. embarrassment associated with odor of ostomy drainage;
g. sterility associated with removal of prostate and seminal vesicles (if a total cystectomy was performed) and loss of ejaculatory function (may occur if sympathetic and parasympathetic fibers are damaged during removal of bladder neck).

---

* This diagnostic label includes the nursing diagnoses of body image disturbance and self-esteem disturbance.

DESIRED OUTCOMES	NURSING ACTIONS AND *SELECTED RATIONALES*

5. The client will demonstrate beginning adaptation to changes in appearance, body functioning, and life style as evidenced by:
a. verbalization of feelings of self-worth and sexual adequacy
b. maintenance of relationships with significant others
c. active participation in activities of daily living
d. active interest in personal appearance
e. willingness to participate in social activities
f. verbalization of a beginning plan for integrating management of the ileal conduit into life style.
	5.a. Determine the meaning of changes in appearance, body functioning, and life style to the client by encouraging him/her to verbalize feelings and by noting nonverbal responses to the changes experienced.
	b. Assess for signs and symptoms of a disturbance in self-concept (e.g. verbal or nonverbal cues denoting a negative response to change[s] in body functioning or appearance such as denial of or preoccupation with change[s] that have occurred, refusal to look at or touch stoma, or withdrawal from significant others).
	c. Implement measures to facilitate the grieving process (see Postoperative Nursing Diagnosis 7, action d).
	d. Assist client to identify strengths and qualities that have a positive effect on self-concept.
	e. Implement measures to assist client *to increase self-esteem* (e.g. limit negative self-criticism, encourage positive comments about self, give positive feedback about accomplishments).
	f. Reinforce actions to assist client to cope with effects of the urinary diversion (see Postoperative Nursing Diagnosis 6, action d).
	g. Reinforce actions that may assist client to adjust to alterations in sexual functioning (see Postoperative Nursing Diagnosis 4, actions c–o).
	h. Instruct and assist client in ways *to decrease odor of ostomy drainage and pouch:*
	  1. use odorproof pouches and change appliance regularly
	  2. use disposable appliances or clean reusable items thoroughly
	  3. empty appliance regularly
	  4. perform actions to ensure an adequate pouch seal (see Postoperative Nursing Diagnosis 1, action b.4.h.4)
	  5. instruct client to avoid foods that cause urine to have a strong odor (e.g. asparagus, onions)
	  6. use room or pouch deodorizers
	  7. change bed linens and clothing as soon as they become soiled.
	i. Assure client that once the edema and discomfort associated with the surgery have resolved, he/she will be able to dress as before with minor, or no, modifications.
	j. Show client and significant others some of the attractive ostomy appliances (e.g. opaque or patterned pouches, pouch covers) that are available.
	k. Assist client with usual grooming and makeup habits if necessary.
	l. Encourage active participation in care of ostomy *in order to assist client to incorporate altered pattern of urinary elimination into body image.*

m. Demonstrate acceptance of client using techniques such as therapeutic touch and frequent visits. Encourage significant others to do the same.

n. Assess for and support behaviors suggesting positive adaptation to changes experienced (e.g. willingness to care for ostomy, compliance with the treatment plan).

o. Encourage significant others to allow client to do what he/she is able *so that independence can be re-established and/or self-esteem redeveloped.*

p. Assist client's and significant others' adjustment by listening, facilitating communication, and providing information.

q. Encourage visits and support from significant others.

r. Encourage client to continue involvement in social activities and to pursue interests. Assure him/her that an ostomy need not alter life style (only contact sports are contraindicated).

s. Provide information about and encourage utilization of community agencies or support groups (e.g. ostomy groups; sexual, family, individual, and/or financial counseling services).

t. Consult physician about psychological counseling if client desires or if he/she seems unwilling or unable to adapt to changes resulting from the urinary diversion.

6. NURSING DIAGNOSIS

Ineffective individual coping related to:

a. fear, anxiety, and depression associated with possibility of rejection by significant others, loss of control over urinary elimination, diagnosis, and prognosis;

b. difficulty in caring for ostomy;

c. need for lifelong medical supervision;

d. inadequate support system.

DESIRED OUTCOMES	NURSING ACTIONS AND *SELECTED RATIONALES*
6. The client will demonstrate the use of effective coping skills and beginning acceptance of effects of the urinary diversion as evidenced by: a. willingness to participate in treatment plan and self-care activities b. verbalization of ability to cope with the urinary diversion and its effects c. identification of stressors d. utilization of appropriate problem-solving techniques e. recognition and utilization of available support systems.	6.a. Assess effectiveness of client's coping strategies by observing behavior and noting strengths, weaknesses, ability to express feelings and concerns, and willingness to participate in treatment plan. b. Assess for and report signs and symptoms that may indicate ineffective coping (e.g. sleep disturbances, increasing fatigue, difficulty concentrating, irritability, decreased tolerance for pain, verbalization of inability to cope, inability to problem-solve). c. Allow time for client to adjust psychologically to the urinary diversion. d. Implement measures *to promote effective coping:* 　1. arrange for a visit with an ostomate of similar age and same sex who has successfully adjusted to a urinary diversion 　2. perform actions to reduce fear and anxiety (see Standardized Postoperative Care Plan, Nursing Diagnosis 1, action c) 　3. perform actions to promote a positive self-concept (see Postoperative Nursing Diagnosis 5, actions c–s) 　4. maintain consistency of approaches and explanations 　5. do not overload client with information irrelevant to present stage of ostomy management unless client is questioning or expressing an interest 　6. encourage participation in ostomy care as soon as possible 　7. use appliances that client is expected to use when discharged 　8. ensure adequate time for and privacy during ostomy care 　9. include client in planning of care, encourage maximum participation in ostomy care, and allow choices whenever possible *to allow him/her to maintain a sense of control*

10. instruct client in effective problem-solving techniques (e.g. accurate identification of stressors, determination of various options to solve problem)
11. assist client to maintain usual daily routines whenever possible
12. discuss with significant others the fear of rejection client may be experiencing and encourage their support
13. provide diversional activities according to client's interests
14. assist client to identify and utilize available support systems; provide information about available community resources that can assist client and significant others in coping with effects of urinary diversion and the underlying disease process (e.g. United Ostomy Association, American Cancer Society, counseling services, local ostomy support groups, community health agencies).

e. Encourage continued emotional support from significant others.
f. Encourage the client to share with significant others the kind of support that would be most beneficial (e.g. listening, inspiring hope, providing reassurance and accurate information).
g. Assess for and support behaviors suggesting positive adaptation to changes experienced (e.g. willingness to participate in self-care, verbalization of ability to cope, recognition and use of available support systems, utilization of effective problem-solving strategies).
h. Consult physician about psychological counseling if appropriate. Initiate a referral if necessary.

□ ▐▬▬▬▬▬▬▬▬▬▬▬▬▬▬▬▬▬▬▬▬▬▬▬▬▬▬▬▬▬▬▬▬▐

7. NURSING DIAGNOSIS

Grieving* related to loss of bladder and the ability to urinate normally, change in appearance, and effects of the surgery on sexual functioning.

_____

* This diagnostic label includes anticipatory grieving and grieving following the actual losses/changes.

□ ▐▬▬▬▬▬▬▬▬▬▬▬▬▬▬▬▬▬▬▬▬▬▬▬▬▬▬▬▬▬▬▬▬▐

DESIRED OUTCOMES	NURSING ACTIONS AND *SELECTED RATIONALES*

7. The client will demonstrate beginning progression through the grieving process as evidenced by:
a. verbalization of feelings about the urinary diversion and its effects
b. expression of grief
c. participation in treatment plan and self-care activities
d. utilization of available support systems
e. verbalization of a plan for integrating ostomy care into life style.
	7.a. Determine client's perception of the impact of the urinary diversion on his/her future.
	b. Determine how client usually expresses grief.
	c. Observe for signs of grieving (e.g. changes in eating habits, insomnia, anger, noncompliance, denial).
	d. Implement measures *to facilitate the grieving process:*
	  1. assist client to acknowledge the losses and changes experienced *so grief work can begin;* assess for factors that may hinder or facilitate acknowledgment
	  2. discuss the grieving process and assist client to accept the stages of grieving as an expected response to actual and anticipated losses; support the realization that grief may recur *because of the extended period of adjustment to the urinary diversion and, if diversion was performed for cancer, subsequent treatment*
	  3. allow time for client to progress through the stages of grieving (denial, anger, bargaining, depression, acceptance [Kübler-Ross, 1969]); be aware that not every stage is experienced or expressed by all individuals
	  4. provide an atmosphere of care and concern (e.g. provide privacy, be available and nonjudgmental, display empathy and respect) *so that client will feel free to verbalize both positive and negative feelings and concerns*
	  5. perform actions *to promote trust* (e.g. answer questions honestly, provide requested information)

6. encourage the expression of anger and sadness about the losses and changes experienced
7. encourage client to express his/her feelings in whatever ways are comfortable (e.g. writing, drawing, conversation)
8. perform actions to facilitate effective coping (see Postoperative Nursing Diagnosis 6, action d)
9. support realistic hope about the effects of the surgery on his/her life (e.g. increased comfort, improved urinary elimination ability).
   e. Assess for and support behaviors suggesting successful resolution of grief (e.g. verbalizing feelings about the urinary diversion and loss of sexual functioning, expressing sorrow, focusing on ways to adapt to changes/losses that have occurred).
   f. Explain the stages of the grieving process to significant others. Encourage their support and understanding.
   g. Provide information regarding counseling services and support groups that might assist client in working through grief.
   h. Arrange for visit from clergy if desired by client.
   i. Monitor for therapeutic and nontherapeutic effects of antidepressants if administered.
   j. Consult physician about referral for counseling if signs of dysfunctional grieving (e.g. persistent denial of losses or changes, excessive anger or sadness, hysteria, suicidal behaviors, phobias) occur.

□ ▬▬▬▬▬▬▬▬▬▬▬▬▬▬▬▬▬▬▬▬▬▬▬▬▬▬▬▬▬▬

8. NURSING DIAGNOSIS

Knowledge deficit regarding follow-up care.

□ ▬▬▬▬▬▬▬▬▬▬▬▬▬▬▬▬▬▬▬▬▬▬▬▬▬▬▬▬▬▬

DESIRED OUTCOMES	NURSING ACTIONS AND *SELECTED RATIONALES*
8.a. The client will verbalize a basic understanding of the anatomical changes that have occurred as a result of the surgery.	8.a. Reinforce teaching about the anatomical changes that have occurred as a result of the cystectomy and urinary diversion. Use appropriate teaching aids (e.g. pictures, videotapes, anatomical models).
8.b. The client will demonstrate ways to maintain stomal and peristomal skin integrity.	8.b.1. Demonstrate correct application of the ostomy appliance. 2. Provide instructions on ways *to maintain stomal and peristomal skin integrity:* a. patch test all adhesives, sprays, solvents, and skin barriers before using for the first time; avoid any product that causes redness, itching, or burning b. change appliance only when necessary (should be able to remain in place for 5–7 days after the initial postoperative period) c. shave peristomal skin regularly with an electric razor d. remove appliance carefully (e.g. loosen adhesive with warm water or solvent, remove appliance in direction of hair growth) e. prevent skin contact with urine (e.g. change appliance when the ostomy is least active; place a wick [rolled gauze pad], vaginal tampon, or tissue on stoma when appliance is off; utilize skin sealants; accurately fit and apply pouch; ensure an adequate appliance seal; empty pouch when ⅓ full; position pouch properly; utilize a bedside collection system when lying down for extended periods) f. prevent urine crystals from forming on peristomal skin: 1. maintain acidity of urine (see action d.2.c in this diagnosis) 2. cleanse equipment thoroughly; replace equipment from which urine crystals cannot be completely removed

3. be sure that opening on pouch is only ⅛ inch larger than diameter of stoma

g. remove urine crystals from peristomal skin if they occur by removing flange or stoma pouch every 2–3 days and applying a vinegar and water (1:1) compress to affected area for 30 minutes; compress should be remoistened frequently

h. follow special precautions for products used (e.g. inert, moldable skin barriers must be kept in airtight container; skin sealants should be used only on healthy peristomal skin *because they can further irritate reddened and excoriated skin)*.

3. Allow time for questions, clarification, practice, and return demonstration of appliance application and appropriate care of the stoma and peristomal skin.

8.c. The client will demonstrate proper technique for cleansing reusable ostomy equipment.

8.c.1. Discuss recommended method of cleansing reusable ostomy equipment based on manufacturer's recommendations.

2. Demonstrate appropriate cleansing technique. Emphasize importance of:
   a. washing and rinsing pouch thoroughly upon removal
   b. soaking pouch according to manufacturer's instructions
   c. allowing pouch to dry thoroughly
   d. storing pouch according to manufacturer's instructions (e.g. apply powder or cornstarch to inside and store in a clean, dry place).

3. Allow time for questions, clarification, and return demonstration.

8.d. The client will verbalize ways to prevent excessive skin growth over the stoma and peristomal area.

8.d.1. Explain that excessive skin growth over the stoma and peristomal area is thought to be due to prolonged skin contact with urine (particularly alkaline urine).

2. Instruct client in ways *to prevent excessive skin growth over the stoma and peristomal area:*
   a. instruct client to check pH of his/her urine as directed *to be sure acidity is being maintained*
   b. reduce contact of stoma and periostomal area with urine by:
      1. using a pouch with an antireflux valve
      2. utilizing skin barriers that fit properly
      3. applying and fitting pouch correctly
   c. maintain urine acidity by:
      1. increasing intake of foods/fluids that form an acid ash (e.g. cranberry and prune juice, meat, eggs, poultry, fish, grapes, whole grains)
      2. limiting intake of milk, carbonated beverages, and citrus fruit
      3. taking medications *that acidify the urine* (e.g. ascorbic acid) as prescribed
      4. preventing urinary tract infection (see action f in this diagnosis)
   d. prevent or, if present, remove urine crystals (see actions b.2.f and g in this diagnosis).

8.e. The client will identify ways to control odor of ostomy drainage and pouch.

8.e. Provide instructions on ways *to control odor of ostomy drainage and pouch:*
   1. drink at least 10 glasses of liquid/day; increase volume of liquid if urine appears concentrated
   2. avoid foods that cause urine to have a strong odor (e.g. asparagus, onions)
   3. place a small amount of deodorizer or vinegar in bottom of pouch
   4. change appliance at appropriate intervals and cleanse it thoroughly
   5. rinse appliance with a vinegar and water solution (1:1)
   6. prevent urinary tract infections (see action f in this diagnosis)
   7. use odor-proof pouch and empty appliance regularly.

8.f. The client will identify ways to prevent urinary tract infection.

8.f. Provide instructions on ways *to prevent urinary tract infection:*
   1. drink at least 10 glasses of liquid/day
   2. prevent reflux of urine by:
      a. emptying pouch when it is ⅓ full (approximately every 2–3 hours)
      b. attaching a bedside collection system when lying down for an extended period
      c. using a pouch with an antireflux valve
   3. maintain urine acidity (see action d.2.c in this diagnosis)

4. clean reusable equipment thoroughly (see action c.2 in this diagnosis) *in order to reduce risk of bacterial contamination*
5. take prophylactic anti-infectives as prescribed.

8.g. The client will state signs and symptoms to report to the health care provider.	8.g.1. Refer to Standardized Postoperative Care Plan, Nursing Diagnosis 20, action c, for signs and symptoms to report to the health care provider. 2. Instruct client to also report: a. dark red, blue-black, magenta, or pale stoma b. change in color, consistency, or odor of urine that is not readily identified as a response to food or fluid intake; emphasize that mucous shreds in urine are normal with an ileal conduit and that an increased amount of mucus should be expected for several weeks postoperatively c. absence of or reduction in urinary output despite an adequate fluid intake d. excessive bleeding of stoma or bloody drainage from ostomy e. excessive mucus drainage from urinary meatus (some drainage should be expected for several weeks postoperatively) f. change in contour of stoma (use diagrams and descriptive terms *so client does not confuse decreasing stoma size due to resolving edema with actual stoma retraction*) g. persistent skin irritation or breakdown of peristomal skin h. persistent presence of urine crystals on stoma or peristomal skin i. persistent leakage of ostomy appliance j. fever, irregular pulse, drowsiness, nausea, vomiting, diarrhea, muscle weakness (may indicate hyperchloremic acidosis) k. inability to maintain an acidic urine l. signs and symptoms of urinary tract infection (e.g. fever; chills; cloudy, foul-smelling urine) m. signs and symptoms of renal calculi (e.g. dull, aching or severe, colicky flank pain; blood in urine; nausea; vomiting); stone formation, a late complication of a urinary diversion, may result from persistent urinary stasis, urinary tract infection, and inadequate fluid intake n. difficulty coping with ostomy care or altered urinary elimination pattern.
8.h. The client will identify appropriate community resources that can assist with home management and adjustment to changes resulting from the urinary diversion.	8.h.1. Provide information about community resources that can assist the client and significant others with home management and adjustment to changes resulting from urinary diversion (e.g. local ostomy support groups; American Cancer Society; community health agencies; enterostomal therapist; home health agencies; Visiting Nurse Association; financial, individual, and family counseling services). 2. Initiate a referral if indicated.
8.i. The client will verbalize an understanding of and a plan for adhering to recommended follow-up care including future appointments with health care provider, wound care, activity level, and medications prescribed.	8.i.1. Refer to Standardized Postoperative Care Plan, Nursing Diagnosis 20, for routine postoperative instructions and measures to improve client compliance. 2. Reinforce the physician's instructions regarding activity limitations: a. avoid lifting objects over 10 pounds until permitted by physician b. avoid participating in contact sports *to prevent stomal damage.* 3. Explain the rationale for, side effects of, and importance of taking medications prescribed (e.g. anti-infectives, ascorbic acid).

□ ▬▬▬

Reference

Kübler-Ross, E. On death and dying. New York: Macmillan, 1969.

UNIT X

Nephrectomy

Nephrectomy is the surgical removal of the kidney. Renal conditions that are commonly treated by nephrectomy include malignancy and irreparable kidney damage caused by trauma, hypertension, polycystic disease, or calculi. The kidney may also be removed for the purpose of donation. The most common approach utilized for a simple nephrectomy is the subcostal flank approach. Other approaches (i.e. thoracoabdominal, transabdominal, dorsolumbar) may be utilized when greater visualization, improved access, or a more radical procedure is necessary.

This care plan focuses on the adult client hospitalized for a unilateral nephrectomy. Preoperatively, the goals of care are to reduce fear and anxiety and prepare the client for the surgical experience. Postoperative goals of care are to maintain comfort, prevent complications, and educate the client regarding follow-up care. The care plan will need to be individualized according to the client's diagnosis, prognosis, and plans for subsequent treatment.

DISCHARGE CRITERIA

Prior to discharge, the client will:

- verbalize ways to maintain health of the remaining kidney
- state signs and symptoms to report to the health care provider
- share thoughts and feelings about the loss of the kidney
- verbalize an understanding of and a plan for adhering to recommended follow-up care including future appointments with health care provider, medications prescribed, activity level, wound care, and plans for subsequent treatment of the underlying disorder.

NURSING/COLLABORATIVE DIAGNOSES

Postoperative
1. Ineffective breathing patterns:
   a. hypoventilation
   b. hyperventilation ☐ 529
2. Potential complications:
   a. hypovolemic shock
   b. pneumothorax ☐ 529
3. Grieving ☐ 530
4. Knowledge deficit regarding follow-up care ☐ 531

Preoperative

Use in conjunction with the Standardized Preoperative Care Plan.

Postoperative

Use in conjunction with the Standardized Postoperative Care Plan.

1. NURSING DIAGNOSIS

Ineffective breathing patterns:

a. **hypoventilation** related to depressant effects of anesthesia and some medications (e.g. narcotic analgesics, muscle relaxants), reluctance to breathe deeply due to chest incision pain if thoracoabdominal or subcostal approach was used and fear of dislodging chest tube(s) if in place, weakness, and pressure on the diaphragm resulting from abdominal distention;

b. **hyperventilation** related to pain, fear, and anxiety.

DESIRED OUTCOMES	NURSING ACTIONS AND *SELECTED RATIONALES*
1. The client will maintain an effective breathing pattern (see Standardized Postoperative Care Plan, Nursing Diagnosis 3, for outcome criteria).	1.a. Refer to Standardized Postoperative Care Plan, Nursing Diagnosis 3, for measures related to assessment and management of ineffective breathing patterns. b. If client has chest tube(s), assure him/her that deep breathing will not dislodge the tube(s).

2. COLLABORATIVE DIAGNOSIS

Potential complications:

a. **hypovolemic shock** related to:
   1. massive blood loss (the renal area is highly vascular)
   2. fluid volume deficit associated with excessive fluid loss and inadequate fluid replacement;

b. **pneumothorax** related to surgical opening of pleura and/or malfunction of chest tube(s) if thoracic approach was used.

DESIRED OUTCOMES	NURSING ACTIONS AND *SELECTED RATIONALES*
2.a. The client will not develop hypovolemic shock (see Standardized Postoperative Care Plan, Collaborative Diagnosis 19, outcome a, for outcome criteria).	2.a.1. Refer to Standardized Postoperative Care Plan, Collaborative Diagnosis 19, action a, for measures related to assessment, prevention, and management of hypovolemic shock. 2. Implement additional measures *to prevent hemorrhage in order to decrease risk of hypovolemic shock:* a. anchor nephrostomy tube securely to flank or abdomen *in order to avoid tissue irritation and subsequent bleeding caused by movement of the tube*

b. perform actions *to reduce strain on the suture line:*
   1. instruct client to splint incisional area with hands or pillow when turning, coughing, and deep breathing
   2. maintain patency of urinary catheters and wound drains
   3. implement measures to prevent nausea and vomiting (see Standardized Postoperative Care Plan, Nursing Diagnosis 7.C, action 2).
3. Prepare client for immediate surgical ligation of bleeding vessels if indicated.

2.b. The client will experience normal lung re-expansion if a thoracic approach was utilized as evidenced by:
1. normal breath sounds and percussion note by the 3rd or 4th postoperative day
2. unlabored respirations at 16–20/minute
3. blood gases returning toward normal
4. chest x-ray showing lung re-expansion.

2.b.1. Assess for and immediately report signs and symptoms of:
   a. malfunction of the chest drainage system (e.g. respiratory distress, sudden cessation of drainage, excessive bubbling in water seal chamber, significant increase in subcutaneous emphysema)
   b. further lung collapse (e.g. extended area of absent breath sounds and hyperresonant percussion note; rapid, shallow, or labored respirations; tachycardia; increased chest pain; cyanosis; restlessness; confusion).
2. Monitor blood gases. Report values that have worsened.
3. Monitor chest x-ray results. Report findings of delayed lung re-expansion.
4. Implement measures *to prevent further lung collapse and promote lung re-expansion:*
   a. perform actions *to maintain patency and integrity of chest drainage system if present:*
      1. maintain water seal and suction levels as ordered
      2. maintain air occlusive dressing over chest tube insertion site(s)
      3. tape all connections securely
      4. milk or strip chest tube(s) if ordered
      5. keep chest drainage and suction tubing free of kinks
      6. keep drainage system below level of client's chest at all times
   b. perform actions to improve breathing pattern (see Postoperative Nursing Diagnosis 1) and facilitate airway clearance (see Standardized Postoperative Care Plan, Nursing Diagnosis 4, action b).
5. If signs and symptoms of further lung collapse occur:
   a. maintain client on bedrest in a semi- to high Fowler's position
   b. maintain oxygen therapy as ordered
   c. assess for and immediately report signs and symptoms of mediastinal shift (e.g. severe dyspnea, increased restlessness and agitation, rapid and/or irregular pulse rate, cyanosis, shift in point of apical impulse and trachea toward unaffected side)
   d. assist with clearing of existing chest tube(s) and/or insertion of a new tube
   e. provide emotional support to client and significant others.

☐ ▬▬▬▬▬▬▬▬▬▬▬▬▬▬▬▬▬▬▬▬▬▬▬▬▬▬▬▬▬▬▬

3. NURSING DIAGNOSIS

Grieving* related to loss of a major body organ.

---

 * This diagnostic label includes anticipatory grieving and grieving following the actual losses or changes.

☐ ▬▬▬▬▬▬▬▬▬▬▬▬▬▬▬▬▬▬▬▬▬▬▬▬▬▬▬▬▬▬▬

DESIRED OUTCOMES	NURSING ACTIONS AND *SELECTED RATIONALES*

3. The client will demonstrate beginning progression through the grieving process as evidenced by:
   a. verbalization of feelings about the loss of a kidney

3.a. Determine the client's perception of the impact of the loss of a kidney on his/her life style and future.
   b. Determine how client usually expresses grief.
   c. Observe for signs of grieving (e.g. changes in eating habits, insomnia, anger, noncompliance, denial).
   d. Implement measures *to facilitate the grieving process:*

b. expression of grief
c. participation in treatment plan and self-care activities
d. utilization of available support systems.

1. assist client to acknowledge the changes resulting from loss of the kidney *so grief work can begin;* assess for factors that may hinder or facilitate acknowledgment
2. discuss the grieving process and assist client to accept the stages of grieving as an expected response to his/her loss
3. allow time for client to progress through the stages of grieving (denial, anger, bargaining, depression, acceptance [Kübler-Ross, 1969]); be aware that not every stage is experienced or expressed by all individuals
4. provide an atmosphere of care and concern (e.g. provide privacy, be available and nonjudgmental, display empathy and respect) *so that client will feel free to verbalize both positive and negative feelings and concerns*
5. perform actions *to promote trust* (e.g. answer questions honestly, provide requested information)
6. encourage the expression of anger and sadness about the loss of the kidney
7. encourage client to express his/her feelings in whatever ways are comfortable (e.g. writing, drawing, conversation)
8. assist client to identify personal strengths that have helped him/her to cope in previous situations of loss
9. support realistic hope about the ability to resume his/her usual activities; reassure client that one functional kidney is sufficient to meet body needs.
e. Assess for and support behaviors suggesting successful resolution of grief (e.g. verbalizing feelings about loss of the kidney, expressing sorrow).
f. Explain the stages of the grieving process to significant others. Encourage their support and understanding.
g. Provide information regarding counseling services that might assist client in working through grief.
h. Arrange for visit from clergy if desired by client.
i. Monitor for therapeutic and nontherapeutic effects of antidepressants if administered.
j. Consult physician about referral for counseling if signs of dysfunctional grieving (e.g. persistent denial of loss and necessary changes in life style, excessive anger or sadness, hysteria, suicidal behaviors, phobias) occur.

UNIT
X

4. NURSING DIAGNOSIS

Knowledge deficit regarding follow-up care.

DESIRED OUTCOMES	NURSING ACTIONS AND *SELECTED RATIONALES*

4.a. The client will verbalize ways to maintain health of the remaining kidney.

4.a. Instruct client regarding ways *to maintain health of the remaining kidney:*
1. adhere to precautions *to prevent a urinary tract infection:*
   a. perform actions *to prevent urinary stasis:*
      1. drink at least 10 glasses of liquid/day
      2. void whenever the urge is felt
      3. avoid long periods of inactivity (if unable to maintain a program of moderate activity, be sure to change positions frequently)
   b. perform actions *to maintain acidic urine:*
      1. include foods/fluids in diet that form an acid ash (e.g. cranberry and prune juice, meat, eggs, poultry, fish, grapes, whole-grain products)
      2. limit intake of milk, carbonated beverages, and citrus fruit
      3. take acidifying agents (e.g. ascorbic acid) as prescribed
   c. wipe from front to back after urinating and defecating if female
   d. keep perineal area clean and dry
   e. take prophylactic anti-infectives as prescribed

2. immediately report signs and symptoms of a urinary tract infection (e.g. chills; fever; urgency, frequency, or burning on urination; cloudy, foul-smelling urine)
3. notify physician if a cold or other infection persists for more than 3 days or if unable to maintain an adequate fluid intake
4. inform other health care providers about the nephrectomy so that prophylactic anti-infective therapy may be initiated before invasive procedures such as dental work, cystoscopy, and minor surgeries
5. avoid activities that might cause trauma to the remaining kidney (e.g. contact sports, horseback riding)
6. consult health care provider before taking any prescription and nonprescription medications that may be toxic to the remaining kidney (e.g. aminoglycosides, salicylates, cyclophosphamide, ibuprofen, sulfonamides)
7. if nephrectomy was performed for renal calculi, reinforce physician's instructions on diet, drug therapy, and daily fluid requirements *to prevent formation of stones in the remaining kidney*
8. if surgery was necessary because of renal hypertension, reinforce the physician's instructions about methods of controlling B/P (e.g. dietary modifications, medication therapy, stress management).

4.b. The client will state signs and symptoms to report to the health care provider.

4.b.1. Refer to Standardized Postoperative Care Plan, Nursing Diagnosis 20, action c, for signs and symptoms to report to the health care provider.
2. Instruct client to report these additional signs and symptoms:
a. unexplained weight gain
b. decreased urine output
c. flank pain on the unoperative side
d. blood in the urine.

4.c. The client will verbalize an understanding of and a plan for adhering to recommended follow-up care including future appointments with health care provider, medications prescribed, activity level, wound care, and plans for subsequent treatment of underlying disorder.

4.c.1. Refer to Standardized Postoperative Care Plan, Nursing Diagnosis 20, for routine postoperative instructions and measures to improve client compliance.
2. Reinforce physician's instructions regarding activity:
a. gauge activity according to tolerance and allow adequate rest periods
b. avoid lifting heavy objects for at least 6 months *to allow complete healing of incised muscles.*
3. Clarify plans for subsequent treatment of underlying disorder (e.g. chemotherapy, radiation therapy) if appropriate.

Reference

Kübler-Ross, E. On death and dying. New York: Macmillan, 1969.

Renal Calculi with Lithotomy

Renal calculi (stones) are formed when substances normally dissolved in the urine precipitate out and aggregate or become bound to particles such as blood, devitalized tissue, or mucus that may be present in the urine. Renal calculi can be composed of substances such as calcium, oxalate, struvite (the triple salt of magnesium, ammonium, and phosphate), urate, or cystine, but the types that occur most often are calcium oxalate and calcium phosphate. Calculi usually form in the pelvis or calyx of the kidney and, if small enough, travel with urine and smooth muscle contraction through the ureters, bladder, and urethra. They may be bilateral or unilateral, solitary or multiple, smooth and round or irregularly shaped, and very small or large enough to fill the renal calyx ("staghorn" calculi). Conditions that predispose a person to renal calculi formation include urinary stasis, urinary tract infection, dehydration, increased loss of bone calcium (occurs with prolonged immobility and diseases such as multiple myeloma and hyperparathyroidism), excessive calcium and/or vitamin D intake, inflammatory bowel disease, and gout. Often, however, the exact cause of calculi formation is unknown.

Conservative management aimed at facilitating passage or dissolution of the stones involves increased hydration, chemolytic irrigations, and medication therapy. If the calculus is too large to travel through the urinary tract, ureteral and/or urethral catheters may be inserted to dilate the passageways. Endourological methods of litholapaxy or ultrasonic or electrohydraulic lithotripsy may be used to break up a large stone. A newer procedure being performed to treat renal calculi is extracorporeal shock wave lithotripsy (ESWL). This procedure is noninvasive and utilizes high-energy electrical shock waves to break the stone into tiny fragments, which are then excreted in the urine. If nonsurgical methods are contraindicated or unsuccessful, surgery is necessary to remove calculi that are causing pain, infection, obstruction of urine flow, and/or renal damage. The surgical procedure is determined by the location, number, and size of the stones. Usually a nephrolithotomy, pyelolithotomy, or ureterolithotomy is performed, but a nephrectomy may be necessary in persons with multiple kidney stones, "staghorn" calculi, or extensive kidney damage.

This care plan focuses on the adult client with renal calculi who is hospitalized for a lithotomy.* The goals of preoperative care are to reduce fear, anxiety, pain, nausea, and vomiting and maintain urine flow. Postoperatively, goals of care are to maintain comfort, prevent complications, and educate the client regarding follow-up care.

_____

*If a nephrectomy is planned, refer also to the Nephrectomy Care Plan.

DISCHARGE CRITERIA

Prior to discharge, the client will:

- identify ways to prevent the recurrence of renal calculi
- demonstrate the proper procedure for straining urine and determining the pH of urine if indicated
- state signs and symptoms to report to the health care provider
- verbalize an understanding of and a plan for adhering to recommended follow-up care including future appointments with health care provider, medications prescribed, activity level, and wound care.

UNIT
X

NURSING/COLLABORATIVE DIAGNOSES

Preoperative
1. Anxiety □ *534*
2A. Altered comfort: renal colic □ *534*
2B. Altered comfort: nausea and vomiting □ *535*
3. Potential complication: obstruction of urine flow □ *536*

Postoperative
1. Potential for infection: urinary tract □ *537*
2. Potential complications:
   a. hypovolemic shock
   b. peritonitis □ *537*
3. Knowledge deficit regarding follow-up care □ *538*

☐

Preoperative

Use in conjunction with the Standardized Preoperative Care Plan.

☐

1. NURSING DIAGNOSIS

Anxiety related to unfamiliar environment, pain, and lack of understanding of diagnostic tests and planned surgical procedure.

☐

DESIRED OUTCOMES	NURSING ACTIONS AND *SELECTED RATIONALES*

1. The client will experience a reduction in fear and anxiety (see Standardized Preoperative Care Plan, Nursing Diagnosis 1, for outcome criteria).	1.a. Refer to Standardized Preoperative Care Plan, Nursing Diagnosis 1, for measures related to assessment and reduction of fear and anxiety.
	b. Implement additional measures *to reduce fear and anxiety:*
	  1. perform actions to reduce renal colic (see Preoperative Nursing Diagnosis 2.A, action 5)
	  2. explain diagnostic tests that may be done to locate the calculi, evaluate renal function, and/or determine possible composition or cause of calculi:
	    a. x-ray of kidneys, ureters, and bladder (KUB)
	    b. intravenous pyelography
	    c. cystoscopy
	    d. ultrasonography and/or computed tomography (CT) of abdomen
	    e. blood studies (e.g. electrolytes, BUN, uric acid, creatinine)
	    f. urine studies (e.g. culture and sensitivity, pH, 24-hour collection for volume and content).

☐

2.A. NURSING DIAGNOSIS

Altered comfort:* **renal colic** related to:

1. partial or complete ureteral obstruction (the blockage of urine flow causes pressure behind the calculi and increased frequency and force of contractions of the ureter);
2. kidney and/or ureteral tissue trauma associated with passage or lodging of the calculi.

---

* In this care plan, the nursing diagnosis "pain" is included under the diagnostic label of altered comfort.

☐

DESIRED OUTCOMES	NURSING ACTIONS AND *SELECTED RATIONALES*

2.A. The client will experience diminished renal colic as evidenced by:
  1. verbalization of a reduction in pain
	2.A.1. Determine how the client usually responds to pain.
	  2. Assess for nonverbal signs of renal colic (e.g. wrinkled brow, clenched fists, rubbing lower back and flank area, frequent position changes, reluctance to ambulate, diaphoresis, facial pallor or flushing, change in B/P, tachycardia).

2. relaxed facial expression and body positioning
3. increased participation in activities
4. stable vital signs.

3. Assess verbal complaints of pain. Ask client to be specific about location, severity, and type of pain. (The pain is usually described as occurring in the flank area and being dull and aching or severe and colicky.)
4. Assess for factors that seem to aggravate and alleviate pain.
5. Implement measures *to reduce renal colic:*
   a. monitor for therapeutic and nontherapeutic effects of analgesics if administered
   b. encourage client to use patient-controlled analgesia (PCA) device as instructed
   c. perform actions *to facilitate passage of the stone:*
      1. encourage a fluid intake of at least 2500 cc/day unless contraindicated *in order to increase hydrostatic pressure behind stone*
      2. assist client to ambulate for 5–10 minutes each hour while awake if tolerated *in order to promote movement of stone*
      3. monitor for therapeutic and nontherapeutic effects of antispasmodics (e.g. atropine, methantheline bromide) if administered
   d. if ureter is obstructed, assist with insertion of a nephrostomy tube if indicated *to reduce pressure behind the obstruction*
   e. provide or assist with nonpharmacological measures for pain relief (e.g. moist heat to flank area, warm bath, back rub, position change, relaxation techniques, guided imagery, quiet conversation, restful environment, diversional activities).
6. Consult physician if:
   a. renal colic persists or worsens
   b. calculi are eliminated through the urethra or urinary catheter and/or renal colic suddenly ceases *(may indicate that surgery is no longer necessary).*

2.B. NURSING DIAGNOSIS

Altered comfort: nausea and vomiting related to stimulation of the vomiting center associated with:

1. vagal and/or sympathetic stimulation resulting from distention of the kidney pelvis, ureteral spasm, and abdominal distention (kidney irritation stimulates the renointestinal reflex, which inhibits intestinal activity);
2. cortical stimulation due to pain and stress.

DESIRED OUTCOMES	NURSING ACTIONS AND *SELECTED RATIONALES*

2.B. The client will experience relief of nausea and vomiting as evidenced by:
1. verbalization of relief of nausea
2. absence of vomiting.
	2.B.1. Assess client to determine factors that contribute to nausea and vomiting (e.g. severe pain or spasms, abdominal distention).
	2. Implement measures *to reduce nausea and vomiting:*
	  a. perform actions to reduce renal colic (see Preoperative Nursing Diagnosis 2.A, action 5)
	  b. perform actions to reduce fear and anxiety (see Preoperative Nursing Diagnosis 1)
	  c. eliminate noxious sights and smells from the environment *(noxious stimuli cause cortical stimulation of the vomiting center)*
	  d. encourage client to take deep, slow breaths when nauseated
	  e. encourage client to change positions slowly *(movement stimulates the chemoreceptor trigger zone)*
	  f. provide oral hygiene after each emesis and before meals
	  g. provide small, frequent meals rather than 3 large ones

h. instruct client to ingest food and fluids slowly
i. encourage client to eat dry foods (e.g. toast, crackers) and avoid drinking liquids with meals if nauseated
j. instruct client to rest after eating with head of bed elevated
k. monitor for therapeutic and nontherapeutic effects of antiemetics and gastrointestinal stimulants (e.g. metoclopramide) if administered
l. if bowel sounds are hypoactive or absent:
    1. maintain food and fluid restrictions as ordered
    2. insert nasogastric tube and maintain suction as ordered.
3. Consult physician if above measures fail to control nausea and vomiting.

□ ▬▬▬▬▬▬▬▬▬▬▬▬▬▬▬▬▬▬▬▬▬▬▬▬▬▬▬

3. COLLABORATIVE DIAGNOSIS

Potential complication: obstruction of urine flow related to:

a. presence of calculi;
b. ureteral inflammation associated with trauma to the mucosa;
c. ureteral spasms associated with mucosal irritation resulting from movement of or pressure from the calculi;
d. sympathetic stimulation of urinary sphincter associated with anxiety and pain.

□ ▬▬▬▬▬▬▬▬▬▬▬▬▬▬▬▬▬▬▬▬▬▬▬▬▬▬▬

DESIRED OUTCOMES	NURSING ACTIONS AND *SELECTED RATIONALES*

3. The client will not experience obstruction of urine flow as evidenced by:
  a. no complaints of increasing flank pain and pressure
  b. no complaints of urgency, bladder fullness, and suprapubic discomfort
  c. absence of suprapubic distention
  d. balanced intake and output.
	3.a. Assess for and report signs and symptoms of:
	    1. ureteral obstruction (e.g. increased complaints of flank pain or pressure, output less than intake)
	    2. urethral obstruction (e.g. complaints of bladder fullness and suprapubic discomfort, suprapubic distention, output less than intake).
	  b. Implement measures *to prevent obstruction of urine flow:*
	    1. perform actions to facilitate passage of the stone (see Preoperative Nursing Diagnosis 2.A, action 5.c)
	    2. perform actions to reduce fear and anxiety (see Preoperative Nursing Diagnosis 1) and renal colic (see Preoperative Nursing Diagnosis 2.A, action 5) *in order to prevent excessive sympathetic stimulation of the urinary sphincter.*
	  c. If signs and symptoms of obstruction of urine flow occur:
	    1. assist with insertion of a urethral or ureteral catheter and/or nephrostomy tube if indicated
	    2. implement measures *to maintain patency of urinary catheter if inserted* (e.g. keep tubing free of kinks, irrigate as ordered)
	    3. prepare client for surgical removal of calculi if indicated (surgery may need to be performed before the scheduled time)
	    4. provide emotional support to client and significant others.

□ ▬▬▬▬▬▬▬▬▬▬▬▬▬▬▬▬▬▬▬▬▬▬▬▬▬▬▬

Postoperative

Use in conjunction with the Standardized Postoperative Care Plan.

1. NURSING DIAGNOSIS

Potential for infection: urinary tract related to instrumentation of the urinary tract during surgery, fluid volume deficit, and urinary catheterization.

DESIRED OUTCOMES	NURSING ACTIONS AND *SELECTED RATIONALES*
1. The client will remain free of urinary tract infection (see Standardized Postoperative Care Plan, Nursing Diagnosis 16, outcome c, for outcome criteria).	1. Refer to Standardized Postoperative Care Plan, Nursing Diagnosis 16, action c, for measures related to assessment, prevention, and treatment of urinary tract infection.

2. COLLABORATIVE DIAGNOSIS

Potential complications:

a. **hypovolemic shock** related to:
   1. hemorrhage (hemorrhage can readily occur during or following a nephrolithotomy because the kidney is a highly vascular organ)
   2. fluid volume deficit associated with excessive fluid loss and inadequate fluid replacement;
b. **peritonitis** related to leakage of urine into the peritoneal cavity (the ureteral suture line does not become watertight for about 48 hours) and wound infection.

DESIRED OUTCOMES	NURSING ACTIONS AND *SELECTED RATIONALES*

2.a. The client will not develop hypovolemic shock (see Standardized Postoperative Care Plan, Collaborative Diagnosis 19, outcome a, for outcome criteria).	2.a.1. Assess for and report:
	  a. persistent bloody drainage on dressings or from urinary catheter(s) or wound drain (urine should be slightly blood-tinged to clear amber within 48 hours after surgery)
	  b. persistent vomiting
	  c. difficulty maintaining intravenous or oral fluid intake
	  d. significant decline in RBC, Hct., and Hgb. levels
	  e. signs and symptoms of hypovolemic shock (see Standardized Postoperative Care Plan, Collaborative Diagnosis 19, action a.3).
	  2. Refer to Standardized Postoperative Care Plan, Collaborative Diagnosis 19, actions a.4 and 5, for measures related to prevention and management of hypovolemic shock.
	  3. Implement additional measures *to prevent hypovolemic shock:*
	    a. perform actions *to prevent hemorrhage:*
	     1. anchor the nephrostomy tube securely to flank or abdomen *in order to prevent irritation of kidney tissue*
	     2. implement measures *to prevent excessive strain on suture lines:*
	      a. instruct client to support incision site with hands or pillow when turning and deep breathing (coughing is usually contraindicated)

UNIT
X

b. perform actions to prevent nausea and vomiting (see Standardized Postoperative Care Plan, Nursing Diagnosis 7.C, action 2)

c. maintain patency of urinary catheter(s) and wound drain if present

b. prepare client for immediate surgical ligation of bleeding vessels if indicated.

2.b. The client will not develop peritonitis as evidenced by:
1. gradual resolution of abdominal pain
2. soft, nondistended abdomen
3. temperature declining toward normal
4. stable vital signs
5. gradual return of normal bowel sounds
6. WBC count declining toward normal.

2.b.1. Assess for and report signs and symptoms of peritonitis (e.g. increase in severity of abdominal pain; generalized abdominal pain; rebound tenderness; tense, rigid abdomen; increase in temperature; tachycardia; tachypnea; hypotension; failure of bowel sounds to return to normal).

2. Monitor WBC counts. Report levels that increase or fail to decline toward normal.

3. Implement measures *to prevent peritonitis:*
   a. perform actions to prevent and treat wound infection (see Standardized Postoperative Care Plan, Nursing Diagnosis 16, actions b.4 and 5)
   b. perform actions *to prevent increased pressure on suture lines:*
      1. implement measures *to prevent accumulation of drainage:*
         a. maintain patency of urinary catheter(s) and wound drain (e.g. keep tubing free of kinks, empty collection device as often as necessary, keep collection device below the level of bladder, irrigate as ordered) if present
         b. perform actions *to prevent inadvertent removal of urinary catheter(s) and wound drain if present:*
            1. use caution when changing dressings surrounding catheter(s) and drain
            2. provide extension tubing if necessary *to enable client to move without placing tension on catheter(s) and drain*
            3. instruct client not to pull on catheter(s), drain, and drainage tubings
      2. if irrigation of the urinary catheter is ordered, irrigate gently using only the prescribed amount of solution.
   4. If signs and symptoms of peritonitis occur:
      a. withhold all food and fluid as ordered
      b. place client on bedrest in a semi-Fowler's position *to assist in pooling or localizing the urine in the pelvis rather than under the diaphragm*
      c. insert a nasogastric or intestinal tube and maintain suction as ordered
      d. monitor for therapeutic and nontherapeutic effects of anti-infectives if administered
      e. monitor for therapeutic and nontherapeutic effects of intravenous fluids and/or blood volume expanders if administered *to prevent or treat shock (shock can occur as a result of the escape of protein, fluid, and electrolytes into the peritoneal cavity)*
      f. prepare client for surgical repair of site of leakage if indicated
      g. provide emotional support to client and significant others.

☐ ▬▬▬▬▬▬▬▬▬▬▬▬▬▬▬▬▬▬▬▬▬▬▬▬▬▬▬▬▬▬▬▬

3. NURSING DIAGNOSIS

Knowledge deficit regarding follow-up care.

☐ ▬▬▬▬▬▬▬▬▬▬▬▬▬▬▬▬▬▬▬▬▬▬▬▬▬▬▬▬▬▬▬▬

DESIRED OUTCOMES	NURSING ACTIONS AND *SELECTED RATIONALES*

3.a. The client will identify ways to prevent the recurrence of renal calculi.

3.a.1. Instruct client regarding ways *to prevent recurrence of renal calculi:*
   a. prevent dehydration by:
      1. drinking at least 10 glasses of liquid/day

    2. increasing intake of liquid during hot weather and during and after episodes of fever, diarrhea, and strenuous physical activity

b. prevent urinary stasis by:
    1. voiding whenever the urge is felt, right before bedtime, and once in the middle of the night
    2. avoiding prolonged periods of inactivity (if unable to maintain a program of moderate activity, be sure to change positions frequently)
    3. drinking at least 10 glasses of liquid/day

c. space liquid intake evenly throughout the day and drink 2 glasses of water at bedtime and another 1 in the middle of the night *in order to maintain constant dilution of urine*

d. prevent urinary tract infection by:
    1. continuing with above measures to prevent stasis
    2. wiping from front to back after urinating and defecating (if female)
    3. keeping perineal area clean and dry
    4. taking prophylactic anti-infectives as prescribed

e. if composition of stone is known before client's discharge, provide these additional instructions if appropriate:
    1. if stone is composed of calcium oxalate:
        a. decrease intake of foods/fluids high in calcium (e.g. dairy products)
        b. avoid excessive intake of foods/fluids high in oxalate (e.g. tea, instant coffee, colas, nuts, chocolate, rhubarb, spinach)
        c. take the following medications as prescribed:
            1. anion-exchange resins (e.g. cholestyramine) *to bind oxalate and increase its excretion from the bowel*
            2. calcium-binding resins (e.g. cellulose sodium phosphate) *to decrease absorption of calcium from the intestine*
            3. thiazide diuretics (e.g. hydrochlorothiazide) *to decrease calcium content in urine*
    2. if stone is composed of calcium phosphate or struvite, maintain acidic urine by:
        a. including foods/fluids in diet that form an acid ash (e.g. cranberry or prune juice, meat, eggs, poultry, fish, grapes, whole grains)
        b. limiting intake of milk, citrus fruits, and carbonated beverages *(these tend to alkalinize the urine)*
        c. taking acidifying agents (e.g. ascorbic acid) as prescribed
        d. preventing urinary tract infection (see action a.1.d in this diagnosis) *because the infection causes the urine to become alkaline*
    3. if stone is composed of uric acid, oxalate, or cystine, maintain alkaline urine by:
        a. including foods/fluids in diet that leave an alkaline ash (e.g. milk; vegetables, especially legumes and green vegetables; fruits except prunes, plums, and cranberries)
        b. taking medications that alkalinize the urine (e.g. sodium bicarbonate, citrate preparations) as prescribed
    4. if stone is composed of calcium:
        a. decrease intake of dairy products and salt *(salt increases calcium excretion in the urine)*
        b. take calcium-binding resins (e.g. cellulose sodium phosphate) and thiazide diuretics (e.g. hydrochlorothiazide) as prescribed
        c. maintain acidic urine (see action a.1.e.2 in this diagnosis)
    5. if stone is composed of uric acid:
        a. maintain alkaline urine (see action a.1.e.3 in this diagnosis)
        b. take xanthine oxidase inhibitor (allopurinol) as prescribed *to decrease uric acid production*
        c. reduce intake of foods/fluids high in purine (e.g. liver, kidney, goose, venison, seafood, meat soups and gravies, anchovies)
    6. if stone is composed of oxalate:
        a. maintain alkaline urine (see action a.1.e.3 in this diagnosis)
        b. avoid excessive intake of foods/fluids high in oxalate (e.g. tea, instant coffee, colas, nuts, chocolate, rhubarb, spinach)
        c. take anion-exchange resins (e.g. cholestyramine) as prescribed *to bind oxalate and increase its excretion from the bowel*

UNIT
X

   7. if stone is composed of cystine:
      a. maintain alkaline urine (see action a.1.e.3 in this diagnosis)
      b. take penicillamine as prescribed *to lower urinary cystine level*
   8. if stone is composed of phosphate:
      a. maintain acidic urine (see action a.1.e.2 in this diagnosis)
      b. reduce intake of foods/fluids high in phosphorus (e.g. nuts, poultry, milk, peas, cheese, corn)
      c. take aluminum-containing gels (e.g. Amphojel, Basaljel) as prescribed *to bind phosphorus*
   f. continue with medical follow-up and treatment of conditions that may cause or contribute to calculi formation (e.g. hyperparathyroidism, gout, inflammatory bowel disease).
2. Stress importance of complying with the treatment plan *in order to prevent repeated episodes of renal calculi and irreversible kidney damage*.
3. Obtain a dietary consult to assist client in planning ways to meet recommended dietary restrictions.

3.b. The client will demonstrate the proper procedure for straining urine and determining the pH of urine if indicated.

3.b. If physician wants client to strain urine and/or monitor urine pH at home:
1. explain the rationale for straining urine *(to verify passage of stones and collect stones for analysis)* and monitoring urine pH *(provides a guide for assessing effectiveness of treatment plan)*
2. instruct client to strain urine at home by voiding into a container and then pouring urine through cheesecloth or gauze
3. instruct client regarding the correct procedure for testing urine pH using nitrazide paper or the dipstick test:
   a. use fresh urine only
   b. dip test strip into urine and remove quickly *to avoid washing off the reagent*
   c. immediately compare color on test strip to color on pH color chart
4. allow time for questions, clarification, and return demonstration.

3.c. The client will state signs and symptoms to report to the health care provider.

3.c. 1. Refer to Standardized Postoperative Care Plan, Nursing Diagnosis 20, action c, for signs and symptoms to report to health care provider.
2. Instruct client to also report:
   a. increased blood in urine (inform client that a slight pink tinge to urine may occur following increased activity but that this should clear with rest and increased intake of liquids)
   b. presence of sediment in urine or passage of more stones
   c. abdominal pain, tenderness, or distention
   d. recurrence of colicky flank pain (pain may also radiate to genital area)
   e. persistent feeling of pressure over kidney or bladder
   f. decreased urine output
   g. prolonged episodes of decreased intake
   h. inability to maintain pH of urine within prescribed range.

3.d. The client will verbalize an understanding of and a plan for adhering to recommended follow-up care including future appointments with health care provider, medications prescribed, activity level, and wound care.

3.d. 1. Refer to Standardized Postoperative Care Plan, Nursing Diagnosis 20, for routine postoperative instructions and measures to improve client compliance.
2. Reinforce the physician's instructions regarding temporary activity restrictions (these activities may be restricted for a few weeks to months depending on the extensiveness of surgery):
   a. avoid lifting objects over 10 pounds
   b. avoid strenuous exercise.

Renal Failure

Renal failure is a reduction in renal function to the extent that it interferes with biological homeostasis. It is classified as acute or chronic. Acute renal failure is a rapid loss of renal function that, with proper management, is usually reversible. Its causes are generally categorized as prerenal, intrarenal (intrinsic or parenchymal renal disease), and postrenal. Prerenal causes include conditions such as dehydration, prolonged shock, and renal vascular obstruction that result in decreased renal blood flow. Intrarenal causes are those conditions that directly damage the renal tissue (e.g. glomerulonephritis, pyelonephritis, polycystic kidney disease, interstitial nephritis). Postrenal causes of acute renal failure include conditions such as urinary calculi, prostatic enlargement, or tumors that obstruct urine outflow. The usual pattern of reversible acute renal failure includes an initial oliguric phase followed by a diuretic phase and then a convalescent phase. Prognosis depends on the cause, extent of renal damage, and effectiveness of treatment.

Chronic renal failure is a progressive reduction in functioning renal tissue. It can develop gradually over years or can result from irreversible acute renal failure. Causes of chronic renal failure are systemic diseases such as diabetes, hypertension, and lupus erythematosus or those conditions known to cause acute renal failure. The glomerular filtration rate (GFR) is the basis for the staging of chronic renal failure; the lower the GFR, the greater the loss of kidney function. The beginning stages of chronic renal failure are often characterized by a large urine output, and as the renal failure progresses, the urine output usually diminishes. The stages are identified as diminished renal reserve in which the kidneys are able to compensate for any loss of renal function, renal insufficiency (at this point nitrogenous wastes begin to accumulate in the blood and mild anemia occurs), and uremia or end-stage renal disease (ESRD). In ESRD, the GFR is reduced by over 90% and the kidneys are no longer able to maintain homeostasis. At this point, hemodialysis, peritoneal dialysis, or kidney transplantation is necessary for survival.

This care plan focuses on the adult client with chronic renal insufficiency who is experiencing progressive symptoms and is hospitalized for evaluation of kidney function and modification of his/her treatment plan.* The goals of care are to control symptoms, prevent complications, and educate the client regarding follow-up care.

---

* If hemodialysis or peritoneal dialysis is indicated, refer to nephrology or medical-surgical nursing textbooks for appropriate nursing care. If a nephrectomy is planned, refer also to the Nephrectomy Care Plan.

UNIT
X

DISCHARGE CRITERIA

Prior to discharge, the client will:

- verbalize a basic understanding of renal failure
- identify ways to reduce the risk of further kidney damage
- verbalize an understanding of fluid restrictions and dietary modifications
- demonstrate the ability to accurately weigh self and measure fluid intake and output
- identify precautions necessary to prevent bleeding
- identify ways to reduce the risk of infection
- identify ways to manage problems that often occur as a result of renal failure
- share feelings and concerns about the effects of chronic renal failure on life style, roles, and self-concept
- state signs and symptoms to report to the health care provider
- identify community resources that can assist with adjustment to changes resulting from chronic renal failure
- verbalize an understanding of and a plan for adhering to recommended follow-up care including future appointments with health care provider and medications prescribed.

Use in conjunction with the Care Plan on Immobility.

NURSING/COLLABORATIVE DIAGNOSES

1. Anxiety □ 543
2. Altered fluid and electrolyte balance:
   a. fluid volume deficit
   b. fluid volume excess
   c. hyponatremia
   d. hypernatremia
   e. hypokalemia
   f. hyperkalemia
   g. hypocalcemia
   h. hypercalcemia
   i. hyperphosphatemia
   j. hypermagnesemia
   k. metabolic acidosis □ 543
3. Altered nutrition: less than body requirements □ 548
4A. Altered comfort: nausea and vomiting □ 549
4B. Altered comfort:
   1. muscle cramps
   2. paresthesias (burning, numbness, tingling, and restless leg syndrome [crawling, prickling, itching sensations]) □ 550
4C. Altered comfort: pruritus □ 551
5. Impaired skin integrity: irritation and breakdown □ 551
6. Altered oral mucous membrane:
   a. dryness
   b. stomatitis □ 552
7. Activity intolerance □ 553
8. Impaired physical mobility □ 554
9. Self-care deficit □ 554
10. Constipation □ 555
11. Diarrhea □ 555
12. Altered thought processes: shortened attention span; inability to concentrate; impaired memory, reasoning ability, and judgment; irritability; confusion; and hallucinations □ 556
13. Sleep pattern disturbance □ 557
14. Potential for infection □ 557
15. Potential for trauma □ 558
16. Potential complications:
   a. uremia (uremic syndrome)
   b. arrhythmias
   c. hypertension
   d. pericarditis
   e. congestive heart failure (CHF) and pulmonary edema
   f. bleeding
   g. pathologic fractures □ 559
17. Sexual dysfunction:
   a. decreased libido
   b. impotence □ 563
18. Disturbance in self-concept □ 563
19. Grieving □ 564
20. Noncompliance □ 565
21. Knowledge deficit regarding follow-up care □ 566

1. NURSING DIAGNOSIS

Anxiety related to unfamiliar environment; lack of understanding of diagnostic tests, diagnosis, treatment plan, and prognosis; current symptoms; and the effect of chronic renal failure on life style and roles.

DESIRED OUTCOMES	NURSING ACTIONS AND *SELECTED RATIONALES*

1. The client will experience a reduction in fear and anxiety (see Care Plan on Immobility, Nursing Diagnosis 1, for outcome criteria).	1.a. Refer to Care Plan on Immobility, Nursing Diagnosis 1, for measures related to assessment and reduction of fear and anxiety.
	b. Implement additional measures *to reduce fear and anxiety:*
	  1. explain diagnostic tests performed to determine the extensiveness of kidney damage:
	    a. urine studies (e.g. creatinine clearance, routine urinalysis, protein, osmolality)
	    b. blood studies (e.g. BUN, creatinine, Hct., Hgb., electrolytes, osmolality)
	    c. computed tomography of kidneys
	    d. retrograde pyelography, intravenous pyelogram
	    e. renal angiography, renal venography
	    f. renogram, renal scan
	    g. renal ultrasonography
	    h. renal biopsy
	  2. inform client that treatment measures should relieve or control some of the symptoms currently being experienced.

2. NURSING/COLLABORATIVE DIAGNOSIS

Altered fluid and electrolyte balance:

a. **fluid volume deficit** related to:
  1. decreased fluid intake associated with nausea and anorexia
  2. increased fluid loss associated with:
      a. inability of the hypertrophied nephrons (the functioning nephrons hypertrophy in an effort to maintain homeostasis) to concentrate urine in nonoliguric chronic renal failure
      b. decreased ability of renal tubules to reabsorb electrolytes (urine then contains large amounts of sodium, which causes increased loss of fluid) in nonoliguric chronic renal failure
      c. vomiting and diarrhea associated with retention of nitrogenous wastes (results in irritation of gastrointestinal mucosa)
      d. diuretic therapy;
b. **fluid volume excess** related to:
  1. retention of sodium and water in oliguric chronic renal failure due to a decrease in number of functioning nephrons and decreased glomerular filtration rate
  2. increased aldosterone output associated with diminished renal blood flow (a reduction in renal blood flow causes an increased output of renin; this is converted to angiotension, which then stimulates aldosterone output);
c. **hyponatremia** related to:
  1. loss of sodium associated with vomiting, diarrhea, impaired reabsorption resulting from damage to the tubules (in nonoliguric phase), and/or diuretic therapy

2. excessive fluid intake in relation to output (causes a relative hyponatremia)
3. reduced intake of dietary sodium;

d. **hypernatremia** related to increased aldosterone output, decreased ability of the kidneys to excrete sodium, and/or excessive intake of dietary sodium;

e. **hypokalemia** related to:
1. loss of potassium associated with vomiting, diarrhea, and/or diuretic therapy
2. decreased intake of potassium;

f. **hyperkalemia** related to:
1. decreased ability of the kidneys to excrete potassium
2. increased cellular release of potassium associated with progressive renal tissue damage, metabolic acidosis, and hemolysis (hemolysis is caused by high serum levels of nitrogenous wastes)
3. excessive intake of dietary potassium or potassium supplements;

g. **hypocalcemia** related to:
1. decreased absorption of calcium associated with inability of the kidneys to activate vitamin D (vitamin D is needed to stimulate calcium absorption from the intestine)
2. increased retention of phosphorus (an inverse relationship exists between calcium and phosphorus)
3. rapid correction of acidosis (as the serum pH increases, there is decreased ionization of calcium);

h. **hypercalcemia** related to:
1. increased release of calcium from the bone associated with hyperparathyroidism (the parathyroids secrete increased amounts of parathyroid hormone in an attempt to maintain adequate calcium levels) and decreased activity
2. increased intestinal absorption of calcium associated with vitamin D therapy
3. excessive intake of dietary calcium or calcium-containing antacids;

i. **hyperphosphatemia** related to decreased ability of the kidneys to excrete phosphorus;

j. **hypermagnesemia** related to:
1. decreased ability of the kidneys to excrete magnesium
2. excessive intake of magnesium-containing antacids and laxatives;

k. **metabolic acidosis** related to:
1. decreased ability of the kidneys to excrete hydrogen ions, phosphates, sulfates, and the end products of protein metabolism
2. excessive loss of bicarbonate associated with diarrhea and a decreased ability of the kidneys to reabsorb bicarbonate
3. hyperkalemia (high serum potassium levels cause hydrogen ions to shift into the vascular space)
4. hyponatremia.

DESIRED OUTCOMES	NURSING ACTIONS AND *SELECTED RATIONALES*
2.a. The client will not experience a fluid volume deficit as evidenced by: 1. normal skin turgor 2. moist mucous membranes 3. weight loss no greater than 0.5 kg/day 4. B/P and pulse within normal range for client and stable with position change.	2.a.1. Assess for and report signs and symptoms of fluid volume deficit: a. decreased skin turgor b. dry mucous membranes, thirst c. weight loss greater than 0.5 kg/day d. low B/P and/or decline in systolic B/P of at least 15 mm Hg with concurrent rise in pulse when client sits up e. weak, rapid pulse. 2. Implement measures *to prevent or treat fluid volume deficit:* a. encourage maximum fluid intake allowed (usually 500 cc plus the amount of urine output) b. maintain intravenous fluid therapy as ordered if client is unable to tolerate oral fluids c. perform actions to prevent vomiting (see Nursing Diagnosis 4.A, action 2) d. perform actions to control diarrhea (see Nursing Diagnosis 11, action d).

3. Consult physician if signs and symptoms of fluid volume deficit persist or worsen.

2.b. The client will not experience fluid volume excess as evidenced by:
1. stable weight
2. stable B/P and pulse
3. absence of gallop rhythms
4. usual mental status
5. normal breath sounds
6. absence of dyspnea, peripheral edema, distended neck veins
7. CVP within normal range.

2.b.1. Assess for and report signs and symptoms of fluid volume excess:
   a. significant weight gain (greater than 0.5 kg/day)
   b. elevated B/P and pulse (B/P may not be elevated if fluid has shifted out of vascular space)
   c. development of an S_3 and/or S_4 gallop rhythm
   d. change in mental status
   e. crackles and diminished or absent breath sounds
   f. dyspnea, orthopnea
   g. peripheral edema
   h. distended neck veins
   i. elevated CVP (use internal jugular vein pulsation method to estimate CVP if monitoring device not present).
2. Monitor chest x-ray results. Report findings of vascular congestion, pleural effusion, and pulmonary edema.
3. Implement measures *to prevent or treat fluid volume excess:*
   a. maintain fluid restrictions as ordered (intake allowed is usually 500 cc plus the amount of urine output)
   b. restrict sodium intake as ordered
   c. monitor for therapeutic and nontherapeutic effects of the following medications if administered:
      1. diuretics
      2. arterial vasodilators *to improve renal blood flow and subsequently increase urine output.*
4. Consult physician if signs and symptoms of fluid volume excess persist or worsen and prepare client for dialysis if planned.

2.c. The client will maintain a safe serum sodium level as evidenced by:
1. usual mental status
2. usual strength and muscle tone
3. moist mucous membranes
4. absence of fever, nausea, vomiting, abdominal cramps, twitching, seizure activity
5. serum sodium within usual range for client.

2.c.1. Assess for and report signs and symptoms of:
   a. hyponatremia (e.g. lethargy, confusion, weakness, nausea, vomiting, abdominal cramps, twitching, seizures)
   b. hypernatremia (e.g. restlessness; lethargy; weakness; thirst; dry, sticky mucous membranes; elevated temperature; seizures).
2. Monitor serum sodium results. Report values that are not within a safe range for client (clients with renal failure have sodium levels that normally range from 125–150 mEq/liter).
3. Implement measures *to prevent or treat hyponatremia:*
   a. perform actions to reduce nausea and vomiting (see Nursing Diagnosis 4.A, action 2)
   b. perform actions to control diarrhea (see Nursing Diagnosis 11, action d)
   c. maintain fluid restrictions as ordered *to prevent dilutional hyponatremia*
   d. increase dietary allotment of sodium if ordered
   e. monitor for therapeutic and nontherapeutic effects of hypertonic or isotonic saline infusions if administered (if ordered, these must be administered very slowly and cautiously *to prevent fluid volume excess).*
4. Implement measures *to prevent or treat hypernatremia:*
   a. maintain maximum fluid intake allowed
   b. maintain dietary sodium restrictions if ordered
   c. monitor for therapeutic and nontherapeutic effects of hypotonic solutions and diuretics if administered.
5. Consult physician if unsafe serum sodium levels persist.

2.d. The client will maintain a safe serum potassium level as evidenced by:
1. regular pulse at 60–100 beats/minute
2. usual muscle tone and strength
3. normal bowel sounds
4. serum potassium within usual range for client.

2.d.1. Assess for and report signs and symptoms of:
   a. hypokalemia (e.g. irregular pulse; muscle weakness and cramping; paresthesias; nausea and vomiting; hypoactive or absent bowel sounds; drowsiness; EKG reading showing ST depression, T wave inversion or flattening, and presence of U waves)
   b. hyperkalemia (e.g. slow or irregular pulse; paresthesias; muscle weakness and flaccidity; hyperactive bowel sounds with diarrhea and intestinal colic; EKG reading showing peaked T wave, prolonged PR interval, and/or widened QRS).
2. Monitor serum potassium results. Report values that are not within a safe range for client.

UNIT
X

3. Implement measures *to prevent or treat hypokalemia:*
   a. perform actions to reduce nausea and vomiting (see Nursing Diagnosis 4.A, action 2)
   b. perform actions to control diarrhea (see Nursing Diagnosis 11, action d)
   c. maintain intravenous and oral potassium replacements as ordered (monitor serum potassium and urine output closely when giving supplemental potassium and consult physician if potassium level increases above normal and/or urine output is less than usual)
   d. encourage intake of foods/fluids high in potassium (e.g. bananas, potatoes, raisins, figs, apricots, dates, Gatorade, fruit juices).
4. Implement measures *to prevent or treat hyperkalemia:*
   a. maintain dietary restrictions of potassium as ordered
   b. perform actions *to reduce the cellular release of potassium:*
      1. implement measures *to spare body proteins and prevent excessive tissue breakdown:*
         a. encourage client to consume the amount of dietary protein allotted
         b. provide allotted amount of carbohydrates *(spares the protein by providing a quick energy source)*
         c. restrict activity as ordered *to reduce energy requirements*
      2. implement measures to reduce accumulation of serum nitrogenous wastes (see Collaborative Diagnosis 16, action a.4) *in order to reduce the rate of hemolysis (high serum levels of nitrogenous wastes decrease the life span of RBCs)*
      3. implement measures to prevent or treat metabolic acidosis (see action h.2 in this diagnosis)
   c. consult physician before administering prescribed potassium supplements if signs and symptoms of hyperkalemia are present
   d. request fresh blood if transfusions are necessary *(the potassium content of stored blood is higher than that of fresh blood)*
   e. monitor for therapeutic and nontherapeutic effects of the following medications if administered:
      1. loop diuretics (e.g. ethacrynic acid, furosemide) *to increase renal excretion of potassium*
      2. cation-exchange resins (e.g. Kayexalate) *to increase potassium excretion via the intestines (act by exchanging sodium for potassium)*
      3. intravenous insulin and hypertonic glucose solutions *to enhance transport of potassium back into cells*
   f. prepare client for dialysis if planned *to reduce serum potassium levels.*
5. Consult physician if unsafe serum potassium levels persist.

2.e. The client will maintain a safe serum calcium level as evidenced by:
1. usual mental status
2. regular pulse at 60–100 beats/minute
3. negative Chvostek's and Trousseau's signs
4. absence of paresthesias, nausea, vomiting, anorexia, muscle cramps, tetany, seizure activity
5. serum calcium within usual range for client.

2.e.1. Assess for and report signs and symptoms of:
   a. hypocalcemia (e.g. change in mental status; cardiac arrhythmias; positive Chvostek's and Trousseau's signs; numbness and tingling of fingers, toes, and circumoral area; muscle cramps; tetany; seizures)
   b. hypercalcemia (e.g. change in mental status, cardiac arrhythmias, muscle weakness and flaccidity, nausea, vomiting, anorexia, constipation).
2. Monitor serum calcium results. Report values that are not within a safe range for client.
3. Implement measures *to prevent or treat hypocalcemia:*
   a. provide sources of calcium (e.g. dairy products) in diet
   b. administer activated vitamin D and calcium supplements as ordered
   c. request fresh blood if transfusions are necessary *(citrate in stored blood binds the calcium)*
   d. perform actions to prevent or treat hyperphosphatemia (see action f.2 in this diagnosis)
   e. avoid rapid or aggressive treatment of acidosis *in order to prevent a reduction in calcium ionization.*
4. If signs and symptoms of hypocalcemia occur:
   a. institute seizure precautions
   b. have intravenous calcium preparation readily available.

5. Implement measures *to prevent or treat hypercalcemia:*
   a. maintain dietary restrictions of calcium as ordered
   b. avoid giving calcium-containing antacids (e.g. Os-Cal, Tums, Titralac)
   c. mobilize client as much as possible *(weight-bearing reduces calcium loss from bones)*
   d. monitor for therapeutic and nontherapeutic effects of the following medications if administered:
      1. calcitonin *to inhibit bone resorption and increase renal clearance of calcium*
      2. loop diuretics (e.g. ethacrynic acid, furosemide) *to increase renal excretion of calcium*
      3. corticosteroids *to promote urinary calcium excretion and decrease absorption of calcium from the intestine*
      4. mithramycin *to inhibit loss of calcium from bones*
      5. etidronate *to decrease bone resorption*
   e. prepare client for dialysis if planned *to reduce serum calcium levels*
   f. prepare client for a parathyroidectomy if planned.
6. Consult physician if unsafe serum calcium levels persist.

2.f. The client will maintain a safe serum phosphorus level as evidenced by:
1. absence of paresthesias, muscle cramps, tetany, seizure activity
2. serum phosphorus within usual range for client.

2.f.1. Assess for and report signs and symptoms of hyperphosphatemia (e.g. paresthesias, muscle cramps, tetany, seizures, higher than usual serum phosphorus level).
2. Implement measures *to prevent or treat hyperphosphatemia:*
   a. restrict dietary intake of phosphorus as ordered by limiting foods/fluids such as fish, red meat, poultry, milk, eggs, and dried beans and peas
   b. monitor for therapeutic and nontherapeutic effects of phosphate-binding preparations such as aluminum hydroxide (e.g. Amphojel, ALternaGEL) and aluminum carbonate gel (e.g. Basaljel) if administered.
3. If serum phosphorus remains at an unsafe level, consult physician and prepare client for dialysis if planned.

2.g. The client will maintain a safe serum magnesium level as evidenced by:
1. usual mental status
2. usual sensory and motor function
3. vital signs within normal range for client
4. serum magnesium within usual range for client.

2.g.1. Assess for and report signs and symptoms of hypermagnesemia (e.g. decreasing level of consciousness; muscle weakness; flushed, warm skin; nausea and vomiting; hypotension; depressed respirations; bradycardia; higher than usual serum magnesium level).
2. Implement measures *to prevent or treat hypermagnesemia:*
   a. avoid giving laxatives and antacids that contain magnesium (e.g. Milk of Magnesia, Gelusil, Mylanta, Maalox)
   b. maintain dietary restrictions of magnesium as ordered by limiting intake of foods/fluids such as nuts, whole-grain breads and cereals, meat, legumes, and instant coffee.
3. If serum magnesium remains at an unsafe level, consult physician and prepare client for dialysis if planned.

2.h. The client will maintain acid-base balance as evidenced by:
1. usual mental status
2. unlabored respirations at 16–20/minute
3. absence of headache, nausea, vomiting
4. blood gases within safe range for client
5. anion gap less than 16 mEq/liter.

2.h.1. Assess for and report signs and symptoms of metabolic acidosis (e.g. drowsiness; disorientation; stupor; rapid, deep respirations; headache; nausea; vomiting; lower than usual pH and CO_2 content and negative base excess; anion gap greater than 16 mEq/liter).
2. Implement measures *to prevent or treat metabolic acidosis:*
   a. perform actions to prevent and treat hyperkalemia and hyponatremia (see actions d.4 and c.3 in this diagnosis)
   b. perform actions to control diarrhea (see Nursing Diagnosis 11, action d)
   c. perform actions to maintain an adequate nutritional status (see Nursing Diagnosis 3, action e) *in order to decrease the release of acid end products associated with catabolism of body proteins*
   d. monitor for therapeutic and nontherapeutic effects of sodium bicarbonate if administered (reserved for use in severe acidosis when plasma bicarbonate is below 16 mEq/liter or client is symptomatic)
   e. prepare client for dialysis if planned *(dialysis will remove excess phosphates and sulfates).*
3. Consult physician if signs and symptoms of acidosis persist or worsen.

□ ▋▋▋▋▋▋▋▋▋▋▋▋▋▋▋▋▋▋▋▋▋▋▋

3. NURSING DIAGNOSIS

Altered nutrition: less than body requirements related to:

a. decreased oral intake associated with:
   1. anorexia resulting from depression, constipation, taste alterations (may experience a metallic, bitter, or ammonia taste due to accumulation of serum nitrogenous wastes), and early satiety (can occur as a result of slowed gastrointestinal motility due to hypercalcemia and decreased activity)
   2. dislike of prescribed diet
   3. prescribed dietary modifications (especially protein restrictions that are necessary in order to control the serum levels of nitrogenous wastes)
   4. fatigue
   5. nausea
   6. oral pain and dysphagia resulting from stomatitis;
b. loss of nutrients associated with vomiting and diarrhea.

□ ▋▋▋▋▋▋▋▋▋▋▋▋▋▋▋▋▋▋▋▋▋▋▋

DESIRED OUTCOMES	NURSING ACTIONS AND *SELECTED RATIONALES*
3. The client will maintain an adequate nutritional status as evidenced by: a. dry weight within normal range for client's age, height, and build b. serum albumin, protein, Hct., Hgb., cholesterol, and lymphocyte levels within client's usual range c. triceps skinfold measurements within normal range d. usual or improved strength and activity tolerance e. healthy oral mucous membrane.	3.a. Assess the client for signs and symptoms of malnutrition: 1. dry weight below normal for client's age, height, and build (dry weight is achieved after fluid volume excess has been resolved) 2. low serum albumin, protein, Hct., Hgb., cholesterol, and lymphocyte levels (many of these values may be abnormal as a result of decreased renal function) 3. triceps skinfold measurement less than normal for build 4. weakness and fatigue (may also be a reflection of decreased renal function) 5. stomatitis (may also be a reflection of decreased renal function). b. Reassess nutritional status on a regular basis and report decline. c. Monitor percentage of meals eaten. d. Assess client to determine causes of inadequate intake (e.g. anorexia, nausea, fatigue, mouth discomfort, prescribed dietary modifications). e. Implement measures *to improve nutritional status:* 1. perform actions *to improve oral intake:* a. implement measures to reduce nausea and vomiting (see Nursing Diagnosis 4.A, action 2) b. implement measures to reduce discomfort resulting from stomatitis (see Nursing Diagnosis 6, actions c and e) c. implement measures to prevent constipation (see Nursing Diagnosis 10) d. implement measures to decrease serum calcium levels if elevated (see Nursing Diagnosis 2, action e.5) e. implement measures to reduce the accumulation of serum nitrogenous wastes (see Collaborative Diagnosis 16, action a.4) *in order to reduce taste alterations* f. provide oral care before meals g. serve small portions of nutritious foods/fluids that are appealing to client h. provide a clean, relaxed, pleasant atmosphere i. obtain a dietary consult if necessary to assist client in selecting foods/fluids that meet nutritional needs as well as preferences j. encourage significant others to bring in client's favorite foods that meet dietary modifications k. encourage a rest period before meals *to minimize fatigue* l. provide extra sweeteners for foods if client desires *(may improve taste of foods)*

m. encourage client to experiment with spices and other seasonings (e.g. lemon, garlic, onion) *to mask taste distortion and make diet more palatable*

n. allow adequate time for meals; reheat food if necessary

o. increase activity as tolerated *(activity stimulates appetite)*

2. encourage client to eat the maximum amount of protein allowed; instruct him/her to satisfy protein requirements with foods/fluids that also contain essential amino acids (e.g. eggs, milk, meat, poultry, fish) rather than foods such as rice, dried beans, and macaroni

3. perform actions to prevent diarrhea (see Nursing Diagnosis 11, action d)

4. monitor for therapeutic and nontherapeutic effects of vitamins, minerals, and hematinics if administered.

f. Perform a 72-hour calorie count if nutritional status declines.

g. Consult physician regarding alternative methods of providing nutrition (e.g. parenteral nutrition, tube feedings) if client does not consume enough food or fluids to meet nutritional needs.

4.A. NURSING DIAGNOSIS

Altered comfort: nausea and vomiting related to stimulation of the vomiting center associated with:

1. chemoreceptor trigger zone stimulation resulting from high serum levels of nitrogenous wastes and acid-base and electrolyte imbalances;
2. vagal and/or sympathetic stimulation resulting from irritation of the gastric mucosa by increased serum levels of nitrogenous wastes;
3. cortical stimulation due to stress.

DESIRED OUTCOMES	NURSING ACTIONS AND *SELECTED RATIONALES*
4.A. The client will experience relief of nausea and vomiting as evidenced by: 1. verbalization of relief of nausea 2. absence of vomiting.	4.A.1. Assess client to determine factors that contribute to nausea and vomiting (e.g. electrolyte imbalances, increasing serum levels of nitrogenous wastes, fear, anxiety). 2. Implement measures *to reduce nausea and vomiting:* a. perform actions to prevent or treat hyponatremia, hypokalemia, hypercalcemia, hypermagnesemia, and metabolic acidosis (see Nursing Diagnosis 2, actions c.3, d.3, e.5, g.2 and 3, and h.2) b. perform actions to reduce fear and anxiety (see Nursing Diagnosis 1) c. perform actions to reduce accumulation of serum nitrogenous wastes (see Collaborative Diagnosis 16, action a.4) d. eliminate noxious sights and smells from the environment *(noxious stimuli cause cortical stimulation of the vomiting center)* e. encourage client to change positions slowly *(movement stimulates the chemoreceptor trigger zone)* f. encourage client to take deep, slow breaths when nauseated g. provide oral hygiene after each emesis and before meals h. provide small, frequent meals rather than 3 large ones i. instruct client to ingest foods and fluids slowly j. provide non-cola carbonated beverages for client to sip if nauseated (cola beverages are usually contraindicated *because they have high potassium and sodium content*) k. instruct client to avoid foods/fluids that irritate the gastric mucosa (e.g. spicy foods; citrus fruits or juices; caffeine-containing items such as chocolate, coffee, tea, or colas) l. encourage client to eat dry foods (e.g. toast, crackers) and avoid drinking liquids with meals if nauseated

UNIT X

      m. instruct client to rest after eating with head of bed elevated

      n. assist client to schedule food/fluid allotments over a 24-hour period *in order to reduce morning nausea and vomiting* (the serum level of nitrogenous wastes increases in the morning *because protein catabolism is more apt to occur after client has fasted through the night)*

      o. monitor for therapeutic and nontherapeutic effects of antiemetics if administered.

   3. Consult physician if above measures fail to control nausea and vomiting.

☐ ▬▬▬▬▬▬▬▬▬▬▬▬▬▬▬▬▬▬▬▬▬▬▬▬▬▬▬▬▬

4.B. NURSING DIAGNOSIS

Altered comfort:*

1. **muscle cramps** related to electrolyte imbalances and irritation of the nerves by high serum levels of nitrogenous wastes;
2. **paresthesias (burning, numbness, tingling, and restless leg syndrome [crawling, prickling, itching sensations])** related to peripheral neuropathies associated with electrolyte imbalances and high serum levels of nitrogenous wastes.

---

   * In this care plan, the nursing diagnosis "pain" is included under the diagnostic label of altered comfort.

☐ ▬▬▬▬▬▬▬▬▬▬▬▬▬▬▬▬▬▬▬▬▬▬▬▬▬▬▬▬▬

DESIRED OUTCOMES	NURSING ACTIONS AND *SELECTED RATIONALES*

4.B. The client will experience a reduction in muscle cramping and paresthesias as evidenced by:
1. verbalization of same
2. relaxed facial expression and body positioning
3. increased participation in activities.

4.B.1. Determine how the client usually responds to discomfort.

   2. Assess for nonverbal signs of discomfort (e.g. wrinkled brow, clenched fists, reluctance to move, rubbing affected areas, restlessness).

   3. Assess verbal complaints of muscle cramps and numbness, tingling, burning, crawling, prickling, and itching sensations (neuropathies most often occur in the extremities). Ask client to be specific about location, severity, and type of discomfort.

   4. Assess for factors that seem to aggravate and alleviate discomfort.

   5. Implement measures *to reduce discomfort:*

     a. perform actions *to control muscle cramps:*

       1. implement measures to prevent or treat hyponatremia, hypokalemia, hypocalcemia, and hyperphosphatemia (see Nursing Diagnosis 2, actions c.3, d.3, e.3, and f.2 and 3)

       2. place footboard on bed and instruct client to push feet against the board when cramps in foot and calf occur

       3. consult physician regarding application of warm packs to affected areas

       4. monitor for therapeutic and nontherapeutic effects of muscle relaxants and quinine sulfate if administered

     b. perform actions *to reduce discomfort associated with paresthesias:*

       1. implement measures to prevent or treat hyperkalemia, hypocalcemia, and hyperphosphatemia (see Nursing Diagnosis 2, actions d.4, e.3, and f.2 and 3)

       2. provide bed cradle or footboard to keep linens off involved extremities

       3. if client experiences restless leg syndrome, instruct him/her to move legs while in bed or chair or to ambulate *(movement of the legs relieves symptoms)*

     c. perform actions to reduce the accumulation of serum nitrogenous wastes (see Collaborative Diagnosis 16, action a.4)

     d. provide or assist with nonpharmacological measures to reduce discomfort (e.g. position change, relaxation techniques, guided imagery, diversional activities)

   e. monitor for therapeutic and nontherapeutic effects of analgesics if administered.
  6. Consult physician if above measures fail to provide adequate relief of discomfort.

4.C. NURSING DIAGNOSIS

Altered comfort: pruritus related to:

1. dry skin associated with atrophy of sweat glands;
2. subcutaneous precipitation of calcium phosphate crystals;
3. presence of urate crystals on the skin (uremic frost) associated with high serum levels of nitrogenous wastes (can occur in advanced renal failure).

DESIRED OUTCOMES	NURSING ACTIONS AND *SELECTED RATIONALES*
4.C. The client will experience relief of pruritus as evidenced by: 1. verbalization of same 2. no scratching or rubbing of skin.	4.C.1. Assess pruritus including onset, characteristics, location, factors that aggravate or alleviate it, and client tolerance. 2. Instruct client in and/or implement measures *to relieve pruritus:* a. perform actions to prevent or treat hypercalcemia and hyperphosphatemia (see Nursing Diagnosis 2, actions e.5 and f.2 and 3) b. perform actions to reduce accumulation of serum nitrogenous wastes (see Collaborative Diagnosis 16, action a.4) c. remove "uremic frost" (white powdery substance composed mainly of urates) with soap and water d. apply cool, moist compresses to pruritic areas e. apply emollients to skin *to help alleviate dryness* f. add emollients, cornstarch, baking soda, or oatmeal to bath water g. use tepid water and mild soaps for bathing h. pat skin dry making sure to dry thoroughly i. maintain a cool environment j. encourage participation in diversional activity k. utilize relaxation techniques l. utilize cutaneous stimulation techniques (e.g. pressure, massage, vibration, stroking with a soft brush) at the sites of itching or acupressure points m. encourage client to wear loose cotton garments. 3. Monitor for therapeutic and nontherapeutic effects of antihistamines and antipruritic lotions if administered. 4. Consult physician if above measures fail to alleviate pruritus or if skin becomes excoriated.

UNIT
X

5. NURSING DIAGNOSIS

Impaired skin integrity: irritation and breakdown related to:

a. prolonged pressure on tissues associated with decreased mobility;
b. frequent contact with irritants associated with diarrhea;
c. increased fragility of the skin associated with edema, malnutrition, tissue hypoxia (resulting from anemia), and dryness;
d. scratching associated with pruritus.

DESIRED OUTCOMES	NURSING ACTIONS AND *SELECTED RATIONALES*

5. The client will maintain skin integrity as evidenced by:
   a. absence of redness and irritation
   b. no skin breakdown.

5.a. Inspect the skin (especially bone prominences, dependent and pruritic areas, and perineum) for pallor, redness, and breakdown.
  b. Refer to Care Plan on Immobility, Nursing Diagnosis 7, action b, for measures to prevent skin breakdown associated with decreased mobility.
  c. Implement measures *to decrease skin irritation and prevent breakdown resulting from diarrhea:*
     1. perform actions to control diarrhea (see Nursing Diagnosis 11, action d)
     2. instruct and assist client to thoroughly cleanse and dry perineal area after each bowel movement; apply a protective ointment or cream (e.g. Sween cream, Desitin, Karaya gel, A & D ointment, Vaseline)
     3. use soft tissue to cleanse perianal area
     4. avoid direct contact of skin with Chux (e.g. place turn sheet or bed pad over Chux).
  d. Implement measures *to prevent skin breakdown associated with edema:*
     1. perform actions to prevent and treat fluid volume excess (see Nursing Diagnosis 2, action b.3)
     2. perform actions *to reduce fluid accumulation in dependent areas:*
        a. instruct client in and assist with range of motion exercises
        b. instruct and assist client to turn at least every 2 hours
        c. elevate affected extremities whenever possible
        d. apply elastic wraps or antiembolic hose to lower extremities as ordered
        e. apply a scrotal support if scrotal edema is present
     3. handle edematous areas carefully.
  e. Implement measures *to prevent drying of the skin:*
     1. avoid use of harsh soaps and hot water
     2. apply skin moisturizers or emollient creams to skin at least once a day.
  f. Implement measures *to prevent skin breakdown associated with scratching:*
     1. perform actions to relieve pruritus (see Nursing Diagnosis 4.C, actions 2 and 3)
     2. keep nails trimmed and/or apply mittens if necessary
     3. instruct client to apply firm pressure to pruritic areas rather than scratching.
  g. Maintain an optimal nutritional status (see Nursing Diagnosis 3, action e).
  h. If skin breakdown occurs:
     1. notify physician
     2. continue with above measures to prevent further irritation and breakdown
     3. perform decubitus care as ordered or per standard hospital policy
     4. monitor client closely and report signs and symptoms of infection (e.g. elevated temperature; redness, warmth, and edema around area of breakdown; unusual drainage from site).

6. NURSING DIAGNOSIS

Altered oral mucous membrane:

a. **dryness** related to restricted fluid intake;
b. **stomatitis** related to increased serum levels of nitrogenous wastes (the excessive salivary urea is converted to ammonia by the enzyme urease that is present in bacteria on teeth; the ammonia irritates the mucosa).

DESIRED OUTCOMES	NURSING ACTIONS AND *SELECTED RATIONALES*

6. The client will maintain a healthy oral cavity as evidenced by:

6.a. Assess client for dryness of the oral mucosa and signs and symptoms of stomatitis (e.g. inflamed and/or ulcerated oral mucosa, leukoplakia, complaints of oral dryness and/or burning, dysphagia, viscous saliva).

a. absence of inflammation and ulcerations
b. pink, moist, intact mucosa
c. absence of oral dryness and burning
d. ability to swallow without discomfort
e. usual consistency of saliva.

b. Obtain cultures from suspicious oral lesions as ordered. Report positive results.
c. Implement measures *to relieve discomfort associated with dryness and/or prevent or reduce the severity of stomatitis:*
   1. perform actions to reduce accumulation of serum nitrogenous wastes (see Collaborative Diagnosis 16, action a.4) *in order to reduce amount of salivary urea*
   2. maintain the maximum fluid intake allowed
   3. reinforce importance of and assist client with oral hygiene after meals and snacks and as often as needed
   4. instruct client to rinse mouth frequently with a solution of 25% acetic acid and cool water *in order to neutralize ammonia*
   5. instruct client to avoid products such as lemon-glycerin swabs and commercial mouthwashes containing alcohol *(these products have a drying or irritating effect on oral mucous membrane)*
   6. instruct or assist client to use a soft bristle brush or low-pressure power spray for oral care
   7. encourage client to breathe through nose *in order to reduce mouth dryness*
   8. encourage client to use artificial saliva (e.g. Moi-stir, Salivart) *to lubricate the mucous membrane*
   9. encourage client not to smoke *(smoking irritates and dries the mucosa)*
   10. encourage client to lubricate lips with Vaseline, K-Y jelly, ChapStick, Blistex, or mineral oil when oral care is given
   11. instruct client to avoid substances that might further irritate oral mucosa (e.g. extremely hot, spicy, or acidic foods/fluids)
   12. consult physician about an order for a prophylactic antifungal or antibacterial agent.
d. If stomatitis is not controlled:
   1. increase frequency of oral hygiene
   2. if client has dentures, remove and replace only for meals.
e. Monitor for therapeutic and nontherapeutic effects of topical anesthetics, oral protective pastes, and topical and systemic analgesics if administered.
f. Consult physician if signs and symptoms of dryness and/or stomatitis persist or worsen.

□ ▮▮▮▮▮▮▮▮▮▮▮▮▮▮▮▮▮▮▮▮▮▮▮▮

7. NURSING DIAGNOSIS

Activity intolerance related to:

a. inadequate tissue oxygenation associated with anemia resulting from decreased production of erythropoietin, decreased production and shortened life span of RBCs (the accumulated nitrogenous wastes have a toxic effect on the bone marrow and destroy the RBCs), malnutrition, and blood loss (bleeding can occur as a result of reduced platelet number and platelet dysfunction);
b. inadequate nutritional status;
c. difficulty resting and sleeping associated with discomfort, fear, anxiety, hallucinations, nightmares, and frequent assessments and treatments.

□ ▮▮▮▮▮▮▮▮▮▮▮▮▮▮▮▮▮▮▮▮▮▮▮▮

DESIRED OUTCOMES	NURSING ACTIONS AND *SELECTED RATIONALES*

7. The client will demonstrate an increased tolerance for activity (see Care Plan on Immobility, Nursing Diagnosis 8, for outcome criteria).	7.a. Refer to Care Plan on Immobility, Nursing Diagnosis 8, for measures related to assessment and improvement of activity tolerance.
	b. Implement additional measures *to promote rest and improve activity tolerance:*
	  1. perform actions to reduce fear and anxiety (see Nursing Diagnosis 1)
	  2. perform actions to promote sleep (see Nursing Diagnosis 13)

   3. perform actions to reduce discomfort (see Nursing Diagnoses 4.A, action 2; 4.B, action 5; and 4.C, actions 2 and 3)
   4. perform actions to improve nutritional status (see Nursing Diagnosis 3, action e)
   5. perform actions *to improve tissue oxygenation:*
      a. implement measures to reduce the accumulation of serum nitrogenous wastes (see Collaborative Diagnosis 16, action a.4) *in order to promote RBC production and reduce the rate of hemolysis*
      b. implement measures to prevent bleeding (see Collaborative Diagnosis 16, action f.4)
      c. maintain oxygen therapy as ordered
      d. discourage smoking *(smoking decreases oxygen availability)*
      e. monitor for therapeutic and nontherapeutic effects of the following if administered:
         1. androgens *to stimulate RBC production*
         2. whole blood or packed red cells (transfusions are avoided whenever possible *because they further suppress erythropoiesis and increase risk of infection).*

8. NURSING DIAGNOSIS

Impaired physical mobility related to weakness and fatigue, nausea, muscle cramps, and prescribed activity restrictions.

DESIRED OUTCOMES	NURSING ACTIONS AND *SELECTED RATIONALES*
8.a. The client will maintain an optimal level of physical mobility within prescribed activity restrictions and physical limitations.	8.a.1. Assess for factors that impair physical mobility (e.g. weakness, fatigue, nausea, muscle cramps, restrictions imposed by treatment plan). 2. Implement measures *to increase mobility:* a. perform actions to relieve nausea (see Nursing Diagnosis 4.A, action 2) b. perform actions to maintain sodium and potassium balance and prevent or treat hypercalcemia and hypermagnesemia (see Nursing Diagnosis 2, actions c.3 and 4, d.3 and 4, e.5, and g.2 and 3) *in order to improve muscle strength* c. perform actions to control muscle cramps (see Nursing Diagnosis 4.B, actions 5.a and c) d. perform actions to improve strength and activity tolerance (see Nursing Diagnosis 7) e. instruct client in and assist with correct use of mobility aids (e.g. cane, walker) if appropriate. 3. Increase activity and participation in self-care activities as allowed and tolerated. 4. Provide praise and encouragement for all efforts to increase physical mobility. 5. Encourage the support of significant others. Allow them to assist with activity if desired.
8.b. The client will not experience problems associated with immobility.	8.b. Refer to Care Plan on Immobility for actions to prevent problems associated with immobility.

9. NURSING DIAGNOSIS

Self-care deficit related to impaired physical mobility associated with weakness, fatigue, discomfort, and prescribed activity restrictions.

DESIRED OUTCOMES	NURSING ACTIONS AND *SELECTED RATIONALES*
9. The client will demonstrate increased participation in self-care activities within physical limitations and activity restrictions imposed by the treatment plan.	9.a. Refer to Care Plan on Immobility, Nursing Diagnosis 9, for measures related to assessment of, planning for, and meeting the client's self-care needs. b. Implement measures to increase mobility (see Nursing Diagnosis 8, action a.2) *in order to further facilitate the client's ability to perform self-care activities.*

□ ▬▬▬▬▬▬▬▬▬▬▬▬▬▬▬▬▬▬▬▬▬

10. NURSING DIAGNOSIS

Constipation related to decreased mobility, fluid restrictions, dietary modifications, use of antacids containing aluminum or calcium, and electrolyte imbalances.

□ ▬▬▬▬▬▬▬▬▬▬▬▬▬▬▬▬▬▬▬▬▬

DESIRED OUTCOMES	NURSING ACTIONS AND *SELECTED RATIONALES*

10. The client will maintain usual bowel elimination pattern.	10.a. Refer to Care Plan on Immobility, Nursing Diagnosis 11, for measures related to assessment, prevention, and management of constipation.
	b. Implement additional measures *to prevent constipation:*
	  1. perform actions to prevent or treat hypokalemia and hypercalcemia (see Nursing Diagnosis 2, actions d.3 and e.5)
	  2. encourage client to increase intake of bran (bran is recommended *because it is a good source of fiber and is low in phosphorus*)
	  3. consult physician about alternating antacids that are constipating (e.g. Amphojel, Rolaids, Tums) with those that have a laxative effect (e.g. Milk of Magnesia, Gelusil, Mylanta, Maalox).

□ ▬▬▬▬▬▬▬▬▬▬▬▬▬▬▬▬▬▬▬▬▬

11. NURSING DIAGNOSIS

Diarrhea related to electrolyte imbalances, use of antacids containing magnesium, inflammation and ulceration of the gastrointestinal mucosa (associated with high serum levels of nitrogenous wastes), and extreme fear and anxiety.

□ ▬▬▬▬▬▬▬▬▬▬▬▬▬▬▬▬▬▬▬▬▬

DESIRED OUTCOMES	NURSING ACTIONS AND *SELECTED RATIONALES*

11. The client will have fewer bowel movements and more formed stool.	11.a. Ascertain client's usual bowel elimination habits.
	b. Assess for signs and symptoms of diarrhea (e.g. frequent, loose stools; abdominal pain and cramping).
	c. Assess bowel sounds regularly. Report an increase in frequency and/or a higher pitch of bowel sounds.
	d. Implement measures *to control diarrhea:*
	  1. perform actions *to rest the bowel:*
	    a. instruct client to avoid foods/fluids that are:
	      1. extremely hot or cold
	      2. spicy or high in fat
	      3. high in caffeine (e.g. coffee, tea, chocolate, colas)
	      4. diarrhea- or gas-producing (e.g. cabbage, onions, popcorn, licorice, prunes, chili, baked beans, carbonated beverages)

UNIT X

    b. provide small, frequent meals
    c. implement measures to reduce fear and anxiety (see Nursing
       Diagnosis 1)
    d. discourage smoking *(nicotine has a stimulant effect on the
       gastrointestinal tract)*
  2. perform actions to prevent or treat hyperkalemia and hypocalcemia (see
     Nursing Diagnosis 2, actions d.4 and e.3)
  3. perform actions to reduce accumulation of serum nitrogenous wastes
     (see Collaborative Diagnosis 16, action a.4) *in order to reduce
     inflammation and ulceration of gastrointestinal mucosa*
  4. consult physician about alternating antacids that have a laxative effect
     (e.g. Milk of Magnesia, Gelusil, Mylanta, Maalox) with those that are
     constipating (e.g. Amphojel, Rolaids, Tums)
  5. monitor for therapeutic and nontherapeutic effects of the following
     medications if administered:
     a. opiate or opiate-like substances (e.g. loperamide) *to decrease
        gastrointestinal motility*
     b. bulk-forming agents (e.g. methylcellulose, psyllium hydrophilic
        mucilloid) *to absorb water in bowel and produce a soft, formed
        stool.*
e. Consult physician if diarrhea persists.

12. NURSING DIAGNOSIS

**Altered thought processes: shortened attention span; inability to concentrate;
impaired memory, reasoning ability, and judgment; irritability; confusion;
and hallucinations** related to:

a. irritation and/or depression of the central nervous system associated with high
   serum levels of nitrogenous wastes, acidosis, and fluid and electrolyte imbalances;
b. cerebral hypoxia associated with inadequate tissue oxygenation.

DESIRED OUTCOMES	NURSING ACTIONS AND *SELECTED RATIONALES*

12. The client will experience improvement in thought processes as evidenced by:
a. usual or improved attention span, memory, reasoning ability, and judgment
b. orientation to person, place, and time.
	12.a. Assess client for alterations in thought processes (e.g. shortened attention span, decreased ability to concentrate, impaired memory, poor judgment, irritability, confusion).
	b. Ascertain from significant others client's usual level of intellectual functioning.
	c. Implement measures *to improve thought processes:*
	  1. perform actions to reduce accumulation of serum nitrogenous wastes (see Collaborative Diagnosis 16, action a.4)
	  2. perform actions to prevent or treat fluid and electrolyte imbalances (see appropriate actions in Nursing Diagnosis 2)
	  3. perform actions to improve tissue oxygenation (see Nursing Diagnosis 7, actions b.4 and 5).
	d. If client shows evidence of altered thought processes:
	  1. reorient to person, place, and time as necessary
	  2. allow adequate time for communication and performance of activities
	  3. repeat instructions as necessary using clear, simple language
	  4. keep environmental stimuli to a minimum
	  5. write out schedule of activities for client to refer to if desired
	  6. encourage client to make lists of planned activities and questions or concerns he/she may have
	  7. assist client to problem-solve if necessary
	  8. maintain realistic expectations of client's ability to learn, comprehend, and remember information provided

9. if client is experiencing hallucinations, allow significant others or a sitter to remain with client *in order to provide constant reassurance*
10. encourage significant others to be supportive of client; instruct them in methods of dealing with the alterations in thought processes
11. discuss physiological basis for alterations in thought processes with client and significant others; inform them that thought processes are expected to improve during treatment of renal failure
12. consult physician if alterations in thought processes persist or worsen.

13. NURSING DIAGNOSIS

Sleep pattern disturbance related to frequent assessments and treatments, decreased physical activity, fear, anxiety, muscle cramps, paresthesias, pruritus, nausea, nocturia (in nonoliguric renal failure), and hallucinations and nightmares (due to high serum levels of nitrogenous wastes).

DESIRED OUTCOMES	NURSING ACTIONS AND *SELECTED RATIONALES*

13. The client will attain optimal amounts of sleep within the parameters of the treatment regimen (see Care Plan on Immobility, Nursing Diagnosis 12, for outcome criteria).	13.a. Refer to Care Plan on Immobility, Nursing Diagnosis 12, for measures related to assessment and promotion of sleep.
	b. Implement additional measures *to promote sleep:*
	  1. perform actions to reduce discomfort (see Nursing Diagnoses 4.A, action 2; 4.B, action 5; and 4.C, actions 2 and 3)
	  2. perform actions to reduce accumulation of serum nitrogenous wastes (see Collaborative Diagnosis 16, action a.4)
	  3. if client is experiencing hallucinations and nightmares, allow significant others or a sitter to remain with client throughout the night *in order to provide constant reassurance.*

14. NURSING DIAGNOSIS

Potential for infection related to lowered natural resistance associated with:

a. depressed immune response resulting from high serum levels of nitrogenous wastes;
b. malnutrition, anemia, and general debilitation.

DESIRED OUTCOMES	NURSING ACTIONS AND *SELECTED RATIONALES*

14. The client will remain free of infection as evidenced by:
a. absence of chills and fever
b. pulse within normal limits
c. normal breath sounds
d. voiding clear, yellow urine without complaints of
	14.a. Assess for and report signs and symptoms of infection:
	  1. elevated temperature
	  2. chills
	  3. pattern of increased pulse or pulse rate greater than 100 beats/minute
	  4. adventitious breath sounds
	  5. cloudy or foul-smelling urine
	  6. complaints of frequency, urgency, or burning when urinating

UNIT
X

frequency, urgency, and burning
e. absence of redness, swelling, and unusual drainage in any area where there is a break in skin integrity
f. intact oral mucous membrane
g. WBC and differential counts within normal range
h. negative results of cultured specimens.

7. presence of WBCs, bacteria, and/or nitrites in urine
8. redness, swelling, or unusual drainage in any area where there is a break in skin integrity
9. irritation or ulceration of oral mucous membrane
10. elevated WBC count and/or significant change in differential.

b. Obtain culture specimens (e.g. urine, vaginal, mouth, sputum, blood) as ordered. Report positive results.
c. Implement measures *to reduce the risk of infection:*
1. perform actions to reduce accumulation of serum nitrogenous wastes (see Collaborative Diagnosis 16, action a.4)
2. maintain the maximum fluid intake allowed
3. use good handwashing technique and encourage client to do the same
4. maintain meticulous aseptic technique during all invasive procedures (e.g. catheterizations, venous and arterial punctures, injections)
5. protect client from others who have an infection
6. maintain an optimal nutritional status (see Nursing Diagnosis 3, action e)
7. reinforce importance of good oral care
8. provide proper balance of exercise and rest
9. perform actions *to prevent respiratory tract infection:*
   a. instruct and assist client to turn, cough, and deep breathe at least every 2 hours if activity is limited
   b. instruct and assist client in use of inspiratory exerciser at least every 2 hours if indicated
   c. encourage client to stop smoking
   d. increase activity as allowed and tolerated
10. perform actions *to prevent urinary tract infection:*
    a. instruct and assist female client to wipe from front to back following urination and defecation
    b. keep perianal area clean.
d. Monitor for therapeutic and nontherapeutic effects of anti-infectives if administered.

---

15. NURSING DIAGNOSIS

Potential for trauma related to:

a. falls associated with:
1. weakness resulting from anemia, fluid and electrolyte imbalances, and malnutrition
2. altered thought processes;
b. burns associated with paresthesias resulting from peripheral neuropathies.

DESIRED OUTCOMES	NURSING ACTIONS AND *SELECTED RATIONALES*
15. The client will not experience falls or burns.	15.a. Determine whether conditions predisposing client to falls or burns (e.g. weakness, decreased sensation in extremities, confusion) exist. b. Implement measures to reduce accumulation of serum nitrogenous wastes (see Collaborative Diagnosis 16, action a.4) and prevent or treat fluid and electrolyte imbalances (see appropriate actions in Nursing Diagnosis 2) *in order to minimize the conditions that predispose client to falls and burns.* c. Implement measures *to prevent falls:* 1. keep bed in low position with side rails up when client is in bed 2. keep needed items within easy reach 3. encourage client to request assistance whenever needed; have call signal within easy reach

4. use lap belt when client is in chair if indicated
5. instruct client to wear shoes with nonskid soles and low heels when ambulating
6. avoid unnecessary clutter in room
7. accompany client during ambulation utilizing a transfer safety belt if necessary
8. provide ambulatory aids (e.g. walker, cane) if client is weak or unsteady on feet
9. instruct client to ambulate in well-lit areas and to use handrails if needed
10. do not rush client; allow adequate time for activities such as trips to the bathroom and ambulation in hallway
11. perform actions to increase strength and activity tolerance (see Nursing Diagnosis 7).

d. Implement measures *to prevent burns:*
1. let hot foods and fluids cool slightly before serving *to reduce risk of burns if spills occur*
2. supervise client while smoking if indicated
3. assess temperature of bath water and heating pad before and during use.

e. If client is confused or irrational, implement additional measures *to reduce risk of injury:*
1. reorient frequently to surroundings and necessity of adhering to safety precautions
2. provide constant supervision (e.g. staff member, significant other) if indicated
3. use jacket or wrist restraints or safety alarm device if necessary *to reduce the risk of client's getting out of bed or chair unattended*
4. monitor for therapeutic and nontherapeutic effects of antianxiety and antipsychotic medications if administered.

f. Include client and significant others in planning and implementing measures to prevent injury.

g. If injury does occur, initiate appropriate first aid and notify physician.

16. COLLABORATIVE DIAGNOSIS

Potential complications:

a. **uremia (uremic syndrome)** related to accumulation of toxic serum levels of nitrogenous wastes (e.g. creatinine, urea, phenols) associated with progressive loss of renal function (uremic syndrome develops when glomerular filtration rate [GFR] falls to 10% or below);

b. **arrhythmias** related to altered myocardial conductivity associated with fluid and electrolyte imbalances and accumulation of serum nitrogenous wastes;

c. **hypertension** related to fluid overload (with oliguric renal failure) and increased plasma renin levels (occurs when there is diminished renal blood flow);

d. **pericarditis** related to irritation of the pericardium by the accumulated serum nitrogenous wastes:

e. **congestive heart failure (CHF) and pulmonary edema** related to pump failure associated with a sustained increase in cardiac workload resulting from fluid overload, anemia, arrhythmias, and hypertension;

f. **bleeding** related to decreased number of platelets and platelet dysfunction associated with high serum levels of nitrogenous wastes;

g. **pathologic fractures** related to osteodystrophy associated with impaired calcium absorption in the gastrointestinal tract (the kidneys are unable to activate vitamin D) and decreased calcium reabsorption by the kidney.

DESIRED OUTCOMES	**NURSING ACTIONS AND *SELECTED RATIONALES***

16.a. The client will not experience uremia as evidenced by:
   1. pulse regular at 60–100 beats/minute
   2. usual or improved mental status
   3. improved skin color
   4. improved strength and activity tolerance
   5. decreased complaints of nausea, itching, muscle cramping, paresthesias, unusual taste in mouth
   6. absence of or reduction in episodes of vomiting, diarrhea, and bleeding
   7. intact oral mucous membrane
   8. absence of asterixis and seizure activity
   9. decreasing serum levels of nitrogenous wastes
   10. increased creatinine clearance.

16.a.1. Assess for signs and symptoms of uremia:
   a. arrhythmias
   b. increased difficulty concentrating, lethargy, confusion, or hallucinations
   c. episodes of paranoid delusions
   d. sallow or grayish-bronze skin color
   e. increased weakness and fatigue
   f. increased complaints of nausea, itching, muscle cramps, paresthesias, and/or metallic or bitter taste in mouth
   g. increased episodes of vomiting, diarrhea, and/or bleeding
   h. stomatitis
   i. asterixis, seizures.
2. Monitor BUN and serum creatinine results. Report levels that increase or fail to return to client's usual level (client's usual BUN level may be 50–80 mg/dl and usual serum creatinine level may be as high as 13 mg/dl).
3. Collect a 24-hour urine specimen if ordered. Report creatinine clearance levels that decrease or fail to return to client's usual level.
4. Implement measures *to reduce accumulation of serum nitrogenous wastes in order to prevent uremia:*
   a. perform actions to improve nutritional status (see Nursing Diagnosis 3, action e) *in order to reduce catabolism of body proteins*
   b. perform actions as ordered to control disease conditions that have caused or contributed to renal failure (e.g. diabetes, hypertension, atherosclerosis, lupus erythematosus)
   c. consult physician before administering the following medications that are known to be nephrotoxic:
      1. aminoglycosides (e.g. gentamicin, kanamycin, tobramycin, streptomycin)
      2. sulfonamides (e.g. furosemide, probenecid, sulfasalazine)
      3. nonsteroidal anti-inflammatory drugs (e.g. salicylates, phenylbutazone, indomethacin, ibuprofen, naproxen).
5. If signs and symptoms of uremia occur:
   a. consult physician
   b. initiate seizure precautions (e.g. have plastic airway readily available, pad side rails)
   c. prepare client for hemodialysis or peritoneal dialysis if planned
   d. provide emotional support to client and significant others.

16.b. The client will not experience cardiac arrhythmias as evidenced by:
   1. regular apical pulse at 60–100 beats/minute
   2. equal apical and radial pulses
   3. absence of syncope and palpitations
   4. EKG reading showing normal sinus rhythm.

16.b.1. Assess for and report signs and symptoms of arrhythmias (e.g. irregular apical pulse; pulse rate below 60 or above 100 beats/minute; apical-radial pulse deficit; syncope; palpitations; abnormal rate, rhythm, or configurations on EKG).
2. Implement measures *to prevent arrhythmias:*
   a. perform actions to prevent or treat hypokalemia, hyperkalemia, hypocalcemia, hypercalcemia, and hypermagnesemia (see Nursing Diagnosis 2, actions d.3 and 4, e.3 and 5, and g.2 and 3)
   b. perform actions to reduce accumulation of serum nitrogenous wastes (see action a.4 in this diagnosis).
3. If arrhythmias occur:
   a. initiate cardiac monitoring if not already being done
   b. monitor for therapeutic and nontherapeutic effects of the following medications if administered:
      1. antiarrhythmics (e.g. propranolol, procainamide, disopyramide, quinidine, phenytoin, lidocaine, bretylium)
      2. anticholinergic agents (e.g. atropine) or sympathomimetics (e.g. ephedrine, isoproterenol) *to increase heart rate*
      3. cardiac glycosides (e.g. digitalis) *to decrease heart rate*
   c. restrict client's activity based on his/her tolerance and the severity of arrhythmia
   d. maintain oxygen therapy as ordered
   e. assist with cardioversion if performed
   f. assess cardiovascular status closely and report signs and symptoms of inadequate tissue perfusion (e.g. decline in B/P; cool, clammy, mottled

skin; cyanosis; diminished peripheral pulses; further decline in urine output; restlessness and agitation; shortness of breath)
    g. have emergency cart readily available for cardiopulmonary resuscitation.

16.c. The client will maintain B/P within a safe range as evidenced by:
1. systolic pressure of 140 mm Hg or less; diastolic pressure of 90 mm Hg or less
2. no complaints of headache or dizziness
3. no increase in nausea and vomiting.

16.c.1. Assess for and report signs and symptoms of hypertension (e.g. systolic pressure of 140 mm Hg or greater, diastolic pressure of 90 mm Hg or greater, headache, dizziness, increased nausea and vomiting).
    2. Implement measures *to prevent or control hypertension:*
      a. perform actions to prevent or treat fluid volume excess and hypernatremia (see Nursing Diagnosis 2, actions b.3 and c.4)
      b. perform actions to reduce fear and anxiety (see Nursing Diagnosis 1)
      c. monitor for therapeutic and nontherapeutic effects of antihypertensives if administered.
    3. If sustained or severe hypertension occurs:
      a. continue with above actions
      b. assess for and report signs and symptoms of:
        1. myocardial infarction (e.g. sudden, severe, persistent chest pain; significant increase in cardiac enzymes; significant ST elevation, T wave changes, and/or pathological Q wave on EKG reading)
        2. cerebrovascular accident (e.g. decreased level of consciousness, alteration in usual sensory and motor function)
      c. refer to Care Plan on Hypertension for additional care measures.

16.d. The client will not experience pericarditis as evidenced by:
1. no complaints of substernal or precordial pain
2. absence of pericardial friction rub
3. unlabored respirations at 16–20/minute
4. stable temperature
5. WBC count and sedimentation rate within normal range.

16.d.1. Assess for and report signs and symptoms of pericarditis:
    a. substernal or precordial pain that frequently radiates to left shoulder, neck, and arm; is intensified during deep inspiration; and usually is relieved by sitting up
    b. pericardial friction rub (may be transient)
    c. dyspnea, tachypnea
    d. elevated temperature
    e. elevated WBC count and sedimentation rate
    f. chest x-ray and echocardiography results showing cardiomegaly and pericardial effusion.
    2. Implement measures to prevent accumulation of serum nitrogenous wastes (see action a.4 in this diagnosis) *in order to reduce risk of development of pericarditis.*
    3. If signs and symptoms of pericarditis occur:
      a. allay client's anxiety (client may believe that symptoms indicate a heart attack)
      b. monitor for therapeutic and nontherapeutic effects of medications that may be administered *to reduce inflammation* (e.g. corticosteroids)
      c. assess for and immediately report signs of cardiac tamponade (e.g. rapid and continual decline in B/P; narrowed pulse pressure; pulsus paradoxus; weak, rapid pulse; distant or muffled heart sounds; neck vein distention on inspiration; decreased amplitude of waves on EKG; increased CVP and pulmonary pressures)
      d. prepare client for and assist with pericardiocentesis if performed.

16.e. The client will not develop CHF and pulmonary edema as evidenced by:
1. vital signs within normal range for client
2. audible heart sounds without an S_3 or S_4 or softening of pre-existing murmurs
3. normal breath sounds
4. absence of or no increase in dyspnea and orthopnea
5. palpable peripheral pulses and strong carotid pulse amplitude

16.e.1. Assess for and report signs and symptoms of CHF:
    a. tachycardia
    b. softened or muffled heart sounds
    c. development of an S_3 and/or S_4 gallop rhythm
    d. crackles and diminished or absent breath sounds
    e. dyspnea, orthopnea
    f. displaced apical impulse
    g. diminished or absent peripheral pulses
    h. decreased amplitude of carotid pulse
    i. elevated CVP
    j. peripheral edema
    k. distended neck veins
    l. tender, enlarged liver.
    2. Monitor chest x-ray results. Report findings of cardiomegaly, pleural effusion, and pulmonary edema.
    3. Implement measures *to prevent CHF:*

6. CVP within normal range
7. absence of peripheral edema; distended neck veins; enlarged, tender liver.

a. perform actions to prevent or treat arrhythmias and hypertension (see actions b.2 and 3 and c.2 and 3 in this diagnosis) *because these conditions contribute to development of CHF*
b. perform additional actions *to reduce cardiac workload:*
   1. implement measures to promote physical and emotional rest
   2. place client in a semi- to high-Fowler's position
   3. instruct client to avoid activities that create a Valsalva response (e.g. straining to have a bowel movement, bending at the waist, holding breath while moving)
   4. maintain oxygen therapy as ordered
   5. discourage smoking *(smoking has a cardiostimulatory effect, causes vasoconstriction, and reduces myocardial oxygen availability)*
   6. discourage intake of foods/fluids high in caffeine such as coffee, tea, chocolate, and colas *(caffeine is a myocardial stimulant and increases myocardial oxygen consumption)*
   7. provide small, frequent meals rather than 3 large ones *(large meals require an increase in blood supply to gastrointestinal tract for digestion)*
   8. implement measures to prevent or treat fluid overload (see Nursing Diagnosis 2, action b.3)
   9. increase activity gradually as allowed and tolerated.
4. If signs and symptoms of CHF occur:
   a. continue with above actions
   b. monitor for therapeutic and nontherapeutic effects of medications that may be administered *to reduce vascular congestion and/or cardiac workload* (e.g. diuretics, cardiotonics, vasodilators, morphine sulfate)
   c. apply rotating tourniquets according to hospital policy if ordered *to reduce pulmonary vascular congestion*
   d. refer to Care Plan on Congestive Heart Failure for additional care measures.

16.f. The client will not experience unusual bleeding as evidenced by:
1. skin and mucous membranes free of bleeding, petechiae, and ecchymosis
2. absence of unusual joint pain and swelling
3. no increase in abdominal girth
4. absence of frank or occult blood in stool, urine, and vomitus
5. usual menstrual flow
6. vital signs within normal range for client
7. stable or improved Hct. and Hgb.
8. usual mental status.

16.f.1. Assess client for and report signs and symptoms of unusual bleeding:
   a. petechiae
   b. multiple ecchymotic areas
   c. bleeding gums
   d. frequent or uncontrollable episodes of epistaxis
   e. unusual oozing from injection sites
   f. unusual joint pain or swelling
   g. increase in abdominal girth
   h. hematemesis, melena, red or smoke-colored urine
   i. hypermenorrhea
   j. significant drop in B/P accompanied by an increased pulse rate
   k. further decline in client's usual Hct. and Hgb. levels
   l. restlessness, confusion.
2. Monitor coagulation test results (e.g. platelet count, bleeding time). Report abnormal values.
3. If coagulation test results are abnormal or Hct. and Hgb. levels decline, test all stools, urine, and vomitus for occult blood. Report positive results.
4. Implement measures *to prevent bleeding:*
   a. perform actions to reduce the levels of serum nitrogenous wastes (see action a.4 in this diagnosis)
   b. use the smallest gauge needle possible when giving injections and performing venous or arterial punctures
   c. apply gentle, prolonged pressure after injections and venous or arterial punctures
   d. take B/P only when necessary and avoid overinflating cuff
   e. caution client to avoid activities that increase potential for trauma (e.g. shaving with a straight-edge razor, cutting nails, using stiff bristle toothbrush or dental floss)
   f. pad side rails if client is confused or restless
   g. perform actions to prevent falls (see Nursing Diagnosis 15, action c)
   h. instruct client to avoid blowing nose forcefully or straining to have a bowel movement; consult physician regarding order for decongestants, stool softeners, and/or laxatives if indicated
   i. monitor for therapeutic and nontherapeutic effects of platelets if administered.

5. If bleeding occurs and does not subside spontaneously:
    a. apply firm, prolonged pressure to bleeding area if possible
    b. if epistaxis occurs, place client in high Fowler's position and apply pressure and ice packs to nasal area
    c. maintain oxygen therapy as ordered
    d. perform iced water or saline lavage as ordered *to control gastric bleeding*
    e. administer blood products (usually platelets and/or fresh frozen plasma) as ordered
    f. prepare client for surgical repair of bleeding vessels if indicated
    g. provide emotional support to client and significant others.

16.g. The client will not experience pathologic fractures (see Care Plan on Immobility, Collaborative Diagnosis 14, outcome e, for outcome criteria).	16.g.1. Refer to Care Plan on Immobility, Collaborative Diagnosis 14, action e, for measures related to assessment, prevention, and treatment of pathologic fractures. 2. Implement measures to prevent hypocalcemia (see Nursing Diagnosis 2, action e.3) *in order to prevent excessive parathyroid hormone output (parathyroid hormone increases bone resorption, which further increases the risk of pathologic fractures).*

□ ▬▬▬▬▬▬▬▬▬▬▬▬▬▬▬▬▬▬▬▬▬▬▬▬▬▬▬

17. NURSING DIAGNOSIS

Sexual dysfunction:

a. **decreased libido** related to weakness, fatigue, anxiety, depression, and discomfort;
b. **impotence** related to effects of certain medications (e.g. antihypertensives) and neuropathies associated with fluid and electrolyte imbalances and high serum levels of nitrogenous wastes.

□ ▬▬▬▬▬▬▬▬▬▬▬▬▬▬▬▬▬▬▬▬▬▬▬▬▬▬▬

DESIRED OUTCOMES	NURSING ACTIONS AND *SELECTED RATIONALES*
17. The client will perceive self as sexually adequate and acceptable (see Care Plan on Immobility, Nursing Diagnosis 15, for outcome criteria).	17.a. Refer to Care Plan on Immobility, Nursing Diagnosis 15, for measures related to assessment and management of sexual dysfunction. b. Implement additional measures *to promote optimal sexual functioning:* 1. perform actions to reduce accumulation of serum nitrogenous wastes (see Collaborative Diagnosis 16, action a.4) 2. instruct client to allow adequate rest periods before and after sexual activity 3. if impotence is a problem, encourage client to discuss it with physician if desired.

□ ▬▬▬▬▬▬▬▬▬▬▬▬▬▬▬▬▬▬▬▬▬▬▬▬▬▬▬

18. NURSING DIAGNOSIS

Disturbance in self-concept* related to:

a. changes in appearance (e.g. pale, grayish-bronze skin color; dry skin; multiple ecchymotic areas; thin, brittle and/or discolored nails; brittle, dry hair that falls out easily; subcutaneous nodules [composed of calcium phosphate]);

---

* This diagnostic label includes the nursing diagnoses of body image disturbance and self-esteem disturbance.

UNIT X

b. altered reproductive function (infertility in males due to decreased sperm count, sterility in females due to cessation of menses) associated with high serum levels of nitrogenous wastes;

c. dependence on others to meet self-care needs;

d. changes in life style and roles resulting from the treatment regimen and effects of renal failure on body functioning.

☐ ▰▰▰▰▰▰▰▰▰▰▰▰▰▰▰▰▰▰▰▰▰▰▰▰▰▰

DESIRED OUTCOMES	NURSING ACTIONS AND *SELECTED RATIONALES*

18. The client will demonstrate beginning adaptation to changes in appearance, body functioning, life style, roles, and level of independence (see Care Plan on Immobility, Nursing Diagnosis 16, for outcome criteria).

18.a. Refer to Care Plan on Immobility, Nursing Diagnosis 16, for measures related to assessment and promotion of a positive self-concept.

  b. Implement additional measures *to promote a positive self-concept:*

    1. perform actions *to assist client to adapt to changes in appearance, body functioning, life style, and roles:*

      a. discuss alternative forms of becoming a parent (e.g. artificial insemination, adoption) if of concern to client

      b. implement measures *to assist client to minimize changes in appearance:*

        1. offer suggestions regarding appropriate makeup and color of clothing that will minimize changes in skin color

        2. reinforce use of mild soaps and lanolin-based lotions and avoidance of hot baths *in order to reduce skin dryness*

        3. instruct client in ways to avoid bumps and falls *in order to decrease incidence of ecchymosis*

        4. instruct client in ways *to reduce hair loss:*

          a. avoid use of harsh shampoos

          b. use hair conditioners that strengthen hair

          c. brush hair gently using a soft bristle brush

        5. if hair loss is occurring, assist with hair styling that disguises loss and/or encourage wearing of wig or scarf if desired

        6. instruct client in or assist with nail care

      c. instruct client in ways *to adapt to changes in thought processes* (e.g. keeping lists to aid memory, minimizing environmental stimuli to aid concentration)

    2. teach client the rationale for treatments and encourage maximum participation in treatment regimen *to enable him/her to maintain a sense of control over life*

    3. encourage significant others to allow client to do what he/she is able *so that independence can be re-established and/or self-esteem redeveloped.*

  c. Ensure that client and significant others have similar expectations and understanding of future life style.

  d. Assist client and significant others to identify ways that personal and family goals can be adjusted rather than abandoned.

☐ ▰▰▰▰▰▰▰▰▰▰▰▰▰▰▰▰▰▰▰▰▰▰▰▰▰▰

19. NURSING DIAGNOSIS

Grieving* related to progressive loss of normal function of a major organ, possible changes in life style and roles, and uncertainty of prognosis.

---

* This diagnostic label includes anticipatory grieving and grieving following the actual losses/changes.

☐ ▰▰▰▰▰▰▰▰▰▰▰▰▰▰▰▰▰▰▰▰▰▰▰▰▰▰

DESIRED OUTCOMES	**NURSING ACTIONS AND *SELECTED RATIONALES***

19. The client will demonstrate beginning progression through the grieving process as evidenced by:
    a. verbalization of feelings about having chronic renal failure
    b. expression of grief
    c. participation in treatment plan and self-care activities
    d. utilization of available support systems
    e. verbalization of a plan for integrating prescribed follow-up care into life style.

19.a. Determine client's perception of the impact of chronic renal failure on his/her future.
   b. Determine how the client usually expresses grief.
   c. Observe for signs of grieving (e.g. changes in eating habits, insomnia, anger, noncompliance, denial).
   d. Implement measures *to facilitate the grieving process:*
     1. assist client to acknowledge the losses and changes experienced *so grief work can begin;* assess for factors that may hinder or facilitate acknowledgment
     2. discuss the grieving process and assist client to accept the stages of grieving as an expected response to actual and/or anticipated changes or losses; support the realization that grief may recur *because of the chronic, progressive nature of the disease*
     3. allow time for client to progress through the stages of grieving (denial, anger, bargaining, depression, acceptance [Kübler-Ross, 1969]); be aware that not every stage is experienced or expressed by all individuals
     4. provide an atmosphere of care and concern (e.g. provide privacy, be available and nonjudgmental, display empathy and respect) *so that client will feel free to verbalize both positive and negative feelings and concerns*
     5. perform actions *to promote trust* (e.g. answer questions honestly, provide requested information)
     6. encourage the expression of anger and sadness about the losses and changes experienced; recognize displacement of anger and assist client to see actual cause of angry feelings and resentment; establish limits on abusive behavior
     7. encourage client to express his/her feelings in whatever ways are comfortable (e.g. writing, drawing, conversation)
     8. assist client to identify personal strengths that have helped him/her to cope in previous situations of loss or change
     9. support realistic hope about the effect of the treatment plan on prognosis.
   e. Assess for and support behaviors suggesting successful resolution of grief (e.g. verbalizing feelings about changes, expressing sorrow, focusing on ways to adapt to changes).
   f. Explain the stages of the grieving process to significant others. Encourage their support and understanding.
   g. Provide information regarding counseling services and support groups that might assist client in working through grief.
   h. Arrange for visit from clergy if desired by client.
   i. Monitor for therapeutic and nontherapeutic effects of antidepressants if administered.
   j. Consult physician regarding referral for counseling if signs of dysfunctional grieving (e.g. persistent denial of losses or changes, excessive anger or sadness, hysteria, suicidal behaviors, phobias) occur.

☐ ██

20. NURSING DIAGNOSIS

Noncompliance* related to lack of understanding of the implications of not following the prescribed treatment plan, altered thought processes, difficulty integrating necessary treatments into life style, lack of financial resources, and dysfunctional grieving.

---

* This diagnostic label includes both an informed decision by client not to comply and an inability to comply due to circumstances beyond the client's control.

☐ ██

UNIT X

DESIRED OUTCOMES	NURSING ACTIONS AND *SELECTED RATIONALES*

20. The client will demonstrate probability of future compliance with the prescribed treatment plan as evidenced by:
  a. willingness to learn about and participate in treatments and care
  b. statements reflecting ways to modify personal habits and integrate treatments into life style
  c. statements reflecting an understanding of the implications of not following the prescribed treatment plan.

20.a. Assess for indications that the client may be unwilling or unable to comply with the prescribed treatment plan:
  1. statements reflecting that he/she was unable to manage care at home
  2. failure to adhere to treatment plan while in the hospital (e.g. not adhering to dietary modifications and fluid restrictions, refusing medications)
  3. statements reflecting a lack of understanding of factors that will cause further renal damage
  4. statements reflecting an unwillingness or inability to modify personal habits and integrate necessary treatments into life style
  5. statements reflecting view that kidney damage will reverse itself or that the situation is hopeless and efforts to comply with treatments are useless.
  b. Implement measures *to improve client compliance:*
    1. explain renal failure in terms client can understand; stress the fact that it is a chronic disease and that adherence to treatment plan is necessary *in order to delay and/or prevent complications*
    2. initiate and reinforce discharge teaching outlined in Nursing Diagnosis 21 *in order to promote a sense of control and self-reliance*
    3. encourage client to participate in treatments (e.g. monitoring intake and output, calculating allowed fluid intake, selecting foods and fluids within dietary restrictions, performing good oral and skin care)
    4. assist client to identify ways he/she can incorporate treatments into life style; focus on modifications of life style rather than complete change
    5. obtain a dietary consult to assist client in planning a dietary program based on prescribed modifications and client's likes, dislikes, and daily routines
    6. encourage questions and allow time for reinforcement and clarification of information provided; recognize that repeated teaching sessions may be needed due to client's alterations in thought processes
    7. provide client with written instructions about future appointments with health care provider, ways to prevent further kidney damage, dietary modifications, fluid restrictions, medications, safety measures, and signs and symptoms to report
    8. encourage client to discuss his/her financial concerns about the cost of medications and dialysis treatments if necessary; obtain a social service consult to assist client with financial planning and to obtain aid if indicated
    9. provide information about and encourage utilization of community resources that can assist client to make necessary life-style changes (e.g. local chapter of the American Kidney Association, vocational rehabilitation, stress management classes, counseling services).
  c. Assess for and reinforce behaviors suggesting future compliance with prescribed treatments (e.g. statements reflecting plan for integrating treatments into life style, changes in personal habits, active participation in treatment plan).
  d. Include significant others in explanations and teaching sessions and encourage their support.
  e. Reinforce need for client to assume responsibility for managing as much of care as possible.
  f. Consult physician regarding referrals to community health agencies if continued instruction, support, or supervision is needed.

☐ ▄▄▄▄▄▄▄▄▄▄▄▄▄▄▄▄▄▄▄▄▄▄▄▄▄▄▄▄

21. NURSING DIAGNOSIS

Knowledge deficit regarding follow-up care.

☐ ▄▄▄▄▄▄▄▄▄▄▄▄▄▄▄▄▄▄▄▄▄▄▄▄▄▄▄▄

DESIRED OUTCOMES	**NURSING ACTIONS AND *SELECTED RATIONALES***

21.a. The client will verbalize a basic understanding of renal failure.

21.a. Explain renal failure in terms the client can understand. Utilize appropriate teaching aids (e.g. pictures, videotapes, kidney models).

21.b. The client will identify ways to reduce the risk of further kidney damage.

21.b.1. Provide instructions regarding ways *to reduce risk of further kidney damage:*
    a. control hypertension by adhering to dietary modifications, taking medications as prescribed, and reducing stress
    b. reduce the risk of urinary tract infection:
        1. cleanse perianal area thoroughly after each bowel movement
        2. maintain allowed fluid intake
        3. wipe from front to back after urination and defecation (if female)
        4. take prophylactic anti-infectives if prescribed
    c. reduce the risk of nephrotoxic reactions by:
        1. consulting the health care provider before:
            a. taking any additional prescription and nonprescription drugs
            b. receiving any vaccines
            c. resuming any occupation or hobby involving exposure to chemicals or fumes
        2. avoiding contact with products such as antifreeze, insecticides, carbon tetrachloride, mercuric chloride, lead, arsenic, and creosote.
  2. With client and significant others, discuss ways in which above health care measures can be incorporated into life style.

21.c. The client will verbalize an understanding of fluid restrictions and dietary modifications.

21.c.1. Reinforce the importance of adhering to prescribed fluid restrictions and dietary modifications *in order to reduce risk of complications.*
  2. Reinforce physician's instructions about specific fluid restrictions and dietary modifications.
  3. Reinforce dietician's instructions on how to calculate and measure dietary allotments and use an exchange list. Have client develop sample menus.
  4. If client is on a protein- and sodium-restricted diet, inform him/her that numerous salt-free and protein-free products are available. Provide names of local stores that carry these products.
  5. If client is on fluid restrictions, instruct to:
    a. take oral medications with soft foods (e.g. applesauce, pudding) rather than liquids
    b. reduce thirst by:
        1. sucking on sour, hard candy or ice cubes made with favorite juices (caution client that the fluid volume of the ice cubes must be considered as oral fluid intake)
        2. spacing fluids evenly over a 24-hour period
    c. set out the 24-hour allotment of liquids in the morning *in order to visualize the amount allowed for the day (may help him/her to adhere to restrictions).*

21.d. The client will demonstrate the ability to accurately weigh self and measure fluid intake and output.

21.d.1. If client is supposed to monitor weight, instruct him/her to weigh at the same time, on the same scale, and with similar amounts of clothing on.
  2. Demonstrate how to measure and record fluid intake and urinary output if indicated. Stress that any substance that is liquid at room temperature is counted as fluid intake.
  3. Allow time for questions, clarification, and practice sessions. Have client return demonstrate how to weigh self and record weight and how to calculate and record intake and output.

21.e. The client will identify precautions necessary to prevent bleeding.

21.e.1. Instruct client about ways *to minimize the risk of bleeding:*
    a. avoid taking aspirin, aspirin-containing compounds, and ibuprofen
    b. use an electric rather than a straight-edge razor
    c. floss and brush teeth gently
    d. cut nails carefully
    e. avoid situations that could result in injury (e.g. contact sports)
    f. avoid blowing nose forcefully
    g. avoid straining to have a bowel movement.
  2. Instruct client to control any bleeding by applying firm, prolonged pressure to the area if possible.

UNIT X

21.f. The client will identify ways to reduce the risk of infection.

21.f. Instruct client in ways *to reduce the risk of infection:*
1. continue with coughing and deep breathing or use of inspiratory exerciser every 2 hours while awake as long as activity level is limited
2. increase activity as tolerated
3. avoid contact with persons who have an infection
4. avoid crowds during the flu or cold season
5. decrease or stop smoking if possible
6. drink allotted amounts of liquids
7. maintain good personal hygiene
8. take vitamin and mineral supplements and hematinics as prescribed.

21.g. The client will identify ways to manage problems that often occur as a result of renal failure.

21.g. Provide instructions regarding ways *to manage problems that often occur as a result of renal failure:*
1. if client is experiencing pruritus:
   a. reinforce instructions identified in Nursing Diagnosis 4.C, action 2 to reduce pruritus
   b. instruct client to apply antipruritic lotions as needed
   c. instruct client to consult health care provider regarding a prescription for an antihistamine if above measures fail to control itching adequately
2. if client is experiencing stomatitis:
   a. reinforce instructions identified in Nursing Diagnosis 6, actions c.3–11 and d, to reduce stomatitis
   b. stress importance of consuming the maximum amount of liquids allowed
   c. instruct clients with dentures to remove them except at mealtime if stomatitis is not controlled
   d. instruct client how and when to apply topical anesthetics, oral protective pastes, and topical analgesics if prescribed
3. if morning nausea and vomiting occur, instruct client to:
   a. schedule food/fluid allotments evenly over a 24-hour period
   b. take antiemetics as prescribed
4. if client is experiencing muscle cramps, instruct to:
   a. push feet against the wall or end of the bed if cramping occurs in lower extremities
   b. take a warm bath or apply warm pack to affected area
   c. take muscle relaxants and quinine sulfate as prescribed
5. if client is experiencing restless leg syndrome, instruct to move legs while in bed or chair or to ambulate *in order to obtain relief of the symptoms*
6. if client is experiencing alterations in appearance and thought processes, reinforce instructions provided in Nursing Diagnosis 18, actions b.1.b and c, to assist in adaptation to these changes
7. reinforce the need to schedule adequate rest periods *in order to reduce fatigue and weakness.*

21.h. The client will state signs and symptoms to report to the health care provider.

21.h. Instruct client to report the following:
1. weight gain of more than 0.5 kg (1 pound)/day or a continued weight loss
2. uncontrolled nausea or vomiting
3. increasing fatigue and weakness
4. increasing difficulty concentrating and making decisions
5. confusion
6. severe headache
7. palpitations
8. any blood in stools, urine, or vomitus; persistent bleeding from nose, mouth, or any cut; prolonged or excessive menses; excessive bruising; sudden abdominal or back pain
9. skin breakdown
10. itching that is not relieved by prescribed methods
11. increasing oral pain or breakdown of oral mucous membrane
12. shortness of breath
13. increased muscle cramping
14. twitching, tremors, seizures.

21.i. The client will identify community resources that can assist with adjustment to changes resulting from chronic renal failure.

21.i.1. Provide information about community resources that can assist the client and significant others to adjust to changes resulting from chronic renal failure (e.g. local chapter of the American Kidney Association, vocational rehabilitation, social services, counseling services).
   2. Initiate a referral if indicated.

21.j. The client will verbalize an understanding of and a plan for adhering to recommended follow-up care including future appointments with health care provider and medications prescribed.

21.j.1. Reinforce the importance of keeping follow-up appointments with health care provider.
   2. Explain the rationale for, side effects of, and importance of taking prescribed medications (e.g. antihypertensives, antacids, vitamins, hematinics, electrolyte supplements, diuretics).
   3. Refer to Nursing Diagnosis 20, action b, for measures to improve client compliance.

Reference

Kübler-Ross, E. On death and dying. New York: Macmillan, 1969.

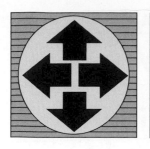
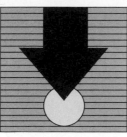
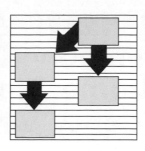
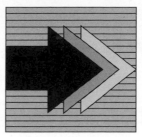
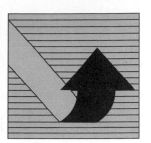

Unit XI

Nursing Care of the Client with Disturbances of Hematopoietic and Lymphatic Function

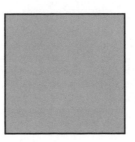
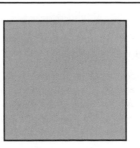
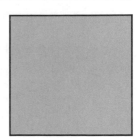

Acquired Immune Deficiency Syndrome: Human Immunodeficiency Virus Infection

Human immunodeficiency virus (HIV) infection is a clinical spectrum consisting of an underlying immunodeficiency that predisposes the host to certain opportunistic infections, unusual malignancies, and/or neurological impairments. HIV is a retrovirus that has a particular affinity for cells in the body that have a CD4 molecule, the largest group of which is the T4-lymphocytes. Other body cells that have this molecule are some macrophages and their precursors (monocytes) and tissue-dendritic cells found in the skin, mucous membranes, lymph nodes, liver, spleen, and brain. The behavior of the virus seems to depend on the host cell. The virus ultimately destroys the T4-lymphocytes and results in severely impaired cell-mediated immunity in the host. Humoral immune function is also impaired in that B-cells are unable to respond appropriately to the presence of a new antigen without the help of normal T4-cells. The effect of HIV and altered T4-lymphocyte function on macrophage activity further depresses immune function.

The virus has been isolated from blood, semen, vaginal secretions, saliva, tears, breast milk, cerebrospinal fluid, amniotic fluid, and urine. It is transmitted sexually and parenterally and tends to occur in distinct groups of people: homosexually/bisexually active males, intravenous drug abusers, recipients of blood/blood products (particularly hemophiliacs who receive Factor VIII concentrates), sexual partners of those infected, and infants born to infected mothers.

Three to 6 weeks following infection with the virus, the client may develop an acute, transitory, flu-like illness with symptoms such as fever, chills, myalgias, or rash that may persist for as long as 3 weeks. Most clients, however, show no overt signs of infection. Serum conversion typically occurs 8–12 weeks following the initial exposure. The client may then experience a latent period that can range from 2 months to 10 years depending on the rapidity with which the T4-cells are destroyed. For the majority of clients, the first sign that something is wrong is the development of chronically enlarged lymph nodes. This occurs because of overstimulation of B-lymphocytes by the continuous presence of HIV in the body. As the T4-cell count continues to decline, the client will begin to develop the first overt signs of inadequate cell-mediated immunity (e.g. persistent viral or fungal infections). Some will go on to develop symptoms such as fever, malaise, unexplained weight loss, night sweats, and persistent diarrhea. This group of symptoms has been referred to as AIDS-related complex or ARC. Acquired immune deficiency syndrome (AIDS), the end-stage manifestation of HIV infection, is associated with the development of chronic or disseminated opportunistic infections at sites other than the skin and mucous membranes (e.g. *Pneumocystis carinii* pneumonia [PCP], cryptococcosis, toxoplasmosis, strongyloidiasis, cytomegalovirus infection, candidiasis), HIV-related cancers (e.g. Kaposi's sarcoma [KS], non-Hodgkin's lymphoma, primary CNS lymphoma), and/or HIV encephalopathy, which results from the direct effect of HIV on the central nervous system. Because there is no known cure at this time for HIV infection or the underlying immunodeficiency, treatment is aimed primarily at prevention and control of the potentially fatal opportunistic diseases to which the infected person is particularly susceptible.

This care plan focuses on the adult client hospitalized with signs and symptoms of an opportunistic infection and probable AIDS. Goals of care are to assist with measures to treat the infection, reduce fear and anxiety, maintain comfort, assist the client to cope with the diagnosis, and educate him/her regarding follow-up care. A major concern while caring for the client with AIDS is prevention of the spread of infection to others. It is the responsibility of each health care provider to carry out appropriate precautions as defined by hospital policy to prevent disease transmission. If the client is admitted with an opportunistic infection involving the respiratory system, this care plan should be used in conjunction with the Care Plan on Pneumonia.

DISCHARGE CRITERIA

Prior to discharge, the client will:

- identify ways to prevent the spread of HIV
- identify ways to decrease the risk of opportunistic infections
- state signs and symptoms to report to the health care provider
- share feelings about change in self-concept and the social isolation that may result from the diagnosis

- identify community resources that can assist in adjustment to changes resulting from the diagnosis of AIDS
- verbalize an understanding of and a plan for adhering to recommended follow-up care including future appointments with health care provider and medications prescribed.

NURSING DIAGNOSES

1. Anxiety ☐ *573*
2. Altered nutrition: less than body requirements ☐ *574*
3. Altered comfort: chills and excessive diaphoresis ☐ *575*
4. Hyperthermia ☐ *576*
5. Altered oral mucous membrane: stomatitis, pharyngitis, and esophagitis ☐ *576*
6. Activity intolerance ☐ *577*
7. Self-care deficit ☐ *578*
8. Diarrhea ☐ *579*
9. Altered thought processes: slowed verbal responses, inability to concentrate, memory loss, impaired reasoning ability and judgment, apathy toward personal and professional responsibilities, disorientation, and hallucinations ☐ *580*
10. Sleep pattern disturbance ☐ *581*
11. Potential for infection: opportunistic ☐ *582*
12. Potential for trauma ☐ *583*
13. Sexual dysfunction:
    a. alteration in usual sexual activities
    b. decreased libido
    c. impotence ☐ *584*
14. Ineffective individual coping ☐ *584*
15. Powerlessness ☐ *585*
16. Grieving ☐ *586*
17. Social isolation ☐ *587*
18. Altered family processes ☐ *588*
19. Knowledge deficit regarding follow-up care ☐ *589*

UNIT XI

---

1. NURSING DIAGNOSIS

Anxiety related to unfamiliar environment; current signs and symptoms; lack of understanding of diagnostic tests, diagnosis of AIDS and its implications, and treatment plan; disclosure of diagnosis; and probability of premature death.

DESIRED OUTCOMES	NURSING ACTIONS AND *SELECTED RATIONALES*
1. The client will experience a reduction in fear and anxiety	1.a. Assess client for signs and symptoms of fear and anxiety (e.g. verbalization of fears and concerns; tenseness; tremors; irritability; restlessness;

as evidenced by:
a. verbalization of feeling less anxious or fearful
b. relaxed facial expression and body movements
c. stable vital signs
d. usual skin color
e. verbalization of an understanding of hospital routines, diagnostic tests, diagnosis, treatment plan, and prognosis.

diaphoresis; tachypnea; tachycardia; elevated blood pressure; facial tension, pallor, or flushing; noncompliance with treatments and isolation precautions). Validate perceptions carefully, remembering that some behavior may be due to neurological changes resulting from HIV infection.

b. Ascertain the effectiveness of current coping skills.
c. Implement measures *to reduce fear and anxiety:*
   1. orient to hospital environment, equipment, and routines
   2. introduce staff who will be participating in his/her care; if possible, maintain consistency in staff assigned to his/her care *to provide feelings of stability and comfort with the environment*
   3. assure client that staff members are nearby; respond to call signal as soon as possible
   4. maintain a calm, confident manner when interacting with client
   5. encourage verbalization of fear and anxiety; provide feedback
   6. explain all tests that may be performed to diagnose HIV infection and/or concurrent diseases:
      a. blood studies (e.g. enzyme-linked immunosorbent assay [ELISA], immunofluorescence assay [IFA], and Western Blot *to detect and confirm presence of antibodies to HIV*; T4:T8 ratio; total lymphocyte counts; monocyte analysis)
      b. magnetic resonance imaging [MRI] for suspected cerebral toxoplasmosis
      c. bronchoscopy and chest x-rays for suspected PCP
      d. skin lesion biopsy for KS
   7. reinforce physician's explanation about HIV infection including mode of transmission, effects on immune system, and prognosis; encourage questions and clarify misconceptions
   8. provide a calm, restful environment
   9. instruct in relaxation techniques and encourage participation in quiet diversional activities
   10. perform actions to assist client to cope with the diagnosis and its implications (see Nursing Diagnosis 14, action d)
   11. encourage significant others to project a caring, concerned attitude without obvious anxiousness
   12. monitor for therapeutic and nontherapeutic effects of antianxiety agents if administered.
d. Include significant others in orientation and teaching sessions and encourage their continued support of the client. Assist them to understand the client's fears and to express theirs.
e. Provide information based on current needs of client and significant others at a level they can understand. Encourage questions and clarification of information provided.
f. Consult physician if above actions fail to control fear and anxiety.

2. NURSING DIAGNOSIS

Altered nutrition: less than body requirements related to:

a. decreased oral intake associated with:
   1. anorexia resulting from malaise, fatigue, fear, anxiety, and depression
   2. oral pain and/or dysphagia resulting from stomatitis, pharyngitis, and esophagitis;
b. increased utilization of nutrients associated with increased basal metabolic rate that is present in infections;
c. decreased absorption of nutrients associated with chronic diarrhea.

DESIRED OUTCOMES	NURSING ACTIONS AND *SELECTED RATIONALES*

2. The client will maintain an adequate nutritional status as evidenced by:
a. weight within normal range for client's age, height, and build
b. normal BUN and serum albumin, protein, Hct., Hgb., and cholesterol levels
c. triceps skinfold measurements within normal range
d. usual strength and activity tolerance
e. healthy oral mucous membrane.
	2.a. Assess the client for signs and symptoms of malnutrition:
	  1. weight below normal for client's age, height, and build
	  2. abnormal BUN and low serum albumin, protein, Hct., Hgb., and cholesterol levels
	  3. triceps skinfold measurement less than normal for build
	  4. weakness and fatigue
	  5. stomatitis.
	b. Reassess nutritional status on a regular basis and report decline.
	c. Monitor percentage of meals eaten.
	d. Assess the client to determine the causative factors of inadequate intake (e.g. anorexia, oral pain, dysphagia).
	e. Implement measures *to improve nutritional status:*
	  1. perform actions *to improve oral intake:*
	    a. implement measures to reduce discomfort associated with stomatitis, pharyngitis, and esophagitis (see Nursing Diagnosis 5, actions d and f)
	    b. implement measures to reduce fear and anxiety (see Nursing Diagnosis 1, action c)
	    c. assist client to select foods that are easily chewed and swallowed
	    d. provide oral care before meals
	    e. eliminate noxious stimuli from environment
	    f. obtain a dietary consult if necessary to assist client in selecting foods/fluids that meet nutritional needs as well as preferences
	    g. serve small portions of nutritious foods/fluids that are appealing to the client
	    h. encourage significant others to bring in client's favorite foods and eat with him/her *to make eating more of a familiar social experience*
	    i. encourage a rest period before meals *to minimize fatigue*
	    j. allow adequate time for meals; reheat food if necessary
	    k. increase activity as allowed and tolerated *(activity stimulates appetite)*
	  2. perform actions to control diarrhea (see Nursing Diagnosis 8, action f)
	  3. encourage and instruct client to increase intake of foods high in protein (e.g. meats, poultry, legumes, fish, dairy products) and carbohydrates (e.g. pasta, fruits, some vegetables) *in order to meet increased nutritional needs*
	  4. ensure that meals are well balanced and high in essential nutrients
	  5. monitor for therapeutic and nontherapeutic effects of vitamins and minerals if administered.
	f. Perform a 72-hour calorie count if nutritional status declines or fails to improve.
	g. Consult physician about alternative methods of providing nutrition (e.g. parenteral nutrition, tube feedings) if client does not consume enough food or fluids to meet nutritional needs.

3. NURSING DIAGNOSIS

Altered comfort: chills and excessive diaphoresis related to persistent or recurrent fever associated with HIV and opportunistic infection(s).

DESIRED OUTCOMES	NURSING ACTIONS AND *SELECTED RATIONALES*
3. The client will not experience discomfort associated with	3.a. Monitor client for chills and excessive diaphoresis. b. Implement measures to reduce fever (see Nursing Diagnosis 4, action b).

UNIT XI

chills and diaphoresis as evidenced by:
a. verbalization of comfort
b. ability to rest.

c. Implement measures *to promote comfort if client is having chills:*
   1. maintain a room temperature that is comfortable for client
   2. protect client from drafts
   3. provide extra blankets and clothing as needed
   4. provide warm liquids to drink as tolerated.
d. Implement measures *to promote comfort if excessive diaphoresis is present:*
   1. change linen and clothing whenever damp
   2. bathe client and sponge his/her face as needed.
e. Consult physician if client continues to have chills and excessive diaphoresis.

☐ ▬▬▬▬▬▬▬▬▬▬▬▬▬▬▬▬▬▬▬▬▬▬▬▬▬

4. NURSING DIAGNOSIS

Hyperthermia related to stimulation of the thermoregulatory center in the hypothalamus by endogenous pyrogens that are released in an infectious process.

☐ ▬▬▬▬▬▬▬▬▬▬▬▬▬▬▬▬▬▬▬▬▬▬▬▬▬

DESIRED OUTCOMES	NURSING ACTIONS AND *SELECTED RATIONALES*

4. The client will experience resolution of hyperthermia as evidenced by:
   a. skin usual color and temperature
   b. pulse rate between 60–100 beats/minute
   c. respirations 16–20/minute
   d. normal body temperature.

4.a. Assess for signs and symptoms of hyperthermia (e.g. warm, flushed skin; tachycardia; tachypnea; elevated temperature).
b. Implement measures *to reduce fever:*
   1. perform actions *to resolve the infectious process:*
      a. implement measures to promote rest (see Nursing Diagnosis 6, action b.1)
      b. implement measures to maintain an optimal nutritional status (see Nursing Diagnosis 2, action e)
      c. monitor for therapeutic and nontherapeutic effects of anti-infectives if administered
   2. administer tepid sponge bath
   3. apply cooling blanket as ordered
   4. monitor for therapeutic and nontherapeutic effects of antipyretics if administered.
c. Consult physician if temperature remains higher than 38°C.

☐ ▬▬▬▬▬▬▬▬▬▬▬▬▬▬▬▬▬▬▬▬▬▬▬▬▬

5. NURSING DIAGNOSIS

Altered oral mucous membrane: stomatitis, pharyngitis, and esophagitis related to malnutrition, hairy leukoplakia of the tongue, and infection associated with *Candida albicans* and/or herpes simplex (commonly occurs with an incompetent immune system).

☐ ▬▬▬▬▬▬▬▬▬▬▬▬▬▬▬▬▬▬▬▬▬▬▬▬▬

DESIRED OUTCOMES	NURSING ACTIONS AND *SELECTED RATIONALES*

5. The client will maintain a healthy oral cavity as evidenced by:
   a. absence of inflammation and ulcerations
   b. pink, moist, intact mucosa

5.a. Assess client for and report signs and symptoms of stomatitis, pharyngitis, and esophagitis (e.g. inflamed and/or ulcerated oral mucosa; leukoplakia; complaints of oral, pharyngeal, or esophageal dryness and burning; changes in quality of voice; dysphagia; viscous saliva).
b. Obtain cultures from suspicious oral lesions as ordered. Report positive results.

c. absence of oral, pharyngeal, and esophageal dryness and burning

d. ability to swallow without discomfort

e. usual consistency of saliva.

c. Prepare client for and assist with endoscopy if performed to obtain culture specimens from esophagus. Report positive results.

d. Implement measures *to prevent or reduce the severity of stomatitis, pharyngitis, and esophagitis:*
   1. reinforce importance of and assist client with oral hygiene after meals and snacks
   2. have client rinse mouth frequently with warm saline or baking soda and water
   3. instruct client to avoid products such as lemon-glycerin swabs and commercial mouthwashes containing alcohol *(these products have a drying or irritating effect on oral mucous membrane)*
   4. encourage client to breathe through nose *in order to reduce mouth dryness*
   5. encourage a fluid intake of at least 2500 cc/day unless contraindicated
   6. maintain an optimal nutritional status (see Nursing Diagnosis 2, action e)
   7. encourage client not to smoke *(smoking further irritates and dries the mucosa)*
   8. lubricate client's lips with Vaseline, K-Y jelly, ChapStick, Blistex, or mineral oil when oral care is given
   9. assist with selection of soft, nonspicy, and nonacidic foods
   10. instruct client to avoid extremely hot or cold foods/fluids
   11. use a soft bristle brush or low-pressure power spray for oral care
   12. monitor for therapeutic and nontherapeutic effects of antifungal (e.g. clotrimazole troches, nystatin suspension, ketoconazole) and antiviral (e.g. acyclovir) agents if administered.

e. If stomatitis is not controlled:
   1. increase frequency of oral hygiene
   2. if client has dentures, remove and replace only for meals.

f. Monitor for therapeutic and nontherapeutic effects of antacids, topical anesthetics, oral protective pastes, and topical and systemic analgesics if administered.

g. Consult physician if signs and symptoms of stomatitis, pharyngitis, and esophagitis persist or worsen.

□ ▬▬▬▬▬▬▬▬▬▬▬▬▬▬▬▬▬▬▬▬▬▬▬▬

6. NURSING DIAGNOSIS

Activity intolerance related to:

a. inability to rest and sleep;

b. increased energy utilization associated with the elevated basal metabolic rate that is present in infection;

c. malnutrition;

d. tissue hypoxia associated with impaired alveolar gas exchange if respiratory infection is present.

□ ▬▬▬▬▬▬▬▬▬▬▬▬▬▬▬▬▬▬▬▬▬▬▬▬

DESIRED OUTCOMES	NURSING ACTIONS AND *SELECTED RATIONALES*
6. The client will demonstrate an increased tolerance for activity as evidenced by: a. verbalization of feeling less fatigued and weak b. ability to perform activities of daily living without	6.a. Assess for signs and symptoms of activity intolerance: 1. statements of fatigue and weakness 2. exertional dyspnea, chest pain, increased diaphoresis, or dizziness 3. decrease in pulse rate or an increase in rate of 20 beats/minute above resting rate 4. pulse rate not returning to preactivity level within 5 minutes after stopping activity

exertional dyspnea, chest pain, increased diaphoresis, dizziness, or a significant change in vital signs.

5. decreased blood pressure or an increase in diastolic pressure of 15 mm Hg with activity.
   b. Implement measures *to improve activity tolerance:*
   1. perform actions *to promote rest:*
      a. maintain activity restrictions if ordered
      b. minimize environmental activity and noise
      c. schedule nursing care and diagnostic procedures to allow periods of uninterrupted rest
      d. limit the number of visitors and their length of stay
      e. assist client with self-care activities as needed
      f. keep supplies and personal articles within easy reach
      g. implement measures to reduce fear and anxiety (see Nursing Diagnosis 1, action c)
      h. implement measures to promote sleep (see Nursing Diagnosis 10, action c)
   2. perform actions to resolve the infectious process (see Nursing Diagnosis 4, action b.1)
   3. instruct client in energy-saving techniques (e.g. using shower chair when showering, sitting to brush teeth or comb hair)
   4. perform actions to improve nutritional status (see Nursing Diagnosis 2, action e)
   5. increase client's activity as allowed and tolerated.
   c. Instruct client to:
   1. report a decreased tolerance for activity
   2. stop any activity that causes chest pain, shortness of breath, dizziness, or extreme fatigue or weakness.
   d. Consult physician if signs and symptoms of activity intolerance persist or worsen.

☐ ▬▬▬▬▬▬▬▬▬▬▬▬▬▬▬▬▬▬▬▬▬▬▬▬

7. NURSING DIAGNOSIS

Self-care deficit related to activity intolerance, altered thought processes, and activity restrictions imposed by the treatment plan.

☐ ▬▬▬▬▬▬▬▬▬▬▬▬▬▬▬▬▬▬▬▬▬▬▬▬

DESIRED OUTCOMES	NURSING ACTIONS AND *SELECTED RATIONALES*

7. The client will demonstrate increased participation in self-care activities within activity tolerance level and restrictions imposed by the treatment plan.	7.a. Assess for factors that interfere with the client's ability to perform self-care (e.g. fatigue, weakness, disorientation).
	b. With client, develop a realistic plan for meeting daily physical needs.
	c. Encourage maximum independence within limitations imposed by fatigue, weakness, altered thought processes, and treatment plan.
	d. Implement measures *to facilitate the client's ability to perform self-care activities:*
	  1. perform actions to improve activity tolerance (see Nursing Diagnosis 6, action b)
	  2. schedule care at a time when client is most likely to be able to participate (e.g. after rest periods, not immediately after meals or treatments)
	  3. keep needed objects within easy reach
	  4. allow adequate time for accomplishment of self-care activities.
	e. Provide positive feedback for all efforts and accomplishments of self-care.
	f. Assist the client with those activities he/she is unable to perform independently.
	g. Inform significant others of client's abilities to perform own care. Explain the importance of encouraging and allowing client to maintain an optimal level of independence within prescribed activity restrictions and his/her activity tolerance level and level of orientation.

□ �

8. NURSING DIAGNOSIS

Diarrhea related to:

a. enterocolitis associated with bacterial, parasitic, and/or viral infection(s);
b. increased gastrointestinal motility associated with extreme fear and anxiety;
c. possible direct effect of HIV on cells of intestinal mucosa.

□ �

DESIRED OUTCOMES	NURSING ACTIONS AND *SELECTED RATIONALES*

8. The client will have fewer bowel movements and more formed stool.	8.a. Ascertain client's usual bowel elimination habits.
	b. Assess for signs and symptoms of diarrhea (e.g. frequent, loose stools; abdominal pain and cramping).
	c. Assess bowel sounds regularly. Report an increase in frequency of and/or high-pitched bowel sounds.
	d. Obtain stool specimens for bacterial culture and/or examination for parasites. Report positive results.
	e. Prepare client for anoscopy, proctoscopy, sigmoidoscopy, and/or colonoscopy if planned *to examine mucosa, obtain specimens for culture, and/or perform biopsies.*
	f. Implement measures *to control diarrhea:*
	  1. perform actions *to rest the bowel:*
	    a. instruct client to avoid foods/fluids that are poorly digested or act as irritants to the inflamed bowel:
	      1. milk (client may have a milk intolerance due to a deficiency of lactase)
	      2. those high in fat (e.g. butter, cream, oils, whole milk, ice cream, pork, fried foods, gravies, nuts)
	      3. those with high fiber content (e.g. whole-grain cereals, nuts, raw fruits and vegetables)
	      4. those known to cause diarrhea or be gas-producers (e.g. cabbage, onions, popcorn, licorice, prunes, chili, baked beans, carbonated beverages)
	      5. those high in caffeine (e.g. chocolate, coffee, tea, colas)
	      6. spicy foods
	      7. extremely hot or cold foods/fluids
	    b. provide small, frequent meals
	    c. implement measures to reduce fear and anxiety (see Nursing Diagnosis 1, action c)
	    d. discourage smoking *(nicotine has a stimulant effect on the gastrointestinal tract)*
	  2. monitor for therapeutic and nontherapeutic effects of the following medications if administered:
	    a. opiate or opiate-like substances (e.g. loperamide, diphenoxylate hydrochloride) *to decrease gastrointestinal motility*
	    b. bulk-forming agents (e.g. methylcellulose, psyllium hydrophilic mucilloid, calcium polycarbophil) *to absorb water in the bowel and produce a soft, formed stool*
	    c. antiviral agents (e.g. acyclovir, ganciclovir [DHPG], zidovudine [AZT]), antibiotics (e.g. penicillin, tetracycline), and antifungal agents (e.g. amphotericin B, metronidazole, ketoconazole) *to treat the infectious process.*
	g. Consult physician if:
	  1. diarrhea persists or worsens
	  2. signs and symptoms of fluid volume deficit (e.g. decreased skin turgor, significant weight loss, dry mucous membranes, decreased B/P, increased pulse) and/or electrolyte imbalances (e.g. confusion, muscle or abdominal cramps, irregular pulse) occur.

9. NURSING DIAGNOSIS

Altered thought processes: slowed verbal responses, inability to concentrate, memory loss, impaired reasoning ability and judgment, apathy toward personal and professional responsibilities, disorientation, and hallucinations related to:

a. HIV encephalopathy associated with direct effect of HIV on nervous system (encephalopathy may be present with or without the other characteristics of HIV infection, usually begins insidiously, and gradually progresses);

b. cerebral toxoplasmosis, cryptococcal or tuberculous meningitis, herpes simplex, herpes zoster, cytomegalovirus (CMV) encephalitis, and/or neoplasms of the central nervous system;

c. excessive or inappropriate use of psychoactive drugs in client with HIV encephalopathy (may initiate or aggravate delirium).

DESIRED OUTCOMES	NURSING ACTIONS AND *SELECTED RATIONALES*

9. The client will experience improvement in thought processes as evidenced by:
  a. improved verbal response time
  b. longer attention span
  c. improved memory
  d. improved reasoning ability and judgment
  e. decreased apathy
  f. improved level of orientation
  g. absence of hallucinations.
	9.a. Assess client for alterations in thought processes (e.g. slowed verbal responses, inability to concentrate, memory loss, impaired reasoning ability and judgment, apathy, disorientation, hallucinations).
	  b. Ascertain from significant others client's usual level of intellectual functioning.
	  c. Prepare client for computed tomography, EEG, neuropsychiatric testing, and/or MRI if indicated *to determine specific cause of mental decline.*
	  d. Monitor for therapeutic and nontherapeutic effects of the following medications if administered *to treat conditions that can alter thought processes:*
	    1. anti-infectives (e.g. penicillin, tetracycline, pyrimethamine, sulfadiazine, amphotericin B, acyclovir, DHPG, AZT) *to treat infectious processes*
	    2. cytotoxic agents *to treat neoplastic conditions affecting nervous system*
	    3. antipsychotic agents (e.g. haloperidol, thioridazine) *to treat restlessness, agitation, or hallucinations* or central nervous system stimulants (e.g. amphetamine sulfate) *to reduce apathy and withdrawn behavior* (psychoactive drugs should be used very cautiously and in small, titrated doses *because of their potential to initiate or aggravate delirium in the client with HIV encephalopathy).*
	  e. If client shows evidence of altered thought processes:
	    1. reorient to person, place, and time as necessary
	    2. allow adequate time for communication and performance of activities
	    3. repeat instructions as necessary using clear, simple language
	    4. keep environmental stimuli to a minimum
	    5. write out schedule of activities for client to refer to if desired
	    6. encourage client to make lists of planned activities and questions or concerns he/she may have
	    7. assist client to problem-solve if necessary
	    8. maintain realistic expectations of client's ability to learn, comprehend, and remember information provided
	    9. if client is experiencing hallucinations, allow significant others or sitter to remain with client *in order to provide constant reassurance*
	    10. encourage significant others to be supportive of client; instruct them in methods of dealing with alterations in thought processes
	    11. discuss physiological basis for alterations in thought processes with client and significant others
	    12. consult physician if alterations in thought processes worsen.

10. NURSING DIAGNOSIS

Sleep pattern disturbance related to fear, anxiety, frequent assessments and treatments, chills, diarrhea, night sweats, dyspnea (may occur if respiratory infection is present), decreased physical activity, and unfamiliar environment.

DESIRED OUTCOMES	NURSING ACTIONS AND *SELECTED RATIONALES*

10. The client will attain optimal amounts of sleep within the parameters of the treatment regimen as evidenced by:
a. statements of feeling well rested
b. usual behavior
c. absence of frequent yawning, thick speech, dark circles under eyes.
	10.a. Assess for signs and symptoms of a sleep pattern disturbance:
	  1. verbal complaints of difficulty falling asleep, not feeling well rested, sleep interruptions, or awakening earlier or later than desired
	  2. behavior changes (e.g. irritability, increased disorganization, lethargy)
	  3. frequent yawning, thick speech, dark circles under eyes, slight hand tremors).
	b. Determine the client's usual sleep habits.
	c. Implement measures *to promote sleep:*
	  1. perform actions to reduce fear and anxiety (see Nursing Diagnosis 1, action c)
	  2. perform actions to reduce discomfort associated with chills and excessive diaphoresis (see Nursing Diagnosis 3, actions c and d)
	  3. perform actions to control diarrhea (see Nursing Diagnosis 8, action f)
	  4. if dyspnea is present:
	    a. assist client to assume a comfortable sleep position (e.g. bed in reverse Trendelenburg position with client in usual recumbent sleep position, head of bed elevated with arms supported on pillows, resting forward on overbed table with good pillow support, sitting in chair)
	    b. maintain oxygen therapy during sleep
	  5. allow client to continue usual sleep practices (e.g. position, time, bedtime rituals) if possible
	  6. determine measures that have been helpful to the client in the past (e.g. milk, warm drinks, warm bath) and incorporate in plan of care
	  7. discourage long periods of sleep during the day unless sleep deprivation exists or daytime sleep is usual for client
	  8. encourage participation in relaxing diversional activities in early evening hours
	  9. provide a quiet, restful atmosphere
	  10. discourage intake of foods and fluids high in caffeine (e.g. chocolate, coffee, tea, colas), especially in the evening
	  11. satisfy basic needs such as hunger, comfort, and warmth before sleep
	  12. have client empty bladder just before bedtime
	  13. utilize relaxation techniques (e.g. progressive relaxation exercises, back massage, meditation, soft music) before sleep
	  14. perform actions *to provide for periods of uninterrupted sleep (90- to 120-minute periods of uninterrupted sleep are considered essential)*
	    a. restrict visitors during rest periods
	    b. group care (e.g. medications, treatments, physical care, assessments) whenever possible
	  15. monitor for therapeutic and nontherapeutic effects of sedatives and hypnotics if administered.
	d. Consult physician if signs of sleep deprivation persist or worsen.

UNIT
XI

11. NURSING DIAGNOSIS

Potential for infection: opportunistic related to decreased natural resistance associated with:

a. cellular and humoral immune deficiencies present in HIV infection;
b. general debilitation and malnutrition;
c. treatment of current infection with anti-infectives;
d. depletion of immune mechanisms associated with the presenting infection.

DESIRED OUTCOMES	NURSING ACTIONS AND *SELECTED RATIONALES*

11. The client will remain free of opportunistic infection as evidenced by:
    a. return of temperature toward normal
    b. decrease in episodes of chills and diaphoresis
    c. pulse returning toward normal range
    d. normal or improved breath sounds
    e. absence or resolution of dyspnea and cyanosis
    f. voiding clear, yellow urine without complaints of frequency, urgency, and burning
    g. absence of painful, pruritic skin lesions
    h. stable or gradual increase in body weight
    i. increased strength and activity tolerance
    j. absence of visual disturbances
    k. absence of redness, swelling, and unusual drainage in any area where there is a break in skin integrity
    l. resolution of oral mucous membrane irritation and ulceration
    m. ability to swallow without difficulty
    n. WBC and differential counts returning toward normal range
    o. negative results of cultured specimens.

11.a. Assess for and report signs and symptoms of opportunistic infection:
    1. increase in temperature above client's usual level
    2. increase in episodes of chills and diaphoresis
    3. pattern of increased pulse or pulse rate greater than 100 beats/minute
    4. development or worsening of adventitious breath sounds
    5. development or worsening of dyspnea and cyanosis
    6. cloudy or foul-smelling urine
    7. complaints of frequency, urgency, or burning when urinating
    8. presence of WBCs, bacteria, and/or nitrites in urine
    9. extensive vesicular lesions particularly on face, lips, and perianal area
    10. complaints of pain in and/or itching of skin lesions and surrounding tissue
    11. further increase in weight loss, fatigue, and weakness
    12. visual disturbances
    13. redness, swelling, or unusual drainage in any area where there is a break in skin integrity
    14. irritation or ulceration of oral mucous membrane
    15. dysphagia
    16. significant change in WBC count and/or differential.
b. Obtain culture specimens (e.g. urine, vaginal, rectal, mouth, sputum, blood, skin lesions) as ordered. Report positive results.
c. Implement measures *to treat existing and prevent further infection:*
    1. monitor for therapeutic and nontherapeutic effects of the following medications if administered:
        a. antibiotic and antifungal agents
        b. immune system stimulators (e.g. interleukin-2, alpha and gamma interferon, Ampligen)
        c. antiviral agents such as acyclovir *to treat opportunistic infection* or AZT *to prevent replication of HIV*
    2. maintain a fluid intake of at least 2500 cc/day unless contraindicated
    3. use good handwashing technique and encourage client to do the same
    4. protect client from others with infection
    5. instruct client to avoid use of shared eating utensils
    6. maintain an optimal nutritional status (see Nursing Diagnosis 2, action e)
    7. perform actions to prevent or reduce severity of stomatitis, pharyngitis, and esophagitis (see Nursing Diagnosis 5, actions d–f)
    8. maintain meticulous aseptic technique during all invasive procedures (e.g. catheterization, venous and arterial punctures, injections)
    9. perform actions to promote rest (see Nursing Diagnosis 6, action b.1)
    10. perform actions *to prevent respiratory tract infection:*
        a. instruct and assist client to turn, cough, and deep breathe at least every 2 hours if activity is limited
        b. instruct and assist client in use of inspiratory exerciser at least every 2 hours if indicated

c. encourage client to stop smoking
d. increase activity as allowed and tolerated
11. perform actions *to prevent urinary tract infection:*
a. instruct and assist female client to wipe from front to back following urination and defecation
b. keep perianal area clean.

☐ ▬▬▬▬▬▬▬▬▬▬▬▬▬▬▬▬▬▬▬▬▬▬▬▬▬▬

12. NURSING DIAGNOSIS

Potential for trauma related to falls associated with:

a. weakness and fatigue;
b. confusion and/or impaired motor function resulting from HIV encephalopathy.

☐ ▬▬▬▬▬▬▬▬▬▬▬▬▬▬▬▬▬▬▬▬▬▬▬▬▬▬

DESIRED OUTCOMES	NURSING ACTIONS AND *SELECTED RATIONALES*

12. The client will not experience falls.	12.a. Determine whether conditions predisposing client to falls (e.g. confusion, weakness, fatigue, impaired motor function) exist.
	b. Implement measures *to prevent falls:*
	  1. keep bed in low position with side rails up when client is in bed
	  2. keep needed items within easy reach
	  3. encourage client to request assistance whenever needed; have call signal within easy reach
	  4. use lap belt when client is in chair if indicated
	  5. instruct client to wear shoes with nonskid soles and low heels when ambulating
	  6. avoid unnecessary clutter in room
	  7. accompany client during ambulation utilizing a transfer safety belt if he/she is weak or unsteady on feet
	  8. provide ambulatory aids (e.g. walker, cane) if client is weak or unsteady on feet
	  9. reinforce instructions from physical therapist regarding correct transfer and ambulation techniques
	  10. instruct client to ambulate in well-lit areas and to utilize handrails if needed
	  11. do not rush client; allow adequate time for trips to the bathroom and ambulation in hallway
	  12. perform actions to improve strength and activity tolerance (see Nursing Diagnosis 6, action b)
	  13. if client is confused or irrational, implement additional measures *to reduce the risk of falls:*
	    a. reorient frequently to surroundings and necessity of adhering to safety precautions
	    b. provide constant supervision (e.g. staff member, significant other) if indicated
	    c. use jacket or wrist restraints or safety alarm device if necessary *to reduce the risk of client's getting out of bed or chair unattended*
	    d. monitor for therapeutic and nontherapeutic effects of antianxiety and antipsychotic medications if administered.
	c. Include client and significant others in planning and implementing measures to prevent falls.
	d. If falls occur, initiate appropriate first aid measures and notify physician.

13. NURSING DIAGNOSIS

Sexual dysfunction:

a. **alteration in usual sexual activities** related to limitations imposed by the treatment plan;
b. **decreased libido** related to fatigue, weakness, depression, fear, and anxiety;
c. **impotence** related to ineffective coping and fear of rejection by desired partner(s) and/or transmission of HIV to others.

DESIRED OUTCOMES	NURSING ACTIONS AND *SELECTED RATIONALES*
13. The client will perceive self as sexually adequate and acceptable as evidenced by: a. verbalization of same b. maintenance of relationships with significant others c. statements reflecting beginning adjustment to altered modes of expression of sexuality.	13.a. Assess for signs and symptoms of sexual dysfunction (e.g. verbalization of sexual concerns, failure to maintain relationships with significant others). b. Determine attitudes, knowledge, and concerns about AIDS in relation to sexual functioning. c. Communicate interest, understanding, and respect for the values of the client and his/her partner. d. Provide accurate information to significant others about transmission of HIV during intimate contact. Encourage questions and clarify any misconceptions and fears. e. Facilitate communication between client and his/her partner(s). Assist them to identify factors that may affect their sexual relationship. f. Arrange for uninterrupted privacy during hospital stay if desired by the couple. g. Discuss various options (e.g. masturbation, safe sexual activity with partner[s]) for meeting sexual needs. h. Discuss ways to be creative in expressing sexuality (e.g. massage, fantasies, cuddling). i. Encourage client to keep current on new information about how HIV is spread. j. Provide information on support groups and professional counselors that can assist client in adjusting to effects of AIDS on sexuality. k. Consult physician if counseling appears indicated.

14. NURSING DIAGNOSIS

Ineffective individual coping related to:

a. depression, fear, and anxiety associated with the diagnosis and poor prognosis;
b. effect of the altered immune response and diagnosis of AIDS on usual life style and roles;
c. fear of rejection by others;
d. guilt associated with past behavior or style of living and possibility of having transmitted HIV to others;
e. drug withdrawal if HIV infection developed as a result of parenteral substance abuse;
f. inadequate support system.

DESIRED OUTCOMES	NURSING ACTIONS AND *SELECTED RATIONALES*

14. The client will demonstrate the use of effective coping skills as evidenced by:
   a. willingness to participate in treatment plan and self-care activities
   b. verbalization of ability to cope with the diagnosis and its implications
   c. identification of stressors
   d. utilization of appropriate problem-solving techniques
   e. recognition and utilization of available support systems.

14.a. Assess effectiveness of client's coping strategies by observing behavior and noting strengths, weaknesses, ability to express feelings and concerns, and willingness to participate in treatment plan.
   b. Assess for and report signs and symptoms that may indicate ineffective coping (e.g. sleep disturbances, increasing fatigue, difficulty concentrating, irritability, verbalization of inability to cope, inability to problem-solve).
   c. Allow time for client to adjust psychologically to the diagnosis and its implications.
   d. Implement measures *to promote effective coping:*
      1. arrange for a visit with another who is successfully living with AIDS
      2. perform actions to reduce fear and anxiety (see Nursing Diagnosis 1, action c)
      3. include client in planning of care, encourage maximum participation in the treatment plan, and allow choices when possible *to enable client to maintain a sense of control*
      4. instruct client in effective problem-solving techniques (e.g. accurate identification of stressors, determination of various options to solve problem)
      5. assist client to maintain usual daily routines whenever possible
      6. assist client as he/she starts to plan for necessary life-style and role changes after discharge; provide input related to realistic prioritization of problems that need to be dealt with
      7. assist client and significant others to identify ways that personal and family goals can be adjusted rather than abandoned
      8. discuss ways to maintain health despite a defective immune system; focus on methods of altering rather than changing life style
      9. assist client through methods such as role playing to prepare for negative reactions because of diagnosis of AIDS
      10. assist client to identify and utilize available support systems; provide information about community resources and support groups that can assist client and significant others in coping with effects of AIDS (e.g. Phoenix Rising, Cascade AIDS Project, National Gay Task Force, drug abuse programs, hot lines).
   e. Encourage continued emotional support from significant others. Provide them with current, accurate information about HIV infection *in order to reduce risk of their rejection of the client.*
   f. Encourage client to share with significant others the kind of support that would be most beneficial (e.g. listening, inspiring hope, providing reassurance and accurate information).
   g. Assess for and support behaviors suggesting positive adaptation to changes experienced (e.g. verbalization of ability to cope with diagnosis of AIDS, utilization of available support systems and effective problem-solving strategies).
   h. Consult physician about psychological counseling if appropriate.

UNIT
XI

15. NURSING DIAGNOSIS

Powerlessness related to:

a. feeling of loss of control over health and life;
b. terminal nature of AIDS;
c. increasing dependence on others to meet basic needs;
d. changes in roles, relationships, and future plans.

DESIRED OUTCOMES	NURSING ACTIONS AND *SELECTED RATIONALES*

15. The client will demonstrate increasing feelings of control over his/her situation as evidenced by:
  a. verbalization of same
  b. active participation in planning of care
  c. participation in self-care within physical limitations.
	15.a. Assess client for feelings of powerlessness (e.g. verbalization of lack of control, anger, apathy, hostility, lack of participation in care planning or self-care).
	  b. Obtain information from client and significant others regarding client's usual response to situations in which he/she has had limited control (e.g. loss of job, financial stress).
	  c. Encourage client to verbalize feelings about self and current situation.
	  d. Reinforce physician's explanation about AIDS and the treatment plan. Clarify any misconceptions.
	  e. Encourage client to ask questions about his/her condition, prognosis, and treatment regimen.
	  f. Support client's efforts to increase knowledge of and control over condition. Provide relevant pamphlets, audiovisual materials, and information about available community support for persons with HIV infection.
	  g. Include client in the planning of care, encourage maximum participation in the treatment plan, and allow choices whenever possible *to enable him/her to maintain a sense of control.*
	  h. Consult physical or occupational therapist if indicated about adaptive devices that would allow client more independence in performing activities of daily living.
	  i. Encourage significant others to allow client to do as much as he/she is able *so that a feeling of independence can be maintained as long as possible.*
	  j. Assist client to establish realistic short- and long-term goals.
	  k. Encourage client's participation in support groups if indicated.
	  l. Provide continuity of care through written individualized care plans to ensure that client can maintain appropriate control over his/her environment for as long as possible.

☐ ▉▉▉▉▉▉▉▉▉▉▉▉▉▉▉▉▉▉▉▉▉▉▉▉▉▉▉▉▉▉

16. NURSING DIAGNOSIS

Grieving* related to:

a. changes in body functioning, life style, and roles associated with the disease process;

b. probable premature death.

---

* This diagnostic label includes anticipatory grieving and grieving following the actual losses/changes.

☐ ▉▉▉▉▉▉▉▉▉▉▉▉▉▉▉▉▉▉▉▉▉▉▉▉▉▉▉▉▉▉

DESIRED OUTCOMES	NURSING ACTIONS AND *SELECTED RATIONALES*

16. The client will demonstrate beginning progression through the grieving process as evidenced by:
  a. verbalization of feelings about AIDS and its implications
  b. expression of grief
  c. participation in treatment plan and self-care activities
	16.a. Determine the client's perception of the impact of AIDS on his/her future.
	  b. Determine how client usually expresses grief.
	  c. Observe for signs of grieving (e.g. changes in eating habits, insomnia, anger, noncompliance, denial).
	  d. Implement measures *to facilitate the grieving process:*
	    1. assist client to acknowledge the changes resulting from the diagnosis of AIDS *so grief work can begin;* assess for factors that may hinder or facilitate acknowledgment
	    2. discuss the grieving process and assist client to accept the stages of grieving as an expected response to actual and/or anticipated changes or losses

d. utilization of available support systems
e. verbalization of a plan for integrating prescribed follow-up care into life style.

3. allow time for client to progress through the stages of grieving (denial, anger, bargaining, depression, acceptance [Kübler-Ross, 1969]); be aware that not every stage is experienced or expressed by all individuals

4. provide an atmosphere of care and concern (e.g. provide privacy, be available and nonjudgmental, display empathy and respect) *so that client will feel free to verbalize both positive and negative feelings and concerns*

5. perform actions *to promote trust* (e.g. answer questions honestly, provide requested information)

6. encourage the expression of anger and sadness about the diagnosis of AIDS; recognize displacement of anger and assist client to see actual cause of angry feelings and resentment; establish limits on abusive behavior

7. encourage client to express his/her feelings in whatever ways are comfortable (e.g. writing, drawing, conversation)

8. perform actions to facilitate effective coping (see Nursing Diagnosis 14, action d)

9. support realistic hope by providing accurate information about extensive research currently being done on HIV infection and the possibility of more effective treatment and discovery of a cure.

e. Assess for and support behaviors suggesting successful resolution of grief (e.g. verbalizing feelings about changes and losses, expressing sorrow, focusing on ways to adapt to changes and losses that have occurred).

f. Explain stages of the grieving process to significant others. Encourage their support, understanding, and presence.

g. Provide information regarding counseling services and support groups that might assist client in working through grief.

h. Arrange for visit from clergy if desired by client.

i. Monitor for therapeutic and nontherapeutic effects of antidepressants if administered.

j. Consult physician about referral for counseling if signs of dysfunctional grieving (e.g. persistent denial of losses or changes, excessive anger or sadness, hysteria, suicidal behaviors, phobias) occur.

□ ▬▬▬▬▬▬▬▬▬▬▬▬▬▬▬▬▬▬▬▬

17. NURSING DIAGNOSIS

Social isolation related to:

a. stigma associated with the diagnosis and others' fear of contracting HIV infection;
b. precautions necessary to prevent spread of disease;
c. client's fear of contracting an infection from others.

□ ▬▬▬▬▬▬▬▬▬▬▬▬▬▬▬▬▬▬▬▬

DESIRED OUTCOMES	NURSING ACTIONS AND *SELECTED RATIONALES*

17. The client will experience a decreased sense of isolation as evidenced by:
a. maintenance of relationships with significant others and casual acquaintances
b. verbalization of decreasing loneliness and feeling of rejection.
	17.a. Ascertain the client's usual degree of social interaction.
	b. Assess for and report behaviors indicative of social isolation (e.g. decreased interaction with significant others and staff; expression of feelings of rejection, abandonment, or being different from others; hostility; sad affect).
	c. Encourage client to express feelings of rejection and aloneness. Provide feedback and support.
	d. Implement measures *to decrease social isolation:*
	  1. reinforce physician's explanation about the immune deficiency; assure client that continued social contact with healthy adults will not cause disease or infection
	  2. assure significant others that HIV does not spread through ordinary physical contact and encourage them to visit client

3. facilitate staff acceptance of client by conferencing about constructive approaches to care
4. set up a schedule of visiting times so that client will not go for long periods without visitors
5. encourage telephone contact with significant others, local or national support groups, and hotlines
6. schedule time each day to sit and talk with client
7. assist client to identify a few persons he/she feels comfortable with and encourage interactions with them
8. support any appropriate movement away from social isolation.

18. NURSING DIAGNOSIS

Altered family processes related to:

a. diagnosis of terminal, communicable disease in family member;
b. fear of disclosure of diagnosis to others with subsequent rejection of family unit;
c. change in family roles and structure associated with progressive disability and eventual death of family member;
d. financial burden associated with extended illness and progressive disability of client;
e. fear of contracting disease from client.

DESIRED OUTCOMES	NURSING ACTIONS AND *SELECTED RATIONALES*
18. The family members* will demonstrate beginning adjustment to diagnosis of HIV infection in client and changes in family roles and structure as evidenced by: a. verbalization of ways to adapt to required role and life-style changes b. active participation in decision making and in client's care c. positive interactions with one another.	18.a. Identify components of the family and their patterns of communication and role expectations. b. Assess for signs and symptoms of alterations in family processes (e.g. statements of not being able to accept client's diagnosis or make necessary role and life-style changes, inability to make decisions, inability or refusal to participate in client's care, negative family interactions). c. Implement measures *to facilitate family members' adjustment to client's diagnosis and changes in family life style, roles, and structure:* 1. encourage and assist family members to verbalize feelings about client's diagnosis and its effect on their life style and family structure 2. reinforce physician's explanation about HIV infection, how it is transmitted, and planned treatment program 3. provide privacy *so that family members and client can share their feelings with one another;* stress the importance of and facilitate the use of good communication techniques 4. assist family members to progress through their own grieving process; explain that during this progression, they may encounter times when they need to focus on meeting their own rather than the client's needs 5. emphasize the need for family members to obtain adequate rest and nutrition and to identify and utilize stress management techniques *so that they are better able to emotionally and physically deal with the changes that are being experienced, physical care of the client, and reactions of others when diagnosis is known* 6. encourage and assist family members to identify coping strategies for dealing with the client's diagnosis and its effect on the family 7. include family members in decision making about client and his/her care; convey appreciation for their input and continued support of the client 8. encourage and allow family members to participate in client's care as appropriate

---

* The term "family members" is being used here to include client's significant others.

9. assist family members to identify sources that could assist them in coping with their feelings and meeting their immediate and long-term needs (e.g. counseling and social services; pastoral care; service, church, and AIDS support groups); initiate a referral if indicated.

d. Consult physician if family members continue to demonstrate difficulty adjusting to client's diagnosis and changes in roles and family structure.

☐ ▬▬▬▬▬▬▬▬▬▬▬▬▬▬▬▬▬▬▬▬▬▬▬▬▬▬▬▬▬▬

19. NURSING DIAGNOSIS

Knowledge deficit regarding follow-up care.

☐ ▬▬▬▬▬▬▬▬▬▬▬▬▬▬▬▬▬▬▬▬▬▬▬▬▬▬▬▬▬▬

DESIRED OUTCOMES	NURSING ACTIONS AND *SELECTED RATIONALES*

19.a. The client will identify ways to prevent the spread of HIV.

19.a. Instruct client in ways *to prevent spread of HIV to others:*
1. wash hands before handling food
2. cleanse hands carefully after using bathroom and after contact with body fluids such as semen, mucus, and blood
3. wash dishes in very hot, soapy water (disinfectant is not necessary)
4. if a spill of urine or other body fluids occurs, cleanse area with hot, soapy water and then disinfect with a solution of 1 part bleach to 9 parts water *(this solution is sufficient to kill HIV and other organisms)*
5. do not rinse mops and sponges used to clean up body fluid spills in sinks where food is prepared; dirty mop water should be disposed of in the toilet
6. do not share eating utensils, towels, wash cloths, toothbrushes, razors, enema equipment, and sexual devices
7. cover mouth when coughing and sneezing
8. if sexually active with a partner, instruct to:
   a. avoid multiple sexual partners and sexual contact with promiscuous persons
   b. choose healthy partners
   c. be honest with desired partner about AIDS
   d. modify techniques so that body fluids are not shared
   e. avoid unsafe sexual practices (e.g. rimming, fisting, urinating in mouth or anus or on skin, sharing dildos and sex toys)
   f. utilize the following guidelines in relation to condom use:
      1. always use a condom during anal, vaginal, and oral penetration (condom should be applied every time a body orifice is entered *because HIV is found in preseminal fluid)*
      2. use only latex condoms *(HIV can penetrate other types of materials)*
      3. use only condoms with a reservoir tip *to reduce the risk of spillage of semen*
      4. use additional lubricant inside condom if desired *to increase comfort and satisfaction*
      5. lubricate outside of condom and area to be penetrated *to minimize possibility of condom breakage*
      6. avoid lubricants made of mineral oil or petroleum distillates such as Vaseline or baby oil *(these products dissolve latex)*
      7. use a water-based lubricant such as K-Y jelly or a spermicidal compound containing nonoxynol-9 *(spermicidal lubricants containing 4-5% nonoxynol-9 kill HIV in the laboratory setting)*
      8. use caution during removal of condom *to prevent spillage of semen* (penis should be withdrawn and condom removed before the penis has totally relaxed)
      9. dispose of condom immediately after use (a new one should be used for subsequent sexual activity)

UNIT XI

10. store condoms in a cool place *to prevent them from drying out and breaking during use*
9. do not donate blood, sperm, or body organs.

19.b. The client will identify ways to decrease the risk of opportunistic infections.	19.b. Instruct client in ways *to decrease risk of contracting an opportunistic infection:*

      1. cleanse kitchen and bathroom surfaces (particularly floor of shower) regularly with a disinfectant *to prevent fungal growth*
      2. use gloves when cleaning bird cages and cat litter boxes *to avoid exposure to psittacosis and toxoplasmosis respectively*
      3. avoid cleaning tropical fish tanks *(may contain Mycobacterium organisms)*
      4. cleanse hands carefully after contact with body fluids such as semen, mucus, and blood
      5. do not share eating utensils, towels, wash cloths, toothbrushes, razors, enema equipment, and sexual devices
      6. keep living quarters well ventilated *to reduce exposure to airborne disease*
      7. avoid contact with persons who have an infection (particularly viral) and those who have been recently vaccinated
      8. maintain an adequate balance between activity and rest
      9. be alert for and promptly report signs and symptoms of infection (see action c in this diagnosis)
     10. caution client to inform all health care providers of his/her diagnosis *so that drugs that further suppress the immune system (e.g. corticosteroids, immunosuppressants) will not be prescribed unnecessarily*
     11. maintain an optimal nutritional status
     12. drink at least 10 glasses of liquid/day.

19.c. The client will state signs and symptoms to report to the health care provider.	19.c. Stress importance of notifying the health care provider if the following signs and symptoms occur:

      1. fever, chills
      2. night sweats
      3. persistent headache
      4. swollen glands
      5. painful, itchy skin lesions
      6. reddish-purple patches or nodules on any body area
      7. white patches or ulcerations in the mouth
      8. perianal itching and/or pain
      9. frequency, urgency, or burning on urination
     10. cloudy, foul-smelling urine
     11. dry cough or a cough productive of purulent, green, or rust-colored sputum
     12. progressive shortness of breath
     13. increasing weakness and unexplained fatigue or weight loss.

19.d. The client will identify community resources that can assist in adjustment to changes resulting from the diagnosis of AIDS.	19.d.1. Provide information to client and significant others about resources that can assist in adjustment to the diagnosis of AIDS (e.g. Phoenix Rising, Cascade AIDS Project, National Gay Task Force, AIDS hotlines, Public Health Service, Centers for Disease Control, counselors).

     2. Initiate a referral if indicated.

19.e. The client will verbalize an understanding of and a plan for adhering to recommended follow-up care including future appointments with health care provider and medications prescribed.	19.e.1. Reinforce the importance of keeping scheduled follow-up appointments with health care provider.

     2. Explain the rationale for, side effects of, and importance of taking medications prescribed.
     3. If trimethoprim-sulfamethoxazole is prescribed prophylactically to prevent PCP, provide the following instructions:
        a. take the medication with a large glass of water at least 1 hour before or 2 hours after a meal
        b. drink at least 10 glasses of liquid/day
        c. report development of a rash, sore throat, fever, and sensitivity to light (many clients are unable to tolerate the drug because of these effects)

    d. report a sudden reduction in daily urine output
    e. avoid sun exposure and use of sunscreen preparations containing PABA.
4. If client is discharged on AZT, instruct him/her to:
    a. avoid taking acetaminophen (*may increase toxicity of drug by impairing its metabolism by the liver*)
    b. follow schedule of drug administration carefully (usually every 4 hours around the clock)
    c. avoid taking any other medications for AIDS unless approved by physician (*other "cures" may interfere with the effectiveness of AZT*)
    d. report immediately any signs and symptoms of bone marrow depression such as unusual bleeding and excessive fatigue (it is not uncommon for clients taking this drug to require blood transfusions as a result of the drug's bone marrow depressant effects).
5. Implement measures *to improve client compliance:*
    a. include significant others in discharge teaching sessions if possible
    b. encourage questions and allow time for reinforcement and clarification of information provided
    c. provide written instructions regarding scheduled appointments with health care provider, medications prescribed, signs and symptoms to report, and ways to prevent infection.

Reference

Kübler-Ross, E. On death and dying. New York: Macmillan, 1969.

Anemia

Anemia is a hematological disorder that results when there is a reduction in the volume of red cells and/or a decreased concentration of hemoglobin. The decreased erythrocyte or hemoglobin levels result in hypoxia, which is the major manifestation of anemia. Signs and symptoms of anemia are a result of the decreased oxygen-carrying capacity of the blood and the body's compensatory responses to the hypoxia. Anemia can be classified as primary or secondary depending on the etiology. Primary anemia is due to decreased erythrocyte production (hypoproliferative), increased erythrocyte destruction (hemolytic), or blood loss. Megaloblastic anemias (e.g. pernicious anemia), which usually result from a vitamin B_{12} or folic acid deficiency, are a primary anemia considered by many to be a combination hypoproliferative and hemolytic anemia. This type results from a maturational defect in the erythrocyte associated with impaired DNA synthesis followed by early hemolysis of the defective cell. Secondary anemia is associated with conditions such as renal disease, chronic infection or inflammation, or cirrhosis. Another common classification system is based on red cell morphology (i.e. normochromic, hypochromic, hyperchromic) and red cell size or structure (i.e. normocytic, microcytic, macrocytic). Anemia may be further classified as mild (hemoglobin greater than 10 gm), moderate (hemoglobin between 6–10 gm), or severe (hemoglobin less than 6 gm). Signs and symptoms of anemia are not usually evident until the hemoglobin falls below 10 gm.

This care plan focuses on the adult client hospitalized for diagnosis and initiation of treatment of a hypoproliferative anemia associated with an iron, folic acid, or vitamin B_{12} deficiency. The goals of care are to ensure adequate rest, initiate replacement therapy, improve nutritional status, and educate the client regarding follow-up care.

DISCHARGE CRITERIA

Prior to discharge, the client will:

- verbalize an understanding of the rationale for and constituents of the recommended diet
- verbalize an understanding of medication therapy including rationale for, side effects of, and importance of taking as prescribed
- identify ways to minimize the risk of infection
- identify ways to prevent injury associated with weakness and neurological deficits
- state signs and symptoms to report to the health care provider
- verbalize an understanding of and a plan for adhering to recommended follow-up care including activity level and future appointments with health care provider and for laboratory studies.

Use in conjunction with the Care Plan on Immobility.

NURSING/COLLABORATIVE DIAGNOSES

1. Anxiety ☐ 592
2. Altered nutrition: less than body requirements ☐ 593
3A. Altered comfort: dyspepsia ☐ 594
3B. Altered comfort: coldness and chills ☐ 595
4. Impaired skin integrity: irritation and breakdown ☐ 595
5. Altered oral mucous membrane: glossitis and cheilitis ☐ 595
6. Activity intolerance ☐ 596
7. Impaired physical mobility ☐ 597
8. Self-care deficit ☐ 597
9. Altered thought processes: slowed verbal responses, impaired memory, irritability, shortened attention span, confusion, and personality changes ☐ 598
10. Potential for infection ☐ 598
11. Potential for trauma ☐ 599
12. Potential complications:
    a. congestive heart failure (CHF)
    b. arrhythmias ☐ 600
13. Knowledge deficit regarding follow-up care ☐ 602

1. NURSING DIAGNOSIS

Anxiety related to unfamiliar environment; current symptoms; and lack of understanding of diagnostic tests, diagnosis, treatment plan, and prognosis.

DESIRED OUTCOMES	NURSING ACTIONS AND *SELECTED RATIONALES*

1. The client will experience a reduction in fear and anxiety (see Care Plan on Immobility, Nursing Diagnosis 1, for outcome criteria).	1.a. Refer to Care Plan on Immobility, Nursing Diagnosis 1, for measures related to assessment and reduction of fear and anxiety.
	b. Implement additional measures *to reduce fear and anxiety:*
	  1. explain all diagnostic tests:
	    a. blood studies (e.g. RBCs, Hct., Hgb., RBC indices, RDW, iron, total iron-binding capacity, reticulocyte count, vitamin B_{12}, folate, ferritin, transferrin, ferrokinetic profile)
	    b. Schilling test (a urine test performed *to determine whether vitamin B_{12} deficiency is due to absence of intrinsic factor*)
	    c. bone marrow biopsy or aspiration *to reveal information about erythrocyte production*
	    d. gastric analysis and/or biopsy *to determine activity of the parietal cells that secrete hydrochloric acid and intrinsic factor*
	    e. stool examination for occult blood
	  2. assure client that most of current symptoms will resolve with treatment.

□ ▬▬▬▬▬▬▬▬▬▬▬▬▬▬▬▬▬▬▬

2. NURSING DIAGNOSIS

Altered nutrition: less than body requirements related to:

a. iron deficiency associated with inadequate iron intake, malabsorption of iron, or blood loss;

b. vitamin B_{12} deficiency associated with inadequate intake or malabsorption of B_{12};

c. folic acid deficiency associated with inadequate intake or impaired absorption or utilization of folic acid;

d. decreased oral intake associated with cheilitis, glossitis, dyspepsia, anorexia, fatigue, and weakness.

□ ▬▬▬▬▬▬▬▬▬▬▬▬▬▬▬▬▬▬▬

UNIT XI

DESIRED OUTCOMES	NURSING ACTIONS AND *SELECTED RATIONALES*

2. The client will have an improved nutritional status as evidenced by:
  a. weight increasing toward normal range for client's age, height, and build
  b. improved BUN and serum albumin, protein, Hct., Hgb., B_{12}, folate, cholesterol, lymphocyte, and ferritin levels
  c. triceps skinfold measurements approaching normal range
  d. improved strength and activity tolerance
  e. healthy oral mucous membrane.
	2.a. Assess client for signs and symptoms of malnutrition:
	  1. weight below normal for client's age, height, and build
	  2. abnormal BUN and low serum albumin, protein, Hct., Hgb., B_{12}, folate, cholesterol, lymphocyte, and ferritin levels
	  3. triceps skinfold measurement less than normal for build
	  4. weakness and fatigue
	  5. stomatitis.
	b. Reassess nutritional status on a regular basis and report decline.
	c. Monitor percentage of meals eaten.
	d. Assess client to determine causes of inadequate intake (e.g. dyspepsia, fatigue, weakness, glossitis, anorexia).
	e. Implement measures *to improve nutritional status:*
	  1. perform actions *to improve oral intake:*
	    a. implement measures to relieve dyspepsia (see Nursing Diagnosis 3.A, action 2)
	    b. implement measures to prevent or reduce the severity of glossitis and cheilitis (see Nursing Diagnosis 5, action b)
	    c. provide oral care before meals
	    d. eliminate noxious stimuli from environment
	    e. serve small portions of nutritious foods/fluids that are appealing to client and easy to chew
	    f. obtain a dietary consult if necessary to assist client in selecting foods/fluids that meet nutritional needs as well as preferences

    g. encourage significant others to bring in client's favorite foods
    h. encourage a rest period before meals *to minimize fatigue*
    i. allow adequate time for meals; reheat food if necessary
    j. increase activity as allowed and tolerated *(activity stimulates appetite)*

2. instruct and assist client to select foods/fluids that meet his/her specific dietary needs (determined by the cause of the anemia and the specific deficiency):
    a. foods/fluids that comprise a well-balanced diet
    b. foods high in iron (e.g. organ meats, apricots, figs, green leafy vegetables, whole-grain and enriched breads and cereals)
    c. foods/fluids high in vitamin C (e.g. citrus fruits and juices) *to increase iron absorption*
    d. foods/fluids high in vitamin B_{12} (e.g. organ meats, whole milk, eggs, fresh shrimp, pork, chicken)
    e. foods high in folic acid (e.g. green leafy vegetables, asparagus, organ meats, lima beans, nuts, fruits)

3. instruct client to decrease intake of substances that reduce iron absorption (e.g. tea, bran cereals, milk, antacids) for 1 hour before and after taking oral iron preparation and eating meals that consist of foods high in iron

4. monitor for therapeutic and nontherapeutic effects of the following medications if administered:
    a. iron preparations (e.g. iron-dextran, ferrous sulfate, ferrous gluconate)
    b. vitamin B_{12} (e.g. cyanocobalamin, hydroxocobalamin); if client has pernicious anemia, vitamin B_{12} must be given parenterally or in combination with intrinsic factor *in order to be absorbed*
    c. folic acid (e.g. Folvite, sodium folate)
    d. ascorbic acid (vitamin C) *to increase absorption of iron.*

f. Perform a 72-hour calorie count if nutritional status declines or fails to improve.

g. Consult physician about alternative methods of providing nutrition (e.g. parenteral nutrition, tube feedings) if client does not consume enough food or fluids to meet nutritional needs.

3.A. NURSING DIAGNOSIS

Altered comfort: dyspepsia related to impaired digestion and absorption of foods associated with decreased amounts of hydrochloric acid resulting from gastric atrophy (occurs with prolonged iron deficiency and pernicious anemia) and changes in the intestinal epithelium resulting from vitamin B_{12} or folate deficiency.

DESIRED OUTCOMES	NURSING ACTIONS AND *SELECTED RATIONALES*

3.A. The client will verbalize relief of dyspepsia.	3.A.1. Assess client for verbal complaints of dyspepsia and determine if particular foods contribute to dyspepsia.
	2. Implement measures *to reduce dyspepsia:*
	  a. provide small, frequent meals rather than 3 large ones
	  b. instruct client to ingest foods and fluids slowly
	  c. instruct client to avoid foods/fluids that irritate gastric mucosa (e.g. spicy foods; citrus fruits or juices; caffeine-containing items such as chocolate, coffee, tea, or colas)
	  d. instruct client to eat dry foods (e.g. toast, crackers) and avoid drinking liquids with meals if nauseated
	  e. instruct client to rest after eating with head of bed elevated
	  f. administer oral iron preparations with or immediately after meals *to prevent gastric irritation*

    g. monitor for therapeutic and nontherapeutic effects of antacids and mucosal barrier fortifiers (e.g. sucralfate) if administered *to protect the gastric mucosa.*

  3. Consult physician if above measures fail to control dyspepsia.

3.B. NURSING DIAGNOSIS

Altered comfort: coldness and chills related to a compensatory decrease in blood flow to the skin in an attempt to adequately perfuse and oxygenate the major organs.

DESIRED OUTCOMES	NURSING ACTIONS AND *SELECTED RATIONALES*

3.B. The client will not experience chills and a feeling of being cold.	3.B.1. Assess client for chills, cool skin, and statements of feeling cold.
	2. Implement measures *to prevent chills and feeling of being cold:*
	  a. eliminate drafts in room as possible
	  b. maintain a room temperature that is comfortable for client
	  c. provide client with extra blankets and clothing as needed
	  d. provide warm liquids to drink.

4. NURSING DIAGNOSIS

Impaired skin integrity: irritation and breakdown related to:

a. increased skin fragility associated with malnutrition and inadequate tissue oxygenation;

b. prolonged pressure on tissues associated with decreased mobility.

DESIRED OUTCOMES	NURSING ACTIONS AND *SELECTED RATIONALES*

4. The client will maintain skin integrity (see Care Plan on Immobility, Nursing Diagnosis 7, for outcome criteria).	4.a. Refer to Care Plan on Immobility, Nursing Diagnosis 7, for measures related to assessment, prevention, and management of skin irritation and breakdown.
	b. Implement additional measures *to reduce the risk of skin breakdown:*
	  1. perform actions to improve tissue oxygenation (see Nursing Diagnosis 6, action b.4)
	  2. perform actions to improve nutritional status (see Nursing Diagnosis 2, action e).

5. NURSING DIAGNOSIS

Altered oral mucous membrane: glossitis and cheilitis related to epithelial atrophy associated with iron, vitamin B_{12}, or folate deficiency.

UNIT XI

DESIRED OUTCOMES	NURSING ACTIONS AND *SELECTED RATIONALES*

5. The client will maintain a healthy oral mucous membrane as evidenced by:
a. normal-appearing tongue
b. absence of tongue pain
c. absence of inflamed, painful fissures in lips and at corners of mouth.
	5.a. Assess client for and report signs and symptoms of glossitis and cheilitis (e.g. glossy, beefy red tongue; complaints of a sore, burning tongue; painful, reddened fissures in lips or at corners of mouth).
	b. Implement measures *to prevent or reduce the severity of glossitis and cheilitis:*
	  1. reinforce importance of and assist client with oral hygiene after meals and snacks
	  2. have client rinse mouth frequently with warm saline or baking soda and water
	  3. instruct client to avoid products such as lemon-glycerin swabs and commercial mouthwashes containing alcohol *(these products have a drying or irritating effect on oral mucous membrane)*
	  4. encourage a fluid intake of at least 2500 cc/day unless contraindicated
	  5. maintain an optimal nutritional status (see Nursing Diagnosis 2, action e)
	  6. encourage client not to smoke *(smoking irritates and dries the mucosa)*
	  7. lubricate client's lips with Vaseline, K-Y jelly, ChapStick, Blistex, or mineral oil when oral care is given
	  8. assist with selection of soft, nonspicy, and nonacidic foods
	  9. instruct client to avoid extremely hot or cold foods/fluids
	  10. use a soft bristle brush or low-pressure power spray for oral care
	  11. consult physician about an order for a prophylactic antifungal or antibacterial agent.
	c. Monitor for therapeutic and nontherapeutic effects of topical anesthetics, oral protective pastes, and topical and systemic analgesics if administered.
	d. Consult physician if signs and symptoms of glossitis and cheilitis persist or worsen.

6. NURSING DIAGNOSIS

Activity intolerance related to malnutrition and tissue hypoxia associated with anemia and the cardiac deconditioning that may result from prolonged inactivity (decreased cardiac output may also be present due to a prolonged increase in cardiac workload associated with persistent tissue hypoxia).

DESIRED OUTCOMES	NURSING ACTIONS AND *SELECTED RATIONALES*

6. The client will demonstrate an increased tolerance for activity (see Care Plan on Immobility, Nursing Diagnosis 8, for outcome criteria).	6.a. Refer to Care Plan on Immobility, Nursing Diagnosis 8, for measures related to assessment and improvement of activity tolerance.
	b. Implement additional measures *to promote rest and improve activity tolerance:*
	  1. maintain activity restrictions as ordered
	  2. perform actions to reduce fear and anxiety (see Nursing Diagnosis 1)
	  3. perform actions to improve nutritional status (see Nursing Diagnosis 2, action e)
	  4. perform actions *to improve tissue oxygenation:*
	    a. maintain oxygen therapy as ordered
	    b. discourage smoking *(smoking decreases oxygen availability)*
	    c. monitor for therapeutic and nontherapeutic effects of whole blood or packed red cells if administered; administer blood slowly if any evidence of cardiac decompensation is present
	  5. increase client's activity gradually as allowed and tolerated.

7. NURSING DIAGNOSIS

Impaired physical mobility related to:

a. weakness, fatigue, and fear of falls;
b. balance and gait disturbances associated with the neurological changes resulting from vitamin B_{12} deficiency;
c. activity restrictions imposed by the treatment plan.

DESIRED OUTCOMES	NURSING ACTIONS AND *SELECTED RATIONALES*

7.a. The client will maintain an optimal level of physical mobility within physical limitations and activity restrictions imposed by the treatment plan.	7.a.1. Assess for factors that impair physical mobility (e.g. loss of balance, gait disturbances, weakness, fatigue, activity restrictions imposed by treatment plan).
	 2. Implement measures *to increase mobility:*
	   a. perform actions to improve strength and activity tolerance (see Nursing Diagnosis 6)
	   b. monitor for therapeutic and nontherapeutic effects of vitamin B_{12} (e.g. cyanocobalamin, hydroxocobalamin) injections if administered *to prevent further neurological changes*
	   c. perform actions to prevent falls (see Nursing Diagnosis 11, action b) *in order to decrease client's fear of injury*
	   d. instruct client in and assist with correct use of mobility aids (e.g. cane, walker) if appropriate.
	 3. Increase activity and participation in self-care activities as allowed and tolerated.
	 4. Provide praise and encouragement for all efforts to increase physical mobility.
	 5. Encourage the support of significant others. Allow them to assist with activity if desired.

7.b. The client will not experience problems associated with immobility.	7.b. Refer to Care Plan on Immobility for actions to prevent problems associated with immobility if client is on bedrest for longer than 48 hours.

UNIT XI

8. NURSING DIAGNOSIS

Self-care deficit related to:

a. altered thought processes;
b. impaired physical mobility associated with weakness, fatigue, fear of falls, neurological impairments, and prescribed activity restrictions.

DESIRED OUTCOMES	NURSING ACTIONS AND *SELECTED RATIONALES*

8. The client will demonstrate increased participation in self-care activities within prescribed activity restrictions and/or physical limitations.	8.a. Refer to Care Plan on Immobility, Nursing Diagnosis 9, for measures related to assessment of, planning for, and meeting the client's self-care needs.
	 b. Implement additional measures *to facilitate the client's ability to perform self-care activities:*
	   1. perform actions to increase mobility (see Nursing Diagnosis 7, action a.2)
	   2. perform actions to maintain optimal thought processes (see Nursing Diagnosis 9, action c).

9. NURSING DIAGNOSIS

Altered thought processes: slowed verbal responses, impaired memory, irritability, shortened attention span, confusion, and personality changes related to:

a. cerebral hypoxia associated with decreased oxygen-carrying capacity of the blood;
b. cerebral degeneration associated with vitamin B_{12} deficiency.

DESIRED OUTCOMES	NURSING ACTIONS AND *SELECTED RATIONALES*

9. The client will experience an improvement in thought processes as evidenced by:
  a. improved verbal response time
  b. improved memory
  c. longer attention span
  d. absence of confusion and personality changes.
	9.a. Assess client for alterations in thought processes (e.g. slowed verbal response time, impaired memory, irritability, shortened attention span, confusion).
	  b. Ascertain from significant others client's usual level of intellectual functioning and whether personality changes have occurred.
	  c. Implement measures *to maintain optimal thought processes:*
	    1. perform actions to improve nutritional status (see Nursing Diagnosis 2, action e)
	    2. monitor for therapeutic and nontherapeutic effects of vitamin B_{12} (e.g. hydroxocobalamin, cyanocobalamin) injections if administered *to prevent further neurological degeneration*
	    3. maintain oxygen therapy as ordered.
	  d. If client shows evidence of altered thought processes:
	    1. allow adequate time for communication and performance of activities
	    2. repeat instructions as necessary using clear, simple language
	    3. reorient client to person, place, and time as necessary
	    4. write out a schedule of daily activities for client to refer to
	    5. maintain realistic expectations of client's ability to learn, comprehend, and remember information provided
	    6. encourage significant others to be supportive of client; instruct them in methods of dealing with the alterations in thought processes
	    7. inform client and significant others that intellectual and emotional functioning usually improve once the anemia has been adequately treated
	    8. consult physician if alterations in thought processes persist or worsen.

10. NURSING DIAGNOSIS

Potential for infection related to lowered natural resistance associated with:

a. tissue hypoxia;
b. decreased production of leukocytes in megaloblastic anemias associated with impaired synthesis of DNA;
c. inadequate nutritional status.

DESIRED OUTCOMES	NURSING ACTIONS AND *SELECTED RATIONALES*
10. The client will remain free of infection as evidenced by:	10.a. Assess for and report signs and symptoms of infection: 1. elevated temperature

a. absence of chills and fever
b. pulse within normal limits
c. normal breath sounds
d. voiding clear, yellow urine without complaints of frequency, urgency, and burning
e. absence of redness, swelling, and unusual drainage in any area where there is a break in skin integrity
f. intact oral mucous membrane
g. WBC and differential counts within normal range
h. negative results of cultured specimens.

2. chills
3. pattern of increased pulse or pulse rate greater than 100 beats/minute
4. adventitious breath sounds
5. cloudy or foul-smelling urine
6. complaints of frequency, urgency, or burning when urinating
7. presence of WBCs, bacteria, and/or nitrites in urine
8. redness, swelling, or unusual drainage in any area where there is a break in skin integrity
9. irritation or ulceration of oral mucous membrane
10. elevated WBC count and/or significant change in differential.
b. Obtain culture specimens (e.g. urine, vaginal, mouth, sputum, blood) as ordered. Report positive results.
c. Implement measures *to reduce risk of infection:*
   1. maintain a fluid intake of at least 2500 cc/day unless contraindicated
   2. use good handwashing technique and encourage client to do the same
   3. maintain meticulous aseptic technique during all invasive procedures (e.g. catheterizations, venous and arterial punctures, injections)
   4. protect client from others with infection
   5. maintain an optimal nutritional status (see Nursing Diagnosis 2, action e)
   6. perform actions to prevent or reduce severity of glossitis and cheilitis (see Nursing Diagnosis 5, action b)
   7. provide proper balance of exercise and rest
   8. perform actions *to prevent respiratory tract infection:*
      a. instruct and assist client to turn, cough, and deep breathe at least every 2 hours while mobility is limited
      b. instruct and assist client in the use of inspiratory exerciser at least every 2 hours if indicated
      c. encourage client to stop smoking
      d. increase activity as allowed and tolerated
   9. perform actions *to prevent urinary tract infection:*
      a. instruct and assist female client to wipe from front to back following urination and defecation
      b. keep perianal area clean.
d. Monitor for therapeutic and nontherapeutic effects of anti-infectives if administered.

11. NURSING DIAGNOSIS

Potential for trauma related to:

a. falls associated with:
   1. dizziness resulting from cerebral hypoxia
   2. impaired proprioception resulting from neurological changes associated with vitamin B_{12} deficiency
   3. weakness resulting from tissue hypoxia
   4. altered thought processes
   5. gait disturbances resulting from the demyelinating neuropathy that occurs with a vitamin B_{12} deficiency;
b. cuts and burns associated with:
   1. altered thought processes
   2. paresthesias and uncoordinated movements resulting from the demyelinating neuropathy that occurs with vitamin B_{12} deficiency.

DESIRED OUTCOMES	NURSING ACTIONS AND *SELECTED RATIONALES*
11. The client will not experience falls, burns, or cuts.	11.a. Determine whether conditions predisposing the client to falls, burns, or cuts exist:

UNIT XI

      1. dizziness
      2. weakness and fatigue
      3. uncoordinated movements
      4. gait disturbances
      5. decreased sensation in extremities
      6. altered thought processes.

b. Implement measures *to prevent falls:*
    1. keep bed in low position with side rails up when client is in bed
    2. keep needed items within easy reach
    3. encourage client to request assistance whenever needed; have call signal within easy reach
    4. use lap belt when client is in chair if indicated
    5. instruct client to wear shoes with nonskid soles and low heels when ambulating
    6. avoid unnecessary clutter in room
    7. accompany client during ambulation utilizing a transfer safety belt if indicated
    8. provide ambulatory aids (e.g. walker, cane) if client is weak or unsteady on feet
    9. instruct client to ambulate in well-lit areas and to utilize handrails if needed
    10. do not rush client; allow adequate time for trips to the bathroom and ambulation in hallway
    11. perform actions to improve strength and activity tolerance (see Nursing Diagnosis 6).

c. Implement measures *to prevent burns:*
    1. let hot foods and fluids cool slightly before serving *to reduce risk of burns if spills occur*
    2. supervise client while smoking if indicated
    3. assess temperature of bath water and heating pad before and during use.

d. Assist client with tasks that require fine motor skills (e.g. shaving) *in order to prevent cuts.*

e. If client is confused or irrational, implement additional measures *to reduce risk of injury:*
    1. reorient frequently to surroundings and necessity of adhering to safety precautions
    2. provide constant supervision (e.g. staff member, significant other) if indicated
    3. use jacket or wrist restraints or safety alarm device if necessary *to reduce the risk of client's getting out of bed or chair unattended*
    4. monitor for therapeutic and nontherapeutic effects of antianxiety and antipsychotic medications if administered.

f. Include client and significant others in planning and implementing measures to prevent injury.

g. If injury does occur, initiate appropriate first aid and notify physician.

12. COLLABORATIVE DIAGNOSIS

Potential complications:

a. **congestive heart failure (CHF)** related to a prolonged increase in cardiac workload resulting from the heart's attempt to compensate for decreased oxygen levels;

b. **arrhythmias** related to myocardial hypoxia (hypoxia alters the normal conductivity and contractility of the heart).

DESIRED OUTCOMES	NURSING ACTIONS AND *SELECTED RATIONALES*

12.a. The client will not develop CHF as evidenced by:
1. B/P and pulse stable with position change
2. audible heart sounds without an S_3 or S_4 or softening of pre-existing murmurs
3. normal breath sounds
4. absence of or no increase in dyspnea and orthopnea
5. palpable peripheral pulses
6. balanced intake and output
7. stable weight
8. CVP within normal range
9. absence of peripheral edema; distended neck veins; enlarged, tender liver
10. BUN and serum creatinine and alkaline phosphatase levels within normal range.

12.a.1. Assess for and report the following:
  a. signs and symptoms of a hyperkinetic circulatory state (a compensatory increase in cardiac output):
    1. bounding pulse with a further increase in pulse rate
    2. increase in B/P with widened pulse pressure
    3. palpitations
    4. development of or intensified systolic murmurs
    5. buzzing in head or high-pitched tinnitus
    6. pounding headache
    7. increased amplitude of carotid pulse
  b. signs and symptoms of CHF:
    1. decline in systolic B/P of at least 15 mm Hg with a concurrent rise in pulse when client changes from a lying to sitting or standing position
    2. softened or muffled heart sounds
    3. development of or intensified S_3 and/or S_4 gallop rhythm
    4. crackles and diminished or absent breath sounds
    5. development of or increase in dyspnea and orthopnea
    6. displaced apical impulse
    7. diminished or absent peripheral pulses
    8. intake greater than output
    9. weight gain
    10. elevated CVP
    11. peripheral edema
    12. distended neck veins
    13. enlarged, tender liver
    14. elevated BUN and serum creatinine and alkaline phosphatase levels.
  2. Monitor chest x-ray results. Report findings of cardiomegaly, pleural effusion, and pulmonary edema.
  3. Implement measures *to prevent CHF:*
    a. perform actions *to reduce cardiac workload:*
      1. implement measures to promote physical and emotional rest
      2. caution client to avoid activities that create a Valsalva response (e.g. straining to have a bowel movement, bending at the waist, holding breath while moving)
      3. place client in a semi- to high Fowler's position
      4. maintain oxygen therapy as ordered
      5. discourage smoking *(smoking has a cardiostimulatory effect, causes vasoconstriction, and reduces myocardial oxygen availability)*
      6. provide small, frequent meals rather than 3 large ones *(large meals require an increase in blood supply to gastrointestinal tract for digestion)*
      7. discourage intake of foods/fluids high in caffeine such as coffee, tea, chocolate, and colas *(caffeine is a myocardial stimulant and increases myocardial oxygen consumption)*
      8. increase activity gradually
    b. perform actions as ordered to treat arrhythmias and hypertension if present *(these conditions contribute to the development of CHF).*
  4. If signs and symptoms of CHF occur:
    a. continue with above actions
    b. monitor for therapeutic and nontherapeutic effects of medications that may be administered *to reduce vascular congestion and/or cardiac workload* (e.g. diuretics, cardiotonics, vasodilators, morphine sulfate)
    c. apply rotating tourniquets according to hospital policy if ordered *to reduce pulmonary vascular congestion*
    d. refer to Care Plan on Congestive Heart Failure for additional care measures.

12.b. The client will have resolution of cardiac

12.b.1. Assess for and report signs and symptoms of arrhythmias (e.g. irregular apical pulse; pulse rate below 60 or above 100 beats/minute; apical-

UNIT XI

arrhythmias if they occur as evidenced by:
1. regular apical pulse at 60–100 beats/minute
2. equal apical and radial pulses
3. absence of syncope and palpitations
4. EKG reading showing normal sinus rhythm.

radial pulse deficit; syncope; palpitations; abnormal rate, rhythm, or configurations on EKG).

2. If arrhythmias occur:
   a. initiate cardiac monitoring if not already being done
   b. monitor for therapeutic and nontherapeutic effects of the following medications if administered:
      1. antiarrhythmics (e.g. propranolol, procainamide, disopyramide, quinidine, phenytoin, lidocaine, bretylium)
      2. anticholinergic agents (e.g. atropine) or sympathomimetics (e.g. ephedrine, isoproterenol) *to increase heart rate*
      3. cardiac glycosides (e.g. digitalis) *to decrease the heart rate*
   c. restrict client's activity based on his/her tolerance and the severity of the arrhythmia
   d. maintain oxygen therapy as ordered
   e. assist with cardioversion if performed
   f. assess cardiovascular status closely and report signs and symptoms of inadequate tissue perfusion (e.g. decline in B/P; cool, clammy, mottled skin; cyanosis; diminished peripheral pulses; declining urine output; increased restlessness and agitation; shortness of breath)
   g. have emergency cart readily available for cardiopulmonary resuscitation.

13. NURSING DIAGNOSIS

Knowledge deficit regarding follow-up care.

DESIRED OUTCOMES	NURSING ACTIONS AND *SELECTED RATIONALES*
13.a. The client will verbalize an understanding of the rationale for and constituents of the recommended diet.	13.a.1. Explain the importance of diet therapy in the treatment of anemia. 2. Reinforce appropriate dietary instructions (see Nursing Diagnosis 2, actions e.2 and 3). Instructions will vary according to the type of anemia. 3. Instruct client to increase intake of foods high in iron such as organ meats, apricots, figs, green leafy vegetables, and whole-grain enriched breads and cereals. *(Even in anemias other than iron deficiency anemia, increased iron is needed when treatment is initiated because it is picked up by new erythrocytes as they form.)* 4. Obtain a dietary consult to assist client in menu planning if appropriate.
13.b. The client will verbalize an understanding of medication therapy including rationale for, side effects of, and importance of taking as prescribed.	13.b.1. Explain the rationale for, side effects of, and importance of taking medications prescribed. 2. If client is discharged on an iron preparation, instruct to: a. take medication between meals if tolerated *to promote maximum absorption*; if gastric upset occurs, take iron with or immediately after meals b. substantially increase intake of vitamin C (e.g. citrus fruits) or take a vitamin C preparation while taking iron *in order to increase iron absorption* c. avoid taking iron with tea, milk, antacids, or bran cereal *because each impairs iron absorption* d. dilute liquid preparations, drink solution through a straw, and rinse mouth well after taking *to avoid staining teeth* e. expect stools to be dark green or black f. report diarrhea or constipation g. keep iron preparations out of reach of children.

3. If client is discharged on parenteral vitamin B$_{12}$:
   a. demonstrate appropriate injection technique and location of possible injection sites
   b. allow time for questions, clarification, and return demonstration.
4. If client is discharged on a folic acid preparation:
   a. instruct client to restrict alcohol intake to a minimum *because it impairs folic acid utilization*
   b. instruct the client to inform physician if taking any other medications (many medications such as phenytoin, oral contraceptives, antineoplastic agents, primidone, and pyrimethamine inhibit folic acid utilization)
   c. reinforce the need to continue intake of foods high in folic acid content; caution that cooking meats and vegetables for longer than 15 minutes destroys folic acid content.

13.c. The client will identify ways to minimize the risk of infection.

13.c. Instruct client in ways *to reduce risk of infection:*
1. continue with coughing and deep breathing or use of inspiratory exerciser every 2 hours while awake as long as activity level is limited
2. increase activity as recommended
3. avoid contact with persons with infection
4. avoid crowds during the flu or cold season
5. decrease or stop smoking if possible
6. drink at least 10 glasses of liquid/day
7. adhere to recommended diet
8. maintain good personal hygiene especially oral care, handwashing, and perineal care.

13.d. The client will identify ways to prevent injury associated with weakness and neurological deficits.

13.d. Provide the following instructions on ways *to reduce risk of injury until weakness and neurological deficits have improved:*
1. obtain assistance or utilize a cane or walker when ambulating until steadiness has returned
2. avoid use of heating pads, hot water bottles, and ice packs until normal sensation is regained
3. wear shoes or slippers with nonskid soles and low heels *to prevent falls*
4. use an electric rather than straight-edge razor for shaving *to prevent cuts*
5. reduce risk of burns by:
   a. letting hot foods and fluids cool slightly before consuming
   b. testing bath water with thermometer before use
6. do not hurry; allow ample time for all actions.

13.e. The client will state signs and symptoms to report to the health care provider.

13.e. Instruct client to report the following signs and symptoms:
1. increased weakness and fatigue
2. shortness of breath and chest pain
3. increased heartburn, indigestion, or nausea
4. progressive loss of sensation or motor function
5. increasing loss of memory, difficulty concentrating or making decisions, behavior changes
6. skin breakdown
7. cracked, painful lips and/or tongue.

13.f. The client will verbalize an understanding of and a plan for adhering to recommended follow-up care including activity level and future appointments with health care provider and for laboratory studies.

13.f.1. Reinforce the importance of keeping follow-up appointments with health care provider and for laboratory studies.
2. Reinforce the need to adhere to planned rest periods and avoid strenuous activity until anemia has improved.
3. Implement measures *to improve client compliance:*
   a. include significant others in teaching sessions if possible
   b. encourage questions and allow time for reinforcement and clarification of information provided
   c. provide written instructions on future appointments with health care provider, medications prescribed, diet therapy, signs and symptoms to report, and future laboratory studies.

UNIT XI

Multiple Myeloma

Multiple myeloma is a neoplastic condition of unknown etiology in which a single clone of plasma cells proliferates and replaces normal bone marrow with eventual invasion and destruction of the skeletal structure. The skull, spine, sternum, ribs, proximal ends of the humerus, and pelvis are the areas most commonly affected. Essential diagnostic criteria include a greater than 10% infiltration of the bone marrow by abnormal or premature plasma cells, the presence of an M component immunoglobulin (monoclonal immunoglobulin and/or monoclonal free light chains) in the urine or serum, and characteristic diffuse osteoporosis or osteolytic bone lesions. The disease is also characterized by a deficiency of normal immunoglobulins. Multiple myeloma usually occurs in people over 40 and has a very gradual onset (can be over a period of several years).

The clinical picture can vary, but most frequently the client presents with the classic symptoms of anemia, bone pain, and proteinuria and a history of frequent infection. A small percentage of persons with a high concentration of M proteins (particularly IgG and IgA) may experience a hyperviscosity syndrome. The treatment of multiple myeloma is primarily symptomatic with the major emphasis being on reducing the tumor burden with cytotoxic drugs and radiation to localized areas.

This care plan focuses on the adult client hospitalized for staging, initiation of treatment, and control of symptoms of multiple myeloma. The goals of care are to reduce fear and anxiety, relieve discomfort, prevent complications, and educate the client regarding follow-up care.

DISCHARGE CRITERIA

Prior to discharge, the client will:

- identify ways to minimize the risk of infection
- verbalize ways to improve appetite and nutritional status
- verbalize ways to manage and cope with persistent fatigue
- verbalize ways to prevent urinary calculi and maintain adequate renal function
- identify ways to minimize the risk of bleeding
- identify ways to prevent pathologic fractures
- identify ways to prevent injury associated with weakness and neurological impairments
- state signs and symptoms to report to the health care provider
- share thoughts and feelings about the diagnosis of multiple myeloma; prognosis; and effects of the disease process and its treatment on self-concept, life style, and roles
- identify community resources that can assist with home management and adjustment to changes resulting from the diagnosis and effects of treatment
- verbalize an understanding of and a plan for adhering to recommended follow-up care including future appointments with health care provider and for laboratory studies, medications prescribed, and plans for subsequent treatment.

Use in conjunction with the Care Plans on Immobility, Chemotherapy, and/or External Radiation Therapy.

NURSING/COLLABORATIVE DIAGNOSES

1. Anxiety □ *605*
2. Altered fluid and electrolyte balance:
    a. hypercalcemia
    b. fluid volume deficit, hyponatremia, hypokalemia, and hypochlore-mia
    c. metabolic acidosis
    d. metabolic alkalosis □ *606*
3. Altered nutrition: less than body requirements □ *607*
4. Pain □ *608*
5. Sensory-perceptual alteration: visual □ *609*
6. Fatigue □ *610*
7. Activity intolerance □ *610*
8. Impaired physical mobility □ *611*
9. Self-care deficit □ *612*
10. Constipation □ *612*
11. Altered thought processes: slowed verbal responses, impaired memory, irritability, shortened attention span, and/or confusion □ *612*
12. Potential for infection □ *613*
13. Potential for trauma □ *614*
14. Potential complications:
    a. renal calculi
    b. impaired renal function
    c. septic shock
    d. thromboembolism
    e. bleeding
    f. pathologic fractures □ *615*
15. Disturbance in self-concept □ *617*
16. Ineffective individual coping □ *618*
17. Grieving □ *618*
18. Knowledge deficit regarding follow-up care □ *618*

1. NURSING DIAGNOSIS

Anxiety related to:

a. unfamiliar environment;
b. lack of understanding of the diagnosis, staging procedures, and treatment plan;
c. severe bone pain;
d. anticipated effects of cancer and its treatment on body functioning and usual life style and roles;
e. poor prognosis associated with multiple myeloma (median survival time following diagnosis is approximately 2–3 years).

DESIRED OUTCOMES	NURSING ACTIONS AND *SELECTED RATIONALES*
1. The client will experience a reduction in fear and anxiety as evidenced by:	1.a. Assess client on admission for: 1. fears, misconceptions, and level of understanding about multiple myeloma, tests to stage the disease, and possible treatment modes

a. verbalization of feeling less anxious or fearful

b. relaxed facial expression and body movements

c. stable vital signs

d. usual skin color

e. verbalization of an understanding of hospital routines, diagnosis, staging procedures, treatment plan and its effects, and prognosis.

2. perception of anticipated results of diagnostic tests and planned treatment

3. significance of diagnosis of multiple myeloma

4. availability of an adequate support system

5. past experiences with cancer and its treatment

6. signs and symptoms of fear and anxiety (e.g. verbalization of fears and concerns; tenseness; tremors; irritability; restlessness; diaphoresis; tachypnea; tachycardia; elevated blood pressure; facial tension, pallor, or flushing; noncompliance with treatment plan); validate perceptions carefully, remembering that some signs and symptoms may be the result of factors such as pain, anemia, and infection.

b. Ascertain effectiveness of current coping skills.

c. Refer to Care Plan on Immobility, Nursing Diagnosis 1, action c, for measures to reduce fear and anxiety.

d. Implement additional measures *to reduce fear and anxiety:*

1. explain all tests performed to stage multiple myeloma:
   a. bone marrow aspiration and biopsy
   b. x-rays of entire skeleton
   c. blood studies (e.g. complete blood count and chemistry analysis, immunoglobulin assay, serum protein electrophoresis)
   d. electrophoresis of 24-hour urine specimen for M component, particularly Bence-Jones protein

2. refer to Nursing Diagnosis 1, action c, in Care Plans on Chemotherapy and/or External Radiation for measures to reduce fear and anxiety associated with planned treatment

3. perform actions to reduce pain (see Nursing Diagnosis 4, action e)

4. perform actions to assist the client to cope with the diagnosis and its implications (see Care Plan on Chemotherapy, Nursing Diagnosis 22, action d).

e. Include significant others in orientation and teaching sessions and encourage their continued support of client.

f. Provide information based on current needs of client and significant others at a level they can understand. Encourage questions and clarification of information provided.

g. Consult physician if above actions fail to control fear and anxiety.

□ ▬▬▬▬▬▬▬▬▬▬▬▬▬▬▬▬▬▬

2. NURSING/COLLABORATIVE DIAGNOSIS

Altered fluid and electrolyte balance:

a. **hypercalcemia** related to:
   1. uncontrolled osteolysis associated with the secretion of osteoclast-activating factors (OAFs) by myeloma cells
   2. increased bone resorption associated with immobility;

b. **fluid volume deficit, hyponatremia, hypokalemia, and hypochloremia** related to:
   1. decreased oral intake associated with:
      a. anorexia
      b. dysphagia and oral, pharyngeal, and esophageal pain resulting from mucositis due to chemotherapy
      c. nausea
   2. excessive loss of fluid and electrolytes associated with:
      a. persistent vomiting resulting from radiation therapy and/or treatment with cytotoxic drugs
      b. diarrhea resulting from treatment with cytotoxic drugs and/or radiation therapy if the lower bowel is included in the radiation treatment field;

c. **metabolic acidosis** related to hyponatremia and persistent diarrhea associated with side effects of radiation therapy and/or chemotherapy;

d. **metabolic alkalosis** related to hypokalemia, hypochloremia, and persistent vomiting associated with side effects of radiation therapy and/or chemotherapy.

□ ▬▬▬▬▬▬▬▬▬▬▬▬▬▬▬▬▬▬

DESIRED OUTCOMES	NURSING ACTIONS AND *SELECTED RATIONALES*
2.a. The client will maintain a safe serum calcium level (see Care Plan on Immobility, Collaborative Diagnosis 5, for outcome criteria).	2.a.1. Refer to Care Plan on Immobility, Collaborative Diagnosis 5, for measures related to assessment, prevention, and treatment of hypercalcemia. 2. Monitor for therapeutic and nontherapeutic effects of the following medications if administered as additional treatment of hypercalcemia: a. corticosteroids (e.g. prednisone) b. cytotoxic agents (e.g. melphalan, cyclophosphamide) *to reduce tumor volume and amount of OAFs produced by the myeloma cells.*
2.b. The client will maintain fluid, electrolyte, and acid-base balance (see Care Plan on Chemotherapy, Nursing Diagnosis 2, outcomes a and b, for outcome criteria).	2.b. Refer to Care Plan on Chemotherapy, Nursing Diagnosis 2, actions a and b, for measures related to assessment and management of fluid, electrolyte, and acid-base balance.

□ ▉▉▉▉▉▉▉▉▉▉▉▉▉▉▉▉▉▉▉▉▉▉▉▉▉▉▉▉▉

3. NURSING DIAGNOSIS

Altered nutrition: less than body requirements related to:*

a. decreased oral intake associated with:
   1. anorexia resulting from:
      a. depression, fear, and anxiety
      b. fatigue and discomfort
      c. taste alteration associated with:
         1. change in the sense of smell and the threshold for bitter, sweet, sour, and salt taste (particularly red meat, coffee, tea, tomatoes, and chocolate) related to the release of tumor byproducts into the bloodstream
         2. zinc, copper, nickel, niacin, and vitamin A deficiency and increased serum levels of calcium and lactate resulting from the disease process
      d. alteration in the metabolism of proteins, fats, and carbohydrates
      e. early satiety associated with direct stimulation of the satiety center by anorexigenic factors (e.g. peptides) secreted by tumor cells
      f. increased concentration of neurotransmitters in the brain and/or derangements in the serotoninergic system associated with the disease process
      g. hyperviscosity syndrome
   2. dysphagia and oral, pharyngeal, and esophageal pain resulting from mucositis associated with the effects of cytotoxic drugs on the gastrointestinal mucosa
   3. nausea;
b. loss of nutrients associated with persistent vomiting and diarrhea resulting from effects of radiation therapy and/or chemotherapy;
c. malabsorption associated with loss of absorptive surface of the intestinal mucosa resulting from mucositis due to effects of radiation therapy and/or chemotherapy;
d. elevated metabolic rate associated with an increased and continuous energy utilization by rapidly proliferating myeloma cells;
e. utilization of available nutrients by the malignant cells rather than the host;
f. failure of feeding center to induce a sufficient increase in the intake of food to match metabolic needs;
g. inefficient and accelerated metabolism of proteins, fats, and carbohydrates associated with the disease process.

---

* Some of the etiologic factors presented here are currently under investigation.

□ ▉▉▉▉▉▉▉▉▉▉▉▉▉▉▉▉▉▉▉▉▉▉▉▉▉▉▉▉▉

UNIT XI

DESIRED OUTCOMES	NURSING ACTIONS AND *SELECTED RATIONALES*
3. The client will maintain an adequate nutritional status (see Care Plan on Chemotherapy, Nursing Diagnosis 3, for outcome criteria).	3. Refer to Care Plan on Chemotherapy, Nursing Diagnosis 3, for measures related to assessment and promotion of an optimal nutritional status.

□ ▇▇▇▇▇▇▇▇▇▇▇▇▇▇▇▇▇▇▇▇▇▇▇▇▇▇

4. NURSING DIAGNOSIS

Pain related to erosion of the marrow cavity and cortex of the bone, intraosseous pressure created by the tumor, muscle spasms in involved areas, pathologic fractures, and compression or displacement of nerve roots by extraosseous tumor or collapsed vertebrae.

□ ▇▇▇▇▇▇▇▇▇▇▇▇▇▇▇▇▇▇▇▇▇▇▇▇▇▇

DESIRED OUTCOMES	NURSING ACTIONS AND *SELECTED RATIONALES*

4. The client will experience diminished pain as evidenced by:
a. verbalization of reduction in pain
b. relaxed facial expression and body positioning
c. increased participation in activities
d. stable vital signs.
	4.a. Determine how the client usually responds to pain.
	b. Assess for nonverbal signs of pain (e.g. guarding of affected areas, wrinkled brow, clenched fists, reluctance to move, restlessness, diaphoresis, facial pallor or flushing, change in B/P, tachycardia).
	c. Assess verbal complaints of pain. Ask client to be specific regarding location, severity, and type of pain. (Back and rib pain is very common.)
	d. Assess for factors that seem to aggravate and alleviate pain.
	e. Implement measures *to reduce pain:*
	  1. perform actions to reduce fear and anxiety about the pain experience (e.g. assure client that his/her needs for pain relief will be met)
	  2. medicate prior to any painful treatments or procedures and before pain is severe
	  3. maintain activity restrictions as ordered
	  4. provide firm mattress or place a bed board under mattress for added support
	  5. avoid jarring the bed
	  6. place alternating pressure pad, eggcrate mattress, or sheepskin on bed
	  7. consult physician about use of a kinetic bed if client is immobile
	  8. encourage and assist client to apply brace or corset if ordered and use ambulatory aids (e.g. walker with seat, cane) when up *in order to relieve pressure on painful limbs and back*
	  9. if a bedpan is needed, use a fracture pan
	  10. utilize a bed cradle or footboard *to eliminate weight of linens on painful areas*
	  11. keep affected limbs well supported
	  12. perform actions *to reduce pain associated with movement of affected areas:*
	    a. instruct and assist client to support affected limbs with hands or pillow when changing position
	    b. use smooth movements and allow client to move at his/her own pace *in order to avoid paroxysmal spasms*
	    c. instruct and assist client to keep body in good alignment
	    d. caution client to avoid sudden twisting and turning
	    e. avoid pulling or tugging on extremities and torso when positioning client
	    f. administer analgesics before planned physical activities

13. consult physician about management of cough or cold *(sneezing and coughing can greatly aggravate pain)*
14. provide or assist with nonpharmacological measures for pain relief (e.g. cutaneous stimulation techniques such as massage, heat and cold applications, transcutaneous electrical nerve stimulation, or vibration; relaxation techniques such as progressive relaxation exercises or meditation; distraction by quiet conversation, rhythmic massage, or diversional activities; guided imagery; position change)
15. plan methods for achieving pain relief with client *in order to assist him/her to maintain a sense of control over the pain experience*
16. prepare client for radiation therapy and/or chemotherapy *in order to reduce the tumor burden and pressure in the painful areas*
17. monitor for therapeutic and nontherapeutic effects of the following medications if administered:
    a. analgesics
    b. muscle relaxants
    c. nonsteroidal anti-inflammatory agents
    d. corticosteroids *to reduce inflammation and tumor burden* (corticosteroids have an antilymphocytic effect that is useful in reducing tumor size in malignancies of lymphoid origin)
18. consult physician about order for patient-controlled analgesia (PCA) if adequate pain relief cannot be achieved with usual pain control methods.
f. Consult physician if above measures fail to provide adequate pain relief.

5. NURSING DIAGNOSIS

Sensory-perceptual alteration: visual related to retinopathy and retinal hemorrhages associated with occlusion of small blood vessels resulting from hyperviscosity syndrome.

DESIRED OUTCOMES	NURSING ACTIONS AND *SELECTED RATIONALES*
5. The client will experience gradual improvement in vision as evidenced by: a. increased participation in activities b. verbalization of improved vision.	5.a. Assess for visual disturbances (e.g. blurred vision, partial or total blindness). b. Implement measures *to reduce blood viscosity in order to reduce vascular congestion and the resultant changes in retinal vessels:* 1. assist with treatment measures to reduce tumor burden *in order to decrease production of abnormal immunoglobulins* 2. assist with plasmapheresis if performed. c. If vision is impaired: 1. implement measures *to prevent injury:* a. orient client to surroundings, room, and arrangement of furniture b. keep side rails up and call signal within reach c. place desired personal articles within reach and assist client to identify their location d. instruct client to request assistance as needed e. assist client with ambulation by walking a half step ahead of client and describing approaching objects and obstacles; instruct client to grasp back of nurse's arm during ambulation f. avoid unnecessary clutter in room g. provide adequate lighting in room 2. avoid startling client (e.g. speak client's name and identify yourself when entering room and before any physical contact, describe activities and reasons for various noises in the room) 3. assist client with personal hygiene he/she is unable to perform independently

4. identify where items are placed on plate or tray, cut food, open packages, or feed if necessary
5. assist with activities that require reading (e.g. menu selection, mail, legal documents)
6. provide auditory rather than visual diversionary activities
7. inform client of resources available if he/she desires additional information about visual aids (e.g. publications such as Aids for the Blind; American Foundation for the Blind).
d. Reinforce physician's explanation about permanency of visual disturbances.
e. Consult physician if visual disturbances persist or worsen.

6. NURSING DIAGNOSIS

Fatigue related to:

a. accumulation of cellular waste products associated with rapid lysis of cancerous and normal cells exposed to radiation and/or cytotoxic drugs;
b. inability to rest and sleep;
c. anxiety and depression associated with the diagnosis, the treatment regimen and its effects, the need to alter usual activities, and the inability to fulfill usual roles;
d. increased energy expenditure associated with an increase in the basal metabolic rate resulting from continuous, active tumor growth.

DESIRED OUTCOMES	NURSING ACTIONS AND *SELECTED RATIONALES*
6. The client will experience a reduction in fatigue (see Care Plan on Chemotherapy, Nursing Diagnosis 10, for outcome criteria).	6. Refer to Care Plan on Chemotherapy, Nursing Diagnosis 10, for measures related to assessment and management of fatigue.

7. NURSING DIAGNOSIS

Activity intolerance related to:

a. tissue hypoxia associated with severe anemia resulting from:
   1. replacement of erythrocyte-producing marrow by neoplastic plasma cells
   2. chemotherapy- and radiation-induced bone marrow suppression
   3. decreased erythrocyte survival time resulting from disease process
   4. nutritional deficits
   5. chronic blood loss associated with impaired clotting ability and the increased hydrostatic pressure resulting from hyperviscosity syndrome if present;
b. inability to rest and sleep associated with severe pain, persistent vomiting, fear, and anxiety;
c. cardiac deconditioning associated with prolonged inactivity (decreased cardiac output may also be present due to a prolonged increase in cardiac workload associated with tissue hypoxia);
d. malnutrition.

DESIRED OUTCOMES	**NURSING ACTIONS AND *SELECTED RATIONALES***

7. The client will demonstrate an increased tolerance for activity (see Care Plan on Chemotherapy, Nursing Diagnosis 11, for outcome criteria).

7.a. Refer to Care Plan on Chemotherapy, Nursing Diagnosis 11, for measures related to assessment and improvement of activity tolerance.
  b. Implement additional measures *to promote rest and improve activity tolerance:*
   1. perform actions to reduce pain (see Nursing Diagnosis 4, action e)
   2. perform actions to reduce fear and anxiety (see Nursing Diagnosis 1, actions c and d)
   3. perform actions *to improve tissue oxygenation:*
      a. maintain oxygen therapy as ordered
      b. discourage smoking *(smoking decreases oxygen availability)*
      c. monitor for therapeutic and nontherapeutic effects of whole blood or packed red cells if administered.

8. NURSING DIAGNOSIS

Impaired physical mobility related to:

a. sensory and motor impairments associated with spinal cord or nerve root compression resulting from extension of myeloma from the marrow of the vertebrae to the extradural space;
b. muscle weakness associated with hypercalcemia and prolonged disuse;
c. reluctance to move due to severe pain, fear of injury, and visual disturbances;
d. activity intolerance associated with anemia, nutritional deficits, and inability to rest and sleep.

DESIRED OUTCOMES	**NURSING ACTIONS AND *SELECTED RATIONALES***

8.a. The client will maintain an optimal level of physical mobility within the limitations imposed by the disease process.

8.a.1. Assess for factors that impair physical mobility (e.g. sensory, motor, and visual impairments; reluctance to move because of severe pain or fear of injury; fatigue; weakness).
   2. Implement measures *to increase mobility:*
      a. perform actions to control pain (see Nursing Diagnosis 4, action e)
      b. perform actions to reduce fatigue and improve activity tolerance (see Nursing Diagnoses 6 and 7)
      c. perform actions to prevent and treat hypercalcemia (see Care Plan on Immobility, Collaborative Diagnosis 5, action b) *in order to help maintain normal neuromuscular function*
      d. instruct client in and assist with correct use of mobility aids (e.g. cane, walker) if appropriate
      e. perform actions to prevent falls (see Nursing Diagnosis 13, actions b and c) *in order to reduce fear of injury*
      f. reinforce instructions regarding activities and exercise plan recommended by physical and/or occupational therapists.
   3. Increase activity and participation in self-care activities as tolerated. Encourage client to use unaffected extremities in carrying out activities of daily living.
   4. Provide praise and encouragement for all efforts to increase physical mobility.
   5. Encourage the support of significant others. Allow them to assist with range of motion exercises, positioning, and activity if desired.
   6. Consult physician if client is unable to maintain or achieve expected level of mobility.

UNIT XI

8.b. The client will not experience problems associated with immobility.

8.b. Refer to Care Plan on Immobility for actions to prevent problems associated with immobility.

9. NURSING DIAGNOSIS

Self-care deficit related to altered thought processes, visual impairments, and impaired physical mobility associated with motor deficits, activity intolerance, pain, and fear of injury.

DESIRED OUTCOMES	NURSING ACTIONS AND *SELECTED RATIONALES*

9. The client will demonstrate increased participation in self-care activities within limitations imposed by the disease process.	9.a. Refer to Care Plan on Immobility, Nursing Diagnosis 9, for measures related to assessment of, planning for, and meeting client's self-care needs.
	b. Implement measures *to further facilitate client's ability to perform self-care activities:*
	  1. perform actions to increase mobility (see Nursing Diagnosis 8, action a.2)
	  2. if client has a visual impairment, identify where items are placed on his/her plate and tray.

10. NURSING DIAGNOSIS

Constipation related to:

a. decreased intake of fluids and foods high in fiber;
b. reluctance to use a bedpan;
c. weakened abdominal and perineal muscles associated with a generalized loss of muscle tone resulting from prolonged immobility;
d. decreased gastrointestinal motility associated with decreased activity, use of narcotic analgesics, the neuromuscular depressant effects of hypercalcemia if present, and increased sympathetic nervous system activity resulting from anxiety.

DESIRED OUTCOMES	NURSING ACTIONS AND *SELECTED RATIONALES*
10. The client will maintain usual bowel elimination pattern.	10. Refer to Care Plan on Immobility, Nursing Diagnosis 11, for measures related to assessment, prevention, and management of constipation.

11. NURSING DIAGNOSIS

Altered thought processes: slowed verbal responses, impaired memory, irritability, shortened attention span, and/or confusion related to:

a. cerebral hypoxia associated with decreased oxygen-carrying capacity of the blood (due to severe anemia) and decreased tissue perfusion associated with delayed circulation time if hyperviscosity syndrome is present;
b. depressant effects of hypercalcemia on the central nervous system.

DESIRED OUTCOMES	NURSING ACTIONS AND *SELECTED RATIONALES*
11. The client will experience an improvement in thought processes as evidenced by: a. improved verbal response time b. longer attention span c. improved memory d. absence of irritability and confusion.	11.a. Assess client for alterations in thought processes (e.g. slowed verbal responses to questions, shortened attention span, impaired memory, irritability, confusion). b. Ascertain from significant others client's usual level of intellectual functioning. c. Implement measures *to maintain optimal thought processes:* 1. maintain oxygen therapy as ordered 2. perform actions to prevent and treat hypercalcemia (see Care Plan on Immobility, Collaborative Diagnosis 5, action b) 3. assist with plasmapheresis if performed *to decrease serum viscosity.* d. If client shows evidence of altered thought processes: 1. allow adequate time for communication and performance of activities 2. repeat instructions as necessary using clear, simple language 3. reorient client to person, place, and time as necessary 4. write out a schedule of activities for client to refer to if desired 5. encourage significant others to be supportive of client; instruct them to reorient client as necessary 6. inform client and significant others that intellectual and emotional functioning usually improve once the serum calcium levels have returned to normal, plasmapheresis is complete, and/or anemia has improved 7. consult physician if alterations in thought processes persist or worsen.

UNIT XI

12. NURSING DIAGNOSIS

Potential for infection related to:

a. lowered natural resistance associated with:
   1. immunosuppressive effects of radiation therapy, chemotherapy, and long-term corticosteroid use
   2. decreased production of and increased catabolism of normal immunoglobulins (B-cell deficiency is present at diagnosis in the majority of clients and persists through remissions)
   3. impaired neutrophil opsonization and phagocytosis associated with the disease process
   4. reduction in bone marrow production of leukocytes resulting from infiltration of the marrow by myeloma cells
   5. malnutrition, anemia, and general debilitation;
b. break in integrity of the skin associated with placement of a central venous catheter (e.g. Groshong) or implanted infusion device (e.g. Port-a-Cath) and/or radiation-induced desquamation.

DESIRED OUTCOMES	NURSING ACTIONS AND *SELECTED RATIONALES*

12. The client will remain free of infection (see Care Plan on Chemotherapy, Nursing Diagnosis 17, for outcome criteria).

12. Refer to Care Plan on Chemotherapy, Nursing Diagnosis 17, for measures related to assessment, prevention, and management of infection.

□ ▉▉▉▉▉▉▉▉▉▉▉▉▉▉▉▉▉▉▉▉▉▉▉▉▉▉▉▉

13. NURSING DIAGNOSIS

Potential for trauma related to:

a. falls associated with:
   1. weakness and fatigue resulting from tissue hypoxia, malnutrition, difficulty resting and sleeping, and side effects of chemotherapy and/or radiation therapy
   2. motor and sensory impairments resulting from spinal cord or nerve root compression, hypercalcemia, and effects of certain cytotoxic drugs (e.g. vinca alkaloids)
   3. altered thought processes resulting from cerebral hypoxia and hypercalcemia
   4. visual impairments and vertigo resulting from increased serum viscosity
   5. depressant effects of certain medications (e.g. narcotics, sedatives) on the central nervous system;
b. cuts and burns associated with altered thought processes and sensory and motor impairments.

□ ▉▉▉▉▉▉▉▉▉▉▉▉▉▉▉▉▉▉▉▉▉▉▉▉▉▉▉▉

DESIRED OUTCOMES	NURSING ACTIONS AND *SELECTED RATIONALES*

13. The client will not experience falls, burns, or cuts.

13.a. Determine whether conditions predisposing client to falls, burns, or cuts exist:
   1. weakness and fatigue
   2. sensory and motor impairments
   3. altered thought processes
   4. visual disturbances.
  b. Refer to Care Plan on Chemotherapy, Nursing Diagnosis 18, action b, for measures related to prevention of falls.
  c. Implement additional measures *to prevent falls:*
   1. perform actions to prevent or treat hypercalcemia (see Care Plan on Immobility, Collaborative Diagnosis 5, action b) *in order to help maintain mental alertness and normal neuromuscular function*
   2. perform actions to prevent injury associated with visual impairments if present (see Nursing Diagnosis 5, action c.1)
   3. perform actions to maintain optimal thought processes (see Nursing Diagnosis 11, action c).
  d. Implement measures *to prevent burns:*
   1. let hot foods and fluids cool slightly before serving *to reduce risk of burns if spills occur*
   2. supervise client while smoking if indicated
   3. assess temperature of bath water and heating pad before and during use.
  e. Assist client with tasks that require fine motor skills (e.g. shaving) *in order to prevent cuts.*
  f. If client is confused or irrational, implement additional measures *to reduce risk of injury:*

    1. reorient frequently to surroundings and necessity of adhering to safety precautions
    2. provide constant supervision (e.g. staff member, significant other) if indicated
    3. use jacket or wrist restraints or safety alarm device if necessary *to reduce the risk of client's getting out of bed or chair unattended*
    4. monitor for therapeutic and nontherapeutic effects of antianxiety and antipsychotic medications if administered.
  g. Administer central nervous system depressants such as narcotics and sedatives judiciously.
  h. Include client and significant others in planning and implementing measures to prevent injury.
  i. If injury does occur, initiate appropriate first aid and notify physician.

14. COLLABORATIVE DIAGNOSIS

Potential complications:

a. **renal calculi** related to:
    1. urinary stasis associated with decreased mobility
    2. increased renal excretion of calcium associated with uncontrolled bone destruction resulting from the disease process and prolonged immobility
    3. increased renal excretion of uric acid associated with rapid lysis of tumor cells resulting from the initiation of treatment;
b. **impaired renal function** related to:
    1. nephrotoxic effects of increased urinary light chains (Bence-Jones protein) and some cytotoxic agents
    2. excessive deposits of uric acid crystals and calcium salts associated with increased serum uric acid and calcium levels
    3. decreased renal blood flow associated with fluid volume deficit
    4. infiltration of the kidney by myeloma cells
    5. inadequate glomerular oxygenation associated with anemia and increased serum viscosity
    6. amyloidosis (occurs in approximately 7–10% of clients and is manifested by nephrotic syndrome);
c. **septic shock** related to septicemia associated with overwhelming bacterial invasion and proliferation due to decreased resistance and ability to fight infection;
d. **thromboembolism** related to venous stasis associated with increased serum viscosity (due to fluid volume deficit and hyperviscosity syndrome if present) and decreased mobility;
e. **bleeding** related to:
    1. thrombocytopenia associated with replacement of hematopoietic tissue of bone marrow with neoplastic plasma cells and radiation- or chemotherapy-induced bone marrow suppression
    2. abnormalities in platelet function (may occur in a few clients) associated with the disease process
    3. increased hydrostatic pressure associated with the hyperviscosity syndrome if present
    4. reduced levels of one or more coagulation factors (e.g. I, II, V, VII, VIII, X) associated with the disease process;
f. **pathologic fractures** related to osteolytic lesions and/or diffuse osteoporosis associated with secretion of OAFs by myeloma cells (prolonged immobility may further accelerate osteoporosis).

DESIRED OUTCOMES	NURSING ACTIONS AND *SELECTED RATIONALES*

14.a. The client will not develop renal calculi (see Care Plan on Chemotherapy, Collaborative Diagnosis 19, outcome b, for outcome criteria).

14.a.1. Assess for and report signs and symptoms of renal calculi (e.g. dull, aching or severe, colicky flank pain; hematuria; urinary frequency or urgency; nausea; vomiting).
2. Monitor serum calcium and uric acid levels and report elevations.
3. Obtain a urine specimen for analysis if ordered. Report the presence of crystals and/or high levels of calcium and uric acid.
4. Refer to Care Plan on Immobility, Collaborative Diagnosis 14, action c.4, for measures to prevent calcium stone formation.
5. Refer to Care Plan on Chemotherapy, Collaborative Diagnosis 19, action b.4, for measures to prevent uric acid stone formation.
6. If signs and symptoms of renal calculi occur:
   a. strain all urine carefully and save any calculi for analysis; report finding to physician
   b. encourage a minimum fluid intake of 3000 cc/day unless contraindicated
   c. administer analgesics as ordered
   d. refer to Care Plan on Renal Calculi for additional care measures.

14.b. The client will maintain adequate renal function (see Care Plan on Chemotherapy, Collaborative Diagnosis 19, outcome c, for outcome criteria).

14.b.1. Refer to Care Plan on Chemotherapy, Collaborative Diagnosis 19, action c, for measures related to assessment and maintenance of adequate renal function.
2. Implement additional measures *to maintain adequate renal function:*
   a. perform actions to prevent renal calculi (see actions a.4 and 5 in this diagnosis)
   b. perform actions to prevent fluid volume deficit (see Care Plan on Chemotherapy, Nursing Diagnosis 2, actions a.3.a–e)
   c. encourage fluid intake of at least 3000 cc/day *in order to prevent precipitation of uric acid, calcium, and Bence-Jones protein*
   d. prepare client for the following if planned:
      1. plasmapheresis *(more effective than peritoneal dialysis in removing light chain proteins)*
      2. chemotherapy *to reduce production of monoclonal free light chains by myeloma cells.*

14.c. The client will not develop septic shock as evidenced by:
1. usual mental status
2. stable vital signs
3. skin warm and usual color
4. urine output at least 30 cc/hour
5. blood gases within normal range.

14.c.1. Assess for and report signs and symptoms of septic shock:
   a. early or hyperdynamic stage (e.g. confusion; chills and fever; warm, flushed skin; lower extremity mottling; tachycardia; tachypnea)
   b. hypodynamic stage (e.g. cool, clammy skin; severe hypotension; tachycardia; thready pulse; cyanosis; low pH and CO_2 content; oliguria or anuria; respiratory insufficiency or failure).
2. Implement measures to prevent and treat infection (see Care Plan on Chemotherapy, Nursing Diagnosis 17, actions c and d) *in order to decrease risk of septic shock.*
3. If signs and symptoms of septic shock occur:
   a. maintain intravenous fluid therapy as ordered
   b. monitor vital signs frequently
   c. administer oxygen therapy as ordered
   d. obtain cultures from all possible sites of infection (e.g. urine, infusion sites, wounds, blood, sputum) as ordered; report abnormal results
   e. monitor for therapeutic and nontherapeutic effects of the following medications if administered:
      1. vasopressors (may be given for a short period *to maintain mean arterial pressure)*
      2. positive inotropic agents (e.g. dopamine) *to increase cardiac output and improve blood flow to major organs*
      3. anti-infectives *to control the precipitating infection*
   f. provide emotional support to client and significant others.

14.d. The client will not develop a venous thrombus or pulmonary embolism (see Care Plan on Immobility,

14.d.1. Refer to Care Plan on Immobility, Collaborative Diagnosis 14, actions a.1 and 2, for measures related to assessment, prevention, and treatment of a venous thrombus and pulmonary embolism.
2. Implement measures *to reduce blood viscosity in order to further reduce*

Collaborative Diagnosis 14, outcomes a.1 and 2, for outcome criteria).

the risk of venous thrombus:
   a. assist with treatment measures to reduce tumor burden *in order to reduce production of M proteins causing the hyperviscosity syndrome*
   b. assist with plasmapheresis if performed.

14.e. The client will not experience unusual bleeding (see Care Plan on Chemotherapy, Collaborative Diagnosis 19, outcome a, for outcome criteria).

14.e.1. Refer to Care Plan on Chemotherapy, Collaborative Diagnosis 19, action a, for measures related to assessment, prevention, and management of bleeding.
    2. Assist with plasmapheresis if performed *to reduce serum viscosity and the resultant increase in hydrostatic pressure.*
    3. Assist with treatment measures to reduce tumor burden *in order to allow increased production of normal platelets.*

14.f. The client will not experience pathologic fractures (see Care Plan on Immobility, Collaborative Diagnosis 14, outcome e, for outcome criteria).

14.f.1. Refer to Care Plan on Immobility, Collaborative Diagnosis 14, action e for measures related to assessment, prevention, and treatment of pathologic fractures.
    2. Implement additional measures *to prevent pathologic fractures:*
      a. prepare client for:
        1. radiation therapy and/or chemotherapy *to reduce the tumor burden*
        2. surgical stabilization of involved weight-bearing bones
      b. monitor for therapeutic and nontherapeutic effects of sodium fluoride and calcium carbonate if administered *to increase bone calcification.*

---

15. NURSING DIAGNOSIS

Disturbance in self-concept* related to:

a. dependence on others to meet self-care needs;
b. changes in appearance (e.g. alopecia, excessive weight loss, skin changes) associated with the side effects of chemotherapy and/or radiation therapy;
c. reduction in height (can lose up to 5 inches in height) due to loss of bone mass resulting from the disease process;
d. altered thought processes;
e. alteration in usual sexual functioning associated with weakness, fatigue, depression, and side effects of cytotoxic drugs;
f. stigma associated with diagnosis of cancer;
g. changes in life style and roles associated with the effects of the disease process and its treatment.

---

* This diagnostic label includes the nursing diagnoses of body image disturbance and self-esteem disturbance.

DESIRED OUTCOMES	NURSING ACTIONS AND *SELECTED RATIONALES*

15. The client will demonstrate beginning adaptation to changes in appearance, body functioning, life style, and roles (see Care Plan on Chemotherapy, Nursing Diagnosis 21, for outcome criteria).

15.a. Refer to Care Plan on Chemotherapy, Nursing Diagnosis 21, for measures related to assessment and maintenance of a positive self-concept.
   b. Discuss techniques client can use *to adapt to alterations in thought processes:*
    1. encourage client to make lists and jot down messages and refer to these notes rather than relying on his/her memory
    2. encourage client to place self in a calm environment when making decisions
    3. encourage client to validate decisions, clarify information, and seek assistance to problem-solve if indicated.

☐ ▐▀▀▀▀▀▀▀▀▀▀▀▀▀▀▀▀▀▀▀▀▀▀▀▀▀

16. NURSING DIAGNOSIS

Ineffective individual coping related to:

a. inadequate support system;
b. discomfort and chronic fatigue associated with the disease process and side effects of treatment;
c. depression, fear, and anxiety associated with the diagnosis, prognosis, and effects of the disease process and its treatment on usual body functioning and life style.

☐ ▐▀▀▀▀▀▀▀▀▀▀▀▀▀▀▀▀▀▀▀▀▀▀▀▀▀

DESIRED OUTCOMES	NURSING ACTIONS AND *SELECTED RATIONALES*
16. The client will demonstrate the use of effective coping skills (see Care Plan on Chemotherapy, Nursing Diagnosis 22, for outcome criteria).	16. Refer to Care Plan on Chemotherapy, Nursing Diagnosis 22, for measures related to assessment and management of ineffective coping.

☐ ▐▀▀▀▀▀▀▀▀▀▀▀▀▀▀▀▀▀▀▀▀▀▀▀▀▀

17. NURSING DIAGNOSIS

Grieving* related to:

a. diagnosis of cancer with potential for premature death;
b. changes in body image and usual life style and roles associated with multiple myeloma and its treatment.

———————————

 * This diagnostic label includes anticipatory grieving and grieving following the actual losses/changes.

☐ ▐▀▀▀▀▀▀▀▀▀▀▀▀▀▀▀▀▀▀▀▀▀▀▀▀▀

DESIRED OUTCOMES	NURSING ACTIONS AND *SELECTED RATIONALES*
17. The client will demonstrate beginning progression through the grieving process (see Care Plan on Chemotherapy, Nursing Diagnosis 23, for outcome criteria).	17. Refer to Care Plan on Chemotherapy, Nursing Diagnosis 23, for measures related to assessment and facilitation of grieving.

☐ ▐▀▀▀▀▀▀▀▀▀▀▀▀▀▀▀▀▀▀▀▀▀▀▀▀▀

18. NURSING DIAGNOSIS

Knowledge deficit regarding follow-up care.

☐ ▐▀▀▀▀▀▀▀▀▀▀▀▀▀▀▀▀▀▀▀▀▀▀▀▀▀

DESIRED OUTCOMES	NURSING ACTIONS AND *SELECTED RATIONALES*

18.a. The client will identify ways to minimize the risk of infection.

18.a.1. Refer to Care Plan on Chemotherapy, Nursing Diagnosis 24, action a, for instructions related to preventing infection.
   2. Reinforce the need for client to continue with measures to prevent infection even if remission has been achieved *because increased susceptibility to infection will persist.*

18.b. The client will verbalize ways to improve appetite and nutritional status.

18.b. Refer to Care Plan on Chemotherapy, Nursing Diagnosis 24, action e, for instructions related to improving appetite and nutritional status.

18.c. The client will verbalize ways to manage and cope with persistent fatigue.

18.c. Refer to Care Plan on Chemotherapy, Nursing Diagnosis 24, action f, for instructions regarding ways to manage and cope with persistent fatigue.

18.d. The client will verbalize ways to prevent urinary calculi and maintain adequate renal function.

18.d.1. Refer to Care Plan on Chemotherapy, Nursing Diagnosis 24, action g, for instructions related to prevention of uric acid stone formation.
   2. Provide instructions regarding ways to prevent urinary calcium stone formation (see Care Plan on Immobility, Nursing Diagnosis 19, action a.3).

18.e. The client will identify ways to minimize the risk of bleeding.

18.e. Refer to Care Plan on Chemotherapy, Nursing Diagnosis 24, action h, for instructions related to minimizing risk of and controlling bleeding.

18.f. The client will identify ways to prevent pathologic fractures.

18.f. Provide instructions regarding ways *to prevent pathologic fractures:*
   1. avoid coughing, sneezing, trauma to bones, lifting heavy objects, and straining to have a bowel movement
   2. apply corset, brace, or splint correctly and wear as prescribed
   3. use good body mechanics
   4. maintain the maximum activity and exercise level tolerated *to reduce calcium loss from the bones*
   5. use ambulatory aids (e.g. cane, walker) if necessary *to prevent falls and further trauma to the bone.*

18.g. The client will identify ways to prevent injury associated with weakness and neurological impairments.

18.g. Provide the following instructions on ways *to reduce risk of injury resulting from weakness and neurological impairments:*
   1. obtain assistance or utilize a cane or walker when ambulating
   2. wear shoes or slippers with nonskid soles and low heels *to prevent falls*
   3. use an electric rather than straight-edge razor for shaving *to prevent cuts*
   4. *reduce risk of burns by:*
     a. letting hot foods and fluids cool slightly before consuming
     b. testing bath water with thermometer before use
     c. avoiding use of heating pads and hot water bottles
   5. do not hurry; allow ample time for all actions.

18.h. The client will state signs and symptoms to report to the health care provider.

18.h.1. Refer to Care Plan on Chemotherapy, Nursing Diagnosis 24, action l, for signs and symptoms to report.
   2. Instruct client to report these additional signs and symptoms:
     a. decreased urine output
     b. excessive pain or swelling in any body area
     c. progressive loss of sensation and/or ability to move extremities
     d. loss of bowel or bladder control
     e. change in or loss of vision
     f. dizziness
     g. increased fatigue and weakness
     h. increasing loss of memory, difficulty concentrating or making decisions, behavior changes
     i. loss of appetite, nausea, vomiting, constipation, increased thirst, increased urination, drowsiness (may indicate calcium excess).

18.i. The client will identify community resources that

18.i.1. Provide information about community resources that can assist the client and significant others with home management and adjustment to the

can assist with home management and adjustment to changes resulting from the diagnosis and effects of treatment.

diagnosis and effects of treatment (e.g. American Cancer Society, Meals on Wheels, counselors, support groups, Hospice, Visiting Nurse Association, home health agencies, Make Today Count).

2. Initiate a referral if indicated.

18.j. The client will verbalize an understanding of and a plan for adhering to recommended follow-up care including future appointments with health care provider and for laboratory studies, medications prescribed, and plans for subsequent treatment.

18.j.1. Reinforce physician's explanation of planned chemotherapy and/or radiation therapy if appropriate. Stress importance of strictly following the prescribed protocol for chemotherapy and/or radiation therapy and keeping all appointments for follow-up supervision and laboratory work.

2. Explain the rationale for, side effects of, and importance of taking medications prescribed (e.g. allopurinol, corticosteroids, cytotoxic agents, anti-infectives).

3. Implement measures *to improve client compliance:*
   a. include significant others in teaching sessions if possible
   b. encourage questions and allow time for reinforcement and clarification of information provided
   c. provide written instructions regarding scheduled appointments with health care provider and for chemotherapy, radiation therapy, and laboratory work; medications prescribed; and signs and symptoms to report.

☐☐

Splenectomy

Splenectomy is the surgical removal of the spleen. The most common indications for the surgery are rupture of the spleen and splenomegaly. Causes of rupture include trauma to the spleen, accidental tearing of the splenic capsule during surgery on nearby organs, and softening of or damage to the spleen as a result of disease (e.g. infectious mononucleosis). Splenomegaly occurs with disease conditions such as idiopathic thrombocytopenic purpura, some hemolytic anemias, leukemia, lymphoma, and cirrhosis of the liver. A splenectomy may also be performed prior to organ transplantation (believed by some to reduce the risk of rejection of the transplanted organ); to stage Hodgkin's disease; and as treatment for splenic aneurysm, cysts, and neoplasm. When feasible, a partial splenectomy or splenic autotransplantation (transplantation of a small portion of the spleen into another area of the abdomen) may be done so that some of the spleen's immunological function is maintained.

This care plan focuses on the adult client hospitalized with a suspected splenic rupture resulting from trauma. Preoperatively, goals of care are to maintain adequate systemic tissue perfusion and prepare the client for surgery. Postoperative goals of care are to maintain comfort, prevent complications, and educate the client regarding follow-up care.

DISCHARGE CRITERIA

Prior to discharge, the client will:

• identify ways to prevent infection
• state signs and symptoms of complications to report to the health care provider
• verbalize an understanding of and a plan for adhering to recommended follow-up care including future appointments with health care provider, medications prescribed, wound care, and activity level.

NURSING/COLLABORATIVE DIAGNOSES

Preoperative
1. Potential complication: hypovolemic shock □ *621*
Postoperative
1. Potential for infection □ *622*
2. Potential complications:
   a. pancreatitis
   b. subphrenic abscess
   c. thromboembolism
   d. postsplenectomy sepsis □ *623*
3. Knowledge deficit regarding follow-up care □ *624*

Preoperative

Use in conjunction with the Standardized Preoperative Care Plan.

1. COLLABORATIVE DIAGNOSIS

Potential complication: hypovolemic shock related to blood loss resulting from rupture of the spleen.

UNIT
XI

DESIRED OUTCOMES	NURSING ACTIONS AND *SELECTED RATIONALES*

1. The client will not develop hypovolemic shock as evidenced by:
  a. usual mental status
  b. stable vital signs
  c. skin warm and usual color
  d. palpable peripheral pulses
  e. capillary refill time less than 3 seconds
  f. urine output at least 30 cc/hour.
	1.a. Assess for and report:
	   1. signs and symptoms of splenic rupture (e.g. left upper abdominal pain and tenderness, referred pain in left shoulder, shifting dullness noted during percussion of abdomen)
	   2. declining RBC, Hct., and Hgb. levels
	   3. signs and symptoms of hypovolemic shock:
	     a. restlessness, agitation, confusion
	     b. significant decrease in B/P
	     c. decline in B/P of at least 15 mm Hg with concurrent rise in pulse when client changes from lying to sitting or standing position
	     d. resting pulse rate greater than 100 beats/minute
	     e. rapid or labored respirations
	     f. cool, pale, or cyanotic skin
	     g. diminished or absent peripheral pulses
	     h. capillary refill time greater than 3 seconds
	     i. urine output less than 30 cc/hour.
	  b. Monitor for therapeutic and nontherapeutic effects of blood products and/or volume expanders if administered *to prevent hypovolemic shock.*

c. If signs and symptoms of hypovolemic shock occur:
  1. continue to administer blood products and/or volume expanders as ordered
  2. place client flat in bed with legs elevated unless contraindicated
  3. monitor vital signs frequently
  4. administer oxygen as ordered
  5. monitor for therapeutic and nontherapeutic effects of vasopressors if administered (may be given for a short period *to maintain mean arterial pressure*)
  6. assist with application of military antishock trousers (MAST) if indicated
  7. prepare client for splenectomy (surgery may need to be performed before scheduled time)
  8. provide emotional support to client and significant others.

□ ▬▬▬▬▬▬▬▬▬▬▬▬▬▬▬▬▬▬▬▬▬▬▬▬▬▬▬▬

Postoperative

Use in conjunction with the Standardized Postoperative Care Plan.

□ ▬▬▬▬▬▬▬▬▬▬▬▬▬▬▬▬▬▬▬▬▬▬

1. NURSING DIAGNOSIS

Potential for infection related to removal of the spleen (the spleen is part of the reticuloendothelial system and the rest of the system cannot immediately compensate for its loss).

□ ▬▬▬▬▬▬▬▬▬▬▬▬▬▬▬▬▬▬▬▬▬▬

DESIRED OUTCOMES	NURSING ACTIONS AND *SELECTED RATIONALES*

1. The client will remain free of infection as evidenced by:
  a. temperature 38.3°C or less
  b. absence of chills
  c. pulse within normal limits
  d. normal breath sounds
  e. voiding clear, yellow urine without complaints of frequency, urgency, and burning
  f. absence of redness, swelling, and unusual drainage in any area where there is a break in skin integrity
  g. intact oral mucous membrane
  h. WBC and differential counts returning toward normal
  i. negative results of cultured specimens.
	1.a. Assess for and report signs and symptoms of infection:
	  1. increase in temperature above 38.3°C (after splenectomy, a temperature of up to 38.3°C is often present for at least 10 days)
	  2. chills
	  3. pattern of increased pulse or pulse rate greater than 100 beats/minute
	  4. adventitious breath sounds
	  5. cloudy or foul-smelling urine
	  6. complaints of frequency, urgency, or burning when urinating
	  7. presence of WBCs, bacteria, and/or nitrites in urine
	  8. redness, swelling, or unusual drainage in any area where there is a break in skin integrity
	  9. irritation or ulceration of oral mucous membrane
	  10. WBC level that increases or fails to decline toward normal and/or significant change in differential.
	b. Obtain culture specimens (e.g. wound, urine, vaginal, mouth, sputum, blood) as ordered. Report positive results.
	c. Implement measures *to reduce risk of infection:*
	  1. maintain a fluid intake of at least 2500 cc/day unless contraindicated
	  2. use good handwashing technique and encourage client to do the same
	  3. maintain meticulous aseptic technique during all invasive procedures (e.g. catheterizations, venous and arterial punctures, injections)
	  4. protect client from others with infection

5. perform actions to maintain and improve nutritional status (see Standardized Postoperative Care Plan, Nursing Diagnosis 6, action f)
6. reinforce importance of good oral care
7. provide proper balance of exercise and rest
8. perform actions to prevent pneumonia and wound and urinary tract infections (see Standardized Postoperative Care Plan, Nursing Diagnosis 16, actions a.6, b.4, and c.4).

    d. Monitor for therapeutic and nontherapeutic effects of anti-infectives if administered.

2. COLLABORATIVE DIAGNOSIS

Potential complications:

a. **pancreatitis** related to injury to the pancreas during surgery;
b. **subphrenic abscess** related to suppuration in the inflamed area and increased susceptibility to infection;
c. **thromboembolism** related to:
    1. hypercoagulability associated with:
        a. fluid volume deficit due to excessive fluid loss and inadequate fluid replacement
        b. temporary increase in RBCs and platelets (the spleen normally destroys RBCs and platelets)
    2. venous stasis associated with decreased activity and abdominal distention
    3. trauma to vein walls during surgery;
d. **postsplenectomy sepsis** related to decreased resistance to infection (does not occur commonly, but in clients with mild infections, sepsis can develop within hours).

DESIRED OUTCOMES	NURSING ACTIONS AND *SELECTED RATIONALES*

2.a. The client will experience resolution of pancreatitis if it occurs as evidenced by:
1. gradual resolution of abdominal pain
2. temperature declining toward normal
3. stable B/P and pulse
4. serum amylase and lipase levels declining toward normal
5. renal amylase/creatinine clearance ratio returning toward normal
6. WBC count declining toward normal.
	2.a.1. Assess for and report signs and symptoms of pancreatitis (e.g. extension of abdominal pain to midepigastric area or back, increased left upper quadrant pain, increase in temperature, tachycardia, hypotension, elevated serum amylase and lipase levels).
	2. Collect a timed (usually 2-hour) urine specimen if ordered. Report an elevated renal amylase/creatinine clearance ratio.
	3. Monitor WBC counts. Report levels that increase or fail to decline toward normal.
	4. If signs and symptoms of pancreatitis occur:
	  a. asssist client to assume position of greatest comfort (usually side-lying with knees flexed)
	  b. maintain food and fluid restrictions as ordered
	  c. insert nasogastric tube and maintain suction as ordered *(removal of gastric juices reduces the pancreatic stimulation normally caused by these juices)*
	  d. monitor for therapeutic and nontherapeutic effects of the following medications if administered:
	    1. analgesics and smooth muscle relaxants (e.g. nitroglycerin) *to reduce pain*
	    2. antacids and histamine$_2$ receptor antagonists *to neutralize and/or reduce output of hydrochloric acid and thereby reduce pancreatic stimulation*
	  e. refer to Care Plan on Pancreatitis for additional care measures.

2.b. The client will experience resolution of a subphrenic abscess if it develops as evidenced by:
   1. decrease in abdominal pain
   2. temperature declining toward normal
   3. WBC count declining toward normal.

2.b.1. Assess for and report signs and symptoms of a subphrenic abscess (e.g. increased, persistent abdominal pain; increase in temperature and pulse rate).
   2. Monitor WBC count and report levels that increase or fail to decline toward normal.
   3. If signs and symptoms of subphrenic abscess occur:
      a. monitor for therapeutic and nontherapeutic effects of anti-infectives if administered
      b. prepare client for surgical intervention (e.g. incision and drainage)
      c. assess for and report signs and symptoms of peritonitis (e.g. further increase in temperature; tense, rigid abdomen; increased severity of abdominal pain; rebound tenderness; failure of bowel sounds to return to normal; tachycardia; tachypnea; hypotension)
      d. provide emotional support to client and significant others.

2.c. The client will not experience signs and symptoms of a venous thrombus or pulmonary embolism (see Standardized Postoperative Care Plan, Collaborative Diagnosis 19, outcomes c.1 and 2, for outcome criteria).

2.c.1. Refer to Standardized Postoperative Nursing Care Plan, Collaborative Diagnosis 19, actions c.1 and 2, for measures related to assessment, prevention, and treatment of a venous thrombus and pulmonary embolism.
   2. In addition to the above assessments, monitor for and report:
      a. platelet count above 450,000 μl and/or elevated RBC levels (indicate that client has an increased risk for thromboembolism)
      b. increasing abdominal distention and pain (may indicate portal system thrombus or mesenteric embolism).

2.d. The client will not experience postsplenectomy sepsis as evidenced by:
   1. absence of nausea, vomiting, and headache
   2. usual mental status
   3. stable vital signs.

2.d.1. Assess for and report signs and symptoms of postsplenectomy sepsis (e.g. nausea, vomiting, headache, confusion, significant decrease in B/P, tachycardia, rapid or labored respirations).
   2. Implement measures to reduce risk of infection (see Postoperative Nursing Diagnosis 1, actions c and d) *in order to prevent postsplenectomy sepsis.*
   3. If signs and symptoms of postsplenectomy sepsis occur:
      a. notify physician immediately *(shock usually develops rapidly)*
      b. maintain intravenous fluid therapy as ordered
      c. monitor vital signs frequently
      d. obtain cultures from all possible sites of infection (e.g. urine, infusion sites, wounds, blood, sputum) as ordered; report abnormal results
      e. monitor for therapeutic and nontherapeutic effects of anti-infectives if administered *to control the precipitating infection* (usually respiratory tract infection)
      f. provide emotional support to client and significant others.

3. NURSING DIAGNOSIS

Knowledge deficit regarding follow-up care.

DESIRED OUTCOMES	NURSING ACTIONS AND *SELECTED RATIONALES*

3.a. The client will identify ways to prevent infection.

3.a.1. Explain to client that he/she will be more prone to infection for a while following splenectomy *(the rest of the reticuloendothelial system cannot immediately compensate for the loss of the spleen).*
   2. Instruct client in ways to prevent postoperative infection (see Standardized Postoperative Care Plan, Nursing Diagnosis 20, action a).
   3. Encourage client to consult health care provider about receiving vaccinations to reduce the risk of pneumonia and influenza.
   4. Reinforce the importance of taking anti-infectives if prescribed (may be prescribed for prophylaxis).

3.b. The client will state signs and symptoms of complications to report to the health care provider.

3.b.1. Refer to Standardized Postoperative Care Plan, Nursing Diagnosis 20, action c, for signs and symptoms to report to the health care provider.

2. In addition, instruct client to report nausea, vomiting, headache, and confusion (could be indicative of postsplenectomy sepsis).

3.c. The client will verbalize an understanding of and a plan for adhering to recommended follow-up care including future appointments with health care provider, medications prescribed, wound care, and activity level.

3.c. Refer to Standardized Postoperative Care Plan, Nursing Diagnosis 20, for routine postoperative instructions and measures to improve client compliance.

UNIT
XI

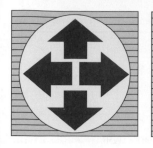
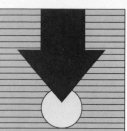
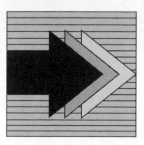
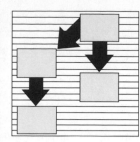
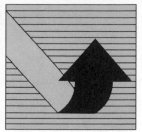

Unit XII

Nursing Care of the Client with Disturbances of the Gastrointestinal Tract

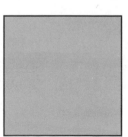

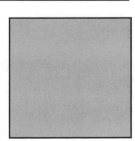

Appendectomy

An appendectomy is the surgical removal of the vermiform appendix (a small tubular projection of unknown function at the end of the cecum just below the ileocecal valve). It is performed to treat appendicitis, which occurs as a result of obstruction of the lumen of the appendix by a fecalith, parasites, bowel adhesions or fibrosis, tumor, foreign body, or lymphoid hyperplasia associated with infections. The increased intraluminal pressure and accumulation of mucosal fluid eventually exceed venous pressure. This results in a decreased blood supply to the area, mucosal ulceration, and bacterial invasion. Infection causes further inflammation, which leads to increased ischemia. Untreated, the appendix will rupture and peritonitis will result.

This care plan focuses on the adult client with appendicitis who is hospitalized for an appendectomy. Preoperative goals of care are to reduce fear and anxiety, control discomfort, and prevent rupture of the appendix. The goals of postoperative care are to maintain comfort, prevent complications, and educate the client regarding follow-up care.

DISCHARGE CRITERIA

Prior to discharge, the client will:

- state signs and symptoms of complications to report to the health care provider
- verbalize an understanding of and a plan for adhering to recommended follow-up care including future appointments with health care provider, medications prescribed, activity level, and wound care.

NURSING/COLLABORATIVE DIAGNOSES

Preoperative
1A. Altered comfort: abdominal pain particularly in the periumbilical area or right lower quadrant ☐ 629
1B. Altered comfort: nausea and vomiting ☐ 629
 2. Potential complication: peritonitis ☐ 630
Postoperative
 1. Potential complications:
    a. abscess formation
    b. peritonitis ☐ 631
 2. Knowledge deficit regarding follow-up care ☐ 631

Preoperative

Use in conjunction with the Standardized Preoperative Care Plan.

1.A. NURSING DIAGNOSIS

Altered comfort:* abdominal pain particularly in the periumbilical area or right lower quadrant related to obstruction and inflammation of the appendix.

---

* In this care plan, the nursing diagnosis "pain" is included under the diagnostic label of altered comfort.

DESIRED OUTCOMES	NURSING ACTIONS AND *SELECTED RATIONALES*

1.A. The client will experience diminished abdominal pain as evidenced by:
1. verbalization of reduction of pain
2. relaxed facial expression and body positioning
3. stable vital signs.
	1.A.1. Determine how client usually responds to pain.
	2. Assess for nonverbal signs of pain (e.g. guarding or rubbing of abdomen, wrinkled brow, clenched fists, reluctance to move, restlessness, diaphoresis, facial pallor or flushing, change in B/P, tachycardia).
	3. Assess verbal complaints of pain. Ask client to be specific about location, severity, and type of pain.
	4. Assess for factors that seem to aggravate and alleviate pain.
	5. Implement measures *to reduce abdominal pain:*
	  a. apply ice packs to painful area as ordered *in order to reduce inflammation*
	  b. assist client to assume a comfortable position (e.g. side-lying with right knee flexed)
	  c. monitor for therapeutic and nontherapeutic effects of analgesics if administered.
	6. Consult physician if above measures fail to provide adequate pain relief.

1.B. NURSING DIAGNOSIS

Altered comfort: nausea and vomiting related to stimulation of the vomiting center associated with:

1. vagal and/or sympathetic stimulation resulting from visceral irritation associated with inflammation and abdominal distention (due to decreased gastrointestinal motility);
2. cortical stimulation due to pain and stress.

DESIRED OUTCOMES	NURSING ACTIONS AND *SELECTED RATIONALES*

1.B. The client will experience relief of nausea and vomiting as evidenced by:
1. verbalization of relief of nausea
2. absence of vomiting.
	1.B.1. Assess client to determine factors that contribute to nausea and vomiting (e.g. abdominal distention, pain, movement, fear, anxiety).
	2. Implement measures *to reduce nausea and vomiting:*
	  a. perform actions to reduce pain (see Preoperative Nursing Diagnosis 1.A, action 5)
	  b. perform actions to reduce fear and anxiety (see Standardized Preoperative Care Plan, Nursing Diagnosis 1, action d)
	  c. eliminate noxious sights and smells from the environment *(noxious stimuli cause cortical stimulation of the vomiting center)*
	  d. encourage client to take deep, slow breaths when nauseated
	  e. encourage client to change positions slowly *(movement stimulates chemoreceptor trigger zone)*

   f. provide oral hygiene every 2 hours and after each emesis
   g. maintain food and fluid restrictions as ordered
   h. monitor for therapeutic and nontherapeutic effects of antiemetics if administered.
3. If above measures fail to control nausea and vomiting:
   a. consult physician
   b. be prepared to insert a nasogastric tube and maintain suction as ordered.

2. COLLABORATIVE DIAGNOSIS

Potential complication: peritonitis related to release of intestinal contents into the peritoneal cavity associated with rupture of the appendix.

DESIRED OUTCOMES	NURSING ACTIONS AND *SELECTED RATIONALES*

2. The client will not develop peritonitis as evidenced by:
a. no further increase in temperature
b. soft, nondistended abdomen
c. no increase in abdominal pain and tenderness
d. normal bowel sounds
e. stable vital signs
f. no further increase in WBC count.
	2.a. Assess frequently for and report signs and symptoms of peritonitis (e.g. further increase in temperature; tense, rigid abdomen; increase in severity of abdominal pain; rebound tenderness; diminished or absent bowel sounds; tachycardia; tachypnea; hypotension).
	b. Monitor WBC counts. Report increasing levels.
	c. Implement measures *to prevent rupture of the appendix:*
	   1. perform actions *to prevent a further increase in intraluminal pressure:*
	      a. maintain food and fluid restrictions as ordered
	      b. insert a nasogastric tube and maintain suction as ordered
	      c. do not administer an enema
	   2. avoid use of laxatives *(may cause excessive peristalsis)*
	   3. do not apply heat to abdomen *(may speed up the suppurative process and precipitate rupture).*
	d. If signs and symptoms of peritonitis occur:
	   1. withhold all food and fluid as ordered
	   2. place client on bedrest in a semi-Fowler's position *to assist in pooling or localizing gastrointestinal contents in the pelvis rather than under the diaphragm*
	   3. insert nasogastric tube and maintain suction as ordered
	   4. monitor for therapeutic and nontherapeutic effects of anti-infectives if administered
	   5. monitor for therapeutic and nontherapeutic effects of intravenous fluids and/or blood volume expanders if administered *to prevent or treat shock (shock can occur as a result of the escape of protein, fluid, and electrolytes into the peritoneal cavity)*
	   6. provide emotional support to client and significant others.

Postoperative

Use in conjunction with the Standardized Postoperative Care Plan.

1. COLLABORATIVE DIAGNOSIS

Potential complications:

a. **abscess formation** related to suppuration in the inflamed or infected area;
b. **peritonitis** related to wound infection, leakage from an abscess, and/or release of intestinal contents into the peritoneal cavity associated with preoperative or intraoperative rupture of the appendix and leakage of suture lines postoperatively.

DESIRED OUTCOMES	NURSING ACTIONS AND *SELECTED RATIONALES*

1.a. The client will experience resolution of an abscess if it occurs as evidenced by:
1. temperature declining toward normal
2. absence of abdominal cramping
3. resolution of abdominal pain
4. WBC count declining toward normal.

1.a.1. Assess for and report signs and symptoms of abscess formation (e.g. increase in temperature, abdominal cramping, increased and more constant abdominal pain, further increase in WBC count).
  2. If signs and symptoms of an abscess occur:
    a. monitor for therapeutic and nontherapeutic effects of anti-infectives if administered
    b. prepare client for surgical drainage of the abscess if indicated
    c. provide emotional support to client and significant others.

1.b. The client will not have or will have resolution of peritonitis as evidenced by:
1. temperature declining toward normal
2. soft, nondistended abdomen
3. gradual resolution of abdominal pain
4. gradual return of normal bowel sounds
5. stable vital signs
6. WBC count declining toward normal.

1.b.1. Refer to Preoperative Collaborative Diagnosis 2, actions a and d, for measures related to assessment and treatment of peritonitis.
  2. Monitor WBC counts. Report levels that increase or fail to return to normal.
  3. Implement measures *to prevent or control existing peritonitis:*
    a. perform actions to treat an abscess if it occurs (see action a.2 in this diagnosis)
    b. perform actions *to maintain patency of wound drain(s) if present in order to prevent increased pressure on the suture line:*
      1. keep tubing free of kinks
      2. empty collection device as often as necessary
      3. maintain suction as ordered
    c. perform actions *to prevent inadvertent removal of wound drain(s) if present:*
      1. use caution when changing dressings surrounding drain(s)
      2. provide extension tubing if necessary *to enable client to move without placing tension on the drain(s)*
      3. instruct client not to pull on drain(s) or drainage tubing
    d. maintain aseptic technique during dressing changes and wound care
    e. keep dressings clean and dry
    f. monitor for therapeutic and nontherapeutic effects of anti-infectives if administered.

2. NURSING DIAGNOSIS

Knowledge deficit regarding follow-up care.

DESIRED OUTCOMES	NURSING ACTIONS AND *SELECTED RATIONALES*
2.a. The client will state signs and symptoms of complications to report to the health care provider.	2.a. Refer to Standardized Postoperative Care Plan, Nursing Diagnosis 20, action c, for signs and symptoms to report to the health care provider.
2.b. The client will verbalize an understanding of and a plan for adhering to recommended follow-up care including future appointments with health care provider, medications prescribed, activity level, and wound care.	2.b. Refer to Standardized Postoperative Care Plan, Nursing Diagnosis 20, for routine postoperative instructions and measures to improve client compliance.

■ ■

Bowel Diversion: Ileostomy

An ileostomy is the diversion of the ileum from the abdominal cavity through an opening created in the abdominal wall. It may be performed to treat conditions such as familial polyposis, intestinal cancer, and, most commonly, inflammatory bowel disease that is refractory to conservative management. A proctocolectomy (removal of the colon and rectum) may be done at the same time to prevent future bowel changes due to recurrent inflammatory bowel disease or cancer of the colon.

Ileostomies can be temporary or permanent. The most common permanent one is the conventional type (end ileostomy). It drains intermittently, and because it cannot be regulated, a collection device needs to be worn over the stoma at all times. Another type of permanent ileal diversion is the continent ileostomy in which the terminal ileum is used to construct an intra-abdominal reservoir (Kock pouch). This reservoir is drained at in-tervals by inserting a catheter through a valve that has been surgically constructed or inserted beneath the stoma. A temporary ileostomy may be created to rest the bowel following traumatic abdominal injury or during the first stage of an ileoanal anastomosis in order to allow healing of the newly constructed ileal pouch or reservoir.

This care plan focuses on the adult client with inflammatory bowel disease hospitalized for bowel diversion with creation of a permanent ileostomy. Preoperatively, goals of care are to reduce fear and anxiety and begin to educate the client about the ileostomy. The postoperative goals of care are to maintain integrity of the stoma and peristomal and perianal skin, prevent complications, facilitate psychological adjustment to the ileostomy, and educate the client regarding follow-up care.

DISCHARGE CRITERIA

Prior to discharge, the client will:

- verbalize a basic understanding of the anatomical changes that have occurred as a result of the surgery
- identify ways to maintain fluid and electrolyte balance
- identify methods of controlling odor and noise associated with ostomy drainage and gas
- demonstrate ways to maintain integrity of the stoma and peristomal and perianal skin
- demonstrate proper use and care of ostomy equipment

- demonstrate proper techniques for draining and irrigating a continent ileostomy if present
- identify ways to prevent blockage of the stoma
- state signs and symptoms to report to the health care provider
- share thoughts and feelings about the effect of altered bowel function on self-concept and life style
- identify appropriate community resources that can assist with home management and adjustment to changes resulting from the bowel diversion
- verbalize an understanding of and a plan for adhering to recommended follow-up care including future appointments with health care provider, wound care, activity level, and medications prescribed.

NURSING/COLLABORATIVE DIAGNOSES

Preoperative
1. Anxiety □ *634*
2. Knowledge deficit □ *634*

Postoperative
1. Altered fluid and electrolyte balance:
   a. fluid volume deficit, hyponatremia, hypokalemia, and hypochloremia
   b. metabolic alkalosis
   c. metabolic acidosis □ *635*
2. Impaired skin integrity:
   a. surgical incision
   b. impaired wound healing
   c. irritation or breakdown around suture lines and wound drains
   d. peristomal irritation or breakdown
   e. perianal irritation or breakdown □ *636*
3. Potential complications:
   a. peritonitis
   b. stomal changes:
      1. necrosis
      2. excessive bleeding or irritation
      3. prolapse
   c. stomal obstruction □ *639*
4. Disturbance in self-concept □ *641*
5. Ineffective individual coping □ *642*
6. Grieving □ *644*
7. Knowledge deficit regarding follow-up care □ *644*

UNIT XII

Preoperative

Use in conjunction with the Care Plan on Inflammatory Bowel Disease and the Standardized Preoperative Care Plan.

1. NURSING DIAGNOSIS

Anxiety related to unfamiliar environment; lack of understanding of planned surgery; and anticipated postoperative discomfort, changes in body image and functioning, and effects of the ileostomy on life style.

DESIRED OUTCOMES	NURSING ACTIONS AND *SELECTED RATIONALES*
1. The client will experience a reduction in fear and anxiety (see Standardized Preoperative Care Plan, Nursing Diagnosis 1, for outcome criteria).	1.a. Refer to Standardized Preoperative Care Plan, Nursing Diagnosis 1, for measures related to assessment and reduction of fear and anxiety. b. Implement additional measures *to reduce fear and anxiety:* 1. show client a picture of a stoma *so that he/she will know what to expect;* explain that every attempt will be made to place the stoma in an area that will be easily accessible for self-care and enable the appliance to lie flat and be unobtrusive (the tentative stoma site is mapped out preoperatively by the physician and/or enterostomal therapist) 2. show client the ostomy appliances that he/she will be using in the immediate postoperative period; allow client to handle the appliances; assure him/her that current ostomy collection devices are odorproof and available in sizes that fit various body contours 3. inform client that the stoma will shrink in size as edema resolves during the 6 weeks after surgery 4. explain that slight bleeding of the stoma is expected 5. assure client that the stoma has no pain receptors and will not be painful when touched 6. emphasize that the liquid drainage that will come from the stoma 1–3 days after surgery will decrease in amount to 400–800 cc/day (about ½–¾ quart/day) and will have a more paste-like consistency within 3–6 months 7. explain that the occasional feelings of pressure that may occur in the rectal area after a proctectomy are not unusual and will subside as postoperative swelling decreases 8. focus on activities that the client will be able to do or resume once the ileostomy is established (the discomfort, diarrhea, and prescribed medication therapy associated with inflammatory bowel disease frequently have limited client's activities) 9. arrange for a visit with a person of similar age and same sex who has successfully adjusted to his/her ileostomy.

2. NURSING DIAGNOSIS

Knowledge deficit regarding hospital routines associated with the surgery, physical preparation for the bowel diversion, and postoperative care and management of the ileostomy.

DESIRED OUTCOMES	NURSING ACTIONS AND *SELECTED RATIONALES*
2.a. The client will verbalize an understanding of usual preoperative and	2.a.1. Refer to Standardized Preoperative Care Plan, Nursing Diagnosis 4, actions a.1–4, for information to include in preoperative teaching. 2. Provide additional information regarding specific preoperative and

postoperative care and routines.

postoperative care and routines for clients having a bowel diversion with ileostomy:
a. explain the preoperative bowel preparation (e.g. low-residue diet, enemas, anti-infective therapy)
b. if proctocolectomy is planned, inform client that perineal wound drains will be present after surgery
c. if a continent ileostomy is planned, inform client that:
1. a temporary drainage catheter will be in the stoma for at least 10–14 days after surgery and an external collection device will need to be worn during this time
2. an intermittent catheter clamping regimen will begin 10–14 days after surgery and catheter irrigations will be done periodically; then, when physician allows, the catheter will be removed and inserted only for short periods (usually 10–15 minutes) at scheduled intervals throughout the day and night to drain the internal reservoir
d. offer basic information regarding postoperative care of the stoma and peristomal and perianal skin, ways to control intestinal gas and odor of the ostomy drainage (effluent), and use of various types of appliances.
3. Allow time for questions and clarification of information provided.

2.b. The client will demonstrate the ability to perform techniques designed to prevent postoperative complications.

2.b. Refer to Standardized Preoperative Care Plan, Nursing Diagnosis 4, action b, for instructions on ways to prevent postoperative complications.

□ ▬▬▬▬▬▬▬▬▬▬▬▬▬▬▬▬▬▬▬▬▬▬▬▬▬▬▬

Postoperative

Use in conjunction with the Standardized Postoperative Care Plan.

□ ▬▬▬▬▬▬▬▬▬▬▬▬▬▬▬▬▬▬▬▬▬▬▬▬▬▬▬

1. NURSING/COLLABORATIVE DIAGNOSIS

Altered fluid and electrolyte balance:

a. **fluid volume deficit, hyponatremia, hypokalemia, and hypochloremia** related to excessive loss of fluid and electrolytes associated with vomiting, nasogastric tube and/or profuse wound drainage, and ileostomy drainage (effluent contains fluid and electrolytes that would normally be absorbed throughout the large intestine);
b. **metabolic alkalosis** related to excessive loss of hydrochloric acid associated with vomiting and nasogastric tube drainage;
c. **metabolic acidosis** related to loss of bicarbonate ions associated with ileostomy drainage (effluent contains bicarbonate ions that would normally be absorbed throughout the large intestine).

□ ▬▬▬▬▬▬▬▬▬▬▬▬▬▬▬▬▬▬▬▬▬▬▬▬▬▬▬

DESIRED OUTCOMES	NURSING ACTIONS AND *SELECTED RATIONALES*
1. The client will maintain fluid and electrolyte balance as evidenced by: a. normal skin turgor	1.a. Assess for and report: 1. signs and symptoms of fluid volume deficit, hyponatremia, hypokalemia, hypochloremia, and metabolic alkalosis (see Standardized Postoperative Care Plan, Nursing Diagnosis 5, action a.1)

b. moist mucous membranes
c. stable weight
d. B/P and pulse within normal range for client and stable with position change
e. usual rate and depth of respirations
f. urine specific gravity between 1.010–1.030
g. no evidence of confusion, irritability, lethargy, excessive thirst, headache, nausea, vomiting, ileus, cardiac arrhythmias, muscle weakness
h. normal serum osmolality, electrolytes, and blood gases.

2. excessive ileostomy output (after the return of bowel activity, output may be as high as 2000 cc/day but should gradually decrease to 400–800 cc/day)
3. signs and symptoms of metabolic acidosis (e.g. drowsiness; disorientation; stupor; rapid, deep respirations; headache; nausea; vomiting).
b. Monitor serum osmolality, electrolyte, and blood gas results. Report abnormal values.
c. Refer to Standardized Postoperative Care Plan, Nursing Diagnosis 5, action a.3, for measures to prevent and treat fluid and electrolyte imbalances.
d. Implement additional measures *to prevent and treat fluid and electrolyte imbalances:*
   1. when the ileostomy begins to function (usually 1–3 days postoperatively), perform actions *to prevent excessive ileostomy output:*
      a. instruct client to avoid excessive intake of foods/fluids that may cause diarrhea (e.g. prunes, iced or hot fluids, whole milk, raw fruits)
      b. monitor for therapeutic and nontherapeutic effects of antidiarrheal agents if administered
   2. monitor for therapeutic and nontherapeutic effects of sodium bicarbonate if administered *to prevent or treat metabolic acidosis (reserved for use in severe acidosis when pH is less than 7.1).*

---

2. NURSING DIAGNOSIS

Impaired skin integrity:

a. **surgical incision;**
b. **impaired wound healing** related to inadequate nutritional status, inadequate blood supply to wound area, stress on wound area, infection, and increased levels of glucocorticoids (levels usually rise with stress);
c. **irritation or breakdown around suture lines and wound drains** related to contact of the skin with wound drainage, pressure from drainage tubes, and use of tape;
d. **peristomal irritation or breakdown** related to:
   1. chemical irritation associated with contact of peristomal skin with intestinal drainage (the effluent is rich in proteolytic enzymes), soap residue and perspiration under the appliance, and allergic reaction to substances used to secure the appliance
   2. mechanical irritation associated with frequent and/or improper removal of adhesives, skin cements, and tape; aggressive cleansing of peristomal area; and pressure from appliance belt and drainage valves or clamps on the appliance;
e. **perianal irritation or breakdown** related to contact of skin with mucous drainage from the anus (occurs if the rectal mucosa and anus were left intact) and/or wound drainage from perianal incision(s) and drain(s) if proctocolectomy was performed.

DESIRED OUTCOMES	NURSING ACTIONS AND *SELECTED RATIONALES*
2.a. The client will experience normal healing of surgical wounds (see Standardized Postoperative Care Plan, Nursing Diagnosis 9, outcome a, for outcome criteria).	2.a. Refer to Standardized Postoperative Care Plan, Nursing Diagnosis 9, action a, for measures related to assessment and promotion of normal wound healing.

2.b. The client will maintain skin integrity (see Standardized Postoperative Care Plan, Nursing Diagnosis 9, outcome b, for outcome criteria).

2.b.1. Inspect skin areas that are in contact with wound drainage, tape, and drainage tubings for signs of irritation and breakdown.

2. Assess for signs and symptoms of:
   a. peristomal irritation and breakdown (e.g. redness, inflammation, and/or excoriation of peristomal skin; complaints of itching and burning under the appliance; inability to keep appliance on)
   b. perianal irritation and breakdown (e.g. redness, inflammation, and/or excoriation of perianal skin; complaints of itching or burning in perianal area).

3. Refer to Standardized Postoperative Care Plan, Nursing Diagnosis 9, action b.2, for measures to prevent skin irritation and breakdown resulting from wound drainage, tape, and drainage tubings.

4. Implement measures *to prevent peristomal irritation and breakdown:*
   a. patch test all adhesives, sprays, solvents, and skin barriers before initial use; do not use products that cause redness, itching, burning, or inflammation
   b. change appliance only when necessary (e.g. as ordered, if appliance or seal is leaking, if stoma size changes, if client complains of burning or itching under the seal)
   c. always use a skin barrier (e.g. karaya, ReliaSeal, Stomahesive) on the peristomal area *to protect the skin from the proteolytic enzymes that are in the effluent*
   d. when the appliance is expected to need frequent changing, use a 2-piece appliance (faceplate and pouch, barrier/flange and pouch) *so that the adhesive does not have to be removed with each pouch change*
   e. use a 1-piece drainable appliance unless contraindicated *(the 1-piece appliance combines the skin barrier and pouch, which eliminates the possibility of effluent leaking out between them)*
   f. remove hair from peristomal skin using an electric or safety razor *to help maintain an adequate seal and to reduce irritation when the appliance is removed*
   g. perform actions *to reduce peristomal irritation during removal of appliance:*
      1. apply warm water or solvent to edge of adhesive disc if necessary *to dissolve adhesive* (allow time for adhesive to loosen before pulling appliance off)
      2. remove appliance gently and in direction of hair growth
      3. if solvent was used, gently wash skin with mild soap and warm water and rinse thoroughly after pouch is removed
      4. do not forcefully remove protective skin barrier paste residues *(reapplications are less irritating than vigorous cleansing)*
   h. perform actions *to prevent effluent from coming in contact with the skin when changing appliance:*
      1. change appliance when the ostomy is least active (usually before meals or 2–4 hours after eating)
      2. place a "wick" (rolled gauze pad), vaginal tampon, or tissue on the stoma opening when the appliance is off
   i. cleanse peristomal skin thoroughly with mild soap and water and rinse completely; use tepid rather than hot water *to prevent burns*
   j. if using skin cement, allow it to dry thoroughly before applying pouch *in order to prevent severe chemical burns*
   k. if indicated, apply skin sealants (e.g. United Skin Prep, Hollister Skin Gel) before applying adhesive or barrier *in order to protect peristomal area*
   l. perform actions *to prevent effluent from contacting the skin when appliance is on:*
      1. measure the diameter of the stoma; cut skin barrier the same size as stoma and select a pouch with an opening that is no more than 0.3 cm (⅛ inch) larger than the stoma (it may be necessary to create a pattern to use for cutting barrier and pouch opening if stoma has an irregular shape and cannot be measured using appliance manufacturer's standard measuring guide)
      2. instruct and assist client to remeasure the stoma size frequently during the first 6 weeks after surgery and to alter skin barrier and pouch openings as stomal edema decreases

UNIT XII

3. implement measures *to ensure an adequate seal:*
   a. avoid use of ointments or creams on peristomal skin *(these can interfere with adequate adhesive binding)*
   b. follow manufacturer's instructions carefully when applying skin barrier and appliances
   c. use products such as ostomy paste (e.g. Stomahesive paste, Premium paste) to fill in irregularities around stoma site (e.g. body folds, previous scars, retention sutures) before applying collection device
   d. apply firm pressure and remove all air pockets when applying barrier and appliance
   e. use products with a flexible or convex backing or medical adhesive if needed *to achieve an adequate seal*
   f. empty pouch when it is about ⅓ full of effluent *(a heavy pouch is more likely to separate from the skin or faceplate)*
4. position pouch so gravity flow facilitates drainage away from stoma and skin
5. cleanse bottom of drainable appliance after emptying it and close appliance properly *to prevent leakage*
6. use drainable or 2-piece appliance or appliance with release valve if gas is a problem; the pouch should never be punctured or cut to release gas *because effluent can seep out of the opening*

m. if a belted appliance is used, fasten the belt so that 2 fingers can slip easily between belt and skin *in order to prevent excessive pressure on skin*
n. check appliance periodically to ensure that clamps or valves are not placing pressure on the skin.

5. Implement measures *to prevent perianal irritation and breakdown:*
   a. keep perianal area clean and dry
   b. instruct client to perform anal sphincter strengthening exercises (e.g. contracting the anal sphincter for 20 seconds at least 6 times/day) as ordered *to improve sphincter tone and reduce the risk of mucus leakage*
   c. place perineal pads in client's underwear if needed and change pads when they become damp
   d. expose perianal area to air for 20–30 minutes 1–4 times/day if possible
   e. apply petroleum-based ointments to perianal area as ordered *to protect skin.*

6. If signs and symptoms of peristomal and/or perianal skin irritation or breakdown occur:
   a. cleanse area gently with warm water
   b. avoid use of any skin barrier and topical medication that can cause further irritation to affected skin (e.g. plain tincture of benzoin)
   c. perform skin care according to physician's order or hospital protocol; skin care may include the following:
      1. application of aluminum acetate (Burow's solution) compresses for 20–30 minutes 3 times/day
      2. exposure of affected area to light or heat for 20–30 minutes 1–4 times/day; heat source (e.g. hair dryer on lukewarm setting, heat lamp) should be kept about 30 cm (12 inches) away from skin; cover stoma with a damp gauze pad *to prevent burns and decrease the risk of stomal swelling due to heat-induced increased blood flow*
      3. application of hypoallergenic skin barrier
   d. avoid changing appliance unless there are signs of leakage or skin care is ordered
   e. monitor for therapeutic and nontherapeutic effects of the following if applied:
      1. nystatin powder *to treat fungal infections*
      2. corticosteroids (e.g. triamcinolone) *to reduce inflammation associated with severe skin reactions*
   f. consult physician and/or enterostomal therapist if:
      1. areas of irritation or breakdown do not gradually improve
      2. signs and symptoms of infection (e.g. elevated temperature; redness, warmth, and edema around area of breakdown; unusual drainage from site) are present.

□

3. COLLABORATIVE DIAGNOSIS

Potential complications:

a. **peritonitis** related to:
1. wound infection (these clients may be more susceptible to infection due to immunosuppression associated with long-term corticosteroid use and/or malnutrition due to persistent diarrhea in the preoperative period)
2. leakage of bowel contents into the peritoneum during surgery or postoperatively associated with failure of the surgical anastomosis or retraction of the peristomal skin (retraction can occur with slippage of the sutures or shrinkage of the supporting tissues)
3. abscess formation;

b. **stomal changes:**
1. **necrosis** related to intraoperative and/or postoperative interruption of blood supply to the stoma
2. **excessive bleeding or irritation** related to aggressive cleansing or poor appliance fit
3. **prolapse** related to loss of integrity of the sutures;

c. **stomal obstruction** related to edema and/or blockage by food.

□

DESIRED OUTCOMES	NURSING ACTIONS AND *SELECTED RATIONALES*

3.a. The client will not develop peritonitis as evidenced by:
1. gradual resolution of abdominal pain
2. soft, nondistended abdomen
3. temperature declining toward normal
4. stable vital signs
5. gradual return of normal bowel sounds
6. WBC count declining toward normal.

3.a.1. Assess for and report signs and symptoms of peritonitis (e.g. increase in severity of abdominal pain; generalized abdominal pain; rebound tenderness; tense, rigid abdomen; increase in temperature; tachycardia; tachypnea; hypotension; continued absent or diminished bowel sounds).

2. Monitor WBC counts. Report levels that increase or fail to decline toward normal.

3. Implement measures *to prevent peritonitis:*
   a. perform actions to prevent and treat wound infection (see Standardized Postoperative Care Plan, Nursing Diagnosis 16, actions b.4 and 5)
   b. perform actions *to prevent overdistention of the intestine and resultant strain on and leakage from the suture line:*
      1. implement measures to prevent obstruction of the stoma (see action c.2 in this diagnosis)
      2. instruct client to avoid activities that can cause air swallowing (e.g. chewing gum, sucking on hard candy, smoking)
   c. perform actions *to maintain patency of wound drain(s) if present:*
      1. keep tubing free of kinks
      2. empty collection device as often as necessary
      3. maintain suction as ordered
   d. perform actions *to prevent inadvertent removal of wound drain(s) if present:*
      1. use caution when changing dressings surrounding drain(s)
      2. provide extension tubing if necessary *to enable client to move without placing tension on drain(s)*
      3. instruct client not to pull on drain(s) or drainage tubing
   e. if client has a continent ileostomy:
      1. perform actions *to prevent overdistention of the reservoir and resultant strain on and leakage from the suture line:*
         a. maintain stomal catheter suction as ordered *to keep the reservoir decompressed*
         b. when suction is discontinued, keep drainage bag below level of reservoir *to maintain gravity drainage*

UNIT XII

     c. keep stomal catheter free of kinks and dependent loops

     d. irrigate the reservoir as ordered using only a minimal amount of irrigating solution (usually 20–30 cc of normal saline)

  2. do not reposition the stomal catheter *(repositioning may damage or disrupt the suture line)*

f. if peristomal skin is retracted, perform wound care as ordered *to facilitate the formation of granulation tissue in retracted area.*

4. If signs and symptoms of peritonitis occur:

  a. withhold all food and fluid as ordered

  b. place client on bedrest in a semi-Fowler's position *to assist in pooling or localizing gastrointestinal contents in the pelvis rather than under the diaphragm*

  c. insert a nasogastric tube and maintain suction as ordered

  d. monitor for therapeutic and nontherapeutic effects of anti-infectives if administered

  e. monitor for therapeutic and nontherapeutic effects of intravenous fluids and/or blood volume expanders if administered *to prevent or treat shock (shock can occur as a result of escape of protein, fluid, and electrolytes into peritoneal cavity)*

  f. prepare client for surgical intervention (e.g. repair of site of anastomosis or peristomal skin retraction, drainage of abscess) if indicated

  g. provide emotional support to client and significant others.

3.b. The client will maintain integrity of the stoma as evidenced by:

1. red or dark pink stomal coloring
2. expected stomal height
3. absence of excessive bleeding and increasing edema of the stoma.

3.b.1. Assess for and report signs and symptoms of impaired stomal integrity (e.g. pale, dark red, blue-black, or magenta color of stoma; increased height of stoma; increased stomal edema or bleeding). Use only clear appliances during the immediate postoperative period *to allow easy visibility of stoma.*

2. Implement measures *to maintain integrity of stoma:*

  a. ensure that openings of the adhesive disc, skin barrier, faceplate, and/or pouch are not too small and carefully center stoma in the openings *in order to maintain adequate stomal circulation*

  b. anchor faceplate and pouch securely *to prevent a shearing action across stoma*

  c. cleanse stoma gently using a soft cloth, gauze, or tissue.

3. If signs and symptoms of impaired stomal integrity occur, prepare client for surgical revision of stoma if indicated.

3.c. The client will not develop stomal obstruction as evidenced by:

1. expected amount and consistency of ileostomy output
2. no complaints of abdominal cramping, nausea, increased feeling of fullness
3. absence of vomiting.

3.c.1. Assess for and report signs and symptoms of stomal obstruction:

  a. less than expected amount of ileostomy output (after return of peristalsis, output may be as high as 2000 cc/day and will gradually decrease to about 400–800 cc/day)

  b. change in effluent consistency from a thicker consistency to a thin, watery liquid (postoperatively, effluent gradually becomes thicker; a return to thin, watery consistency may indicate a stomal blockage)

  c. complaints of abdominal cramping, nausea, increased feeling of fullness

  d. vomiting.

2. Implement measures *to prevent stomal obstruction:*

  a. if stomal catheter is present:

    1. perform actions *to prevent inadvertent removal* (e.g. secure tubing, instruct client not to pull on catheter)

    2. perform actions *to maintain patency of catheter* (e.g. avoid kinks in tubing, irrigate as ordered [usually 20–30 cc of normal saline every 2 hours])

  b. monitor for therapeutic and nontherapeutic effects of corticosteroids if administered *to reduce stomal edema*

  c. administer oral medications in liquid form *(undigested pills can block stoma)*

  d. when oral intake is allowed, perform actions *to prevent blockage of stoma by food:*

    1. slowly advance diet as ordered and tolerated

    2. instruct client to chew food thoroughly

    3. instruct client to avoid or eat only small amounts of foods that are hard to digest (e.g. popcorn, coconut, celery, bean sprouts, bamboo

shoots, whole kernel corn, raw carrots, nuts, granola, mushrooms, vegetable and fruit skins).
3. If food blockage occurs, implement measures *to aid in evacuation of effluent:*
   a. perform actions *to promote peristalsis* (e.g. gently massage abdomen, apply warm water to stoma, apply warm compresses to abdomen)
   b. perform actions *to break up or shift food blockage:*
      1. encourage fluid intake if nausea or vomiting is not a problem
      2. instruct and assist client to assume a knee-chest position and gently massage abdominal area under the stoma
      3. if client is performing intermittent clamping of temporary catheter in a continent ileostomy (usually begins 10–14 days after surgery), instruct and assist him/her to unclamp catheter and irrigate with or instill normal saline as ordered
   c. encourage participation in relaxing activities (e.g. reading, listening to music) *in order to reduce muscle tension*
   d. assist with irrigation of the ileostomy if indicated.
4. If signs and symptoms of stomal obstruction persist:
   a. withhold all food and fluid as ordered
   b. insert a nasogastric tube and maintain suction as ordered
   c. prepare client for surgical intervention to relieve obstruction if indicated
   d. provide emotional support to client and significant others.

□ ▬▬▬▬▬▬▬▬▬▬▬▬▬▬▬▬▬▬▬▬▬▬▬▬▬▬

4. NURSING DIAGNOSIS

Disturbance in self-concept* related to:

a. change in appearance resulting from presence of a stoma;
b. embarrassment associated with noise and odor resulting from gas and effluent;
c. dependence on others for assistance with ostomy management;
d. alteration in life style associated with altered bowel elimination.

---

* This diagnostic label includes the nursing diagnoses of body image disturbance and self-esteem disturbance.

□ ▬▬▬▬▬▬▬▬▬▬▬▬▬▬▬▬▬▬▬▬▬▬▬▬▬▬

UNIT
XII

DESIRED OUTCOMES	NURSING ACTIONS AND *SELECTED RATIONALES*
4. The client will demonstrate beginning adaptation to changes in appearance and body functioning as evidenced by: a. verbalization of feelings of self-worth and sexual adequacy b. maintenance of relationships with significant others c. active participation in activities of daily living d. active interest in personal appearance e. willingness to participate in social activities f. verbalization of a plan for	4.a. Determine the meaning of changes in appearance and body functioning to the client by encouraging him/her to verbalize feelings and by noting nonverbal responses to the changes experienced. b. Assess for signs and symptoms of a disturbance in self-concept (e.g. verbal or nonverbal cues denoting a negative response to change in body functioning or appearance such as denial of or preoccupation with changes that have occurred, refusal to look at or touch stoma, or withdrawal from significant others). c. Assist client to identify strengths and qualities that have a positive effect on self-concept. d. Implement measures *to assist client to improve self-esteem* (e.g. limit negative self-criticism, encourage positive comments about self, give positive feedback about accomplishments). e. Implement measures to facilitate the grieving process (see Postoperative Nursing Diagnosis 6, action d). f. Reinforce actions to assist client to cope with effects of the ileostomy (see Postoperative Nursing Diagnosis 5, action d). g. Clarify misconceptions about future limitations on usual activities.

integrating changes in appearance and bowel elimination into life style.

h. Instruct client in ways *to reduce gas formation:*
   1. avoid activities that can cause air swallowing (e.g. chewing gum, drinking through a straw, sucking on hard candy, smoking)
   2. eat small, frequent meals and chew food well
   3. limit intake of gas-producing foods/fluids (e.g. cabbage, onions, beans, carbonated beverages, sauerkraut)
   4. increase intake of foods/fluids that decrease gas formation (e.g. yogurt, buttermilk).
i. Instruct client in and assist with measures *to reduce odor resulting from ileostomy drainage:*
   1. use odorproof pouches and/or pouch deodorizers
   2. empty pouch regularly; rinse inside of pouch and clean off any effluent before closing pouch
   3. drain the reservoir of continent ileostomy as ordered *to reduce possibility of leakage*
   4. use disposable appliances or clean reusable items thoroughly
   5. perform actions to ensure an adequate pouch seal (see Postoperative Nursing Diagnosis 2, action b.4.l.3)
   6. limit intake of foods that cause effluent to have a stronger odor (e.g. onions, garlic, fish, eggs, cheese, asparagus)
   7. increase intake of foods/fluids that control odor (e.g. spinach, parsley, yogurt, buttermilk)
   8. take charcoal tablets or antiflatulents such as bismuth subgallate or bismuth subcarbonate *(the bismuth combines with sulfur in intestine to reduce odor).*
j. Assure client that the pouch and clothing will muffle sounds of bowel activity.
k. Assure client that once the stomal edema and surgical discomfort have resolved, he/she will be able to dress as before with minor, or no, modifications.
l. If client is concerned about the presence of the stoma and appliance, discuss the possibility of:
   1. using attractive ostomy appliances (e.g. opaque or patterned pouches, pouch covers)
   2. wearing underwear with the crotch removed (for females), boxer shorts (for males), or abdominal binders during sexual activity.
m. Assist client with usual grooming and makeup habits if necessary.
n. Demonstrate acceptance of client using techniques such as therapeutic touch and frequent visits. Encourage significant others to do the same.
o. Assess for and support behaviors suggesting positive adaptation to changes experienced (e.g. willingness to care for ileostomy, compliance with treatment plan).
p. Encourage significant others to allow client to do what he/she is able *so that independence can be re-established and/or self-esteem redeveloped.*
q. Assist client's and significant others' adjustment by listening, facilitating communication, and providing information.
r. Encourage visits and support from significant others.
s. Encourage client to continue involvement in social activities and to pursue interests.
t. Provide information about and encourage utilization of community agencies or support groups (e.g. ostomy groups; sexual, family, individual, and/or financial counseling).
u. Consult physician about psychological counseling if client desires or if he/she seems unwilling or unable to adapt to changes resulting from the ileostomy.

☐ ▄▄▄

5. NURSING DIAGNOSIS

Ineffective individual coping related to fear, anxiety, change in usual method of bowel elimination, difficulty in caring for ileostomy, fear of rejection by others, and inadequate support system.

☐ ▄▄▄

DESIRED OUTCOMES	NURSING ACTIONS AND *SELECTED RATIONALES*

5. The client will demonstrate the use of effective coping skills as evidenced by:
   a. willingness to participate in treatment plan and self-care activities
   b. verbalization of ability to cope with the ileostomy
   c. identification of stressors
   d. utilization of appropriate problem-solving techniques
   e. recognition and utilization of available support systems.

5.a. Assess effectiveness of client's coping strategies by observing behavior and noting strengths, weaknesses, ability to express feelings and concerns, and willingness to participate in treatment plan.
   b. Assess for and report signs and symptoms that may indicate ineffective coping (e.g. sleep disturbances, increasing fatigue, difficulty concentrating, irritability, decreased tolerance for pain, verbalization of inability to cope, inability to problem-solve).
   c. Allow time for client to adjust psychologically to the ileostomy (many clients welcome the bowel diversion because it means an end to the pain and diarrhea that occur with inflammatory bowel disease).
   d. Implement measures *to promote effective coping:*
      1. arrange for a visit from a person of similar age and same sex who has successfully adjusted to an ileostomy
      2. perform actions to reduce fear and anxiety (see Standardized Postoperative Care Plan, Nursing Diagnosis 1, action c)
      3. perform actions to promote a positive self-concept (see Postoperative Nursing Diagnosis 4, actions c–t)
      4. perform actions *to assist client to adapt to his/her new method of bowel elimination:*
         a. maintain consistency of approaches and explanations
         b. do not overload client with information irrelevant to present stage of ostomy management unless client is questioning or expressing an interest
         c. encourage participation in ostomy care as soon as possible
         d. use appliances that client is expected to use when discharged
         e. ensure adequate time and privacy for ostomy care
      5. include client in planning of care, encourage maximum participation in ostomy care, and allow choices whenever possible *to enable him/her to maintain a sense of control*
      6. instruct client in effective problem-solving techniques (e.g. accurate identification of stressors, determination of various options to solve problem)
      7. assist client to maintain usual daily routines whenever possible
      8. assist client through methods such as role playing to prepare for negative reactions from others because of ileostomy
      9. provide diversional activities according to client's interests
      10. instruct client to carry extra ostomy appliances on his/her person so they will be readily available if needed
      11. assist client to identify and utilize available support systems; provide information about available community resources that can assist client and significant others in coping with effects of the ileostomy (e.g. stress management classes, local ostomy support groups, United Ostomy Association, counseling services).
   e. Implement measures *to decrease possibility of rejection by partner:*
      1. provide support for the partner by helping him/her to acknowledge both positive and negative feelings about changes in the client
      2. if appropriate, involve partner in ostomy care *to facilitate adjustment to and integration of his/her partner's new body image.*
   f. Encourage continued emotional support from significant others.
   g. Encourage the client to share with significant others the kind of support that would be most beneficial (e.g. listening, inspiring hope, providing reassurance and accurate information).
   h. Assess for and support behaviors suggesting positive adaptation to changes (e.g. willingness to participate in self-care, verbalization of ability to cope, recognition and use of available support systems).
   i. Consult physician about psychological counseling if appropriate. Initiate a referral if necessary.

UNIT
XII

□ ▬▬▬▬▬▬▬▬▬▬▬▬▬▬▬▬▬

6. NURSING DIAGNOSIS

Grieving* related to loss of usual manner of bowel elimination and resultant change in body image.

_____

* This diagnostic label includes anticipatory grieving and grieving following the actual losses/changes.

□ ▬▬▬▬▬▬▬▬▬▬▬▬▬▬▬▬▬

DESIRED OUTCOMES	NURSING ACTIONS AND *SELECTED RATIONALES*

6. The client will demonstrate beginning progression through the grieving process as evidenced by:
   a. verbalization of feelings about the ileostomy
   b. expression of grief
   c. participation in treatment plan and self-care activities
   d. utilization of available support systems
   e. verbalization of a plan for integrating ostomy care into life style.

6.a. Determine client's perception of the impact of the ileostomy on his/her future.
  b. Determine how client usually expresses grief.
  c. Observe for signs of grieving (e.g. changes in eating habits, insomnia, anger, noncompliance, denial).
  d. Implement measures *to facilitate the grieving process:*
    1. assist client to acknowledge losses and changes experienced *so grief work can begin*; assess for factors that may hinder or facilitate acknowledgment
    2. discuss the grieving process and assist client to accept the stages of grieving as an expected response to the actual and/or anticipated changes or losses
    3. allow time for client to progress through the stages of grieving (denial, anger, bargaining, depression, acceptance [Kübler-Ross, 1969]); be aware that not every stage is experienced or expressed by all individuals
    4. provide an atmosphere of care and concern (e.g. provide privacy, be available and nonjudgmental, display empathy and respect) *so that client will feel free to verbalize both positive and negative feelings and concerns*
    5. perform actions *to promote trust* (e.g. answer questions honestly, provide requested information)
    6. encourage the expression of anger and sadness about the losses/changes experienced
    7. encourage client to express his/her feelings in whatever ways are comfortable (e.g. writing, drawing, conversation)
    8. perform actions to facilitate effective coping (see Postoperative Nursing Diagnosis 5, action d)
    9. support realistic hope about effects of the bowel diversion on his/her life (e.g. increased comfort).
  e. Assess for and support behaviors suggesting successful resolution of grief (e.g. verbalizing feelings about ileostomy, expressing sorrow, focusing on ways to adapt to changes).
  f. Explain the stages of the grieving process to significant others. Encourage their support and understanding.
  g. Provide information regarding counseling services and support groups that might assist client in working through grief.
  h. Arrange for visit from clergy if desired by client.
  i. Monitor for therapeutic and nontherapeutic effects of antidepressants if administered.
  j. Consult physician regarding referral for counseling if signs of dysfunctional grieving (e.g. persistent denial of losses or changes, excessive anger or sadness, hysteria, suicidal behaviors, phobias) occur.

□ ▬▬▬▬▬▬▬▬▬▬▬▬▬▬▬▬▬

7. NURSING DIAGNOSIS

Knowledge deficit regarding follow-up care.

□ ▬▬▬▬▬▬▬▬▬▬▬▬▬▬▬▬▬

DESIRED OUTCOMES	NURSING ACTIONS AND *SELECTED RATIONALES*

7.a. The client will verbalize a basic understanding of the anatomical changes that have occurred as a result of the surgery.

7.a. Reinforce teaching regarding the anatomical changes that have occurred as a result of the ileostomy. Use appropriate teaching aids (e.g. pictures, videotapes, anatomical models).

7.b. The client will identify ways to maintain fluid and electrolyte balance.

7.b. Provide the following instructions on ways *to maintain fluid and electrolyte balance:*
1. instruct client to perform the following actions *to prevent excessive ileostomy output and/or watery effluent* (e.g. avoid intake of foods/fluids such as prunes, iced or hot fluids, and raw fruits; take antidiarrheal agents as prescribed)
2. if ileostomy output increases or becomes more watery, instruct client to:
   a. increase intake of strained fruit juices, Gatorade, potatoes, soups, bouillon, and cured meats *to maintain electrolyte balance*
   b. drink a mixture of baking soda and water (¼–½ teaspoon baking soda and 1 cup of water) as prescribed by physician *to maintain acid-base balance.*

7.c. The client will identify methods of controlling odor and noise associated with ostomy drainage and gas.

7.c.1. Reinforce instructions regarding ways to reduce gas formation and odor associated with ileostomy drainage and gas (see Postoperative Nursing Diagnosis 4, actions h and i).
2. Inform client that the ostomy pouch and clothing will tend to muffle the noises.

7.d. The client will demonstrate ways to maintain integrity of the stoma and peristomal and perianal skin.

7.d.1. Instruct client in ways to prevent peristomal and perianal skin irritation and breakdown and maintain integrity of the stoma (see Postoperative Nursing Diagnosis 2, actions b.4 and 5 and Collaborative Diagnosis 3, action b.2, for appropriate measures).
2. Support client's efforts to decrease odor of effluent and gas but discourage excessive changing and emptying of appliance.
3. Instruct and assist client to establish a routine time and system for emptying and changing appliance or emptying continent ileostomy *in order to reduce risk of leakage of effluent.*
4. Instruct client to follow special precautions for products used (e.g. inert, moldable skin barriers must be kept in airtight container; skin sealants should be used only on healthy peristomal skin *because they can further irritate reddened and excoriated skin).*
5. Allow time for questions, clarification, and practice of appropriate stoma and skin care.

7.e. The client will demonstrate proper use and care of ostomy equipment.

7.e.1. Instruct client regarding proper use of appliances he/she will be using after discharge.
2. Discuss recommended methods of cleansing and storing ostomy equipment based on manufacturer's recommendations.
3. Demonstrate appropriate cleansing techniques. Emphasize importance of:
   a. rinsing inside of collection pouch each time it is emptied
   b. soaking pouch according to manufacturer's instructions and allowing it to dry thoroughly if it is to be reused.
4. Allow time for questions, clarification, and return demonstration.

7.f. The client will demonstrate proper techniques for draining and irrigating a continent ileostomy if present.

7.f.1. Explain the gradual and progressive clamping routine if catheter will be in the stoma of continent ileostomy at time of discharge.
2. When the clamping routine is complete, inform client that he/she will be instructed in the correct method of and schedule for catheter insertion (initially the reservoir will need to be drained for 10–15 minutes every 3–4 hours, but after about 6 months, it may need emptying only 2–3 times/day).
3. Demonstrate correct technique for irrigating a continent ileostomy. Caution client to use only the prescribed amount of irrigant (usually 20–30 cc) *in order to avoid overdistending and damaging reservoir.*
4. Allow time for questions, clarification, and return demonstration of clamping and irrigating techniques.

UNIT XII

7.g. The client will identify ways to prevent blockage of the stoma.

7.g.1. Instruct client in ways *to prevent food from blocking the stoma:*
    a. chew food thoroughly
    b. avoid or eat only small amounts of foods that are hard to digest (e.g. popcorn, coconut, celery, bean sprouts, bamboo shoots, whole kernel corn, raw carrots, nuts, granola, mushrooms, vegetable and fruit skins).
  2. Instruct client to do the following if stoma seems blocked:
    a. apply warm water to stoma and warm compresses to abdomen and/or gently massage abdomen *in order to stimulate peristalsis*
    b. participate in relaxing activities (e.g. warm bath, reading) *in order to reduce muscle tension*
    c. reinforce actions to break-up or shift food blockage (e.g. increase fluid intake, assume a knee-chest position and gently massage abdomen, irrigate stoma via catheter).

7.h. The client will state signs and symptoms to report to the health care provider.

7.h.1. Refer to Standardized Postoperative Care Plan, Nursing Diagnosis 20, action c, for signs and symptoms to report to the health care provider.
  2. Instruct client to also report:
    a. dark red, blue-black, magenta, or pale stoma
    b. change in color, consistency, or odor of effluent that is not readily identified as a response to food or fluid intake
    c. absence of or persistent increase in ileostomy output
    d. change in contour of stoma (use diagrams or descriptive terms *so client does not confuse decreasing stoma size due to resolving edema with actual stomal retraction*)
    e. difficulty accomplishing ostomy care
    f. persistent skin irritation
    g. skin breakdown
    h. persistent thirst, dry mucous membranes, decreased urine output *(may indicate fluid volume deficit)*
    i. signs and symptoms of hypokalemia (e.g. irregular pulse, muscle weakness and cramping, nausea, vomiting)
    j. signs and symptoms of hyponatremia (e.g. headache, abdominal cramps, fatigue, irritability)
    k. thin, watery ileostomy output; absence of ileostomy output; unusual foul odor of gas; abdominal distention; and/or nausea and vomiting that does not resolve within 2 hours of implementing measures to relieve stomal blockage
    l. difficulty draining continent ileostomy or persistent leakage of effluent.

7.i. The client will identify appropriate community resources that can assist with home management and adjustment to changes resulting from the bowel diversion.

7.i.1. Provide information about community resources that can assist the client and significant others with home management and adjustment to changes resulting from bowel diversion (e.g. local ostomy support groups; community health agencies; enterostomal therapist; home health agencies; Visiting Nurse Association; financial, individual, and family counseling services).
  2. Initiate a referral if appropriate.

7.j. The client will verbalize an understanding of and a plan for adhering to recommended follow-up care including future appointments with health care provider, wound care, activity level, and medications prescribed.

7.j.1. Refer to Standardized Postoperative Care Plan, Nursing Diagnosis 20, for routine postoperative instructions and measures to improve client compliance.
  2. Reinforce physician's instructions regarding activity limitations:
    a. avoid lifting objects over 10 pounds for at least 6 weeks
    b. avoid participating in contact sports.
  3. Explain the rationale for, side effects of, and importance of taking medications prescribed (e.g. electrolyte supplements, bismuth subcarbonate).
  4. Stress the fact that oral medications should be in liquid, chewable, uncoated, or sugar-coated form rather than enteric-coated tablets or timed-release spansules *so absorption can take place before the medication is excreted.*

Reference

Kübler-Ross, E. On death and dying. New York: Macmillan, 1969.

□□□□□□□□□□□□□□□□□□□□□□□□□□□□□□□□□□□□□

Gastrectomy

Gastrectomy is the surgical removal of all or part of the stomach. A subtotal gastrectomy involves removal of the distal 65–80% of the stomach. The area excised contains gastrin-secreting cells and some of the parietal (oxyntic) cells, which secrete hydrochloric acid and the intrinsic factor. A subtotal gastrectomy is commonly performed to treat peptic ulcer disease that continues to be symptomatic despite conservative management. It is also indicated when complications of peptic ulcer disease (e.g. perforation, gastric outlet obstruction, hemorrhage) develop or if ulcerated lesions are believed to be precancerous. In a subtotal gastrectomy, gastrointestinal continuity is re-established by an anastomosis of the remaining stomach to the duodenum (gastroduodenostomy or Billroth I) or jejunum (gastrojejunostomy or Billroth II). In the latter procedure, the duodenal stump remains intact to preserve the flow of bile and pancreatic juices into the jejunum. A vagotomy is usually performed at the same time to further reduce gastric acid secretion. If a total gastrectomy is performed, gastrointestinal continuity is re-established by an esophagojejunostomy (anastomosis of the esophagus to the jejunum). This extensive surgery may be performed to treat cancer of the stomach, which is usually quite advanced at time of diagnosis, and advanced cases of Zollinger-Ellison syndrome or hemorrhagic gastritis. Total gastrectomy is not done frequently because it is difficult to maintain an adequate nutritional status postoperatively.

This care plan focuses on the adult client with intractable peptic ulcer disease who is hospitalized for a gastroduodenostomy or gastrojejunostomy. Preoperatively, the goals of care are to maintain comfort, reduce fear and anxiety, assist the client to achieve an optimal nutritional status, and prevent and/or treat complications of peptic ulcer disease. Postoperative goals of care are to maintain comfort, assist the client to maintain or achieve an optimal nutritional status, prevent complications, and educate the client regarding follow-up care.

DISCHARGE CRITERIA

Prior to discharge, the client will:

- identify ways to prevent recurrence of peptic ulcers
- identify ways to control dumping syndrome and postprandial hypoglycemia
- state signs and symptoms to report to the health care provider
- verbalize an understanding of and a plan for adhering to recommended follow-up care including future appointments with health care provider, medications prescribed, activity level, and wound care.

NURSING/COLLABORATIVE DIAGNOSES

Postoperative
1. Altered nutrition: less than body requirements □ *648*
2. Potential complications:

Preoperative

Use in conjunction with the Care Plan on Peptic Ulcer and the Standardized Preoperative Care Plan.

Postoperative

Use in conjunction with the Standardized Postoperative Care Plan.

1. NURSING DIAGNOSIS

Altered nutrition: less than body requirements related to:

a. decreased oral intake associated with prescribed dietary modifications, fear of experiencing recurrent ulcer pain or symptoms of dumping syndrome and postprandial hypoglycemia (especially with a gastrojejunostomy), incisional pain, and early satiety due to decreased stomach size;

b. decreased absorption of nutrients associated with impaired digestion resulting from:
   1. decreased hydrochloric acid secretion due to vagotomy if performed and removal of gastrin-secreting cells (gastrin stimulates parietal cells to produce hydrochloric acid) and some of the parietal cells
   2. rapid entry of food into the small intestine
   3. decreased stimulation and secretion of pancreatic juice and bile associated with:
      a. reduction in hydrochloric acid and gastrin secretion (hydrochloric acid and gastrin stimulate pancreatic enzyme secretion and gallbladder contraction)
      b. absence of food moving through the duodenum following gastrojejunostomy (the presence of food in the duodenum causes the release of secretin and cholecystokinin-pancreozymin, which stimulate gallbladder contraction and pancreatic enzyme secretion);

   c. decreased absorption of:
     1. vitamin B_{12} associated with the removal of gastrin-secreting cells (gastrin is needed to stimulate the parietal cells to secrete the intrinsic factor) and some of the parietal cells (the intrinsic factor is necessary for absorption of vitamin B_{12} from the small intestine)
     2. iron associated with bypassing of the duodenum with a gastrojejunostomy;
  d. increased nutritional needs associated with increased metabolic rate that occurs during normal wound healing.

DESIRED OUTCOMES	NURSING ACTIONS AND *SELECTED RATIONALES*

1. The client will maintain an adequate nutritional status (see Standardized Postoperative Care Plan, Nursing Diagnosis 6, for outcome criteria).	1.a. Refer to Standardized Postoperative Care Plan, Nursing Diagnosis 6, for measures related to assessment and maintenance of nutritional status.
	b. Implement additional measures *to maintain and improve nutritional status when oral intake is allowed:*
	  1. provide small, frequent meals *to compensate for early satiety*
	  2. perform actions to prevent or reduce the severity of dumping syndrome and postprandial hypoglycemia (see Postoperative Collaborative Diagnosis 2, action e.2) *in order to reduce the client's fear of precipitating these conditions and to promote increased absorption of nutrients*
	  3. monitor for therapeutic and nontherapeutic effects of the following medications if administered:
	    a. pancreatic enzymes *to aid digestion*
	    b. iron preparations, vitamin B_{12} injections, and fat-soluble vitamins
	    c. medium-chain triglycerides (MCT) in an oil medium *to provide an absorbable source of fatty acids.*

---

2. COLLABORATIVE DIAGNOSIS

Potential complications:

a. **peritonitis** related to:
  1. wound infection
  2. leakage from an abscess in or around surgical area
  3. leakage of gastric contents into the peritoneal cavity associated with loss of integrity of the suture line at the duodenal stump (with gastrojejunostomy) or the site of anastomosis;

b. **pancreatitis** related to obstruction of flow of pancreatic secretions associated with trauma to the pancreas or pancreatic ducts during surgery;

c. **afferent loop syndrome** related to partial obstruction of the duodenal loop associated with factors such as edema or presence of a kink in the efferent jejunal limb after gastrojejunostomy;

d. **recurrent peptic ulcer** related to:
  1. delayed gastric emptying while edema resolves
  2. reflux of the alkaline pancreatic secretions and bile into the remaining stomach as a result of excessive secretions and/or absence of the pyloric sphincter (the sphincter may be bypassed or removed during surgery)
  3. continued secretion of hydrochloric acid (especially with gastroduodenostomy and/or if vagotomy was not performed);

e. **dumping syndrome** related to rapid emptying of hypertonic food into the jejunum especially after a gastrojejunostomy (the bolus of food pulls fluid from the vascular space; this distends the bowel lumen and increases intestinal peristalsis and motility);

f. **postprandial hypoglycemia** related to rapid emptying of food/fluid high in carbohydrates into the jejunum (results in hyperglycemia, increased insulin secretion, and subsequent hypoglycemia).

☐ ▇▇

DESIRED OUTCOMES	NURSING ACTIONS AND *SELECTED RATIONALES*

2.a. The client will not develop peritonitis as evidenced by:
1. gradual resolution of abdominal pain
2. soft, nondistended abdomen
3. temperature declining toward normal
4. stable vital signs
5. bowel sounds returning to normal
6. WBC count declining toward normal.

2.a.1. Assess for and report signs and symptoms of peritonitis (e.g. increase in severity of abdominal pain; generalized abdominal pain; rebound tenderness; tense, rigid abdomen; increase in temperature; tachycardia; tachypnea; hypotension; continued diminished or absent bowel sounds).
2. Monitor WBC counts. Report levels that increase or fail to decline toward normal.
3. Implement measures *to prevent peritonitis:*
   a. perform actions to prevent and treat wound infection (see Standardized Postoperative Care Plan, Nursing Diagnosis 16, actions b.4 and 5)
   b. perform actions *to maintain patency of wound drain if present:*
      1. keep tubing free of kinks
      2. empty collection device as often as necessary
      3. maintain suction as ordered
   c. perform actions *to prevent inadvertent removal of wound drain if present:*
      1. use caution when changing dressings surrounding drain
      2. provide extension tubing if necessary *to enable client to move without placing tension on the drain*
      3. instruct client not to pull on drain or drainage tubing
   d. perform actions *to prevent stress on and leakage from the suture line at site of anastomosis:*
      1. do not change position of the nasogastric or gastrostomy tube unless ordered *(the tube is positioned during surgery and change could traumatize suture line)*
      2. implement measures to prevent nausea and vomiting (see Standardized Postoperative Care Plan, Nursing Diagnosis 7.C, action 2)
      3. when oral fluids are allowed, instruct client to avoid drinking ice cold beverages *in order to prevent gastric spasms*
      4. implement measures *to prevent overdistention of the remaining stomach:*
         a. perform actions to reduce the accumulation of gastrointestinal gas and fluid (see Standardized Postoperative Care Plan, Nursing Diagnosis 7.B, action 3)
         b. as diet progresses, instruct client to avoid drinking fluid with meals
      5. if gastric distention occurs:
         a. maintain food and fluid restrictions as ordered
         b. assist physician to reposition nasogastric or gastrostomy tube if indicated.
4. If signs and symptoms of peritonitis occur:
   a. withhold all food and fluid as ordered
   b. place client on bedrest in a semi-Fowler's position *to assist in pooling or localizing gastrointestinal contents in the pelvis rather than under the diaphragm*
   c. assist physician with insertion of a nasogastric or gastrostomy tube if not already present and maintain suction as ordered
   d. monitor for therapeutic and nontherapeutic effects of anti-infectives if administered
   e. monitor for therapeutic and nontherapeutic effects of intravenous fluids and/or blood volume expanders if administered *to prevent or treat shock (shock can occur as a result of escape of protein, fluid, and electrolytes into the peritoneal cavity)*

f. prepare client for surgical intervention (e.g. repair of anastomosis, drainage of abscess) if indicated

g. provide emotional support to client and significant others.

2.b. The client will experience resolution of pancreatitis if it occurs as evidenced by:
1. gradual resolution of abdominal pain
2. temperature declining toward normal
3. stable B/P and pulse
4. serum amylase and lipase levels declining toward normal
5. renal amylase/creatinine clearance ratio returning toward normal
6. WBC count declining toward normal.

2.b.1. Assess for and report signs and symptoms of pancreatitis (e.g. extension of pain to left upper quadrant or back, increase in temperature, tachycardia, hypotension, elevated serum amylase and lipase levels).

2. Collect a timed (usually 2-hour) urine specimen if ordered. Report an elevated renal amylase/creatinine clearance ratio.

3. Monitor WBC counts. Report levels that increase or fail to decline toward normal.

4. If signs and symptoms of pancreatitis occur:
   a. assist client to assume position of greatest comfort (usually side-lying with knees flexed)
   b. maintain food and fluid restrictions as ordered
   c. assist physician with the insertion of a nasogastric or gastrostomy tube if not already present and maintain suction as ordered (*removal of gastric juices reduces the pancreatic stimulation normally caused by these juices*)
   d. monitor for therapeutic and nontherapeutic effects of the following medications if administered:
      1. analgesics and smooth muscle relaxants (e.g. nitroglycerin) *to reduce pain*
      2. antacids and histamine$_2$ receptor antagonists (e.g. cimetidine, famotidine, ranitidine) *to neutralize and/or reduce output of hydrochloric acid and thereby reduce pancreatic stimulation*
   e. refer to Care Plan on Pancreatitis for additional care measures.

2.c. The client will have resolution of the afferent loop syndrome if it occurs as evidenced by:
1. no complaints of intense nausea and epigastric discomfort immediately after eating
2. no episodes of vomiting bile 1–2 hours after eating.

2.c.1. Assess for and report signs and symptoms of the afferent loop syndrome (e.g. intense nausea and/or epigastric discomfort immediately after eating, forceful vomiting of large amounts of bile 1–2 hours after eating).

2. If signs and symptoms of afferent loop syndrome occur:
   a. maintain food and fluid restrictions as ordered
   b. assist physician with insertion of a nasogastric or gastrostomy tube if not already present and maintain suction as ordered
   c. if oral intake is allowed:
      1. provide small, frequent meals rather than 3 large ones
      2. provide a low-fat diet *to reduce the secretion of bile and pancreatic enzymes (foods/fluids containing fat will further stimulate bile and pancreatic secretion and increase pressure in the afferent loop)*
   d. monitor for therapeutic and nontherapeutic effects of anti-infectives if administered (*infection can develop due to stasis of secretions in the afferent loop*)
   e. assist with endoscopy if performed
   f. prepare client for surgical intervention if obstruction is due to kinking of the efferent jejunal limb.

2.d. The client will not develop a recurrent peptic ulcer as evidenced by:
1. gradual resolution of epigastric discomfort
2. absence of frank or occult blood in stool and gastric contents within 3–4 days after surgery
3. stable or improved RBC, Hct., and Hgb. levels.

2.d.1. Assess for and report signs and symptoms of:
   a. delayed gastric emptying (e.g. increasing epigastric discomfort and distention, anorexia, nausea)
   b. alkaline reflux gastritis (e.g. complaints of epigastric burning or aching that is aggravated by meals, frequent vomiting or eructation of bile and food particles)
   c. peptic ulceration (e.g. continued epigastric discomfort, persistent or increased amount of frank or occult blood in stool or gastric drainage [drainage should change from bright red to dark red or brown within 6–12 hours after surgery and to greenish yellow within 24–36 hours after surgery]).

2. Monitor RBC, Hct., and Hgb. levels. Report decreasing values.

3. Implement measures *to prevent recurrent ulcer development*:
   a. maintain patency of nasogastric or gastrostomy tube if present *in order to remove gastric secretions and any alkaline pancreatic secretions and bile that may be present because of reflux*
   b. when oral intake is allowed, instruct client to:
      1. avoid foods/fluids high in fat (e.g. milk, cheese, pork, fried foods) *in order to avoid excessive stimulation of pancreatic secretions and bile*

      2. avoid foods/fluids known to directly irritate the gastric mucosa and/or stimulate hydrochloric acid secretion (e.g. extremely hot or cold foods/fluids; fresh fruits; rich pastries; caffeine-containing items such as chocolate, tea, coffee, or colas)

  c. provide a calm, quiet environment

  d. assist client to identify and manage stressors

  e. monitor for therapeutic and nontherapeutic effects of the following medications if administered:

      1. histamine$_2$ receptor antagonists (e.g. cimetidine, famotidine, ranitidine) *to inhibit gastric acid secretions*

      2. antacids *to neutralize gastric contents*

      3. mucosal barrier fortifiers (e.g. sucralfate)

      4. cholestyramine resins *to bind with the bile salts that are present with reflux gastritis (the bile salts cause mucosal irritation).*

4. If signs and symptoms of peptic ulcer occur:

  a. withhold food and fluid as ordered

  b. assist physician with insertion of nasogastric or gastrostomy tube and maintain suction as ordered

  c. continue with above medication therapy as ordered

  d. prepare client for surgical intervention to resect ulcerated area or convert gastroduodenostomy to gastrojejunostomy if indicated

  e. provide emotional support to client and significant others

  f. refer to Care Plan on Peptic Ulcer for additional care measures.

2.e. The client will not experience dumping syndrome after eating as evidenced by:
1. no complaints of epigastric fullness and abdominal cramping
2. normal bowel sounds
3. skin dry and usual color
4. absence of weakness, dizziness, and diarrhea
5. stable vital signs.

2.e.1. Assess for signs and symptoms of dumping syndrome (e.g. complaints of epigastric fullness and abdominal cramping, hyperactive bowel sounds, diaphoresis, pallor, generalized weakness, dizziness, diarrhea, tachycardia, tachypnea, and/or decreased B/P within 1 hour after eating).

2. Implement measures *to prevent dumping syndrome:*

  a. instruct client to avoid intake of simple carbohydrates (e.g. fruit juices, milkshakes, candy) *because they are hypertonic and tend to rapidly draw fluid into the intestine*

  b. encourage intake of foods containing moderate amounts of fats and proteins such as fish, poultry, meat, and eggs *(these foods leave the stomach more slowly and are less hypertonic)*

  c. instruct client in ways *to delay gastric emptying:*

      1. eat small, frequent, dry meals

      2. eat meals slowly

      3. drink fluids between rather than with meals; avoid fluids for at least 1 hour before and after meals

      4. avoid foods/fluids that are extremely hot or cold

      5. eat in a semi-recumbent position, then lie down for at least 30 minutes after each meal unless contraindicated.

3. If signs and symptoms of dumping syndrome occur:

  a. continue with above measures

  b. assure client that these symptoms usually subside within a few months (if symptoms are not controlled, surgical revision [conversion of a gastrojejunostomy to a gastroduodenostomy] may be necessary *to delay gastric emptying).*

2.f. The client will not experience postprandial hypoglycemia 2–3 hours after eating as evidenced by:
1. usual mental status
2. no complaints of hunger, nausea, palpitations, and feeling faint
3. usual strength and activity tolerance
4. absence of diaphoresis and tremors.

2.f.1. Assess for and report signs and symptoms of postprandial hypoglycemia (e.g. anxiety; complaints of hunger, nausea, palpitations, or feeling faint; weakness; diaphoresis; tremors) occurring 2–3 hours after meals.

2. Monitor results of postprandial serum glucose levels as ordered. Report levels below 60 mg/dl.

3. Implement measures to prevent dumping syndrome (see action e.2 in this diagnosis) *because these measures will also reduce risk of postprandial hypoglycemia.*

4. If signs and symptoms of postprandial hypoglycemia occur:

  a. provide client with a rapid-acting carbohydrate (e.g. orange juice, hard candy, sugar-containing soft drink, Monogel, Glutose)

  b. review dietary management and revise as necessary (e.g. shorten intervals between meals, reduce sugar intake)

  c. assure client that these symptoms usually subside within a few months (if symptoms are not controlled, further dietary modifications or surgical revision may be necessary *to delay gastric emptying).*

3. NURSING DIAGNOSIS

Knowledge deficit regarding follow-up care.

DESIRED OUTCOMES	**NURSING ACTIONS AND *SELECTED RATIONALES***

3.a. The client will identify ways to prevent recurrence of peptic ulcers.

3.a.1. Instruct the client in ways *to prevent peptic ulcer recurrence:*
  a. drink decaffeinated or caffeine-free beverages rather than those containing caffeine
  b. avoid drinking excessive amounts of alcohol (2 ounces or more of ethanol/day)
  c. avoid ingestion of foods known to irritate gastric mucosa directly or by stimulating gastric acid production (e.g. whole grains, chocolate, rich pastries, fresh fruits, raw vegetables, spicy foods, meat extracts, extremely hot or cold foods)
  d. eliminate any other foods/fluids that cause gastric distress
  e. adhere to low-fat diet if recommended *to reduce risk of alkaline reflux gastritis*
  f. eat small, frequent meals and snacks; do not skip meals
  g. eat slowly and chew food thoroughly
  h. maintain a calm, relaxed atmosphere at mealtime and whenever possible
  i. stop smoking
  j. maintain a balance of physical activity and rest
  k. avoid stressful situations
  l. avoid ingestion of ulcerogenic medications such as aspirin, aspirin-containing products, and ibuprofen
  m. take medications (e.g. antacids, histamine$_2$ receptor antagonists, cholestyramine resins) as prescribed
  n. continue with prescribed treatment of any condition that may be contributing to mucosal irritation and ulceration (e.g. hormone imbalance, chronic obstructive pulmonary disease).
2. Obtain a dietary consult if client needs assistance in planning meals that incorporate dietary modifications.
3. Provide information on community resources that can assist the client in making life-style changes (e.g. stress management classes, stop smoking programs, vocational rehabilitation, counseling services). Initiate a referral if indicated.

3.b. The client will identify ways to control dumping syndrome and postprandial hypoglycemia.

3.b.1. Explain the mechanisms responsible for dumping syndrome and postprandial hypoglycemia and emphasize that these conditions are usually temporary.
2. Instruct client to be alert for signs and symptoms of:
  a. dumping syndrome (e.g. epigastric fullness, abdominal cramping, weakness, dizziness, and/or diarrhea within an hour after eating)
  b. postprandial hypoglycemia (e.g. anxiety, hunger, nausea, palpitations, faintness, weakness, sweating, and/or shakiness 2–3 hours after meals).
3. Reinforce teaching regarding ways to prevent dumping syndrome and postprandial hypoglycemia (see Postoperative Collaborative Diagnosis 2, action e.2).
4. Instruct client to drink fluids with high sugar content (e.g. orange juice, sugar-containing soft drinks) or eat candy that contains sugar if signs and symptoms of postprandial hypoglycemia occur.

3.c. The client will state signs and symptoms to report to the health care provider.

3.c.1. Refer to Standardized Postoperative Care Plan, Nursing Diagnosis 20, action c, for signs and symptoms to report to the health care provider.
2. Instruct client to also report:
  a. persistent nausea and/or vomiting
  b. persistent diarrhea

c. weight loss
d. foul-smelling, greasy bowel movements that float
e. black or tarry bowel movements
f. bloody or coffee-ground vomitus
g. increasing fatigue and weakness
h. increased epigastric discomfort or back pain
i. difficulty controlling physical and emotional stresses
j. persistent signs and symptoms of dumping syndrome and/or postprandial hypoglycemia (see action b.2 in this diagnosis).

3.d. The client will verbalize an understanding of and a plan for adhering to recommended follow-up care including future appointments with health care provider, medications prescribed, activity level, and wound care.	3.d.1. Refer to Standardized Postoperative Care Plan, Nursing Diagnosis 20, for routine postoperative instructions and measures to improve client compliance. 2. Explain the rationale for, side effects of, schedule for taking, and importance of taking medications prescribed (e.g. antacids, histamine$_2$ receptor antagonists, cholestyramine resins, fat-soluble vitamins, vitamin B$_{12}$ injections).

Gastric Partitioning

Gastric partitioning (gastroplasty) is a surgical procedure performed to reduce the size of the stomach in some persons with morbid obesity. The procedure involves altering the capacity of the stomach from approximately 1000 cc to about 50 cc by creating a small pouch distal to the gastroesophageal junction. Initially, the popular method of creating this pouch was to place a row of staples horizontally along the proximal portion of the stomach, leaving a small opening in the staple line through which food and fluid could empty into the distal portion of the stomach. Because of problems with eventual widening of the channel and disruption of the staple line, vertical-banded partitioning has become a more popular technique. With this approach, the pouch is formed by a vertical staple line on the lesser curvature side of the stomach because it stretches less easily. The channel between the pouch and the rest of the stomach is often reinforced with mesh or constructed using silicone tubing to further reduce the risk of channel widening. Another surgical procedure that incorporates gastric partitioning is the gastric bypass in which the stomach is partitioned to form a pouch and a channel is created between the proximal portion of the stomach and the jejunum.

Clients are carefully screened physically and psychologically and must meet certain criteria before undergoing this surgery. The criteria include massive obesity for at least 3–5 years, inability to reduce weight using other forms of treatment, weight that is at least 100 pounds or 100% over ideal weight, and obesity resulting from a caloric intake greater than the body's needs rather than an underlying metabolic problem. The client must also be free of medical conditions that would affect the surgical outcome (e.g. liver, cardiovascular, or pulmonary disease), be psychologically and socially stable, and have access to adequate follow-up medical care.

This care plan focuses on the adult client hospitalized for gastric partitioning. Postoperatively, the goals of care are to maintain comfort, prevent complications, assist the client to adjust to changes in eating habits, and educate the client regarding follow-up care.

DISCHARGE CRITERIA

Prior to discharge, the client will:

- identify ways to prevent excessive stretching of the gastric pouch and/or disruption of the staple line

- verbalize an understanding of ways to maintain an adequate nutritional status
- identify ways to reduce the risk of consuming excessive amounts of food, fluid, and calories
- demonstrate the ability to accurately calculate and measure the allotted amounts of food and fluid
- state signs and symptoms to report to the health care provider
- identify community resources that can assist in the adjustment to prescribed dietary modifications and future changes in body image
- verbalize an understanding of and a plan for adhering to recommended follow-up care including future appointments with health care provider, activity level, medications prescribed, and wound care.

NURSING/COLLABORATIVE DIAGNOSIS

Preoperative
1. Disturbance in self-concept □ *655*
Postoperative
1. Ineffective breathing patterns:
   a. hypoventilation
   b. hyperventilation □ *656*
2. Altered nutrition: less than body requirements □ *657*
3. Impaired skin integrity:
   a. surgical incision
   b. impaired wound healing
   c. irritation or breakdown □ *657*
4. Potential complications:
   a. overdistention of the pouch
   b. peritonitis
   c. thromboembolism
   d. atelectasis □ *658*
5. Noncompliance □ *660*
6. Knowledge deficit regarding follow-up care □ *661*

UNIT
XII

Preoperative

Use in conjunction with the Standardized Preoperative Care Plan.

1. NURSING DIAGNOSIS

Disturbance in self-concept* related to embarrassment associated with obesity and feeling of failure resulting from inability to lose weight by more conventional methods.

---

* This diagnostic label includes the nursing diagnoses of body image disturbance and self-esteem disturbance.

DESIRED OUTCOMES	NURSING ACTIONS AND *SELECTED RATIONALES*

1. The client will demonstrate a positive self-concept as evidenced by:
   a. verbalization of feelings of self-worth
   b. positive statements regarding anticipated effects of surgical procedure
   c. maintenance of relationships with significant others
   d. active interest in personal appearance
   e. active participation in preoperative care.

1.a. Determine the meaning of obesity and anticipated effects of the gastric partitioning on client's self-concept by encouraging him/her to verbalize feelings and by noting nonverbal behavior.
   b. Assess for signs and symptoms of a disturbance in self-concept (e.g. verbal or nonverbal cues denoting a negative response to self, withdrawal from significant others, refusal to participate in preoperative care or accept responsibility for self-care).
   c. Assist the client to identify strengths and qualities that have a positive effect on self-concept.
   d. Implement measures *to assist client to increase self-esteem* (e.g. limit negative self-criticism, encourage positive comments about self, give positive feedback about accomplishments, provide positive reinforcement regarding his/her decision to have the surgery and lose weight).
   e. Implement measures *to reduce client's embarrassment about his/her obesity:*
      1. before admission, obtain information from physician regarding client's height and weight so that oversized equipment and supplies (e.g. bed, chair, commode, blood pressure cuff, gowns, bathrobes) can be obtained if necessary; allow client to wear own clothes rather than hospital gown before and after surgery if desired
      2. remove unnecessary furniture and equipment from room *so client can move around easily*
      3. provide privacy when weighing client
      4. transfer client to and from operating room in own hospital bed rather than using regular-sized gurney.
   f. Identify personal habits or grooming that are important to client's body image (e.g. use of makeup, particular hair styling or clothing). Assure client that he/she will be assisted with usual grooming and makeup habits after surgery if necessary.
   g. Demonstrate acceptance of client using techniques such as therapeutic touch and frequent visits. Encourage significant others to do the same.
   h. Arrange for a visit from another who has achieved weight loss after gastric partitioning if client desires.
   i. Consult physician if client has unrealistic expectations of postoperative weight loss and dietary management.

☐ ▬▬▬▬▬▬▬▬▬▬▬▬▬▬▬▬▬▬▬▬▬▬▬▬▬

Postoperative

Use in conjunction with the Standardized Postoperative Care Plan.

☐ ▬▬▬▬▬▬▬▬▬▬▬▬▬▬▬▬▬▬▬▬▬▬▬▬▬

1. NURSING DIAGNOSIS

Ineffective breathing patterns:

a. **hypoventilation** related to:
   1. limited diaphragmatic excursion associated with large amounts of abdominal adipose tissue, abdominal distention, and reluctance to breathe deeply due to abdominal pain
   2. depressant effects of anesthesia and some medications (e.g. narcotic analgesics)
   3. decreased activity;
b. **hyperventilation** related to fear, anxiety, and pain.

☐ ▬▬▬▬▬▬▬▬▬▬▬▬▬▬▬▬▬▬▬▬▬▬▬▬▬

DESIRED OUTCOMES	**NURSING ACTIONS AND *SELECTED RATIONALES***
1. The client will maintain an effective breathing pattern (see Standardized Postoperative Care Plan, Nursing Diagnosis 3, for outcome criteria).	1.a. Refer to Standardized Postoperative Care Plan, Nursing Diagnosis 3, for measures related to assessment and improvement of breathing pattern. b. Implement additional measures *to improve breathing pattern:* 　1. position client with head of bed elevated at least 30° at all times 　2. instruct and assist client to use trapeze and turn at least every 2 hours 　3. add extensions to tubings if necessary *to enable client to turn and move without fear of dislodging tubes* 　4. assist with ambulation the evening of surgery and at least 4 times/day as ordered.

□ ▰▰▰▰▰▰▰▰▰▰▰▰▰▰▰▰▰▰▰▰▰▰▰▰▰▰▰▰▰▰

2. NURSING DIAGNOSIS

Altered nutrition: less than body requirements related to:

a. decreased oral intake associated with nausea, prescribed dietary modifications, and early satiety due to small pouch size;
b. increased nutritional needs associated with increased metabolic rate that occurs during wound healing.

□ ▰▰▰▰▰▰▰▰▰▰▰▰▰▰▰▰▰▰▰▰▰▰▰▰▰▰▰▰▰▰

DESIRED OUTCOMES	**NURSING ACTIONS AND *SELECTED RATIONALES***
2. The client will maintain an adequate nutritional status (see Standardized Postoperative Care Plan, Nursing Diagnosis 6, for outcome criteria).	2.a. Refer to Standardized Postoperative Care Plan, Nursing Diagnosis 6, for measures related to assessment and maintenance of an adequate nutritional status. b. When oral intake is allowed, implement additional measures *to maintain nutritional status:* 　1. stress the need to adhere to prescribed eating/drinking schedule 　2. provide high-protein liquid nourishment as part of fluid allotment when allowed 　3. consult dietician regarding food/fluid selections that have high nutritional value and meet dietary restrictions and client preferences. c. Consult physician if client is unable to tolerate or adhere to prescribed diet.

UNIT
XII

□ ▰▰▰▰▰▰▰▰▰▰▰▰▰▰▰▰▰▰▰▰▰▰▰▰▰▰▰▰▰▰

3. NURSING DIAGNOSIS

Impaired skin integrity:

a. **surgical incision**;
b. **impaired wound healing** related to inadequate nutritional status, inadequate blood supply to wound area, stress on wound area, infection, and increased levels of glucocorticoids (levels usually rise with stress);
c. **irritation or breakdown** related to difficulty keeping deep skin fold areas dry, contact of skin with wound drainage, pressure from drainage tubes, and use of tape.

□ ▰▰▰▰▰▰▰▰▰▰▰▰▰▰▰▰▰▰▰▰▰▰▰▰▰▰▰▰▰▰

DESIRED OUTCOMES	NURSING ACTIONS AND *SELECTED RATIONALES*

3.a. The client will experience normal healing of surgical wounds (see Standardized Postoperative Care Plan, Nursing Diagnosis 9, outcome a, for outcome criteria).

3.a. Refer to Standardized Postoperative Care Plan, Nursing Diagnosis 9, action a, for measures related to assessment and promotion of normal wound healing.

3.b. The client will maintain skin integrity (see Standardized Postoperative Care Plan, Nursing Diagnosis 9, outcome b, for outcome criteria).

3.b.1. Inspect the skin for areas of irritation and breakdown with particular attention to:
    a. skin folds of abdomen and groin and under breasts
    b. skin areas in contact with wound drainage, tape, and drainage tubings.
2. Refer to Standardized Postoperative Care Plan, Nursing Diagnosis 9, action b.2, for measures to prevent skin irritation and breakdown resulting from wound drainage, tape, and drainage tubings.
3. Assist client to thoroughly cleanse and dry opposing skin surfaces of deep skin folds as often as needed *in order to further reduce the risk of skin irritation and breakdown.*
4. If skin irritation or breakdown occurs:
    a. notify physician
    b. continue with above measures to prevent further irritation and breakdown
    c. perform wound care as ordered or per standard hospital policy
    d. expose opposing skin folds to the air if possible and/or apply protective ointment or cream (e.g. Sween cream, Desitin) as ordered
    e. monitor client closely and report signs and symptoms of infection (e.g. elevated temperature; redness, warmth, and edema around incision or area of breakdown; unusual drainage from site).

4. COLLABORATIVE DIAGNOSIS

Potential complications:

a. **overdistention of the pouch** related to:
    1. accumulation of gas and fluid in the pouch associated with decreased peristalsis
    2. obstruction of the channel between the pouch and distal stomach (or pouch and jejunum if gastric bypass performed) associated with edema and/or presence of large food particles
    3. excessive food/fluid intake;
b. **peritonitis** related to:
    1. wound infection
    2. leakage from an abscess
    3. leakage of gastric contents into the peritoneum associated with disruption of the staple line;
c. **thromboembolism** related to:
    1. venous stasis associated with decreased activity and pressure on abdominal vessels from excessive adipose tissue and intestinal distention
    2. hypercoagulability associated with fluid volume deficit
    3. trauma to vein walls during surgery;
d. **atelectasis** related to hypoventilation and obstruction of the bronchioles associated with retained secretions.

DESIRED OUTCOMES	NURSING ACTIONS AND *SELECTED RATIONALES*

4.a. The client will not experience overdistention of the pouch as evidenced by:
1. decreased complaints of epigastric fullness and nausea
2. absence of vomiting.

4.a.1. Assess for and report signs and symptoms of overdistention of the pouch (e.g. increasing complaints of epigastric fullness and nausea, vomiting).
2. Implement measures *to prevent overdistention of the pouch:*
  a. maintain patency of nasogastric or gastrostomy tube *to reduce gas and fluid accumulation during period of decreased peristalsis*
  b. encourage and assist client with frequent position changes and ambulation as soon as allowed and tolerated (*activity stimulates peristalsis and expulsion of flatus*)
  c. instruct the client to avoid activities such as chewing gum, sucking on hard candy, and smoking *in order to reduce air swallowing*
  d. do not change position of nasogastric or gastrostomy tube unless ordered (*the tube is usually positioned in the pouch during surgery*)
  e. when oral intake is allowed:
    1. adhere strictly to prescribed oral intake schedule (clients usually begin with hourly liquid feedings of 30 cc and, over at least 6 weeks, progress to 5 or 6 small [2-ounce] meals/day with 1–2 ounces of fluid allowed between meals)
    2. provide client with allotted amounts of foods/fluids at the proper times; discard skipped "meals" *so client does not ingest meals too close together*
    3. instruct client to adhere to the liquid or pureed diet as ordered (*foods of thicker consistency can block the channel, which may be narrower in the early postoperative period because of edema*)
    4. crush any oral medication or administer it in liquid form *to prevent blockage of the channel*
  f. encourage client to eructate and expel flatus whenever the urge is felt
  g. encourage use of nonnarcotic analgesics once severe pain has subsided (*narcotic analgesics depress gastrointestinal motility*).
3. If signs and symptoms of overdistention occur:
  a. withhold all food and fluid as ordered
  b. prepare client for abdominal x-rays to check placement of nasogastric or gastrostomy tube
  c. assist physician with adjustment or reinsertion of the nasogastric or gastrostomy tube if indicated.

4.b. The client will not develop peritonitis as evidenced by:
1. gradual resolution of abdominal pain
2. soft, nondistended abdomen
3. temperature declining toward normal
4. stable vital signs
5. return of normal bowel sounds
6. WBC count declining toward normal.

4.b.1. Assess for and report signs and symptoms of peritonitis (e.g. increase in severity of abdominal pain; generalized abdominal pain; rebound tenderness; tense, rigid abdomen; increase in temperature; tachycardia; tachypnea; hypotension; continued diminished or absent bowel sounds).
2. Monitor WBC counts. Report levels that increase or fail to decline toward normal.
3. Implement measures *to prevent peritonitis:*
  a. perform actions to prevent and treat wound infection (see Standardized Postoperative Care Plan, Nursing Diagnosis 16, actions b.4 and 5)
  b. perform actions *to maintain patency of wound drain(s) if present:*
    1. keep tubing free of kinks
    2. empty collection device as often as necessary
    3. maintain suction as ordered
  c. perform actions *to prevent inadvertent removal of wound drain(s) if present:*
    1. use caution when changing dressings surrounding drain(s)
    2. provide extension tubing if necessary *to enable client to move without placing tension on the drain(s)*
    3. instruct client not to pull on drain(s) or drainage tubing
  d. perform actions *to prevent stress on the staple line:*
    1. implement measures to prevent overdistention of pouch (see action a.2 in this diagnosis)
    2. implement measures to prevent nausea and vomiting (see Standardized Postoperative Care Plan, Nursing Diagnosis 7.C, action 2)
    3. do not adjust position of nasogastric or gastrostomy tube unless ordered (*adjustment may cause disruption of staples*).

UNIT XII

4. If signs and symptoms of peritonitis occur:
   a. withhold all food and fluid as ordered
   b. place client on bedrest in a semi-Fowler's position *to assist in pooling or localizing gastric contents in the pelvis rather than under the diaphragm*
   c. assist physician with insertion of a nasogastric or gastrostomy tube if not already present and maintain suction as ordered
   d. monitor for therapeutic and nontherapeutic effects of anti-infectives if administered
   e. monitor for therapeutic and nontherapeutic effects of intravenous fluids and/or blood volume expanders if administered *to prevent or treat shock (shock can occur as a result of the escape of protein, fluid, and electrolytes into the peritoneal cavity)*
   f. prepare client for surgical repair of perforation or drainage of abscess if indicated
   g. provide emotional support to client and significant others.

4.c. The client will not develop a venous thrombus and pulmonary embolism (see Standardized Postoperative Care Plan, Collaborative Diagnosis 19, outcomes c.1 and 2, for outcome criteria).

4.c. Refer to Standardized Postoperative Care Plan, Collaborative Diagnosis 19, actions c.1 and 2, for measures related to assessment, prevention, and treatment of a venous thrombus and pulmonary embolism.

4.d. The client will not develop atelectasis (see Standardized Postoperative Care Plan, Collaborative Diagnosis 19, outcome b, for outcome criteria).

4.d.1. Refer to Standardized Postoperative Care Plan, Collaborative Diagnosis 19, action b, for measures related to assessment, prevention, and treatment of atelectasis.
2. Implement additional measures to improve breathing pattern (see Postoperative Nursing Diagnosis 1, action b) *in order to further reduce the risk of development of atelectasis.*

□ ▬▬▬▬▬▬▬▬▬▬▬▬▬▬▬▬▬▬▬▬▬▬▬▬▬▬▬▬▬▬

5. NURSING DIAGNOSIS

Noncompliance* related to lack of understanding of the implications of not following the prescribed treatment plan and difficulty integrating prescribed dietary modifications into life style.

---

* This diagnostic label includes both an informed decision by client not to comply and an inability to comply due to circumstances beyond the client's control.

□ ▬▬▬▬▬▬▬▬▬▬▬▬▬▬▬▬▬▬▬▬▬▬▬▬▬▬▬▬▬▬

DESIRED OUTCOMES	NURSING ACTIONS AND *SELECTED RATIONALES*

5. The client will demonstrate the probability of future compliance with the prescribed treatment plan as evidenced by:
   a. willingness to learn about and participate in treatments and care
   b. statements reflecting ways to modify personal habits and integrate treatments into life style

5.a. Assess for indications that the client may be unwilling or unable to comply with the prescribed treatment plan:
1. failure to adhere to treatment plan while in hospital (e.g. not adhering to dietary modifications and fluid restrictions, refusing to increase activity)
2. statements reflecting a lack of understanding of dietary modifications and factors that will cause stretching of the gastric pouch or disruption of staple line
3. statements reflecting an unwillingness or inability to modify personal habits and integrate necessary dietary modifications and exercise program into life style
4. statements reflecting view that the surgical procedure will provide

c. statements reflecting an understanding of the implications of not following the prescribed treatment plan.

continued weight loss even without adherence to the prescribed dietary modifications or that he/she will return to preoperative weight despite adherence to dietary modifications.

b. Implement measures *to improve client compliance:*
  1. explain the surgical procedure and importance of dietary modifications and a balanced exercise program in terms the client can understand; emphasize that adherence to the treatment program is necessary if he/she is to attain an optimal weight
  2. inform the client that prescribed food and fluid modifications are not as strict after the surgical area has healed (usually 6–8 weeks)
  3. stress the positive effects of compliance with dietary modifications and exercise program (e.g. weight loss resulting in change in appearance; decreased risk of development of health-related problems such as diabetes mellitus, cardiovascular disease, respiratory dysfunction, and osteoarthritis)
  4. focus on modifications of life style rather than complete change (e.g. schedule meetings after rather than at lunch, meet friends at a park rather than a restaurant)
  5. provide a dietary consult to assist client in planning a dietary program based on prescribed modifications and client's likes, dislikes, and daily routines
  6. encourage the development and use of techniques other than eating to cope with stress (e.g. relaxation, guided imagery, diversion, exercise)
  7. initiate discharge teaching outlined in Postoperative Nursing Diagnosis 6 *in order to promote a sense of control and self-reliance*
  8. encourage questions and allow time for reinforcement and clarification of information provided
  9. provide written instructions about future appointments with health care provider, dietary modifications, and signs and symptoms to report
  10. provide information about and encourage utilization of available community resources that can assist client to make necessary life-style changes (e.g. weight reduction groups, counseling services, support groups of persons who have had the same or similar surgery, stress management classes).

c. Assess for and reinforce behaviors suggesting future compliance with prescribed treatments (e.g. statements reflecting plans for integrating treatments into life style, participation in planning dietary program, changes in personal habits).

d. Include significant others in explanations and teaching sessions and encourage their support.

e. Reinforce the need for the client to assume responsibility for managing as much of care as possible.

f. Consult physician regarding referrals to community agencies and/or support groups if continued instruction, support, or supervision is needed.

□ ▬▬▬▬▬▬▬▬▬▬▬▬▬▬▬▬▬▬▬▬▬▬▬

6. NURSING DIAGNOSIS

Knowledge deficit regarding follow-up care.

□ ▬▬▬▬▬▬▬▬▬▬▬▬▬▬▬▬▬▬▬▬▬▬▬

DESIRED OUTCOMES	NURSING ACTIONS AND *SELECTED RATIONALES*
6.a. The client will identify ways to prevent excessive stretching of the gastric pouch and/or disruption of the staple line.	6.a. Instruct client in ways *to prevent excessive stretching of the gastric pouch and/or disruption of the staple line:* 1. decrease risk of channel blockage by: a. limiting oral intake to liquids and pureed foods for about 6–8 weeks after surgery as recommended

     b. taking all prescription and nonprescription medications crushed or in liquid form

     c. chewing foods thoroughly

2. do not exceed prescribed volume of food/fluid intake
3. do not make up for skipped meals while on an hourly drinking/eating schedule
4. eat and drink slowly
5. consume fluids between rather than with meals (recommended intake is usually 50 ounces [1500 cc] of water or low-calorie beverages each day).

6.b. The client will verbalize an understanding of ways to maintain an adequate nutritional status.	**6.b.1.** Instruct client regarding ways *to maintain an adequate nutritional status:*
	  a. do not skip meals
	  b. eat foods from each food group daily
	  c. consume adequate amounts of protein (e.g. blenderized drinks containing peanut butter, pureed meats and fish, creamed cottage cheese)
	  d. take vitamin and mineral supplements as ordered.
	  2. Obtain dietary consult if indicated to assist client in planning meals.

6.c. The client will identify ways to reduce the risk of consuming excessive amounts of food, fluid, and calories.	**6.c.** Instruct client in ways *to reduce the risk of consuming excessive amounts of food, fluid, and calories:*
	  1. limit food/fluid intake to prescribed volume
	  2. prepare foods ahead of time, freeze in 2-ounce portions using plastic ice cube trays or plastic bags, and then reheat only allowed amounts at mealtime
	  3. have jars of prepared strained baby food products rather than high-calorie puddings or snacks on hand
	  4. have only low-calorie drinks available (other than the required high-protein supplements)
	  5. decrease the risk of hunger by adhering to a schedule of 5 or 6 meals/day as diet advances (meals usually will consist of 2–4 tablespoons of food)
	  6. serve food on a small plate and use a salad rather than dinner fork when eating *(this provides an illusion that meals are larger than they really are and also helps client to eat more slowly)*
	  7. eat and drink very slowly (utilize techniques such as putting fork down between bites of food, putting glass down between sips of fluids, and, as diet advances, eating foods that are chewy rather than soft)
	  8. if going out to dinner, order an appetizer and have it served with everyone else's entree
	  9. avoid excessive intake of high-calorie foods/fluids *(it is possible to maintain or gain weight if only high-calorie substances are consumed).*

6.d. The client will demonstrate the ability to accurately calculate and measure the allotted amounts of food and fluid.	**6.d.1.** Demonstrate ways to measure foods/fluids accurately using measuring spoons and a cup with 1-ounce markings. 2. Allow time for questions, clarification, and return demonstration.

6.e. The client will state signs and symptoms to report to the health care provider.	**6.e.1.** Refer to Standardized Postoperative Care Plan, Nursing Diagnosis 20, action c, for signs and symptoms to report to the health care provider.
	  2. Instruct client to also report:
	    a. nausea and vomiting after consuming prescribed amounts of foods/fluids
	    b. inability to adhere to dietary modifications
	    c. weight gain
	    d. inability to lose weight or excessive weight loss (expected weight loss is usually about 10 pounds/month for the 1st year or 35% of preoperative body weight through the 1st year).

6.f. The client will identify community resources that can assist in the adjustment to prescribed dietary modifications and future changes in body image.	**6.f.1.** Provide information about community resources that can assist the client with the adjustment to prescribed dietary modifications and future changes in body image (e.g. weight reduction groups, counseling services, support groups of persons who have had the same or similar surgery). 2. Initiate a referral if indicated.

6.g. The client will verbalize an understanding of and a plan for adhering to recommended follow-up care including future appointments with health care provider, activity level, medications prescribed, and wound care.

6.g.1. Refer to Standardized Postoperative Care Plan, Nursing Diagnosis 20, for routine postoperative instructions.
2. Reinforce the physician's instructions regarding activity:
   a. avoid lifting, pushing, or pulling objects over 10 pounds for at least 3 weeks
   b. adhere to a schedule of moderate exercise (clients are usually instructed to begin a walking program and should be walking 1–2 miles/day by 4th week after discharge).
3. Refer to Postoperative Nursing Diagnosis 5, action b, for measures to improve client compliance.

Hemorrhoidectomy

A hemorrhoidectomy is the removal of hemorrhoids (varicosities of the veins draining the anal canal and rectum). It can be accomplished by methods such as rubber band ligation, cryosurgery, injection of a sclerosing agent, or actual surgical excision. A hemorrhoidectomy is performed when conservative measures have been unsuccessful in controlling pain and bleeding and marked protrusion and/or thrombosis of the hemorrhoidal vessels exist.

This care plan focuses on the adult client hospitalized for the surgical excision of hemorrhoids. Preoperatively, goals of care are to reduce discomfort and educate the client regarding postoperative expectations and management. Postoperative goals of care are to reduce discomfort, prevent constipation, prevent complications, and educate the client regarding follow-up care.

DISCHARGE CRITERIA

Prior to discharge, the client will:

- identify ways to prevent recurrence of hemorrhoids
- identify ways to prevent anorectal strictures
- identify ways to maintain perianal hygiene and comfort
- state signs and symptoms to report to the health care provider
- verbalize an understanding of and a plan for adhering to recommended follow-up care including future appointments with health care provider, medications prescribed, activity level, and wound care.

NURSING/COLLABORATIVE DIAGNOSES

Preoperative
1. Pain: anorectal □ *664*
Postoperative
1. Pain: anorectal □ *665*
2. Urinary retention □ *665*
3. Constipation □ *666*
4. Potential for infection: wound □ *666*
5. Potential complications:
   a. rectal hemorrhage
   b. anorectal stricture □ *666*
6. Knowledge deficit regarding follow-up care □ *667*

Preoperative

Use in conjunction with the Standardized Preoperative Care Plan.

1. NURSING DIAGNOSIS

Pain: anorectal related to pressure in the anal and rectal vessels associated with dilation, thrombosis, and/or strangulation of the vessels.

DESIRED OUTCOMES

1. The client will experience diminished anorectal pain as evidenced by:
   a. verbalization of diminished pain
   b. relaxed facial expression and body positioning
   c. stable vital signs.

NURSING ACTIONS AND *SELECTED RATIONALES*

1.a. Determine how the client usually responds to pain.
   b. Assess for nonverbal signs of pain (e.g. wrinkled brow, clenched fists, reluctance to sit, restlessness, diaphoresis, facial pallor or flushing, change in B/P, tachycardia).
   c. Assess verbal complaints of pain. Ask client to be specific about location, severity, and type of pain.
   d. Assess for factors that seem to aggravate and alleviate pain.
   e. Implement measures *to reduce anorectal pain:*
      1. perform actions *to reduce venous congestion in anal and rectal vessels:*
         a. instruct client to avoid prolonged sitting and standing
         b. instruct client to avoid straining to have a bowel movement
         c. instruct client to lie in a prone position as tolerated
      2. provide a pillow or foam pad or ring for client to sit on if desired
      3. if cleansing enemas are to be administered preoperatively, lubricate enema tubing well and insert gently
      4. consult physician about application of cold and/or heat to anal area
      5. provide or assist with nonpharmacological measures for pain relief (e.g. position change, relaxation techniques, quiet conversation, restful environment, diversional activities)
      6. monitor for therapeutic and nontherapeutic effects of the following medications if administered:
         a. anesthetic ointments or creams (e.g. Americaine, Corticaine, Nupercainal, Tronolane)
         b. anesthetic suppositories (e.g. Tronolane, Corticaine)
         c. astringents (e.g. witch hazel)
         d. analgesics.
   f. Consult physician if above measures fail to provide adequate pain relief or if pain increases significantly *(may indicate severe thrombosis or strangulation of a hemorrhoid).*

Postoperative

Use in conjunction with the Standardized Postoperative Care Plan.

1. NURSING DIAGNOSIS

Pain: anorectal related to surgical trauma, reflex spasms of the anal and/or rectal sphincter, and edema in and irritation of the surgical area.

DESIRED OUTCOMES	NURSING ACTIONS AND *SELECTED RATIONALES*
1. The client will experience diminished anorectal pain (see Standardized Postoperative Care Plan, Nursing Diagnosis 7.A, for outcome criteria).	1.a. Refer to Standardized Postoperative Care Plan, Nursing Diagnosis 7.A, for measures related to assessment and reduction of pain. b. Implement additional measures *to reduce anorectal pain:* 1. perform actions *to reduce venous congestion and edema in the surgical area:* a. apply ice packs to anal area for first 24–48 hours after surgery b. have client lie in a prone position at regular intervals c. apply witch hazel soaks (e.g. Tucks) as ordered d. instruct client to avoid prolonged sitting and standing 2. assist client to assume a comfortable position (e.g. prone, side-lying) 3. apply warm, moist compresses and/or assist with sitz baths beginning 24–48 hours after surgery 4. provide a pillow or foam pad or ring for client to sit on if desired 5. use a T-binder or snug-fitting underwear to secure any rectal drain, packing, or dressing in place *in order to reduce the risk of surgical site irritation and trauma* 6. instruct and assist client to clean and dry perianal area gently 7. apply protective ointments (e.g. petrolatum, zinc oxide) to perianal area *in order to protect the skin from maceration associated with frequent sitz baths and moist soaks* 8. monitor for therapeutic and nontherapeutic effects of anesthetic ointments or creams (e.g. Nupercainal, Americaine, Corticaine, Tronolane) if administered. c. Consult physician if above measures fail to provide adequate pain relief.

2. NURSING DIAGNOSIS

Urinary retention related to reflex spasms of the bladder outlet sphincter, guarding of the pelvic muscles, reluctance to void associated with tenderness and pain in the perineal area, and depressant effects of some medications (e.g. anesthetics, narcotic analgesics) on bladder muscle tone.

DESIRED OUTCOMES	NURSING ACTIONS AND *SELECTED RATIONALES*
2. The client will not experience urinary retention (see Standardized Postoperative Care Plan, Nursing Diagnosis 13, for outcome criteria).	2.a. Refer to Standardized Postoperative Care Plan, Nursing Diagnosis 13, for measures related to assessment and management of urinary retention. b. Implement additional measures *to prevent and manage urinary retention:* 1. perform actions to reduce anorectal pain (see Postoperative Nursing Diagnosis 1) 2. assist with sitz baths as soon as allowed and encourage client to void while in sitz bath if still having difficulty urinating.

UNIT
XII

3. NURSING DIAGNOSIS

Constipation related to reluctance to defecate associated with anorectal pain and decreased gastrointestinal motility resulting from depressant effects of anesthesia and narcotic analgesics.

DESIRED OUTCOMES	NURSING ACTIONS AND *SELECTED RATIONALES*
3. The client will have a soft, formed stool by the 3rd postoperative day.	3.a. Refer to Standardized Postoperative Care Plan, Nursing Diagnosis 14, for measures related to assessment and prevention of constipation. b. Administer an analgesic before client attempts to have a bowel movement *in order to ease the pain associated with passage of stool.*

4. NURSING DIAGNOSIS

Potential for infection: wound related to contamination of the incision by feces.

DESIRED OUTCOMES	NURSING ACTIONS AND *SELECTED RATIONALES*
4. The client will remain free of wound infection (see Standardized Postoperative Care Plan, Nursing Diagnosis 16, outcome b, for outcome criteria).	4.a. Refer to Standardized Postoperative Care Plan, Nursing Diagnosis 16, action b, for measures related to assessment, prevention, and management of wound infection. b. Implement additional measures *to prevent wound infection:* 1. perform actions to prevent trauma to and pressure on the incision (see Postoperative Collaborative Diagnosis 5, action a.2.b) 2. cleanse and dry anal area thoroughly after each bowel movement.

5. COLLABORATIVE DIAGNOSIS

Potential complications:

a. **rectal hemorrhage** related to trauma to the anal and rectal vessels associated with surgery;
b. **anorectal stricture** related to granulation and fibrotic tissue formation in the surgical area.

DESIRED OUTCOMES	NURSING ACTIONS AND *SELECTED RATIONALES*
5.a. The client will not experience rectal hemorrhage as evidenced	5.a.1. Assess for and report signs of rectal hemorrhage (e.g. excessive or prolonged rectal bleeding, significant decline in B/P and increase in pulse rate).

by:
1. absence of excessive or prolonged rectal bleeding
2. stable vital signs.

2. Implement measures *to prevent rectal hemorrhage:*
   a. ensure that local hemostatic agents (e.g. Gelfoam, Oxycel) are secured in or over anal wound as ordered
   b. perform actions *to prevent trauma to and pressure on the incision:*
      1. implement measures to prevent constipation (see Postoperative Nursing Diagnosis 3)
      2. instruct client to avoid straining to have a bowel movement
      3. instruct client to avoid vigorous wiping of anal area
      4. if suppositories or enemas are ordered, lubricate suppository or tubing well and insert gently using extreme caution
   c. perform actions *to reduce venous congestion in the anal and rectal vessels:*
      1. apply ice packs to anal area for first 24–48 hours after surgery
      2. have client lie in a prone position at regular intervals
      3. instruct client to avoid prolonged sitting and standing.
3. If rectal hemorrhage occurs:
   a. maintain client on bedrest in a flat position
   b. prepare client for surgical repair of bleeding vessels if planned.

5.b. The client will not develop stricture of the anorectal canal as evidenced by the ability to pass stool of normal size and shape.

5.b.1. Monitor bowel movements including occurrence of the first bowel movement and size and shape of stool.
2. Implement measures *to promote the passage of soft, formed stools that act as dilators and help maintain the normal size of the lumen of the anorectal canal:*
   a. perform actions to prevent constipation (see Postoperative Nursing Diagnosis 3)
   b. monitor for therapeutic and nontherapeutic effects of bulk-forming laxatives (e.g. methylcellulose, psyllium hydrophilic mucilloid) if administered.
3. If client has not had a bowel movement by the 3rd postoperative day:
   a. notify physician
   b. assist with rectal dilation if performed.

□ ▆▆▆▆▆▆▆▆▆▆▆▆▆▆▆▆▆▆▆▆▆▆▆▆▆▆▆▆▆▆▆

6. NURSING DIAGNOSIS

Knowledge deficit regarding follow-up care.

□ ▆▆▆▆▆▆▆▆▆▆▆▆▆▆▆▆▆▆▆▆▆▆▆▆▆▆▆▆▆▆▆

DESIRED OUTCOMES	NURSING ACTIONS AND *SELECTED RATIONALES*

6.a. The client will identify ways to prevent recurrence of hemorrhoids.

6.a. Provide the following instructions on ways *to prevent recurrence of hemorrhoids:*
1. adhere to following measures *to prevent constipation in order to reduce straining to have a bowel movement:*
   a. drink at least 10 glasses of liquid/day
   b. increase intake of high-fiber foods (e.g. nuts, bran, whole grains, raw fruits and vegetables, dried fruits)
   c. defecate whenever the urge is felt
   d. take stool softeners and gentle laxatives as prescribed; caution client to avoid strong laxatives, *which can cause propulsive, liquid bowel movements and subsequent trauma to operative area*
   e. adhere to a program of regular exercise
2. avoid prolonged standing and sitting *to prevent venous stasis in the anal and rectal vessels.*

6.b. The client will identify ways to prevent anorectal strictures.

6.b. Instruct client in ways *to reduce risk of anorectal stricture formation:*
1. adhere to measures to prevent constipation (see action a.1 in this diagnosis) *in order to promote normal passage of stool*

2. avoid strong laxatives *to prevent liquid bowel movements (formed stool acts as a dilator and helps maintain normal lumen size of anorectal canal)*
3. take bulk-forming laxatives as prescribed.

6.c. The client will identify ways to maintain perianal hygiene and comfort.

6.c. Provide the following instructions regarding ways *to maintain perianal hygiene and comfort:*
1. gently cleanse anal area with warm water after each bowel movement; dry area with clean, soft, cotton towel
2. take 2–4 sitz baths/day for first week or two after surgery
3. apply astringents (e.g. Tucks) to anal area if approved by physician.

6.d. The client will state signs and symptoms to report to the health care provider.

6.d.1. Refer to Standardized Postoperative Care Plan, Nursing Diagnosis 20, action c, for signs and symptoms to report to the health care provider.
2. Instruct client to report these additional signs and symptoms:
   a. rectal bleeding
   b. inability to have a bowel movement at least every 3 days.

6.e. The client will verbalize an understanding of and a plan for adhering to recommended follow-up care including future appointments with health care provider, medications prescribed, activity level, and wound care.

6.e. Refer to Standardized Postoperative Care Plan, Nursing Diagnosis 20, for routine postoperative instructions and measures to improve client compliance.

Hiatal Hernia Repair

A hiatal (hiatus) hernia occurs when the abdominal portion of the esophagus and/or a portion of the stomach herniates through the esophageal hiatus in the diaphragm. The most common type of hiatal hernia is the direct or "sliding" type in which the esophagogastric junction and a portion of the stomach slip through the hiatus into the thoracic cavity when the client is horizontal or when intra-abdominal pressure is increased. With the paraesophageal or "rolling" type of hiatal hernia, the esophagogastric junction remains below the diaphragm but a portion of the stomach rolls up through the weakened area in the diaphragm and forms a pocket next to the esophagus. The third type is the esophagogastric hernia that is a combination of the direct and paraesophageal types. A hiatal hernia can result from changes in the esophageal hiatus due to increased intra-abdominal pressure resulting from obesity, pregnancy, ascites, or continued lifting of heavy objects; muscle stretching or weakening; congenital abnormalities; or abdominal trauma. Most people with a hiatal hernia also have a lower esophageal sphincter (LES) pressure that is less than the gastric pressure, so reflux of gastric contents is common. The signs and symptoms of hiatal her-

nia are mainly the result of delayed emptying of the herniated portion of the stomach and reflux of gastric contents.

Surgical intervention becomes necessary when conservative management is no longer effective in controlling symptoms or if complications such as strictures, incarceration, chronic esophagitis, or bleeding occur. The aim of the surgery is to secure the herniated portion below the diaphragm and stop the reflux of gastric contents. This is accomplished by surgical procedures such as the Nissen fundoplication, Hill operation, or Belsey operation, which involve wrapping the gastric fundus partially or completely around the portion of the esophagus that is below the level of the diaphragm. Although an abdominal approach is used most frequently, a thoracic approach is sometimes utilized.

This care plan focuses on the adult client hospitalized for surgical repair of a hiatal hernia. Preoperative goals of care are to control discomfort and prevent complications. Postoperatively, the goals of care are to maintain comfort, prevent complications, and educate the client regarding follow-up care.

DISCHARGE CRITERIA

Prior to discharge, the client will:

- identify ways to prevent gastric distention
- state signs and symptoms of complications to report to the health care provider
- verbalize an understanding of and a plan for adhering to recommended follow-up care including future appointments with health care provider, medications prescribed, activity level, and wound care.

□

NURSING/COLLABORATIVE DIAGNOSES

Preoperative
1. Impaired swallowing □ *669*
2. Altered comfort:
    a. pyrosis (heartburn)
    b. substernal pain
    c. bloated feeling or feeling of fullness □ *670*
3. Potential complications:
    a. esophageal bleeding
    b. gastric obstruction □ *671*
Postoperative
1. Altered nutrition: less than body requirements □ *672*
2A. Altered comfort:
    1. chest pain
    2. abdominal pain □ *673*
2B. Altered comfort: abdominal discomfort (distention and gas pain) □ *673*
3. Potential complications:
    a. pneumothorax
    b. peritonitis □ *674*
4. Knowledge deficit regarding follow-up care □ *675*

UNIT
XII

□

Preoperative

Use in conjunction with the Standardized Preoperative Care Plan.

□

1. NURSING DIAGNOSIS

Impaired swallowing related to esophageal irritation and muscle spasm associated with reflux of gastric contents.

□

DESIRED OUTCOMES	NURSING ACTIONS AND *SELECTED RATIONALES*

1. The client will experience an improvement in swallowing as evidenced by verbalization of the same.	1.a. Assess for signs and symptoms of impaired swallowing (e.g. statements that food gets stuck in the esophagus, complaints of increased esophageal pressure or discomfort when eating).
	 b. Implement measures *to improve ability to swallow:*
	   1. perform actions to prevent reflux of gastric contents and to reduce esophageal irritation if reflux occurs (see Preoperative Nursing Diagnosis 2, actions e.1 and 2)
	   2. perform actions *to facilitate passage of foods/fluids through the esophagus:*
	     a. place client in high Fowler's position during meals and snacks
	     b. assist client to select foods that are easy to swallow (e.g. custard, cottage cheese, ground meat)
	     c. moisten dry foods with gravy or sauces (e.g. catsup, salad dressing, sour cream)
	     d. encourage client to swallow frequently when eating
	     e. encourage client to drink fluids with meals.
	 c. Consult physician if swallowing difficulties worsen.

☐ ▐██▌

2. NURSING DIAGNOSIS

Altered comfort:*

a. **pyrosis (heartburn)** related to irritation of the esophageal mucosa associated with reflux of gastric contents resulting from increased gastric and/or intra-abdominal pressure and decreased lower esophageal sphincter (LES) pressure;

b. **substernal pain** related to distention of the herniated portion of the stomach and esophageal spasm;

c. **bloated feeling or feeling of fullness** related to distention of the herniated portion of the stomach.

---

* In this care plan, the nursing diagnosis "pain" is included under the diagnostic label of altered comfort.

☐ ▐██▌

DESIRED OUTCOMES	NURSING ACTIONS AND *SELECTED RATIONALES*

2. The client will experience diminished discomfort as evidenced by:
 a. verbalization of relief of heartburn, substernal pain, and bloated or full feeling
 b. relaxed facial expression and body positioning
 c. stable vital signs.
	2.a. Determine how the client usually responds to discomfort.
	 b. Assess for nonverbal signs of discomfort (e.g. wrinkled brow, reluctance to move, rubbing substernal area, restlessness, diaphoresis, facial pallor or flushing, change in B/P, tachycardia).
	 c. Assess verbal complaints of discomfort. Ask client to be specific about location, severity, and type of discomfort.
	 d. Assess for factors that seem to aggravate and alleviate discomfort.
	 e. Implement measures *to reduce discomfort:*
	   1. perform actions *to prevent reflux of gastric contents:*
	     a. implement measures *to prevent an increase in intra-abdominal pressure:*
	       1. instruct client to avoid coughing and straining to have a bowel movement; consult physician about an order for an antitussive, laxative, and/or stool softener if indicated
	       2. place needed items within easy reach *so client does not need to twist or bend at the waist*
	       3. instruct client to avoid wearing clothing that is tight around the waist or abdomen

   4. instruct client to avoid activities such as chewing gum, sucking on hard candy, drinking through a straw, and smoking *in order to reduce air swallowing*
   5. provide small, frequent meals rather than 3 large ones
   6. instruct client to avoid gas-producing foods/fluids (e.g. cabbage, onions, beans, carbonated beverages)
   b. instruct client to eat in a sitting position and avoid lying down for at least 2–3 hours after eating
   c. keep head of the bed elevated 20–25 cm (8–10 inches); bed is often put in reverse Trendelenburg position to accomplish this
   d. implement measures *to prevent a further decrease in LES pressure:*
      1. encourage client to stop smoking *(smoking has been found to immediately decrease LES pressure)*
      2. instruct client to avoid foods/fluids known to decrease LES pressure (e.g. chocolate, peppermint, coffee)
      3. instruct client to avoid foods/fluids high in fat such as butter, cream, oils, whole milk, ice cream, pork, fried foods, gravies, and nuts *(fatty foods stimulate the release of cholecystokinin, which decreases LES pressure)*
   e. monitor for therapeutic and nontherapeutic effects of the following medications if administered:
      1. gastrointestinal stimulants (e.g. metoclopramide) *to hasten gastric emptying and increase LES pressure*
      2. cholinergics (e.g. bethanechol) *to increase LES pressure*
   2. perform actions *to reduce irritation of the esophageal mucosa if reflux occurs:*
      a. provide a bland diet as ordered
      b. instruct client to avoid spicy foods; citrus fruits or juices; and caffeine-containing items such as chocolate, coffee, tea, or colas
      c. instruct client to drink water after meals or episodes of reflux *in order to cleanse the esophagus*
      d. if client is receiving ulcerogenic medications (e.g. corticosteroids, aspirin, indomethacin), administer them with meals or snacks
      e. monitor for therapeutic and nontherapeutic effects of antacids and histamine$_2$ receptor antagonists (e.g. cimetidine, famotidine, ranitidine) if administered *to reduce the acidity of gastric contents*
   3. provide or assist with nonpharmacological measures for relief of discomfort (e.g. position change, relaxation techniques, guided imagery, quiet conversation, restful environment, diversional activities)
   4. monitor for therapeutic and nontherapeutic effects of analgesics if administered.
   f. Consult physician if above measures fail to provide adequate relief of discomfort.

UNIT XII

3. COLLABORATIVE DIAGNOSIS

Potential complications:

a. **esophageal bleeding** related to ulceration of the esophagus associated with persistent reflux of gastric contents;
b. **gastric obstruction** related to incarceration of the herniated portion of the stomach.

DESIRED OUTCOMES	NURSING ACTIONS AND *SELECTED RATIONALES*
3.a. The client will not experience esophageal bleeding as evidenced by:	3.a.1. Assess for and report signs and symptoms of esophageal bleeding (e.g. complaints of increased substernal discomfort or fullness, frank or occult blood in stool or gastric contents, decreased B/P, increased pulse).

1. no complaints of increased substernal discomfort and fullness
2. absence of occult or frank blood in stool and gastric contents
3. B/P and pulse within normal range for client
4. RBC, Hct., and Hgb. levels within normal range.

2. Monitor RBC, Hct., and Hgb. levels. Report declining values.
3. Implement measures to prevent gastric reflux and reduce irritation of esophageal mucosa if reflux occurs (see Preoperative Nursing Diagnosis 2, actions e.1 and 2).
4. If signs and symptoms of esophageal bleeding occur:
   a. maintain food and fluid restrictions as ordered
   b. administer antacids hourly as ordered
   c. insert a nasogastric tube and maintain suction as ordered *to decrease the amount of gastric contents and further reduce reflux*
   d. assess for and immediately report signs and symptoms of hypovolemic shock (e.g. restlessness; agitation; significant decline in B/P; resting pulse rate greater than 100 beats/minute; rapid or labored respirations; cool, pale, or cyanotic skin; diminished or absent peripheral pulses; urine output less than 30 cc/hour)
   e. assist with transendoscopic electrocoagulation, selective arterial embolization, endoscopic laser photocoagulation, and/or intra-arterial administration of vasopressors (e.g. vasopressin) if ordered
   f. monitor for therapeutic and nontherapeutic effects of blood products and/or volume expanders if administered
   g. provide emotional support to client and significant others.

3.b. The client will not experience gastric obstruction as evidenced by:
1. no complaints of increased fullness, bloating, and substernal pain
2. absence of nausea and vomiting.

3.b.1. Assess for and report signs and symptoms of gastric obstruction (e.g. complaints of increased fullness, bloating, or substernal pain; nausea; vomiting).
2. Implement measures *to prevent herniation of a portion of the stomach:*
   a. instruct client to always avoid the horizontal position *(an upright or semi-recumbent posture helps maintain the stomach in its proper position)*
   b. perform actions to prevent an increase in intra-abdominal and gastric pressure (see Preoperative Nursing Diagnosis 2, action e.1.a–c) *in order to avoid increased pressure on weakened area of diaphragm.*
3. If signs and symptoms of gastric obstruction occur:
   a. maintain food and fluid restrictions as ordered
   b. prepare client for early surgery if planned (immediate surgical repair of the hiatal hernia is often necessary *to prevent strangulation and subsequent gangrene of the herniated portion)*
   c. provide emotional support to client and significant others.

Postoperative

Use in conjunction with the Standardized Postoperative Care Plan.

1. NURSING DIAGNOSIS

Altered nutrition: less than body requirements related to:

a. decreased oral intake associated with:
   1. anorexia resulting from discomfort, fatigue, constipation, and decreased activity
   2. dislike of prescribed diet
   3. nausea;
b. inadequate nutritional replacement therapy;

c. increased nutritional needs associated with:
1. decreased nutritional status preoperatively resulting from decreased oral intake if symptoms such as heartburn, odynophagia, epigastric bloating, and substernal pain were severe
2. increased metabolic rate that occurs during wound healing.

DESIRED OUTCOMES	NURSING ACTIONS AND *SELECTED RATIONALES*

1. The client will maintain an adequate nutritional status (see Standardized Postoperative Care Plan, Nursing Diagnosis 6, for outcome criteria).

1. Refer to Standardized Postoperative Care Plan, Nursing Diagnosis 6, for measures related to assessment and promotion of an optimal nutritional status.

2.A. NURSING DIAGNOSIS

Altered comfort:*

1. **chest pain** related to tissue trauma, reflex muscle spasm, and tissue irritation associated with presence of chest tubes (with thoracic approach);
2. **abdominal pain** related to tissue trauma and reflex muscle spasm (with abdominal approach).

---

* In this care plan, the nursing diagnosis "pain" is included under the diagnostic label of altered comfort.

DESIRED OUTCOMES	NURSING ACTIONS AND *SELECTED RATIONALES*

2.A. The client will experience diminished pain (see Standardized Postoperative Care Plan, Nursing Diagnosis 7.A, for outcome criteria).

2.A.1. Refer to Standardized Postoperative Care Plan, Nursing Diagnosis 7.A, for measures related to assessment and management of postoperative pain.
2. If a thoracic approach was utilized, implement additional measures *to reduce pain:*
a. securely anchor or fasten chest tube(s) *to decrease discomfort resulting from movement of the tube(s)*
b. provide adequate support (e.g. pillows) for arm and shoulder on operative side.

2.B. NURSING DIAGNOSIS

Altered comfort: abdominal discomfort (distention and gas pain) related to accumulation of gas and fluid associated with:

1. decreased peristalsis resulting from manipulation of the bowel during surgery (if abdominal approach was utilized), depressant effects of anesthesia and some medications (e.g. narcotic analgesics, antiemetics), and decreased activity;
2. inability to eructate (the surgical technique that prevents reflux also results in decreased ability or inability to eructate).

UNIT
XII

DESIRED OUTCOMES	NURSING ACTIONS AND *SELECTED RATIONALES*
2.B. The client will experience diminished abdominal distention and gas pain (see Standardized Postoperative Care Plan, Nursing Diagnosis 7.B, for outcome criteria).	2.B. Refer to Standardized Postoperative Care Plan, Nursing Diagnosis 7.B, for measures related to assessment of abdominal distention and gas pain and measures to reduce the accumulation of gastrointestinal gas and fluid.

□ ▬▬

3. COLLABORATIVE DIAGNOSIS

Potential complications:

a. **pneumothorax** related to surgical opening of pleura and chest tube malfunction (chest tube[s] will be present if thoracic approach was utilized);
b. **peritonitis** related to:
   1. leakage of lower esophageal or gastric contents into the peritoneal cavity associated with loss of integrity of esophageal or gastric sutures
   2. leakage from an abscess
   3. wound infection (especially if the abdominal approach was utilized).

□ ▬▬

DESIRED OUTCOMES	NURSING ACTIONS AND *SELECTED RATIONALES*

3.a. The client will experience normal lung re-expansion postoperatively as evidenced by:
1. normal breath sounds and percussion note by 3rd–4th postoperative day
2. unlabored respirations at 16–20/minute
3. blood gases returning toward normal
4. chest x-ray showing lung re-expansion.
	3.a.1. Assess for and immediately report signs and symptoms of:
	a. malfunction of the chest drainage system (e.g. respiratory distress, sudden cessation of drainage, excessive bubbling in water seal chamber, significant increase in subcutaneous emphysema)
	b. further lung collapse (e.g. extended area of absent breath sounds with hyperresonant percussion note; rapid, shallow, and/or labored respirations; tachycardia; sudden, sharp chest pain; cyanosis; restlessness; confusion).
	2. Monitor blood gases. Report values that have worsened.
	3. Monitor chest x-ray results. Report findings of delayed lung re-expansion.
	4. Implement measures *to prevent further lung collapse and promote lung re-expansion:*
	a. perform actions *to maintain patency and integrity of chest drainage system:*
	  1. maintain water seal and suction levels as ordered
	  2. maintain an air occlusive dressing over chest tube insertion site(s)
	  3. tape all connections securely
	  4. milk or strip tube(s) if ordered
	  5. keep chest drainage and suction tubing free of kinks
	  6. keep drainage system below level of client's chest at all times
	b. perform actions to improve breathing pattern and facilitate airway clearance (see Standardized Postoperative Care Plan, Nursing Diagnoses 3, action d and 4, action b).
	5. If signs and symptoms of further lung collapse occur:
	a. maintain client on bedrest in a semi- to high Fowler's position
	b. maintain oxygen therapy as ordered
	c. assess for and immediately report signs and symptoms of mediastinal shift (e.g. severe dyspnea, increased restlessness and agitation, rapid and/or irregular pulse rate, cyanosis, shift in point of apical impulse and trachea toward unaffected side)
	d. assist with clearing of existing chest tube(s) and/or insertion of a new tube
	e. provide emotional support to client and significant others.

3.b. The client will not develop peritonitis as evidenced by:
1. gradual resolution of abdominal pain
2. soft, nondistended abdomen
3. temperature declining toward normal
4. stable vital signs
5. bowel sounds returning to normal
6. WBC count declining toward normal.

3.b.1. Assess for and report signs and symptoms of peritonitis (e.g increase in severity of abdominal pain; generalized abdominal pain; rebound tenderness; tense, rigid abdomen; increase in temperature; tachycardia; tachypnea; hypotension; continued diminished or absent bowel sounds).
2. Monitor WBC counts. Report levels that increase or fail to decline toward normal.
3. Implement measures *to prevent peritonitis:*
   a. perform actions to prevent and treat wound infection (see Standardized Postoperative Care Plan, Nursing Diagnosis 16, actions b.4 and 5)
   b. perform actions *to maintain patency of wound drain(s) if present:*
      1. keep tubing free of kinks
      2. empty collection device as often as necessary
      3. maintain suction as ordered
   c. perform actions *to prevent inadvertent removal of wound drain(s) if present:*
      1. use caution when changing dressings surrounding drain(s)
      2. provide extension tubing if necessary *to enable client to move without placing tension on drain(s)*
      3. instruct client not to pull on drain(s) or drainage tubing
   d. perform actions *to prevent stress on and leakage from the suture lines:*
      1. do not adjust position of nasogastric tube unless ordered *(adjustment may cause disruption of the suture line)*
      2. implement measures to reduce accumulation of gastrointestinal gas and fluid and prevent or control nausea, vomiting attempts, and hiccoughs (see Standardized Postoperative Care Plan, Nursing Diagnoses 7.B, action 3; 7.C, action 2; and 7.D) *in order to prevent increased intra-abdominal pressure.*
4. If signs and symptoms of peritonitis occur:
   a. withhold all food and fluid as ordered
   b. place client on bedrest in a semi-Fowler's position *to assist in pooling or localizing the gastrointestinal contents in the pelvis rather than under the diaphragm*
   c. assist physician with insertion of a nasogastric tube if not already present or an intestinal tube and maintain suction as ordered
   d. monitor for therapeutic and nontherapeutic effects of anti-infectives if administered
   e. monitor for therapeutic and nontherapeutic effects of intravenous fluids and/or blood volume expanders if administered *to prevent or treat shock (shock can occur as a result of the escape of protein, fluid, and electrolytes into the peritoneal cavity)*
   f. prepare client for surgical repair of perforation or drainage of an abscess if indicated
   g. provide emotional support to client and significant others.

□ ▮▮▮▮▮▮▮▮▮▮▮▮▮▮▮▮▮▮▮▮▮▮▮▮▮▮▮▮▮▮

4. NURSING DIAGNOSIS

Knowledge deficit regarding follow-up care.

□ ▮▮▮▮▮▮▮▮▮▮▮▮▮▮▮▮▮▮▮▮▮▮▮▮▮▮▮▮▮▮

DESIRED OUTCOMES	NURSING ACTIONS AND *SELECTED RATIONALES*

4.a. The client will identify ways to prevent gastric distention.

4.a.1. Explain that gastric distention can occur because the surgery has resulted in a smaller stomach size and a decreased ability or inability to eructate or vomit (the lower esophageal sphincter was strengthened to prevent reflux).
2. Instruct the client in ways *to prevent gastric distention:*
   a. eat slowly and chew food thoroughly
   b. avoid eating large meals

c. decrease intake of gas-producing foods/fluids (e.g. cabbage, onions, beans, carbonated beverages)

d. stop smoking and avoid gum chewing and drinking through a straw *to reduce risk of air swallowing.*

4.b. The client will state signs and symptoms of complications to report to the health care provider.

4.b.1. Refer to Standardized Postoperative Care Plan, Nursing Diagnosis 20, action c, for signs and symptoms to report to the health care provider.

2. Instruct client to report these additional signs and symptoms:

a. regurgitation or sensation of hot liquid or sour, bitter taste in back of throat

b. persistent difficulty swallowing

c. persistent epigastric fullness or bloating.

4.c. The client will verbalize an understanding of and a plan for adhering to recommended follow-up care including future appointments with health care provider, medications prescribed, activity level, and wound care.

4.c.1. Refer to Standardized Postoperative Care Plan, Nursing Diagnosis 20, for routine postoperative instructions and measures to improve client compliance.

2. Reinforce the physician's instructions regarding the need to avoid lifting objects over 10 pounds for 4–6 weeks after surgery.

Inflammatory Bowel Disease: Ulcerative Colitis and Crohn's Disease

Crohn's disease and ulcerative colitis are the most common forms of inflammatory bowel disease. Both conditions commonly affect young adults, are of unknown etiology, can have very similar symptoms, and are characterized by periods of remission and exacerbation. Extraintestinal manifestations such as liver and joint involvement and skin, eye, and oral lesions may occur in both diseases and often subside once the intestinal inflammation resolves. Crohn's disease and ulcerative colitis differ as to the area and extent of bowel involved and the depth of inflammation and ulceration of bowel tissue. Ulcerative colitis involves the mucosa and submucosa of the bowel wall, typically starts in the distal colon, and progresses in a regular pattern throughout the colon with minimal involvement of the small intestine. Crohn's disease, on the other hand, involves the entire thickness of the bowel wall, begins anywhere in the intestinal tract, usually involves the terminal ileum, and has an unusual pattern of progression. Complications differ somewhat between the two in that clients with ulcerative colitis have a greater predisposition to cancer and a higher incidence of rectal bleeding whereas those with Crohn's disease have a higher incidence of anorectal fissures.

This care plan focuses on the adult client with longstanding ulcerative colitis or Crohn's disease hospitalized for control of an acute exacerbation of the disease. The goals of care are to increase comfort, rest the bowel, maintain adequate nutrition and hydration, prevent complications, and educate the client regarding effective home management of the disease.

DISCHARGE CRITERIA

Prior to discharge, the client will:

- identify ways to reduce the incidence of disease exacerbation
- verbalize ways to maintain an optimal nutritional status

- state ways to prevent perianal skin breakdown
- identify ways to minimize the risk of bleeding
- verbalize an understanding of medication therapy including rationale for, side effects of, schedule for taking, and importance of taking as prescribed
- state signs and symptoms to report to the health care provider
- identify community resources that can assist in the adjustment to changes resulting from inflammatory bowel disease and its treatment
- share feelings and thoughts about the effects of inflammatory bowel disease on life style and self-concept
- verbalize an understanding of and a plan for adhering to recommended follow-up care including future appointments with health care provider and activity level.

Use in conjunction with the Care Plan on Immobility.

NURSING/COLLABORATIVE DIAGNOSES

1. Anxiety □ *678*
2. Altered fluid and electrolyte balance:
   a. fluid volume deficit, hypokalemia, hyponatremia, hypochloremia, hypomagnesemia, and hypocalcemia
   b. metabolic acidosis □ *678*
3. Altered nutrition: less than body requirements □ *680*
4A. Altered comfort:
   1. abdominal cramping and pain
   2. joint pain
   3. anorectal pain
   4. oral pain
   5. skin tenderness and pain □ *681*
4B. Altered comfort: nausea and vomiting □ *682*
5. Impaired skin integrity: irritation or breakdown □ *683*
6. Altered oral mucous membrane:
   a. stomatitis
   b. oral lesions (aphthous ulcers) □ *684*
7. Activity intolerance □ *685*
8. Impaired physical mobility □ *685*
9. Self-care deficit □ *686*
10. Diarrhea □ *686*
11. Sleep pattern disturbance □ *687*
12. Potential for infection □ *687*
13. Potential for trauma □ *688*
14. Potential complications:
   a. renal calculi
   b. impaired renal function
   c. ocular manifestations: uveitis, iritis, episcleritis
   d. impaired liver function
   e. bleeding
   f. perirectal, rectovaginal, enterovesical, and intra-abdominal abscesses, fissures, and fistulas
   g. toxic megacolon

UNIT
XII

□ ▬▬▬▬▬▬▬▬▬▬▬▬▬▬▬▬▬▬▬▬▬▬

1. NURSING DIAGNOSIS

Anxiety related to unfamiliar environment; discomfort; persistent diarrhea; lack of understanding of diagnosis, diagnostic tests, and treatments; uncertain prognosis; and possibility of surgery.

□ ▬▬▬▬▬▬▬▬▬▬▬▬▬▬▬▬▬▬▬▬▬▬

DESIRED OUTCOMES	NURSING ACTIONS AND *SELECTED RATIONALES*

1. The client will experience a reduction in fear and anxiety (see Care Plan on Immobility, Nursing Diagnosis 1, for outcome criteria).	1.a. Refer to Care Plan on Immobility, Nursing Diagnosis 1, for measures related to assessment and reduction of fear and anxiety.
	b. Implement additional measures *to reduce fear and anxiety:*
	   1. explain all diagnostic tests (e.g. blood studies, barium enema, proctosigmoidoscopy, stool analysis, rectal biopsy, colonoscopy, upper gastrointestinal series with small bowel follow through)
	   2. perform actions to reduce discomfort (see Nursing Diagnoses 4.A, action 5 and 4.B, action 2)
	   3. perform actions to control diarrhea (see Nursing Diagnosis 10, action d)
	   4. perform actions to assist the client to cope with the diagnosis and its implications (see Nursing Diagnosis 16, action c)
	   5. begin preoperative teaching if surgical intervention is planned.

□ ▬▬▬▬▬▬▬▬▬▬▬▬▬▬▬▬▬▬▬▬▬▬

2. NURSING/COLLABORATIVE DIAGNOSIS

Altered fluid and electrolyte balance:

a. **fluid volume deficit, hypokalemia, hyponatremia, hypochloremia, hypomagnesemia, and hypocalcemia** related to:
   1. prolonged inadequate oral intake associated with pain, nausea, fatigue, fear of precipitating an attack, and prescribed dietary restrictions
   2. impaired absorption of fluid and electrolytes associated with inflammation and ulceration of the small intestine (particularly in Crohn's disease)
   3. impaired absorption of calcium and magnesium (particularly in Crohn's disease) associated with decreased absorption of vitamin D and fat from the inflamed small intestine (excess fats then bind calcium and magnesium and are excreted in the stool)
   4. excessive loss of fluid and electrolytes associated with vomiting and persistent diarrhea;

    b. **metabolic acidosis** related to hyponatremia and excessive loss of bicarbonate associated with persistent diarrhea.

DESIRED OUTCOMES	NURSING ACTIONS AND *SELECTED RATIONALES*

2. The client will maintain fluid and electrolyte balance as evidenced by:
   a. normal skin turgor
   b. moist mucous membranes
   c. stable weight
   d. B/P and pulse within normal range for client and stable with position change
   e. balanced intake and output
   f. urine specific gravity between 1.010–1.030
   g. usual sensory and motor function
   h. no evidence of dizziness, confusion, irritability, lethargy, headache, excessive thirst, ileus, cardiac arrhythmias
   i. negative Chvostek's and Trousseau's signs
   j. normal serum osmolality, electrolytes, and blood gases.

2.a. Assess for and report signs and symptoms of:
  1. fluid volume deficit:
    a. decreased skin turgor, dry mucous membranes, thirst
    b. weight loss greater than 0.5 kg/day
    c. low B/P and/or decline in systolic B/P of at least 15 mm Hg with concurrent rise in pulse when client sits up
    d. weak, rapid pulse
    e. output less than intake with urine specific gravity higher than 1.030 (reflects an actual rather than potential fluid volume deficit)
  2. hypokalemia (e.g. irregular pulse, muscle weakness and cramping, paresthesias, nausea and vomiting, hypoactive or absent bowel sounds, drowsiness)
  3. hyponatremia (e.g. nausea and vomiting, abdominal cramps, weakness, twitching, lethargy, confusion, seizures)
  4. hypochloremia (e.g. twitching, tetany, depressed respirations)
  5. hypomagnesemia (e.g. change in mental status, muscle cramps, numbness and tingling in extremities, tremors, positive Chvostek's and Trousseau's signs, tachycardia)
  6. hypocalcemia (e.g. change in mental status; cardiac arrhythmias; numbness and tingling of fingers, toes, and circumoral area; positive Chvostek's and Trousseau's signs; muscle cramps; tetany; seizures)
  7. metabolic acidosis (e.g. drowsiness; disorientation; stupor; rapid, deep respirations; headache; nausea and vomiting).
  b. Monitor serum osmolality, electrolyte, and blood gas results. Report abnormal values.
  c. Implement measures *to prevent and treat fluid and electrolyte imbalances:*
    1. perform actions to control diarrhea (see Nursing Diagnosis 10, action d)
    2. perform actions to reduce nausea and vomiting (see Nursing Diagnosis 4.B, action 2)
    3. perform actions to improve oral intake (see Nursing Diagnosis 3, action c.4)
    4. maintain a fluid intake of at least 2500 cc/day unless contraindicated
    5. monitor for therapeutic and nontherapeutic effects of intravenous fluid and electrolyte therapy if administered
    6. when oral intake is allowed:
      a. assist client to select foods/fluids within the prescribed dietary regimen that would replenish electrolytes (be aware that most foods/fluids high in potassium and sodium are contraindicated on a low-residue diet):
        1. foods/fluids high in potassium (e.g. bananas, apricots, potatoes, Gatorade)
        2. foods/fluids high in sodium (e.g. processed cheese, soups, canned vegetables, bouillon)
        3. foods/fluids high in calcium (e.g. dairy products)
        4. foods/fluids high in magnesium (e.g. legumes, seafood)
      b. encourage a low-fat diet *to reduce binding and subsequent loss of calcium and magnesium*
    7. monitor for therapeutic and nontherapeutic effects of the following medications if administered *to treat specific electrolyte deficiencies:*
      a. electrolyte replacements (e.g. potassium chloride, potassium gluconate, magnesium sulfate, calcium gluconate, sodium chloride, sodium bicarbonate)
      b. vitamin D preparations *to increase intestinal absorption of calcium.*
  d. If signs and symptoms of hypomagnesemia, hyponatremia, or hypocalcemia occur, institute seizure precautions.
  e. Consult physician if signs and symptoms of fluid and electrolyte imbalances persist or worsen.

UNIT
XII

3. NURSING DIAGNOSIS

Altered nutrition: less than body requirements related to:

a. decreased oral intake associated with pain, nausea, fatigue, taste alterations resulting from zinc deficiency, prescribed dietary restrictions, and the knowledge that eating often precipitates cramping and diarrhea;

b. decreased absorption of nutrients associated with persistent diarrhea and impaired absorptive function of the bowel due to inflammation and ulceration;

c. loss of nutrients associated with vomiting;

d. decreased intake of folic acid and other vitamins resulting from treatment with a low-residue diet (this type of diet is low in vitamins and folic acid);

e. impaired folic acid absorption resulting from treatment with sulfasalazine;

f. catabolic effects of long-term treatment with corticosteroids.

DESIRED OUTCOMES	NURSING ACTIONS AND *SELECTED RATIONALES*

3. The client will have an improved nutritional status as evidenced by:
a. weight approaching a normal range for client's age, height, and build
b. improved BUN and serum albumin, protein, Hct., Hgb., folate, cholesterol, lymphocyte, and ferritin levels
c. increased triceps skinfold measurements
d. increased strength and activity tolerance
e. healthy oral mucous membrane.
	3.a. Assess the client for signs and symptoms of malnutrition:
	  1. weight below normal for client's age, height, and build
	  2. abnormal BUN and low serum albumin, protein, Hct., Hgb., folate, cholesterol, lymphocyte, and ferritin levels
	  3. triceps skinfold measurement less than normal for build
	  4. weakness and fatigue
	  5. stomatitis.
	b. When oral intake is allowed:
	  1. monitor percentage of meals eaten
	  2. assess the client to determine causes of inadequate intake (e.g. nausea, fear of precipitating an attack, pain, dietary restrictions).
	c. Implement measures *to improve nutritional status:*
	  1. monitor for therapeutic and nontherapeutic effects of total parenteral nutrition if administered
	  2. administer tube feedings of elemental formulas as ordered (these formulas are low in fat and residue, are high in calories and nitrogen content, and are absorbed in the jejunum)
	  3. perform actions to reduce inflammation and hyperactivity of the bowel (see Nursing Diagnosis 10, action d) *in order to reduce episodes of diarrhea and increase absorption of nutrients*
	  4. perform actions *to improve oral intake when allowed:*
	    a. implement measures to reduce pain (see Nursing Diagnosis 4.A, action 5)
	    b. implement measures to reduce nausea and vomiting (see Nursing Diagnosis 4.B, action 2)
	    c. encourage a rest period before meals *to minimize fatigue*
	    d. provide oral care before meals
	    e. provide a quiet, relaxed atmosphere for meals
	    f. implement measures *to improve palatability of elemental formulas* (e.g. offer a variety of flavors, serve chilled)
	    g. serve small portions of nutritious foods/fluids that are appealing to client
	    h. obtain a dietary consult if necessary to assist the client in selecting foods/fluids that meet nutritional needs as well as preferences
	  5. assist client in and provide instructions regarding ways *to meet nutritional needs:*
	    a. avoid skipping meals
	    b. consume a diet high in calories, protein, vitamins, and minerals
	    c. increase intake of foods high in iron within prescribed dietary regimen (e.g. organ meats, apricots, cooked green leafy vegetables, enriched breads)
	    d. increase intake of foods high in folic acid (e.g. cooked green leafy vegetables, asparagus, organ meats, lima beans)

      e. increase intake of foods/fluids high in vitamin B$_{12}$ (e.g. organ meats, whole milk, eggs, fresh shrimp, pork, chicken)

      f. drink supplemental elemental formulas as ordered

  6. monitor for therapeutic and nontherapeutic effects of the following medications if administered:

      a. iron preparations (oral iron preparations may not be effective during an acute attack *because they may be poorly absorbed from the inflamed bowel)*

      b. ascorbic acid *to improve iron absorption and promote healing of ulcerations in the bowel*

      c. elemental zinc *to replenish deficient levels and improve appetite (zinc enhances sense of taste and smell)*

      d. vitamin preparations (e.g. fat-soluble vitamins, cyanocobalamin, folic acid)

      e. medium-chain triglycerides (MCT) in an oil medium *to provide an absorbable source of fatty acids*

      f. lactase enzyme supplements (e.g. LactAid, Lactrase) *to aid lactose digestion and enable client to tolerate an increased intake of calcium-rich dairy products.*

  d. Perform a 72-hour calorie count if nutritional status declines or fails to improve.

  e. Reassess nutritional status on a regular basis and report decline.

4.A. NURSING DIAGNOSIS

Altered comfort:*

1. **abdominal cramping and pain** related to inflammation and ulceration of the intestinal wall;
2. **joint pain** related to extraintestinal involvement of the musculoskeletal system (arthritis of large joints and ankylosing spondylitis are the most common);
3. **anorectal pain** related to irritation and breakdown associated with persistent diarrhea and anorectal fissures;
4. **oral pain** related to oral lesions (aphthous ulcers sometimes occur as extraintestinal manifestations of the disease process) and stomatitis;
5. **skin tenderness and pain** related to presence of skin lesions (e.g. erythema nodosum, pyoderma gangrenosum).

---

* In this care plan, the nursing diagnosis "pain" is included under the diagnostic label of altered comfort.

DESIRED OUTCOMES	NURSING ACTIONS AND *SELECTED RATIONALES*

4.A. The client will experience diminished pain as evidenced by:
1. verbalization of pain relief
2. relaxed facial expression and body positioning
3. increased participation in activities
4. stable vital signs.
	4.A.1. Determine how the client usually responds to pain.
	  2. Assess for nonverbal signs of pain (e.g. wrinkled brow, clenched fists, reluctance to move, rubbing joints, restlessness, diaphoresis, facial pallor or flushing, change in B/P, tachycardia).
	  3. Assess verbal complaints of pain. Ask client to be specific about location, severity, and type of pain.
	  4. Assess for factors that seem to aggravate and alleviate pain.
	  5. Implement measures *to reduce pain:*
	    a. perform actions to reduce inflammation and hyperactivity of the bowel (see Nursing Diagnosis 10, action d) *in order to reduce abdominal cramping and pain*
	    b. perform actions *to reduce joint pain:*
	      1. maintain activity restrictions as ordered
	      2. implement measures *to protect affected joint from trauma, pressure, or excessive movement:*

       a. avoid jarring the bed

       b. use a bed cradle or footboard *to relieve pressure of bedding*

       c. instruct or assist client to support affected extremity with hands or pillows when changing positions

       d. instruct client to move affected extremity slowly and cautiously

       e. apply a splint to the affected joint if indicated

    3. consult physician regarding application of heat to affected joint

    4. monitor for therapeutic and nontherapeutic effects of anti-inflammatory medications if administered

  c. perform actions *to relieve anorectal pain:*

    1. implement measures to control diarrhea (see Nursing Diagnosis 10, action d)

    2. wash and dry anal area thoroughly after each bowel movement

    3. provide a foam pad for client to sit on

    4. consult physician about order for sitz baths

    5. apply protective ointment (e.g. Sween cream, A & D ointment, Desitin, Vaseline) to anal area after each bowel movement

    6. monitor for therapeutic and nontherapeutic effects of the following medications if administered or applied to anorectal area:

       a. corticosteroid foam, suppository, or enema

       b. anesthetic ointment or cream (e.g. Nupercainal, Tronolane)

  d. perform actions *to relieve oral pain:*

    1. implement measures to prevent and reduce the severity of stomatitis and promote healing of oral lesions (see Nursing Diagnosis 6, action c)

    2. monitor for therapeutic and nontherapeutic effects of topical anesthetics, oral protective pastes, and topical analgesics if administered

  e. perform actions *to relieve tenderness and pain associated with skin lesions:*

    1. use a bed cradle over affected areas (lesions usually develop on arms and lower legs) *to relieve pressure from bedding*

    2. apply wet compresses (e.g. Burow's or potassium permanganate solution) to lesions as ordered

    3. monitor for therapeutic and nontherapeutic effects of medications that may be used to treat pyoderma gangrenosum (e.g. clofazimine, dapsone, sulfasalazine) or erythema nodosum (e.g. potassium iodide)

  f. provide or assist with nonpharmacological measures for pain relief (e.g. position change, relaxation techniques, guided imagery, quiet conversation, restful environment, diversional activities)

  g. monitor for therapeutic and nontherapeutic effects of analgesics if administered (narcotic analgesics must be administered judiciously *because they slow gastrointestinal motility and can cause a bowel obstruction).*

6. Consult physician if above measures fail to provide adequate pain relief.

□ ▬▬▬▬▬▬▬▬▬▬▬▬▬▬▬▬▬▬▬▬▬▬▬▬▬▬▬▬▬

4.B. NURSING DIAGNOSIS

Altered comfort: nausea and vomiting related to stimulation of the vomiting center associated with:

1. vagal and/or sympathetic stimulation resulting from visceral irritation associated with intestinal inflammation;
2. cortical stimulation due to stress and pain.

□ ▬▬▬▬▬▬▬▬▬▬▬▬▬▬▬▬▬▬▬▬▬▬▬▬▬▬▬▬▬

DESIRED OUTCOMES	NURSING ACTIONS AND *SELECTED RATIONALES*
4.B. The client will experience relief of nausea and	4.B.1. Assess client to determine factors that contribute to nausea and vomiting (e.g. pain, eating, certain positions, particular foods, anxiety).

vomiting as evidenced by:
1. verbalization of relief of nausea
2. absence of vomiting.

2. Implement measures *to reduce nausea and vomiting:*
   a. maintain patency of nasogastric tube (e.g. keep tubing free of kinks, irrigate as ordered, maintain suction as ordered) if present
   b. perform actions to reduce bowel inflammation and hyperactivity (see Nursing Diagnosis 10, action d)
   c. perform actions to reduce fear and anxiety (see Nursing Diagnosis 1)
   d. perform actions to reduce pain (see Nursing Diagnosis 4.A, action 5)
   e. eliminate noxious sights and smells from the environment (*noxious stimuli cause cortical stimulation of the vomiting center*)
   f. encourage client to take deep, slow breaths when nauseated
   g. encourage client to change positions slowly (*movement stimulates chemoreceptor trigger zone*)
   h. provide oral hygiene every 2 hours and after each emesis
   i. when oral intake is allowed:
      1. advance diet as tolerated
      2. provide small, frequent meals rather than 3 large ones
      3. instruct client to ingest foods and fluids slowly
      4. instruct client to eat dry foods (e.g. toast, crackers) and avoid drinking liquids with meals if nauseated
      5. instruct client to avoid foods/fluids that irritate gastric mucosa (e.g. spicy foods; citrus fruits or juices; caffeine-containing items such as chocolate, coffee, tea, and colas)
      6. instruct client to rest after eating with head of bed elevated
   j. monitor for therapeutic and nontherapeutic effects of antiemetics if administered.
3. Consult physician if above measures fail to control nausea and vomiting.

□ ▬▬▬▬▬▬▬▬▬▬▬▬▬▬▬▬▬▬▬▬▬▬

5. NURSING DIAGNOSIS

Impaired skin integrity: irritation or breakdown related to:

a. prolonged pressure on tissues associated with decreased mobility;
b. frequent contact with irritants associated with persistent diarrhea;
c. ulceration of extraintestinal skin lesions;
d. increased fragility of skin associated with malnutrition.

□ ▬▬▬▬▬▬▬▬▬▬▬▬▬▬▬▬▬▬▬▬▬▬

DESIRED OUTCOMES	NURSING ACTIONS AND *SELECTED RATIONALES*

5. The client will maintain skin integrity as evidenced by:
   a. absence of redness and irritation
   b. no skin breakdown.

5.a. Inspect the skin (especially bone prominences, dependent areas, perianal area, and areas where skin lesions have developed) for pallor, redness, and breakdown.
 b. Refer to Care Plan on Immobility, Nursing Diagnosis 7, action b, for measures to prevent skin breakdown associated with decreased mobility.
 c. Implement additional measures *to prevent skin breakdown:*
   1. perform actions *to decrease skin irritation and prevent breakdown resulting from diarrhea:*
      a. implement measures to control diarrhea (see Nursing Diagnosis 10, action d)
      b. provide soft toilet tissue for wiping after bowel movements
      c. instruct and assist client to thoroughly cleanse and dry perineal area after each bowel movement; apply a protective ointment or cream (e.g. Sween cream, Desitin, karaya gel, A & D ointment, Vaseline)
      d. avoid direct contact of skin with Chux (e.g. place turn sheet or bed pad over Chux)
      e. apply a perianal pouch if diarrhea is severe
   2. use a bed cradle over areas where skin lesions are present *to prevent irritation and pressure from bedding*

3. maintain an optimal nutritional status (see Nursing Diagnosis 3, action c).
d. If skin breakdown occurs:
   1. notify physician
   2. continue with above measures to prevent further irritation and breakdown
   3. perform decubitus care as ordered or per standard hospital policy
   4. monitor client closely and report signs and symptoms of infection (e.g. elevated temperature; redness, warmth, and edema around area of breakdown; unusual drainage from site).

☐ ▮▮▮▮▮▮▮▮▮▮▮▮▮▮▮▮▮▮▮▮▮▮▮▮▮▮▮▮▮▮▮▮▮▮▮

6. NURSING DIAGNOSIS

Altered oral mucous membrane:

a. **stomatitis** related to malnutrition and fluid volume deficit;
b. **oral lesions (aphthous ulcers)** related to extraintestinal involvement of the oral cavity.

☐ ▮▮▮▮▮▮▮▮▮▮▮▮▮▮▮▮▮▮▮▮▮▮▮▮▮▮▮▮▮▮▮▮▮▮▮

DESIRED OUTCOMES	NURSING ACTIONS AND *SELECTED RATIONALES*

6. The client will maintain a healthy oral cavity as evidenced by:
   a. absence of inflammation and ulcerations
   b. pink, moist, intact mucosa
   c. absence of oral pain
   d. ability to swallow without discomfort.

6.a. Assess client for and report signs and symptoms of stomatitis and/or oral lesions (e.g. inflamed and/or ulcerated oral mucosa, complaints of oral pain, dysphagia).
   b. Culture suspicious oral lesions as ordered. Report positive results.
   c. Implement measures *to prevent or reduce severity of stomatitis and promote healing of oral lesions:*
      1. reinforce importance of and assist client with oral hygiene after meals and snacks; avoid products such as lemon-glycerin swabs and commercial mouthwashes containing alcohol *(these products have a drying or irritating effect on the oral mucous membrane)*
      2. lubricate client's lips with Vaseline, K-Y jelly, ChapStick, Blistex, or mineral oil when oral care is given
      3. use a soft bristle brush or low-pressure power spray for oral care
      4. have client rinse mouth frequently with warm saline or baking soda and water
      5. encourage client to breathe through nose *in order to reduce mouth dryness*
      6. encourage a fluid intake of at least 2500 cc/day unless contraindicated
      7. maintain an optimal nutritional status (see Nursing Diagnosis 3, action c)
      8. encourage client not to smoke *(smoking irritates and dries the mucosa)*
      9. encourage client to use artificial saliva (e.g. Moi-stir, Salivart) *to lubricate the oral mucous membrane*
      10. assist with selection of soft, nonspicy, and nonacidic foods
      11. instruct client to avoid extremely hot or cold foods/fluids
      12. if oral lesions are present or stomatitis is severe, remove dentures and replace only for meals
      13. consult physician regarding an order for a prophylactic antifungal or antibacterial agent.
   d. Monitor for therapeutic and nontherapeutic effects of topical anesthetics, oral protective pastes, and topical and systemic analgesics if administered.
   e. Consult physician if signs and symptoms of stomatitis and oral lesions persist or worsen.

7. NURSING DIAGNOSIS

Activity intolerance related to:

a. inadequate nutritional status;
b. difficulty resting and sleeping associated with discomfort, frequent need to defecate, fear, and anxiety;
c. tissue hypoxia associated with anemia resulting from impaired absorption of vitamin B_{12}, folic acid, and iron; blood loss; bone marrow depression that occurs in many chronic inflammatory conditions; and hemolysis associated with sulfonamide therapy.

DESIRED OUTCOMES	NURSING ACTIONS AND *SELECTED RATIONALES*
7. The client will demonstrate an increased tolerance for activity (see Care Plan on Immobility, Nursing Diagnosis 8, for outcome criteria).	7.a. Refer to Care Plan on Immobility, Nursing Diagnosis 8, for measures related to assessment and improvement of activity tolerance. b. Implement additional measures *to promote rest and improve activity tolerance:* 1. maintain activity restrictions as ordered 2. perform actions to reduce fear and anxiety (see Nursing Diagnosis 1) 3. perform actions to promote sleep (see Nursing Diagnosis 11) 4. perform actions to reduce discomfort (see Nursing Diagnoses 4.A, action 5 and 4.B, action 2) 5. perform actions to improve nutritional status (see Nursing Diagnosis 3, action c) 6. monitor for therapeutic and nontherapeutic effects of whole blood or packed red cells if administered 7. increase client's activity gradually as allowed and tolerated.

8. NURSING DIAGNOSIS

Impaired physical mobility related to activity intolerance, discomfort, sensory and motor deficits associated with fluid and electrolyte imbalances, fear that movement will precipitate cramping and diarrhea, and activity restrictions imposed by the treatment plan.

DESIRED OUTCOMES	NURSING ACTIONS AND *SELECTED RATIONALES*
8.a. The client will maintain an optimal level of physical mobility within physical limitations and activity restrictions imposed by the treatment plan.	8.a.1. Assess for factors that impair physical mobility (e.g. weakness, fatigue, pain, fear of precipitating an attack, activity restrictions imposed by treatment plan). 2. Implement measures *to increase mobility:* a. perform actions to reduce discomfort (see Nursing Diagnoses 4.A, action 5 and 4.B, action 2) b. perform actions to reduce fear and anxiety (see Nursing Diagnosis 1) c. perform actions to improve strength and activity tolerance (see Nursing Diagnosis 7) d. perform actions to maintain fluid and electrolyte balance (see Nursing Diagnosis 2, action c) *in order to prevent sensory and motor deficits* e. instruct and assist client in use of mobility aids (e.g. cane, walker) if indicated.

UNIT
XII

3. Increase activity and participation in self-care activities as allowed and tolerated.
4. Provide praise and encouragement for all efforts to increase physical mobility.

8.b. The client will not experience problems associated with immobility.

8.b. Refer to Care Plan on Immobility for actions to prevent problems associated with immobility if client is to remain on bedrest for longer than 48 hours.

☐ ▬▬▬▬▬▬▬▬▬▬▬▬▬▬▬▬▬▬▬▬▬▬▬▬

9. NURSING DIAGNOSIS

Self-care deficit related to impaired physical mobility associated with fatigue, sensory and motor deficits, discomfort, fear, and activity restrictions.

☐ ▬▬▬▬▬▬▬▬▬▬▬▬▬▬▬▬▬▬▬▬▬▬▬▬

DESIRED OUTCOMES	NURSING ACTIONS AND *SELECTED RATIONALES*
9. The client will demonstrate increased participation in self-care activities within prescribed activity restrictions and/or physical limitations.	9.a. Refer to Care Plan on Immobility, Nursing Diagnosis 9, for measures related to assessment of, planning for, and meeting the client's self-care needs. b. Implement measures to increase mobility (see Nursing Diagnosis 8, action a.2) *in order to facilitate the client's ability to perform self-care activities.*

☐ ▬▬▬▬▬▬▬▬▬▬▬▬▬▬▬▬▬▬▬▬▬▬▬▬

10. NURSING DIAGNOSIS

Diarrhea related to intestinal hyperactivity and diminished water absorption from the bowel associated with inflammation and irritation of the bowel wall.

☐ ▬▬▬▬▬▬▬▬▬▬▬▬▬▬▬▬▬▬▬▬▬▬▬▬

DESIRED OUTCOMES	NURSING ACTIONS AND *SELECTED RATIONALES*

10. The client will have fewer bowel movements and more formed stool.	10.a. Ascertain client's usual bowel elimination habits.
	b. Assess for signs and symptoms of diarrhea (e.g. frequent, loose stools; abdominal pain and cramping).
	c. Assess bowel sounds regularly. Report an increase in frequency of and/or higher pitch of bowel sounds.
	d. Implement measures *to reduce inflammation and hyperactivity of the bowel in order to control diarrhea:*
	  1. perform actions *to rest the bowel:*
	    a. maintain food and fluid restrictions as ordered (usually NPO during acute stage)
	    b. implement measures to promote physical and emotional rest
	    c. discourage smoking *(nicotine has a stimulant effect on gastrointestinal tract)*
	    d. when oral intake is allowed:
	      1. instruct client to avoid foods/fluids that are poorly digested or act as irritants to the inflamed bowel:
	        a. dairy products *(clients with Crohn's disease may have an intolerance to lactose-rich foods due to a deficiency of lactase)*
	        b. those high in fat (e.g. butter, cream, oils, whole milk, ice cream, pork, fried foods, gravies, nuts)
	        c. those high in fiber or residue (e.g. whole-grain cereals, nuts, raw fruits and vegetables)
	        d. those known to cause diarrhea or be gas-producers (e.g.

cabbage, onions, popcorn, licorice, prunes, chili, baked beans, carbonated beverages)
    e. those high in caffeine (e.g. chocolate, coffee, tea, colas)
    f. spicy foods
    g. extremely hot or cold foods/fluids
  2. instruct client to add new foods one at a time
  3. provide small, frequent meals
2. monitor for therapeutic and nontherapeutic effects of the following medications if administered:
    a. corticosteroids or ACTH *to reduce inflammation*
    b. immunosuppressives (e.g. azathioprine, 6-mercaptopurine) *to reduce inflammation associated with an immune reaction (it has been theorized that both conditions may be autoimmune diseases)*
    c. anticholinergic agents (e.g. propantheline bromide, dicyclomine hydrochloride) and opiate or opiate-like medications (e.g. opium tincture, loperamide, diphenoxalate hydrochloride) *to decrease intestinal spasms and motility* (use of these agents is controversial *because of their tendency to cause toxic megacolon)*
    d. sulfasalazine *(used primarily for its anti-inflammatory action; the sulfapyridine component may provide some antibacterial effect also)*
    e. adsorbent and protectant agents (e.g. kaolin, pectin) *to absorb bacteria and toxins and coat the intestinal mucosa*
    f. cholestyramine and/or aluminum hydroxide *to bind bile salts (diarrhea may occur as a result of irritation of intestines by excessive bile salts)*
    g. bulk-forming agents (e.g. methylcellulose, psyllium hydrophilic mucilloid, calcium polycarbophil) *to absorb water in the bowel and produce a soft, formed stool.*
  e. Consult physician if diarrhea persists.

---

11. NURSING DIAGNOSIS

Sleep pattern disturbance related to frequent need to defecate, discomfort, decreased activity, fear, and anxiety.

DESIRED OUTCOMES	NURSING ACTIONS AND *SELECTED RATIONALES*
11. The client will attain optimal amounts of sleep within the parameters of the treatment regimen (see Care Plan on Immobility, Nursing Diagnosis 12, for outcome criteria).	11.a. Refer to Care Plan on Immobility, Nursing Diagnosis 12, for measures related to assessment and promotion of sleep. b. Implement additional measures *to promote sleep:* 1. perform actions to reduce inflammation and hyperactivity of the bowel (see Nursing Diagnosis 10, action d) *in order to reduce abdominal cramping and pain and the frequency of bowel movements* 2. perform actions to reduce discomfort (see Nursing Diagnoses 4.A, action 5 and 4.B, action 2).

UNIT
XII

---

12. NURSING DIAGNOSIS

Potential for infection related to:

a. ulcerations in bowel wall;
b. lowered natural resistance associated with malnutrition, anemia, alterations in immune system (it is postulated that these clients have impaired cell-mediated immunity and impaired phagocytosis), and long-term treatment with corticosteroids and/or immunosuppressives.

DESIRED OUTCOMES	NURSING ACTIONS AND *SELECTED RATIONALES*

12. The client will remain free of infection as evidenced by:
   a. temperature declining toward normal
   b. absence of chills
   c. pulse within normal limits
   d. normal breath sounds
   e. voiding clear, yellow urine without complaints of frequency, urgency, and burning
   f. no increase in episodes of diarrhea and abdominal cramping and pain
   g. absence of redness, swelling, and unusual drainage in any area where there is a break in skin integrity
   h. intact oral mucous membrane
   i. WBC and differential counts declining toward normal
   j. negative results of cultured specimens.

12.a. Assess for and report signs and symptoms of infection:
   1. significant increase in temperature (a low-grade temperature may be present in some clients due to the inflammation)
   2. chills
   3. pattern of increased pulse or pulse rate greater than 100 beats/minute
   4. adventitious breath sounds
   5. cloudy or foul-smelling urine
   6. complaints of frequency, urgency, or burning when urinating
   7. presence of WBCs, bacteria, and/or nitrites in urine
   8. increase in episodes of diarrhea and abdominal cramping and pain
   9. redness, swelling, or unusual drainage in any area where there is a break in skin integrity
   10. irritation or ulceration of oral mucous membrane
   11. increase in WBC count above previous levels (WBC count will usually be elevated as a result of inflammation) and/or significant change in differential.

   b. Obtain culture specimens (e.g. urine, vaginal, stool, mouth, sputum, blood) as ordered. Report positive results.

   c. Implement measures *to reduce risk of infection:*
   1. maintain a fluid intake of at least 2500 cc/day unless contraindicated
   2. use good handwashing technique and encourage client to do the same
   3. maintain meticulous aseptic technique during all invasive procedures (e.g. catheterizations, venous and arterial punctures, injections)
   4. protect client from others with infection and instruct client to continue this after discharge
   5. maintain an optimal nutritional status (see Nursing Diagnosis 3, action c)
   6. reinforce importance of good oral care
   7. provide proper balance of exercise and rest within current activity restrictions
   8. perform actions to prevent or reduce the severity of stomatitis and promote healing of oral lesions (see Nursing Diagnosis 6, action c)
   9. perform actions to maintain skin integrity (see Nursing Diagnosis 5, actions b and c)
   10. perform actions *to prevent respiratory tract infection:*
      a. instruct and assist client to turn, cough, and deep breathe at least every 2 hours if mobility is limited
      b. instruct and assist client in use of inspiratory exerciser at least every 2 hours if indicated
      c. encourage client to stop smoking
      d. increase activity as allowed and tolerated
   11. perform actions *to prevent urinary tract infection:*
      a. instruct and assist female client to wipe from front to back following urination and defecation
      b. keep perianal area clean
   12. perform actions to reduce inflammation and hyperactivity of the bowel (see Nursing Diagnosis 10, action d) *in order to prevent further ulceration and reduce the risk of intestinal infection.*

   d. Monitor for therapeutic and nontherapeutic effects of anti-infectives if administered.

☐ ▪▪▪▪▪▪▪▪▪▪▪▪▪▪▪▪▪▪▪▪▪▪▪▪▪▪▪▪▪▪

13. NURSING DIAGNOSIS

Potential for trauma related to falls associated with:

a. weakness resulting from anemia, malnutrition, fluid and electrolyte imbalances, and prolonged inactivity;
b. dizziness resulting from orthostatic hypotension due to fluid volume deficit.

☐ ▪▪▪▪▪▪▪▪▪▪▪▪▪▪▪▪▪▪▪▪▪▪▪▪▪▪▪▪▪▪

DESIRED OUTCOMES	NURSING ACTIONS AND *SELECTED RATIONALES*

13. The client will not experience falls.

13.a. Determine whether conditions predisposing client to falls (e.g. weakness, fatigue, orthostatic hypotension) exist.
  b. Implement measures *to prevent falls:*
    1. keep bed in low position with side rails up when client is in bed
    2. keep needed items within easy reach
    3. encourage client to request assistance whenever needed; have call signal within easy reach
    4. instruct and assist client to change positions slowly *in order to reduce dizziness associated with orthostatic drop in B/P*
    5. use lap belt when client is in chair if indicated
    6. instruct client to wear shoes with nonskid soles and low heels when ambulating
    7. avoid unnecessary clutter in room
    8. accompany client during ambulation utilizing a transfer safety belt if indicated
    9. provide ambulatory aids (e.g. walker, cane) if client is weak or unsteady on feet
    10. instruct client to ambulate in well-lit areas and to utilize handrails if needed
    11. do not rush client; allow adequate time for trips to the bathroom and ambulation in hallway
    12. leave commode or bedpan next to the bed *in case assistance is not readily available and he/she has an urgent need to defecate*
    13. perform actions to increase strength and activity tolerance (see Nursing Diagnosis 7)
    14. perform actions to maintain fluid and electrolyte balance (see Nursing Diagnosis 2, action c).
  c. Include client and significant others in planning and implementing measures to prevent falls.
  d. If falls occur, initiate appropriate first aid measures and notify physician.

□ ▬▬▬▬▬▬▬▬▬▬▬▬▬▬▬▬▬▬▬▬▬▬▬▬▬▬

14. COLLABORATIVE DIAGNOSIS

Potential complications:

a. **renal calculi** related to:
  1. increased serum oxalate (dietary oxalate normally binds with calcium in the intestine and is excreted in the stool; in these clients, calcium is bound with the poorly absorbed fat and oxalate becomes available for absorption)
  2. fluid volume deficit
  3. treatment with sulfasalazine (this medication may crystallize and precipitate in acidic urine)
  4. urinary stasis associated with decreased mobility;
b. **impaired renal function** related to development of calculi, obstructive hydronephrosis (may result from entrapment of a ureter by an abscess or intestinal and lymphatic inflammation), amyloidosis, and diminished renal blood flow resulting from fluid volume deficit;
c. **ocular manifestations: uveitis, iritis, episcleritis** (occur with extraintestinal involvement);
d. **impaired liver function** related to extraintestinal involvement of the liver associated with processes such as fatty infiltration, cholangitis, or hepatitis;
e. **bleeding** related to:
  1. decreased production of prothrombin associated with liver involvement and vitamin K deficiency (results from decreased oral intake and malabsorption)
  2. erosion of intestinal blood vessels;
f. **perirectal, rectovaginal, enterovesical, and intra-abdominal abscesses, fissures, and fistulas** related to inflammation, ulceration, and the presence of increased intraluminal pressure;

UNIT XII

g. **toxic megacolon** related to loss of colonic muscle tone associated with widespread inflammation, use of opiates and anticholinergics, and hypokalemia;

h. **bowel obstruction** related to inflammation and fibrosis;

i. **peritonitis** related to colonic perforation or leakage from an abscess or fistula;

j. **thromboembolism** related to:
   1. hypercoagulability associated with increased levels of certain clotting factors, thrombocytosis (a frequent manifestation of acute inflammation), and increased blood viscosity (may result from fluid volume deficit)
   2. venous stasis associated with decreased mobility and pelvic inflammation;

k. **shock** related to septicemia (septic shock) and hemorrhage (hypovolemic shock).

DESIRED OUTCOMES	NURSING ACTIONS AND *SELECTED RATIONALES*

14.a. The client will not develop renal calculi as evidenced by:
1. absence of flank pain, hematuria, urinary frequency and urgency, nausea, vomiting
2. clear urine without calculi.

14.a.1. Assess for and report signs and symptoms of renal calculi (e.g. dull, aching or severe, colicky flank pain; hematuria; urinary frequency or urgency; nausea; vomiting).

2. Obtain a urine specimen for analysis if ordered. Report hyperoxaluria and/or crystalluria.

3. Implement measures *to prevent renal calculi:*
   a. perform actions *to prevent urinary stasis:*
      1. encourage a minimum fluid intake of 2500 cc/day unless contraindicated
      2. assist client to change positions at least every 2 hours
      3. progress activity as allowed and tolerated
      4. implement measures *to facilitate voiding* (e.g. provide privacy, allow client to assume normal voiding position unless contraindicated, run warm water over perineum)
      5. instruct client to void whenever the urge is felt
      6. maintain patency of urinary catheter if present
   b. if client is taking sulfasalazine:
      1. monitor pH of urine every day and report levels below 6 (*sulfasalazine tends to precipitate in acidic urine*)
      2. administer medications that alkalinize the urine (e.g. sodium bicarbonate, citrate preparations) as ordered
   c. perform actions *to decrease absorption of oxalate from the intestine:*
      1. encourage client to decrease intake of foods/fluids high in oxalate (e.g. instant coffee, tea, chocolate, colas, spinach, rhubarb)
      2. encourage client to adhere to a low-fat diet (*this reduces the amount of fat available to bind calcium, thereby freeing calcium to bind with oxalate*)
      3. monitor for therapeutic and nontherapeutic effects of cholestyramine if administered *to bind oxalate and increase its excretion from the bowel*
   d. perform actions to prevent and treat fluid volume deficit (see Nursing Diagnosis 2, actions c.1–5).

4. If signs and symptoms of renal calculi occur:
   a. strain all urine carefully and save any calculi for analysis; report finding to physician
   b. encourage a minimum fluid intake of 2500 cc/day unless contraindicated
   c. administer analgesics as ordered
   d. refer to Care Plan on Renal Calculi for additional care measures.

14.b. The client will maintain adequate renal function as evidenced by:
1. urine output at least 30 cc/hour
2. urine specific gravity between 1.010–1.030
3. BUN and serum

14.b.1. Assess for and report signs and symptoms of impaired renal function (e.g. urine output less than 30 cc/hour, urine specific gravity fixed at or less than 1.010, elevated BUN and serum creatinine levels).

2. Collect a 24-hour urine specimen if ordered. Report decreased creatinine clearance.

3. Implement measures *to maintain adequate renal function:*
   a. perform actions to prevent renal calculi (see action a.3 in this diagnosis)

creatinine levels within normal range.

    b. perform actions to reduce inflammation and hyperactivity of the bowel (see Nursing Diagnosis 10, action d) *in order to decrease bowel and lymphatic inflammation (control of the inflammatory response will reduce incidence of obstructive hydronephrosis)*

    c. perform actions to prevent a fluid volume deficit (see Nursing Diagnosis 2, actions c.1–5).

4. If signs and symptoms of impaired renal function occur:
    a. continue with above actions
    b. administer diuretics as ordered
    c. assess for and report signs of acute renal failure (e.g. oliguria or anuria; weight gain; edema; elevated B/P; lethargy and confusion; increasing BUN and serum creatinine, phosphorus, and potassium levels)
    d. prepare client for surgery to unsheath the involved ureter if indicated
    e. prepare client for dialysis if indicated
    f. refer to Care Plan on Renal Failure for additional care measures.

14.c. The client will experience remission of ocular manifestations if they occur as evidenced by:
1. statements of diminished eye pain and photophobia
2. improved vision.

14.c.1. Assess for signs and symptoms of ocular lesions (e.g. eye pain, photophobia, loss of vision).

2. Implement measures to reduce inflammation and hyperactivity of the bowel (see Nursing Diagnosis 10, action d) *because remission of ocular manifestations is often simultaneous with control of inflammation of the bowel.*

3. If vision is impaired:
    a. perform actions to prevent falls (see Nursing Diagnosis 13, action b)
    b. orient client to surroundings, room, and arrangement of furniture
    c. avoid startling client (e.g. speak client's name and identify yourself when entering room and before any physical contact, describe activities and reasons for various noises in room)
    d. assist client with personal hygiene he/she is unable to perform independently
    e. identify where items are placed on his/her plate or tray, cut food, open packages, or feed if necessary
    f. assist with activities that require reading (e.g. menu selection, mail, legal documents).

4. Avoid use of bright lights if client has photophobia.

5. Consult physician if eye pain, photophobia, or visual disturbances worsen.

14.d. The client will maintain adequate liver function as evidenced by:
1. no unusual bleeding
2. stable mental status
3. absence of jaundice, asterixis, fetor hepaticus
4. serum bilirubin, GGT, ALT (SGPT), alkaline phosphatase (ALP), ammonia, albumin, and prothrombin levels within client's usual range.

14.d.1. Assess for and report signs and symptoms of impaired liver function:
    a. unusual bleeding
    b. jaundice
    c. elevated serum bilirubin, GGT, ALT (SGPT), alkaline phosphatase (ALP), and ammonia levels
    d. decreasing serum albumin
    e. increasing prothrombin time.

2. Implement measures to reduce inflammation and hyperactivity of the bowel (see Nursing Diagnosis 10, action d) *because control of extraintestinal manifestations is often simultaneous with control of inflammation of the bowel.*

3. If signs and symptoms of impaired liver function occur:
    a. institute bleeding precautions (see action e.4 in this diagnosis)
    b. consult physician before administering known or potential hepatotoxins (e.g. isoniazid, methyldopa, acetaminophen)
    c. assess for and report signs and symptoms of hypokalemia (see Nursing Diagnosis 2, action a.2, for a list of signs and symptoms); *hypokalemia may precipitate hepatic coma*
    d. assess for and report signs and symptoms of hepatic encephalopathy (e.g. decline in mental status and motor skills, slurred speech, asterixis, fetor hepaticus)
    e. refer to Care Plan on Cirrhosis for additional care measures.

14.e. The client will not experience unusual bleeding as evidenced by:
1. skin and mucous membranes free of

14.e.1. Assess client for and report signs and symptoms of unusual bleeding:
    a. petechiae
    b. multiple ecchymotic areas
    c. bleeding gums
    d. frequent or uncontrollable episodes of epistaxis

UNIT
XII

bleeding, petechiae, and ecchymosis
2. absence of unusual joint pain and swelling
3. no increase in abdominal girth
4. absence of frank or occult blood in stool, urine, and vomitus
5. usual menstrual flow
6. vital signs within normal range for client
7. stable or improved Hct. and Hgb.
8. usual mental status.

    e. unusual oozing from injection sites
    f. unusual joint pain or swelling
    g. increase in abdominal girth
    h. hematemesis, melena, red or smoke-colored urine
    i. hypermenorrhea
    j. significant drop in B/P accompanied by an increased pulse rate
    k. decline in Hct. and Hgb. levels
    l. restlessness, confusion.
2. Monitor prothrombin times (PT). Report values greater than 2½ times the control.
3. If prothrombin times are abnormal or Hct. and Hgb. levels decline, test all stools, urine, and vomitus for occult blood. Report positive results.
4. Implement measures *to prevent bleeding:*
    a. use the smallest gauge needle possible when giving injections and performing venous or arterial punctures
    b. apply gentle, prolonged pressure following injections and venous or arterial punctures
    c. take B/P only when necessary and avoid overinflating the cuff
    d. caution client to avoid activities that increase potential for trauma (e.g. shaving with a straight-edge razor, cutting nails, using stiff bristle toothbrush or dental floss)
    e. pad side rails if client is confused or restless
    f. perform actions to prevent falls (see Nursing Diagnosis 13, action b)
    g. instruct client to avoid blowing nose forcefully or straining to have a bowel movement; consult physician about order for decongestants, stool softeners, and/or laxatives if indicated
    h. instruct client to increase intake of foods high in vitamin K (e.g. cooked green leafy vegetables, liver, tomatoes)
    i. monitor for therapeutic and nontherapeutic effects of the following if administered *to improve clotting ability:*
        1. vitamin K injections
        2. fresh frozen plasma or whole blood *to replace clotting factors.*
5. If bleeding occurs and does not subside spontaneously:
    a. apply firm, prolonged pressure to bleeding area if possible
    b. if epistaxis occurs, place client in a high Fowler's position and apply pressure and ice packs to nasal area
    c. maintain oxygen therapy as ordered
    d. perform iced water or saline lavage as ordered *to control gastric bleeding*
    e. administer fresh frozen plasma, whole blood, and/or vitamin K (e.g. phytonadione) injections as ordered
    f. prepare client for surgical repair of bleeding vessels if planned
    g. provide emotional support to client and significant others.

14.f. The client will have resolution of any abscesses, fissures, and fistulas that develop as evidenced by:
1. temperature declining toward normal
2. resolution of rectal pain and abdominal pain and cramping
3. clear, yellow urine
4. WBC count declining toward normal.

14.f.1. Assess for and report signs and symptoms of abscess and/or fistula formation (e.g. further increase in temperature, increased abdominal cramping, increased and more constant abdominal or rectal pain, fecaluria, further increase in WBC count).
2. Observe for perianal fissures.
3. Implement measures to reduce inflammation and hyperactivity of the bowel (see Nursing Diagnosis 10, action d) *in order to decrease risk of development of abscesses, fissures, and fistulas and promote healing of any that exist.*
4. If signs and symptoms of fissures, abscesses, or fistulas occur:
    a. monitor for therapeutic and nontherapeutic effects of anti-infectives if administered
    b. perform wound care as ordered
    c. prepare client for surgical intervention (e.g. incision and drainage, fistulectomy, colectomy, ileostomy) if indicated
    d. provide emotional support to client and significant others.

14.g. The client will not develop toxic megacolon as evidenced by:
1. gradual resolution of

14.g.1. Assess for and report signs and symptoms of toxic megacolon:
    a. severe abdominal pain, tenderness, and distention
    b. hypoactive or absent bowel sounds with tympanic percussion note
    c. sudden decrease in episodes of diarrhea

abdominal discomfort
2. absence of abdominal distention
3. active bowel sounds
4. gradual resolution of diarrhea
5. temperature and WBC count declining toward normal.

d. high fever (usually 40–40.5°C)
e. increase in WBC count.
2. Monitor abdominal x-ray results. Report findings of colonic dilation.
3. Implement measures *to prevent development of toxic megacolon:*
   a. perform actions to reduce inflammation and hyperactivity of the bowel (see Nursing Diagnosis 10, action d)
   b. administer narcotics, opiates or opiate-like medications, and anticholinergics judiciously *(all decrease intestinal motility)*
   c. perform actions to prevent and treat hypokalemia (see Nursing Diagnosis 2, action c).
4. If signs and symptoms of toxic megacolon occur:
   a. continue with above actions
   b. insert nasogastric tube and maintain suction as ordered
   c. monitor for therapeutic and nontherapeutic effects of the following if administered:
      1. intravenous fluid and electrolyte therapy *to maintain adequate vascular volume (third-space fluid shifting occurs as a result of increased capillary permeability associated with increased intraluminal pressure)*
      2. high-dose parenteral corticosteroids *to reduce intestinal inflammation*
      3. anti-infectives *to prevent infection (the risk of perforation is increased when toxic megacolon develops)*
   d. prepare client for surgical intervention (e.g. proctocolectomy with ileostomy, colectomy with ileorectal anastomosis) if indicated
   e. provide emotional support to client and significant others.

14.h. The client will not develop a bowel obstruction as evidenced by:
1. absence of vomiting and abdominal distention
2. gradual return of normal bowel sounds.

14.h.1. Assess for and report signs and symptoms of a bowel obstruction:
   a. vomiting (vomitus initially contains gastric juices and bile and, eventually, fecal material)
   b. abdominal distention
   c. change in bowel sounds (in mechanical obstruction, bowel sounds are initially high-pitched and hyperactive; in paralytic ileus, bowel sounds are absent).
2. Monitor abdominal x-ray results. Report findings of partial or complete bowel obstruction.
3. Implement measures to reduce inflammation and hyperactivity of the bowel (see Nursing Diagnosis 10, action d) *in order to reduce risk of obstruction.*
4. If signs and symptoms of a bowel obstruction occur:
   a. withhold all food and fluid
   b. insert a nasogastric tube and maintain suction as ordered
   c. monitor for therapeutic and nontherapeutic effects of intravenous fluid and electrolytes if administered *to maintain an adequate vascular volume (relative hypovolemia occurs due to third-spacing associated with the increased capillary permeability that results from increased intraluminal pressure in a bowel obstruction)*
   d. prepare client for surgical intervention (e.g. colectomy, colostomy, ileostomy) if indicated
   e. provide emotional support to client and significant others.

14.i. The client will not develop peritonitis as evidenced by:
1. temperature declining toward normal
2. soft, nondistended abdomen
3. gradual resolution of abdominal pain
4. gradual return of normal bowel sounds
5. stable vital signs
6. WBC count declining toward normal.

14.i.1. Assess for and report signs and symptoms of peritonitis (e.g. further increase in temperature; tense, rigid abdomen; severe abdominal pain; rebound tenderness; diminished or absent bowel sounds; tachycardia; tachypnea; hypotension).
2. Monitor WBC counts. Report levels that increase or fail to decline toward normal.
3. Implement measures to prevent and treat abscesses, fistulas, toxic megacolon, and/or bowel obstruction (see actions f.3 and 4, g.3 and 4, and h.3 and 4 in this diagnosis) *in order to prevent peritonitis.*
4. If signs and symptoms of peritonitis occur:
   a. withhold all food and fluid as ordered
   b. place client on bedrest in a semi-Fowler's position *to assist in pooling or localizing gastrointestinal contents in the pelvis rather than under the diaphragm*

UNIT
XII

c. insert nasogastric tube and maintain suction as ordered
d. monitor for therapeutic and nontherapeutic effects of anti-infectives if administered
e. monitor for therapeutic and nontherapeutic effects of intravenous fluids and/or blood volume expanders if administered *to prevent or treat shock (shock can occur as a result of the escape of protein, fluid, and electrolytes into the peritoneal cavity)*
f. prepare client for surgical intervention (e.g. fistulectomy, incision and drainage, colectomy) if indicated
g. provide emotional support to client and significant others.

14.j. The client will not develop a venous thrombus and pulmonary embolism (see Care Plan on Immobility, Collaborative Diagnosis 14, outcomes a.1 and 2, for outcome criteria).

14.j. Refer to Care Plan on Immobility, Collaborative Diagnosis 14, actions a.1 and 2, for measures related to assessment, prevention, and treatment of a venous thrombus and pulmonary embolism.

14.k. The client will not develop shock as evidenced by:
1. usual mental status
2. stable vital signs
3. skin warm and usual color
4. palpable peripheral pulses
5. capillary refill time less than 3 seconds
6. urine output at least 30 cc/hour.

14.k.1. Assess for and report signs and symptoms of:
a. bleeding (see action e.1 in this diagnosis)
b. early or hyperdynamic stage of septic shock (e.g. confusion; chills and fever; warm, flushed skin; tachycardia; tachypnea; lower extremity mottling)
c. shock:
1. restlessness, agitation, confusion
2. significant decrease in B/P
3. decline in B/P of at least 15 mm Hg with concurrent rise in pulse when client changes from lying to sitting or standing position
4. resting pulse rate greater than 100 beats/minute
5. rapid or labored respirations
6. cool, pale, or cyanotic skin
7. diminished or absent peripheral pulses
8. capillary refill time greater than 3 seconds
9. urine output less than 30 cc/hour.
2. Implement measures *to prevent septicemia:*
a. perform actions to prevent and treat infection (see Nursing Diagnosis 12, actions c and d)
b. perform actions to prevent and treat abscesses, fistulas, and peritonitis (see actions f.3 and 4 and i.3 and 4 in this diagnosis).
3. Implement measures *to prevent hemorrhage:*
a. perform actions to prevent and control bleeding (see actions e.4 and 5 in this diagnosis)
b. perform actions to reduce inflammation and hyperactivity of the bowel (see Nursing Diagnosis 10, action d) *in order to prevent ulceration.*
4. If signs and symptoms of shock occur:
a. continue with above measures to treat infection and control bleeding
b. place client flat in bed with legs elevated unless contraindicated
c. monitor vital signs frequently
d. administer oxygen as ordered
e. monitor for therapeutic and nontherapeutic effects of the following if administered:
1. blood products and/or volume expanders
2. vasopressors (may be given for a short time *to maintain mean arterial pressure*)
f. assist with the application of military antishock trousers (MAST) if indicated
g. provide emotional support to client and significant others.

15. NURSING DIAGNOSIS

Disturbance in self-concept* related to:

a. dependence on others to meet self-care needs;
b. changes in appearance associated with long-term corticosteroid therapy and extraintestinal manifestations such as skin lesions and arthritic changes;
c. embarrassment associated with diarrhea;
d. changes in sexual functioning associated with pain, fatigue, and weakness;
e. changes in life style imposed by inflammatory bowel disease and its treatment;
f. stigma of having a chronic illness.

---

* This diagnostic label includes the nursing diagnoses of body image disturbance and self-esteem disturbance.

DESIRED OUTCOMES	NURSING ACTIONS AND *SELECTED RATIONALES*

15. The client will demonstrate beginning adaptation to changes in appearance, body functioning, life style, and roles (see Care Plan on Immobility, Nursing Diagnosis 16, for outcome criteria).	15.a. Refer to Care Plan on Immobility, Nursing Diagnosis 16, for measures related to assessment and promotion of a positive self-concept.
	b. Implement additional measures *to assist client to adapt to changes in appearance, body functioning, level of independence, life style, and roles:*
	  1. reinforce actions to assist the client to cope with the effects of the disease (see Nursing Diagnosis 16, action c)
	  2. perform actions to facilitate the client's ability to meet self-care needs (see Nursing Diagnosis 9) *in order to reduce feelings of dependency*
	  3. perform actions *to reduce embarrassment associated with diarrhea:*
	    a. provide a private room if possible
	    b. keep commode or bedpan within easy reach
	    c. utilize room deodorizers and empty bedpan or commode as soon as possible after each bowel movement *to reduce odor*
	  4. encourage client to discuss concerns about sexual functioning; offer suggestions to assist client to regain optimal level of sexual functioning (e.g. adequate rest periods before and after sexual activity)
	  5. ensure that client and significant others have similar expectations and understanding of future life style
	  6. teach client rationale for treatments and encourage maximum participation in treatment regimen *to enable him/her to maintain a sense of control over life*
	  7. provide information about and encourage utilization of community resources (e.g. colitis support groups; sexual, family, and individual counseling).

UNIT XII

16. NURSING DIAGNOSIS

Ineffective individual coping related to:

a. chronicity of condition and need for repeated hospitalization;
b. effect of disease on life style;
c. fear of an eventual need for an ileostomy;
d. inadequate support systems.

DESIRED OUTCOMES	NURSING ACTIONS AND *SELECTED RATIONALES*

16. The client will demonstrate the use of effective coping skills as evidenced by:
    a. willingness to participate in treatment plan and self-care activities
    b. verbalization of ability to cope with inflammatory bowel disease and its effects
    c. identification of stressors
    d. utilization of appropriate problem-solving techniques
    e. recognition and utilization of available support systems.

16.a. Assess effectiveness of client's coping strategies by observing behavior and noting strengths, weaknesses, ability to express feelings and concerns, and willingness to participate in the treatment plan.
   b. Assess for and report signs and symptoms that may indicate ineffective coping (e.g. sleep disturbances, increasing fatigue, difficulty concentrating, irritability, decreased tolerance for pain, verbalization of inability to cope, inability to problem-solve).
   c. Implement measures *to promote effective coping:*
      1. arrange for a visit with another who has successfully adjusted to inflammatory bowel disease
      2. provide consistency in caregiving; inform client if there will be a change in caregivers *so he/she will not interpret the change as rejection*
      3. include client in planning of care, encourage maximum participation in treatment plan, and allow choices when possible *to enable him/her to maintain a sense of control*
      4. instruct client in effective problem-solving techniques (e.g. accurate identification of stressors, determination of various options to solve problem)
      5. assist client to maintain usual daily routines whenever possible
      6. encourage diversional activities according to client's interests
      7. assist client as he/she starts to plan for necessary life-style changes after discharge; provide input related to realistic prioritization of problems that need to be dealt with
      8. assist the client and significant others to identify ways that personal and family goals can be adjusted rather than abandoned
      9. assist client to prepare for negative reactions from others because of diarrhea and odor of flatus
      10. assist client to identify and utilize available support systems; provide information regarding available community resources that can assist client and significant others in coping with the disease (e.g. colitis support groups, counseling services)
      11. monitor for therapeutic and nontherapeutic effects of antidepressants if administered.
   d. Encourage continued emotional support from significant others. Reinforce the importance of maintaining a calm, nonstressful atmosphere during visits.
   e. Assess for and support behaviors suggesting positive adaptation to changes experienced (e.g. increased participation in self-care activities and treatment plan, verbalization of ways to adapt to necessary changes in life style).
   f. Consult physician about psychological counseling if appropriate. Initiate a referral if necessary.

17. NURSING DIAGNOSIS

Knowledge deficit regarding follow-up care.

DESIRED OUTCOMES	NURSING ACTIONS AND *SELECTED RATIONALES*

17.a. The client will identify ways to reduce the incidence of disease exacerbation.

17.a.1. Reinforce the importance of adhering to the prescribed treatment regimen in order to keep condition in a state of remission.
   2. Instruct the client regarding ways *to reduce bowel irritation:*

a. avoid eating foods likely to be poorly digested or that irritate the bowel (see Nursing Diagnosis 10, action d.1.d.1, for a list of foods/fluids to avoid)

b. avoid use of laxatives

c. avoid over-the-counter medications that are gastrointestinal irritants (e.g. aspirin, ibuprofen)

d. avoid alcohol intake.

3. Explain to client that stress can precipitate periods of exacerbation. Provide information about stress management classes and counseling services that may assist him/her to manage stress.

17.b. The client will verbalize ways to maintain an optimal nutritional status.	17.b. Provide instructions regarding ways *to maintain an optimal nutritional status:* 1. reinforce instructions in Nursing Diagnosis 3, action c.5, regarding ways to meet nutritional needs 2. stress the importance of taking medium-chain triglycerides, vitamins, and minerals as prescribed.
17.c. The client will state ways to prevent perianal skin breakdown.	17.c. Provide the following instructions about ways *to prevent perianal skin breakdown:* 1. use soft toilet tissue for wiping after each bowel movement 2. cleanse perianal area with a mild soap and warm water after each bowel movement 3. apply a protective ointment or cream (e.g. Sween cream, Desitin, Vaseline, A & D ointment) to perianal area after skin has been cleansed.
17.d. The client will identify ways to minimize the risk of bleeding.	17.d.1. Instruct client about ways *to minimize risk of bleeding:* a. avoid taking aspirin, aspirin-containing products, and ibuprofen b. use an electric rather than a straight-edge razor c. floss and brush teeth gently d. cut nails carefully e. do not blow nose forcefully f. avoid straining to have a bowel movement g. avoid situations that could result in injury (e.g. contact sports) h. increase intake of foods high in vitamin K (e.g. cooked green leafy vegetables, liver, tomatoes) i. keep appointments for vitamin K injections if prescribed (some clients may be instructed in self-administration). 2. Instruct client to control any bleeding by applying firm, prolonged pressure to the area if possible.
17.e. The client will verbalize an understanding of medication therapy including rationale for, side effects of, schedule for taking, and importance of taking as prescribed.	17.e.1. Explain rationale for, side effects of, and importance of taking medications prescribed. 2. If client is discharged on sulfasalazine, instruct to: a. drink at least 10 glasses of liquid/day *to reduce risk of kidney stone formation* b. expect that urine might be an orange-yellow color c. avoid exposure to ultraviolet light and excessive sunlight d. take medication with food or after meals e. report a sore throat or mouth, fever, unusual fatigue, continuous headache or aching joint(s), unusual bruising or bleeding, rash, or marked decline in urine output f. notify health care provider if unable to impregnate partner *(sulfasalazine may cause a reduction in sperm count)* g. test urine pH and report decreasing levels (if requested by physician) h. keep scheduled appointments for blood and urine studies. 3. If client is discharged on a corticosteroid preparation, instruct to: a. take medications exactly as prescribed; explain that the reason for taking daily dose or larger dose in the morning is *to simulate the body's normal pattern of steroid secretion* b. adjust dosage only if prescribed by physician c. notify health care provider if unable to tolerate oral medication d. avoid discontinuing medication suddenly or of own accord e. take with food, milk, or antacids *to reduce gastric irritation* f. eat smaller, more frequent meals if gastric irritation occurs g. weigh self twice a week and keep a record of weights

h. expect that certain effects such as facial rounding, slight weight gain and swelling, increased appetite, and slight mood changes may occur

i. report undesirable effects of corticosteroid therapy such as marked swelling in extremities, weight gain of more than 5 pounds in a week, extreme emotional and behavioral changes, extreme weakness, tarry stools, bloody or coffee-ground vomitus, frequent or persistent headaches, insomnia, and lack of menses

j. avoid contact with persons who have an infection *because corticosteroids lower resistance to infection.*

4. If client is to administer corticosteroid enemas at home, instruct in technique and length of time he/she should retain the solution. Allow time for questions, clarification, and return demonstration.

5. Instruct client to inform physician before taking other prescription and nonprescription medications.

6. Instruct client to inform all health care providers of medications being taken.

17.f. The client will state signs and symptoms to report to the health care provider.	17.f. Instruct client to report the following signs and symptoms: 1. recurrent episodes of diarrhea and abdominal cramping 2. increasing abdominal distention 3. persistent vomiting 4. unusual rectal or vaginal drainage 5. rectal pain 6. unusual bleeding from any site 7. yellowing of skin 8. change in vision, eye pain 9. skin breakdown 10. increase in joint pain and swelling 11. pain and swelling in extremities 12. sudden chest pain accompanied by shortness of breath.
17.g. The client will identify community resources that can assist in the adjustment to changes resulting from inflammatory bowel disease and its treatment.	17.g.1. Provide information about community resources that can assist the client and significant others in adjusting to inflammatory bowel disease and its effects (e.g. colitis support groups, counseling services, stress management classes). 2. Initiate a referral if indicated.
17.h. The client will verbalize an understanding of and a plan for adhering to recommended follow-up care including future appointments with health care provider and activity level.	17.h.1. Reinforce importance of keeping follow-up appointments with health care provider. 2. Reinforce importance of frequent rest periods throughout the day. 3. Implement measures *to improve client compliance:* a. include significant others in teaching sessions if possible b. encourage questions and allow time for reinforcement and clarification of information provided c. provide written instructions on future appointments with health care provider, medications prescribed, signs and symptoms to report, and future laboratory studies.

■ ■

Jaw Reconstruction

Surgical reconstruction of the jaw is performed to improve dental occlusion, correct functional problems, and/or improve appearance. Conditions necessitating the surgery include trauma, congenital deformities of the mandible or maxilla, derangement of the fibrocartilaginous disc of the temporomandibular joint, and degenerative joint disorders such as osteoarthritis. Following surgery, the maxilla and mandible need to be immobilized in order to maintain proper jaw positioning during the 4- to 6-week healing process. This immobilization is usually accomplished by intermaxillary fixation (maxillary-mandibular fixation), which involves attaching wires or arch bars along upper and lower teeth and then connecting these with cross wires or rubber bands so that the lower and upper jaws are positioned together. In some instances of jaw reconstruction, the immobilization is accomplished by plates and screws at the surgical site rather than by intermaxillary fixation with wires and bands.

This care plan focuses on the adult client hospitalized for reconstruction of the jaw with intermaxillary fixation. Preoperative goals of care are to educate the client regarding anticipated oral care and alternative methods for communicating following surgery. Postoperatively, the goals of care are to maintain comfort, a patent airway, immobilization of the jaw, and an adequate nutritional status; prevent complications; and educate the client regarding follow-up care.

DISCHARGE CRITERIA

Prior to discharge, the client will:

- identify ways to maintain a patent airway
- demonstrate the ability to perform oral care
- verbalize an understanding of dietary modifications and ways to maintain an adequate nutritional status
- identify ways to prevent constipation that may result from temporary dietary modifications
- state signs and symptoms to report to the health care provider
- share thoughts and feelings regarding temporary alterations in diet, speech, and appearance
- verbalize an understanding of and a plan for adhering to recommended follow-up care including future appointments with health care provider, wound care, activity level, and medications prescribed.

NURSING/COLLABORATIVE DIAGNOSES

Preoperative
1. Anxiety □ *700*
2. Knowledge deficit □ *700*
Postoperative
1. Ineffective airway clearance □ *701*
2. Altered nutrition: less than body requirements □ *702*
3. Altered comfort: nausea and vomiting □ *702*
4. Impaired verbal communication □ *703*
5. Altered oral mucous membrane:
   a. dry, sore lips
   b. irritation of oral mucosa
   c. stomatitis □ *703*
6. Potential for aspiration □ *704*
7. Potential complications:
   a. respiratory distress
   b. osteomyelitis
   c. facial nerve damage □ *705*
8. Disturbance in self-concept □ *706*
9. Knowledge deficit regarding follow-up care □ *707*

Preoperative

Use in conjunction with the Standardized Preoperative Care Plan.

1. NURSING DIAGNOSIS

Anxiety related to unfamiliar environment, lack of understanding of planned surgical procedure, effects of anesthesia, anticipated postoperative discomfort, and anticipated effects of surgery on appearance and ability to communicate verbally and maintain a good nutritional status.

DESIRED OUTCOMES	NURSING ACTIONS AND *SELECTED RATIONALES*

1. The client will experience a reduction in fear and anxiety (see Standardized Preoperative Care Plan, Nursing Diagnosis 1, for outcome criteria).	1.a. Refer to Standardized Preoperative Care Plan, Nursing Diagnosis 1, for measures related to assessment and reduction of fear and anxiety.
	b. Implement additional measures *to reduce fear and anxiety:*
	  1. inform client that the facial edema and ecchymosis that follow surgery usually diminish after 2–3 days
	  2. discuss alternative methods of communicating after surgery (e.g. magic slate, pad and pencil, flash cards); stress that client's difficulty communicating verbally will be temporary and that it will improve as facial edema subsides and resolve when immobilization devices are removed (devices are usually removed 4–6 weeks after surgery)
	  3. discuss ways that the client can maintain a good nutritional status during the period of jaw immobilization (e.g. drinking high-protein liquids and blenderized nutritious foods, taking liquid vitamins).

2. NURSING DIAGNOSIS

Knowledge deficit regarding hospital routines associated with surgery, physical preparation for oral surgery, and postoperative care.

DESIRED OUTCOMES	NURSING ACTIONS AND *SELECTED RATIONALES*
2.a. The client will verbalize an understanding of usual preoperative and postoperative care and routines.	2.a. Refer to Standardized Preoperative Care Plan, Nursing Diagnosis 4, action a, for information to include in preoperative teaching.

2.b. The client will demonstrate the ability to perform techniques designed to prevent postoperative complications.

2.b.1. Refer to Standardized Preoperative Care Plan, Nursing Diagnosis 4, action b.1, for instructions on ways to prevent postoperative complications.
2. Provide additional instructions on ways *to prevent postoperative complications:*
   a. explain the importance of good oral care after surgery
   b. demonstrate proper use of a low-pressure power spray, correct oral suctioning technique, and correct way to rinse mouth thoroughly and brush teeth using a soft bristle toothbrush.
3. Allow time for questions, clarification, and return demonstration of oral care.

Postoperative

Use in conjunction with the Standardized Postoperative Care Plan.

1. NURSING DIAGNOSIS

Ineffective airway clearance related to:

a. stasis of secretions associated with decreased activity and poor cough effort resulting from discomfort, fatigue, and depressant effects of anesthesia and some medications (e.g. narcotic analgesics);
b. increased secretions associated with irritation of the respiratory tract (can result from inhalation anesthetics and endotracheal intubation);
c. tenacious secretions associated with fluid loss and decreased fluid intake;
d. accumulation of oral secretions associated with reluctance to swallow due to oral discomfort (can result in aspiration).

UNIT XII

DESIRED OUTCOMES	NURSING ACTIONS AND *SELECTED RATIONALES*

1. The client will maintain clear, open airways (see Standardized Postoperative Care Plan, Nursing Diagnosis 4, for outcome criteria).

1.a. Refer to Standardized Postoperative Care Plan, Nursing Diagnosis 4, for measures related to assessment and promotion of effective airway clearance.
b. Implement additional measures *to promote effective airway clearance:*
   1. perform actions to reduce discomfort (see Standardized Postoperative Care Plan, Nursing Diagnosis 7.A, action 5 and Postoperative Nursing Diagnosis 3) *in order to improve client's cough effort*
   2. perform actions *to facilitate removal of oral secretions in order to prevent aspiration:*
      a. place client in a side-lying or high Fowler's position with head and shoulders slightly forward
      b. assist client with oral suctioning (if client has natural dentition, there is usually enough room behind the last tooth or between the upper and lower teeth to allow passage of suction catheter).

☐ ▬▬▬▬▬▬▬▬▬▬▬▬▬▬▬▬▬▬▬

2. NURSING DIAGNOSIS

Altered nutrition: less than body requirements related to:

a. decreased oral intake associated with nausea, oral discomfort, prescribed dietary modifications, fear of choking, and dislike of the prescribed diet;
b. inadequate nutritional replacement therapy;
c. loss of nutrients associated with vomiting;
d. increased nutritional needs associated with increased metabolic rate that occurs during wound healing.

☐ ▬▬▬▬▬▬▬▬▬▬▬▬▬▬▬▬▬▬▬

DESIRED OUTCOMES	NURSING ACTIONS AND *SELECTED RATIONALES*

2. The client will maintain an adequate nutritional status (see Standardized Postoperative Care Plan, Nursing Diagnosis 6, for outcome criteria).	2.a. Refer to Standardized Postoperative Care Plan, Nursing Diagnosis 6, for measures related to assessment and maintenance of an adequate nutritional status.
	b. Implement additional measures *to maintain an adequate nutritional status:*
	  1. perform actions *to increase oral intake:*
	    a. implement measures to reduce discomfort and prevent further irritation of the oral mucous membrane (see Postoperative Nursing Diagnosis 5, action b)
	    b. implement measures to prevent nausea and vomiting (see Postoperative Nursing Diagnosis 3)
	    c. allow client to use the technique he/she is most comfortable with when feeding self (e.g. bulb syringe, spoon, straw, cup) *in order to decrease fear of choking*
	  2. advance diet from clear liquids to blenderized foods with high-protein dietary supplements when allowed and tolerated.

☐ ▬▬▬▬▬▬▬▬▬▬▬▬▬▬▬▬▬▬▬

3. NURSING DIAGNOSIS

Altered comfort: nausea and vomiting related to stimulation of the vomiting center associated with:

a. vagal and/or sympathetic stimulation resulting from irritation of the gastric mucosa due to swallowed blood;
b. cortical stimulation due to pain, stress, and the taste of blood.

☐ ▬▬▬▬▬▬▬▬▬▬▬▬▬▬▬▬▬▬▬

DESIRED OUTCOMES	NURSING ACTIONS AND *SELECTED RATIONALES*

3. The client will experience relief of nausea and vomiting (see Standardized Postoperative Care Plan, Nursing Diagnosis 7.C, for outcome criteria).	3.a. Refer to Standardized Postoperative Care Plan, Nursing Diagnosis 7.C, for measures related to assessment and prevention of nausea and vomiting.
	b. Implement additional measures *to prevent nausea and vomiting:*
	  1. keep container of suctioned secretions out of client's sight (e.g. cover it with towel, place it at head of the bed) and empty it frequently *(noxious stimuli cause cortical stimulation of the vomiting center)*
	  2. instruct and assist client to remove blood and saliva from mouth by performing oral suctioning and/or pushing it out through spaces between teeth rather than swallowing it.

4. NURSING DIAGNOSIS

Impaired verbal communication related to accumulation of oral secretions, oral and jaw edema and discomfort, and jaw immobilization.

DESIRED OUTCOMES	NURSING ACTIONS AND *SELECTED RATIONALES*

4. The client will communicate needs and desires effectively.	4.a. Assess for factors that interfere with verbal communication (e.g. jaw or oral edema and discomfort, accumulation of oral secretions, immobilization of the jaw).
	b. Implement measures *to facilitate communication:*
	  1. answer call signal promptly and in person rather than using the intercommunication system
	  2. make frequent rounds to ascertain needs
	  3. try to anticipate needs *in order to minimize necessity of verbal communication*
	  4. ask questions that require short answers or nod of head
	  5. provide materials necessary for communication (e.g. magic slate, pad and pencil, flash cards)
	  6. ensure that intravenous therapy does not interfere with client's ability to write
	  7. instruct and assist client to perform oral suctioning before he/she attempts verbal communication if oral secretions have accumulated
	  8. apply ice to jaw for 24–48 hours postoperatively *in order to decrease edema and promote comfort*
	  9. perform actions to reduce discomfort and prevent further irritation of the oral mucous membrane (see Postoperative Nursing Diagnosis 5, action b)
	  10. maintain a patient, calm approach; avoid interrupting client and allow ample time for communication
	  11. listen carefully when client is speaking *(client will be unable to enunciate clearly because of restricted jaw movement)*
	  12. maintain a quiet environment *so that client does not have to raise voice to be heard.*
	c. Inform significant others and health care personnel of approaches being used to maximize client's ability to communicate.
	d. Consult physician if client experiences increasing impairment of verbal communication.

UNIT XII

5. NURSING DIAGNOSIS

Altered oral mucous membrane:

a. **dry, sore lips** related to stretching of the lips during surgery and difficulty moistening lips with tongue due to jaw immobilization;
b. **irritation of oral mucosa** related to protruding wires;
c. **stomatitis** related to trauma resulting from surgery and inadequate oral hygiene.

DESIRED OUTCOMES	NURSING ACTIONS AND *SELECTED RATIONALES*

5. The client will experience improved health and comfort of the oral mucous membrane as evidenced by:
   a. moist lips
   b. decreased mucosal inflammation
   c. absence of ulcerations
   d. decreasing complaints of oral discomfort.

5.a. Assess for signs and symptoms of impaired integrity of the oral mucous membrane:
   1. dry, cracked lips
   2. mucosal inflammation
   3. ulcerations
   4. increasing or persistent complaints of oral discomfort (be aware that temporary facial nerve injury may cause decreased sensation).
   b. Implement measures *to reduce discomfort and prevent further irritation of the oral mucous membrane:*
   1. instruct client in and assist with prescribed oral care (e.g. rinsing mouth with warm saline, suctioning, brushing teeth with a soft bristle toothbrush, using low-pressure power spray)
   2. stress the importance of performing oral care gently and thoroughly
   3. lubricate client's lips with Vaseline, K-Y jelly, ChapStick, Blistex, or mineral oil when oral care is given
   4. avoid use of products such as lemon-glycerin swabs and commercial mouthwashes containing alcohol *(these products have a drying or irritating effect on the mucous membrane)*
   5. encourage client not to smoke *(smoking dries and irritates the mucosa)*
   6. assist client to select bland, nonacidic beverages
   7. if protruding wires are irritating the oral mucosa, assist client to apply warmed beeswax or oral surgery wax to the ends of the wires (wax should be removed before eating and brushing teeth).
   c. Consult physician about readjustment of wires and/or alternative methods of oral care if irritation of oral mucous membrane persists or worsens.

□ ▬▬▬▬▬▬▬▬▬▬▬▬▬▬▬▬▬▬▬▬▬▬▬

6. NURSING DIAGNOSIS

Potential for aspiration related to:

a. decreased level of consciousness associated with effects of anesthesia and narcotic analgesics;
b. difficulty expectorating secretions and/or vomitus associated with intermaxillary fixation.

□ ▬▬▬▬▬▬▬▬▬▬▬▬▬▬▬▬▬▬▬▬▬▬▬

DESIRED OUTCOMES	NURSING ACTIONS AND *SELECTED RATIONALES*

6. The client will not aspirate secretions and vomitus (see Standardized Postoperative Care Plan, Nursing Diagnosis 10, for outcome criteria).

6.a. Refer to Standardized Postoperative Care Plan, Nursing Diagnosis 10, for measures related to assessment and prevention of aspiration.
   b. Implement additional measures *to prevent aspiration:*
   1. perform actions to prevent nausea and vomiting (see Postoperative Nursing Diagnosis 3)
   2. if vomiting does occur:
      a. position client on his/her side or assist him/her to sit up and lean foward
      b. instruct client to expel vomitus through teeth (there is usually a ¼-inch space left between upper and lower teeth)
      c. assist client to retract cheeks by holding them out and back with fingers *so vomitus does not pool between cheeks and gingiva*
      d. suction oral cavity and perform good oral care *to remove vomitus from mouth.*

□ ▬▬▬▬▬▬▬▬▬▬▬▬▬▬▬▬▬▬▬▬▬▬▬▬▬▬▬▬▬▬

7. COLLABORATIVE DIAGNOSIS

Potential complications:

a. **respiratory distress** related to airway obstruction associated with aspiration and tracheal compression resulting from edema and/or hematoma in the neck and lower jaw area;
b. **osteomyelitis** related to surgical trauma to the jaw and postoperative wound infection;
c. **facial nerve damage** related to trauma during surgery and pressure on the nerve associated with edema and/or hematoma.

□ ▬▬▬▬▬▬▬▬▬▬▬▬▬▬▬▬▬▬▬▬▬▬▬▬▬▬▬▬▬▬

DESIRED OUTCOMES	NURSING ACTIONS AND *SELECTED RATIONALES*
7.a. The client will not experience respiratory distress as evidenced by: 1. unlabored respirations at 16–20/minute 2. absence of stridor and sternocleidomastoid muscle retraction 3. usual skin color 4. usual mental status 5. blood gases within normal range.	7.a.1. Assess for and immediately report: a. increased edema or expanding hematoma in the neck and lower jaw area b. deviation of trachea from midline c. persistent or increased difficulty swallowing d. signs and symptoms of respiratory distress (e.g. rapid and/or labored respirations, stridor, sternocleidomastoid muscle retraction, cyanosis, restlessness, agitation) e. abnormal blood gases f. significant changes in ear oximetry and capnograph results. 2. Have nasal airway, wire cutters or scissors, and tracheostomy and suction equipment readily available. 3. Implement measures *to prevent respiratory distress*: a. perform actions to prevent aspiration (see Postoperative Nursing Diagnosis 6) b. perform actions *to minimize edema and bleeding in the neck and lower jaw area*: 1. keep head of bed elevated at least 30° 2. apply ice to neck and lower jaw during first 24–48 hours after surgery 3. instruct and assist client to perform oral suctioning and oral hygiene gently and carefully *to decrease risk of trauma* c. monitor for therapeutic and nontherapeutic effects of corticosteroids if administered *to reduce operative site edema.* 4. If signs and symptoms of respiratory distress occur: a. place client in a high Fowler's position b. administer oxygen as ordered c. use wire cutters to release wires or scissors to cut bands if absolutely necessary (many physicians will perform a tracheotomy rather than cut the wires or bands) d. prepare client for evacuation of hematoma, surgical repair of bleeding vessel, and/or emergency tracheotomy if indicated e. provide emotional support to client and significant others.
7.b. The client will not develop osteomyelitis as evidenced by: 1. resolution of tenderness, warmth, and redness over involved bone 2. afebrile status 3. return of WBC count toward normal range.	7.b.1. Assess for and report signs and symptoms of osteomyelitis: a. increasing tenderness, warmth, and redness over mandible or maxilla b. fever and chills. 2. Monitor WBC count. Report persistent elevation or increasing values. 3. Obtain cultures of blood, oral secretions, and wound drainage as ordered. Report positive results. 4. Implement measures *to decrease risk of osteomyelitis*: a. perform actions to prevent and treat wound infection (see Standardized Postoperative Care Plan, Nursing Diagnosis 16, actions b.4 and 5)

UNIT
XII

b. perform actions to maintain an adequate nutritional status (see Postoperative Nursing Diagnosis 2)

c. perform actions to prevent further irritation of oral mucous membrane (see Postoperative Nursing Diagnosis 5, action b) *in order to further reduce the risk of infection.*

5. If signs and symptoms of osteomyelitis occur:
   a. maintain client on bedrest with limited movement of head
   b. monitor for therapeutic and nontherapeutic effects of anti-infectives if administered
   c. prepare client for surgery (e.g. incision and drainage of exudate, removal of necrotic bone) if indicated.

7.c. The client will experience resolution of facial nerve damage if it occurs as evidenced by:
1. gradual return of normal facial movements within limitations imposed by jaw immobilization
2. decreasing complaints of circumoral numbness and tingling
3. gradual return of normal taste sensation.

7.c.1. Assess for signs and symptoms of facial nerve damage (e.g. facial droop, uneven smile, complaints of circumoral numbness or tingling, diminished taste sensation).

2. Implement measures *to decrease edema and promote resolution of facial nerve damage:*
   a. keep head of bed elevated at least 30°
   b. apply ice to jaw during first 24–48 hours after surgery
   c. monitor for therapeutic and nontherapeutic effects of corticosteroids if administered.

3. If signs and symptoms of facial nerve damage are present:
   a. instruct client to avoid hot fluids *in order to decrease risk of mouth and lip burns*
   b. inspect oral cavity carefully for signs of irritation (the client may be less aware of discomfort)
   c. encourage client to use a straw when drinking fluids if drooling is a problem
   d. encourage client to use additional seasonings if taste alteration has occurred
   e. reassure client that signs and symptoms usually resolve within a few months
   f. monitor for and report an increase in severity of signs and symptoms.

□ ▬▬▬▬▬▬▬▬▬▬▬▬▬▬▬▬▬▬▬▬▬▬▬▬▬▬

8. NURSING DIAGNOSIS

Disturbance in self-concept* related to impaired verbal communication and change in appearance associated with facial edema, presence of jaw immobilization devices (e.g. arch bars, wires, rubber bands), restricted jaw movement, and damage to the facial nerve.

---

* This diagnostic label includes the nursing diagnoses of body image disturbance and self-esteem disturbance.

□ ▬▬▬▬▬▬▬▬▬▬▬▬▬▬▬▬▬▬▬▬▬▬▬▬▬▬

DESIRED OUTCOMES	NURSING ACTIONS AND *SELECTED RATIONALES*

8. The client will demonstrate beginning adaptation to the temporary changes in appearance and ability to communicate verbally as evidenced by:
a. communication of feelings of self-worth
b. maintenance of

8.a. Determine the meaning of change in appearance and difficulty communicating verbally to the client by encouraging him/her to communicate feelings and by noting nonverbal responses to these changes.

b. Assess for signs and symptoms of a disturbance in self-concept (e.g. verbal or nonverbal cues denoting a negative response to change in appearance such as refusal to look in mirror, reluctance to participate in oral care, or withdrawal from significant others).

c. Assist the client to identify strengths and qualities that have a positive effect on self-concept.

relationships with significant others
c. active participation in activities of daily living
d. active interest in personal appearance
e. willingness to participate in social activities.

d. Implement measures *to assist client to increase self-esteem* (e.g. limit negative self-criticism, encourage positive comments about self).
e. Assist the client to identify and utilize coping techniques that have been helpful in the past.
f. Inform client that facial edema and facial nerve damage will gradually resolve.
g. Stress the temporary nature of jaw immobilization (usually 4–6 weeks) and positive effects of the surgical procedure.
h. Provide privacy during oral care and suctioning.
i. Provide privacy at mealtime if client is embarrassed (client may need to use syringe to feed self and may drool while eating).
j. Assist client with usual grooming and makeup habits if necessary.
k. Assess for and support behaviors suggesting positive adaptation to changes experienced (e.g. willingness to suction and feed self, attempts at verbal communication).
l. Encourage visits and support from significant others.

□ ▬▬▬▬▬▬▬▬▬▬▬▬▬▬▬▬▬▬▬▬▬

9. NURSING DIAGNOSIS

Knowledge deficit regarding follow-up care.

□ ▬▬▬▬▬▬▬▬▬▬▬▬▬▬▬▬▬▬▬▬▬

DESIRED OUTCOMES	NURSING ACTIONS AND *SELECTED RATIONALES*

9.a. The client will identify ways to maintain a patent airway.

9.a.1. Instruct client regarding ways *to maintain a patent airway:*
   a. avoid any situation that might lead to nausea and vomiting (e.g. ingestion of foods/fluids that client has not been able to tolerate in the past, noxious sights and odors)
   b. keep pulmonary secretions thin by:
     1. drinking at least 10 glasses of liquid/day
     2. humidifying inspired air if recommended
   c. reduce the risk of choking by:
     1. sitting up in a chair and leaning forward slightly when eating and drinking
     2. preparing food as recommended (e.g. blenderized, pureed)
     3. taking all oral medications in liquid form
   d. if vomiting does occur:
     1. sit up, lean forward, and expel vomitus through space between upper and lower teeth
     2. hold cheeks out and back with fingers *to facilitate removal of vomitus*
     3. utilize suction equipment if indicated (a soft, small bulb syringe is usually all that is needed after discharge)
   e. perform good oral care after any episode of emesis and after meals *to decrease possibility of aspiration*
   f. have wire cutters (if wires present) or scissors (if bands present) readily available at all times if recommended by physician.
  2. If appropriate, show client and significant others where wires or bands should be cut in case of severe respiratory distress (some physicians prefer that client go to emergency room rather than cutting wires).

9.b. The client will demonstrate the ability to perform oral care.

9.b.1. Stress the importance of performing oral care as prescribed.
  2. Instruct client to avoid drinking alcohol and using products that contain alcohol (e.g. some mouthwashes, liquid decongestants, and analgesics) *in order to avoid irritation of the oral mucous membrane.*
  3. Instruct client to strain and thin blended protein foods *in order to decrease risk of food fibers getting caught under wires.*

UNIT
XII

4. Reinforce the proper method of applying warmed beeswax or oral surgery wax to the protruding wires and removing the wax before meals and oral care.
5. Instruct client in proper oral care techniques (e.g. rinsing mouth with saline, gentle brushing, using low-pressure power spray).
6. Instruct client to use a lip moisturizer if lips are dry.
7. Allow time for questions, clarification, and return demonstration.

9.c. The client will verbalize an understanding of dietary modifications and ways to maintain an adequate nutritional status.

9.c.1. Reinforce prescribed dietary modifications (client usually progresses rapidly from clear liquids to blenderized and pureed low-fiber foods).
2. Instruct client in ways *to maintain an adequate nutritional status:*
   a. plan well-balanced meals that meet caloric needs (food items are then blenderized or pureed)
   b. drink protein supplements between meals
   c. experiment with spices that may make diet more appetizing and enhance taste sensation
   d. take supplemental vitamins and minerals as ordered.
3. Inform client that appetite will be stimulated by seeing and smelling food before it is blenderized.
4. Consult dietician regarding menu planning and food preparation if indicated.

9.d. The client will identify ways to prevent constipation that may result from temporary dietary modifications.

9.d.1. Inform client of the effect that a decrease in dietary fiber will have on bowel habits.
2. Instruct client in ways *to prevent constipation:*
   a. drink at least 10 glasses of liquid/day
   b. continue with measures previously used to stimulate bowel activity (e.g. warm tea in the morning, prune juice)
   c. take liquid stool softeners and laxatives as prescribed
   d. use suppositories or enemas if needed.

9.e. The client will state signs and symptoms to report to the health care provider.

9.e.1. Refer to Standardized Postoperative Care Plan, Nursing Diagnosis 20, action c, for signs and symptoms to report to health care provider.
2. Instruct client to also report:
   a. difficulty breathing
   b. bluish color of lips or nail beds
   c. jaw pain or oral pain unrelieved by prescribed medications and treatment
   d. constipation not controlled by usual techniques, stool softeners, laxatives, suppositories, or enemas
   e. persistent irritation or breakdown of oral mucosa
   f. facial swelling that persists or increases
   g. weight loss of over 10–15 pounds during the first 6 weeks after surgery
   h. increasing weakness and fatigue
   i. inability to adhere to prescribed diet
   j. unusual mouth odor, drainage, or taste
   k. increased numbness and tingling of or around mouth, lips, and chin
   l. temperature elevation that lasts more than 2 days
   m. discoloration of rubber bands (could indicate bands have stretched) and/or loosening of wires or bands.

9.f. The client will verbalize an understanding of and a plan for adhering to recommended follow-up care including future appointments with health care provider, wound care, activity level, and medications prescribed.

9.f.1. Refer to Standardized Postoperative Care Plan, Nursing Diagnosis 20, for routine postoperative instructions and measures to improve client compliance.
2. Explain the rationale for, side effects of, and importance of taking medications prescribed (e.g. laxatives, stool softeners, analgesics, anti-infectives, vitamins, corticosteroids).
3. Instruct client to keep teeth clenched and contact physician immediately if wires or bands are cut or become loose or disconnected.

Peptic Ulcer

A peptic ulcer is a circumscribed lesion of the gastrointestinal mucosa that is exposed to acidic digestive secretions. The areas most often involved are the stomach and duodenum, although ulcers of the lower part of the esophagus and the margin of a gastrojejunal anastomosis may also occur. Erosion of the mucosa occurs when the normal buffering system is altered by increased amounts of gastric secretions; changes in the mucosal barrier resulting from back diffusion of hydrogen ions, decreased cell renewal, decreased mucosal blood flow, or decreased mucosal secretion; and/or changes in the normal gastric emptying time. Factors responsible for these alterations include psychological stressors and personal habits such as smoking, alcohol and caffeine consumption, ingestion of ulcerogenic drugs, irregular mealtimes, and ingestion of foods that irritate the gastric mucosa. Hormone imbalances such as those occurring with menopause, genetic factors such as blood type, and anatomical factors including incompetent cardiac or pyloric sphincters are also implicated in peptic ulcer development. Peptic ulcers may also occur secondary to diseases such as chronic obstructive pulmonary disease and Zollinger-Ellison syndrome or in response to acute medical crises (e.g. severe burns, head injury, shock, trauma).*

Peptic ulcers are classified by location (e.g. gastric, duodenal) or as acute (superficial erosion with minimal inflammation) or chronic (erosion of mucosa and submucosa with scar tissue formation). The epigastric pain experienced in peptic ulcer disease is usually described as burning, aching, gnawing, and/or cramping. The relationship between eating and the presence and intensity of pain is dependent mainly on the location of the ulcer.

This care plan focuses on the adult client hospitalized for treatment of a peptic ulcer that has continued to be symptomatic despite conservative management. The goals of care are to relieve discomfort, maintain an adequate nutritional status, prevent complications, and educate the client regarding follow-up care.

---

* The ulcers occurring in response to medical crises are referred to as stress ulcers and are caused by decreased circulation to the gastric mucosa and/or excessive gastric secretions due to vagal stimulation.

DISCHARGE CRITERIA

Prior to discharge, the client will:

- identify ways to promote healing of the existing ulcer and prevent recurrence of peptic ulcers
- verbalize an understanding of medication therapy including rationale for, side effects of, schedule for taking, and importance of taking as prescribed
- state signs and symptoms to report to the health care provider
- identify community resources that can assist with making life-style changes necessary to prevent peptic ulcer recurrence
- verbalize an understanding of and a plan for adhering to recommended follow-up care including future appointments with health care provider.

UNIT XII

NURSING/COLLABORATIVE DIAGNOSES

1. Anxiety □ 710
2. Altered nutrition: less than body requirements □ 710
3. Pain: epigastric □ 711
4. Activity intolerance □ 712
5. Potential complications:
   a. hypovolemic shock
   b. peritonitis
   c. gastric outlet obstruction □ 713
6. Noncompliance □ 715
7. Knowledge deficit regarding follow-up care □ 716

1. NURSING DIAGNOSIS

Anxiety related to unfamiliar environment; pain; lack of understanding of the diagnosis, diagnostic tests, and treatment plan; and possible changes in life style.

DESIRED OUTCOMES	NURSING ACTIONS AND *SELECTED RATIONALES*

1. The client will experience a reduction in fear and anxiety as evidenced by:
 a. verbalization of feeling less anxious or fearful
 b. relaxed facial expression and body movements
 c. stable vital signs
 d. usual skin color
 e. verbalization of an understanding of hospital routines, diagnosis, diagnostic tests, and treatment plan.
	1.a. Assess client for signs and symptoms of fear and anxiety (e.g. verbalization of fears and concerns; tenseness; tremors; irritability; restlessness; diaphoresis; tachypnea; tachycardia; elevated blood pressure; facial tension, pallor, or flushing; noncompliance with treatment plan).
	 b. Ascertain effectiveness of current coping skills.
	 c. Implement measures *to reduce fear and anxiety:*
	   1. orient to hospital environment, equipment, and routines
	   2. introduce staff who will be participating in his/her care; if possible, maintain consistency in staff assigned to his/her care *in order to provide feelings of stability and comfort with the environment*
	   3. assure client that staff members are nearby; respond to call signal as soon as possible
	   4. maintain a calm, confident manner when interacting with client
	   5. encourage verbalization of fear and anxiety; provide feedback
	   6. reinforce physician's explanations and clarify any misconceptions client may have about peptic ulcers, the treatment plan, and prognosis
	   7. explain all diagnostic tests (e.g. CBC, gastric analysis, stool testing for occult blood, barium swallow, endoscopy)
	   8. perform actions to reduce epigastric pain (see Nursing Diagnosis 3, action e)
	   9. provide a calm, restful environment
	   10. instruct in relaxation techniques and encourage participation in diversional activities
	   11. assist client to identify specific stressors and ways to cope with them
	   12. encourage significant others to project a caring, concerned attitude without obvious anxiousness
	   13. monitor for therapeutic and nontherapeutic effects of antianxiety agents if administered.
	 d. Include significant others in orientation and teaching sessions and encourage their continued support of the client.
	 e. Provide information based on current needs of the client and significant others at a level they can understand. Encourage questions and clarification of information provided.
	 f. Consult physician if above actions fail to control fear and anxiety.

2. NURSING DIAGNOSIS

Altered nutrition: less than body requirements related to:

a. decreased oral intake associated with pain, dislike of the prescribed diet, knowledge that eating precipitates pain (especially with a gastric ulcer), weakness, and fatigue;

b. decreased intake of folic acid and other vitamins as a result of prescribed bland diet or self-imposed dietary modifications.

DESIRED OUTCOMES	NURSING ACTIONS AND *SELECTED RATIONALES*

2. The client will maintain an adequate nutritional status as evidenced by:
a. weight within normal range for client's age, height, and build
b. normal BUN and serum albumin, protein, Hct., Hgb., cholesterol, lymphocyte, and folate levels
c. triceps skinfold measurements within normal range
d. usual strength and activity tolerance
e. healthy oral mucous membrane.
	2.a. Assess the client for signs and symptoms of malnutrition:
	  1. weight below normal for client's age, height, and build
	  2. abnormal BUN and low serum albumin, protein, Hct., Hgb., cholesterol, lymphocyte, and folate levels (Hct. and Hgb. may also be decreased due to bleeding of the ulcerated area)
	  3. triceps skinfold measurement less than normal for build
	  4. weakness and fatigue (may also result from chronic blood loss)
	  5. stomatitis.
	b. Reassess nutritional status on a regular basis and report decline.
	c. Monitor percentage of meals eaten.
	d. Assess client to determine causes of inadequate intake (e.g. pain, fear of precipitating pain, dietary restrictions, dislike of prescribed diet, weakness, fatigue).
	e. Implement measures *to maintain and improve nutritional status:*
	  1. perform actions *to improve oral intake:*
	    a. implement measures to reduce epigastric pain (see Nursing Diagnosis 3, actions e.1.b–f, 2, and 3)
	    b. provide oral care before meals
	    c. eliminate noxious stimuli from the environment
	    d. provide a quiet, unstressful atmosphere for meals
	    e. serve small portions of nutritious foods and fluids that are appealing to the client
	    f. encourage a rest period before meals *to minimize fatigue*
	    g. obtain a dietary consult if necessary to assist client in selecting foods and fluids that meet nutritional needs as well as preferences
	    h. allow adequate time for meals; reheat food if necessary
	  2. ensure that meals are well balanced and high in essential nutrients
	  3. encourage intake of foods high in folic acid (e.g. cooked green leafy vegetables, asparagus, organ meats, lima beans) as allowed
	  4. monitor for therapeutic and nontherapeutic effects of vitamins, minerals, and hematinics if administered.
	f. Perform a 72-hour calorie count if nutritional status declines or fails to improve.
	g. Consult physician regarding the need for parenteral nutrition if client does not consume enough food or fluid to meet nutritional needs.

☐ ▆▆▆▆▆▆▆▆▆▆▆▆▆▆▆▆▆▆▆▆▆▆▆▆▆▆▆▆

3. NURSING DIAGNOSIS

Pain: epigastric related to:

a. inflammation and edema of the ulcerated area;
b. exposure of nerve endings in the ulcerated area;
c. reflex muscle spasms that occur when hydrochloric acid and pepsin come in contact with the ulcerated area.

☐ ▆▆▆▆▆▆▆▆▆▆▆▆▆▆▆▆▆▆▆▆▆▆▆▆▆▆▆▆

DESIRED OUTCOMES	NURSING ACTIONS AND *SELECTED RATIONALES*
3. The client will experience diminished pain as evidenced by: a. verbalization of pain relief b. relaxed facial expression and body positioning	3.a. Determine how the client usually responds to pain. b. Assess for nonverbal signs of pain (e.g. wrinkled brow, rubbing epigastric area, clenched fists, reluctance to move, restlessness, diaphoresis, facial pallor or flushing, change in B/P, tachycardia). c. Assess verbal complaints of pain. Ask client to be specific about location, severity, and type of pain.

c. increased participation in activities

d. stable vital signs.

d. Assess for factors that seem to aggravate and alleviate pain.

e. Implement measures *to reduce epigastric pain:*

1. perform actions *to prevent further irritation and/or promote healing of the ulcerated area:*

    a. insert a nasogastric tube and maintain suction as ordered *to remove gastric secretions*

    b. monitor for therapeutic and nontherapeutic effects of the following medications if administered:

        1. histamine$_2$ receptor antagonists (e.g. cimetidine, famotidine, ranitidine) *to inhibit gastric acid secretion*

        2. antacids *to neutralize gastric secretions*

        3. antimuscarinics (e.g. propantheline bromide, glycopyrrolate) *to reduce gastric acid secretion*

        4. mucosal barrier fortifiers (e.g. sucralfate) *to protect the ulcerated area from further irritation*

        5. carbenoxolone *to increase secretion of protective mucus*

    c. consult physician before administering medications known to be ulcerogenic (e.g. aspirin, corticosteroids, phenylbutazone, indomethacin); if ulcerogenic medications are administered, give them with antacids or foods whenever possible

    d. implement measures *to reduce the stimulation of hydrochloric acid and pepsin secretion:*

        1. perform actions to reduce fear and anxiety (see Nursing Diagnosis 1, action c) *in order to reduce stress (stress stimulates hydrocholoric acid secretion)*

        2. instruct client to:

            a. avoid intake of foods/fluids that contain caffeine (e.g. coffee, tea, chocolate, colas)

            b. chew food thoroughly and eat slowly *(a large bolus of food causes increased output of hydrochloric acid and pepsin)*

            c. avoid intake of extremely hot or cold foods/fluids

            d. adhere to prescribed dietary modifications (bland diet may be ordered)

            e. avoid intake of foods and fluids that produce pain (this is often referred to as a "free-choice" diet)

    e. encourage client to stop smoking

    f. provide regularly scheduled, frequent meals and snacks as ordered *to neutralize gastric acidity*

    g. prepare client for a vagotomy if indicated *to reduce gastric acid production*

2. provide or assist with nonpharmacological measures for pain relief (e.g. relaxation techniques, guided imagery, quiet conversation, restful environment, diversional activities)

3. monitor for therapeutic and nontherapeutic effects of the following if administered:

    a. antimuscarinics (e.g. dicyclomine, oxyphencyclimine) *to reduce spasm of the pyloric sphincter*

    b. analgesics.

f. Consult physician if above measures fail to provide adequate pain relief.

☐ ▬▬▬▬▬▬▬▬▬▬▬▬▬▬▬▬▬▬▬▬▬▬▬▬▬▬▬▬▬▬▬▬▬

4. NURSING DIAGNOSIS

Activity intolerance related to:

a. inadequate nutritional status;

b. tissue hypoxia associated with anemia resulting from chronic blood loss and decreased intake of folic acid (if client is on a bland diet);

c. difficulty resting and sleeping associated with frequent assessments and treatments, pain, fear, and anxiety.

☐ ▬▬▬▬▬▬▬▬▬▬▬▬▬▬▬▬▬▬▬▬▬▬▬▬▬▬▬▬▬▬▬▬▬

DESIRED OUTCOMES	NURSING ACTIONS AND *SELECTED RATIONALES*

4. The client will demonstrate an increased tolerance for activity as evidenced by:
   a. verbalization of feeling less fatigued and weak
   b. ability to perform activities of daily living without exertional dyspnea, chest pain, diaphoresis, dizziness, or a significant change in vital signs.

4.a. Assess for signs and symptoms of activity intolerance:
   1. statements of fatigue and weakness
   2. exertional dyspnea, chest pain, diaphoresis, or dizziness
   3. decrease in pulse rate or an increase in rate of 20 beats/minute above resting rate
   4. pulse rate not returning to preactivity level within 5 minutes after stopping activity
   5. decreased blood pressure or an increase in diastolic pressure of 15 mm Hg with activity.
   b. Implement measures *to improve activity tolerance:*
      1. perform actions *to promote rest:*
         a. maintain activity restrictions if ordered
         b. minimize environmental activity and noise
         c. schedule nursing care and diagnostic procedures to allow periods of uninterrupted rest
         d. limit the number of visitors and their length of stay
         e. assist client with self-care activities as needed
         f. keep supplies and personal articles within easy reach
         g. implement measures to reduce fear and anxiety (see Nursing Diagnosis 1, action c)
      2. perform actions to prevent further gastric irritation and/or promote healing of the ulcerated area (see Nursing Diagnosis 3, action e.1) *in order to reduce blood loss*
      3. instruct client in energy-saving techniques (e.g. using shower chair when showering, sitting to brush teeth or comb hair)
      4. perform actions to improve nutritional status (see Nursing Diagnosis 2, action e)
      5. monitor for therapeutic and nontherapeutic effects of whole blood or packed red cells if administered
      6. increase client's activity gradually as allowed and tolerated.
   c. Instruct client to:
      1. report a decreased tolerance for activity
      2. stop any activity that causes chest pain, shortness of breath, dizziness, or extreme fatigue or weakness.
   d. Consult physician if signs and symptoms of activity intolerance persist or worsen.

☐ ▇▇▇▇▇▇▇▇▇▇▇▇▇▇▇▇▇▇▇▇▇▇

5. COLLABORATIVE DIAGNOSIS

Potential complications:

a. **hypovolemic shock** related to hemorrhage associated with erosion of the ulcer through a major blood vessel (usually the right or left gastric artery) or numerous smaller vessels;

b. **peritonitis** related to perforation of ulcerated area and escape of gastrointestinal contents into the peritoneal cavity;

c. **gastric outlet obstruction** related to inflammation, edema, and spasm of or scar tissue formation in an ulcerated area that is at or near the pyloric sphincter.

☐ ▇▇▇▇▇▇▇▇▇▇▇▇▇▇▇▇▇▇▇▇▇▇

DESIRED OUTCOMES	NURSING ACTIONS AND *SELECTED RATIONALES*

5.a. The client will not develop hypovolemic shock as evidenced by:

5.a.1. Assess for and report signs and symptoms of gastrointestinal hemorrhage (e.g. hematemesis [2000–3000 cc of blood may be vomited], melena, increased epigastric pain, complaints of epigastric fullness).

1. usual mental status
2. stable vital signs
3. skin warm and usual color
4. palpable peripheral pulses
5. capillary refill time less than 3 seconds
6. urine output at least 30 cc/hour.

2. Monitor RBC, Hct., and Hgb. levels. Report declining values.
3. Assess for and report signs and symptoms of hypovolemic shock:
   a. restlessness, agitation, confusion
   b. significant decrease in B/P
   c. decline in B/P of at least 15 mm Hg with concurrent rise in pulse when client changes from lying to sitting or standing position
   d. resting pulse rate greater than 100 beats/minute
   e. rapid or labored respirations
   f. cool, pale, or cyanotic skin
   g. diminished or absent peripheral pulses
   h. capillary refill time greater than 3 seconds
   i. urine output less than 30 cc/hour.
4. Implement measures to prevent further irritation and/or promote healing of the ulcerated area (see Nursing Diagnosis 3, action e.1) *in order to prevent hemorrhage.*
5. If signs and symptoms of gastrointestinal hemorrhage occur, implement the following measures *to control bleeding:*
   a. assist with iced water or saline gastric lavage, selective arterial embolization, endoscopic laser photocoagulation, transendoscopic electrocoagulation, and/or intra-arterial administration of vasopressors (e.g. vasopressin) if ordered
   b. prepare client for surgical intervention (e.g. ligation of bleeding vessels, partial gastrectomy) if indicated.
6. If signs and symptoms of hypovolemic shock occur:
   a. continue with above measures to control bleeding
   b. place client flat in bed with legs elevated unless contraindicated
   c. monitor vital signs frequently
   d. administer oxygen as ordered
   e. monitor for therapeutic and nontherapeutic effects of the following if administered:
      1. blood products and/or volume expanders
      2. vasopressors (may be given for a short time *to maintain mean arterial pressure)*
   f. provide emotional support to client and significant others.

5.b. The client will not develop peritonitis as evidenced by:
1. afebrile status
2. soft, nondistended abdomen
3. no complaints of generalized abdominal pain and tenderness
4. stable vital signs
5. normal bowel sounds
6. WBC count within normal range.

5.b.1. Assess for and report:
   a. signs and symptoms of perforation of a peptic ulcer (e.g. sudden, severe upper abdominal pain; midback and/or right shoulder pain [referred pain resulting from stimulation of the vagus nerve]; abdominal tenderness)
   b. signs and symptoms of peritonitis (e.g. elevated temperature; tense, rigid abdomen; generalized abdominal pain; rebound tenderness; tachycardia; tachypnea; decreased B/P; diminished or absent bowel sounds)
   c. further increase in WBC count.
2. Implement measures to prevent further irritation and/or promote healing of the ulcerated area (see Nursing Diagnosis 3, action e.1) *in order to prevent perforation.*
3. If signs and symptoms of peritonitis occur:
   a. withhold all food and fluid as ordered
   b. place client on bedrest in a semi-Fowler's position *to assist in pooling or localizing the gastrointestinal contents in the pelvis rather than under the diaphragm*
   c. insert a nasogastric or intestinal tube and maintain suction as ordered
   d. monitor for therapeutic and nontherapeutic effects of anti-infectives if administered
   e. monitor for therapeutic and nontherapeutic effects of intravenous fluids and/or blood volume expanders if administered *to prevent or treat shock (shock can occur as a result of the escape of protein, fluid, and electrolytes into the peritoneal cavity)*
   f. prepare client for surgical repair of the perforation if indicated
   g. provide emotional support to client and significant others.

5.c. The client will not experience gastric outlet

5.c.1. Assess for and report signs and symptoms of gastric outlet obstruction (e.g. epigastric distention, complaints of epigastric fullness, nausea, vomiting,

obstruction as evidenced by:
1. soft, nondistended epigastric area
2. no complaints of epigastric fullness
3. absence of nausea and vomiting
4. no unusual odor to breath.

vomitus containing particles of food ingested hours or days before, fetid breath).
2. Implement measures *to prevent gastric outlet obstruction:*
   a. perform actions to prevent further irritation and/or promote healing of the ulcerated area (see Nursing Diagnosis 3, action e.1) *in order to reduce inflammation, edema, spasm, and scar tissue formation*
   b. monitor for therapeutic and nontherapeutic effects of antimuscarinics (e.g. dicyclomine, oxyphencyclimine) if administered *to further reduce spasm of the pyloric sphincter.*
3. If signs and symptoms of gastric outlet obstruction occur:
   a. withhold all food and fluid as ordered
   b. insert a nasogastric tube and maintain suction as ordered
   c. monitor for therapeutic and nontherapeutic effects of intravenous fluid and electrolyte replacements if administered
   d. prepare client for surgical intervention (e.g. vagotomy with antral resection, partial gastrectomy, pyloroplasty) if indicated
   e. provide emotional support to client and significant others.

---

6. NURSING DIAGNOSIS

Noncompliance* related to:

a. lack of understanding of the implications of not following the prescribed treatment plan;
b. difficulty modifying personal habits.

---

* This diagnostic label includes both an informed decision by client not to comply and an inability to comply due to circumstances beyond the client's control.

DESIRED OUTCOMES	NURSING ACTIONS AND *SELECTED RATIONALES*

6. The client will demonstrate the probability of future compliance with the prescribed treatment plan as evidenced by:
   a. willingness to learn about and participate in treatments and care
   b. statements reflecting ways to modify personal habits and integrate treatments into life style
   c. statements reflecting an understanding of the implications of not following the prescribed treatment plan.

6.a. Assess for indications that the client may be unwilling or unable to comply with the prescribed treatment plan:
   1. statements reflecting that he/she was unable to adhere to treatment program at home
   2. failure to adhere to treatment plan while in hospital (e.g. refusing medications, not adhering to dietary modifications)
   3. statements reflecting a lack of understanding of factors that aggravate or cause peptic ulcer disease
   4. statements reflecting an unwillingness or inability to modify personal habits and integrate necessary treatments into life style
   5. statements reflecting the view that the peptic ulcer will resolve without any treatment or that recurrence and complications are inevitable and efforts to comply with treatments are useless.
   b. Implement measures *to improve client compliance:*
   1. explain peptic ulcer disease in terms the client can understand; stress the fact that complications can occur and/or it can develop into a chronic condition if treatment program is not followed
   2. inform client that prescribed dietary restrictions and medication therapy will not be as extensive after the existing ulcer has healed (usually 6–8 weeks)
   3. initiate and reinforce the discharge teaching outlined in Nursing Diagnosis 7 *in order to promote a sense of control over disease progression*
   4. focus on modifications of life style rather than complete change (e.g. drinking alcohol with meals rather than when stomach is empty; drinking decaffeinated rather than caffeine-containing beverages)

5. provide a dietary consult to assist client in planning a dietary program based on the prescribed modifications and his/her likes, dislikes, and daily routines
6. provide information about various antacids available if appropriate; instruct client to alternate antacids *in order to minimize side effects such as diarrhea or constipation*
7. assist client in setting up a medication schedule that he/she can incorporate into daily activities and that maximizes the length of effectiveness of the medication (e.g. antacids taken after rather than before meals have a longer buffering action)
8. encourage questions and allow time for reinforcement and clarification of information provided
9. provide written instructions about future appointments with health care provider, diet, medications, and signs and symptoms to report
10. if client has concerns regarding the cost of medications, obtain a social service consult to assist him/her with financial planning and to obtain financial aid if indicated
11. provide information about and encourage utilization of community resources that can assist client to make necessary life-style changes (e.g. stop smoking programs, stress management classes, vocational rehabilitation, counseling services).

c. Assess for and reinforce behaviors suggesting future compliance with prescribed treatments (e.g. participation in the treatment plan, statements reflecting ways to modify personal habits).

d. Include significant others in explanations and teaching sessions and encourage their support.

☐ ▬▬▬▬▬▬▬▬▬▬▬▬▬▬▬▬▬▬▬▬▬▬▬▬

7. NURSING DIAGNOSIS

Knowledge deficit regarding follow-up care.

☐ ▬▬▬▬▬▬▬▬▬▬▬▬▬▬▬▬▬▬▬▬▬▬▬▬

DESIRED OUTCOMES	NURSING ACTIONS AND *SELECTED RATIONALES*
7.a. The client will identify ways to promote healing of the existing ulcer and prevent recurrence of peptic ulcers.	7.a.1. Instruct the client in ways *to promote healing of the existing ulcer and prevent recurrence of peptic ulcers:* a. drink decaffeinated or caffeine-free beverages rather than those containing caffeine b. avoid drinking excessive amounts of alcohol (2 ounces or more of ethanol/day) c. drink alcohol only during or immediately after eating (not on an empty stomach) d. avoid ingestion of foods that are known to irritate gastric mucosa directly or by increasing gastric acid production (e.g. whole grains, chocolate, rich pastries, fresh fruits, raw vegetables, spicy foods, meat extracts, extremely hot or cold foods) e. eliminate any other foods and fluids that cause gastric distress f. adhere to a bland diet if prescribed g. eat small, frequent meals and snacks; do not skip meals h. eat slowly and chew food thoroughly i. maintain a calm, relaxed atmosphere at mealtime and whenever possible j. stop smoking k. maintain a balance of physical activity and rest l. avoid stressful situations m. avoid ingestion of over-the-counter medications such as aspirin and ibuprofen; if it is necessary to take these or other ulcerogenic

medications (e.g. corticosteroids, indomethacin), take them with antacids or food whenever possible

n. continue medication therapy as prescribed

o. continue with treatment of any condition that may be contributing to mucosal irritation and ulceration of the gastrointestinal tract (e.g. hormone imbalances, chronic obstructive pulmonary disease).

2. Obtain a dietary consult if client needs assistance in planning meals that incorporate dietary modifications with his/her likes, dislikes, and daily routines.

3. Assist client to identify ways he/she can make necessary life-style changes.

7.b. The client will verbalize an understanding of medication therapy including rationale for, side effects of, schedule for taking, and importance of taking as prescribed.	**7.b.1.** Explain the rationale for, side effects of, and importance of taking medications prescribed.
	
	2. If client is discharged on antacid therapy, instruct to:
	  a. take antacids as ordered (usually 1 tablespoon every hour while awake for 2 weeks to 2 months, then 4 times/day [1 hour after each meal and at bedtime] if epigastric discomfort recurs)
	  b. chew tablets thoroughly and follow with a glass of water
	  c. allow effervescent antacids to stop bubbling before drinking *in order to prevent gaseous distention*
	  d. avoid use of flavored antacids (*mint flavoring tends to hasten gastric emptying*)
	  e. incorporate measures *to delay gastric emptying and enhance effectiveness of antacids* (e.g. lying down for an hour after meals)
	  f. inform health care providers of other medications being taken (*antacid therapy can alter the absorption of many other medications*)
	  g. alternate aluminum-containing antacids (e.g. Amphojel, Basaljel) and magnesium-containing antacids (e.g. Maalox, Mylanta) periodically if signs and symptoms of diarrhea or constipation develop
	  h. avoid antacids high in sodium (e.g. Amphojel, Gaviscon, Di-Gel, Titralac liquid, Basaljel ExtraStrength) if conditions such as hypertension and congestive heart failure exist
	  i. avoid use of antacids high in calcium (e.g. Titralac, Tums) and sodium bicarbonate (e.g. Pepto-Bismol, Alka-Seltzer) on a regular basis
	  j. observe for and report:
	    1. flank pain, pain when urinating, blood in urine (*may indicate urinary stones resulting from excessive amounts of calcium-containing antacids*)
	    2. dizziness, confusion, tingling of fingers and toes or around mouth, muscle twitching, seizures (*may indicate metabolic alkalosis resulting from excessive amounts of antacids containing sodium bicarbonate*)
	    3. thirst, dry mouth, weakness, lethargy (*may indicate hypernatremia resulting from excessive amounts of antacids containing sodium*) and/or swelling of extremities and weight gain (*can occur with the subsequent water retention*)
	    4. constipation not resolved by increased fluid intake, laxatives, stool softeners, and alternating antacids
	    5. diarrhea not controlled by antidiarrheal medication and/or change in brand of antacid.
	
	3. If client is discharged on sucralfate, instruct to:
	  a. take it an hour before meals and at bedtime
	  b. avoid taking antacids for at least 30 minutes before and after taking the medication.
	
	4. If client is discharged on a histamine₂ receptor antagonist (e.g. cimetidine, famotidine, ranitidine), instruct to:
	  a. avoid taking antacids within an hour before or after taking the drug
	  b. monitor for and report mental confusion, persistent diarrhea, muscle pain, or breast enlargement (in males).

7.c. The client will state signs and symptoms to report to the health care provider.	**7.c.** Instruct client to report:
	  1. red or black stools
	  2. bloody or coffee-ground vomitus
	  3. increased feeling of epigastric fullness or abdominal distention
	  4. persistent nausea and/or vomiting
	  5. continued weight loss
	  6. persistent or increased epigastric discomfort

UNIT XII

7. sudden, severe abdominal pain
8. epigastric or abdominal pain that radiates to shoulder or back
9. temperature elevation that lasts more than 2 days
10. persistent or increased weakness and fatigue
11. undesirable side effects of medication therapy (see actions b.2.j and b.4.b in this diagnosis)
12. difficulty controlling physical and emotional stress
13. inability to adhere to diet or medication therapy.

7.d. The client will identify community resources that can assist with making life-style changes necessary to prevent peptic ulcer recurrence.	7.d.1. Provide information about community resources that can assist client to make life-style changes necessary to prevent peptic ulcer recurrence (e.g. stop smoking programs, stress management classes, vocational rehabilitation, counseling services). 2. Initiate a referral if indicated.
7.e. The client will verbalize an understanding of and a plan for adhering to recommended follow-up care including future appointments with health care provider.	7.e.1. Reinforce the importance of follow-up appointments with health care provider. 2. Refer to Nursing Diagnosis 6, action b, for measures to improve client compliance.

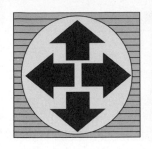
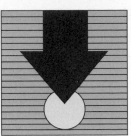
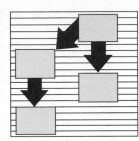
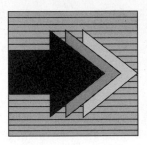
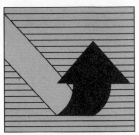

Unit XIII

Nursing Care of the Client with Disturbances of the Liver, Biliary Tract, and Pancreas

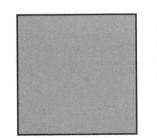
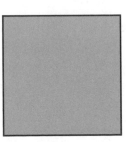
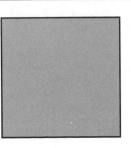

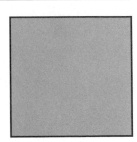

Cholecystectomy

Cholecystectomy is the surgical removal of the gallbladder. It is commonly performed to treat cholecystitis and/or cholelithiasis that have been refractory to conservative management. It may also be performed to treat a malignancy of the gallbladder or surrounding duct system. If stones are present in the common bile duct, a choledocholithotomy will be performed and a T tube will be placed in the common bile duct to maintain adequate flow or drainage of bile until ductal edema has subsided.

This care plan focuses on the adult client hospitalized for a cholecystectomy with common bile duct exploration. Preoperatively, the goals of care are to maintain comfort, reduce fear and anxiety, and prepare the client for the postoperative period. Postoperative goals of care are to maintain comfort, prevent complications, and educate the client regarding follow-up care.

DISCHARGE CRITERIA

Prior to discharge, the client will:

- demonstrate the ability to appropriately care for T tube and surrounding skin if indicated
- verbalize an understanding of the rationale for and constituents of a low- to moderate-fat diet
- state signs and symptoms of complications to report to the health care provider
- verbalize an understanding of and a plan for adhering to recommended follow-up care including future appointments with health care provider, wound care, medications prescribed, and activity level.

NURSING/COLLABORATIVE DIAGNOSES

Postoperative
1. Ineffective breathing patterns:
   a. hypoventilation
   b. hyperventilation □ 721
2. Altered nutrition: less than body requirements □ 721
3. Impaired skin integrity:
   a. surgical incision
   b. impaired wound healing
   c. irritation or breakdown □ 722
4. Potential complications:
   a. hypovolemic shock
   b. abscess and/or fistula formation
   c. peritonitis
   d. pancreatitis
   e. continued obstruction of bile flow □ 722
5. Knowledge deficit regarding follow-up care □ 725

Preoperative

Use in conjunction with the Care Plan on Cholelithiasis/Cholecystitis and the Standardized Preoperative Care Plan.

Postoperative

Use in conjunction with the Standardized Postoperative Care Plan.

1. NURSING DIAGNOSIS

Ineffective breathing patterns:

a. **hypoventilation** related to:
1. reluctance to breathe deeply associated with pain resulting from a high abdominal incision
2. depressant effects of anesthesia and some medications (e.g. narcotic analgesics)
3. weakness and fatigue
4. pressure on the diaphragm resulting from abdominal distention;
b. **hyperventilation** related to pain, fear, and anxiety.

DESIRED OUTCOMES	NURSING ACTIONS AND *SELECTED RATIONALES*
1. The client will maintain an effective breathing pattern (see Standardized Postoperative Care Plan, Nursing Diagnosis 3, for outcome criteria).	1.a. Refer to Standardized Postoperative Care Plan, Nursing Diagnosis 3, for measures related to assessment and management of ineffective breathing patterns. b. Implement additional measures *to improve breathing pattern:* 1. instruct client to bend knees while coughing and deep breathing *in order to relieve tension on abdominal muscles and incision* 2. instruct and assist client to splint incision with hands or pillow when coughing and deep breathing.

2. NURSING DIAGNOSIS

Altered nutrition: less than body requirements related to:

a. loss of nutrients associated with vomiting and nasogastric tube drainage;
b. decreased oral intake associated with nausea, anorexia, and dislike of prescribed diet;
c. increased nutritional needs associated with the increased metabolic rate that occurs during healing;
d. decreased absorption of fats and fat-soluble vitamins associated with excessive loss or obstructed flow of bile.

DESIRED OUTCOMES	NURSING ACTIONS AND *SELECTED RATIONALES*
2. The client will maintain an adequate nutritional status (see Standardized Postoperative Care Plan, Nursing Diagnosis 6, for outcome criteria).	2. Refer to Standardized Postoperative Care Plan, Nursing Diagnosis 6, for measures related to assessment and maintenance of an adequate nutritional status.

3. NURSING DIAGNOSIS

Impaired skin integrity:

a. **surgical incision;**
b. **impaired wound healing** related to inadequate nutritional status, inadequate blood supply to wound area, stress on wound area, infection, and increased levels of glucocorticoids (levels usually rise with stress);
c. **irritation or breakdown** related to contact of skin with wound drainage (bile is extremely irritating to the skin and large amounts of drainage are normal for the first 24–48 hours), pressure from drainage tubes, and use of tape.

DESIRED OUTCOMES	NURSING ACTIONS AND *SELECTED RATIONALES*
3.a. The client will experience normal healing of surgical wounds (see Standardized Postoperative Care Plan, Nursing Diagnosis 9, outcome a, for outcome criteria).	3.a. Refer to Standardized Postoperative Care Plan, Nursing Diagnosis 9, action a, for measures related to assessment and promotion of normal wound healing.
3.b. The client will maintain skin integrity (see Standardized Postoperative Care Plan, Nursing Diagnosis 9, outcome b, for outcome criteria).	3.b. Refer to Standardized Postoperative Care Plan, Nursing Diagnosis 9, action b, for measures related to assessment and prevention of skin irritation and breakdown.

4. COLLABORATIVE DIAGNOSIS

Potential complications:

a. **hypovolemic shock** related to:
   1. increased susceptibility to bleeding associated with decreased production of certain clotting factors resulting from impaired vitamin K absorption preoperatively and in the immediate postoperative period until normal bile flow is restored
   2. fluid volume deficit associated with excessive fluid loss and inadequate fluid replacement;

b. **abscess and/or fistula formation** related to inflammation, presence of increased pressure in the subhepatic space (a result of the accumulation of blood, bile, and lymph), or disruption of the sutures at surgical site;

c. **peritonitis** related to leakage from an abscess or fistula or escape of bile from the cystic or common bile ducts into the peritoneal cavity;

d. **pancreatitis** related to obstruction of the flow of pancreatic secretions as a result of trauma to the pancreatic duct during surgery and inflammation of the common bile duct;

e. **continued obstruction of bile flow** related to residual stones or persistent inflammation and/or strictures of the common bile duct due to surgical trauma.

□ ▮▮▮▮▮▮▮▮▮▮▮▮▮▮▮▮▮▮▮▮▮▮▮▮▮▮▮▮▮▮▮▮▮▮▮

DESIRED OUTCOMES	NURSING ACTIONS AND *SELECTED RATIONALES*
4.a. The client will not develop hypovolemic shock (see Standardized Postoperative Care Plan, Collaborative Diagnosis 19, outcome a, for outcome criteria).	4.a.1. Assess for and report the following: a. excessive bleeding and gastrointestinal and wound drainage, persistent vomiting, and/or difficulty maintaining intravenous fluid intake as ordered b. declining RBC, Hct., and Hgb. levels c. prolonged prothrombin time, partial thromboplastin time, and/or activated partial thromboplastin time d. signs and symptoms of hypovolemic shock (see Standardized Postoperative Care Plan, Collaborative Diagnosis 19, action a.3). 2. Refer to Standardized Postoperative Care Plan, Collaborative Diagnosis 19, actions a.4 and 5, for measures to prevent and treat hypovolemic shock. 3. Monitor for therapeutic and nontherapeutic effects of vitamin K (e.g. phytonadione) injections, whole blood, and/or fresh frozen plasma if administered *to prevent or control bleeding.*
4.b. The client will not develop an abscess and/or fistula as evidenced by: 1. gradual resolution of right upper quadrant pain 2. absence of external bile leakage 3. temperature declining toward normal 4. WBC count declining toward normal.	4.b.1. Assess for and report signs and symptoms of abscess and/or fistula formation (e.g. increased and more constant right upper quadrant pain, bile leakage in wound or around T tube or drain, increase in temperature and pulse rate, further increase in WBC count). 2. Implement measures *to reduce risk of abscess and fistula formation:* a. perform actions *to maintain patency of wound drain and/or T tube if present:* 1. implement measures *to prevent stasis and reflux of drainage:* a. keep drainage tubing free of kinks and dependent loops b. keep drainage apparatus at or below waist level unless ordered otherwise c. empty collection device(s) as necessary and at least every shift 2. implement measures *to prevent inadvertent removal of wound drain and/or T tube:* a. instruct client not to pull on drain(s) or drainage tubing b. use caution when changing dressings surrounding drain(s) c. attach T tube collection device securely to abdominal dressing b. maintain client in a semi-Fowler's position as much as possible when in bed *to reduce accumulation of drainage in the subhepatic space.* 3. If signs and symptoms of an abscess or fistula occur: a. monitor for therapeutic and nontherapeutic effects of anti-infectives if administered b. prepare client for surgical intervention (e.g. incision and drainage, fistulectomy) if planned c. provide emotional support to client and significant others.
4.c. The client will not develop peritonitis as evidenced by: 1. gradual resolution of abdominal pain 2. soft, nondistended abdomen	4.c.1. Assess for and report signs and symptoms of peritonitis (e.g. increase in severity of abdominal pain; generalized abdominal pain; rebound tenderness; tense, rigid abdomen; increase in temperature; tachycardia; tachypnea; hypotension; continued diminished or absent bowel sounds). 2. Monitor WBC counts. Report levels that increase or fail to decline toward normal.

UNIT
XIII

3. temperature declining toward normal
4. stable vital signs
5. gradual return of normal bowel sounds
6. WBC count declining toward normal.

3. Implement measures *to prevent peritonitis:*
   a. question any order for morphine sulfate *(may cause an increase in ductal pressure due to ductal spasm and contraction of the sphincter of Oddi)*
   b. perform actions to reduce risk of abscess and fistula formation (see action b.2 in this diagnosis)
   c. monitor for therapeutic and nontherapeutic effects of anti-infectives if administered.
4. If signs and symptoms of peritonitis occur:
   a. withhold all food and fluid as ordered
   b. place client on bedrest in a semi-Fowler's position *to assist in pooling or localizing gastrointestinal contents in the pelvis rather than under the diaphragm*
   c. insert a nasogastric or intestinal tube and maintain suction as ordered
   d. monitor for therapeutic and nontherapeutic effects of anti-infectives if administered
   e. monitor for therapeutic and nontherapeutic effects of intravenous fluids and/or blood volume expanders if administered *to prevent or treat shock (shock can occur as a result of the escape of protein, fluid, and electrolytes into the peritoneal cavity)*
   f. prepare client for surgical intervention (e.g. repair of leakage site, drainage of abscess, fistulectomy) if planned
   g. provide emotional support to client and significant others.

4.d. The client will experience resolution of pancreatitis if it occurs as evidenced by:
1. gradual resolution of abdominal pain
2. temperature declining toward normal
3. stable B/P and pulse
4. serum amylase and lipase levels declining toward normal
5. renal amylase/creatinine clearance ratio returning toward normal
6. WBC count declining toward normal.

4.d.1. Assess for and report signs and symptoms of pancreatitis (e.g. extension of pain to midepigastric area, left upper quadrant, or back; increase in temperature; tachycardia; hypotension; elevated serum amylase and lipase levels).
2. Collect a timed (usually 2-hour) urine specimen if ordered. Report an elevated renal amylase/creatinine clearance ratio.
3. Monitor WBC counts. Report levels that increase or fail to decline toward normal.
4. If signs and symptoms of pancreatitis occur:
   a. assist client to assume position of greatest comfort (usually side-lying with knees flexed)
   b. maintain food and fluid restrictions as ordered
   c. insert nasogastric tube and maintain suction if ordered *(removal of gastric juices reduces the pancreatic stimulation normally caused by these juices)*
   d. monitor for therapeutic and nontherapeutic effects of the following medications if administered:
      1. analgesics and smooth muscle relaxants (e.g. nitroglycerin) *to reduce pain*
      2. antacids and histamine$_2$ receptor antagonists (e.g. cimetidine, ranitidine, famotidine) *to neutralize and/or reduce output of hydrochloric acid and thereby reduce pancreatic stimulation*
   e. refer to Care Plan on Pancreatitis for additional care measures.

4.e. The client will experience normal bile flow within 7–10 days after surgery as evidenced by:
1. decline in output of bile to 200 cc/day
2. resolution of right upper quadrant pain
3. absence of pain, nausea, and fullness when T tube is clamped
4. absence of jaundice; clay-colored stools; dark, foamy urine.

4.e.1. Assess for and report signs and symptoms of continued bile flow obstruction (e.g. T tube draining more than 1000 cc in 24 hours; T tube drainage of greater than 500 cc/day for longer than 5 days; persistent pain, nausea, or feeling of fullness when T tube is clamped; jaundice; clay-colored stools; dark, foamy urine).
2. If signs and symptoms of bile flow obstruction occur:
   a. leave T tube unclamped
   b. perform actions to maintain patency of T tube (see action b.2.a in this diagnosis)
   c. prepare client for T tube cholangiogram
   d. assist with irrigation of T tube if performed
   e. prepare client for basket removal of stone(s) through T tube, ductal stone removal via endoscopic papillotomy, or surgery if planned
   f. provide emotional support to client and significant others.

5. NURSING DIAGNOSIS

Knowledge deficit regarding follow-up care.

DESIRED OUTCOMES	NURSING ACTIONS AND *SELECTED RATIONALES*
5.a. The client will demonstrate the ability to appropriately care for T tube and surrounding skin if indicated.	5.a.1. If the client is to be discharged with a T tube in place, instruct regarding care of the T tube and surrounding skin: a. cleanse the skin around the T tube insertion site daily and apply a skin protectant (e.g. karaya gel, zinc oxide, petrolatum); cover the site with a dry sterile dressing b. always keep the T tube drainage collection device at or below the insertion site c. keep the tubing pinned to the dressing and avoid any strain or pull on the tubing d. empty the drainage collection device at least twice daily or more often if needed; keep a record of the amount of drainage e. when emptying the drainage collection device, check to see that the tube has not become dislodged (this can be easily monitored if the tube is marked at the skin line before discharge) f. clamp T tube only as instructed. 2. Allow time for questions, clarification, and return demonstration of care of T tube and surrounding skin.
5.b. The client will verbalize an understanding of the rationale for and constituents of a low- to moderate-fat diet.	5.b.1. Explain the rationale for avoiding excessive fat intake for the first 4–6 weeks after surgery (some physicians instruct client to avoid only those foods that cause epigastric discomfort). 2. Instruct client to increase fat intake gradually and introduce foods/fluids high in fat (e.g. butter, cream, oils, whole milk, ice cream, pork, fried foods, gravies, nuts) one at a time.
5.c. The client will state signs and symptoms of complications to report to the health care provider.	5.c.1. Refer to Standardized Postoperative Care Plan, Nursing Diagnosis 20, action c, for signs and symptoms to report to health care provider. 2. Instruct client to report these additional signs and symptoms: a. increased itchiness or yellowing of skin b. clay-colored stools or dark amber urine c. green-brown drainage around T tube or from wound site d. more than 500 cc/day of drainage from T tube e. persistent heartburn and feeling of bloating.
5.d. The client will verbalize an understanding of and a plan for adhering to recommended follow-up care including future appointments with health care provider, wound care, medications prescribed, and activity level.	5.d.1. Refer to Standardized Postoperative Care Plan, Nursing Diagnosis 20, for routine postoperative instructions and measures to improve client compliance. 2. Instruct client to avoid lifting objects over 10 pounds for 4–6 weeks after surgery.

UNIT
XIII

Cholelithiasis/Cholecystitis

Cholelithiasis refers to the presence of gallstones in the gallbladder. Gallstones form when bile becomes supersaturated with insoluble solutes such as cholesterol, calcium bilirubinate or other calcium salts, and bilirubin polymers. Stasis of bile resulting from spasm of the sphincter of Oddi or decreased contractility or delayed emptying of the gallbladder further contributes to the development of gallstones. Stones either remain in the gallbladder or migrate into the duct system where they may cause obstruction. The severity of the symptoms experienced by the client depends on the degree of bile flow obstruction.

Cholecystitis is an inflammation of the gallbladder, usually results from cystic duct obstruction and chemical irritation, and is most commonly associated with gallstones. Scarring occurs following an acute attack and results in loss of function of the gallbladder if large amounts of tissue have become fibrotic.

This care plan focuses on the adult client hospitalized for diagnosis and conservative treatment of cholelithiasis and/or cholecystitis. The goals of treatment are to relieve pain, prevent complications, and educate the client regarding follow-up care.

DISCHARGE CRITERIA

Prior to discharge, the client will:

- verbalize an understanding of the rationale for and constituents of a low- to moderate-fat diet
- identify ways to minimize the risk of bleeding
- state signs and symptoms to report to the health care provider
- verbalize an understanding of and a plan for adhering to recommended follow-up care including future appointments with health care provider and medications prescribed.

NURSING/COLLABORATIVE DIAGNOSES

1. Anxiety □ 727
2. Ineffective breathing patterns:
   a. hypoventilation
   b. hyperventilation □ 727
3. Altered fluid and electrolyte balance: fluid volume deficit, hyponatremia, hypokalemia, hypochloremia, and metabolic alkalosis □ 728
4. Altered nutrition: less than body requirements □ 729
5A. Altered comfort: pain in epigastric area or right upper quadrant of abdomen with radiation to right scapula or shoulder □ 730
5B. Altered comfort: pruritus □ 731
5C. Altered comfort: nausea and vomiting □ 731
5D. Altered comfort: dyspepsia, gas pain, and abdominal distention □ 732
6. Altered oral mucous membrane: dryness □ 733
7. Potential complications:
   a. abscess or fistula formation
   b. peritonitis
   c. pancreatitis
   d. cholangitis
   e. bleeding □ 733
8. Knowledge deficit regarding follow-up care □ 736

1. NURSING DIAGNOSIS

Anxiety related to unfamiliar environment, discomfort, unknown diagnosis, and lack of understanding of diagnostic tests and treatments.

DESIRED OUTCOMES	NURSING ACTIONS AND *SELECTED RATIONALES*

1. The client will experience a reduction in fear and anxiety as evidenced by:
   a. verbalization of feeling less anxious or fearful
   b. relaxed facial expression and body movements
   c. stable vital signs
   d. usual skin color
   e. verbalization of an understanding of hospital routines, diagnostic tests, diagnosis, and treatments.

1.a. Assess client for signs and symptoms of fear and anxiety (e.g. verbalization of fears and concerns; tenseness; tremors; irritability; restlessness; diaphoresis; tachypnea; tachycardia; elevated blood pressure; facial tension, pallor, or flushing; noncompliance with treatment plan).
   b. Ascertain effectiveness of current coping skills.
   c. Implement measures *to reduce fear and anxiety:*
      1. orient to hospital environment, equipment, and routines
      2. introduce staff who will be participating in his/her care; if possible, maintain consistency in staff assigned to his/her care *to provide feelings of stability and comfort with the environment*
      3. assure client that staff members are nearby; respond to call signal as soon as possible
      4. maintain a calm, confident manner when interacting with client
      5. encourage verbalization of fear and anxiety; provide feedback
      6. explain all diagnostic tests (e.g. blood and urine studies, cholecystogram, cholangiogram, endoscopic retrograde cholangiopancreatography [ERCP], radionuclide imaging, ultrasonography)
      7. when the diagnosis has been confirmed, assure client that he/she has not had a "heart attack" (the symptoms of cholelithiasis and cholecystitis often mimic those of a "heart attack")
      8. reinforce physician's explanations and clarify any misconceptions client may have about cholelithiasis and/or cholecystitis and the treatment plan
      9. perform actions to reduce discomfort (see Nursing Diagnoses 5.A, action 5; 5.B, actions 2 and 3; 5.C, action 2; and 5.D, action 3)
      10. provide a calm, restful environment
      11. instruct in relaxation techniques and encourage participation in diversional activities once severe pain has subsided
      12. assist client to identify specific stressors and ways to cope with them
      13. encourage significant others to project a caring, concerned attitude without obvious anxiousness
      14. monitor for therapeutic and nontherapeutic effects of antianxiety agents if administered.
   d. Include significant others in orientation and teaching sessions and encourage their continued support of the client.
   e. Provide information based on current needs of the client and significant others at a level they can understand. Encourage questions and clarification of information provided.
   f. Consult physician if above actions fail to control fear and anxiety.

2. NURSING DIAGNOSIS

Ineffective breathing patterns:

a. **hypoventilation** related to reluctance to breathe deeply associated with severe upper abdominal pain, depressant effects of some medications (e.g. narcotic analgesics), and pressure on the diaphragm associated with abdominal distention;
b. **hyperventilation** related to pain, fear, and anxiety.

UNIT
XIII

DESIRED OUTCOMES	NURSING ACTIONS AND *SELECTED RATIONALES*

2. The client will maintain an effective breathing pattern as evidenced by:
   a. normal rate, rhythm, and depth of respirations
   b. blood gases within normal range.

2.a. Assess for signs and symptoms of ineffective breathing patterns (e.g. shallow, rapid, or slow respirations).
   b. Monitor blood gases. Report abnormal results.
   c. Monitor for and report significant changes in ear oximetry and capnograph results.
   d. Implement measures *to improve breathing pattern:*
      1. perform actions to reduce pain (see Nursing Diagnosis 5.A, action 5)
      2. perform actions to decrease fear and anxiety (see Nursing Diagnosis 1, action c)
      3. instruct client to breathe slowly if he/she is hyperventilating
      4. perform actions to reduce abdominal distention (see Nursing Diagnosis 5.D, action 3) *in order to decrease pressure on the diaphragm*
      5. place client in a semi- to high Fowler's position unless contraindicated
      6. if client is on bedrest, assist him/her to turn at least every 2 hours
      7. instruct client to deep breathe or use inspiratory exerciser at least every 2 hours
      8. administer or assist with IPPB treatments as ordered
      9. increase activity as allowed and tolerated
      10. administer central nervous system depressants (e.g. narcotic analgesics, sedatives) judiciously; hold medication and consult physician if respiratory rate is less than 12/minute.
   e. Consult physician if:
      1. ineffective breathing patterns continue
      2. signs and symptoms of impaired gas exchange (e.g. confusion, restlessness, irritability, cyanosis, decreased PaO_2 and increased $PaCO_2$ levels) are present.

☐ ▬▬▬▬▬▬▬▬▬▬▬▬▬▬▬▬▬▬▬▬▬▬▬▬▬▬▬▬▬

3. NURSING/COLLABORATIVE DIAGNOSIS

Altered fluid and electrolyte balance: fluid volume deficit, hyponatremia, hypokalemia, hypochloremia, and metabolic alkalosis related to decreased oral intake and excessive loss of fluid and electrolytes associated with vomiting and nasogastric tube drainage.

☐ ▬▬▬▬▬▬▬▬▬▬▬▬▬▬▬▬▬▬▬▬▬▬▬▬▬▬▬▬▬

DESIRED OUTCOMES	NURSING ACTIONS AND *SELECTED RATIONALES*

3. The client will maintain fluid and electrolyte balance as evidenced by:
   a. normal skin turgor
   b. moist mucous membranes
   c. stable weight
   d. B/P and pulse within normal range for client and stable with position change
   e. balanced intake and output
   f. urine specific gravity between 1.010–1.030
   g. no evidence of confusion, irritability, lethargy,

3.a. Assess for and report signs and symptoms of:
   1. fluid volume deficit:
      a. decreased skin turgor, dry mucous membranes, thirst
      b. weight loss greater than 0.5 kg/day
      c. low B/P and/or decline in systolic B/P of at least 15 mm Hg with concurrent rise in pulse when client sits up
      d. weak, rapid pulse
      e. output less than intake with urine specific gravity higher than 1.030 (reflects an actual rather than potential fluid volume deficit)
   2. hyponatremia (e.g. nausea and vomiting, abdominal cramps, weakness, lethargy, twitching, confusion, seizures)
   3. hypokalemia (e.g. irregular pulse, muscle weakness and cramping, paresthesias, nausea and vomiting, hypoactive or absent bowel sounds, drowsiness)
   4. hypochloremia (e.g. twitching, tetany, depressed respirations)

excessive thirst, ileus, cardiac arrhythmias, muscle weakness

h. normal serum osmolality, electrolytes, and blood gases.

5. metabolic alkalosis (e.g. dizziness; confusion; bradypnea; tingling of fingers, toes, and circumoral area; muscle twitching; seizures).

b. Monitor serum osmolality, electrolyte, and blood gas results. Report abnormal values.

c. Implement measures *to prevent and treat fluid and electrolyte imbalances*:
1. perform actions to reduce nausea and vomiting (see Nursing Diagnosis 5.C, action 2)
2. if irrigation of nasogastric tube is indicated, use normal saline rather than water
3. monitor for therapeutic and nontherapeutic effects of fluid and electrolyte replacements if administered
4. maintain a fluid intake of at least 2500 cc/day unless contraindicated
5. when oral intake is allowed, assist client to select foods/fluids high in potassium (e.g. bananas, potatoes, raisins, figs, apricots, dates, Gatorade, fruit juices) and sodium (e.g. bouillon, catsup, soups, pickles, processed cheese, canned vegetables).

d. Consult physician if signs and symptoms of fluid and electrolyte imbalances persist or worsen.

---

4. NURSING DIAGNOSIS

Altered nutrition: less than body requirements related to:

a. decreased oral intake associated with nausea, dyspepsia, pain, and self-imposed or prescribed dietary restrictions;
b. loss of nutrients associated with vomiting;
c. decreased absorption of fats and fat-soluble vitamins associated with bile flow obstruction.

DESIRED OUTCOMES	NURSING ACTIONS AND *SELECTED RATIONALES*

4. The client will maintain an adequate nutritional status as evidenced by:
a. weight within normal range for client's age, height, and build
b. normal BUN and serum albumin, protein, Hct., Hgb., cholesterol, and lymphocyte levels
c. triceps skinfold measurements within normal range
d. usual strength and activity tolerance
e. healthy oral mucous membrane.

4.a. Assess the client for signs and symptoms of malnutrition:
1. weight below normal for client's age, height, and build
2. abnormal BUN and low serum albumin, protein, Hct., Hgb., cholesterol, and lymphocyte levels
3. triceps skinfold measurement less than normal for build
4. weakness and fatigue
5. stomatitis.

b. Reassess nutritional status on a regular basis and report decline.
c. Monitor percentage of meals eaten.
d. Assess the client to determine causes of inadequate intake (e.g. nausea, severe pain, dyspepsia, food and fluid restrictions).
e. Implement measures *to improve nutritional status*:
1. when food and fluids are allowed, perform actions *to improve oral intake*:
a. implement measures to reduce nausea, vomiting, and dyspepsia (see Nursing Diagnoses 5.C, action 2 and 5.D, action 3)
b. implement measures to reduce pain (see Nursing Diagnosis 5.A, action 5)
c. provide oral care before meals
d. serve small portions of nutritious foods/fluids that are appealing to the client
e. provide a clean, relaxed, pleasant atmosphere
f. obtain a dietary consult if necessary to assist client in selecting foods/fluids that meet nutritional needs as well as preferences
2. ensure that meals are well balanced and high in essential nutrients (diet

UNIT XIII

> may be advanced from powdered protein and carbohydrate supplements in skim milk to a low- to moderate-fat diet)
>
> 3. monitor for therapeutic and nontherapeutic effects of fat-soluble vitamins if administered.
>
> f. Perform a 72-hour calorie count if nutritional status declines.
> g. Consult physician regarding alternative methods of providing nutrition (e.g. parenteral nutrition, tube feedings) if client does not consume enough food or fluids to meet nutritional needs.

☐ ▅▅▅▅▅▅▅▅▅▅▅▅▅▅▅▅▅▅▅▅▅▅▅▅▅▅▅▅▅▅▅▅

5.A. NURSING DIAGNOSIS

Altered comfort:* pain in epigastric area or right upper quadrant of abdomen with radiation to right scapula or shoulder related to inflammation and distention of the gallbladder and obstruction and spasms of the bile ducts.

---

* In this care plan, the nursing diagnosis "pain" is included under the diagnostic label of altered comfort.

☐ ▅▅▅▅▅▅▅▅▅▅▅▅▅▅▅▅▅▅▅▅▅▅▅▅▅▅▅▅▅▅▅▅

DESIRED OUTCOMES	NURSING ACTIONS AND *SELECTED RATIONALES*

5.A. The client will experience diminished pain in epigastric area, right upper quadrant of abdomen, and right scapula and shoulder as evidenced by:
1. verbalization of pain relief
2. relaxed facial expression and body positioning
3. increased participation in activities
4. stable vital signs.
	5.A.1. Determine how the client usually responds to pain.
	2. Assess for nonverbal signs of pain (e.g. wrinkled brow; clenched fists; reluctance to move; guarding of abdomen; rubbing right shoulder; facial pallor or flushing; rapid, shallow respirations; change in B/P; tachycardia).
	3. Assess verbal complaints of pain. Ask client to be specific about location, severity, and type of pain. (A feeling of increased pain with a transient inspiratory arrest upon deep palpation of the right upper quadrant [Murphy's sign] is indicative of cholecystitis.)
	4. Assess for factors that seem to aggravate and alleviate pain.
	5. Implement measures *to reduce pain:*
	  a. perform actions *to reduce stimulation of gallbladder contractions:*
	    1. maintain NPO status as ordered
	    2. insert nasogastric tube and maintain suction as ordered
	    3. when oral intake is allowed, maintain dietary restrictions of fat as ordered (avoid foods/fluids high in fat such as butter, cream, oils, whole milk, ice cream, pork, fried foods, gravies, and nuts)
	    4. administer anticholinergics as ordered
	  b. monitor for therapeutic and nontherapeutic effects of anti-infectives if administered *to prevent or treat infection and subsequently reduce inflammation*
	  c. monitor for therapeutic and nontherapeutic effects of chenodeoxycholic acid if administered *to dissolve gallstones* (the client will need to continue taking this medication following discharge *because it takes from 6 months to 2 years to dissolve a cholesterol stone when this medication is administered orally*)
	  d. provide or assist with nonpharmacological measures for pain relief (e.g. back rub, position change, relaxation techniques, guided imagery, quiet conversation, restful environment, diversional activities)
	  e. monitor for therapeutic and nontherapeutic effects of the following medications if administered *to relieve pain:*
	    1. analgesics (morphine sulfate should be avoided *because it increases spasms of the sphincter of Oddi*)
	    2. smooth muscle relaxants (e.g. nitroglycerin) *to relieve ductal spasms*
	  f. prepare client for endoscopic ductal stone removal, infusion of cholesterol stone solvent, or extracorporeal shock-wave lithotripsy if planned.
	6. Consult physician if above measures fail to provide adequate pain relief.

5.B. NURSING DIAGNOSIS

Altered comfort: pruritus related to bile salt accumulation underneath the skin associated with obstruction of bile flow.

DESIRED OUTCOMES	NURSING ACTIONS AND *SELECTED RATIONALES*

5.B. The client will experience relief of pruritus as evidenced by:
1. verbalization of same
2. no scratching or rubbing of skin.
	5.B.1. Assess pruritus including onset, characteristics, location, factors that aggravate or alleviate it, and client tolerance.
	2. Instruct client in and/or implement measures *to relieve pruritus:*
	  a. perform actions *to promote capillary constriction:*
	    1. apply cool, moist compresses to pruritic areas
	    2. maintain a cool environment
	  b. apply emollients to skin *to help alleviate dryness*
	  c. add emollients, cornstarch, baking soda, or oatmeal to bath water
	  d. use tepid water and mild soaps for bathing
	  e. pat skin dry, making sure to dry thoroughly
	  f. encourage participation in diversional activity
	  g. utilize cutaneous stimulation techniques (e.g. massage, pressure, vibration, stroking with soft brush) at the site of itching or acupressure points
	  h. encourage client to wear loose cotton garments
	  i. utilize relaxation techniques.
	3. Monitor for therapeutic and nontherapeutic effects of antihistamines, antipruritic lotions, and cholestyramine *(binds bile salts and reduces their accumulation under skin)* if administered *to relieve itching.*
	4. Consult physician if above measures fail to alleviate pruritus or if the skin becomes excoriated.

5.C. NURSING DIAGNOSIS

Altered comfort: nausea and vomiting related to stimulation of the vomiting center associated with:

1. vagal and/or sympathetic stimulation resulting from visceral irritation due to gallbladder and bile duct inflammation and abdominal distention;
2. cortical stimulation due to pain and stress.

UNIT
XIII

DESIRED OUTCOMES	NURSING ACTIONS AND *SELECTED RATIONALES*

5.C. The client will experience relief of nausea and vomiting as evidenced by:
1. verbalization of relief of nausea
2. absence of vomiting.
	5.C.1. Assess client to determine factors that contribute to nausea and vomiting (e.g. eating, particular foods, certain positions, pain).
	2. Implement measures *to reduce nausea and vomiting:*
	  a. maintain patency of nasogastric tube (e.g. keep tubing free of kinks, irrigate and maintain suction as ordered) if present
	  b. eliminate noxious sights and smells from the environment *(noxious stimuli cause cortical stimulation of the vomiting center)*
	  c. instruct client to change positions slowly *(movement stimulates the chemoreceptor trigger zone)*

    d. provide oral hygiene every 2 hours and after each emesis

    e. perform actions to reduce fear and anxiety (see Nursing Diagnosis 1, action c)

    f. perform actions to reduce pain and abdominal distention (see Nursing Diagnoses 5.A, action 5 and 5.D, action 3)

    g. encourage client to take deep, slow breaths when nauseated

    h. when oral intake is allowed:

       1. advance diet as tolerated

       2. instruct client to ingest foods and fluids slowly

       3. instruct client to eat dry foods (e.g. toast, crackers) and avoid drinking liquids with meals if nauseated

       4. provide small, frequent meals rather than 3 large ones

       5. instruct client to avoid the following:

          a. foods/fluids high in fat (e.g. butter, cream, oils, whole milk, ice cream, pork, fried foods, gravies, nuts)

          b. foods/fluids that irritate the gastric mucosa (e.g. spicy foods; citrus fruits or juices; caffeine-containing items such as chocolate, tea, coffee, or colas)

       6. instruct client to rest after eating with head of bed elevated

    i. monitor for therapeutic and nontherapeutic effects of antiemetics if administered (phenothiazines are contraindicated *because of their potential cholestatic effect).*

  3. Consult physician if above measures fail to control nausea and vomiting.

5.D. NURSING DIAGNOSIS

Altered comfort: dyspepsia, gas pain, and abdominal distention related to gas accumulation associated with impaired fat digestion due to bile flow obstruction.

DESIRED OUTCOMES	NURSING ACTIONS AND *SELECTED RATIONALES*

5.D. The client will experience diminished dyspepsia, gas pain, and abdominal distention as evidenced by:
1. verbalization of same
2. relaxed facial expression and body positioning
3. diminished eructation
4. decrease in abdominal distention.
	5.D.1. Assess for nonverbal signs of dyspepsia, gas pain, and abdominal distention (e.g. clutching and guarding of abdomen, restlessness, reluctance to move, grimacing, frequent eructation, increase in abdominal girth, dyspnea).
	2. Assess for verbal complaints of indigestion, gas pain, and abdominal fullness.
	3. Implement measures *to reduce gastrointestinal gas accumulation in order to decrease dyspepsia, gas pain, and abdominal distention:*
	  a. encourage and assist client with frequent position change and ambulation as soon as allowed and tolerated (*activity stimulates expulsion of flatus*)
	  b. instruct client to avoid activities such as gum chewing, sucking on hard candy, and smoking *in order to reduce air swallowing*
	  c. maintain patency of nasogastric tube if present
	  d. when oral intake is allowed, instruct client to avoid the following:
	    1. gas-producing foods/fluids (e.g. cabbage, onions, popcorn, baked beans, carbonated beverages)
	    2. foods/fluids high in fat (e.g. butter, cream, oils, whole milk, ice cream, pork, fried foods, gravies, nuts)
	  e. encourage client to eructate and expel flatus whenever the urge is felt
	  f. monitor for therapeutic and nontherapeutic effects of antiflatulents if administered *to reduce gas accumulation.*
	4. Consult physician if signs and symptoms of dyspepsia, gas pain, and abdominal distention persist or worsen.

6. NURSING DIAGNOSIS

Altered oral mucous membrane: dryness related to:
a. fluid volume deficit associated with fluid loss (resulting from vomiting or naso-gastric tube drainage) and fluid restrictions;
b. decreased salivation associated with fluid volume deficit and treatment with some medications (e.g. narcotic analgesics, anticholinergics);
c. mouth breathing when nasogastric tube is in place.

DESIRED OUTCOMES	NURSING ACTIONS AND *SELECTED RATIONALES*

6. The client will maintain a moist, intact oral mucous membrane.	6.a. Assess client every shift for dryness of the oral mucosa.
	b. Implement measures *to relieve dryness of the oral mucous membrane:*
	  1. instruct and assist client to perform good oral hygiene as often as needed; avoid use of lemon-glycerin swabs and commercial mouthwashes containing alcohol *(these products have a drying or irritating effect on oral mucous membrane)*
	  2. encourage client to rinse mouth frequently with water
	  3. lubricate client's lips with Vaseline, K-Y jelly, ChapStick, Blistex, or mineral oil when oral care is given
	  4. encourage client to breathe through nose if possible
	  5. encourage client not to smoke *(smoking further irritates and dries the mucosa)*
	  6. maintain intravenous fluid administration as ordered *to improve hydration*
	  7. provide sips of water frequently if allowed
	  8. encourage client to use artificial saliva (e.g. Moi-stir, Salivart) *to lubricate the mucous membrane*
	  9. advance oral intake as soon as allowed and tolerated *to improve hydration and stimulate salivation.*
	c. If oral mucosa is irritated or cracked, implement measures *to relieve discomfort and promote healing:*
	  1. assist client to select soft, bland, and nonacidic foods
	  2. instruct client to avoid extremely hot or cold foods/fluids
	  3. use a soft bristle brush or low-pressure power spray for oral care
	  4. monitor for therapeutic and nontherapeutic effects of topical anesthetics, oral protective pastes, and topical and systemic analgesics if administered.
	d. Consult physician if dryness, irritation, and discomfort persist.

UNIT XIII

7. COLLABORATIVE DIAGNOSIS

Potential complications:
a. **abscess or fistula formation** related to inflammation and presence of increased cholecystic and ductal pressure;
b. **peritonitis** related to leakage from an abscess or fistula or escape of bile into the peritoneal cavity associated with rupture of the gallbladder or cystic or common bile duct;
c. **pancreatitis** related to obstruction of the flow of pancreatic secretions as a result of a stone or inflammation in the common bile duct;
d. **cholangitis** related to irritation and inflammation of bile ducts associated with presence of ductal stones;
e. **bleeding** related to decreased production of certain clotting factors associated with impaired vitamin K absorption resulting from bile flow obstruction.

DESIRED OUTCOMES	NURSING ACTIONS AND *SELECTED RATIONALES*

7.a. The client will experience resolution of any abscess and/or fistula that develops as evidenced by:
1. decrease in abdominal pain
2. temperature declining toward normal
3. WBC count declining toward normal.

7.a.1. Assess for and report signs and symptoms of abscess and/or fistula formation (e.g. increased and more constant abdominal pain, further increase in temperature and pulse rate, further increase in WBC count).
2. If signs and symptoms of an abscess or fistula occur:
   a. monitor for therapeutic and nontherapeutic effects of anti-infectives if administered
   b. prepare client for surgical intervention (e.g. incision and drainage, fistulectomy) if indicated
   c. provide emotional support to client and significant others.

7.b. The client will not develop peritonitis as evidenced by:
1. gradual resolution of abdominal pain
2. soft, nondistended abdomen
3. temperature declining toward normal
4. stable vital signs
5. normal bowel sounds
6. WBC count declining toward normal.

7.b.1. Assess for and report signs and symptoms of peritonitis (e.g. increase in severity of abdominal pain; generalized abdominal pain; rebound tenderness; tense, rigid abdomen; further increase in temperature; tachycardia; tachypnea; hypotension; diminished or absent bowel sounds).
2. Monitor WBC counts. Report levels that increase or fail to decline toward normal.
3. Implement measures *to prevent peritonitis:*
   a. perform actions to reduce stimulation of gallbladder contraction (see Nursing Diagnosis 5.A, action 5.a) *in order to reduce the risk of gallbladder and ductal rupture*
   b. if an incision and drainage of an abscess or a fistulectomy was done and drain is present:
     1. keep drain free of kinks
     2. perform actions *to prevent inadvertent removal of drain:*
       a. use caution when changing dressings surrounding drain
       b. instruct client not to pull on drain or drainage tubing
     3. use aseptic technique during dressing changes
     4. keep dressings clean and dry
   c. monitor for therapeutic and nontherapeutic effects of anti-infectives if administered.
4. If signs and symptoms of peritonitis occur:
   a. withhold all food and fluid as ordered
   b. place client on bedrest in a semi-Fowler's position *to assist in pooling or localizing gastrointestinal contents in the pelvis rather than under the diaphragm*
   c. insert a nasogastric or intestinal tube and maintain suction as ordered
   d. monitor for therapeutic and nontherapeutic effects of anti-infectives if administered
   e. monitor for therapeutic and nontherapeutic effects of intravenous fluids and/or blood volume expanders if administered *to prevent or treat shock (shock can occur as a result of the escape of protein, fluid, and electrolytes into the peritoneal cavity)*
   f. prepare client for surgical intervention (e.g. repair of perforation, removal of abscess, fistulectomy) if indicated
   g. provide emotional support to client and significant others.

7.c. The client will experience resolution of pancreatitis if it occurs as evidenced by:
1. gradual resolution of abdominal pain
2. temperature declining toward normal
3. stable B/P and pulse
4. serum amylase and lipase levels declining toward normal
5. renal amylase/creatinine clearance ratio returning toward normal
6. WBC count declining toward normal.

7.c.1. Assess for and report signs and symptoms of pancreatitis (e.g. extension of pain to midepigastric area, left upper quadrant, or back; further increase in temperature; tachycardia; hypotension; elevated serum amylase and lipase levels).
2. Collect a timed (usually 2-hour) urine specimen if ordered. Report an elevated renal amylase/creatinine clearance ratio.
3. Monitor WBC counts. Report levels that increase or fail to decline toward normal.
4. If signs and symptoms of pancreatitis occur:
   a. assist client to assume position of greatest comfort (usually side-lying with knees flexed)
   b. maintain food and fluid restrictions as ordered
   c. insert nasogastric tube and maintain suction as ordered (*removal of gastric juices reduces pancreatic stimulation normally caused by these juices*)
   d. monitor for therapeutic and nontherapeutic effects of the following medications if administered:

1. analgesics and smooth muscle relaxants (e.g. nitroglycerin) *to reduce pain*
2. antacids and histamine₂ receptor antagonists (e.g. cimetidine, ranitidine, famotidine) *to neutralize and/or reduce output of hydrochloric acid and thereby reduce pancreatic stimulation*

e. assist with peritoneal lavage if indicated (may be performed *to remove toxic pancreatic exudate from the peritoneal cavity*)
f. refer to Care Plan on Pancreatitis for additional care measures.

7.d. The client will experience resolution of cholangitis if it occurs as evidenced by:
1. gradual resolution of abdominal pain
2. absence of jaundice and chills
3. temperature declining toward normal.

7.d.1. Assess for signs and symptoms of cholangitis (e.g. increased abdominal pain, jaundice, chills, increase in temperature). Be aware that lethargy, confusion, and hypotension with or without the above signs and symptoms may indicate septic shock, which can develop with suppurative cholangitis.
2. If signs and symptoms of cholangitis occur:
   a. monitor for therapeutic and nontherapeutic effects of anti-infectives if administered
   b. prepare client for endoscopic sphincterotomy or surgical removal of ductal stone if planned
   c. provide emotional support to client and significant others.

7.e. The client will not experience unusual bleeding as evidenced by:
1. skin and mucous membranes free of bleeding, petechiae, and ecchymosis
2. absence of unusual joint pain and swelling
3. no further increase in abdominal girth
4. absence of frank or occult blood in stool, urine, and vomitus
5. usual menstrual flow
6. vital signs within normal range for client
7. stable Hct. and Hgb.
8. usual mental status.

7.e.1. Assess client for and report signs and symptoms of unusual bleeding:
   a. petechiae
   b. multiple ecchymotic areas
   c. bleeding gums
   d. frequent or uncontrollable episodes of epistaxis
   e. unusual oozing from injection sites
   f. unusual joint pain or swelling
   g. further increase in abdominal girth
   h. hematemesis, melena, red or smoke-colored urine
   i. hypermenorrhea
   j. significant drop in B/P accompanied by an increased pulse rate
   k. decline in Hct. and Hgb. levels
   l. restlessness, confusion.
2. Monitor coagulation test results (e.g. activated partial thromboplastin time, prothrombin time). Report values greater than 2½ times the control.
3. If coagulation test results are abnormal or Hct. and Hgb. levels decline, test all stools, urine, and vomitus for occult blood. Report positive results.
4. Implement measures *to prevent bleeding:*
   a. use the smallest gauge needle possible when giving injections and performing venous or arterial punctures
   b. apply gentle, prolonged pressure after injections and venous or arterial punctures
   c. take B/P only when necessary and avoid overinflating the cuff
   d. caution client to avoid activities that increase the potential for trauma (e.g. shaving with a straight-edge razor, cutting nails, using stiff bristle toothbrush or dental floss)
   e. pad side rails if client is confused or restless
   f. remove hazardous objects from pathway *to prevent bumps or falls*
   g. instruct client to avoid blowing nose forcefully or straining to have a bowel movement; consult physician about an order for decongestants, stool softeners, and/or laxatives if indicated
   h. monitor for therapeutic and nontherapeutic effects of vitamin K (e.g. phytonadione) injections if administered *to improve clotting ability.*
5. If bleeding occurs and does not subside spontaneously:
   a. apply firm, prolonged pressure to bleeding area if possible
   b. if epistaxis occurs, place client in a high Fowler's position and apply pressure and ice packs to nasal area
   c. maintain oxygen therapy as ordered
   d. perform iced water or saline lavage as ordered *to control gastric bleeding*
   e. administer whole blood, fresh frozen plasma, and/or vitamin K (e.g. phytonadione) injections as ordered
   f. prepare client for surgical repair of bleeding vessels if planned
   g. provide emotional support to client and significant others.

UNIT XIII

□ ▬▬▬▬▬▬▬▬▬▬▬▬▬▬▬▬▬▬▬▬▬

8. NURSING DIAGNOSIS

Knowledge deficit regarding follow-up care.

□ ▬▬▬▬▬▬▬▬▬▬▬▬▬▬▬▬▬▬▬▬▬

DESIRED OUTCOMES	NURSING ACTIONS AND *SELECTED RATIONALES*
8.a. The client will verbalize an understanding of the rationale for and constituents of a low- to moderate-fat diet.	8.a.1. Explain the purpose of a low- to moderate-fat diet in preventing further gallbladder attacks. 2. Instruct the client to avoid foods/fluids high in fat (e.g. butter, cream, oils, whole milk, ice cream, pork, fried foods, gravies, nuts). 3. Obtain a dietary consult if client needs assistance in planning meals that incorporate dietary modifications.

8.b. The client will identify ways to minimize the risk of bleeding.	8.b.1. Instruct client about ways *to minimize risk of bleeding:*
	  a. avoid taking aspirin, aspirin-containing products, and ibuprofen
	  b. use an electric rather than a straight-edge razor
	  c. floss and brush teeth gently
	  d. cut nails carefully
	  e. avoid situations that could result in injury (e.g. contact sports)
	  f. avoid blowing nose forcefully
	  g. avoid straining to have a bowel movement.
	2. Instruct client to control any bleeding by applying firm, prolonged pressure to the area if possible.

8.c. The client will state signs and symptoms to report to the health care provider.	8.c. Instruct client to report the following signs and symptoms: 1. recurrent temperature elevation 2. persistent nausea, vomiting, or flatulence 3. increased abdominal distention 4. persistent pain or spasms 5. increased itchiness of skin, yellow coloring of skin or eyes, and/or dark urine and clay-colored stools *(indicative of bile flow obstruction)* 6. excessive bruising; prolonged or excessive bleeding from skin, nose, or mouth; blood in urine, vomitus, or stools; prolonged or excessive menses; severe headache; or sudden abdominal or back pain.

8.d. The client will verbalize an understanding of and a plan for adhering to recommended follow-up care including future appointments with health care provider and medications prescribed.	8.d.1. Reinforce importance of keeping follow-up appointments with health care provider.
	2. Explain the rationale for, side effects of, and importance of taking prescribed medications (e.g. fat-soluble vitamins, cholestyramine, chenodeoxycholic acid, anti-infectives).
	3. Implement measures *to improve client compliance:*
	  a. include significant others in teaching sessions if possible
	  b. encourage questions and allow time for reinforcement and clarification of information provided
	  c. provide written instructions on future appointments with health care provider, medications prescribed, and signs and symptoms to report.

Cirrhosis

Cirrhosis is a chronic liver disease characterized by distortion of normal liver structure due to degeneration, abnormal regeneration, and eventual fibrosis of the cell mass. The fibrosis or scarring eventually impairs normal liver function and obstructs the portal blood flow. This results in venous congestion in other organs and systems such as the spleen and gastrointestinal tract. The four types of cirrhosis are Laennec's (e.g. portal, alcoholic, fatty, micronodular), postnecrotic, biliary, and cardiac. Laennec's cirrhosis is the most common type and thought to be due to excessive alcohol intake and/or a dietary protein deficiency. All types of cirrhosis have similar signs and symptoms, which are manifestations of impaired liver function, malnutrition, and/or venous congestion. Alcohol-related cirrhosis has additional manifestations (e.g. demyelinating neuropathies, cerebral degeneration, hypogonadism) that are thought to be a direct result of the toxic effects of alcohol.

This care plan focuses on the adult client with alcohol-related Laennec's cirrhosis hospitalized for management of increasing ascites and peripheral edema. The goals of care are to maintain comfort, improve nutritional status and fluid balance, prevent complications, and educate the client regarding follow-up care.

DISCHARGE CRITERIA

Prior to discharge, the client will:

- identify ways to prevent further liver damage
- verbalize an understanding of the rationale for and constituents of the recommended diet
- identify ways to reduce irritation of and stress on esophageal vessels
- identify ways to prevent bleeding
- identify ways to reduce the risk of infection
- identify ways to relieve pruritus
- state signs and symptoms to report to the health care provider
- identify community resources that can assist with home management and adjustment to life-style changes necessary for effective management of cirrhosis
- share concerns and feelings about the diagnosis of cirrhosis; prognosis; and effects of the disease process and its treatment on self-concept, life style, and roles
- verbalize an understanding of and a plan for adhering to recommended follow-up care including future appointments with health care provider, medications prescribed, and activity level.

**UNIT
XIII**

Use in conjunction with the Care Plan on Immobility.

NURSING/COLLABORATIVE DIAGNOSES

1. Anxiety □ *738*
2. Altered respiratory function:
   a. ineffective breathing patterns:
      1. hyperventilation
      2. hypoventilation

1. NURSING DIAGNOSIS

Anxiety related to unfamiliar environment; difficulty breathing; lack of understanding of diagnosis, diagnostic tests, and treatments; uncertainty of prognosis; and possibility of further changes in life style and roles.

DESIRED OUTCOMES	NURSING ACTIONS AND *SELECTED RATIONALES*
1. The client will experience a reduction in fear and anxiety	1.a. Refer to Care Plan on Immobility, Nursing Diagnosis 1, for measures related to assessment and reduction of fear and anxiety.

(see Care Plan on Immobility, Nursing Diagnosis 1, for outcome criteria).

b. Implement additional measures *to reduce fear and anxiety:*
1. explain tests performed to determine the extensiveness of cirrhosis:
   a. blood studies;
      1. serum enzymes (e.g. AST [SGOT], ALT [SGPT], GGT, LDH, alkaline phosphatase [ALP], LAP, 5'-nucleotidase)
      2. serum proteins and protein electrophoresis
      3. indirect (unconjugated), direct (conjugated), and total serum bilirubin levels
      4. serum cholesterol and triglyceride levels
      5. prothrombin time (PT)
      6. complete blood count (CBC)
      7. ammonia levels
   b. urine studies for bilirubin and urobilinogen levels
   c. liver biopsy
   d. angiography
   e. percutaneous transhepatic portography
   f. radioisotope scans, ultrasonography, computed tomography (CT), and/or magnetic resonance imaging (MRI) of liver
   g. esophagoscopy and/or barium contrast esophagography *to detect varices*
2. perform actions to improve respiratory status (see Nursing Diagnosis 2, action e) *in order to decrease dyspnea.*

2. NURSING DIAGNOSIS

Altered respiratory function:*

a. **ineffective breathing patterns:**
   1. **hyperventilation** related to fear, anxiety, and the respiratory stimulant effects of high serum ammonia
   2. **hypoventilation** related to restricted lung expansion associated with:
      a. prolonged side-lying or recumbent position
      b. pleural effusion resulting from fluid volume excess and third-spacing and passage of ascitic fluid into the pleural space through a probable pressure-related defect in the diaphragm
      c. pressure on the diaphragm resulting from peritoneal fluid accumulation (ascites);
b. **ineffective airway clearance** related to:
   1. fluid accumulation in the alveoli and bronchioles associated with pulmonary edema (may result from fluid volume excess and third-spacing)
   2. poor cough effort associated with weakness and fatigue;
c. **impaired gas exchange** related to ineffective breathing patterns and airway clearance, a thickened alveolar-capillary membrane associated with pulmonary edema, and decreased bronchial blood flow associated with portal hypertension.

---

* This diagnostic label includes the following nursing diagnoses: ineffective breathing pattern, ineffective airway clearance, and impaired gas exchange (Carpenito, 1989).

UNIT
XIII

DESIRED OUTCOMES	NURSING ACTIONS AND *SELECTED RATIONALES*
2. The client will experience adequate respiratory function as evidenced by: a. normal rate, rhythm, and depth of respirations	2.a. Assess for and report signs and symptoms of altered respiratory function: 1. rapid, shallow, slow, or irregular respirations 2. dyspnea, orthopnea 3. use of accessory muscles when breathing 4. adventitious breath sounds (e.g. rhonchi, crackles)

b. decreased dyspnea
c. improved breath sounds
d. usual mental status
e. usual skin color
f. blood gases within normal range.

5. diminished or absent breath sounds
6. persistent cough productive of frothy or blood-tinged sputum
7. restlessness, irritability
8. confusion, somnolence
9. dusky or cyanotic skin color.

b. Monitor blood gases. Report abnormal results.
c. Monitor for and report significant changes in ear oximetry and capnograph results.
d. Monitor chest x-ray results and report abnormalities.
e. Implement measures *to improve respiratory status:*
   1. perform actions to reduce fear and anxiety (see Nursing Diagnosis 1)
   2. perform actions to restore fluid balance (see Nursing Diagnosis 3, action a.4) *in order to reduce fluid accumulation in the lungs and peritoneal cavity*
   3. instruct client to breathe slowly if he/she is hyperventilating
   4. instruct client to avoid gas-producing foods/fluids (e.g. beans, cauliflower, cabbage, onions, carbonated beverages) and large meals *in order to prevent gastric distention and additional pressure on the diaphragm*
   5. place client in a semi-Fowler's position (a high Fowler's position is uncomfortable if ascites is severe)
   6. if client is on bedrest, assist him/her to turn at least every 2 hours
   7. instruct client to deep breathe and use inspiratory exerciser at least every 2 hours
   8. perform actions *to facilitate removal of pulmonary secretions:*
      a. instruct and assist client to cough every 1–2 hours
      b. implement measures *to liquefy tenacious secretions:*
         1. humidify inspired air as ordered
         2. assist with administration of mucolytic agents via nebulizer or IPPB treatment (IPPB may be contraindicated *because it increases intrathoracic pressure, which causes impairment of venous blood flow to the right atrium)*
         3. maintain the maximum fluid intake allowed
      c. assist with or perform postural drainage, percussion, and vibration if ordered
      d. perform tracheal suctioning if needed
      e. monitor for therapeutic and nontherapeutic effects of expectorants if administered
   9. maintain oxygen therapy as ordered (initially, high concentrations may be used *to overcome the pressure barrier caused by alveolar fluid accumulation)*
   10. encourage client to stop smoking *(smoking irritates the respiratory tract, causes an increase in mucus production, impairs ciliary function, and decreases oxygen availability)*
   11. increase activity as allowed and tolerated
   12. administer central nervous system depressants (e.g. narcotic analgesics, sedatives, antianxiety agents) judiciously; hold medication and consult physician if respiratory rate is less than 12/minute
   13. assist with thoracentesis and/or paracentesis if performed *to remove pleural and/or peritoneal fluid in order to allow increased lung expansion.*
f. Consult physician if signs and symptoms of impaired respiratory function persist or worsen.

☐ ▰▰▰▰▰▰▰▰▰▰▰▰▰▰▰▰▰▰▰▰▰▰▰

3. NURSING/COLLABORATIVE DIAGNOSIS

Altered fluid and electrolyte balance:

a. **fluid volume excess** related to high aldosterone and antidiuretic hormone (ADH) levels associated with:
   1. increased output of these hormones as a result of decreased renal blood flow

(inadequate renal blood flow results in increased secretion of aldosterone and ADH)

    2. decreased metabolism of these hormones as a result of liver malfunction;

  b. **third-spacing** related to:

    1. low plasma colloid osmotic pressure associated with decreased plasma proteins (a result of decreased hepatic synthesis of plasma proteins and a possible loss of proteins into the peritoneal cavity due to obstructed hepatic lymph flow and increased hydrostatic pressure in the portal vein)

    2. increased hydrostatic pressure in the hepatic venous and lymph systems associated with fatty infiltration and fibrosis of the liver

    3. generalized increase in hydrostatic pressure associated with a fluid volume excess;

  c. **hypokalemia** related to decreased oral intake and potassium loss associated with an increased aldosterone level (aldosterone causes potassium excretion), diuretic therapy, and diarrhea;

  d. **hyponatremia** related to dietary restriction of sodium, hemodilution associated with fluid volume excess, and sodium loss associated with diuretic therapy and diarrhea.

DESIRED OUTCOMES	**NURSING ACTIONS AND *SELECTED RATIONALES***

3.a. The client will experience resolution of fluid imbalance as evidenced by:
1. decline in weight toward client's normal
2. B/P and pulse within normal range for client and stable with position change
3. resolution of gallop rhythms
4. balanced intake and output
5. CVP within normal range
6. resolution of neck vein distention, ascites, peripheral edema
7. less labored respirations
8. improved breath sounds
9. usual mental status.

3.a.1. Assess for signs and symptoms of the following:
  a. fluid volume excess:
    1. significant weight gain (greater than 0.5 kg/day)
    2. elevated B/P and pulse (B/P may not be elevated if fluid has shifted out of the vascular space)
    3. development or worsening of S_3 and/or S_4 gallop rhythms
    4. intake greater than output
    5. elevated CVP (use internal jugular vein pulsation method to estimate CVP if monitoring device not present)
    6. distended neck veins
  b. third-spacing:
    1. peripheral edema
    2. ascites as evidenced by:
      a. increase in abdominal girth (abdominal girth should be measured daily at the same time and in the same location on the abdomen with client in same position)
      b. dull percussion note over abdomen with finding of shifting dullness
      c. presence of abdominal fluid wave
      d. protruding umbilicus and bulging flanks
    3. dyspnea, orthopnea
    4. crackles and diminished or absent breath sounds
    5. change in mental status
    6. decline in systolic B/P of at least 15 mm Hg with a concurrent rise in pulse when client changes from a supine to sitting position.
  2. Monitor chest x-ray results. Report findings of vascular congestion, pleural effusion, and pulmonary edema.
  3. Monitor serum albumin levels. Report below-normal levels *(albumin maintains plasma colloid osmotic pressure)*.
  4. Implement measures *to restore fluid balance:*
    a. perform actions *to reduce fluid volume excess:*
      1. maintain fluid restrictions as ordered (fluids are often restricted to 1500 cc/day)
      2. restrict sodium intake as ordered (sodium is usually restricted to 500–1000 mg/day)
      3. monitor for therapeutic and nontherapeutic effects of diuretics if administered *to increase excretion of water* (usually a thiazide

UNIT XIII

diuretic or furosemide is given in conjunction with an aldosterone-blocking agent)
   b. perform actions *to promote mobilization of fluid back into the vascular space and prevent further third-spacing:*
      1. implement measures to reduce fluid volume excess (see action a.4.a in this diagnosis)
      2. maintain bedrest if ordered or encourage client to lie down periodically *(lying down promotes reshifting of fluid into vascular space)*
      3. implement measures *to increase colloid osmotic pressure:*
         a. provide a diet high in protein and still within the prescribed sodium restriction (e.g. poultry, fish, protein supplements) *to increase serum protein levels* (this is contraindicated if serum ammonia level is elevated or clinical signs and symptoms of encephalopathy are present)
         b. monitor for therapeutic and nontherapeutic effects of salt-poor albumin infusions if administered
         c. assist with intravenous administration of ascitic fluid if indicated (the fluid is obtained by paracentesis using an ultrafiltration device and then administered intravenously *to replace the albumin that is lost; it is given in conjunction with diuretics to mobilize fluid into the vascular space for diuresis)*
      4. prepare client for surgical insertion of a peritoneovenous shunt (e.g. Denver shunt, LeVeen shunt) if planned.
   5. Consult physician if signs and symptoms of fluid imbalance persist or worsen.

3.b. The client will maintain a safe serum potassium level as evidenced by:
   1. regular pulse at 60–100 beats/minute
   2. usual muscle tone and strength
   3. normal bowel sounds
   4. serum potassium within normal range.

3.b.1. Assess for and report signs and symptoms of hypokalemia (e.g. irregular pulse; muscle weakness and cramping; paresthesias; nausea and vomiting; hypoactive or absent bowel sounds; drowsiness; EKG reading showing ST depression, T wave inversion or flattening, and presence of U waves; low serum potassium level).
   2. Implement measures *to prevent or treat hypokalemia:*
      a. perform actions to prevent and treat diarrhea (see Nursing Diagnosis 10, action d)
      b. maintain intravenous and oral potassium replacements as ordered (monitor serum potassium and urine output closely when giving supplemental potassium and consult physician if potassium level increases above normal and/or urine output is less than 30 cc/hour)
      c. if client is taking a potassium-depleting diuretic or if signs and symptoms of hypokalemia are present, encourage intake of foods/fluids high in potassium (e.g. bananas, potatoes, raisins, figs, apricots, dates, Gatorade, fruit juices).
   3. Consult physician if signs and symptoms of hypokalemia persist or worsen.

3.c. The client will maintain a safe serum sodium level as evidenced by:
   1. usual mental status
   2. usual strength and muscle tone
   3. absence of nausea, vomiting, abdominal cramps, twitching, seizure activity
   4. serum sodium within normal range.

3.c.1. Assess for and report signs and symptoms of hyponatremia (e.g. lethargy, confusion, weakness, nausea, vomiting, abdominal cramps, twitching, seizures, low serum sodium level).
   2. Implement measures *to prevent or treat hyponatremia:*
      a. perform actions to prevent and treat diarrhea (see Nursing Diagnosis 10, action d)
      b. perform actions to reduce fluid volume excess (see action a.4.a in this diagnosis)
      c. monitor for therapeutic and nontherapeutic effects of hypertonic or isotonic saline if administered.
   3. Consult physician if signs and symptoms of hyponatremia persist or worsen.

4. NURSING DIAGNOSIS

Altered nutrition: less than body requirements related to:

a. poor eating habits before admission;
b. decreased oral intake associated with anorexia, abdominal pain, dyspepsia, fatigue, dyspnea, dislike of the prescribed diet, and early satiety (a result of increased intra-abdominal pressure);
c. reduced metabolism and storage of nutrients by the liver associated with a reduction of functional tissue;
d. malabsorption of fats and fat-soluble vitamins associated with impaired bile flow;
e. loss of nutrients associated with diarrhea.

DESIRED OUTCOMES	NURSING ACTIONS AND *SELECTED RATIONALES*

4. The client will have an improved nutritional status as evidenced by:
a. dry weight approaching normal range for client's age, height, and build (dry weight is achieved after fluid volume excess has been resolved)
b. improved serum albumin, protein, Hct., Hgb., B$_{12}$, folate, ferritin, cholesterol, and lymphocyte levels
c. triceps skinfold measurements approaching normal range
d. improved strength and activity tolerance
e. healthy oral mucous membrane.
	4.a. Assess the client for signs and symptoms of malnutrition:
	  1. dry weight below normal for client's age, height, and build
	  2. decreased serum albumin, protein, Hct., Hgb., B$_{12}$, folate, ferritin, cholesterol, and lymphocyte levels (these values are also a reflection of impaired liver function)
	  3. triceps skinfold measurement less than normal for build
	  4. weakness and fatigue
	  5. stomatitis.
	  b. Reassess nutritional status on a regular basis and report decline.
	  c. Monitor percentage of meals eaten.
	  d. Assess client to determine causes of inadequate intake (e.g. dyspepsia, fatigue, dyspnea, anorexia).
	  e. Implement measures *to improve nutritional status:*
	    1. perform actions *to improve oral intake:*
	      a. implement measures to relieve abdominal pain and dyspepsia (see Nursing Diagnoses 5.A, action 5 and 5.C, action 3)
	      b. provide oral care before meals
	      c. serve small portions of nutritious foods/fluids that are appealing to client
	      d. provide a clean, relaxed, pleasant atmosphere
	      e. obtain a dietary consult if necessary to assist the client in selecting foods/fluids that meet nutritional needs as well as preferences
	      f. instruct client to use herbs, spices, and salt substitutes (if approved by physician) *in order to make low-sodium diet more palatable*
	      g. elevate head of bed as tolerated for meals *to help relieve dyspnea* (a high Fowler's position may be too uncomfortable if ascites is severe)
	      h. encourage a rest period before meals *to minimize fatigue*
	      i. allow adequate time for meals; reheat food if necessary
	      j. increase activity as allowed and tolerated *(activity stimulates appetite)*
	    2. perform actions to prevent and treat diarrhea (see Nursing Diagnosis 10, action d)
	    3. assist and instruct client to adhere to the following dietary recommendations:
	      a. avoid skipping meals
	      b. consume a diet high in calories (2500–3000 calories/day) and carbohydrates
	      c. maintain a moderate to high protein intake (generally at least 1 gm of protein/kg of body weight is recommended unless the serum ammonia level is high or clinical evidence of encephalopathy is present) *in order to replace serum proteins and promote liver cell regeneration*
	      d. increase intake of foods high in the following vitamins and minerals:
	        1. vitamin B$_{12}$ (e.g. organ meats, eggs, fresh shrimp, chicken)

   2. folic acid (e.g. green leafy vegetables, asparagus, organ meats, lima beans, fruits)
   3. thiamine (e.g. whole-grain cereals, peas, beans, meat)
   4. iron (e.g. organ meats, apricots, green leafy vegetables, whole-grain and enriched breads)
   e. suck on hard candy and drink fruit juices if unable to tolerate solid food *(these items provide a quick source of energy)*
4. monitor for therapeutic and nontherapeutic effects of the following medications if administered:
   a. elemental zinc *(zinc level is often below normal in alcoholics; zinc is also given to improve appetite because it enhances the sense of taste and smell)*
   b. vitamin preparations (e.g. fat-soluble vitamins, B-complex vitamins, folic acid)
   c. medium-chain triglycerides (MCT) in an oil medium *to provide an absorbable source of fatty acids.*
f. Perform a 72-hour calorie count if nutritional status declines or fails to improve.
g. Consult physician if:
   1. client does not consume enough food or fluids to meet nutritional needs (alternative forms of providing nutrition such as parenteral nutrition or tube feeding may be necessary)
   2. client develops or continues to have steatorrhea or clay-colored stools *(indicates continued bile flow obstruction and malabsorption of fats).*

☐ ▐▬▬▬▬▬▬▬▬▬▬▬▬▬▬▬▬▬▬▬▬▬▬▬▬

5.A. NURSING DIAGNOSIS

Altered comfort:* abdominal pain related to swelling and distention of the liver capsule, spasms of the biliary ducts, and distention of the peritoneum as a result of excessive fluid accumulation.

---

* In this care plan, the nursing diagnosis "pain" is included under the diagnostic label of altered comfort.

☐ ▐▬▬▬▬▬▬▬▬▬▬▬▬▬▬▬▬▬▬▬▬▬▬▬▬

DESIRED OUTCOMES	NURSING ACTIONS AND *SELECTED RATIONALES*

5.A. The client will experience diminished abdominal pain as evidenced by:
1. verbalization of pain relief
2. relaxed facial expression and body positioning
3. increased participation in activities
4. stable vital signs.
	5.A.1. Determine how the client usually responds to pain.
	2. Assess for nonverbal signs of pain (e.g. wrinkled brow, clenched fists, reluctance to move, guarding of abdomen, restlessness, diaphoresis, facial pallor or flushing, change in B/P, tachycardia).
	3. Assess verbal complaints of pain. Ask client to be specific about location, severity, and type of pain.
	4. Assess for factors that seem to aggravate and alleviate pain.
	5. Implement measures *to reduce pain:*
	  a. perform actions to restore fluid balance (see Nursing Diagnosis 3, action a.4) *in order to reduce peritoneal fluid accumulation*
	  b. provide or assist with nonpharmacological measures for pain relief (e.g. position change, relaxation techniques, guided imagery, quiet conversation, restful environment, diversional activities)
	  c. if analgesics are ordered for pain:
	    1. question any order for a normal adult dose of a narcotic analgesic *(the liver cannot detoxify narcotics at its usual rate)* and for an analgesic containing acetaminophen *(acetaminophen is a potential hepatotoxin)*
	    2. monitor for therapeutic and nontherapeutic effects if administered (be alert to the fact that narcotic analgesics may fail to relieve or actually intensify pain *because they can cause biliary spasm).*
	6. Consult physician if above measures fail to provide adequate pain relief.

5.B. NURSING DIAGNOSIS

Altered comfort: pruritus related to bile salt accumulation underneath the skin associated with obstruction of bile flow.

DESIRED OUTCOMES	NURSING ACTIONS AND *SELECTED RATIONALES*

5.B. The client will experience relief of pruritus as evidenced by:
1. verbalization of same
2. no scratching or rubbing of skin.
	5.B.1. Assess pruritus including onset, characteristics, location, factors that aggravate or alleviate it, and client tolerance.
	2. Instruct client in and/or carry out measures *to relieve pruritus:*
	  a. apply cool, moist compresses to pruritic areas
	  b. apply emollients to skin *to help alleviate dryness*
	  c. add emollients, cornstarch, baking soda, or oatmeal to bath water
	  d. use tepid water and mild soaps for bathing
	  e. pat skin dry, making sure to dry thoroughly
	  f. maintain a cool environment
	  g. encourage participation in diversional activity
	  h. utilize relaxation techniques
	  i. utilize cutaneous stimulation techniques (e.g. massage, pressure, vibration, stroking with soft brush) at the site of itching or acupressure points
	  j. encourage client to wear loose cotton garments.
	3. Monitor for therapeutic and nontherapeutic effects of the following if administered *to relieve itching:*
	  a. antihistamines
	  b. antipruritic lotions
	  c. cholestyramine *to bind bile salts and reduce their accumulation under skin.*
	4. Consult physician if above measures fail to alleviate pruritus or if the skin becomes excoriated.

5.C. NURSING DIAGNOSIS

Altered comfort:

1. **dyspepsia** related to impaired fat digestion and gastroesophageal reflux associated with increased intra-abdominal pressure due to ascites;
2. **gas pain** related to gas accumulation associated with impaired fat digestion due to bile flow obstruction.

DESIRED OUTCOMES	NURSING ACTIONS AND *SELECTED RATIONALES*

5.C. The client will experience diminished dyspepsia and gas pain as evidenced by:
1. verbalization of same
2. relaxed facial expression and body positioning
3. diminished eructation.
	5.C.1. Assess for nonverbal signs of dyspepsia and gas pain (e.g. clutching and guarding of abdomen, restlessness, reluctance to move, grimacing, frequent eructation, reluctance to eat).
	2. Assess for verbal complaints of fullness, indigestion, and gas pain.
	3. Implement measures *to reduce dyspepsia and gas pain:*
	  a. perform actions *to reduce gastroesophageal reflux:*
	    1. keep head of bed elevated for 2–3 hours after meals

UNIT XIII

2. implement measures to restore fluid balance (see Nursing Diagnosis 3, action a.4) *in order to reduce ascites*
   b. perform actions *to reduce accumulation of gastrointestinal gas:*
      1. encourage and assist client with frequent position change and ambulation as soon as allowed and tolerated *(activity stimulates expulsion of flatus)*
      2. instruct client to avoid activities such as gum chewing, sucking on hard candy, and smoking *in order to reduce air swallowing*
      3. instruct client to avoid the following:
         a. gas-producing foods/fluids (e.g. cabbage, onions, popcorn, baked beans, carbonated beverages)
         b. foods/fluids high in fat (e.g. butter, cream, oils, whole milk, ice cream, pork, fried foods, gravies, nuts)
      4. encourage client to eructate and expel flatus whenever the urge is felt
      5. monitor for therapeutic and nontherapeutic effects of antiflatulents if administered
   c. monitor for therapeutic and nontherapeutic effects of antacids and histamine$_2$ receptor antagonists (e.g. famotidine, ranitidine) if administered *to reduce acidity of gastric contents and thereby reduce esophageal irritation if reflux occurs.*
4. Consult physician if signs and symptoms of dyspepsia and gas pain persist or worsen.

☐ ▇▇▇▇▇▇▇▇▇▇▇▇▇▇▇▇▇▇▇▇▇▇▇▇▇▇▇▇▇▇▇▇

6. NURSING DIAGNOSIS

Impaired skin integrity: irritation and breakdown related to:

a. prolonged pressure on tissues associated with decreased mobility;
b. increased fragility of the skin associated with edema and malnutrition;
c. excessive scratching associated with pruritus;
d. frequent contact with irritants associated with diarrhea.

☐ ▇▇▇▇▇▇▇▇▇▇▇▇▇▇▇▇▇▇▇▇▇▇▇▇▇▇▇▇▇▇▇▇

DESIRED OUTCOMES	NURSING ACTIONS AND *SELECTED RATIONALES*

6. The client will maintain skin integrity as evidenced by:
a. absence of redness and irritation
b. no skin breakdown.
	6.a. Inspect the skin, especially bone prominences and dependent and pruritic areas, for pallor, redness, and breakdown.
	b. Refer to Care Plan on Immobility, Nursing Diagnosis 7, action b, for measures to prevent skin breakdown associated with decreased mobility.
	c. Implement measures *to prevent skin breakdown associated with edema:*
	  1. perform actions to restore fluid balance (see Nursing Diagnosis 3, action a.4)
	  2. perform actions *to reduce fluid accumulation in dependent areas:*
	    a. assist with range of motion exercises
	    b. turn client at least every 2 hours
	    c. elevate lower extremities
	    d. apply a scrotal support if scrotal edema is present
	    e. apply elastic wraps or hose to lower extremities as ordered
	  3. handle edematous areas carefully.
	d. Implement measures *to prevent skin breakdown associated with scratching:*
	  1. perform actions to relieve pruritus (see Nursing Diagnosis 5.B, actions 2 and 3)
	  2. keep nails trimmed and/or apply mittens if necessary
	  3. instruct client to apply firm pressure to pruritic areas rather than scratching.

e. Implement measures *to decrease skin irritation and prevent breakdown resulting from diarrhea:*
   1. perform actions to prevent and treat diarrhea (see Nursing Diagnosis 10, action d)
   2. assist client to thoroughly cleanse and dry perineal area after each bowel movement; apply a protective ointment or cream (e.g. Sween cream, Desitin, A & D ointment, Vaseline)
   3. use soft toilet tissue to cleanse perianal area.
f. Maintain an optimal nutritional status (see Nursing Diagnosis 4, action e).
g. If skin breakdown occurs:
   1. notify physician
   2. continue with above measures to prevent further irritation and breakdown
   3. perform decubitus care as ordered or per standard hospital policy
   4. monitor client closely and report signs and symptoms of infection (e.g. elevated temperature; redness, warmth, and edema around area of breakdown; unusual drainage from site).

□ ▰▰▰▰▰▰▰▰▰▰▰▰▰▰▰▰▰▰▰▰▰▰▰▰▰▰▰

7. NURSING DIAGNOSIS

Activity intolerance related to:

a. tissue hypoxia associated with:
   1. impaired alveolar gas exchange
   2. anemia resulting from:
      a. decreased production and slow maturation of RBCs resulting from a decreased oral intake of vitamins and minerals; an inability of the liver to store iron, vitamin B_{12}, and folic acid; and toxic effects of alcohol on the bone marrow
      b. excessive RBC destruction resulting from hypersplenism (if venous congestion has resulted in splenomegaly, the spleen will destroy RBCs faster than usual)
      c. blood loss resulting from an increased bleeding tendency and bleeding esophageal varices;
b. inadequate nutritional status;
c. cardiac deconditioning associated with a prolonged decrease in mobility;
d. difficulty resting and sleeping due to dyspnea, discomfort, frequent assessments and treatments, fear, and anxiety.

□ ▰▰▰▰▰▰▰▰▰▰▰▰▰▰▰▰▰▰▰▰▰▰▰▰▰▰▰

UNIT
XIII

DESIRED OUTCOMES	NURSING ACTIONS AND *SELECTED RATIONALES*

7. The client will demonstrate an increased tolerance for activity (see Care Plan on Immobility, Nursing Diagnosis 8, for outcome criteria).	7.a. Refer to Care Plan on Immobility, Nursing Diagnosis 8, for measures related to assessment and improvement of activity tolerance.
	b. Implement additional measures *to promote rest and improve activity tolerance:*
	  1. perform actions to reduce fear and anxiety (see Nursing Diagnosis 1)
	  2. perform actions to promote sleep (see Nursing Diagnosis 13)
	  3. perform actions to reduce discomfort (see Nursing Diagnoses 5.A, action 5; 5.B, actions 2 and 3; and 5.C, action 3)
	  4. maintain an optimal nutritional status (see Nursing Diagnosis 4, action e)
	  5. perform actions to improve respiratory status (see Nursing Diagnosis 2, action e) *in order to decrease dyspnea and improve tissue oxygenation*
	  6. monitor for therapeutic and nontherapeutic effects of whole blood or packed red cells if administered
	  7. increase activity gradually as allowed and tolerated.

8. NURSING DIAGNOSIS

Impaired physical mobility related to:

a. weakness and fatigue;
b. balance and gait disturbances associated with the neurological changes that can result from vitamin B_{12} and thiamine deficiencies and toxic effects of alcohol on the nervous system;
c. activity restrictions imposed by the treatment plan.

DESIRED OUTCOMES	NURSING ACTIONS AND *SELECTED RATIONALES*

8.a. The client will maintain an optimal level of physical mobility within physical limitations and activity restrictions imposed by the treatment plan.	8.a.1. Assess for factors that impair physical mobility (e.g. loss of balance, gait disturbances, weakness and fatigue, activity restrictions imposed by treatment plan).
	2. Implement measures *to increase mobility:*
	  a. perform actions to increase strength and activity tolerance (see Nursing Diagnosis 7)
	  b. monitor for therapeutic and nontherapeutic effects of thiamine and vitamin B_{12} (e.g. cyanocobalamin) if administered *to prevent further neurological manifestations*
	  c. instruct client in and assist with correct use of mobility aids (e.g. cane, walker) if appropriate.
	3. Increase activity and participation in self-care activities as allowed and tolerated.
	4. Provide praise and encouragement for all efforts to increase physical mobility.
	5. Encourage the support of significant others. Allow them to assist with positioning and activity if desired.

8.b. The client will not experience problems associated with immobility.	8.b. Refer to Care Plan on Immobility for actions to prevent problems associated with immobility if client remains on bedrest longer than 48 hours.

9. NURSING DIAGNOSIS

Self-care deficit related to:

a. altered thought processes;
b. impaired physical mobility associated with weakness, fatigue, balance and gait disturbances, and prescribed activity restrictions;
c. dyspnea.

DESIRED OUTCOMES	NURSING ACTIONS AND *SELECTED RATIONALES*
9. The client will demonstrate increased participation in self-care activities within physical and mental limitations and prescribed activity restrictions.	9.a. Refer to Care Plan on Immobility, Nursing Diagnosis 9, for measures related to assessment of, planning for, and meeting the client's self-care needs. b. Implement measures *to further facilitate the client's ability to perform self-care activities:* 1. perform actions to increase mobility (see Nursing Diagnosis 8, action a.2)

2. perform actions to maintain optimal thought processes (see Nursing Diagnosis 12, action c)
3. perform actions to improve respiratory status (see Nursing Diagnosis 2, action e) *in order to decrease dyspnea.*

☐ ▬▬▬▬▬▬▬▬▬▬▬▬▬▬▬▬▬▬▬▬▬▬▬▬▬

10. NURSING DIAGNOSIS

Diarrhea related to decreased absorption of water from the intestines associated with effects of vitamin deficiencies and excessive alcohol intake on intestinal functioning.

☐ ▬▬▬▬▬▬▬▬▬▬▬▬▬▬▬▬▬▬▬▬▬▬▬▬▬

DESIRED OUTCOMES	NURSING ACTIONS AND *SELECTED RATIONALES*

10. The client will maintain usual bowel elimination pattern.	10.a. Ascertain client's usual bowel elimination habits.
	 b. Assess for signs and symptoms of diarrhea (e.g. frequent, loose stools; abdominal pain and cramping).
	 c. Assess bowel sounds regularly. Report an increase in frequency of and/or high-pitched sounds.
	 d. Implement measures *to prevent and treat diarrhea:*
	   1. instruct client to avoid foods/fluids that are:
	     a. extremely hot or cold
	     b. spicy or high in fat content
	     c. high in caffeine (e.g. coffee, tea, chocolate, colas)
	     d. diarrhea or gas-producing (e.g. cabbage, onions, popcorn, licorice, prunes, chili, baked beans)
	   2. provide small, frequent meals
	   3. discourage smoking *(nicotine has a stimulant effect on the gastrointestinal tract)*
	   4. monitor for therapeutic and nontherapeutic effects of the following medications if administered:
	     a. opiate or opiate-like substances (e.g. loperamide) *to decrease gastrointestinal motility*
	     b. bulk-forming agents (e.g. methylcellulose, psyllium hydrophilic mucilloid, calcium polycarbophil) *to absorb water in the bowel and produce a soft, formed stool.*
	 e. Consult physician if diarrhea persists.

☐ ▬▬▬▬▬▬▬▬▬▬▬▬▬▬▬▬▬▬▬▬▬▬▬▬▬

11. NURSING DIAGNOSIS

Constipation related to decreased activity, anxiety, decreased food and fluid intake, and slowed bowel activity associated with vascular congestion in the gastrointestinal tract.

☐ ▬▬▬▬▬▬▬▬▬▬▬▬▬▬▬▬▬▬▬▬▬▬▬▬▬

DESIRED OUTCOMES	NURSING ACTIONS AND *SELECTED RATIONALES*
11. The client will maintain usual bowel elimination pattern.	11.a. Refer to Care Plan on Immobility, Nursing Diagnosis 11, for measures related to assessment, prevention, and treatment of constipation.

UNIT
XIII

b. Implement additional measures *to prevent and treat constipation*:
   1. perform actions to restore fluid balance (see Nursing Diagnosis 3, action a.4) *in order to reduce vascular congestion in the gastrointestinal tract*
   2. monitor for therapeutic and nontherapeutic effects of lactulose if administered *to stimulate catharsis.*

☐ ▬▬▬▬▬▬▬▬▬▬▬▬▬▬▬▬▬▬▬▬▬▬▬

12. NURSING DIAGNOSIS

Altered thought processes: slowed verbal responses, impaired memory, shortened attention span, confusion, and personality changes related to:

a. cerebral hypoxia associated with anemia and impaired alveolar gas exchange;
b. neurological changes associated with thiamine and vitamin B_{12} deficiencies, toxic effects of alcohol on the nervous system, delayed drug detoxification, and impending hepatic coma.

☐ ▬▬▬▬▬▬▬▬▬▬▬▬▬▬▬▬▬▬▬▬▬▬▬

DESIRED OUTCOMES	NURSING ACTIONS AND *SELECTED RATIONALES*

12. The client will demonstrate improvement in thought processes as evidenced by:
   a. improved verbal response time
   b. improved memory
   c. longer attention span
   d. absence of confusion
   e. absence of personality changes.

12.a. Assess client for alterations in thought processes (e.g. slowed verbal responses, impaired memory, shortened attention span, confusion).
   b. Ascertain from significant others the client's usual level of intellectual functioning and whether personality changes have occurred.
   c. Implement measures *to maintain optimal thought processes:*
      1. perform actions *to reduce tissue hypoxia:*
         a. implement measures to improve respiratory status (see Nursing Diagnosis 2, action e)
         b. maintain an optimal nutritional status (see Nursing Diagnosis 4, action e) *in order to prevent anemia*
      2. perform actions to prevent or manage hepatic coma (see Collaborative Diagnosis 16, actions d.3 and 4)
      3. administer central nervous system depressants such as narcotics, sedatives, hypnotics, and antianxiety agents with extreme caution *(many of these agents are metabolized in the liver);* question any order for a normal adult dose of these medications
      4. monitor for therapeutic and nontherapeutic effects of vitamin B_{12} (e.g. cyanocobalamin) or thiamine if administered *to prevent further neurological manifestations.*
   d. If client shows evidence of altered thought processes:
      1. allow adequate time for communication and performance of activities
      2. repeat instructions as necessary using clear, simple language
      3. reorient client to person, place, and time as necessary
      4. write out a schedule of activities for client to refer to if desired
      5. encourage client to make lists of planned activities and questions or concerns he/she may have
      6. assist client to problem-solve if necessary
      7. maintain realistic expectations of client's ability to learn, comprehend, and remember information provided
      8. encourage significant others to be supportive of client; instruct them in methods of dealing with the alterations in thought processes
      9. inform client and significant others that intellectual and emotional functioning should improve once liver function improves
      10. consult physician if alterations in thought processes persist or worsen.

13. NURSING DIAGNOSIS

Sleep pattern disturbance related to unfamiliar environment, frequent assessments and treatments, decreased physical activity, discomfort, fear, anxiety, and inability to assume usual sleep position due to orthopnea.

DESIRED OUTCOMES	NURSING ACTIONS AND *SELECTED RATIONALES*

13. The client will attain optimal amounts of sleep within the parameters of the treatment regimen (see Care Plan on Immobility, Nursing Diagnosis 12, for outcome criteria).	13.a. Refer to Care Plan on Immobility, Nursing Diagnosis 12, for measures related to assessment and promotion of sleep.
	b. Implement additional measures *to promote sleep:*
	  1. assist client to assume a comfortable sleep position (e.g. bed in reverse Trendelenburg position with client in usual recumbent position, head of bed elevated with arms supported on pillows, resting forward on overbed table with good pillow support, sitting in chair)
	  2. maintain oxygen therapy during sleep if indicated
	  3. ensure good room ventilation *to reduce feeling of suffocation*
	  4. perform actions to reduce discomfort (see Nursing Diagnoses 5.A, action 5; 5.B, actions 2 and 3; and 5.C, action 3)
	  5. increase activity as allowed and tolerated
	  6. consult physician about an order for a mild sedative such as diphenhydramine *(considered safer for use in persons with liver disease than many sedatives)* if client is unable to sleep.

14. NURSING DIAGNOSIS

Potential for infection related to lowered natural resistance associated with:

a. diminished function of the Kupffer cells in the liver (these cells normally phago-cytize bacteria);
b. tissue hypoxia resulting from impaired alveolar gas exchange and anemia;
c. malnutrition;
d. leukopenia resulting from hypersplenism (if venous congestion has resulted in splenomegaly, the spleen will destroy leukocytes faster than usual).

DESIRED OUTCOMES	NURSING ACTIONS AND *SELECTED RATIONALES*

14. The client will remain free of infection as evidenced by:
a. absence of chills and fever
b. pulse within normal limits
c. normal breath sounds
d. voiding clear, yellow urine without complaints of frequency, urgency, and burning
e. absence of redness, swelling, and unusual drainage in any area
	14.a. Assess for and report signs and symptoms of infection:
	  1. elevated temperature
	  2. chills
	  3. pattern of increased pulse or pulse rate greater than 100 beats/minute
	  4. adventitious breath sounds
	  5. cloudy or foul-smelling urine
	  6. complaints of frequency, urgency, or burning when urinating
	  7. presence of WBCs, bacteria, and/or nitrites in urine
	  8. redness, swelling, or unusual drainage in any area where there is a break in skin integrity
	  9. irritation or ulceration of oral mucous membrane
	  10. elevated WBC count and/or significant change in differential.

where there is a break in skin integrity

f. intact oral mucous membrane

g. WBC and differential counts within normal range

h. negative results of cultured specimens.

b. Obtain culture specimens (e.g. urine, vaginal, mouth, sputum, blood) as ordered. Report positive results.

c. Implement measures *to reduce risk of infection:*
1. perform actions to prevent skin breakdown (see Nursing Diagnosis 6, actions b–f)
2. maintain the maximum fluid intake allowed
3. use good handwashing technique and encourage client to do the same
4. maintain meticulous aseptic technique during all invasive procedures (e.g. catheterizations, venous and arterial punctures, injections)
5. protect client from others with infection
6. maintain an optimal nutritional status (see Nursing Diagnosis 4, action e)
7. provide or assist with good oral care
8. provide proper balance of exercise and rest
9. perform actions *to prevent respiratory tract infection:*
   a. instruct and assist client to turn, cough, and deep breathe at least every 2 hours while mobility is limited
   b. instruct and assist client in use of inspiratory exerciser at least every 2 hours if indicated
   c. encourage client to stop smoking
   d. increase activity as allowed and tolerated
10. perform actions *to prevent urinary tract infection:*
    a. instruct and assist female client to wipe from front to back following urination and defecation
    b. keep perianal area clean.

d. Monitor for therapeutic and nontherapeutic effects of anti-infectives if administered. (Monitor liver function tests closely *because many anti-infective agents have a hepatotoxic and/or cholestatic effect.*)

☐ ▬▬▬▬▬▬▬▬▬▬▬▬▬▬▬▬

15. NURSING DIAGNOSIS

Potential for trauma related to:

a. falls associated with:
1. fatigue and weakness
2. dizziness resulting from cerebral hypoxia associated with impaired alveolar gas exchange, anemia, and orthostatic hypotension (may occur as a result of third-spacing)
3. impaired proprioception and gait disturbances resulting from neurological changes associated with toxic effects of alcohol and deficiencies of thiamine and vitamin B_{12}
4. altered thought processes
5. delirium tremens ("DTs") resulting from alcohol withdrawal if it occurs;
b. cuts and burns associated with:
1. altered thought processes
2. paresthesias and uncoordinated movements resulting from nutritional and alcohol-induced neuropathies
3. delirium tremens ("DTs") if present.

☐ ▬▬▬▬▬▬▬▬▬▬▬▬▬▬▬▬

DESIRED OUTCOMES	NURSING ACTIONS AND *SELECTED RATIONALES*
15. The client will not experience falls, cuts, or burns.	15.a. Determine whether conditions predisposing the client to falls, cuts, or burns exist: 1. dizziness 2. weakness and fatigue 3. uncoordinated movements

 4. gait disturbances
 5. decreased sensation in extremities
 6. altered thought processes
 7. delirium tremens (signs and symptoms may include insomnia, restlessness, agitation, tremors, hallucinations, and confusion).
 b. Implement measures *to prevent falls:*
 1. keep bed in low position with side rails up when client is in bed
 2. keep needed items within easy reach
 3. encourage client to request assistance whenever needed; have call signal within easy reach
 4. assist and instruct client to move from a horizontal to upright position slowly *in order to reduce dizziness associated with orthostatic hypotension*
 5. use lap belt when client is in chair if indicated
 6. instruct client to wear shoes with nonskid soles and low heels when ambulating
 7. avoid unnecessary clutter in room
 8. accompany client during ambulation utilizing a transfer safety belt
 9. provide ambulatory aids (e.g. walker, cane) if the client is weak or unsteady on feet
 10. instruct client to ambulate in well-lit areas and to utilize handrails if needed
 11. do not rush client; allow adequate time for trips to the bathroom and ambulation in hallway
 12. perform actions to increase strength and activity tolerance (see Nursing Diagnosis 7)
 13. administer central nervous system depressants such as narcotics, sedatives, hypnotics, and antianxiety agents with extreme caution *(many of these agents are metabolized in the liver);* question any order for a normal adult dose of these medications.
 c. Implement measures *to prevent burns:*
 1. let hot foods and fluids cool slightly before serving *to reduce risk of burns if spills occur*
 2. supervise client while smoking if indicated
 3. assess temperature of bath water and heating pad before and during use.
 d. Assist client with tasks that require fine motor skills (e.g. shaving) *in order to prevent cuts.*
 e. If client has signs and symptoms of "DTs" and/or is confused or irrational, implement additional measures *to reduce risk of injury:*
 1. reorient frequently to surroundings and necessity of adhering to safety precautions
 2. provide constant supervision (e.g. staff member, significant other) if indicated
 3. use jacket or wrist restraints or safety alarm device if necessary *to reduce risk of client's getting out of bed or chair unattended*
 4. monitor for therapeutic and nontherapeutic effects of antianxiety and antipsychotic medications if administered, remembering that these agents must be used cautiously (the benzodiazepines are safer than many agents).
 f. Include client and significant others in planning and implementing measures to prevent injury.
 g. If injury does occur, initiate appropriate first aid and notify physician.

☐ ▮▮

16. COLLABORATIVE DIAGNOSIS

Potential complications:

a. **bleeding** related to:
 1. decreased production of clotting factors associated with impaired liver function and impaired vitamin K absorption (normal bile flow is necessary for absorption of vitamin K)

UNIT
XIII

2. splenic platelet pooling and thrombocytopenia associated with hypersplenism (if venous congestion has resulted in splenomegaly, the spleen will pool platelets and also destroy them faster than usual);

b. **renal insufficiency and/or hepatorenal syndrome** related to diminished renal blood flow associated with:
1. hypovolemia resulting from third-spacing and rapid or excessive diuresis
2. renal cortical vessel constriction resulting from activation of the renin-angiotensin axis (a result of diminished renal blood flow), decreased degradation of renin by the failing liver, and/or an alteration in renal prostaglandin output
3. increased intra-abdominal and renal venous pressures;

c. **bleeding esophageal varices** related to:
1. mechanical or chemical trauma to dilated, fragile esophageal vessels (esophageal varices are a result of the development of collateral circulation in the lower esophagus, which is a compensatory response to portal hypertension)
2. increase in intra-abdominal pressure
3. increased bleeding tendency;

d. **hepatic coma (portal systemic encephalophy)** related to cerebral toxicity associated with:
1. high serum ammonia levels resulting from the liver's inability to convert ammonia to urea
2. deficiency of neurotransmitters resulting from an inability of the liver to detoxify certain substances that act as false neurotransmitters (these false neurotransmitters then occupy sites the neurotransmitters normally occupy)
3. increased levels of certain amino acids, short- and medium-chain fatty acids, and mercaptans resulting from the liver's inability to metabolize these substances;

e. **spontaneous bacterial peritonitis** related to stasis of organisms in the ascitic fluid associated with obstructed flow through the reticuloendothelial filtering system due to portal-systemic shunting.

DESIRED OUTCOMES	NURSING ACTIONS AND *SELECTED RATIONALES*

16.a. The client will not experience unusual bleeding as evidenced by:
1. skin and mucous membranes free of bleeding, petechiae, and ecchymosis
2. absence of unusual joint pain and swelling
3. no further increase in abdominal girth
4. absence of frank or occult blood in stool, urine, and vomitus
5. usual menstrual flow
6. vital signs within normal range for client
7. stable or improved Hct. and Hgb.
8. usual mental status.

16.a.1. Assess client for and report signs and symptoms of unusual bleeding:
  a. petechiae
  b. multiple ecchymotic areas
  c. bleeding gums
  d. frequent or uncontrollable episodes of epistaxis
  e. unusual oozing from injection sites
  f. unusual joint pain or swelling
  g. further increase in abdominal girth
  h. hematemesis, melena, red or smoke-colored urine
  i. hypermenorrhea
  j. significant drop in B/P accompanied by an increased pulse rate
  k. decline in Hct. and Hgb. levels
  l. restlessness, confusion.
2. Monitor coagulation test results (e.g. prothrombin time, activated partial thromboplastin time, platelet count, bleeding time). Report abnormal values.
3. If coagulation test results are abnormal or Hct. and Hgb. levels decline, test all stools, urine, and vomitus for occult blood. Report positive results.
4. Implement measures *to prevent bleeding:*
  a. perform actions to reduce risk of bleeding from esophageal varices (see action c.3 in this diagnosis)
  b. use smallest gauge needle possible when giving injections and performing venous or arterial punctures
  c. apply gentle, prolonged pressure after injections and venous or arterial punctures
  d. take B/P only when necessary and avoid overinflating the cuff

e. caution client to avoid activities that increase the potential for trauma (e.g. shaving with a straight-edge razor, cutting nails, using stiff bristle toothbrush or dental floss)

f. pad side rails if client is confused or restless

g. perform actions to prevent falls (see Nursing Diagnosis 15, action b)

h. instruct client to avoid blowing nose forcefully or straining to have a bowel movement; consult physician about an order for decongestants, stool softeners, and/or laxatives if indicated

i. monitor for therapeutic and nontherapeutic effects of the following if administered *to improve clotting ability:*

1. vitamin K (e.g. phytonadione) injections
2. platelets
3. fresh blood or plasma *(the liver cannot detoxify the preservative in stored blood).*

5. If bleeding occurs and does not subside spontaneously:

a. apply firm, prolonged pressure to bleeding area if possible

b. if epistaxis occurs, place client in a high Fowler's position and apply pressure and ice packs to nasal area

c. maintain oxygen therapy as ordered

d. implement measures identified in action c.4 in this diagnosis if gastric or esophageal bleeding occurs

e. administer vitamin K (e.g. phytonadione) injections and blood products (e.g. fresh frozen plasma, whole blood, platelets) as ordered

f. prepare client for surgical repair of bleeding vessels if planned

g. provide emotional support to client and significant others.

16.b. The client will maintain adequate renal function as evidenced by:

1. urine–plasma creatinine and osmolality ratios within normal range
2. normal urine sodium
3. urine output at least 30 cc/hour
4. BUN and serum creatinine levels within normal range.

16.b.1. Assess for and report:

a. factors that may cause volume depletion (e.g. excessive diuresis associated with diuretic therapy, hemorrhage)

b. specific signs and symptoms of the hepatorenal syndrome (e.g. high urine–plasma creatinine ratio, urine–plasma osmolality ratio greater than 1, low urine sodium levels)

c. signs of acute renal failure (e.g. urine output less than 30 cc/hour; weight gain; increasing edema; elevated B/P; lethargy and confusion; increasing BUN and serum creatinine, phosphorus, and potassium levels).

2. Implement measures *to maintain adequate renal blood flow:*

a. perform actions to restore fluid balance (see Nursing Diagnosis 3, action a.4) *in order to prevent fluid volume excess (fluid volume excess results in increased intra-abdominal and renal venous pressures)* and hypovolemia resulting from third-spacing

b. maintain the maximum fluid intake allowed

c. monitor for therapeutic and nontherapeutic effects of plasma volume expanders if administered *to increase renal blood flow*

d. assist with paracentesis if performed *to reduce intra-abdominal and renal venous pressures.*

3. If signs and symptoms of impaired renal function occur:

a. continue with above actions

b. administer diuretics as ordered

c. prepare client for dialysis if indicated

d. refer to Care Plan on Renal Failure for additional care measures.

16.c. The client will not experience bleeding of esophageal varices as evidenced by:

1. absence of hematemesis and melena
2. B/P and pulse within normal range for client
3. stable or improved RBC, Hct., and Hgb. levels.

16.c.1. Assess for and report signs and symptoms of bleeding esophageal varices (e.g. frank or occult blood in vomitus or stool, decreased B/P, increased pulse).

2. Monitor RBC, Hct., and Hgb. levels. Report declining values.

3. Implement measures *to reduce risk of bleeding from esophageal varices:*

a. perform actions to reduce fluid volume excess (see Nursing Diagnosis 3, action a.4.a) *in order to reduce portal hypertension and pressure in esophageal vessels*

b. perform actions *to prevent mechanical and chemical irritation of vessels:*

1. eliminate coarse, highly seasoned, and acidic foods from diet
2. eliminate intake of caffeine-containing items (e.g. coffee, tea, colas, chocolate)

UNIT XIII

3. administer ulcerogenic medications (e.g. corticosteroids, aspirin, phenytoin, indomethacin) with meals, snacks, or an antacid
4. keep head of bed elevated for 2–3 hours after meals *to prevent reflux of acidic gastric contents*
5. monitor for therapeutic and nontherapeutic effects of antacids and histamine$_2$ receptor antagonists (e.g. famotidine, ranitidine) if administered *to reduce acidity of gastric contents in case of esophageal reflux*
   c. instruct client to avoid activities such as straining to have a bowel movement, coughing, sneezing, and bending at the waist *in order to prevent an increase in intra-abdominal pressure;* consult physician about an order for stool softener and/or laxative, antitussive, and decongestant if indicated
   d. monitor for therapeutic and nontherapeutic effects of vitamin K and blood products if administered *to improve clotting ability.*
4. If signs and symptoms of bleeding esophageal varices occur:
   a. place client on his/her side *to reduce risk of aspiration*
   b. maintain oxygen therapy as ordered
   c. assist with insertion of a gastroesophageal balloon tube (e.g. Sengstaken-Blakemore tube, Linton Nachlus tube); maintain balloon pressure and suction and perform iced water or saline lavage as ordered
   d. assist with administration of intravenous or intra-arterial vasopressin (*reduces portal vein congestion by constricting the splanchnic arterioles*)
   e. assist with sclerotherapy if performed
   f. administer vitamin K (e.g. phytonadione) injections and blood products (e.g. fresh frozen plasma, whole blood, platelets) as ordered
   g. assess for and immediately report signs and symptoms of hypovolemic shock (e.g. restlessness; agitation; further decline in B/P and increase in pulse; rapid or labored respirations; cool, pale, or cyanotic skin; diminished or absent peripheral pulses; urine output less than 30 cc/hour)
   h. prepare client for surgery (e.g. transesophageal ligation of bleeding vessels, portal-systemic shunt) if planned
   i. provide emotional support to client and significant others.

16.d. The client will not develop hepatic encephalopathy as evidenced by:
1. usual mental status
2. usual speech and handwriting
3. absence of asterixis and fetor hepaticus
4. serum ammonia level within normal range.

16.d.1. Assess for and report signs and symptoms of hepatic encephalopathy:
   a. emotional lability
   b. lapses in memory, inability to concentrate
   c. agitation, combativeness
   d. lethargy, confusion, decreased responsiveness
   e. slow, slurred speech
   f. change in handwriting, inability to draw simple figures or numbers
   g. asterixis (rhythmic movements of hands when client extends arms and dorsiflexes hands, rhythmic movements of legs with dorsiflexion of feet)
   h. fetor hepaticus (musty, sweet odor on breath)
   i. coma.
2. Monitor serum ammonia results. Report elevated values.
3. Implement measures *to prevent hepatic coma:*
   a. perform actions *to prevent or control the following conditions that can lead to increases in ammonia level:*
      1. constipation (*intestinal bacteria have a longer time and more contents to convert to ammonia*)
      2. gastrointestinal hemorrhage (*intestinal bacteria convert the protein in blood to ammonia*)
      3. hypokalemia and/or metabolic alkalosis (*increase the dissociation of NH$_4$ to the more diffusable NH$_3$; hypokalemia also increases renal production of ammonia*)
      4. renal failure (*results in decreased excretion of ammonia*)
      5. excessive protein intake (*intestinal bacteria convert protein to ammonia*)
   b. perform actions *to prevent further damage to the liver:*
      1. implement measures to prevent and treat third-spacing (see Nursing Diagnosis 3, action a.4.b) and bleeding (see actions a.4 and

5 in this diagnosis) *in order to prevent hypovolemia and maintain an adequate blood flow to the liver*
    2. consult physician before giving known or potential hepatotoxins (e.g. methyldopa, isoniazid, acetaminophen, tetracycline, sulfonamides)
  c. perform actions *to reduce metabolic demands on the liver:*
    1. implement measures to prevent and treat infection (see Nursing Diagnosis 14, actions c and d)
    2. maintain activity restrictions as ordered
  d. administer central nervous system depressants such as narcotics, sedatives, hypnotics, and antianxiety agents with extreme caution *(many of these agents are metabolized in the liver and may precipitate nonnitrogenous coma).*
4. If signs and symptoms of hepatic encephalopathy occur:
  a. maintain client on strict bedrest *to reduce metabolic demands on liver*
  b. maintain dietary protein restrictions as ordered (usually 20–40 gm/day) *to reduce serum ammonia level*
  c. ensure a high carbohydrate intake or administer intravenous glucose or tube feedings as ordered *to provide a rapid energy source and prevent protein catabolism*
  d. administer enemas and/or cathartics as ordered *to hasten expulsion of intestinal contents so that bacteria have less time to convert proteins to ammonia*
  e. monitor for therapeutic and nontherapeutic effects of the following medications if administered:
    1. antibiotics (e.g. neomycin, nonabsorbable sulfonamides) *to destroy intestinal bacteria*
    2. potassium supplements *to decrease renal production of ammonia and the dissociation of NH_4 to NH_3*
    3. lactulose *to stimulate catharsis and create an acidic medium in the intestine (the acidity reduces bacterial growth and the resultant formation of ammonia and also traps ammonia in the colon by favoring the conversion of NH_3 to the poorly absorbed NH_4)*
    4. levodopa *to restore catecholamine neurotransmitter levels (these neurotransmitters may have been replaced by false neurotransmitters, which are normally metabolized by the liver)*
  f. prepare client for and assist with dialysis, exchange transfusions, charcoal hemoperfusion, cross circulation, plasmapheresis, or extracorporeal liver perfusion if performed *to reduce cerebrotoxin (e.g. ammonia) levels*
  g. institute general safety precautions
  h. provide emotional support to client and significant others.

16.e. The client will not develop spontaneous bacterial peritonitis as evidenced by:
1. absence of chills and fever
2. no complaints of severe abdominal pain
3. normal bowel sounds
4. WBC count within normal range.

16.e.1. Assess for and report signs and symptoms of spontaneous bacterial peritonitis (e.g. chills, fever, increase in severity or development of abdominal pain, rebound tenderness, diminished or absent bowel sounds, elevated WBC count).
  2. Implement measures *to reduce the risk of spontaneous bacterial peritonitis:*
    a. perform actions to reduce fluid volume excess and third-spacing (see Nursing Diagnosis 3, action a.4) *in order to decrease portal-systemic shunting and ascites*
    b. perform actions to prevent and treat infection (see Nursing Diagnosis 14, actions c and d) *in order to reduce the risk of bacteremia.*
  3. If signs and symptoms of spontaneous bacterial peritonitis occur:
    a. withhold all food and fluid as ordered
    b. place client on bedrest in a semi-Fowler's position *to assist in pooling or localizing the gastrointestinal contents in the pelvis rather than under the diaphragm*
    c. insert a nasogastric or intestinal tube and maintain suction as ordered
    d. monitor for therapeutic and nontherapeutic effects of anti-infectives if administered
    e. monitor for therapeutic and nontherapeutic effects of intravenous fluids and/or volume expanders if administered *to prevent or treat shock (shock can occur as a result of the escape of protein, fluid, and electrolytes into the peritoneal cavity)*

f. prepare client for paracentesis if planned
g. provide emotional support to client and significant others.

17. NURSING DIAGNOSIS

Sexual dysfunction:

a. **impotence** related to:
   1. inability of the liver to metabolize and inactivate estrogen
   2. low testosterone levels associated with an apparent defect in the hypothalamic-pituitary-gonadal axis in alcohol-related cirrhosis;
b. **diminished libido** related to:
   1. hormone imbalances associated with a decreased ability of liver to metabolize hormones and hypogonadism (thought to be a direct effect of excessive alcohol intake)
   2. weakness and fatigue
   3. altered self-concept.

DESIRED OUTCOMES	NURSING ACTIONS AND *SELECTED RATIONALES*
17. The client will demonstrate beginning acceptance of changes in sexual functioning (see Care Plan on Immobility, Nursing Diagnosis 15, for outcome criteria).	17.a. Refer to Care Plan on Immobility, Nursing Diagnosis 15, for measures related to assessment and management of sexual dysfunction. b. Implement additional measures *to promote optimal sexual functioning:* 　1. inform client that sexual dysfunction may be partially reversed in some persons if alcohol intake is stopped and the liver has a chance to regenerate 　2. encourage client to report continued impotence to physician; provide information regarding penile prosthesis if appropriate 　3. instruct client to allow adequate rest periods before and after sexual activity 　4. perform actions to promote a positive self-concept (see Nursing Diagnosis 18).

18. NURSING DIAGNOSIS

Disturbance in self-concept* related to:

a. changes in appearance (e.g. edema, ascites, jaundice, spider angiomas, palmar erythema, gynecomastia);
b. alterations in sexual functioning;
c. infertility associated with hormone imbalances resulting from the liver's inability to metabolize hormones and alcohol-induced hypogonadism;
d. dependence on others to meet self-care needs;
e. altered thought processes;
f. stigma of having a chronic illness;
g. possible changes in life style and roles.

---

* This diagnostic label includes the nursing diagnoses of body image disturbance and self-esteem disturbance.

DESIRED OUTCOMES	NURSING ACTIONS AND *SELECTED RATIONALES*

18. The client will demonstrate beginning adaptation to changes in appearance, level of independence, body functioning, life style, and roles (see Care Plan on Immobility, Nursing Diagnosis 16, for outcome criteria).	18.a. Refer to Care Plan on Immobility, Nursing Diagnosis 16, for measures related to assessment and promotion of a positive self-concept.
	b. Implement additional measures *to assist client to adapt to changes in appearance, level of independence, body functioning, life style, and roles:*
	1. encourage client to discuss concerns about fertility with physician; discuss options for becoming a parent (e.g. adoption, artificial insemination) if appropriate
	2. inform client that many of changes in appearance may be lessened by adherence to treatment regimen
	3. perform actions to promote optimal sexual functioning (see Nursing Diagnosis 17)
	4. discuss techniques the client can utilize *to adapt to alterations in thought processes:*
	  a. encourage client to make lists and jot down messages and refer to these notes rather than relying on memory
	  b. instruct client to place self in a calm environment when making decisions
	  c. encourage client to validate decisions, clarify information, and seek assistance to problem-solve
	5. assist client *to attain and maintain optimal independence:*
	  a. perform actions to increase client's strength and activity tolerance (see Nursing Diagnosis 7)
	  b. consult social services and occupational therapist about a home visit before discharge *to identify appropriate energy-saving techniques for client's current living situation*
	  c. reinforce benefits of utilizing portable oxygen if it has been prescribed
	6. encourge maximum participation in self-care within the prescribed activity restrictions and encourage significant others to allow client to do what he/she is able *so that independence can be re-established and self-esteem redeveloped.*

□ ▬▬▬▬▬▬▬▬▬▬▬▬▬▬▬▬▬▬

19. NURSING DIAGNOSIS

Grieving* related to loss of normal liver function, possible changes in life style, and uncertainty of prognosis.

---

* This diagnostic label includes anticipatory grieving and grieving following the actual changes/losses.

□ ▬▬▬▬▬▬▬▬▬▬▬▬▬▬▬▬▬▬

DESIRED OUTCOMES	NURSING ACTIONS AND *SELECTED RATIONALES*
19. The client will demonstrate beginning progression through the grieving process as evidenced by: a. verbalization of feelings about cirrhosis and its effect on his/her life b. expression of grief c. participation in treatment plan and self-care activities	19.a. Determine client's perception of the impact of cirrhosis on his/her future. b. Determine how client usually expresses grief. c. Observe for signs of grieving (e.g. changes in eating habits, insomnia, anger, noncompliance, denial). d. Implement measures *to facilitate the grieving process:* 1. assist client to acknowledge the loss of liver function *so grief work can begin;* assess for factors that may hinder or facilitate acknowledgment 2. discuss the grieving process and assist client to accept the stages of grieving as an expected response to the actual and/or anticipated changes; support the realization that grief may recur *because of the chronic nature of the disease*

d. utilization of available support systems

e. verbalization of a plan for integrating prescribed follow-up care into life style.

3. allow time for client to progress through the stages of grieving (denial, anger, bargaining, depression, acceptance [Kübler-Ross, 1969]); be aware that not every stage is experienced or expressed by all individuals

4. provide an atmosphere of care and concern (e.g. provide privacy, be available and nonjudgmental, display empathy and respect) *so that client will feel free to verbalize both positive and negative feelings and concerns*

5. perform actions *to promote trust* (e.g. answer questions honestly, provide requested information)

6. encourage the expression of anger and sadness about the changes experienced

7. encourage client to express his/her feelings in whatever ways are comfortable (e.g. writing, drawing, conversation)

8. assist client to identify personal strengths that have helped him/her to cope in previous situations of loss and change

9. support realistic hope about the success of treatment on disease progression.

e. Assess for and support behaviors suggesting successful resolution of grief (e.g. verbalizing feelings about changes, expressing sorrow, focusing on ways to adapt to changes).

f. Explain the stages of the grieving process to significant others. Encourage their support and understanding.

g. Provide information about counseling services and support groups that might assist client in working through grief.

h. Arrange for a visit from clergy if desired by client.

i. Monitor for therapeutic and nontherapeutic effects of antidepressants if administered.

j. Consult physician about referral for counseling if signs of dysfunctional grieving (e.g. persistent denial of losses or changes, excessive anger or sadness, hysteria, suicidal behaviors, phobias) occur.

☐ ▬▬▬▬▬▬▬▬▬▬▬▬▬▬▬▬▬▬▬▬▬▬▬▬▬▬▬▬

20. NURSING DIAGNOSIS

Noncompliance* related to:

a. lack of understanding of the implications of not following the prescribed treatment plan;
b. difficulty modifying personal habits (e.g. dietary habits, alcohol intake);
c. insufficient financial resources;
d. dysfunctional grieving.

---

* This diagnostic label includes both an informed decision by client not to comply and an inability to comply due to circumstances beyond the client's control.

☐ ▬▬▬▬▬▬▬▬▬▬▬▬▬▬▬▬▬▬▬▬▬▬▬▬▬▬▬▬

DESIRED OUTCOMES	NURSING ACTIONS AND *SELECTED RATIONALES*
20. The client will demonstrate the probability of future compliance with the prescribed treatment plan as evidenced by: a. willingness to learn about and participate in treatments and care b. statements reflecting ways to modify personal habits	20.a. Assess for indications that client may be unwilling or unable to comply with prescribed treatment plan: 1. statements reflecting that he/she was unable to manage care at home 2. failure to adhere to treatment plan while in hospital (e.g. not adhering to dietary modifications and fluid restrictions, refusing medications) 3. statements reflecting a lack of understanding of the factors that will cause further progression of liver failure 4. statements reflecting an unwillingness or inability to modify personal habits and integrate necessary treatments into life style 5. statements reflecting the view that cirrhosis has resolved once he/she is

and integrate treatments into life style

c. statements reflecting an understanding of the implications of not following the prescribed treatment plan.

feeling better or that there is no way to control the disease and efforts to comply with treatments are useless.

b. Implement measures *to improve client compliance:*
1. explain cirrhosis in terms the client can understand; stress the fact that cirrhosis is a chronic disease and adherence to the treatment plan is necessary *in order to delay and/or prevent complications*
2. encourage questions and clarify any misconceptions client has about cirrhosis and its effects
3. encourage client to participate in the treatment plan
4. initiate and reinforce the discharge teaching outlined in Nursing Diagnosis 21 *in order to promote a sense of control and self-reliance*
5. provide instructions on measuring intake and output, weighing self, and calculating dietary sodium and protein content; allow time for return demonstration; determine areas of difficulty and misunderstanding and reinforce teaching as necessary
6. provide client with written instructions about scheduled appointments with health care provider, medications, signs and symptoms to report, measuring intake and output, weighing self, and dietary modifications
7. assist client to identify ways he/she can incorporate treatments into life style; focus on modifications of life style rather than complete change
8. encourage client to discuss his/her concerns about cost of hospitalization, medications, and lifelong follow-up care; obtain a social service consult to assist the client with financial planning and to obtain financial aid if indicated
9. provide information about and encourage utilization of community resources that can assist client to make necessary life-style changes (e.g. drug and alcohol rehabilitation programs).

c. Assess for and reinforce behaviors suggesting future compliance with prescribed treatments (e.g. statements reflecting plans for integrating treatments into life style, participation in diet planning, statements reflecting an understanding of the importance of eliminating alcohol intake).

d. Include significant others in explanations and teaching sessions and encourage their support.

e. Reinforce the need for client to assume responsibility for and manage as much of care as possible.

f. Consult physician about referrals to community health agencies if continued instruction, support, or supervision is needed.

---

21. NURSING DIAGNOSIS

Knowledge deficit regarding follow-up care.

DESIRED OUTCOMES	NURSING ACTIONS AND *SELECTED RATIONALES*

21.a. The client will identify ways to prevent further liver damage.	21.a. Provide the following instructions regarding ways *to prevent further liver damage:*
	1. avoid the following hepatotoxic agents:
	  a. alcohol
	  b. cleaning agents containing carbon tetrachloride (these are toxic even when inhaled)
	2. caution client to take acetaminophen (e.g. Tylenol) only when necessary and not to exceed the recommended dose *because of its potential toxic effect on the liver*
	3. adhere to the following precautions *to prevent hepatitis:*
	  a. wash hands thoroughly after using the bathroom
	  b. use disposable seat covers

> c. eat only in restaurants that have been inspected and approved by health authorities
> d. if blood transfusions are necessary, receive autologous blood or blood from donor known not to have hepatitis
> e. do not drink water or eat shellfish that may be contaminated
> f. avoid intimate contact with known carrier of hepatitis
> g. avoid anal intercourse *since it is one way that hepatitis A can be transmitted*
> 4. adhere to prescribed dietary modifications.

21.b. The client will verbalize an understanding of the rationale for and constituents of the recommended diet.	21.b.1. Explain to client that adherence to the recommended diet will promote healing of the liver and reduce the risk of further liver damage. 2. Reinforce the dietary instructions outlined in Nursing Diagnosis 4, action e.3.
21.c. The client will identify ways to reduce irritation of and stress on esophageal vessels.	21.c.1. Provide the following instructions about *ways to reduce irritation of esophageal vessels:* a. avoid drinking alcohol b. do not take aspirin c. eliminate coarse foods (e.g. chips, nuts, celery) from diet d. avoid highly seasoned and acidic foods and foods/fluids containing caffeine (e.g. chocolate, coffee, tea, colas). 2. Instruct client to decrease stress on esophageal vessels by avoiding activities that increase intra-abdominal pressure (e.g. straining to have a bowel movement, coughing, sneezing, lifting heavy objects, eating large meals).
21.d. The client will identify ways to prevent bleeding.	21.d.1. Instruct client about ways *to minimize risk of bleeding:* a. avoid taking aspirin, aspirin-containing products, and ibuprofen b. use an electric rather than a straight-edge razor c. floss and brush teeth gently d. cut nails carefully e. avoid situations that could result in injury (e.g. contact sports) f. avoid blowing nose forcefully g. avoid straining to have a bowel movement. 2. Instruct client to control any bleeding by applying firm, prolonged pressure to the area if possible.
21.e. The client will identify ways to reduce the risk of infection.	21.e. Instruct client in ways *to reduce risk of infection:* 1. continue with coughing and deep breathing or use of inspiratory exerciser every 2 hours while awake as long as activity is limited 2. increase activity as tolerated 3. avoid contact with persons who have an infection 4. avoid crowds, especially during flu and cold seasons 5. decrease or stop smoking 6. drink at least 10 glasses of liquid/day 7. adhere to recommended diet 8. take supplemental vitamins and minerals as prescribed 9. maintain good personal hygiene.
21.f. The client will identify ways to relieve pruritus.	21.f.1. Reinforce instructions in Nursing Diagnosis 5.B, action 2, regarding ways to relieve itching. 2. Instruct client to take cholestyramine or an antihistamine as prescribed.
21.g. The client will state signs and symptoms to report to the health care provider.	21.g. Stress the importance of reporting the following signs and symptoms: 1. weight gain of more than 1 pound a day for more than 3 days 2. increased swelling of ankles, feet, abdomen 3. increasing shortness of breath 4. increased itchiness or yellowing of skin 5. temperature elevation that lasts more than 2 days 6. any blood in stools, urine, or vomitus; persistent bleeding from nose,

mouth, or skin; prolonged or excessive menses; excessive bruising; severe headache; or sudden abdominal or back pain

7. changes in behavior, speech, handwriting.

21.h. The client will identify community resources that can assist with home management and adjustment to life-style changes necessary for effective management of cirrhosis.

21.h.1. Provide information regarding community resources that can assist client and significant others with home management and adjustment to changes necessary for effective management of cirrhosis (e.g. Visiting Nurse Association, Meals on Wheels, home health agencies, transportation services, drug and alcohol rehabilitation programs, counseling services).
2. Initiate a referral if indicated.

21.i. The client will verbalize an understanding of and a plan for adhering to recommended follow-up care including future appointments with health care provider, medications prescribed, and activity level.

21.i.1. Reinforce the importance of keeping follow-up appointments with health care provider.
2. Explain the rationale for, side effects of, and importance of taking medications prescribed.
3. Reinforce physician's instructions regarding activity level. Stress the importance of rest in relation to the liver's ability to heal.
4. Implement measures outlined in Nursing Diagnosis 20, action b, to improve client compliance.

References

Carpenito, LJ. Handbook of nursing diagnosis (3rd ed.). Philadelphia: J.B. Lippincott Company, 1989.
Kübler-Ross, E. On death and dying. New York: Macmillan, 1969.

Hepatitis

Hepatitis is an inflammation of the liver that results in hepatic venous congestion and a temporary alteration of normal liver function. It is most commonly caused by a virus but may also be caused by bacteria or hepatotoxic agents (e.g. drugs, industrial chemicals). The four types of viral hepatitis that have been identified are hepatitis A (HAV); hepatitis B (HBV); non-A, non-B hepatitis; and delta hepatitis or hepatitis D (HDV). Hepatitis A is often referred to as infectious hepatitis and is transmitted primarily by the fecal-oral route. Hepatitis B is often referred to as serum hepatitis with the major modes of transmission being the parenteral and permucosal routes. It occurs most often in drug abusers; staff and clients in dialysis and oncology units; and persons who work in surgery, clinical laboratories, or dental clinics. Non-A, non-B hepatitis is epidemiologically similar to hepatitis B, occurs most frequently in persons who have received multiple transfusions, and accounts for about 90% of post-transfusion hepatitis. Hepatitis D appears to require the presence of the hepatitis B virus for its replication and is seen only in HBV-infected persons.

Hepatitis is a major public health problem because it is highly communicable, is transmissible prior to the onset of symptoms, and, as yet, has no effective drug treatment. The majority of cases of hepatitis resolve completely; there are instances, however, in which progressive liver degeneration occurs.

This care plan focuses on the adult client with viral hepatitis hospitalized because of unmanageable symptoms. The goals of care are to ensure adequate rest, maintain an optimal nutritional status, reduce discomfort, prevent complications, and educate the client regarding follow-up care. It is the responsibility of each health care provider to maintain appropriate isolation precautions for the type of hepatitis diagnosed in order to prevent the spread of infection to others.

UNIT XIII

DISCHARGE CRITERIA

Prior to discharge, the client will:

- identify ways to prevent the spread of hepatitis to others
- identify ways to prevent further liver damage
- verbalize an understanding of the rationale for and constituents of the recommended diet
- identify ways to reduce the risk of infection and bleeding until the liver has healed completely
- state signs and symptoms to report to the health care provider
- identify community resources that can assist with drug or alcohol rehabilitation if indicated
- verbalize an understanding of and a plan for adhering to recommended follow-up care including future appointments with health care provider, activity level, and medications prescribed.

☐ ▄▄

Use in conjunction with the Care Plan on Immobility.

☐ ▄▄

NURSING/COLLABORATIVE DIAGNOSES

1. Anxiety ☐ 765
2. Altered fluid and electrolyte balance:
   a. fluid volume deficit, hyponatremia, hypokalemia, and hypochloremia
   b. metabolic alkalosis ☐ 765
3. Altered nutrition: less than body requirements ☐ 766
4A. Altered comfort:
   1. upper abdominal pain
   2. flu-like symptoms: arthralgias, myalgias, and sore throat ☐ 767
4B. Altered comfort: pruritus ☐ 768
4C. Altered comfort: nausea and vomiting ☐ 769
4D. Altered comfort: chills and diaphoresis ☐ 769
5. Hyperthermia ☐ 770
6. Activity intolerance ☐ 770
7. Impaired physical mobility ☐ 771
8. Self-care deficit ☐ 771
9. Potential for infection: superinfection ☐ 772
10. Potential complications:
    a. bleeding
    b. third-spacing
    c. hepatic coma (portal systemic encephalopathy)
    d. progressive liver degeneration ☐ 773
11. Disturbance in self-concept ☐ 776
12. Noncompliance ☐ 777
13. Knowledge deficit regarding follow-up care ☐ 778

1. NURSING DIAGNOSIS

Anxiety related to unfamiliar environment; lack of understanding of diagnosis, diagnostic tests, treatments, and prognosis; and anticipated changes in life style and roles as a result of hepatitis and its treatment.

DESIRED OUTCOMES	NURSING ACTIONS AND *SELECTED RATIONALES*

1. The client will experience a reduction in fear and anxiety (see Care Plan on Immobility, Nursing Diagnosis 1, for outcome criteria).	1.a. Refer to Care Plan on Immobility, Nursing Diagnosis 1, for measures related to assessment and reduction of fear and anxiety.
	  b. Implement additional measures *to reduce fear and anxiety:*
	   1. explain tests that may be performed to diagnose the type of hepatitis or degree of liver dysfunction:
	     a. blood studies:
	       1. serum enzymes (e.g. AST [SGOT], ALT [SGPT], GGT, LDH, alkaline phosphatase [ALP], LAP, 5'-nucleotidase)
	       2. serum cholesterol and triglyceride levels
	       3. serum proteins and protein electrophoresis
	       4. indirect (unconjugated), direct (conjugated), and total serum bilirubin levels
	       5. antigen-antibody levels (e.g. IgM-specific anti-HAV, HBsAg, HBeAg, anti-HBc, anti-HDV)
	       6. complete blood count (CBC)
	       7. prothrombin time (PT)
	       8. ammonia levels
	     b. urine studies for bilirubin and urobilinogen levels
	     c. radioisotope scans, ultrasonography, computed tomography (CT), and/or magnetic resonance imaging (MRI) of liver
	   2. clarify misconceptions about necessary changes in life style; reinforce the fact that most limitations are temporary.

2. NURSING/COLLABORATIVE DIAGNOSIS

Altered fluid and electrolyte balance:

a. **fluid volume deficit, hyponatremia, hypokalemia, and hypochloremia** related to:
  1. excessive loss of fluid and electrolytes associated with persistent vomiting
  2. decreased oral intake associated with anorexia, nausea, sore throat, and fatigue;
b. **metabolic alkalosis** related to excessive loss of hydrochloric acid associated with persistent vomiting.

DESIRED OUTCOMES	NURSING ACTIONS AND *SELECTED RATIONALES*

2. The client will maintain fluid and electrolyte balance as evidenced by:
  a. normal skin turgor
  b. moist mucous membranes
  c. stable weight
	2.a. Assess for and report signs and symptoms of:
	   1. fluid volume deficit:
	     a. decreased skin turgor, dry mucous membranes, thirst
	     b. weight loss greater than 0.5 kg/day
	     c. low B/P and/or decline in systolic B/P of at least 15 mm Hg with concurrent rise in pulse when client sits up

d. B/P and pulse within normal range for client and stable with position change

e. balanced intake and output

f. urine specific gravity between 1.010–1.030

g. no evidence of confusion, irritability, lethargy, excessive thirst, ileus, cardiac arrhythmias, muscle weakness

h. normal serum osmolality, electrolytes, and blood gases.

d. weak, rapid pulse

e. output less than intake with urine specific gravity higher than 1.030 (reflects an actual rather than potential fluid volume deficit)

2. hyponatremia (e.g. nausea and vomiting, abdominal cramps, weakness, lethargy, twitching, confusion, seizures)

3. hypokalemia (e.g. irregular pulse, muscle weakness and cramping, paresthesias, nausea and vomiting, hypoactive or absent bowel sounds, drowsiness)

4. hypochloremia (e.g. twitching, tetany, depressed respirations)

5. metabolic alkalosis (e.g. dizziness; confusion; bradypnea; tingling of fingers, toes, and circumoral area; muscle twitching; seizures).

b. Monitor serum osmolality, electrolyte, and blood gas results. Report abnormal values.

c. Implement measures *to prevent and treat fluid and electrolyte imbalances:*
   1. perform actions to prevent nausea and vomiting (see Nursing Diagnosis 4.C, action 2)
   2. perform actions to improve oral intake (see Nursing Diagnosis 3, action e.1)
   3. monitor for therapeutic and nontherapeutic effects of fluid and electrolyte replacements if administered
   4. maintain a fluid intake of at least 2500 cc/day unless contraindicated
   5. assist client to select foods/fluids high in potassium (e.g. bananas, raisins, apricots, potatoes, Gatorade, fruit juices) and sodium (e.g. processed cheese, soups, canned vegetables, pickles, bouillon).

d. Consult physician if signs and symptoms of fluid and electrolyte imbalances persist or worsen.

☐ ▆▆▆▆▆▆▆▆▆▆▆▆▆▆▆▆▆▆▆▆▆▆▆▆▆▆▆▆▆▆

3. NURSING DIAGNOSIS

Altered nutrition: less than body requirements related to:

a. decreased oral intake associated with anorexia, nausea, sore throat, and fatigue;

b. loss of nutrients associated with persistent vomiting;

c. reduced metabolism and storage of nutrients by the liver associated with an alteration in normal liver function as a result of inflammation;

d. malabsorption of fats and fat-soluble vitamins associated with impaired bile flow as a result of inflammation;

e. increased utilization of nutrients associated with the increased basal metabolic rate that is present with infection.

☐ ▆▆▆▆▆▆▆▆▆▆▆▆▆▆▆▆▆▆▆▆▆▆▆▆▆▆▆▆▆▆

DESIRED OUTCOMES	NURSING ACTIONS AND *SELECTED RATIONALES*

3. The client will maintain an adequate nutritional status as evidenced by:

a. weight within normal range for client's age, height, and build

b. normal BUN and serum albumin, protein, Hct., Hgb., B_{12}, folate, cholesterol, and lymphocyte levels

c. triceps skinfold measurements within normal range

d. improved strength and activity tolerance

3.a. Assess the client for signs and symptoms of malnutrition:
   1. weight below normal for client's age, height, and build
   2. abnormal BUN and low serum albumin, protein, Hct., Hgb., B_{12}, folate, cholesterol, and lymphocyte levels (these values are also a reflection of impaired liver function)
   3. triceps skinfold measurement less than normal for build
   4. weakness and fatigue
   5. stomatitis.

b. Reassess nutritional status on a regular basis and report decline.

c. Monitor percentage of meals eaten.

d. Assess client to determine causes of inadequate intake (e.g. nausea, sore throat, fatigue, anorexia).

e. Implement measures *to improve nutritional status:*
   1. perform actions *to improve oral intake:*
      a. implement measures to relieve nausea and vomiting (see Nursing Diagnosis 4.C, action 2)

e. healthy oral mucous membrane.

b. provide oral care before meals
c. serve small portions of nutritious foods/fluids that are appealing to client
d. provide a clean, relaxed, pleasant atmosphere
e. offer larger meals in the morning *since nausea is often not as severe in the morning*
f. implement measures to reduce discomfort associated with sore throat (see Nursing Diagnosis 4.A, action 5.a)
g. obtain a dietary consult if necessary to assist client in selecting foods/fluids that meet nutritional needs as well as preferences
h. encourage a rest period before meals *to minimize fatigue*
i. allow adequate time for meals; reheat food if necessary
j. increase activity as allowed and tolerated *(activity stimulates appetite)*

2. assist and instruct client to adhere to the following dietary recommendations:
   a. avoid skipping meals
   b. consume a diet high in calories (2500–3000 calories/day) and carbohydrates
   c. maintain a moderate to high protein intake (unless the serum ammonia level is high or clinical evidence of encephalopathy is present) *in order to promote normal healing of the liver*
   d. increase intake of foods high in the following vitamins and minerals:
      1. vitamin B_{12} (e.g. organ meats, eggs, fresh shrimp, chicken)
      2. folic acid (e.g. green leafy vegetables, asparagus, organ meats, lima beans, fruits)
      3. iron (e.g. organ meats, apricots, green leafy vegetables, whole-grain and enriched breads)
   e. suck on hard candy and drink fruit juices and carbonated beverages if unable to tolerate solid food *(these items provide a quick source of energy)*

3. monitor for therapeutic and nontherapeutic effects of the following medications if administered:
   a. vitamin preparations (e.g. fat-soluble vitamins, B-complex vitamins, folic acid)
   b. medium-chain triglycerides (MCT) in an oil medium *to provide an absorbable source of fatty acids.*

f. Perform a 72-hour calorie count if nutritional status declines or fails to improve.
g. Consult physician about alternative methods of providing nutrition (e.g. parenteral nutrition, tube feeding) if client does not consume enough food or fluids to meet nutritional needs.

□ ▓▓▓▓▓▓▓▓▓▓▓▓▓▓▓▓▓▓▓▓▓▓▓▓▓

4.A. NURSING DIAGNOSIS

Altered comfort:*

1. **upper abdominal pain** related to inflammation of the liver;
2. **flu-like symptoms: arthralgias, myalgias, and sore throat** related to the systemic effects of a viral infection.

---

* In this care plan, the nursing diagnosis "pain" is included under the diagnostic label of altered comfort.

□ ▓▓▓▓▓▓▓▓▓▓▓▓▓▓▓▓▓▓▓▓▓▓▓▓▓

UNIT XIII

DESIRED OUTCOMES	NURSING ACTIONS AND *SELECTED RATIONALES*
4.A. The client will experience diminished discomfort as evidenced by: 1. verbalization of same	4.A.1. Determine how the client usually responds to discomfort. 2. Assess for nonverbal signs of discomfort (e.g. wrinkled brow, reluctance to move, guarding abdomen, rubbing joints and muscles, restlessness, difficulty swallowing).

2. relaxed facial expression and body positioning
3. increased participation in activities.

3. Assess verbal complaints of discomfort. Ask client to be specific about location, severity, and type of discomfort.
4. Assess for factors that seem to aggravate and alleviate discomfort.
5. Implement measures *to reduce discomfort:*
   a. if sore throat is present:
      1. instruct client to avoid substances that might further irritate the throat (e.g. extremely hot, spicy, or acidic foods/fluids; dry or hard foods; raw fruits and vegetables)
      2. encourage client to stop smoking *(smoke irritates the throat)*
      3. offer cool, soothing liquids such as nonacidic juices, ices, and ice cream
      4. instruct client to gargle with a saline solution at least every 2 hours *to soothe the mucous membrane*
      5. consult physician regarding order for anesthetic throat lozenges or sprays
   b. apply heat to aching muscles and joints as ordered
   c. provide or assist with nonpharmacological measures for relief of discomfort (e.g. back rub, position change, relaxation techniques, quiet conversation, restful environment, diversional activities)
   d. monitor for therapeutic and nontherapeutic effects of analgesics if administered (question any order for a normal adult dose of narcotics and acetaminophen *because the liver cannot detoxify narcotics at its usual rate and acetaminophen is a potential hepatotoxin).*
6. Consult physician if above measures fail to provide adequate relief of discomfort.

4.B. NURSING DIAGNOSIS

Altered comfort: pruritus related to:

1. bile salt accumulation underneath the skin associated with obstruction of bile flow;
2. rash (sometimes occurs as a result of activation of the complement system by the immune complexes formed in response to viruses).

DESIRED OUTCOMES	NURSING ACTIONS AND *SELECTED RATIONALES*

4.B. The client will experience relief of pruritus as evidenced by:
 1. verbalization of same
 2. no scratching or rubbing of skin.
	4.B.1. Assess pruritus including onset, characteristics, location, factors that aggravate or alleviate it, and client tolerance.
	 2. Instruct client in and/or implement measures *to relieve pruritus:*
	   a. apply cool, moist compresses to pruritic areas
	   b. apply emollients to skin *to help alleviate dryness*
	   c. add emollients, cornstarch, baking soda, or oatmeal to bath water
	   d. use tepid water and mild soaps for bathing
	   e. pat skin dry, making sure to dry thoroughly
	   f. maintain a cool environment
	   g. encourage participation in diversional activity
	   h. utilize relaxation techniques
	   i. utilize cutaneous stimulation techniques (e.g. massage, pressure, vibration, stroking with a soft brush) at the site of itching or acupressure points
	   j. encourage client to wear loose cotton garments.
	 3. Monitor for therapeutic and nontherapeutic effects of the following if administered *to relieve itching:*
	   a. antihistamines
	   b. antipruritic lotions

c. cholestyramine *to bind bile salts and reduce their accumulation under skin.*
4. Consult physician if above measures fail to alleviate pruritus or if the skin becomes excoriated.

□ ▬▬▬▬▬▬▬▬▬▬▬▬▬▬▬▬▬▬▬▬▬▬▬▬▬▬

4.C. NURSING DIAGNOSIS

Altered comfort: nausea and vomiting related to stimulation of the vomiting center associated with:

1. vagal and/or sympathetic stimulation resulting from visceral irritation due to:
   a. venous congestion of the gastrointestinal tract (a result of portal hypertension)
   b. gaseous distention resulting from impaired fat digestion
   c. superficial gastritis that may be present with a viral infection;
2. cortical stimulation due to stress.

□ ▬▬▬▬▬▬▬▬▬▬▬▬▬▬▬▬▬▬▬▬▬▬▬▬▬▬

DESIRED OUTCOMES	NURSING ACTIONS AND *SELECTED RATIONALES*

4.C. The client will experience relief of nausea and vomiting as evidenced by:
1. verbalization of relief of nausea
2. absence of vomiting.
	4.C.1. Assess client to determine factors that contribute to nausea and vomiting (e.g. eating, particular foods, certain positions).
	2. Implement measures *to reduce nausea and vomiting:*
	  a. eliminate noxious sights and smells from the environment *(noxious stimuli cause cortical stimulation of the vomiting center)*
	  b. instruct client to change positions slowly *(movement stimulates the chemoreceptor trigger zone)*
	  c. provide oral hygiene every 2 hours and after each emesis
	  d. perform actions to reduce fear and anxiety (see Nursing Diagnosis 1)
	  e. encourage client to take deep, slow breaths when nauseated
	  f. encourage client to limit intake of foods/fluids high in fat (e.g. butter, cream, oils, whole milk, ice cream, pork, fried foods, gravies, nuts) *to reduce nausea associated with impaired fat digestion*
	  g. instruct client to ingest foods and fluids slowly
	  h. instruct client to eat dry foods (e.g. toast, crackers) and avoid drinking liquids with meals if nauseated
	  i. provide small, frequent meals rather than 3 large ones
	  j. instruct client to avoid foods/fluids that irritate the gastric mucosa (e.g. spicy foods; citrus fruits or juices; caffeine-containing items such as chocolate, tea, coffee, or colas)
	  k. instruct client to rest after eating with head of bed elevated
	  l. monitor for therapeutic and nontherapeutic effects of antiemetics if administered (phenothiazines are contraindicated *because of their potential cholestatic and central nervous system depressant effects*).
	3. Consult physician if above measures fail to control nausea and vomiting.

□ ▬▬▬▬▬▬▬▬▬▬▬▬▬▬▬▬▬▬▬▬▬▬▬▬▬▬

4.D. NURSING DIAGNOSIS

Altered comfort: chills and diaphoresis related to persistent fever associated with the infectious process.

□ ▬▬▬▬▬▬▬▬▬▬▬▬▬▬▬▬▬▬▬▬▬▬▬▬▬▬

DESIRED OUTCOMES	NURSING ACTIONS AND *SELECTED RATIONALES*

4.D. The client will not experience discomfort associated with chills and diaphoresis as evidenced by:
1. verbalization of comfort
2. ability to rest.
	4.D.1. Assess client for chills and diaphoresis.
	2. Implement measures to reduce fever (see Nursing Diagnosis 5, action b).
	3. Implement measures *to promote comfort if client is having chills:*
	  a. maintain a room temperature that is comfortable for the client
	  b. protect client from drafts
	  c. provide extra clothing and blankets as needed
	  d. provide warm liquids to drink as tolerated.
	4. Implement measures *to promote comfort if excessive diaphoresis is present:*
	  a. change linen and clothing whenever damp
	  b. bathe client and sponge his/her face as needed.
	5. Consult physician if client continues to have chills and excessive diaphoresis.

☐ ▄▄

5. NURSING DIAGNOSIS

Hyperthermia related to stimulation of the thermoregulatory center in the hypothalamus by endogenous pyrogens that are released in an infectious process.

☐ ▄▄

DESIRED OUTCOMES	NURSING ACTIONS AND *SELECTED RATIONALES*

5. The client will have gradual resolution of hyperthermia as evidenced by:
a. skin usual color and temperature
b. pulse rate between 60–100 beats/minute
c. respirations 16–20/minute
d. normal body temperature.
	5.a. Assess for signs and symptoms of hyperthermia (e.g. warm, flushed skin; tachycardia; tachypnea; elevated temperature).
	b. Implement measures *to reduce fever:*
	  1. perform actions *to resolve the infectious process:*
	    a. implement measures to promote physical and emotional rest
	    b. implement measures to maintain an optimal nutritional status (see Nursing Diagnosis 3, action e)
	  2. administer tepid sponge bath
	  3. apply cooling blanket as ordered
	  4. monitor for therapeutic and nontherapeutic effects of antipyretics if administered.
	c. Consult physician if temperature remains higher than 38°C.

☐ ▄▄

6. NURSING DIAGNOSIS

Activity intolerance related to:

a. tissue hypoxia associated with anemia that may result from:
  1. decreased production and slow maturation of RBCs associated with decreased oral intake of vitamins and minerals and an inability of the liver to store iron, vitamin B_{12}, and folic acid
  2. excessive RBC destruction if venous congestion has resulted in splenomegaly
  3. blood loss associated with an increased bleeding tendency;
b. inadequate nutritional status;
c. increased energy utilization associated with the increased basal metabolic rate present in infectious processes;
d. difficulty resting and sleeping due to frequent assessments and treatments, discomfort, fear, and anxiety.

☐ ▄▄

DESIRED OUTCOMES	NURSING ACTIONS AND *SELECTED RATIONALES*

6. The client will demonstrate an increased tolerance for activity (see Care Plan on Immobility, Nursing Diagnosis 8, for outcome criteria).	6.a. Refer to Care Plan on Immobility, Nursing Diagnosis 8, for measures related to assessment and improvement of activity tolerance.
	   b. Implement additional measures *to promote rest and improve activity tolerance:*
	   1. maintain activity restrictions as ordered
	   2. perform actions to reduce fear and anxiety (see Nursing Diagnosis 1)
	   3. perform actions to reduce discomfort (see Nursing Diagnoses 4.A, action 5; 4.B, actions 2 and 3; 4.C, action 2; and 4.D, actions 3 and 4)
	   4. maintain an optimal nutritional status (see Nursing Diagnosis 3, action e)
	   5. monitor for therapeutic and nontherapeutic effects of whole blood or packed red cells if administered (transfusions are not given unless absolutely necessary *because of the risk of further infection*)
	   6. increase activity gradually as allowed and tolerated.

□ ▬▬▬▬▬▬▬▬▬▬▬▬▬▬▬▬▬▬▬▬

7. NURSING DIAGNOSIS

Impaired physical mobility related to weakness and fatigue, reluctance to move due to arthralgias and/or myalgias, and activity restrictions imposed by the treatment plan.

□ ▬▬▬▬▬▬▬▬▬▬▬▬▬▬▬▬▬▬▬▬

DESIRED OUTCOMES	NURSING ACTIONS AND *SELECTED RATIONALES*

7.a. The client will maintain an optimal level of physical mobility within physical limitations and activity restrictions imposed by the treatment plan.	7.a.1. Assess for factors that impair physical mobility (e.g. weakness, fatigue, reluctance to move because of muscle or joint pain, activity restrictions imposed by the treatment plan).
	   2. Implement measures *to increase mobility:*
	   a. perform actions to increase strength and activity tolerance (see Nursing Diagnosis 6)
	   b. perform actions to reduce joint and muscle discomfort (see Nursing Diagnosis 4.A, actions 5.b–d).
	   3. Increase activity and participation in self-care activities as allowed and tolerated.

7.b. The client will not experience problems associated with immobility.	7.b. Refer to Care Plan on Immobility for actions to prevent problems associated with immobility if client is to remain on bedrest for longer than 48 hours.

□ ▬▬▬▬▬▬▬▬▬▬▬▬▬▬▬▬▬▬▬▬

8. NURSING DIAGNOSIS

Self-care deficit related to impaired physical mobility associated with weakness, fatigue, discomfort, and prescribed activity restrictions.

□ ▬▬▬▬▬▬▬▬▬▬▬▬▬▬▬▬▬▬▬▬

DESIRED OUTCOMES	NURSING ACTIONS AND *SELECTED RATIONALES*
8. The client will demonstrate increased participation in self-	8.a. Refer to Care Plan on Immobility, Nursing Diagnosis 9, for measures related to assessment of, planning for, and meeting the client's self-care needs.

care activities within limitations imposed by the disease condition and the treatment plan.

b. Implement measures to increase mobility (see Nursing Diagnosis 7, action a.2) *in order to further facilitate client's ability to perform self-care activities.*

☐ ▬▬▬▬▬▬▬▬▬▬▬▬▬▬▬▬▬▬▬▬▬▬▬▬▬▬

9. NURSING DIAGNOSIS

Potential for infection: superinfection related to lowered natural resistance associated with:

a. diminished function of the Kupffer cells in the liver (these cells normally phagocytize bacteria);
b. inadequate nutritional status and anemia;
c. leukopenia resulting from the viral infection and hypersplenism (if venous congestion has resulted in splenomegaly, the spleen will destroy leukocytes faster than usual).

☐ ▬▬▬▬▬▬▬▬▬▬▬▬▬▬▬▬▬▬▬▬▬▬▬▬▬▬

DESIRED OUTCOMES	NURSING ACTIONS AND *SELECTED RATIONALES*

9. The client will remain free of a superinfection as evidenced by:
   a. decline in or absence of chills and fever
   b. pulse returning toward normal limits
   c. normal breath sounds
   d. voiding clear, yellow urine without complaints of frequency, urgency, and burning
   e. absence of redness, swelling, and unusual drainage in any area where there is a break in skin integrity
   f. intact oral mucous membrane
   g. WBC and differential counts returning toward normal range
   h. negative results of cultured specimens.

9.a. Assess for and report signs and symptoms of superinfection:
   1. increased temperature
   2. persistent or increased chills
   3. pattern of increased pulse or pulse rate greater than 100 beats/minute
   4. adventitious breath sounds
   5. cloudy or foul-smelling urine
   6. complaints of frequency, urgency, or burning when urinating
   7. presence of WBCs, bacteria, and/or nitrites in urine
   8. redness, swelling, or unusual drainage in any area where there is a break in skin integrity
   9. irritation or ulceration of oral mucous membrane
   10. elevated WBC count and/or significant change in differential.
   b. Obtain culture specimens (e.g. urine, vaginal, mouth, sputum, blood) as ordered. Report positive results.
   c. Implement measures *to reduce risk of superinfection:*
      1. maintain a minimum fluid intake of 2500 cc/day unless contraindicated
      2. use good handwashing technique and encourage client to do the same
      3. maintain meticulous aseptic technique during all invasive procedures (e.g. catheterizations, venous and arterial punctures, injections)
      4. protect client from others with infection
      5. maintain an optimal nutritional status (see Nursing Diagnosis 3, action e)
      6. provide or assist with good oral care
      7. provide proper balance of exercise and rest
      8. perform actions *to prevent respiratory tract infection:*
         a. instruct and assist client to turn, cough, and deep breathe at least every 2 hours while mobility is limited
         b. instruct and assist client in use of inspiratory exerciser at least every 2 hours if indicated
         c. encourage client to stop smoking
         d. increase activity as allowed and tolerated
      9. perform actions *to prevent urinary tract infection:*
         a. instruct and assist female client to wipe from front to back following urination and defecation
         b. keep perianal area clean.
   d. Monitor for therapeutic and nontherapeutic effects of anti-infectives if administered. (Monitor liver function tests closely *because many anti-infective agents have a hepatotoxic and/or cholestatic effect.*)

□ ▬▬▬▬▬▬▬▬▬▬▬▬▬▬▬▬▬▬

10. COLLABORATIVE DIAGNOSIS

Potential complications:

a. **bleeding** related to:
  1. decreased production of clotting factors associated with impaired liver function and impaired vitamin K absorption (normal bile flow is necessary for absorption of vitamin K)
  2. splenic platelet pooling and thrombocytopenia associated with hypersplenism (if venous congestion has resulted in splenomegaly, the spleen will pool platelets and also destroy them faster than usual);
b. **third-spacing** related to:
  1. low plasma colloid osmotic pressure associated with decreased plasma proteins (a result of decreased hepatic synthesis of plasma proteins and possible loss of proteins into the peritoneal cavity due to obstructed hepatic lymph flow and increased hydrostatic pressure in the portal vein)
  2. increased hydrostatic pressure in the hepatic venous and lymph systems associated with hepatic inflammation
  3. generalized increase in hydrostatic pressure associated with fluid volume excess resulting from the liver's inability to metabolize aldosterone and diminished renal blood flow due to venous congestion;
c. **hepatic coma (portal systemic encephalopathy)** related to cerebral toxicity associated with:
  1. high serum ammonia levels resulting from the liver's inability to convert ammonia to urea
  2. deficiency of neurotransmitters resulting from an inability of the liver to detoxify certain substances that act as false neurotransmitters (these false neurotransmitters then occupy sites the neurotransmitters normally occupy)
  3. increased levels of certain amino acids, short- and medium-chain fatty acids, and mercaptans resulting from the liver's inability to metabolize these substances;
d. **progressive liver degeneration** related to fulminant hepatitis or chronic active hepatitis.

□ ▬▬▬▬▬▬▬▬▬▬▬▬▬▬▬▬▬▬

DESIRED OUTCOMES	NURSING ACTIONS AND *SELECTED RATIONALES*
10.a. The client will not experience unusual bleeding as evidenced by: 1. skin and mucous membranes free of bleeding, petechiae, and ecchymosis 2. absence of unusual joint pain and swelling 3. no sudden increase in abdominal girth 4. absence of frank or occult blood in stool, urine, and vomitus 5. usual menstrual flow 6. vital signs within normal range for client 7. stable Hct. and Hgb. 8. usual mental status.	10.a.1. Assess client for and report signs and symptoms of unusual bleeding: a. petechiae b. multiple ecchymotic areas c. bleeding gums d. frequent or uncontrollable episodes of epistaxis e. unusual oozing from injection sites f. unusual joint pain or swelling g. sudden increase in abdominal girth h. hematemesis, melena, red or smoke-colored urine i. hypermenorrhea j. significant drop in B/P accompanied by an increased pulse rate k. decline in Hct. and Hgb. levels l. restlessness, confusion. 2. Monitor coagulation test results (e.g. prothrombin time, activated partial thromboplastin time, platelet count, bleeding time). Report abnormal values. 3. If coagulation test results are abnormal or Hct. and Hgb. levels decline, test all stools, urine, and vomitus for occult blood. Report positive results. 4. Implement measures *to prevent bleeding:* a. use smallest gauge needle possible when giving injections and performing venous or arterial punctures

b. apply gentle, prolonged pressure after injections and venous or arterial punctures
c. take B/P only when necessary and avoid overinflating cuff
d. caution client to avoid activities that increase the potential for trauma (e.g. shaving with a straight-edge razor, cutting nails, using stiff bristle toothbrush or dental floss)
e. pad side rails if client is confused or restless
f. remove hazardous objects from pathway *to prevent bumps or falls*
g. instruct client to avoid blowing nose forcefully or straining to have a bowel movement; consult physician about an order for decongestants, stool softeners, and/or laxatives if indicated
h. monitor for therapeutic and nontherapeutic effects of the following if administered *to improve clotting ability:*
1. vitamin K (e.g. phytonadione) injections
2. platelets
3. fresh blood or plasma (*the liver cannot detoxify the preservative in stored blood*).
5. If bleeding occurs and does not subside spontaneously:
a. apply firm, prolonged pressure to bleeding area if possible
b. if epistaxis occurs, place client in a high Fowler's position and apply pressure and ice packs to nasal area
c. maintain oxygen therapy as ordered
d. if gastric or esophageal bleeding occurs, assist with the following measures *to control bleeding:*
1. insertion and maintenance of gastroesophageal balloon tamponade and performance of iced water or saline lavage
2. intravenous or intra-arterial administration of vasopressin (*reduces portal congestion by constricting the splanchnic arterioles*)
3. sclerotherapy
e. administer vitamin K (e.g. phytonadione) injections and blood products (e.g. fresh frozen plasma, whole blood, platelets) as ordered
f. prepare client for surgical repair of bleeding vessels if planned
g. provide emotional support to client and significant others.

10.b. The client will maintain normal fluid balance without evidence of fluid volume excess or third-spacing as evidenced by:
1. stable weight
2. B/P and pulse within normal range for client and stable with position change
3. absence of gallop rhythms
4. balanced intake and output
5. CVP within normal range
6. absence of neck vein distention, peripheral edema, ascites, dyspnea
7. normal breath sounds
8. usual mental status.

10.b.1. Assess for and report signs and symptoms of:
a. fluid volume excess:
1. significant weight gain (greater than 0.5 kg/day)
2. elevated B/P
3. development of an S_3 and/or S_4 gallop rhythm
4. intake greater than output
5. elevated CVP (use internal jugular vein pulsation method to estimate)
6. distended neck veins
b. third-spacing:
1. peripheral edema
2. ascites as evidenced by:
a. increase in abdominal girth (abdominal girth should be measured daily at the same time and in the same location on abdomen with client in same position)
b. dull percussion note over abdomen with finding of shifting dullness
c. presence of abdominal fluid wave
d. protruding umbilicus and bulging flanks
3. dyspnea, orthopnea
4. crackles and diminished or absent breath sounds
5. change in mental status
6. decline in systolic B/P of at least 15 mm Hg with a concurrent rise in pulse when client changes from a supine to sitting position.
2. Monitor chest x-ray results. Report findings of vascular congestion, pleural effusion, and pulmonary edema.
3. Monitor serum albumin levels. Report below-normal levels (*albumin maintains plasma colloid osmotic pressure*).
4. If signs and symptoms of fluid volume excess or third-spacing occur:
a. implement measures *to reduce fluid volume excess:*
1. maintain fluid restrictions as ordered
2. restrict sodium intake as ordered

3. monitor for therapeutic and nontherapeutic effects of diuretics if administered *to increase excretion of water* (usually a thiazide diuretic or furosemide is given in conjunction with an aldosterone-blocking agent)

b. implement measures *to promote mobilization of fluid back into the vascular space and prevent further third-spacing:*
  1. perform actions to reduce fluid volume excess (see action b.4.a in this diagnosis)
  2. maintain bedrest if ordered or encourage client to lie down periodically *(lying down promotes reshifting of fluid into the vascular space)*
  3. perform actions *to increase colloid osmotic pressure:*
    a. provide a diet high in protein and still within the prescribed sodium restriction (e.g. poultry, fish, protein supplements) *to increase serum protein levels* (not appropriate if serum ammonia level is elevated or clinical signs and symptoms of encephalopathy are present)
    b. monitor for therapeutic and nontherapeutic effects of salt-poor albumin infusions if administered.

5. Consult physician if signs and symptoms of fluid imbalance persist or worsen.

10.c. The client will not develop hepatic encephalopathy as evidenced by:
1. usual mental status
2. usual speech and handwriting
3. absence of asterixis and fetor hepaticus
4. serum ammonia level within normal range.

10.c.1. Assess for and report signs and symptoms of hepatic encephalopathy:
a. emotional lability
b. lapses in memory, inability to concentrate
c. agitation, combativeness
d. lethargy, confusion, decreased responsiveness
e. slow, slurred speech
f. change in handwriting, inability to draw simple figures or numbers
g. asterixis (rhythmic movements of hands when client extends arms and dorsiflexes hands, rhythmic movements of legs with dorsiflexion of feet)
h. fetor hepaticus (musty, sweet odor on breath)
i. coma.

2. Monitor serum ammonia results. Report elevated values.
3. Implement measures *to prevent hepatic coma:*
a. perform actions *to prevent or control the following conditions that can lead to increases in ammonia level:*
  1. constipation *(intestinal bacteria have a longer time and more contents to convert to ammonia)*
  2. gastrointestinal hemorrhage *(the intestinal bacteria convert the protein in blood to ammonia)*
  3. hypokalemia and/or metabolic alkalosis *(increase the dissociation of NH_4 to the more diffusable NH_3; hypokalemia also increases renal production of ammonia)*
  4. renal failure *(results in decreased excretion of ammonia)*
  5. excessive protein intake *(intestinal bacteria convert protein to ammonia)*
b. perform actions *to prevent further damage to the liver:*
  1. implement measures to prevent and treat third-spacing (see action b.4.b in this diagnosis) and bleeding (see actions a.4 and 5 in this diagnosis) *in order to prevent hypovolemia and maintain an adequate blood flow to the liver*
  2. consult physician before administering known or potential hepatotoxins (e.g. methyldopa, isoniazid, acetaminophen, tetracycline, sulfonamides)
c. perform actions *to reduce metabolic demands on the liver:*
  1. implement measures to resolve the infectious process (see Nursing Diagnosis 5, action b.1) and prevent and treat superinfection (see Nursing Diagnosis 9, actions c and d)
  2. maintain activity restrictions as ordered
d. administer central nervous system depressants such as narcotics, sedatives, hypnotics, and antianxiety agents with extreme caution *(many of these agents are metabolized in the liver and may precipitate nonnitrogenous coma).*

UNIT XIII

4. If signs and symptoms of hepatic encephalopathy occur:
   a. maintain client on strict bedrest *to reduce metabolic demands on the liver*
   b. maintain dietary protein restrictions as ordered (usually 20–40 gm/day) *to reduce serum ammonia level*
   c. ensure a high carbohydrate intake or administer intravenous glucose or tube feedings as ordered *to provide a rapid energy source and prevent protein catabolism*
   d. administer enemas and/or cathartics as ordered *to hasten expulsion of intestinal contents so that bacteria have less time to convert proteins to ammonia*
   e. monitor for therapeutic and nontherapeutic effects of the following medications if administered:
      1. antibiotics (e.g. neomycin, nonabsorbable sulfonamides) *to destroy intestinal bacteria*
      2. potassium supplements *to decrease renal production of ammonia and the dissociation of NH_4 to NH_3*
      3. lactulose *to stimulate catharsis and create an acidic medium in the intestine (the acidity reduces bacterial growth and the resultant formation of ammonia and also traps ammonia in the colon by favoring the conversion of NH_3 to the poorly absorbed NH_4)*
      4. levodopa *to restore catecholamine neurotransmitter levels (these neurotransmitters may have been replaced by false neurotransmitters, which would normally be metabolized by the liver)*
   f. prepare client for and assist with dialysis, exchange transfusions, cross circulation, charcoal hemoperfusion, plasmapheresis, or extracorporeal liver perfusion if performed *to reduce cerebrotoxin levels*
   g. institute general safety precautions
   h. provide emotional support to client and significant others.

10.d. The client will not experience progressive liver degeneration as evidenced by:
   1. resolution of signs and symptoms of hepatitis
   2. absence of signs and symptoms of complications
   3. coagulation test results and serum AST (SGOT), ALT (SGPT), GGT, LDH, alkaline phosphatase (ALP), and bilirubin levels returning toward normal.

10.d.1. Assess for signs and symptoms of progressive liver degeneration:
   a. delayed resolution of symptoms of hepatitis (e.g. jaundice, weakness, abdominal pain, nausea, clay-colored stools)
   b. delayed or incomplete resolution of complications
   c. persistent or increased elevation of liver function and coagulation test results.
2. Implement measures identified in this care plan to reduce the infectious process and inflammation and promote healing of the liver.
3. Consult physician if signs and symptoms of progressive liver degeneration occur.

11. NURSING DIAGNOSIS

Disturbance in self-concept* related to:

a. change in appearance (jaundice);
b. dependence on others to meet self-care needs;
c. stigma of having a communicable disease;
d. possible alterations in roles and life style (personal habits such as alcohol consumption, drug use, and exercise need to be restricted and there may be a temporary restriction of sexual activity).

---

* This diagnostic label includes the nursing diagnoses of body image disturbance and self-esteem disturbance.

DESIRED OUTCOMES	NURSING ACTIONS AND *SELECTED RATIONALES*

11. The client will demonstrate beginning adaptation to changes in appearance, level of independence, roles, and life style (see Care Plan on Immobility, Nursing Diagnosis 16, for outcome criteria).

11.a. Refer to Care Plan on Immobility, Nursing Diagnosis 16, for measures related to assessment and promotion of a positive self-concept.
   b. Implement additional measures *to assist client to adapt to changes in appearance, level of independence, roles, and life style:*
     1. clarify misconceptions about future limitations on physical activity, personal habits, and sexual activity; reinforce the fact that limitations are usually temporary
     2. inform client that jaundice is temporary and usually subsides within 3 weeks
     3. encourage maximum participation in self-care within the prescribed activity restrictions and encourage significant others to allow client to do what he/she is able *so that independence can be re-established and/or self-esteem redeveloped*
     4. instruct client and significant others in ways to prevent the spread of hepatitis (see Nursing Diagnosis 13, action a) *in order to reduce the fear of disease transmission and promote interaction with others.*

□ ▬▬▬▬▬▬▬▬▬▬▬▬▬▬▬▬▬▬▬▬

12. NURSING DIAGNOSIS

Noncompliance* related to:

a. lack of understanding of the implications of not following the prescribed treatment plan;
b. difficulty modifying personal habits (e.g. alcohol consumption, drug abuse, exercise regimen, sexual activities).

_____

* This diagnostic label includes both an informed decision by client not to comply and an inability to comply due to circumstances beyond the client's control.

□ ▬▬▬▬▬▬▬▬▬▬▬▬▬▬▬▬▬▬▬▬

DESIRED OUTCOMES	NURSING ACTIONS AND *SELECTED RATIONALES*

12. The client will demonstrate the probability of future compliance with the prescribed treatment plan as evidenced by:
  a. willingness to learn about and participate in treatments and care
  b. statements reflecting ways to modify personal habits
  c. statements reflecting an understanding of the implications of not following the prescribed treatment plan.

12.a. Assess for indications that client may be unwilling or unable to comply with prescribed treatment plan:
     1. statements reflecting that he/she was unable to manage care at home
     2. failure to adhere to treatment plan while in hospital (e.g. not adhering to activity restrictions and isolation precautions)
     3. statements reflecting a lack of understanding of factors that will cause further progression of liver damage
     4. statements reflecting an unwillingness or inability to modify personal habits
     5. statements reflecting the view that hepatitis has resolved once he/she is feeling better or that there is no way to control the disease and efforts to comply with treatments are useless.
   b. Implement measures *to improve client compliance:*
     1. explain hepatitis in terms the client can understand; stress the fact that adherence to treatment plan is necessary *in order to delay and/or prevent complications*
     2. encourage questions and clarify any misconceptions client has about hepatitis and its possible long-range effects
     3. initiate and reinforce discharge teaching outlined in Nursing Diagnosis 13 *in order to promote a sense of control and self-reliance*
     4. encourage client to participate in the treatment plan
     5. provide client with written instructions on scheduled appointments with health care provider, dietary recommendations, activity limitations, ways

UNIT XIII

to prevent further trauma to liver, ways to avoid infecting others, and signs and symptoms to report
6. assist client to identify ways to modify life style and adhere to necessary changes in personal habits
7. encourage questions and allow time for clarification of information provided
8. provide information about and encourage utilization of community resources that can assist client to make necessary life-style changes (e.g. drug and alcohol rehabilitation programs).
c. Assess for and reinforce behaviors suggesting future compliance with prescribed treatment regimen (e.g. statements reflecting plans to modify personal habits, statements reflecting an understanding of and a plan for taking necessary precautions to prevent the spread of hepatitis).
d. Include significant others in explanations and teaching sessions and encourage their support.
e. Reinforce the need for client to assume responsibility for adhering to treatment regimen.

☐ ▬▬▬▬▬▬▬▬▬▬▬▬▬▬▬▬▬▬▬▬▬▬▬▬▬

13. NURSING DIAGNOSIS

Knowledge deficit regarding follow-up care.

☐ ▬▬▬▬▬▬▬▬▬▬▬▬▬▬▬▬▬▬▬▬▬▬▬▬▬

DESIRED OUTCOMES	NURSING ACTIONS AND *SELECTED RATIONALES*

13.a. The client will identify ways to prevent the spread of hepatitis to others.

13.a.1. Provide the following instructions on ways *to prevent the spread of hepatitis to others:*
a. if client has hepatitis A, instruct him/her to adhere to the following precautions for 1–2 weeks after the onset of jaundice:
1. wash hands thoroughly after defecating and before meals
2. use separate toilet facilities if possible; if separate toilet facilities are not available:
   a. use disposable toilet seat covers or clean toilet seat with aqueous iodine after each use
   b. use separate toilet paper roll or individual packets of toilet paper
3. wash bedding and underwear separately in hot, soapy water
4. if any injections (e.g. insulin, vitamin B_{12}) are given at home, use disposable equipment and dispose of it properly *to reduce the risk of others coming in contact with contaminated needles*
5. do not donate blood or work in food services until approved by physician
b. if client has hepatitis B; non-A, non-B; or D, instruct him/her to adhere to the following precautions until certain immunoglobulin tests are negative:
1. wash hands thoroughly after urinating and defecating
2. do not share personal articles (e.g. toothbrush, straight-edge razor, thermometer)
3. use disposable eating utensils or wash utensils in an automatic dishwasher on hot water setting
4. do not share food
5. if any injections (e.g. insulin, vitamin B_{12}) are given at home, use disposable equipment and dispose of it properly *to reduce the risk of others coming in contact with contaminated needles*
6. avoid intimate contact such as kissing or sexual intercourse
7. properly dispose of secretions from nose and mouth immediately
8. do not donate blood.

2. Instruct client to inform persons he/she has had personal contact with to see health care provider for appropriate immunization and testing for early detection of hepatitis.

13.b. The client will identify ways to prevent further liver damage.

13.b. Provide the following instructions regarding ways *to prevent further liver damage:*
  1. avoid the following hepatotoxic agents:
    a. alcohol
    b. cleaning agents containing carbon tetrachloride (these are toxic even when inhaled)
  2. caution client to take acetaminophen (e.g. Tylenol) only when necessary and not to exceed recommended dose *because of its potential toxic effect on the liver*
  3. take precautions *to prevent recurrent hepatitis* (client is immune only to the viral type he/she has had):
    a. if client has hepatitis A, instruct in ways *to prevent occurrence of hepatitis B; non-A, non-B; or D:*
      1. receive autologous blood or blood from donor known not to have hepatitis if transfusions are necessary
      2. avoid intimate contact with known carriers of hepatitis B; non-A, non-B; or D
    b. if client has hepatitis B or D, instruct in ways *to prevent occurrence of hepatitis A:*
      1. wash hands thoroughly after defecating and before meals
      2. use disposable seat covers
      3. eat only in restaurants that have been inspected and approved by health authorities
      4. do not drink water or eat shellfish that may be contaminated
      5. avoid anal intercourse *since it is one way that hepatitis A can be transmitted*
    c. if client has non-A, non-B hepatitis, instruct in ways to prevent hepatitis B, D, and A (see actions b.3.a and b in this diagnosis).

13.c. The client will verbalize an understanding of the rationale for and constituents of the recommended diet.

13.c.1. Explain to client that adherence to the recommended diet will promote healing of the liver and reduce the risk of further liver damage.
  2. Reinforce the dietary instructions outlined in Nursing Diagnosis 3, action e.2.

13.d. The client will identify ways to reduce the risk of infection and bleeding until the liver has healed completely.

13.d.1. Instruct client in ways *to reduce risk of infection:*
  a. continue with coughing and deep breathing or use of inspiratory exerciser every 2 hours while awake as long as activity is limited
  b. increase activity as allowed and tolerated
  c. avoid contact with persons who have an infection
  d. avoid crowds, especially in flu and cold seasons
  e. decrease or stop smoking
  f. drink at least 10 glasses of liquid/day
  g. adhere to recommended diet
  h. take supplemental vitamins and minerals prescribed
  i. maintain good personal hygiene.
  2. Instruct client about ways *to minimize risk of bleeding:*
    a. avoid taking aspirin, aspirin-containing products, and ibuprofen
    b. use an electric rather than a straight-edge razor
    c. floss and brush teeth gently
    d. cut nails carefully
    e. avoid situations that could result in trauma (e.g. contact sports)
    f. avoid blowing nose forcefully
    g. avoid straining to have a bowel movement.
  3. Instruct client to control any bleeding by applying firm, prolonged pressure to the area if possible.

13.e. The client will state signs and symptoms to report to the health care provider.

13.e. Stress the importance of reporting the following signs and symptoms:
  1. weight gain of more than 1 pound a day for more than 3 days
  2. swelling of ankles, feet, abdomen
  3. shortness of breath

UNIT XIII

4. increased itchiness or yellowing of skin
5. elevated temperature that lasts more than 2 days
6. blood in stools, urine, or vomitus; prolonged or excessive bleeding from nose, mouth, or skin; prolonged or excessive menses; excessive bruising; severe headache; or sudden abdominal or back pain
7. changes in behavior, speech, or handwriting.

13.f. The client will identify community resources that can assist with drug or alcohol rehabilitation if indicated.	13.f.1. Provide client with information about and encourage participation in drug and alcohol rehabilitation programs if indicated. 2. Initiate a referral if indicated.
13.g. The client will verbalize an understanding of and plan for adhering to recommended follow-up care including future appointments with health care provider, activity level, and medications prescribed.	13.g.1. Reinforce the importance of keeping follow-up appointments with health care provider. 2. Reinforce physician's instructions regarding activity level. Stress importance of rest during convalescent phase (from 6 weeks to 6 months). 3. Explain the rationale for, side effects of, and importance of taking medications prescribed. 4. Refer to Nursing Diagnosis 12, action b, for measures to improve client compliance.

■ ■

Pancreatitis

Pancreatitis is an inflammation of the pancreas commonly associated with biliary disease and alcohol use. Other causes include external trauma to the abdomen, trauma to the pancreas during abdominal surgery, and, less frequently, infection, hyperlipidemia, and use of certain medications (e.g. corticosteroids, estrogens, thiazide diuretics). The two main classifications are acute pancreatitis, in which the structure and function of the organ is usually restored when the inflammation subsides, and chronic pancreatitis, in which permanent changes occur in pancreatic tissue and function.

Signs and symptoms of pancreatitis are primarily due to autodestruction of pancreatic tissue. This destruction occurs when the normal outflow of pancreatic enzymes into the duodenum is blocked and activation of the enzymes takes place within the pancreas itself. The digestion of fats, proteins, and carbohydrates is impaired because of blockage of the outflow of the pancreatic enzymes and hyperglycemia can occur if beta cells are damaged. As activated pancreatic enzymes escape into the systemic circulation, respiratory, cardiac, and vascular changes can also occur.

This care plan focuses on the adult client hospitalized for diagnosis and treatment of acute pancreatitis. The goals of care are to control pain, maintain an adequate nutritional status, prevent complications, and educate the client regarding follow-up care.

DISCHARGE CRITERIA

Prior to discharge, the client will:

- identify ways to prevent overstimulation of and further trauma to the pancreas
- verbalize an understanding of recommended dietary modifications
- state signs and symptoms to report to the health care provider
- identify community resources that can assist in making life-style changes necessary to prevent recurrence of acute pancreatitis
- verbalize an understanding of and a plan for adhering to recommended follow-up care including future appointments with health care provider and medications prescribed.

NURSING/COLLABORATIVE DIAGNOSES

1. Anxiety □ *781*
2. Ineffective breathing patterns:
   a. hypoventilation
   b. hyperventilation □ *782*
3. Altered fluid and electrolyte balance:
   a. fluid volume deficit, hyponatremia, hypokalemia, and hypochloremia
   b. hypovolemia
   c. hypocalcemia
   d. hyperkalemia
   e. metabolic alkalosis
   f. metabolic acidosis □ *783*
4. Altered nutrition: less than body requirements □ *785*
5A. Altered comfort: pain in epigastric area, back, flank, and left side of chest □ *786*
5B. Altered comfort: nausea and vomiting □ *787*
5C. Altered comfort: gas pain and abdominal distention □ *788*
6. Altered oral mucous membrane: dryness □ *788*
7. Potential complications:
   a. hypovolemic shock
   b. pancreatic pseudocyst or abscess formation
   c. peritonitis
   d. hyperglycemia
   e. pleural effusion
   f. adult respiratory distress syndrome (ARDS)
   g. cardiac dysfunction (arrhythmias, myocardial infarction)
   h. disseminated intravascular coagulation (DIC)
   i. fat necrosis □ *789*
8. Noncompliance □ *793*
9. Knowledge deficit regarding follow-up care □ *794*

1. NURSING DIAGNOSIS

Anxiety related to unfamiliar environment; pain; unknown diagnosis; and lack of understanding of diagnostic tests, treatment plan, and prognosis.

DESIRED OUTCOMES	NURSING ACTIONS AND *SELECTED RATIONALES*

1. The client will experience a reduction in fear and anxiety as evidenced by:
a. verbalization of feeling less anxious or fearful
b. relaxed facial expression and body movements
c. stable vital signs
	1.a. Assess client for signs and symptoms of fear and anxiety (e.g. verbalization of fears and concerns; tenseness; tremors; irritability; restlessness; diaphoresis; tachypnea; tachycardia; elevated blood pressure; facial tension, pallor, or flushing; noncompliance with treatment plan).
	b. Ascertain effectiveness of current coping skills.
	c. Implement measures *to reduce fear and anxiety:*
	   1. perform actions to reduce pain (see Nursing Diagnosis 5.A, action 5)
	   2. orient to hospital environment, equipment, and routines

UNIT XIII

d. usual skin color
e. verbalization of an understanding of hospital routines, diagnostic tests, diagnosis, treatment plan, and prognosis.

3. introduce staff who will be participating in his/her care; if possible, maintain consistency in staff assigned to his/her care *in order to provide feelings of stability and comfort with the environment*
4. assure client that staff members are nearby; respond to call signal as soon as possible
5. maintain a calm, confident manner when interacting with client
6. encourage verbalization of fear and anxiety; provide feedback
7. explain all diagnostic tests:
   a. blood studies (e.g. amylase, pancreatic isoamylase, lipase, electrolytes)
   b. urine studies (e.g. amylase, amylase/creatinine clearance ratio)
   c. stool studies for fat content
   d. ultrasonography, computed tomography
   e. endoscopic retrograde cholangiopancreatography (ERCP)
   f. needle biopsy of the pancreas
8. if cardiac involvement has been ruled out, assure client that the pain may mimic but is not indicative of a "heart attack"
9. reinforce physician's explanations and clarify any misconceptions the client may have about pancreatitis, the treatment plan, and prognosis
10. provide a calm, restful environment
11. instruct in relaxation techniques and encourage participation in diversional activities when pain has subsided
12. assist client to identify specific stressors and ways to cope with them
13. encourage significant others to project a caring, concerned attitude without obvious anxiousness
14. monitor for therapeutic and nontherapeutic effects of antianxiety agents if administered.

d. Include significant others in orientation and teaching sessions and encourage their continued support of client.
e. Provide information based on current needs of client and significant others at a level they can understand. Encourage questions and clarification of information provided.
f. Consult physician if above actions fail to control fear and anxiety.

2. NURSING DIAGNOSIS

Ineffective breathing patterns:

a. **hypoventilation** related to:
   1. reluctance to breathe deeply associated with abdominal pain
   2. restricted lung expansion associated with pleural effusion and pressure on the diaphragm (may result from ascites and accumulation of gastrointestinal gas and fluid)
   3. depressant effects of some medications (e.g. narcotic analgesics);
b. **hyperventilation** related to pain, fear, anxiety, and metabolic acidosis.

DESIRED OUTCOMES	NURSING ACTIONS AND *SELECTED RATIONALES*

2. The client will maintain an effective breathing pattern as evidenced by:
a. normal rate, rhythm, and depth of respirations
b. absence of dyspnea
c. blood gases within normal range.
	2.a. Assess for signs and symptoms of ineffective breathing patterns (e.g. shallow or slow respirations, hyperventilation, dyspnea).
	b. Monitor blood gases. Report abnormal results.
	c. Monitor for and report significant changes in ear oximetry and capnograph results.
	d. Implement measures *to improve breathing pattern:*
	  1. perform actions to reduce pain (see Nursing Diagnosis 5.A, action 5)
	  2. perform actions to reduce fear and anxiety (see Nursing Diagnosis 1, action c)

3. perform actions *to reduce pressure on the diaphragm:*
   a. implement measures to reduce the accumulation of gastrointestinal gas and fluid (see Nursing Diagnosis 5.C, action 3)
   b. administer salt-poor albumin infusions as ordered *to reduce ascites*
4. perform actions to prevent and treat pleural effusion (see Collaborative Diagnosis 7, actions e.3 and 4)
5. perform actions to prevent or treat metabolic acidosis (see Nursing Diagnosis 3, action b.4)
6. place client in a semi- to high Fowler's position unless contraindicated
7. if client is on bedrest, assist him/her to turn at least every 2 hours
8. instruct client to deep breathe or use inspiratory exerciser at least every 2 hours
9. administer or assist with IPPB treatments as ordered
10. instruct client to breathe slowly if he/she is hyperventilating
11. increase activity as allowed and tolerated
12. administer central nervous system depressants (e.g. narcotic analgesics, sedatives) judiciously; hold medication and consult physician if respiratory rate is less than 12/minute.
   e. Consult physician if:
      1. ineffective breathing patterns continue
      2. signs and symptoms of impaired gas exchange (e.g. confusion, restlessness, irritability, cyanosis, decreased PaO_2 and increased $PaCO_2$ levels) are present.

3. NURSING/COLLABORATIVE DIAGNOSIS

Altered fluid and electrolyte balance:

a. **fluid volume deficit, hyponatremia, hypokalemia, and hypochloremia** related to decreased oral intake and excessive loss of fluid and electrolytes associated with vomiting and nasogastric tube drainage;
b. **hypovolemia** related to:
   1. fluid volume deficit associated with restricted oral intake, vomiting, and nasogastric tube drainage
   2. third-space fluid shift associated with increased vascular permeability resulting from the inflammatory response and increased activation of kinin peptides such as kallikrein and bradykinin (these peptides are activated by the pancreatic enzyme trypsin)
   3. blood loss associated with destruction of the elastic fibers of the vessel walls resulting from activation of the pancreatic enzyme elastase;
c. **hypocalcemia** related to:
   1. presence of free fats in the intestine (lipase and phospholipase A are not released into the intestinal tract to digest fats so the calcium binds with the free fats and is excreted in the stool)
   2. loss of albumin into peritoneal cavity with third-spacing
   3. sequestration of calcium in areas of fat necrosis;
d. **hyperkalemia** related to metabolic acidosis and pancreatic tissue destruction (both conditions result in cellular release of potassium);
e. **metabolic alkalosis** related to hypokalemia, hypochloremia, and excessive loss of hydrochloric acid associated with vomiting and nasogastric tube drainage;
f. **metabolic acidosis** related to:
   1. lactic acid accumulation associated with tissue hypoxia resulting from hypovolemia
   2. alteration in the flow and absorption of sodium bicarbonate due to pancreatic tissue damage and obstructed outflow of pancreatic secretions (the pancreas normally secretes sodium bicarbonate to neutralize the highly acidic chyme that enters the duodenum)
   3. accumulation of ketone bodies associated with hyperglycemia.

DESIRED OUTCOMES	NURSING ACTIONS AND *SELECTED RATIONALES*

3.a. The client will maintain fluid and electrolyte balance as evidenced by:
1. normal skin turgor
2. moist mucous membranes
3. stable weight
4. B/P and pulse within normal range for client and stable with position change
5. urine specific gravity between 1.010–1.030
6. no evidence of confusion, irritability, lethargy, excessive thirst, ileus, cardiac arrhythmias, muscle weakness, paresthesias, muscle cramps, tetany, seizure activity
7. negative Chvostek's and Trousseau's signs
8. normal serum osmolality and electrolytes.

3.a.1. Assess for and report signs and symptoms of:
  a. third-space fluid shift (e.g. peripheral edema, ascites, dyspnea, crackles and diminished or absent breath sounds)
  b. fluid volume deficit and/or hypovolemia:
    1. decreased skin turgor, dry mucous membranes, thirst
    2. weight loss greater than 0.5 kg/day
    3. low B/P and/or decline in systolic B/P of at least 15 mm Hg with concurrent rise in pulse when client sits up
    4. weak, rapid pulse
    5. urine specific gravity higher than 1.030 (reflects an actual rather than potential fluid volume deficit)
  c. hyponatremia (e.g. nausea, vomiting, abdominal cramps, weakness, twitching, lethargy, confusion, seizures)
  d. hypokalemia (e.g. irregular pulse; muscle weakness and cramping; paresthesias; nausea; vomiting; hypoactive or absent bowel sounds; drowsiness; EKG reading showing ST depression, T wave inversion or flattening, and presence of U waves)
  e. hyperkalemia (e.g. slow or irregular pulse; paresthesias; muscle weakness and flaccidity; hyperactive bowel sounds with diarrhea and intestinal colic; EKG reading showing peaked T wave, prolonged PR interval, and/or widened QRS)
  f. hypochloremia (e.g. twitching, tetany, depressed respirations)
  g. hypocalcemia (e.g. change in mental status; cardiac arrhythmias; positive Chvostek's and Trousseau's signs; numbness and tingling of fingers, toes, and circumoral area; muscle cramps; tetany; seizures).
2. Monitor serum osmolality and electrolyte results. Report abnormal values.
3. Implement measures *to prevent and treat fluid and electrolyte imbalances:*
  a. perform actions to reduce nausea and vomiting (see Nursing Diagnosis 5.B, action 2)
  b. if irrigation of nasogastric tube is necessary, use normal saline rather than water
  c. maintain a fluid intake of 2500 cc/day unless contraindicated
  d. perform actions to prevent or treat metabolic acidosis (see action b.4 in this diagnosis) *in order to decrease cellular release of potassium*
  e. perform actions to prevent and treat fat necrosis (see Collaborative Diagnosis 7, actions i.2 and 3) *in order to reduce sequestration of calcium in areas of fat necrosis*
  f. monitor for therapeutic and nontherapeutic effects of the following if administered:
    1. salt-poor albumin infusions *to promote mobilization of fluid back into extracellular space if third-spacing has occurred*
    2. fluid and electrolyte replacements (if signs and symptoms of hyperkalemia are present, consult physician before administering prescribed potassium supplements)
    3. pancreatic enzymes (e.g. pancreatin, pancrelipase) *to promote fat digestion (there is then less fat available for the calcium to bind to)*
  g. when oral intake is allowed, assist client to select the following foods/fluids:
    1. those high in potassium (e.g. bananas, potatoes, raisins, figs, apricots, dates, Gatorade, fruit juices) if hyperkalemia is not a problem
    2. those high in sodium (e.g. bouillon, sauces, soups, pickles, processed cheese, cured meats, catsup, canned vegetables)
    3. those high in calcium such as dairy products (if client is on a low-fat diet, dairy products such as ice cream, whole milk, butter, and cream may not be allowed).
4. Consult physician if signs and symptoms of fluid and electrolyte imbalances persist or worsen.

3.b. The client will maintain acid-base balance as evidenced by:

3.b.1. Assess for and report signs and symptoms of:
  a. metabolic alkalosis (e.g. dizziness; confusion; bradypnea; tingling of fingers, toes, and circumoral area; muscle twitching; seizures)

1. mentally alert and oriented
2. unlabored respirations at 16–20/minute
3. absence of dizziness, confusion, headache, nausea, vomiting, paresthesias, muscle twitching, seizure activity
4. blood gases within normal range.

    b. metabolic acidosis (e.g. drowsiness; disorientation; stupor; rapid, deep respirations; headache; nausea; vomiting; anion gap greater than 16 mEq/liter).

2. Monitor blood gases. Report abnormal results.
3. Implement measures *to prevent or treat metabolic alkalosis:*
    a. perform actions to prevent vomiting (see Nursing Diagnosis 5.B, action 2)
    b. monitor for therapeutic and nontherapeutic effects of electrolyte replacements if administered *to maintain serum potassium and chloride levels.*
4. Implement measures *to prevent or treat metabolic acidosis:*
    a. monitor for therapeutic and nontherapeutic effects of the following if administered:
      1. sodium bicarbonate
      2. antacids *to neutralize gastric secretions*
      3. histamine$_2$ receptor antagonists *to reduce secretion of hydrochloric acid*
    b. maintain patency of nasogastric tube (e.g. avoid kinks in tubing, ensure proper suction setting) *to facilitate removal of gastric secretions*
    c. perform actions to reduce fear and anxiety (see Nursing Diagnosis 1, action c) *in order to decrease secretion of hydrochloric acid*
    d. perform actions to prevent and treat hyperglycemia (see Collaborative Diagnosis 7, actions d.3 and 4) *in order to decrease production of ketone bodies.*
5. Consult physician if signs and symptoms of acid-base imbalance persist or worsen.

---

4. NURSING DIAGNOSIS

Altered nutrition: less than body requirements related to:

a. decreased oral intake associated with nausea, discomfort, and prescribed dietary restrictions;
b. loss of nutrients associated with vomiting;
c. decreased utilization of nutrients associated with impaired digestion of fats, proteins, and carbohydrates resulting from obstructed outflow of pancreatic enzymes.

DESIRED OUTCOMES	NURSING ACTIONS AND *SELECTED RATIONALES*

4. The client will maintain an adequate nutritional status as evidenced by:
    a. weight within normal range for client's age, height, and build
    b. normal BUN and serum albumin, protein, Hct., Hgb., cholesterol, and lymphocyte levels
    c. triceps skinfold measurements within normal range
    d. usual strength and activity tolerance
    e. healthy oral mucous membrane.

4.a. Assess the client for signs and symptoms of malnutrition:
    1. weight below normal for client's age, height, and build
    2. abnormal BUN and low serum albumin, protein, Hct., Hgb., cholesterol, and lymphocyte levels
    3. triceps skinfold measurement less than normal for build
    4. weakness and fatigue
    5. stomatitis.
  b. Observe stools for steatorrhea. Send stool specimen for analysis of fat content as ordered.
  c. Monitor percentage of meals eaten.
  d. Assess client to determine the causes of inadequate intake (e.g. nausea, pain, food and fluid restrictions).
  e. Implement measures *to maintain or improve nutritional status:*
    1. administer total parenteral nutrition as ordered
    2. when food and fluids are allowed, perform actions *to improve oral intake:*
      a. implement measures to reduce discomfort (see Nursing Diagnoses 5.A, actions 5.b–e and 5.C, action 3)

UNIT
XIII

b. implement measures to relieve nausea and vomiting (see Nursing Diagnosis 5.B, actions 2.b–j)

c. provide oral care before meals

d. serve small portions of nutritious foods/fluids that are appealing to client

e. provide a clean, relaxed, pleasant atmosphere

f. obtain a dietary consult if necessary to assist client in selecting foods/fluids that meet nutritional needs as well as preferences

3. ensure that meals are well balanced and high in essential nutrients

4. monitor for therapeutic and nontherapeutic effects of the following if administered:

a. fat-soluble vitamins

b. pancreatic enzymes (e.g. pancreatin, pancrelipase) *to facilitate the digestion of proteins, fats, and carbohydrates.*

f. Perform a 72-hour calorie count if nutritional status declines or fails to improve.

g. Reassess nutritional status on a regular basis and report decline.

5.A. NURSING DIAGNOSIS

Altered comfort:* pain in epigastric area, back, flank, and left side of chest related to inflammation and distention of the pancreas and obstruction and spasms of the pancreatic and biliary ducts.

---

* In this care plan, the nursing diagnosis "pain" is included under the diagnostic label of altered comfort.

DESIRED OUTCOMES	NURSING ACTIONS AND *SELECTED RATIONALES*

5.A. The client will experience diminished pain in epigastric area, back, flank, and left side of chest as evidenced by:

1. verbalization of same

2. relaxed facial expression and body positioning

3. increased participation in activities

4. stable vital signs.

5.A.1. Determine how the client usually responds to pain.

2. Assess for nonverbal signs of pain (e.g. wrinkled brow; clenched fists; reluctance to move; guarding of the abdomen; rapid, shallow respirations; rubbing flank or left side of chest; facial pallor or flushing; change in B/P; tachycardia).

3. Assess verbal complaints of pain. Ask client to be specific about location, severity, and type of pain.

4. Assess for factors that seem to aggravate and alleviate pain.

5. Implement measures *to reduce pain:*

a. perform actions *to reduce pancreatic stimulation:*

1. withhold all food and fluid as ordered

2. maintain activity restrictions as ordered (*decreases metabolic rate, which results in decreased pancreatic secretions*)

3. insert nasogastric tube and maintain suction as ordered (an abdominal x-ray may be ordered *to determine placement of the nasogastric tube;* ideally, the tube should be in the greater curvature in the body of the stomach *to keep gastric contents from entering the duodenum and stimulating cholecystokinin-pancreozymin [CCK-PZ] and secretin*)

4. monitor for therapeutic and nontherapeutic effects of the following medications if administered:

a. antacids *to neutralize gastric acid*

b. histamine$_2$ receptor antagonists (e.g. cimetidine, famotidine, ranitidine) *to reduce output of hydrochloric acid*

5. minimize client's exposure to the odor and sight of food until oral intake is allowed (*the smell and sight of food stimulate pancreatic enzyme secretion*)

b. monitor for therapeutic and nontherapeutic effects of the following

medications if administered *to relieve pain:*
1. analgesics (morphine sulfate should be avoided *because it increases spasms of the sphincter of Oddi*)
2. smooth muscle relaxants (e.g. papaverine, nitroglycerin) *to relieve ductal spasms*
3. anti-infectives *to treat infection if present and reduce inflammation*

c. provide or assist with nonpharmacological measures for pain relief (e.g. back rub, positioning client on side with his/her knees flexed, relaxation techniques, guided imagery, quiet conversation, restful environment, diversional activities)
d. assist with a paravertebral block if performed
e. when oral intake is allowed, perform actions *to maintain reduced pancreatic activity:*
1. continue to administer antacids and histamine$_2$ receptor antagonists as ordered
2. advance diet slowly
3. provide small, frequent meals rather than 3 large ones
4. maintain dietary restrictions of fat intake as ordered (avoid foods/fluids high in fat content such as butter, cream, oils, whole milk, ice cream, pork, fried foods, gravies, and nuts).

6. Consult physician if above measures fail to provide adequate pain relief.

5.B. NURSING DIAGNOSIS

Altered comfort: nausea and vomiting related to stimulation of the vomiting center associated with:

1. vagal and/or sympathetic stimulation resulting from visceral irritation associated with abdominal distention and inflammation of the pancreas;
2. cortical stimulation due to pain and stress.

DESIRED OUTCOMES	NURSING ACTIONS AND *SELECTED RATIONALES*

5.B. The client will experience relief of nausea and vomiting as evidenced by:
1. verbalization of relief of nausea
2. absence of vomiting.

5.B.1. Assess client to determine factors that contribute to nausea and vomiting (e.g. eating, particular foods, abdominal distention, pain, anxiety, fear).
2. Implement measures *to reduce nausea and vomiting:*
   a. maintain patency of nasogastric tube (e.g. keep tubing free of kinks, irrigate and maintain suction as ordered) if present
   b. eliminate noxious sights and smells from the environment (*noxious stimuli cause cortical stimulation of the vomiting center*)
   c. encourage client to take deep, slow breaths when nauseated
   d. instruct client to change positions slowly (*movement stimulates the chemoreceptor trigger zone*)
   e. provide oral hygiene every 2 hours and after each emesis
   f. perform actions to reduce fear and anxiety (see Nursing Diagnosis 1, action c)
   g. perform actions to reduce pain (see Nursing Diagnosis 5.A, action 5)
   h. perform actions to reduce the accumulation of gastrointestinal gas and fluid (see Nursing Diagnosis 5.C, action 3)
   i. when oral intake is allowed:
      1. instruct client to ingest food and fluid slowly
      2. instruct client to eat dry foods (e.g. toast, crackers) and avoid drinking liquids with meals if nauseated
      3. instruct client to avoid foods/fluids that irritate the gastric mucosa (e.g. spicy foods; citrus fruits or juices; caffeine-containing items such as chocolate, tea, coffee, or colas)
      4. instruct the client to rest after eating with head of bed elevated

j. monitor for therapeutic and nontherapeutic effects of antiemetics if administered.
3. Consult physician if above measures fail to control nausea and vomiting.

5.C. NURSING DIAGNOSIS

Altered comfort: gas pain and abdominal distention related to:

1. accumulation of gastrointestinal gas associated with an inability to digest fats properly due to obstruction of the flow of lipase;
2. accumulation of gastrointestinal gas and fluid associated with decreased gastrointestinal motility due to some medications (e.g. narcotic analgesics) and decreased activity.

DESIRED OUTCOMES	NURSING ACTIONS AND *SELECTED RATIONALES*

5.C. The client will experience diminished abdominal distention and gas pain as evidenced by:
1. verbalization of same
2. relaxed facial expression and body positioning
3. decrease in abdominal distention.
	5.C.1. Assess for nonverbal signs of abdominal distention and gas pain (e.g. clutching and guarding of abdomen, restlessness, reluctance to move, grimacing, increasing abdominal girth, dyspnea).
	2. Assess for verbal complaints of abdominal fullness and gas pain.
	3. Implement measures *to reduce the accumulation of gastrointestinal gas and fluid in order to decrease gas pain and abdominal distention:*
	  a. encourage and assist client with frequent position change and ambulation as soon as allowed *(activity stimulates peristalsis and the expulsion of flatus)*
	  b. instruct the client to avoid activities such as gum chewing, sucking on hard candy, and smoking *in order to reduce air swallowing*
	  c. maintain patency of nasogastric tube if present
	  d. when oral intake is allowed, instruct client to avoid the following:
	    1. gas-producing foods/fluids (e.g. cabbage, onions, popcorn, baked beans, carbonated beverages)
	    2. foods/fluids high in fat (e.g. butter, cream, oils, whole milk, ice cream, pork, fried foods, gravies, nuts)
	  e. encourage client to eructate and expel flatus whenever the urge is felt
	  f. monitor for therapeutic and nontherapeutic effects of the following medications if administered:
	    1. antiflatulents *to reduce gas accumulation*
	    2. pancreatic enzymes *to improve fat digestion*
	  g. when the client's pain subsides, administer nonnarcotic analgesics as ordered *(narcotic analgesics decrease gastrointestinal motility).*
	4. Consult physician if signs and symptoms of gas pain and abdominal distention persist or worsen.

6. NURSING DIAGNOSIS

Altered oral mucous membrane: dryness related to:

a. fluid volume deficit associated with fluid loss and fluid restrictions:
b. decreased salivation associated with fluid volume deficit, food and fluid restrictions, and some medications (e.g. narcotic analgesics);
c. mouth breathing if nasogastric tube is in place.

DESIRED OUTCOMES	NURSING ACTIONS AND *SELECTED RATIONALES*

6. The client will maintain a moist, intact oral mucous membrane.

6.a. Assess client for dryness of the oral mucosa.
   b. Implement measures *to relieve dryness of the oral mucous membrane:*
      1. instruct and assist client to perform good oral hygiene as often as needed
      2. encourage client to rinse mouth frequently with water
      3. avoid the use of lemon-glycerin swabs and commercial mouthwashes containing alcohol *(these products have a drying or irritating effect on oral mucous membrane)*
      4. lubricate client's lips with Vaseline, K-Y jelly, ChapStick, Blistex, or mineral oil when oral care is given
      5. encourage client to breathe through nose if possible
      6. encourage client not to smoke *(smoking further irritates and dries the mucosa)*
      7. maintain intravenous fluid therapy as ordered *to improve hydration*
      8. encourage client to use artificial saliva (e.g. Moi-stir, Salivart) *to lubricate the mucous membrane*
      9. advance oral intake as allowed and tolerated *to improve hydration and stimulate salivation.*
   c. If oral mucosa is irritated or cracked, implement measures *to relieve discomfort and promote healing:*
      1. assist client to select soft, bland, and nonacidic foods
      2. instruct client to avoid foods/fluids that are extremely hot or cold
      3. use a soft bristle brush or low-pressure power spray for oral care
      4. monitor for therapeutic and nontherapeutic effects of topical anesthetics, oral protective pastes, and topical and systemic analgesics if administered.
   d. Consult physician if dryness, irritation, and discomfort persist.

7. COLLABORATIVE DIAGNOSIS

Potential complications:

a. **hypovolemic shock** related to bleeding, third-spacing, and fluid volume deficit;

b. **pancreatic pseudocyst or abscess formation** related to inflammation and necrosis of or around the pancreas (due to escape of pancreatic enzymes);

c. **peritonitis** related to leakage of pseudocyst, abscess, or pancreatic enzymes into the peritoneum;

d. **hyperglycemia** related to increased release of glucagon from the alpha cells and/or decreased release of insulin due to injury to the beta cells;

e. **pleural effusion** related to increased capillary permeability and passage of pancreatic enzymes through the diaphragmatic lymph channels;

f. **adult respiratory distress syndrome (ARDS)** related to release of pancreatic toxins into systemic circulation (the toxins can cause decreased production of surfactant and alveolar-capillary membrane injury with resultant pulmonary edema, atelectasis, and ventilatory-perfusion imbalance);

g. **cardiac dysfunction (arrhythmias, myocardial infarction)** related to fluid and electrolyte imbalances and release of myocardial depressant factor by the damaged pancreas;

h. **disseminated intravascular coagulation (DIC)** related to release of thromboplastin from damaged cells of the pancreas and from those tissues affected by pancreatic enzyme action and fat necrosis;

i. **fat necrosis** related to escape of pancreatic enzymes from the circulation and lymphatic system (it is believed that lipase and phospholipase A damage fat cells).

UNIT
XIII

DESIRED OUTCOMES	NURSING ACTIONS AND *SELECTED RATIONALES*

7.a. The client will not develop hypovolemic shock as evidenced by:
1. usual mental status
2. stable vital signs
3. skin warm and usual color
4. palpable peripheral pulses
5. capillary refill time less than 3 seconds
6. urine output at least 30 cc/hour.

7.a.1. Assess for and report signs and symptoms of third-spacing, fluid volume deficit, and hypovolemia (see Nursing Diagnosis 3, actions a.1.a and b).
2. Monitor RBC, Hct., and Hgb. levels. Report declining values.
3. Assess for and report signs and symptoms of hypovolemic shock:
   a. restlessness, agitation, confusion
   b. significant decrease in B/P
   c. decline in B/P of at least 15 mm Hg with concurrent rise in pulse when client changes from lying to sitting or standing position
   d. resting pulse rate greater than 100 beats/minute
   e. rapid or labored respirations
   f. cool, pale, or cyanotic skin
   g. diminished or absent peripheral pulses
   h. capillary refill time greater than 3 seconds
   i. urine output less than 30 cc/hour.
4. Implement measures to prevent and treat fluid and electrolyte imbalances (see Nursing Diagnosis 3, action a.3) *in order to prevent hypovolemic shock.*
5. If signs and symptoms of hypovolemic shock occur:
   a. continue with above actions
   b. place client flat in bed with legs elevated unless contraindicated
   c. monitor vital signs frequently
   d. administer oxygen as ordered
   e. monitor for therapeutic and nontherapeutic effects of the following if administered:
      1. blood products and/or volume expanders
      2. vasopressors (may be given for a short period *to maintain mean arterial pressure)*
   f. assist with the application of military antishock trousers (MAST) if indicated
   g. provide emotional support to client and significant others.

7.b. The client will have resolution of a pancreatic pseudocyst or abscess if it develops as evidenced by:
1. decrease in abdominal pain
2. temperature declining toward normal
3. WBC count declining toward normal.

7.b.1. Assess for and report signs and symptoms of pancreatic pseudocyst or abscess formation (e.g. increased and more constant abdominal pain, further increase in temperature and pulse rate, further increase in WBC count).
2. If signs and symptoms of a pancreatic pseudocyst or abscess occur:
   a. monitor for therapeutic and nontherapeutic effects of anti-infectives if administered
   b. prepare client for surgical intervention (e.g. incision and drainage) if indicated
   c. provide emotional support to client and significant others.

7.c. The client will not develop peritonitis as evidenced by:
1. gradual resolution of abdominal pain
2. soft, nondistended abdomen
3. temperature declining toward normal
4. stable vital signs
5. normal bowel sounds
6. WBC count declining toward normal.

7.c.1. Assess for and report signs and symptoms of peritonitis (e.g. increase in severity of abdominal pain; generalized abdominal pain; rebound tenderness; tense, rigid abdomen; further increase in temperature; tachycardia; tachypnea; hypotension; diminished or absent bowel sounds).
2. Monitor WBC counts. Report levels that increase or fail to decline toward normal.
3. Implement measures *to prevent peritonitis:*
   a. perform actions to reduce pancreatic stimulation (see Nursing Diagnosis 5.A, action 5.a) *in order to decrease the secretion of pancreatic enzymes*
   b. if an incision and drainage of a pancreatic pseudocyst or abscess was performed and wound drain is present:
      1. perform actions *to maintain patency of wound drain:*
         a. keep tubing free of kinks
         b. empty collection device as often as necessary
         c. maintain suction as ordered
      2. perform actions *to prevent inadvertent removal of wound drain:*
         a. use caution when changing dressings surrounding drain
         b. instruct client not to pull on drain or drainage tubing
      3. maintain aseptic technique during dressing changes and wound care
      4. keep dressings clean and dry

c. prepare client for and assist with peritoneal lavage if performed *to remove pancreatic enzymes from the peritoneal cavity*

d. monitor for therapeutic and nontherapeutic effects of anti-infectives if administered.

4. If signs and symptoms of peritonitis occur:

a. withhold all food and fluid as ordered

b. place client on bedrest in a semi-Fowler's position *to assist in pooling or localizing of gastrointestinal contents in the pelvis rather than under the diaphragm*

c. insert a nasogastric or intestinal tube and maintain suction as ordered

d. monitor for therapeutic and nontherapeutic effects of anti-infectives if administered

e. monitor for therapeutic and nontherapeutic effects of intravenous fluids and/or blood volume expanders if administered *to prevent or treat shock (shock can occur as a result of escape of protein, fluid, and electrolytes into the peritoneal cavity)*

f. prepare client for and assist with peritoneal dialysis if performed *to remove toxins from the peritoneal cavity*

g. prepare client for surgical intervention (e.g. drainage of pancreatic pseudocyst or abscess) if indicated

h. provide emotional support to client and significant others.

7.d. The client will maintain a safe blood glucose level as evidenced by:
1. absence of polydipsia, polyuria, polyphagia
2. usual mental status
3. usual visual acuity
4. serum glucose between 60–200 mg/dl.

7.d.1. Assess for and report signs and symptoms of hyperglycemia (e.g. polydipsia; polyuria; polyphagia; change in mental status; dimmed or blurred vision).

2. Monitor blood glucose levels (use monitoring strip such as Chemstrip bG or Dextrostix). Report blood glucose values above 200 mg/dl or values as otherwise specified by physician.

3. Implement measures *to prevent hyperglycemia*:

a. perform actions to reduce pancreatic stimulation (see Nursing Diagnosis 5.A, action 5.a) *in order to prevent further damage to the alpha and beta cells*

b. perform actions to reduce fear and anxiety and pain (see Nursing Diagnoses 1, action c and 5.A, action 5) *in order to reduce emotional and physiological stress (stress causes an increased output of epinephrine, norepinephrine, glucagon, and cortisol, resulting in a further increase in blood glucose)*

c. monitor for therapeutic and nontherapeutic effects of insulin or oral hypoglycemic agents if administered.

4. If signs and symptoms of hyperglycemia occur:

a. assess for and report signs and symptoms of ketoacidosis (e.g. Kussmaul respirations, fruity odor on breath, nausea, vomiting, abdominal pain, hypotension, oliguria, confusion, lethargy, stupor, elevated serum glucose and/or urine glucose and acetone, low serum pH and CO_2 content)

b. monitor for therapeutic and nontherapeutic effects of the following if administered:
   1. intravenous fluid and electrolyte replacements
   2. insulin therapy
   3. sodium bicarbonate (reserved for use in severe acidosis when pH is less than 7.1)

c. if client has no history of diabetes or chronic pancreatitis, assure him/her that the hyperglycemia is expected to resolve as the pancreatitis does.

7.e. The client will not experience pleural effusion as evidenced by:
1. unlabored respirations at 16–20/minute
2. usual chest excursion
3. resonant percussion note throughout lung fields
4. normal breath sounds.

7.e.1. Assess for and report signs and symptoms of pleural effusion (e.g. dyspnea; decreased chest movement, dull percussion note, diminished or absent breath sounds, and decreased tactile fremitus over the affected area).

2. Monitor chest x-ray results. Report findings of pleural effusion.

3. Implement measures *to decrease the accumulation of pancreatic enzymes in the peritoneum and reduce capillary permeability in order to prevent pleural effusion*:

a. perform actions to reduce pancreatic stimulation (see Nursing Diagnosis 5.A, action 5.a)

b. prepare client for and assist with peritoneal lavage if performed.

UNIT
XIII

4. If signs and symptoms of pleural effusion occur, prepare client for thoracentesis if indicated.

7.f. The client will not experience ARDS as evidenced by:
1. unlabored respirations at 16–20/minute
2. usual skin color
3. usual mental status
4. blood gases within normal range.

7.f.1. Assess for and report signs and symptoms of ARDS (e.g. rapid, shallow respirations; sternocleidomastoid muscle retraction; dusky or cyanotic skin color; drowsiness; confusion).
2. Monitor blood gas values. Report abnormal results (progressive arterial hypoxemia even when receiving oxygen is indicative of ARDS).
3. Monitor for and report significant changes in ear oximetry and capnograph results.
4. Monitor chest x-ray results. Report presence of atelectasis and pulmonary edema.
5. Implement measures to reduce pancreatic stimulation (see Nursing Diagnosis 5.A, action 5.a) *in order to reduce the amount of pancreatic enzymes in the systemic circulation.*
6. If signs and symptoms of ARDS occur:
   a. monitor for therapeutic and nontherapeutic effects of diuretics if administered *to reduce pulmonary edema*
   b. maintain oxygen therapy as ordered
   c. assist with intubation, mechanical ventilation, and transfer to intensive care unit if indicated
   d. provide emotional support to client and significant others.

7.g. The client will not experience cardiac dysfunction as evidenced by:
1. regular apical pulse at 60–100 beats/minute
2. equal apical and radial pulses
3. absence of syncope and palpitations
4. absence of chest pain
5. normal cardiac enzymes
6. normal EKG readings.

7.g.1. Assess for and report signs and symptoms of:
   a. cardiac arrhythmias (e.g. irregular apical pulse, pulse rate below 60 or above 100 beats/minute, apical-radial pulse deficit, syncope, palpitations)
   b. myocardial infarction (e.g. sudden, severe, persistent chest pain; dyspnea; significant increase in cardiac enzymes).
2. Monitor EKG readings. Report abnormal rate, rhythm, or configurations.
3. Implement measures *to prevent cardiac dysfunction:*
   a. perform actions to prevent and treat fluid and electrolyte imbalances (see Nursing Diagnosis 3, action a.3)
   b. perform actions to reduce pancreatic stimulation (see Nursing Diagnosis 5.A, action 5.a) *in order to prevent further pancreatic damage and continued release of myocardial depressant factor.*
4. If signs and symptoms of cardiac dysfunction occur:
   a. initiate cardiac monitoring if not already being done
   b. maintain client on bedrest in a semi- to high Fowler's position
   c. maintain oxygen therapy as ordered
   d. monitor for therapeutic and nontherapeutic effects of antiarrhythmics, vasodilators, and sympathomimetics if administered *to improve cardiac output*
   e. have emergency cart readily available for cardiopulmonary resuscitation
   f. provide emotional support to client and significant others.

7.h. The client will not develop DIC as evidenced by:
1. absence of petechiae, ecchymosis, and frank or occult bleeding
2. skin warm, dry, and usual color
3. absence of new or intensified pain
4. mentally alert and oriented
5. fibrin degradation products (FDP) and protamine sulfate test within normal range
6. fibrinogen, PT, PTT, APTT, TT, and platelet levels within normal range
7. RBCs, Hct., and Hgb.

7.h.1. Assess for and report signs and symptoms of DIC:
   a. petechiae, ecchymosis
   b. mild to severe, frank or occult bleeding
   c. acrocyanosis (diaphoresis and cold, mottled fingers and toes)
   d. paresthesias or dysthesias of extremities
   e. headache, increased abdominal or back pain
   f. restlessness, agitation, confusion.
2. Assess for and report the following diagnostic test results (be certain that blood samples are not drawn from heparinized lines unless lines have been appropriately cleared):
   a. elevated levels of FDP
   b. positive protamine sulfate test
   c. prolonged prothrombin time (PT), partial thromboplastin time (PTT), activated partial thromboplastin time (APTT), and thrombin time (TT)
   d. reduced fibrinogen level and platelet count.
3. Assess for and report signs and symptoms of hypovolemic shock (see action a.3 in this diagnosis).
4. Implement measures *to prevent further tissue damage in order to reduce the risk of DIC:*

within normal range
8. blood pressure and pulse within normal range for client
9. urine output at least 30 cc/hour.

    a. perform actions to reduce pancreatic stimulation (see Nursing Diagnosis 5.A, action 5.a)
    b. prepare client for and assist with peritoneal lavage if performed *to remove pancreatic enzymes from the peritoneal cavity.*
5. If DIC occurs:
    a. implement safety precautions *to prevent further bleeding* (e.g. use of electric rather than straight-edge razor, use of soft bristle toothbrush, avoidance of injections)
    b. maintain oxygen therapy as ordered
    c. monitor for therapeutic and nontherapeutic effects of volume expanders and/or blood products such as fresh frozen plasma (FFP), platelets, and cryoprecipitate if administered
    d. monitor for therapeutic and nontherapeutic effects of heparin if administered *to prevent further clotting and thereby free clotting factors for control of bleeding*
    e. attempt to determine the amount of blood loss (e.g. weigh dressings, monitor changes in Hct. and Hgb.)
    f. provide emotional support to client and significant others.

7.i. The client will not experience signs and symptoms of fat necrosis as evidenced by:
1. absence of yellow, chalky subcutaneous deposits
2. absence of reddened, inflamed skin over affected areas
3. WBC count within normal range.

7.i.1. Assess for and report signs and symptoms of fat necrosis (e.g. yellow, chalky subcutaneous deposits [usually in the lower extremities]; redness and inflammation over affected areas; further increase in temperature and WBC count).
2. Implement measures to reduce pancreatic stimulation (see Nursing Diagnosis 5.A, action 5.a) *in order to reduce capillary permeability and escape of pancreatic enzymes from lymphatic system.*
3. If signs and symptoms of fat necrosis occur:
    a. monitor for therapeutic and nontherapeutic effects of anti-infectives if administered *to prevent infection in involved areas*
    b. prepare client for incision and drainage or removal of the necrotic areas
    c. provide emotional support to client and significant others.

8. NURSING DIAGNOSIS

Noncompliance* related to lack of understanding of the implications of not following the prescribed treatment plan and difficulty modifying personal habits and life style.

   * This diagnostic label includes both an informed decision by client not to comply and an inability to comply due to circumstances beyond the client's control.

DESIRED OUTCOMES	NURSING ACTIONS AND *SELECTED RATIONALES*

8. The client will demonstrate the probability of future compliance with the prescribed treatment plan as evidenced by:
    a. willingness to learn about and participate in treatments and care
    b. statements reflecting ways to modify personal habits and integrate treatments into life style
    c. statements reflecting an

8.a. Assess for indications that the client may be unwilling or unable to comply with the prescribed treatment plan:
1. failure to adhere to treatment plan while in hospital (e.g. not adhering to dietary modifications, refusing medications)
2. statements reflecting a lack of understanding of factors that will cause attacks of acute pancreatitis or lead to development of chronic pancreatitis
3. statements reflecting an unwillingness or inability to modify personal habits and integrate treatments into life style
4. statements reflecting the view that pancreatitis will not recur or that recurrence is inevitable and efforts to comply with treatments are useless.
    b. Implement measures *to improve client compliance:*
1. explain pancreatitis in terms the client can understand; stress the fact

understanding of the implications of not following the prescribed treatment plan.

that it can recur and develop into a chronic condition if treatment program is not followed
2. initiate and reinforce discharge teaching outlined in Nursing Diagnosis 9 *in order to promote a sense of control and self-reliance*
3. assist the client to identify ways he/she can incorporate treatments into life style; focus on modifications of life style rather than complete change
4. provide a dietary consult to assist the client in planning a diet based on the prescribed modifications and his/her likes, dislikes, and daily routines
5. encourage questions and allow time for reinforcement and clarification of information provided
6. provide written instructions about future appointments with health care provider, ways to prevent recurrence of pancreatitis, dietary modifications, medications, and signs and symptoms to report
7. obtain a social service consult to assist the client with financial planning and to obtain financial aid if indicated (aid may be especially needed for alcohol rehabilitation programs if alcohol was a precipitating factor in development of pancreatitis)
8. provide information about and encourage utilization of community resources that can assist client to make necessary life-style changes (e.g. stop smoking programs, alcohol rehabilitation centers, stress management classes, counseling services).

c. Assess for and reinforce behaviors suggesting future compliance with prescribed treatments (e.g. participation in the treatment plan, statements reflecting ways to modify personal habits and life style, changes in personal habits).

d. Include significant others in explanations and teaching sessions and encourage their support.

e. Consult physician regarding referrals to community health agencies if continued support or supervision is needed.

□ ▬▬▬▬▬▬▬▬▬▬▬▬▬▬▬▬▬▬▬▬▬▬▬▬▬

9. NURSING DIAGNOSIS

Knowledge deficit regarding follow-up care.

□ ▬▬▬▬▬▬▬▬▬▬▬▬▬▬▬▬▬▬▬▬▬▬▬▬▬

DESIRED OUTCOMES	NURSING ACTIONS AND *SELECTED RATIONALES*

9.a. The client will identify ways to prevent overstimulation of and further trauma to the pancreas.	9.a.1. Instruct client in importance of avoiding overstimulation of pancreas for the length of time specified by the physician (may be for a few months or for his/her lifetime depending on underlying cause of the pancreatitis).
	2. Instruct client in ways *to prevent overstimulation of and further trauma to the pancreas:*
	  a. maintain a balanced program of rest and exercise
	  b. avoid stressful situations
	  c. stop smoking
	  d. avoid drinking alcohol
	  e. adhere to recommended dietary modifications
	  f. maintain a relaxed, calm atmosphere during and after meals.
	3. Assist client to identify ways he/she can make necessary changes in personal habits and life style.

9.b. The client will verbalize an understanding of recommended dietary modifications.	9.b.1. Instruct client regarding dietary modifications necessary *to prevent overstimulation of the pancreas:*
	  a. eat small, frequent meals rather than 3 large ones
	  b. avoid foods/fluids high in fat (e.g. butter, cream, oils, whole milk, ice cream, pork, fried foods, gravies, nuts)

c. avoid caffeine-containing foods/fluids (e.g. chocolate, coffee, tea, colas).
2. Obtain a dietary consult if client needs assistance in planning meals that incorporate dietary modifications.

9.c. The client will state signs and symptoms to report to the health care provider.

9.c. Instruct client to report:
1. bowel movements that are frothy, that are foul-odored, and that float
2. severe epigastric or back pain
3. persistent nausea or vomiting
4. abdominal distention or increasing feeling of fullness
5. irritability or confusion
6. continued or unexplained weight loss
7. bluish areas on the back or abdomen
8. elevated temperature that lasts more than 2 days
9. tremors, jerking, seizures.

9.d. The client will identify community resources that can assist in making life-style changes necessary to prevent recurrence of acute pancreatitis.

9.d.1. Provide information regarding community resources that can assist client to make life-style changes necessary to prevent recurrence of acute pancreatitis (e.g. stop smoking programs, alcohol rehabilitation centers, stress management classes, counseling services).
2. Initiate a referral if indicated.

9.e. The client will verbalize an understanding of and a plan for adhering to recommended follow-up care including future appointments with health care provider and medications prescribed.

9.e.1. Reinforce the importance of keeping follow-up appointments with health care provider.
2. Explain the rationale for, side effects of, and importance of taking medications prescribed (e.g. fat-soluble vitamins, antacids, histamine$_2$ receptor antagonists, pancreatic enzymes, anti-infectives).
3. Refer to Nursing Diagnosis 8, action b, for measures to improve client compliance.

UNIT
XIII

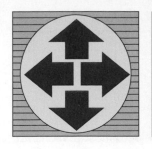
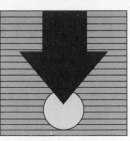
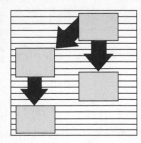
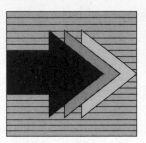
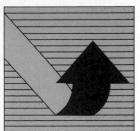

Unit V

Nursing Care of the Client Receiving Treatment for Neoplastic Disorders

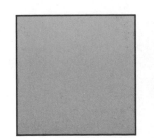

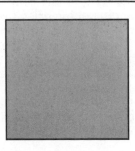
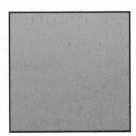

Diabetes Mellitus

Diabetes mellitus is a chronic systemic syndrome characterized by disorders of carbohydrate, fat, and protein metabolism resulting from a relative or absolute deficiency of insulin. It is further characterized by structural and functional abnormalities of the vascular and neurological systems. The atherosclerotic and arteriosclerotic changes that occur in the large vessels (macroangiopathy) affect the cardiac, cerebral, and peripheral circulation. Thickening of the basement membrane of the capillaries (microangiopathy) also occurs and involves vessels of the eyes, skin, and kidneys. Neurological manifestations are thought to be due in part to an insufficient blood supply to the nerves but appear to be primarily a result of a metabolic defect in the polyol pathway leading to an accumulation of byproducts (e.g. sorbitol, fructose) in nerve tissue. These byproducts act as toxins and cause demyelination and decreased nerve conduction.

The two major classifications of diabetes* are insulin-dependent diabetes mellitus (IDDM), also referred to as Type I, and noninsulin-dependent diabetes mellitus (NIDDM), often called Type II. Insulin-dependent diabetics have an absolute insulin deficiency and are dependent on insulin therapy to prevent ketosis. The insulin deficiency is a result of pancreatic beta cell destruction that is thought to be due to the initiation of an immune response by an environmental agent, most often a virus, in a person with a genetic predisposition for diabetes. Noninsulin-dependent diabetics have a relative deficiency of insulin due to faulty insulin secretion (often a delayed and prolonged output), a decreased tissue responsiveness to insulin, and an increased hepatic glucose production. Major factors contributing to the development of Type II diabetes are age (most persons are over 40), heredity, and obesity. Additional classifications of diabetes are related to stage of development or etiology and include (1) impaired glucose tolerance diabetes, (2) gestational diabetes (diabetes that becomes evident during pregnancy), and (3) secondary diabetes, which is associated with other conditions such as pancreatic disease and endocrine disorders (e.g. Cushing's syndrome, acromegaly) or use of medications such as glucocorticoids, estrogens, and thiazides.

Certain pathophysiological events are common to all types of diabetes. When an insulin deficiency exists, glucose cannot be transported into the cells for energy metabolism. As a result, glucose accumulates in the blood (hyperglycemia) and starts to spill into the urine (glucosuria) once the level exceeds 180 mg/dl. Fats and proteins are then mobilized to provide energy for the starving cells. The free fatty acids that are mobilized from adipose tissue are then converted by the liver to ketones (acetoacetate, acetone, β-hydroxybutyrate) to be used as an energy source. The ketones are strong acids and eventually deplete the body's buffer, renal, and respiratory defense systems, leading to a state of acidosis. Continuation of these metabolic derangements results in fluid and electrolyte imbalances and depletion of fat stores, cellular protein, and liver glycogen.

This care plan focuses on the adult client with diabetes mellitus hospitalized to stabilize widely fluctuating blood sugar levels. The goals of care are to maintain glucose levels within a safe range, prevent complications, and educate the client regarding follow-up care. This care plan should be used in conjunction with the care plans on Congestive Heart Failure, Myocardial Infarction, Cerebrovascular Accident, Hypertension, and/or Renal Failure if the client is also being treated for one of these vascular complications of diabetes.

---

* Diabetes mellitus will be referred to as diabetes throughout this care plan.

DISCHARGE CRITERIA

Prior to discharge, the client will:
- verbalize a basic understanding of the pathophysiology of diabetes mellitus
- verbalize an understanding of medication therapy including rationale for, side effects of, schedule for taking, and importance of taking as prescribed
- demonstrate the ability to correctly draw up and administer insulin if prescribed
- verbalize an understanding of the principles of dietary management and be able to calculate and plan meals within the prescribed caloric distribution
- demonstrate the ability to correctly perform blood glucose and urine tests and accurately interpret results
- verbalize an understanding of the role of exercise in the management of diabetes
- identify health care and hygiene practices that should be integrated into life style
- identify appropriate safety measures to follow because of the diagnosis of diabetes
- state signs and symptoms of hypoglycemia and ketoacidosis and appropriate actions for prevention and treatment

- state signs and symptoms to report to the health care provider
- share feelings and concerns about diabetes and its effect on life style
- identify community resources that can assist in the adjustment to and management of diabetes
- verbalize an understanding of and a plan for adhering to recommended follow-up care including future appointments with health care provider and for laboratory studies.

Use in conjunction with the Care Plan on Immobility.

NURSING/COLLABORATIVE DIAGNOSES

1. Anxiety □ *800*
2. Altered systemic tissue perfusion □ *800*
3. Altered fluid and electrolyte balance:
   a. fluid volume deficit, hyponatremia, hypochloremia, hypophosphatemia, and hypomagnesemia
   b. hypokalemia
   c. hyperkalemia
   d. metabolic acidosis □ *802*
4. Altered nutrition: less than body requirements □ *804*
5A. Altered comfort: pain and paresthesias (burning, aching, cramping, numbness, tingling, and/or cold sensation) □ *805*
5B. Altered comfort: gastric fullness and pyrosis □ *806*
5C. Altered comfort: nausea and vomiting □ *807*
6. Sensory-perceptual alteration: visual □ *808*
7. Impaired skin integrity:
   a. irritation or breakdown
   b. ulcerative skin lesions (diabetic dermopathy, necrobiosis lipoidica diabeticorum)
   c. delayed wound healing □ *809*
8. Altered patterns of urinary elimination:
   a. urinary retention
   b. urinary incontinence □ *810*
9. Constipation □ *811*
10. Diarrhea □ *811*
11. Bowel incontinence □ *812*
12. Potential for infection □ *813*
13. Potential for trauma □ *814*
14A. Potential acute metabolic complications:
   1. diabetic ketoacidosis
   2. hypoglycemia (insulin shock)
   3. hyperglycemic, hyperosmolar, nonketotic coma (HHNK)
   4. Somogyi phenomenon □ *815*
14B. Potential complication: thromboembolism □ *818*
15. Sexual dysfunction:
   a. impotence
   b. decreased libido □ *818*
16. Disturbance in self-concept □ *819*
17. Ineffective individual coping □ *819*
18. Grieving □ *820*
19. Noncompliance □ *821*
20. Knowledge deficit regarding follow-up care □ *822*

UNIT XIV

□ ▬▬▬▬▬▬▬▬▬▬▬▬▬▬▬▬▬▬▬▬▬▬▬▬▬▬▬▬

1. NURSING DIAGNOSIS

Anxiety related to unfamiliar environment; current symptoms; lack of understanding of diagnosis, diagnostic tests, treatments, and prognosis; inability to control disease; and possibility of further changes in life style and roles.

□ ▬▬▬▬▬▬▬▬▬▬▬▬▬▬▬▬▬▬▬▬▬▬▬▬▬▬▬▬

DESIRED OUTCOMES	NURSING ACTIONS AND *SELECTED RATIONALES*

1. The client will experience a reduction in fear and anxiety (see Care Plan on Immobility, Nursing Diagnosis 1, for outcome criteria).	1.a. Refer to Care Plan on Immobility, Nursing Diagnosis 1, for measures related to assessment and reduction of fear and anxiety.
	b. Implement additional measures *to reduce fear and anxiety:*
	  1. reinforce explanations of tests that may be performed to monitor effectiveness of treatment and progression of the disease process:
	    a. blood glucose tests:
	      1. glucose tolerance test (GTT)
	      2. fasting blood sugar (FBS)
	      3. 2-hour postprandial (2-hr pp)
	      4. strip or colorimeter measurements using capillary blood (e.g. Chemstrip bG, Dextrostix, Glucometer II)
	    b. tests used as an index of long-term control of blood sugar (glycosylated hemoglobin [HbA_{1c}])
	    c. urine tests for glucose and ketones:
	      1. Clinitest, Tes-Tape, Diastix
	      2. Acetest, Ketostix, Keto-Diastix
	    d. serum studies to determine cholesterol, triglycerides, and lipoprotein profile *(help determine extensiveness of vascular involvement)*
	  2. inform client that some of signs and symptoms may be partially reversed once diabetes is under better control.

□ ▬▬▬▬▬▬▬▬▬▬▬▬▬▬▬▬▬▬▬▬▬▬▬▬▬▬▬▬

2. NURSING DIAGNOSIS

Altered systemic tissue perfusion related to:

a. vascular abnormalities (arteriosclerosis, atherosclerosis, microangiopathies) that develop with diabetes;
b. hypovolemia associated with fluid volume deficit;
c. orthostatic hypotension associated with neuropathy of the autonomic nervous system, peripheral pooling of blood resulting from decreased activity, and hypovolemia.

□ ▬▬▬▬▬▬▬▬▬▬▬▬▬▬▬▬▬▬▬▬▬▬▬▬▬▬▬▬

DESIRED OUTCOMES

NURSING ACTIONS AND *SELECTED RATIONALES*

2. The client will maintain adequate systemic tissue perfusion as evidenced by:
   a. B/P and pulse within normal range for client and stable with position change
   b. unlabored respirations at 16–20/minute
   c. usual mental status
   d. skin warm and usual color
   e. palpable peripheral pulses
   f. capillary refill time less than 3 seconds
   g. urine output at least 30 cc/hour
   h. BUN and serum creatinine levels within normal range.

2.a. Assess for and report signs and symptoms of diminished systemic tissue perfusion:
   1. significant decrease in B/P (be alert to the fact that many diabetics are hypertensive because of vascular changes)
   2. resting pulse rate greater than 100 beats/minute
   3. decline in systolic B/P of at least 15 mm Hg with concurrent rise in pulse when client changes from lying to sitting or standing position
   4. rapid or labored respirations
   5. restlessness, slow responses, confusion
   6. coolness, blanching, pallor, and delayed (longer than 10 seconds) color return in feet and lower legs when legs are returned to a dependent position after being elevated for 60 seconds
   7. dusky red color of lower legs and feet when in dependent position
   8. diminished or absent peripheral pulses
   9. capillary refill time greater than 3 seconds
   10. urine output less than 30 cc/hour
   11. elevated BUN and serum creatinine levels *(may indicate diminished tissue perfusion to kidneys).*
 b. Monitor serum cholesterol, triglycerides, and lipoprotein profiles. Report abnormalities. *(Elevated lipid levels are consistent with atherosclerosis.)*
 c. Implement measures *to maintain adequate systemic tissue perfusion:*
   1. discourage smoking *(smoking causes vasoconstriction)*
   2. maintain a room temperature that is comfortable for client and provide him/her with adequate clothing and blankets *(exposure to cold causes generalized vasoconstriction)*
   3. perform actions *to promote adequate circulation in lower extremities:*
      a. increase activity as allowed; instruct client with intermittent claudication to walk slowly and alternate activity with periods of rest
      b. discourage positions that compromise blood flow (e.g. crossing legs, pillows under knees, use of knee gatch, prolonged sitting or standing)
      c. encourage active foot and leg exercises for 5–10 minutes every 1–2 hours
   4. perform actions *to reduce orthostatic hypotension:*
      a. instruct client to change positions slowly *in order to allow time for autoregulatory mechanisms to adjust to position changes*
      b. keep head of bed elevated 8–12 inches
      c. apply antiembolic hose or elastic wraps as ordered; if applied, remove for 30–60 minutes every shift
      d. monitor for therapeutic and nontherapeutic effects of fludrocortisone acetate if administered *to increase fluid volume and vascular sensitivity to catecholamines*
   5. assist and instruct client to avoid foods high in saturated (animal) fat and cholesterol (e.g. butter, cheese, ice cream, egg yolks, shrimp, cashew nuts, organ meats) *in order to reduce progression of atherogenesis*
   6. perform actions to maintain blood glucose at near-normal level (see Nursing Diagnosis 4, action f); *maintaining blood glucose at near-normal level is thought to delay vascular complications*
   7. perform actions to prevent or treat fluid volume deficit (see Nursing Diagnosis 3, action a.2)
   8. monitor for therapeutic and nontherapeutic effects of the following medications if administered:
      a. peripheral vasodilators (e.g. cyclandelate, papaverine, isoxsuprine) *to improve arterial blood flow*
      b. antihyperlipidemic agents (e.g. clofibrate, nicotinic acid, cholestyramine, probucol) *to prevent further atherogenesis*
      c. pentoxifylline (Trental) *to improve blood flow (increases erythrocyte flexibility and reduces blood viscosity).*
 d. Consult physician if signs and symptoms of decreased tissue perfusion persist or worsen.

UNIT XIV

□ ▬▬▬▬▬▬▬▬▬▬▬▬▬▬▬▬▬

3. NURSING/COLLABORATIVE DIAGNOSIS

Altered fluid and electrolyte balance:

a. **fluid volume deficit, hyponatremia, hypochloremia, hypophosphatemia, and hypomagnesemia** related to excessive loss of fluid and electrolytes associated with diarrhea, vomiting, and osmotic diuresis (results from hyperglycemia);

b. **hypokalemia** related to:
   1. excessive loss of potassium associated with osmotic diuresis, vomiting, diarrhea, and a high aldosterone level (aldosterone output is increased as a result of fluid volume deficit and decreased renal tissue perfusion)
   2. shift of serum potassium into the cells as a result of insulin therapy;

c. **hyperkalemia** related to shift of cellular potassium into the vascular space in exchange for hydrogen in an acidotic state and decreased excretion of potassium if urine output is decreased (urine output can decrease as a result of fluid volume deficit and decreased renal tissue perfusion);

d. **metabolic acidosis** related to:
   1. excess ketone body formation and depletion of available buffers (ketoacidosis) associated with increased mobilization of fatty acids for energy resulting from an inability of cells to use glucose
   2. excessive release of lactic acid from cells (lactic acidosis) associated with cellular hypoxia resulting from inadequate tissue perfusion
   3. excessive loss of bicarbonate associated with diarrhea.

□ ▬▬▬▬▬▬▬▬▬▬▬▬▬▬▬▬▬

DESIRED OUTCOMES	NURSING ACTIONS AND *SELECTED RATIONALES*

3.a. The client will not experience a fluid volume deficit as evidenced by:
1. normal skin turgor
2. moist mucous membranes
3. weight loss no greater than 0.5 kg/day
4. B/P and pulse within normal range for client and stable with position change
5. balanced intake and output
6. urine specific gravity between 1.010–1.030
7. Hct. within normal range.

3.a.1. Assess for and report signs and symptoms of fluid volume deficit:
   a. decreased skin turgor
   b. dry mucous membranes, thirst
   c. weight loss greater than 0.5 kg/day (many clients with diabetes are on weight reduction diets, so some weight loss is expected)
   d. low B/P and/or a decline in systolic B/P of at least 15 mm Hg with a concurrent rise in pulse when client sits up
   e. weak, rapid pulse
   f. output less than intake with urine specific gravity higher than 1.030 (reflects an actual rather than potential water deficit); if client has diabetic nephropathy, specific gravity is not a useful indicator of hydration status
   g. elevated Hct.

2. Implement measures *to prevent or treat fluid volume deficit:*
   a. perform actions to reduce nausea and vomiting (see Nursing Diagnosis 5.C, action 2)
   b. perform actions to control diarrhea (see Nursing Diagnosis 10, action d)
   c. perform actions *to prevent or treat hyperglycemia in order to prevent osmotic diuresis:*
      1. encourage client to adhere to the American Diabetic Association (ADA) diet prescribed
      2. administer insulin as ordered and in an area where it will be absorbed properly *(there is decreased absorption of insulin if it is administered in an area where tissue is hypertrophied);* if client has an insulin pump, maintain prescribed basal infusion rate (usually 0.5–1.2 units/hour) and ensure that client receives preprandial boluses as ordered
      3. administer prescribed oral hypoglycemic agents 30–60 minutes before meals

4. minimize client's exposure to emotional and physiological stress *(stress causes an increased output of epinephrine, norepinephrine, glucagon, and cortisol, all of which increase blood sugar)*
5. consult physician if there is a significant decrease in client's activity level *(this may result in an elevation of blood sugar)*

d. maintain a fluid intake of at least 2500 cc/day unless contraindicated
e. maintain intravenous fluid therapy as ordered.

3. Consult physician if signs and symptoms of fluid volume deficit persist or worsen.

3.b. The client will maintain safe electrolyte levels as evidenced by:
1. regular pulse at 60–100 beats/minute
2. usual mental status
3. usual strength and muscle tone
4. normal bowel sounds
5. absence of nausea, vomiting, abdominal cramps, paresthesias, seizure activity
6. serum sodium, chloride, magnesium, phosphorus, and potassium within normal range.

3.b.1. Assess for and report signs and symptoms of the following electrolyte imbalances:
   a. hyponatremia (e.g. nausea, vomiting, abdominal cramps, weakness, twitching, lethargy, confusion, seizures)
   b. hypochloremia (e.g. twitching, tetany, depressed respirations)
   c. hypomagnesemia (e.g. change in mental status, muscle cramps, numbness and tingling in extremities, tremors, positive Chvostek's and Trousseau's signs, tachycardia)
   d. hypophosphatemia (e.g. confusion, muscle weakness, paresthesias, dysarthria, seizures)
   e. hypokalemia (e.g. irregular pulse, muscle weakness and cramping, paresthesias, nausea and vomiting, hypoactive or absent bowel sounds, drowsiness)
   f. hyperkalemia (e.g. slow or irregular pulse, paresthesias, muscle weakness and flaccidity, hyperactive bowel sounds with diarrhea and intestinal colic).
2. Monitor serum electrolyte results. Report abnormal values.
3. Implement measures *to prevent excessive loss of electrolytes:*
   a. perform actions to reduce nausea and vomiting (see Nursing Diagnosis 5.C, action 2)
   b. perform actions to control diarrhea (see Nursing Diagnosis 10, action d)
   c. perform actions to prevent and treat hyperglycemia (see action a.2.c in this diagnosis) *in order to prevent osmotic diuresis.*
4. If signs and symptoms of electrolyte depletion occur:
   a. continue with above actions to prevent further losses
   b. monitor for therapeutic and nontherapeutic effects of electrolyte replacements (e.g. saline solutions, potassium chloride, potassium phosphate, magnesium sulfate) if administered; monitor serum potassium and urine output closely when giving supplemental potassium and consult physician if potassium level increases above normal and/or urine output is less than 30 cc/hour
   c. when oral intake is allowed, instruct and assist client to select foods/fluids high in the electrolytes in which he/she is deficient:
      1. potassium (e.g. bananas, potatoes, raisins, figs, apricots, dates, Gatorade, fruit juices)
      2. sodium (e.g. processed cheese, soups, catsup, pickles, bouillon)
      3. magnesium (e.g. whole grains, seafood, legumes)
      4. phosphorus (e.g. poultry, milk, peas, cheese, fish, eggs).
5. Implement measures *to prevent or treat hyperkalemia:*
   a. perform actions to prevent or treat acidosis (see action c.2 in this diagnosis)
   b. maintain dietary restrictions of potassium if ordered
   c. perform actions to maintain adequate systemic tissue perfusion (see Nursing Diagnosis 2, action c) *in order to ensure adequate renal blood flow and promote urinary excretion of potassium*
   d. perform actions *to spare body proteins and prevent excessive tissue breakdown:*
      1. encourage client to consume the recommended amount of dietary protein
      2. maintain intravenous glucose infusions as ordered and/or encourage client to consume recommended amount of carbohydrates *(both spare the protein by providing quick energy sources)*
      3. restrict activity as ordered *to reduce energy requirements*
   e. if signs and symptoms of hyperkalemia are present, consult physician before administering prescribed potassium supplements

UNIT
XIV

f. monitor for therapeutic and nontherapeutic effects of the following if administered:
   1. intravenous insulin and hypertonic glucose solutions *to enhance transport of potassium back into cells*
   2. loop diuretics (e.g. ethacrynic acid, furosemide) *to increase renal excretion of potassium*
   3. cation-exchange resins (e.g. Kayexalate) *to increase potassium excretion via the intestines (act by exchanging sodium for potassium)*
g. prepare client for dialysis if planned.
6. Consult physician if signs and symptoms of electrolyte imbalances persist or worsen.

DESIRED OUTCOMES	NURSING ACTIONS AND *SELECTED RATIONALES*
3.c. The client will maintain acid-base balance as evidenced by: 1. usual mental status 2. unlabored respirations at 16–20/minute 3. absence of headache, nausea, vomiting 4. blood gases within normal range 5. anion gap less than 16 mEq/liter.	3.c.1. Assess for and report signs and symptoms of metabolic acidosis (e.g. drowsiness; disorientation; stupor; rapid, deep respirations; headache; nausea; vomiting; low pH and CO_2 content and negative base excess; anion gap greater than 16 mEq/liter). 2. Implement measures *to prevent or treat metabolic acidosis:* a. perform actions to prevent and treat hyperglycemia (see action a.2.c in this diagnosis) *in order to prevent ketoacidosis* b. perform actions to promote adequate tissue perfusion (see Nursing Diagnosis 2, action c) *in order to prevent excessive lactic acid production* c. perform actions to control diarrhea (see Nursing Diagnosis 10, action d) d. monitor for therapeutic and nontherapeutic effects of sodium bicarbonate if administered (reserved for use in severe acidosis when pH is less than 7.1). 3. Consult physician if signs and symptoms of acidosis persist or worsen.

□ ▬▬▬▬▬▬▬▬▬▬▬▬▬▬▬▬▬▬▬▬

4. NURSING DIAGNOSIS

Altered nutrition: less than body requirements related to:

a. defect in glucose metabolism and depletion of fat stores, cellular protein, and liver glycogen associated with an insulin deficiency;
b. decreased oral intake associated with dislike of the prescribed diet, anorexia, gastric fullness, pyrosis, and nausea;
c. hypoglycemia associated with higher insulin levels than the body currently has a need for.

□ ▬▬▬▬▬▬▬▬▬▬▬▬▬▬▬▬▬▬▬▬

DESIRED OUTCOMES	NURSING ACTIONS AND *SELECTED RATIONALES*
4. The client will maintain an adequate nutritional status as evidenced by: a. serum glucose stable at a level between 60–140 mg/dl b. maintenance of or return toward normal weight c. normal BUN and serum albumin, protein, Hct., Hgb., cholesterol, and lymphocyte levels	4.a. Assess the client for signs and symptoms of malnutrition: 1. abnormal weight for client's age, height, and build (many of these clients are overweight) 2. abnormal BUN and low serum albumin, protein, Hct., Hgb., cholesterol, and lymphocyte levels 3. triceps skinfold measurement less than or greater than normal for build 4. weakness and fatigue 5. stomatitis. b. Monitor blood glucose levels using a product such as Glucometer, Chemstrip bG, or Dextrostix. Report values below 60 mg/dl or above 200 mg/dl or outside of the parameters specified by physician. c. Reassess nutritional status on a regular basis and report decline.

d. triceps skinfold measurements within normal range
e. usual strength and activity tolerance
f. healthy oral mucous membrane.

d. Monitor percentage of meals eaten.
e. Assess client to determine causes of inadequate intake (e.g. nausea, feeling of fullness, anorexia, dislike of diet).
f. Implement measures *to maintain blood glucose at near-normal level, achieve ideal weight, and provide necessary nutrients in order to maintain an optimal nutritional status:*
   1. obtain a dietary consult to instruct client about the diet prescribed and ways to adapt it to personal preferences and specific needs (dietary restrictions will vary but are most often prescribed as specific percentages of carbohydrate, fat, and protein within an optimal calorie level; it is recommended that 50–60% of calories be derived from carbohydrate [preferably complex with a low glycemic index], 20–30% from fat [primarily polyunsaturated], and 20% from protein; specific amounts of fiber may also be prescribed *because it slows carbohydrate digestion and absorption and may lower serum lipid levels)*
   2. assist client to calculate and select appropriate foods; utilize the method or combination of methods (e.g. exchange list, glycemic index) that client has been instructed in
   3. reinforce importance of weight loss if client is obese *(studies have shown that obese persons have an increased number of insulin receptors and reduced insulin resistance following weight loss)*
   4. administer insulin or oral hypoglycemic agents as scheduled and provide meals and snacks on time and at evenly spaced intervals *to maintain desired balance between insulin and glucose*
   5. perform actions to prevent and treat hypoglycemia (see Collaborative Diagnosis 14.A, actions 2.b and c)
   6. perform actions *to improve oral intake:*
      a. implement measures to relieve gastric fullness, pyrosis, and nausea (see Nursing Diagnoses 5.B, action 3 and 5.C, action 2)
      b. provide oral care before meals
      c. serve small portions of foods/fluids that are appealing to client and provide snacks as indicated to meet prescribed caloric intake
      d. provide a clean, relaxed, pleasant atmosphere
      e. allow adequate time for meals; reheat food if necessary
      f. increase activity as tolerated *(activity stimulates appetite)*
   7. monitor for therapeutic and nontherapeutic effects of the following medications if administered:
      a. insulin and/or oral hypoglycemic agents *to enhance cellular utilization of glucose and promote normal metabolism of fats and proteins*
      b. vitamins and minerals.
g. Perform a 72-hour calorie count if nutritional status declines or fails to improve.
h. Consult physician about alternative methods of providing nutrition (e.g. parenteral nutrition, tube feedings) if client does not consume enough food or fluid to meet nutritional needs.

5.A. NURSING DIAGNOSIS

Altered comfort:* **pain and paresthesias (burning, aching, cramping, numbness, tingling, and/or cold sensation)** related to peripheral neuropathies and vascular insufficiency associated with peripheral vascular disease.

* In this care plan, the nursing diagnosis "pain" is included under the diagnostic label of altered comfort.

DESIRED OUTCOMES	NURSING ACTIONS AND *SELECTED RATIONALES*

5.A. The client will experience diminished discomfort as evidenced by:
1. verbalization of a reduction of burning, aching, cramping, numbness, tingling, and cold sensation in involved areas
2. relaxed facial expression and body positioning
3. increased participation in activities
4. stable vital signs.

5.A.1. Determine how client usually responds to discomfort.
2. Assess for nonverbal signs of discomfort (e.g. wrinkled brow, clenched fists, reluctance to move, guarding of affected area, restlessness, diaphoresis, facial pallor or flushing, change in B/P, tachycardia).
3. Assess for signs and symptoms of peripheral neuropathies and peripheral vascular insufficiency (can occur anywhere but most often occur in the lower extremities):
   a. persistent burning or aching sensation that often becomes worse at night
   b. numbness, tingling, or lack of sensation
   c. diminished or absent reflexes
   d. constant feeling of coldness in a particular area
   e. cramps, especially in calf muscles, during ambulation (indicative of intermittent claudication).
4. Assess for factors that seem to aggravate or alleviate discomfort.
5. Implement measures *to reduce discomfort:*
   a. provide a bed cradle *to keep bedding off affected extremities*
   b. assist client with ambulation if walking relieves discomfort (walking usually relieves lower extremity discomfort associated with neuropathies); if client is experiencing intermittent claudication, encourage short, more frequent walks *since longer walks exacerbate pain associated with vascular insufficiency*
   c. provide extra blankets if client complains of a cold sensation in affected areas
   d. provide or assist with nonpharmacological measures for relief of discomfort (e.g. position change, transcutaneous electrical nerve stimulation, relaxation techniques, guided imagery, quiet conversation, restful environment, diversional activities)
   e. plan methods for controlling discomfort with client *to enable him/her to maintain a sense of control over the discomfort*
   f. monitor for therapeutic and nontherapeutic effects of the following medications if administered *to control discomfort:*
      1. analgesics (narcotic analgesics are avoided as long as possible *because the pain may be chronic;* some painful neuropathies may, however, subside after a few months)
      2. amitriptyline hydrochloride and fluphenazine hydrochloride (found to be useful in treatment of paresthesias *because they alter the client's sensation of discomfort)*
      3. pentoxifylline (useful for intermittent claudication *because it improves blood flow).*
6. Consult physician if above measures fail to provide adequate relief of discomfort.

5.B. NURSING DIAGNOSIS

Altered comfort: gastric fullness and pyrosis related to accumulation of gas and fluid in the stomach associated with gastroparesis resulting from autonomic neuropathy.

DESIRED OUTCOMES	NURSING ACTIONS AND *SELECTED RATIONALES*

5.B. The client will experience a reduction in gastric fullness

5.B.1. Assess for nonverbal signs of gastric discomfort (e.g. clutching and guarding of stomach, restlessness, reluctance to move, grimacing).

and pyrosis as evidenced by:
1. verbalization of same
2. relaxed facial expression
   and body positioning.

2. Assess verbal complaints of gastric fullness or heartburn.
3. Implement measures *to reduce gastric fullness and pyrosis:*
   a. encourage and assist client with frequent position change and ambulation as tolerated *(activity stimulates gastric motility)*
   b. have client sit up during meals and for 1–2 hours after meals *(gravity will promote passage of food through the gastrointestinal tract)*
   c. provide small, frequent meals
   d. encourage client to drink warm liquids *to stimulate peristalsis*
   e. instruct client to avoid activities such as gum chewing, drinking through a straw, sucking on hard candy, and smoking *in order to reduce air swallowing*
   f. instruct client to avoid:
      1. gas-producing foods/fluids (e.g. cabbage, onions, popcorn, baked beans, carbonated beverages)
      2. foods/fluids that irritate the gastric mucosa (e.g. spicy foods; citrus fruits or juices; caffeine-containing items such as chocolate, coffee, tea, or colas)
   g. monitor for therapeutic and nontherapeutic effects of the following medications if administered:
      1. gastrointestinal stimulants (e.g. metoclopramide)
      2. antiflatulents *to reduce gas accumulation*
      3. antacids and histamine$_2$ receptor antagonists (e.g. cimetidine, ranitidine, famotidine) *to reduce gastric acidity*.
4. Consult physician if gastric discomfort persists or worsens.

5.C. NURSING DIAGNOSIS

Altered comfort: nausea and vomiting related to stimulation of the vomiting center associated with:

1. vagal and/or sympathetic stimulation resulting from visceral irritation due to gastric distention;
2. cortical stimulation due to discomfort and stress;
3. chemoreceptor trigger zone stimulation resulting from acid-base and electrolyte imbalances.

DESIRED OUTCOMES	NURSING ACTIONS AND *SELECTED RATIONALES*

5.C. The client will experience relief of nausea and vomiting as evidenced by:
1. verbalization of relief of nausea
2. absence of vomiting.

5.C.1. Assess client to determine factors that contribute to nausea and vomiting (e.g. gastric fullness, discomfort, anxiety, electrolyte imbalances).
2. Implement measures *to reduce nausea and vomiting:*
   a. perform actions to reduce gastric fullness and pyrosis (see Nursing Diagnosis 5.B, action 3)
   b. perform actions to reduce pain and paresthesias (see Nursing Diagnosis 5.A, action 5)
   c. perform actions to reduce fear and anxiety (see Nursing Diagnosis 1)
   d. perform actions to prevent or treat electrolyte imbalances and metabolic acidosis (see Nursing Diagnosis 3, actions b.3 and 4 and c.2)
   e. eliminate noxious sights and smells from the environment *(noxious stimuli cause cortical stimulation of the vomiting center)*
   f. instruct client to change positions slowly *(movement stimulates the chemoreceptor trigger zone)*
   g. encourage client to take deep, slow breaths when nauseated
   h. provide oral hygiene every 2 hours and after each emesis
   i. instruct client to ingest foods and fluids slowly

> j. instruct client to eat dry foods (e.g. toast, crackers) and avoid drinking liquids with meals if nauseated
> k. monitor for therapeutic and nontherapeutic effects of antiemetics if administered.
> 3. Consult physician if above measures fail to relieve nausea and vomiting.

6. NURSING DIAGNOSIS

Sensory-perceptual alteration: visual related to:

a. neuropathy of cranial nerves III, IV, and VI;
b. retinopathy and/or glaucoma (due to obstruction of usual intraocular fluid flow) associated with vascular changes in the eye;
c. lens changes (metabolic cataracts) associated with the accumulation of fructose and/or sorbitol and fluid in the lens.

DESIRED OUTCOMES	NURSING ACTIONS AND *SELECTED RATIONALES*

6. The client will not experience further progression of visual disturbances.	6.a. Determine the client's baseline visual status upon admission by:
	  1. assessing for the following signs and symptoms:
	    a. blurred vision *(usually associated with a high blood glucose, which can result in accumulation of sugars and fluid in the lens)*
	    b. inability to move eyes in all directions (test by having client follow finger movement with eyes)
	    c. diplopia
	    d. black or red spots in visual field
	    e. distorted vision
	    f. loss of vision
	  2. examining the fundus of the eye for indications of retinal vascular damage (e.g. small retinal hemorrhages, soft exudates).
	b. Prepare client for fluorescein angiography if scheduled *to document type and progression of retinopathy.*
	c. Implement measures *to prevent further visual disturbances:*
	  1. perform actions identified in Nursing Diagnosis 3, action a.2.c, to control hyperglycemia *(maintenance of blood sugar at a stable, near-normal level has been shown to reduce small vessel and nerve involvement and prevent metabolic cataract development)*
	  2. prepare client for photocoagulation or vitrectomy if planned for treatment of retinopathy.
	d. If vision is impaired:
	  1. implement measures to prevent injury (see Nursing Diagnosis 13, actions b–d)
	  2. avoid startling client (e.g. speak client's name and identify yourself when entering room and before any physical contact, describe activities and reasons for various noises in the room)
	  3. assist client with personal hygiene he/she is unable to perform independently
	  4. identify where items are placed on his/her plate or tray, cut food, open packages, or feed client if necessary
	  5. assist with activities that require reading (e.g. menu selection, mail, legal documents)
	  6. instruct client in use of appropriate self-help devices (e.g. magnifier for insulin syringe, dosage monitor for syringe, needle guide for insulin vial, glucometer that displays blood glucose values in bold numbers); monitor client's accuracy in testing urine and blood glucose and administering insulin
	  7. provide auditory rather than visual diversionary activities

8. inform client of resources available if he/she desires additional information about visual aids (e.g. publications such as Aids for Blind; American Foundation for the Blind).

e. Reassess visual status regularly and consult physician if visual status worsens.

7. NURSING DIAGNOSIS

Impaired skin integrity:

a. **irritation or breakdown** related to:
   1. prolonged pressure on tissues associated with decreased mobility
   2. increased fragility of skin associated with protein depletion and inadequate tissue perfusion
   3. abnormal pressure distribution on plantar aspect of feet (results from muscle weakness in feet associated with peripheral neuropathy) and undetected foot injuries associated with diminished sensation (results from vascular insufficiency and neuropathy)
   4. frequent contact with irritants associated with diarrhea and/or incontinence;

b. **ulcerative skin lesions (diabetic dermopathy, necrobiosis lipoidica diabeticorum)**, which sometimes develop in diabetics;

c. **delayed wound healing** related to decreased tissue perfusion, inadequate nutritional status, and impaired protein synthesis (results from insulin deficiency).

DESIRED OUTCOMES	NURSING ACTIONS AND *SELECTED RATIONALES*
7.a. The client will maintain skin integrity (see Care Plan on Immobility, Nursing Diagnosis 7, for outcome criteria).	7.a.1. Inspect skin for areas of pallor, redness, or breakdown with particular attention to: a. skinfolds of abdomen and groin and under breasts b. spaces between toes c. feet and lower legs d. dependent areas e. bone prominences f. buttocks and perianal area g. areas where sensation is diminished *(client may be unaware of development of blisters and ulcerations).* 2. Refer to Care Plan on Immobility, Nursing Diagnosis 7, action b, for measures to prevent skin breakdown associated with decreased mobility. 3. Implement measures *to decrease skin irritation and prevent breakdown resulting from incontinence or diarrhea:* a. perform actions to reduce episodes of urinary incontinence (see Nursing Diagnosis 8, actions b.2 and 3) b. perform actions to control diarrhea and prevent incontinence of stool (see Nursing Diagnoses 10, action d and 11, action b) c. assist client to thoroughly cleanse and dry perineal area after each bowel movement and episode of incontinence; apply a protective ointment or cream (e.g. Sween cream, Desitin, karaya gel, A & D ointment, Vaseline) d. use soft tissue to cleanse perianal area e. avoid direct contact of skin with Chux (e.g. place turn sheet or bed pad over Chux) f. apply a perianal pouch if incontinence of stool is a persistent problem. 4. Implement measures *to reduce risk of skin breakdown associated with vascular insufficiency and neuropathy:* a. perform actions to maintain adequate tissue perfusion (see Nursing Diagnosis 2, action c) b. perform meticulous foot care:

       1. wash feet daily with warm water and a mild soap
       2. dry feet thoroughly using a soft towel or cloth, paying particular attention to interdigital spaces
       3. apply a drying powder or place lamb's wool between toes
       4. massage feet daily with a lubricating lotion (do not apply between toes)
   c. prevent trauma to feet:
       1. cut nails carefully (soften nails by soaking in warm water, then cut straight across using nail clippers); if there are thickened folds of skin on either side of nail, consult physician about a referral to a podiatrist
       2. caution client to always wear socks and shoes or sturdy slippers when ambulating
       3. do not place heating pads or hot water bottles on feet
       4. check the temperature of bath water before client immerses feet.
  5. Maintain an optimal nutritional status (see Nursing Diagnosis 4, action f).
  6. If skin breakdown occurs:
   a. notify physician
   b. continue with above measures to prevent further irritation and breakdown
   c. perform care of decubitus and/or ulcerative skin lesions as ordered or per hospital policy
   d. monitor client closely and report signs and symptoms of infection (e.g. elevated temperature; redness, warmth, and edema around area of breakdown; unusual drainage from site).

7.b. The client will experience normal healing of any wound as evidenced by:
  1. gradual reduction in redness and swelling at wound site
  2. presence of granulation tissue in wound healing by secondary intention
  3. intact, approximated wound edges if wound is healing by primary intention.

7.b.1. Assess for and report signs and symptoms of impaired wound healing (e.g. increasing redness and swelling at wound site, pale or necrotic tissue in wound, separation of wound edges).
  2. Implement measures *to promote normal wound healing:*
   a. perform actions to promote protein anabolism and maintain an optimal nutritional status (see Nursing Diagnosis 4, action f)
   b. perform actions *to maintain adequate circulation to wound area:*
       1. implement measures to maintain adequate systemic tissue perfusion (see Nursing Diagnosis 2, action c)
       2. do not apply dressings tightly *(excessive pressure impairs circulation to the area)*
   c. perform actions *to protect the wound from mechanical injury:*
       1. ensure that dressings are secure enough to keep them from rubbing and irritating the wound
       2. carefully remove tape and dressings when performing wound care
       3. remind client to keep hands away from wound area
       4. utilize bed cradle *to prevent linens from touching wounds not covered by dressings*
       5. implement measures to prevent falls (see Nursing Diagnosis 13, action b)
   d. perform actions to prevent wound infection (see Nursing Diagnosis 12, action c.8).
  3. If signs and symptoms of impaired wound healing occur:
   a. assist with wound debridement if performed
   b. provide emotional support to client and significant others.

8. NURSING DIAGNOSIS

Altered patterns of urinary elimination:

a. **urinary retention** related to loss of bladder sensation and diminished contractility of the bladder detrusor muscles associated with neuropathy of the autonomic nervous system;
b. **urinary incontinence** related to overflow associated with urinary retention and loss of sphincter control associated with autonomic neuropathy.

DESIRED OUTCOMES	NURSING ACTIONS AND *SELECTED RATIONALES*
8.a. The client will not experience urinary retention (see Care Plan on Immobility, Nursing Diagnosis 10, for outcome criteria).	8.a.1. Refer to Care Plan on Immobility, Nursing Diagnosis 10, for measures related to assessment, prevention, and management of urinary retention. 2. Assist with urodynamic studies (e.g. cystometrogram) if ordered.
8.b. The client will maintain optimal urinary control as evidenced by absence of or decreased episodes of incontinence.	8.b.1. Assess for and report urinary incontinence. 2. Implement measures *to maintain urinary continence:* a. perform actions to prevent urinary retention (see Care Plan on Immobility, Nursing Diagnosis 10, action d) *in order to prevent incontinence resulting from urinary overflow* b. offer bedpan or urinal or assist client to commode or bathroom every 2–3 hours c. allow client to assume a normal position for voiding unless contraindicated *in order to promote complete bladder emptying* d. instruct client to perform perineal exercises (e.g. stopping and starting stream during voiding, pressing buttocks together and then relaxing the muscles) *in order to improve urinary sphincter tone* e. limit oral fluid intake in the evening *to decrease possibility of nighttime incontinence* f. instruct client to avoid drinking beverages containing caffeine *(caffeine is a mild diuretic and may make urinary control more difficult)* g. monitor for therapeutic and nontherapeutic effects of alpha-adrenergic agonists (e.g. ephedrine) if administered *to increase urinary sphincter tone.* 3. If urinary incontinence persists: a. consult physician about intermittent catheterization, insertion of indwelling catheter, or use of external catheter or penile clamp b. provide emotional support to client and significant others.

9. NURSING DIAGNOSIS

Constipation related to decreased intake of fluids and foods high in fiber and decreased gastrointestinal motility associated with decreased activity, anxiety, and autonomic neuropathy.

DESIRED OUTCOMES	NURSING ACTIONS AND *SELECTED RATIONALES*
9. The client will maintain usual bowel elimination pattern.	9. Refer to Care Plan on Immobility, Nursing Diagnosis 11, for measures related to assessment and prevention of constipation.

10. NURSING DIAGNOSIS

Diarrhea related to autonomic neuropathy; severe anxiety; and possible intestinal bacterial overgrowth, bile salt malabsorption, and/or pancreatic insufficiency.

UNIT XIV

DESIRED OUTCOMES	NURSING ACTIONS AND *SELECTED RATIONALES*
10. The client will maintain usual bowel elimination pattern.	10.a. Ascertain client's usual bowel elimination habits. b. Assess for and report signs and symptoms of diarrhea (e.g. frequent, loose stools; abdominal pain and cramping). c. Assess bowel sounds regularly. Report an increase in frequency of and/or high-pitched bowel sounds. d. Implement measures *to control diarrhea:* 　1. perform actions *to rest the bowel:* 　　a. instruct client to avoid foods/fluids that are: 　　　1. extremely hot or cold 　　　2. spicy or high in fat content 　　　3. high in caffeine (e.g. coffee, tea, chocolate, colas) 　　　4. diarrhea or gas-producing (e.g. cabbage, onions, popcorn, licorice, prunes, chili, baked beans) 　　b. provide small, frequent meals 　　c. discourage smoking *(nicotine has a stimulant effect on the gastrointestinal tract)* 　　d. implement measures to reduce fear and anxiety (see Nursing Diagnosis 1) 　2. monitor for therapeutic and nontherapeutic effects of the following medications if administered: 　　a. opiate or opiate-like substances (e.g. loperamide, diphenoxylate hydrochloride) if administered *to decrease gastrointestinal motility* 　　b. bulk-forming agents (e.g. methylcellulose, psyllium hydrophilic mucilloid, calcium polycarbophil) *to absorb water in bowel and produce a soft, formed stool* 　　c. antibiotics *to treat bacterial overgrowth.* e. Consult physician if diarrhea persists or worsens.

11. NURSING DIAGNOSIS

Bowel incontinence related to loss of anal sphincter control associated with autonomic neuropathy.

DESIRED OUTCOMES	NURSING ACTIONS AND *SELECTED RATIONALES*
11. The client will maintain optimal bowel control as evidenced by absence of or decreased episodes of incontinence.	11.a. Assess for incontinence of stool. b. Implement measures *to reduce risk of bowel incontinence:* 　1. instruct client to perform perineal exercises (e.g. relaxing and tightening perineal and gluteal muscles) regularly *in order to strengthen the anal sphincter* 　2. have commode or bedpan readily available to client 　3. with client, establish a routine time for defecation; try to schedule it 20–30 minutes after a meal *in order to take advantage of gastrocolic reflex* 　4. perform actions to control diarrhea (see Nursing Diagnosis 10, action d). c. If bowel incontinence persists: 　1. consult physician about the use of a rectal tube or perianal pouch if client is experiencing constant drainage of liquid stool 　2. provide client with absorbent undergarments (e.g. Attends) 　3. provide emotional support to client and significant others.

12. NURSING DIAGNOSIS

Potential for infection related to:

a. high glucose levels that create a good medium for bacterial or fungal growth;
b. depression of leukocyte function associated with hyperglycemia;
c. delayed healing of any break in the skin;
d. malnutrition.

DESIRED OUTCOMES	NURSING ACTIONS AND *SELECTED RATIONALES*

12. The client will remain free of infection as evidenced by:
a. absence of chills and fever
b. pulse within normal limits
c. normal breath sounds
d. absence of any unusual vaginal discharge
e. voiding clear, yellow urine without complaints of frequency, urgency, and burning
f. absence of redness, swelling, and unusual drainage in any area where there is a break in skin integrity
g. absence of red, raised, painful lesion (furuncle) in any area
h. intact oral mucous membrane
i. WBC and differential counts within normal range
j. negative results of cultured specimens.

12.a. Assess for and report signs and symptoms of infection:
  1. elevated temperature
  2. chills
  3. pattern of increased pulse or pulse rate greater than 100 beats/minute
  4. adventitious breath sounds
  5. unusual vaginal discharge and pruritus in vulvovaginal area
  6. cloudy or foul-smelling urine
  7. complaints of frequency, urgency, or burning when urinating
  8. presence of WBCs, bacteria, and/or nitrites in urine
  9. redness, swelling, or unusual drainage in any area where there is a break in skin integrity
  10. red, raised, painful lesion (furuncle) in any area
  11. irritation or ulceration of oral mucous membrane
  12. elevated WBC count and/or significant change in differential.
b. Obtain culture specimens (e.g. urine, vaginal, mouth, sputum, blood) as ordered. Report positive results.
c. Implement measures *to reduce risk of infection:*
  1. maintain a fluid intake of at least 2500 cc/day unless contraindicated
  2. perform actions to maintain an optimal nutritional status and a near-normal blood glucose level (see Nursing Diagnosis 4, action f)
  3. instruct and assist client with good oral hygiene
  4. use good handwashing technique and encourage client to do the same
  5. maintain meticulous aseptic technique during all invasive procedures (e.g. catheterizations, venous and arterial punctures, injections)
  6. protect client from others with infection
  7. perform actions to prevent and treat skin breakdown (see Nursing Diagnosis 7, actions a.2–6)
  8. perform actions *to prevent infection in any existing wound:*
    a. implement measures to promote normal wound healing (see Nursing Diagnosis 7, action b.2)
    b. instruct client to avoid touching dressings or open wounds
    c. maintain meticulous aseptic technique during all dressing changes and wound care
    d. monitor for therapeutic and nontherapeutic effects of anti-infectives if administered prophylactically
  9. provide proper balance of exercise and rest
  10. perform actions *to prevent respiratory tract infection:*
    a. instruct and assist client to turn, cough, and deep breathe at least every 2 hours while mobility is limited
    b. instruct and assist client in use of inspiratory exerciser at least every 2 hours if indicated
    c. encourage client to stop smoking
    d. increase activity as allowed and tolerated
  11. perform actions *to prevent urinary tract infection:*
    a. instruct and assist female client to wipe from front to back after urination and defecation
    b. keep perianal area clean

UNIT XIV

      c. implement measures to prevent urinary retention (see Care Plan on Immobility, Nursing Diagnosis 10, action d) *in order to prevent stasis of urine, which provides an ideal medium for bacterial growth*

    12. assist female client to maintain meticulous perineal care *in order to reduce risk of vaginal infection.*

  d. If signs and symptoms of infection occur:

    1. assess for and immediately report any local signs of gangrene (e.g. severe pain and tenderness; skin color changes progressing from white to bronze, brown, or black; crepitus in surrounding tissues; drainage of frothy fluid with a foul or sweet odor) if infection occurs in an extremity

    2. monitor for therapeutic and nontherapeutic effects of anti-infectives if administered.

---

13. NURSING DIAGNOSIS

Potential for trauma related to:

a. falls associated with:
1. gait abnormalities, inability to perceive position or movement of a body part, and diminished or absent reflexes resulting from motor and sensory neuropathies
2. muscle weakness and atrophy resulting from peripheral neuropathy
3. dizziness and syncope resulting from orthostatic hypotension (due to neuropathy of the autonomic nervous system, decreased activity, and hypovolemia)
4. visual disturbances;

b. burns associated with paresthesias that occur with sensory neuropathy;

c. cuts associated with visual disturbances and inability to perceive position of a body part (results from neuropathy of proprioceptive fibers).

DESIRED OUTCOMES	NURSING ACTIONS AND *SELECTED RATIONALES*

13. The client will not experience falls, burns, or cuts.	13.a. Determine whether conditions predisposing the client to falls, burns, or cuts exist:
	 1. gait disturbances
	 2. diminished or absent reflexes
	 3. muscle weakness or atrophy in lower extremities
	 4. decreased sensation in extremities
	 5. episodes of dizziness or syncope
	 6. visual disturbances.
	 b. Implement measures *to prevent falls:*
	 1. keep bed in low position with side rails up when client is in bed
	 2. keep needed items within easy reach
	 3. encourage client to request assistance whenever needed; have call signal within easy reach
	 4. instruct and assist client to change positions slowly *in order to prevent dizziness and syncope associated with orthostatic hypotension*
	 5. use lap belt when client is in chair if indicated
	 6. instruct client to wear shoes with nonskid soles and low heels when ambulating
	 7. if vision is impaired:
	   a. orient client to surroundings, room, and arrangement of furniture
	   b. assist client with ambulation by walking a half step ahead of client and describing approaching objects or obstacles; instruct client to grasp back of nurse's arm during ambulation

8. avoid unnecessary clutter in room
9. accompany client during ambulation utilizing a transfer safety belt if indicated
10. provide ambulatory aids (e.g. walker, cane) if client is weak or unsteady on feet
11. instruct client to ambulate in well-lit areas and to utilize handrails if needed
12. do not rush client; allow adequate time for trips to the bathroom and ambulation in hallway.

  c. Implement measures *to prevent burns:*
1. let hot foods and fluids cool slightly before serving *to reduce risk of burns if spills occur*
2. supervise client while smoking if indicated
3. assess temperature of bath water and heating pad before and during use
4. warn client not to touch test tube if testing urine using reagent tablets such as Clinitest *(the test tube gets hot from the chemical reaction).*

  d. Assist client with tasks that require fine motor skills (e.g. shaving) *in order to prevent cuts.*
  e. Include client and significant others in planning and implementing measures to prevent injury.
  f. If injury does occur, initiate appropriate first aid measures and notify physician.

14.A. COLLABORATIVE DIAGNOSIS

Potential acute metabolic complications:

1. **diabetic ketoacidosis** related to an acute insulin deficiency and the resultant hyperglycemia and ketosis associated with administration of an inadequate amount of insulin, excessive food intake, significant decrease in activity, and stress;
2. **hypoglycemia (insulin shock)** related to an oversupply of insulin for the available glucose associated with too little food intake, administration of too much insulin or oral hypoglycemic agent, and excessive exercise;
3. **hyperglycemic, hyperosmolar, nonketotic coma (HHNK)** related to a relative insulin deficiency and the resultant hyperglycemia and osmotic diuresis;
4. **Somogyi phenomenon** related to the body's compensatory response to hypoglycemia (occurs when a higher dose of insulin than needed causes hypoglycemia, which results in the release of glucagon and catecholamines; these hormones then promote gluconeogenesis and glycogenolysis, which leads to a state of hyperglycemia).

DESIRED OUTCOMES	NURSING ACTIONS AND *SELECTED RATIONALES*

UNIT XIV

14.A.1. The client will not experience ketoacidosis as evidenced by:
  a. unlabored respirations at 16–20/minute
  b. absence of fruity odor on breath, nausea, vomiting, abdominal pain, extreme weakness, soft eyeballs

14.A.1.a. Assess for signs and symptoms of the following conditions that may indicate impending ketoacidosis:
1. hyperglycemia (e.g. polyuria; polydipsia; polyphagia; dimmed, blurred vision; fasting blood sugar greater than 140 mg/dl)
2. fluid volume deficit (see Nursing Diagnosis 3, action a.1, for signs and symptoms).

  b. Assess for and report signs and symptoms of ketoacidosis:
1. Kussmaul respirations accompanied by a fruity odor on breath
2. nausea, vomiting, abdominal pain
3. extreme weakness
4. soft eyeballs

c. usual skin color and temperature
d. usual mental status
e. stable B/P
f. urine output at least 30 cc/hour
g. blood glucose less than 300 mg/dl
h. absence of ketones in serum and urine
i. anion gap less than 16 mEq/liter
j. blood gases within normal range.

5. warm, flushed, dry skin
6. confusion, lethargy, stupor
7. hypotension
8. urine output less than 30 cc/hour
9. blood glucose above 300 mg/dl
10. presence of serum and urine ketones
11. anion gap greater than 16 mEq/liter
12. low serum pH and CO_2 content.

c. Implement measures *to prevent ketoacidosis:*
   1. perform actions to prevent or treat hyperglycemia (see Nursing Diagnosis 3, action a.2.c)
   2. initiate a thorough teaching plan regarding prevention and early recognition of ketoacidosis (see Nursing Diagnosis 20, action i.3).
d. If signs and symptoms of ketoacidosis occur:
   1. maintain client on bedrest
   2. monitor for therapeutic and nontherapeutic effects of the following if administered:
      a. insulin (usually an intravenous bolus of regular insulin is administered followed by a low-dose continuous infusion)
      b. intravenous fluid and electrolyte replacements:
         1. isotonic or half-strength normal saline (usually rapidly infused until B/P is stabilized and urine output is adequate)
         2. combination saline and glucose solutions once blood sugar falls to 250–300 mg/dl *to prevent hypoglycemia from the rapid drop in blood sugar*
         3. potassium chloride once urine output is at least 30 cc/hour *(hypokalemia results from osmotic diuresis and a shift of extracellular potassium into the cells during insulin therapy and treatment of acidosis)*
         4. potassium phosphate if serum phosphorus levels are low *(insulin shifts phosphorus into the cells, resulting in low serum phosphorus)*
         5. sodium bicarbonate if the serum pH drops below 7.1
      c. vasopressors and/or volume expanders *to maintain mean arterial pressure if hypotension is unresponsive to intravenous fluid replacement*
   3. assess for and report significant worsening of vital signs, mental status, blood glucose, serum electrolytes, blood gases, and EKG readings
   4. provide emotional support to client and significant others.

14.A.2. The client will not experience hypoglycemia as evidenced by:
a. pulse rate between 60–100 beats/minute
b. absence of palpitations
c. warm, dry skin
d. usual mental status
e. absence of slurred speech, incoordination, mood swings
f. blood glucose above 50 mg/dl.

14.A.2.a. Assess for and report signs and symptoms of hypoglycemia (clients at greatest risk are insulin-dependent diabetics, those having adjustments in insulin dosages or having difficulty maintaining an adequate oral intake, and clients with liver disease or end-stage renal failure):
   1. tachycardia; palpitations; cool, clammy skin; diaphoresis; nervousness; tremors *(these signs and symptoms reflect increased sympathetic nervous system activity);* caregivers, clients, and significant others should be aware that early sympathetic warning symptoms may not be present in some clients *because of a decreased glucagon and epinephrine output that may occur with Type I diabetes;* early warning symptoms may also be diminished if client is taking a beta-adrenergic blocking agent
   2. lethargy, inability to concentrate, slurred speech, incoordination, numbness of the tongue and lips, mood swings, visual changes *(these signs and symptoms reflect lack of glucose in the cerebrum)*
   3. nightmares, crying out in sleep, sleepwalking
   4. blood glucose below 50 mg/dl (be aware that hypoglycemic reactions can also occur with normal or above-normal blood glucose values if the glucose has decreased rapidly).
b. Implement measures *to prevent hypoglycemia:*
   1. administer insulin as ordered being careful to inject it into an area that has adequate subcutaneous tissue and is free from atrophy
   2. perform actions *to ensure that client has adequate caloric intake:*
      a. provide meals within 1 hour after administering a rapid-acting insulin (especially routine morning doses)

b. provide protein snacks in midafternoon and at bedtime if client is receiving an intermediate or long-acting insulin

c. consult dietician about appropriate supplements if client does not eat all of the meals and snacks provided

3. consult physician about altering prescribed insulin dose and/or providing alternative forms of intake (e.g. parenteral nutrition) if client is to receive nothing by mouth in preparation for diagnostic tests or is unable to maintain an adequate oral intake

4. maintain activity at a fairly constant level.

c. If signs and symptoms of hypoglycemia occur:

1. administer a rapid-acting source of carbohydrate:

a. if client is able to swallow, give him/her 10–12 gm of simple carbohydrate (e.g. 4 oz of orange juice, regular soft drink, or apple juice; 2 teaspoons of honey or Karo syrup; 2 lumps of sugar; 5–6 Lifesavers) or glucose tablets or paste (e.g. Glutose, Monogel); repeat in 15 minutes if still symptomatic

b. if client is unresponsive or unable to swallow, follow hospital protocol or physician's order and administer the following:

1. subcutaneous or intramuscular glucagon

2. subcutaneous epinephrine

3. intravenous 50% glucose solution

4. additional glucose (10–20 gm of a simple carbohydrate) once client is alert and able to swallow

2. once hypoglycemia is controlled, give client a complex carbohydrate and protein supplement (e.g. crackers and cheese or glass of skim milk)

3. provide emotional support to client and significant others.

14.A.3. The client will not experience HHNK as evidenced by:

a. absence of signs and symptoms of fluid volume deficit (see Nursing Diagnosis 3, outcome a, for outcome criteria)

b. absence of motor and sensory deficits and seizure activity

c. blood glucose less than 600 mg/dl.

14.A.3.a. Assess for and report signs and symptoms of HHNK (clients at greatest risk are persons over 50 years of age; noninsulin-dependent diabetics; clients with inadequate fluid intake; those who are under unusual emotional or physical stress [e.g. acute illness, infection, surgery]; and clients receiving corticosteroids, thiazide diuretics, phenytoin, hyperalimentation, or dialysis treatments):

1. severe fluid volume deficit (see Nursing Diagnosis 3, action a.1, for signs and symptoms)

2. extremely high serum osmolality (usually above 340 mOsm/liter)

3. neurological signs such as hemiparesis, aphasia, lethargy, confusion, and seizures

4. blood glucose above 600 mg/dl with absent or only slight elevation of ketones in urine or serum.

b. Implement measures *to prevent HHNK:*

1. perform actions to prevent and treat hyperglycemia (see Nursing Diagnosis 3, action a.2.c)

2. notify physician if client is unable to take in an adequate amount of oral fluids or if he/she is experiencing diarrhea or unusual emotional stress.

c. If signs and symptoms of HHNK occur:

1. monitor for therapeutic and nontherapeutic effects of the following if administered:

a. fluid replacement (isotonic or half-strength saline is infused rapidly until B/P is stabilized and urine output is adequate; once blood sugar falls to 250–300 mg/dl, 5% glucose is added)

b. insulin (usually an intravenous bolus of regular insulin is administered followed by a low-dose continuous infusion)

c. intravenous potassium chloride or phosphate *(hypokalemia and hypophosphatemia result from osmotic diuresis and a shift of both into the cells during insulin therapy)*

2. provide emotional support to client and significant others.

14.A.4. The client will not experience the Somogyi phenomenon as evidenced by:

a. blood glucose within

14.A.4.a. Assess for and report the following indications of the Somogyi phenomenon:

1. signs and symptoms of hypoglycemia at night, which may only be evidenced as nightmares, night sweats, and a headache upon awakening

desirable range (60–140 mg/dl) at all times
b. absence of signs and symptoms of hypoglycemia or hyperglycemia (see outcomes 1 and 2 in this diagnosis for outcome criteria).

2. signs and symptoms of hyperglycemia in the morning (see action 1.a.1 in this diagnosis)
3. urine and blood glucose values indicating a pattern of hypoglycemia at night and hyperglycemia in the morning.
b. Ensure that client eats 100% of meals and snacks *in order to reduce risk of the Somogyi phenomenon.*
c. If Somogyi phenomenon occurs:
   1. consult dietician about additional protein in bedtime snack
   2. consult physician about changes in insulin dosage and schedule (the usual treatment is to reduce the total insulin dosage or divide a once-daily dose into more frequent doses).

14.B. COLLABORATIVE DIAGNOSIS

Potential complication: thromboembolism related to:

1. hypercoagulability associated with an increased platelet adhesiveness and aggregation present in diabetes;
2. venous stasis associated with decreased mobility and vascular changes present with diabetes.

DESIRED OUTCOMES	NURSING ACTIONS AND *SELECTED RATIONALES*
14.B. The client will not develop a venous thrombus or pulmonary embolism (see Care Plan on Immobility, Collaborative Diagnosis 14, outcomes a.1 and 2 for outcome criteria).	14.B. Refer to Care Plan on Immobility, Collaborative Diagnosis 14, actions a.1 and 2, for measures related to assessment, prevention, and treatment of a venous thrombus and pulmonary embolism.

15. NURSING DIAGNOSIS

Sexual dysfunction:

a. **impotence** related to neuropathy of the sacral parasympathetic nerves that stimulate erection and decreased penile blood flow associated with vascular changes that occur;
b. **decreased libido** related to depression, fear of incontinence during sexual activity, and an altered self-concept.

DESIRED OUTCOMES	NURSING ACTIONS AND *SELECTED RATIONALES*
15. The client will demonstrate beginning acceptance of changes in sexual functioning (see Care Plan on Immobility, Nursing Diagnosis 15, for outcome criteria).	15.a. Refer to Care Plan on Immobility, Nursing Diagnosis 15, for measures related to assessment and management of sexual dysfunction. b. Implement additional measures *to promote optimal sexual functioning:* 1. inform client that sexual dysfunction related to diabetes may be partially reversed in some persons once the diabetes is under better control 2. perform actions to improve self-concept (see Nursing Diagnosis 16)

3. if impotence is a problem, encourage client to discuss the possibility of a penile prosthesis with physician
4. if incontinence is a concern:
   a. reinforce the importance of performing perineal exercises *to improve sphincter control*
   b. encourage client to void and/or defecate just before sexual activity.

---

16. NURSING DIAGNOSIS

Disturbance in self-concept* related to:

a. urinary and/or bowel incontinence;
b. changes in sexual functioning;
c. infertility (may occur in males as a result of retrograde ejaculation associated with pelvic autonomic neuropathy);
d. further changes in body functioning (e.g. progression of visual disturbances, sensory and motor deficits);
e. increasing dependence on others to meet self-care needs;
f. changes in life style imposed by diabetes and its treatment;
g. stigma of having a chronic illness.

---

* This diagnostic label includes the nursing diagnoses of body image disturbance and self-esteem disturbance.

DESIRED OUTCOMES	NURSING ACTIONS AND *SELECTED RATIONALES*
16. The client will demonstrate beginning adaptation to changes in body functioning, level of independence, life style, and roles (see Care Plan on Immobility, Nursing Diagnosis 16, for outcome criteria).	16.a. Refer to Care Plan on Immobility, Nursing Diagnosis 16, for measures related to assessment and promotion of a positive self-concept. b. Implement additional measures *to assist client to adapt to changes in body functioning, level of independence, life style, and roles:* 　1. encourage maximum participation in self-care and encourage significant others to allow client to do what he/she is able *so that independence can be re-established and/or self-esteem redeveloped* 　2. if client is unable to impregnate partner, discuss possibility of fertility studies and options for becoming a parent (e.g. adoption) 　3. perform actions to promote optimal sexual functioning (see Nursing Diagnosis 15) 　4. perform actions to prevent and manage urinary and bowel incontinence (see Nursing Diagnoses 8, actions b.2 and 3 and 11, actions b and c) 　5. if incontinence is not well controlled, instruct client in ways to minimize the problem *so that socialization is possible* (e.g. wear an external catheter with leg collection device, place waterproof disposable liners in underwear) 　6. initiate and reinforce the discharge teaching outlined in Nursing Diagnosis 20 *in order to promote a sense of control and self-reliance.*

UNIT
XIV

---

17. NURSING DIAGNOSIS

Ineffective individual coping related to fear of complications and ability to manage them; discomfort; need to alter life style; knowledge that condition is chronic and will require lifelong medical supervision, dietary regulation, and medication therapy; and an inadequate support system.

DESIRED OUTCOMES	NURSING ACTIONS AND *SELECTED RATIONALES*

17. The client will demonstrate the use of effective coping skills as evidenced by:
    a. willingness to participate in treatment plan and self-care activities
    b. verbalization of ability to cope with diabetes and its management
    c. identification of stressors
    d. utilization of appropriate problem-solving techniques
    e. recognition and utilization of available support systems.

17.a. Assess effectiveness of client's coping strategies by observing behavior and noting strengths, weaknesses, ability to express feelings and concerns, and willingness to participate in the treatment plan.
   b. Assess for and report signs and symptoms that may indicate ineffective coping (e.g. sleep disturbances, increasing fatigue, difficulty concentrating, irritability, decreased tolerance of discomfort, verbalization of inability to cope, inability to problem-solve).
   c. Allow time for client to adjust psychologically to planned treatment and anticipated life-style and role changes.
   d. Implement measures *to promote effective coping:*
      1. arrange for a visit with another person of same sex and similar age who has successfully adjusted to diabetes
      2. perform actions to reduce fear and anxiety (see Nursing Diagnosis 1)
      3. include client in planning of care, encourage maximum participation in treatment plan, and allow choices when possible *to enable him/her to maintain a sense of control*
      4. assist client to maintain usual daily routines whenever possible
      5. perform actions to reduce discomfort (see Nursing Diagnoses 5.A, action 5; 5.B, action 3; and 5.C, action 2)
      6. instruct client in effective problem-solving techniques (e.g. identification of stressors, determination of various options to solve problems)
      7. initiate and reinforce the discharge teaching outlined in Nursing Diagnosis 20 *in order to assist client to develop adaptive strategies before a crisis occurs and promote a sense of control and self-reliance*
      8. assist client as he/she starts to plan for necessary life-style and role changes after discharge; provide input on realistic prioritization of problems that need to be dealt with
      9. assist client and significant others to identify ways that personal and family goals can be adjusted rather than abandoned
      10. assist client to identify and utilize available support systems; provide information regarding available community resources that can assist client in coping with effects of diabetes (e.g. counseling services, diabetic education classes, diabetes support groups).
   e. Encourage client to share with significant others the kind of support that would be most beneficial (e.g. listening, inspiring hope, providing reassurance and accurate information).
   f. Encourage continued emotional support from significant others.
   g. Assess for and support behaviors suggesting positive adaptation to changes experienced (e.g. active participation in the treatment plan, verbalization of plans for altering life style).
   h. Consult physician about psychological counseling if appropriate. Initiate a referral if necessary.

☐ ▬▬▬▬▬▬▬▬▬▬▬▬▬▬▬▬▬▬▬▬▬▬▬

18. NURSING DIAGNOSIS

Grieving* related to changes in life style, progressive changes in or loss of normal body functioning, and uncertainty of future disabilities and losses associated with diabetes.

---

* This diagnostic label includes anticipatory grieving and grieving following the actual losses/changes.

☐ ▬▬▬▬▬▬▬▬▬▬▬▬▬▬▬▬▬▬▬▬▬▬▬

DESIRED OUTCOMES	NURSING ACTIONS AND *SELECTED RATIONALES*

18. The client will demonstrate beginning progression

18.a. Determine client's perception of the impact of diabetes on his/her future.
   b. Determine how client usually expresses grief.

through the grieving process as evidenced by:
a. verbalization of feelings about diabetes and its effect on life style
b. expression of grief
c. participation in treatment plan and self-care activities
d. utilization of available support systems
e. verbalization of a plan for integrating prescribed treatments into life style.

c. Observe for signs of grieving (e.g. changes in eating habits, insomnia, anger, noncompliance, denial).
d. Implement measures *to facilitate the grieving process:*
 1. assist client to acknowledge the changes/losses experienced *so grief work can begin;* assess for factors that may hinder or facilitate acknowledgment
 2. discuss the grieving process and assist client to accept the stages of grieving as an expected response to the actual and/or anticipated changes/losses; explain that grieving may recur *because of the chronicity of the condition*
 3. allow time for client to progress through the stages of grieving (denial, anger, bargaining, depression, acceptance [Kübler-Ross, 1969]); be aware that not every stage is experienced or expressed by all individuals and that the denial stage may be prolonged in many persons *because there are few, if any, visible physical changes*
 4. provide an atmosphere of care and concern (e.g. provide privacy, be available and nonjudgmental, display empathy and respect) *so that client will feel free to verbalize both positive and negative feelings and concerns*
 5. perform actions *to promote trust* (e.g. answer questions honestly, provide requested information)
 6. encourage the expression of anger and sadness about the actual and/or anticipated changes/losses
 7. encourage client to express his/her feelings in whatever ways are comfortable (e.g. writing, drawing, conversation)
 8. perform actions to facilitate effective coping (see Nursing Diagnosis 17, action d)
 9. support realistic hope regarding client's ability to live a useful, productive life and maintain some control over development of complications.
e. Assess for and support behaviors suggesting successful resolution of grief (e.g. verbalizing feelings about changes, expressing sorrow, focusing on ways to adapt to changes and losses).
f. Explain the stages of the grieving process to significant others. Encourage their support and understanding.
g. Provide information about counseling services and support groups that might assist client in working through grief.
h. Arrange for a visit from clergy if desired by client.
i. Monitor for therapeutic and nontherapeutic effects of antidepressants if administered.
j. Consult physician about referral for counseling if signs of dysfunctional grieving (e.g. persistent denial of losses or changes, excessive anger or sadness, hysteria, suicidal behaviors, phobias) occur.

19. NURSING DIAGNOSIS

Noncompliance* related to:

a. lack of understanding of the implications of not following the prescribed treatment plan;
b. difficulty modifying personal habits and integrating necessary treatments and dietary regimen into life style;
c. insufficient financial resources;
d. dysfunctional grieving.

---

* This diagnostic label includes both an informed decision by client not to comply and an inability to comply due to circumstances beyond the client's control.

DESIRED OUTCOMES	NURSING ACTIONS AND *SELECTED RATIONALES*

19. The client will demonstrate the probability of future compliance with the prescribed treatment plan as evidenced by:
   a. willingness to learn about and participate in treatments and care
   b. statements reflecting ways to modify personal habits and integrate treatments into life style
   c. statements reflecting an understanding of the implications of not following the prescribed treatment plan.

19.a. Assess for indications that client may be unwilling or unable to comply with prescribed treatment plan:
   1. statements reflecting that he/she was unable to manage care at home
   2. failure to adhere to treatment plan while in hospital (e.g. refusing medications, not adhering to dietary restrictions)
   3. statements reflecting a lack of understanding of factors that contribute to acute and chronic complications
   4. statements reflecting an unwillingness or inability to modify personal habits and integrate necessary treatments into life style
   5. statements reflecting the view that diabetes is curable or that the situation is hopeless and that efforts to comply with treatments are useless.
   b. Implement measures *to improve client compliance:*
   1. explain diabetes in terms the client can understand; stress the fact that diabetes is a chronic condition and adherence to the treatment plan is necessary *in order to delay and/or prevent complications;* caution client that some complications may occur despite strict adherence to treatment plan
   2. encourage questions and clarify any misconceptions client has about diabetes and its effects
   3. encourage client to participate in assessments and treatments (e.g. blood glucose monitoring, selection of diet, insulin administration)
   4. provide instructions on drawing up and administering insulin, testing blood for glucose and urine for glucose and ketones, and menu selection; allow time for practice and return demonstration; determine areas of difficulty and misunderstanding and reinforce teaching as necessary
   5. provide client with written instructions about future appointments with health care provider, diet, medications, activity level, and signs and symptoms to report
   6. assist client to identify ways he/she can incorporate treatments into life style; focus on modifications of life style rather than complete change
   7. encourage client to discuss his/her concerns about the cost of medications, food, and supplies; obtain a social service consult to assist client with financial planning and obtain financial aid if indicated
   8. perform actions to promote effective coping and facilitate grieving (see Nursing Diagnoses 17, action d and 18, action d)
   9. initiate and reinforce the discharge teaching outlined in Nursing Diagnosis 20 *in order to promote a sense of control and self-reliance*
   10. encourage client to attend follow-up diabetic education classes
   11. provide information about and encourage utilization of community resources and information sources that can assist client to make necessary life-style changes (e.g. diabetes support groups, counseling services, American Diabetes Association, diabetic cookbooks, publications such as Forecast and Diabetes in the News).
   c. Assess for and reinforce behaviors suggesting future compliance with prescribed treatments (e.g. participation in the treatment plan, statements reflecting plans for integrating treatments into life style).
   d. Include significant others in explanations and teaching sessions and encourage their support.
   e. Reinforce the need for client to assume responsibility for managing as much care as possible.
   f. Consult physician about referrals to community health agencies if continued instruction or supervision is needed.

20. NURSING DIAGNOSIS

Knowledge deficit regarding follow-up care.

DESIRED OUTCOMES	NURSING ACTIONS AND *SELECTED RATIONALES*

20.a. The client will verbalize a basic understanding of the pathophysiology of diabetes mellitus.

20.a. Explain the basic pathophysiology of diabetes mellitus in terms the client can understand. Have client paraphrase the explanation *in order to validate his/her understanding.*

20.b. The client will verbalize an understanding of medication therapy including rationale for, side effects of, schedule for taking, and importance of taking as prescribed.

20.b.1. Explain the rationale for, side effects of, and importance of taking medications prescribed.

2. Provide the following instructions if client is to administer own insulin injections after discharge:
   a. store the bottle(s) of insulin currently being used at room temperature unless the room temperature is above 75°F
   b. store unopened bottle(s) of insulin in refrigerator
   c. periodically check expiration date and discard outdated bottle(s) of insulin
   d. do not use insulin that has changed color or contains granules or clumped particles
   e. do not administer cold insulin
   f. rotate injection sites using the following guidelines:
      1. no site should be used more than once a month
      2. there should be at least 2.5 cm (1 inch) between sites
      3. avoid giving injections right at the waistline or within 2.5 cm (1 inch) of the umbilicus
      4. rotate injection sites within an area until the whole area has been used, then move on to a new area
      5. avoid using an area that will be heavily exercised that day *(causes more rapid absorption of insulin from that area)*
      6. do not give injections into areas where the skin appears raised, thickened, or wasted
   g. sterilize reusable glass syringes at least once a week by placing syringe and plunger in boiling water for 15 minutes; store in a sterile container or soak in alcohol between injections
   h. plan meals and snacks keeping the onset, peak action, and length of action of the insulin(s) prescribed in mind
   i. adjust insulin dosage according to blood sugar results (some physicians may not allow clients this degree of independence)
   j. consult health care provider immediately if unable to tolerate food and fluid for 4 hours
   k. if itching, redness, and tenderness appear after injections, allow area to dry more completely after cleaning with alcohol; if problem persists, consult health care provider
   l. always have rapid-acting carbohydrate readily available (e.g. glucose tablets, hard candy, sugar lumps, commercial preparations such as Glutose or Monojel) and take when initial symptoms of hypoglycemia occur; if symptoms do not subside after taking a rapid-acting carbohydrate 2–3 times within 30 minutes, contact health care provider immediately
   m. consult health care provider if repeated episodes of sweating, irritability, weakness, hunger, shakiness, slurred speech, incoordination, and drowsiness occur *(may indicate need to reduce insulin dose)*
   n. consult health care provider if experiencing unusual emotional or physical stress (e.g. acute illness, physical trauma, pregnancy) *so that insulin dose can be increased to provide adequate coverage.*

3. If client is discharged with a button infuser or an insulin pump device, provide instructions regarding its management (e.g. changing the subcutaneous needle every 1–3 days, filling syringes, changing batteries in pump). Allow time for practice and return demonstration.

4. If client is discharged on an oral hypoglycemic agent, instruct to:
   a. take medication exactly as prescribed (the once-daily dose should be taken before breakfast and divided doses should be taken before meals)
   b. report if unable to tolerate food and fluid
   c. limit alcohol intake to small amounts and be aware that an

       intolerance to alcohol as evidenced by nausea, vomiting, headache, sweating, weakness, and confusion sometimes develops when taking an oral hypoglycemic agent

    d. adhere strictly to the prescribed diet *(oral hypoglycemics are not a substitute for good dietary management)*

    e. consult health care provider if experiencing unusual emotional or physical stress (e.g. acute illness, physical injury) *so that dosage may be adjusted to provide adequate coverage.*

  5. Instruct client to consult health care provider before taking other prescription and nonprescription medications.

  6. Instruct client to inform all health care providers of medications being taken.

20.c. The client will demonstrate the ability to correctly draw up and administer insulin if prescribed.

20.c. If client is to be discharged on insulin, provide the following instructions regarding preparation and administration:

  1. mix insulin before use by gently rotating or rolling bottle between palms or palm and thigh; do not vigorously shake the bottle

  2. read the label carefully, making sure the syringe and insulin concentrations match and that it is the correct type of insulin (e.g. regular, NPH)

  3. clean the top of the bottle(s) with alcohol

  4. withdraw the correct amount of insulin

  5. if mixing two insulins, withdraw in the same order every time (usually recommended that the rapid-acting insulin be drawn up first *in order to reduce the risk of contaminating the vial of rapid-acting insulin with a longer-acting insulin)*

  6. insert needle into subcutaneous tissue or into the space between the fat and muscle, aspirate to make sure needle is not in a blood vessel, and inject insulin (the recommended technique for insulin administration may vary from institution to institution and should be reviewed before patient teaching)

  7. following insulin injection, apply gentle pressure to site rather than rubbing it.

20.d. The client will verbalize an understanding of the principles of dietary management and be able to calculate and plan meals within the prescribed caloric distribution.

20.d.1. Reinforce dietary instruction regarding the prescribed ADA diet and method of calculating the foods/fluids allowed (e.g. exchange list, glycemic index).

  2. Have client select sample menus before discharge *to ensure that he/she is able to calculate the diet correctly.*

  3. Explain the purpose of weight reduction if client has been placed on a reducing diet. Reinforce importance of avoiding "crash" or fad diets.

  4. Instruct client on appropriate dietary adjustments that should be made if meal schedule or activity level has been significantly altered.

  5. Reinforce the following principles of good dietary management:

    a. eat 3 or more regularly spaced meals each day and do not skip meals

    b. weigh or measure foods rather than estimating serving sizes

    c. avoid foods/fluids high in concentrated carbohydrate (e.g. sugar, candy, syrups, jams, jellies, cakes, pies, pastries, soft drinks, fruits packed in syrup) and saturated fat (e.g. butter, egg yolks, cheese, ice cream, organ meats)

    d. read processed food/fluid labels and avoid those foods/fluids that contain sugar, sorbitol, and mannitol

    e. incorporate any alcoholic beverages consumed into total calorie and carbohydrate restrictions.

20.e. The client will demonstrate the ability to correctly perform blood glucose and urine tests and accurately interpret results.

20.e.1. Teach client how to perform the following tests that may be utilized *to monitor effectiveness of measures being used to control diabetes:*

    a. tests to determine blood sugar using a lancet and skin puncturing device such as an Autolet or Autoclix with a glucose monitoring strip (e.g. Dextrostix, Chemstrip bG) and/or a machine that reads the color strip (e.g. Glucometer II, Accu-Chek bG, Glucoscan)

    b. tests to determine urine sugar (e.g. 2-drop Clinitest, Diastix, Clinistix, Tes-Tape)

    c. tests to detect ketone levels in the urine (e.g. Ketostix, Acetest).

2. Reinforce the following general instructions about urine testing if client will be doing urine testing following discharge:
   a. test urine before rather than after meals
   b. test second-voided specimen
   c. keep testing agents in a dry, airtight container
   d. avoid touching the pills or the reagent part of the testing strip
   e. keep a record of any medications being taken (*many medications such as salicylates, ascorbic acid, cephalosporins, L-dopa, probenecid, streptomycin, and those in a syrup base alter test results*).
3. Demonstrate the correct way to record urine and blood test results. Instruct client to keep a record of test results.
4. Have client demonstrate blood and urine tests *in order to assess his/her technique and accuracy in interpreting results*. Reinforce teaching as necessary.
5. Provide instructions on actions client should take when test results are abnormal (some clients are allowed to adjust insulin dose and dietary intake; others are instructed to notify appropriate health care provider).

20.f. The client will verbalize an understanding of the role of exercise in the management of diabetes.	20.f.1. Explain how exercise affects blood sugar levels. 2. Provide the following instructions about exercise: a. maintain a regular, daily exercise program b. exercise 1–3 hours after meals when blood sugar is higher c. avoid exercising during insulin peak action time d. adjust dietary intake if there are significant changes in activity level (insulin-dependent diabetics should eat a 10–15 gm carbohydrate snack before planned increases in activity) e. perform blood glucose tests more frequently during periods of significant variation in activity level f. remember that sexual intercourse is a form of exercise g. stop any activity that causes nausea, trembling, extreme breathlessness, chest pain, or throbbing headache h. do not engage in any unusually strenuous activities.

20.g. The client will identify health care and hygiene practices that should be integrated into life style.	20.g.1. Teach client the importance of adhering to the following health care practices:
	a. daily oral hygiene including brushing and flossing teeth
	b. regular dental appointments
	c. frequent eye examinations
	d. not smoking (*smoking contributes to the risk of cardiovascular complications*)
	e. meticulous care of cuts, burns, and scratches
	f. yearly influenza vaccinations.
	2. Provide instructions about foot care:
	a. inspect feet daily for cuts, redness, cracks, blisters, corns, and calluses; use a mirror to check bottoms of feet if necessary
	b. wash feet daily with a mild soap and warm water and dry gently but thoroughly
	c. apply lanolin or other lubricating lotion to feet (except between toes) daily
	d. keep feet dry by:
	  1. applying a mild powder
	  2. placing lamb's wool between toes
	  3. wearing clean, absorbent socks
	  4. avoiding shoes with rubber or plastic soles (*cause feet to sweat*)
	e. cut nails straight across
	f. see a podiatrist rather than using home remedies to manage corns, calluses, and ingrown nails
	g. avoid wearing socks, stockings, or garters that are tight and avoid sitting with legs crossed (*may further compromise peripheral blood flow*)
	h. buy shoes that fit well and break them in gradually
	i. wear shoes or slippers when walking *to protect feet from injury*
	j. do not use a heating pad or hot water bottle on feet (*if paresthesias are present, burns may occur*)
	k. protect feet from extreme cold *to prevent vasoconstriction and possible frostbite*.

UNIT XIV

20.h. The client will identify appropriate safety measures to follow because of the diagnosis of diabetes.

20.h. Teach client the following safety precautions:
1. always carry an identification card and wear a Medic-Alert tag
2. always carry a rapid-acting carbohydrate such as Lifesavers, sugar lumps, or glucose tablets
3. if insulin-dependent, always have insulin readily available (carry in purse or briefcase)
4. consult physician about plans for pregnancy and maintain close prenatal supervision
5. avoid home permanents or coloring of hair; inform hair stylist of diabetes if any chemicals will be used on hair *because of possible increased susceptibility to burns*
6. inform all health care providers of diabetic condition.

20.i. The client will state signs and symptoms of hypoglycemia and ketoacidosis and appropriate actions for prevention and treatment.

20.i.1. Teach client the following information about hypoglycemia:
a. factors that precipitate hypoglycemia (e.g. too much insulin or oral hypoglycemic agent, insufficient oral intake, excessive exercise, heavy alcohol intake)
b. signs and symptoms of hypoglycemia (e.g. shakiness, nervousness, weakness, hunger, sweating, drowsiness, unsteadiness, confusion)
c. actions to take if signs and symptoms of hypoglycemia occur:
  1. immediately take a rapid-acting carbohydrate (e.g. half a glass of fruit juice or regular soft drink, 2 teaspoons of honey or syrup, 2 lumps of sugar, 5–6 Lifesavers, glucose tablets, Glutose or Monojel)
  2. if symptoms persist, take the same amount of carbohydrate again every 15 minutes; consult health care provider if symptoms persist longer than 30 minutes
  3. after the hypoglycemic episode, consume a complex carbohydrate and protein snack (e.g. crackers and cheese or glass of skim milk).
2. Teach significant others how to prepare and administer glucagon in case client has lost consciousness.
3. Teach client the following information about ketoacidosis:
a. factors that precipitate ketoacidosis (e.g. emotional stress, infection, failure to take insulin or oral hypoglycemic agent, dietary excess)
b. signs and symptoms of ketoacidosis (e.g. unusual thirst; excessive urination; weakness; blurred vision; very warm, flushed skin; urine sugar higher than 1%; blood sugar higher than 300; ketones in urine; abdominal pain; nausea and vomiting)
c. immediate actions to take if signs and symptoms of ketoacidosis occur:
  1. drink a cup or more of broth or tea if able to tolerate it
  2. administer insulin (if previously instructed in insulin coverage based on blood or urine test results)
  3. consult health care provider.

20.j. The client will state signs and symptoms to report to the health care provider.

20.j. Instruct client to report the following:
1. unexplained episodes of hypoglycemia and ketoacidosis (see actions i.1.b and 3.b in this diagnosis for signs and symptoms)
2. great variations in blood or urine glucose results
3. frequent nightmares and headaches upon awakening
4. a cut, scratch, or burn that becomes red, swollen, tender, or does not start to heal within 24 hours
5. nausea and vomiting that lasts more than a few hours
6. temperature elevation that lasts more than 2 days
7. persistent cough especially if productive of green or rust-colored sputum
8. change in vision.

20.k. The client will identify community resources that can assist in the adjustment to and management of diabetes.

20.k.1. Provide information about community resources and information sources that can assist client and significant others in adjustment to and management of diabetes (e.g. American Diabetes Association, diabetic education classes, weight loss programs, diabetes support groups, stop smoking programs, counseling services, diabetic clinics, publications such as Forecast and Diabetes in the News).
2. Initiate a referral if indicated.

20.l. The client will verbalize an understanding of and a

20.l.1. Reinforce the importance of keeping follow-up appointments with health care provider and for laboratory studies.

plan for adhering to recommended follow-up care including future appointments with health care provider and for laboratory studies.

2. Refer to Nursing Diagnosis 19, action b, for measures to improve client compliance.

□ ▐██

Reference

Kübler-Ross, E. On death and dying. New York: Macmillan, 1969.

■ ■

Hypophysectomy

Hypophysectomy is the surgical removal of the pituitary gland. It is performed most commonly to remove adenomas that are causing signs and symptoms of hyperpituitarism, hypopituitarism, and/or visual deficits such as unilateral blindness or field cuts. The surgery may also be performed to halt the advance of diabetic retinopathy; remove a necrotic pituitary gland; or slow the metastasis and reduce bone pain associated with endocrine-dependent neoplasms of the breast, ovary, or prostate. The surgery can be performed using an intracranial approach (usually transfrontal) or, more frequently, a transsphenoidal approach. In the transsphenoidal approach, access to the sella turcica, the bony cavity that houses the pituitary gland, is obtained through the floor of the nose and sphenoid sinuses via an incision in the inner aspect of the upper lip and gingiva. In order to prevent cerebral spinal fluid leakage following surgery, the sella turcica is packed with a piece of muscle or fascia from the anterior thigh and/or pieces of bone and cartilage that were removed during surgery.

The nose is then packed with petrolatum gauze to control bleeding. Usually a portion of the pituitary gland is left intact and the client does not require lifelong hormone replacement therapy. If most or all of the gland is removed or nonfunctioning, lifelong replacement of adrenocorticotropic and thyrotropic hormones will be necessary.

This care plan focuses on the adult client hospitalized for removal of a benign adenoma of the pituitary gland via the transsphenoidal approach.* Preoperatively, goals of care are to reduce fear and anxiety, maintain comfort, and prevent injury associated with partial loss of vision if it has occurred. Postoperative goals of care are to manage visual impairments if present, maintain comfort, prevent complications, and educate the client regarding follow-up care.

---

* If an intracranial approach is planned, use in conjunction with the Care Plan on Intracranial Surgery.

UNIT
XIV

DISCHARGE CRITERIA

Prior to discharge, the client will:

- identify ways to promote healing of the operative site
- state signs and symptoms to report to the health care provider
- verbalize an understanding of and a plan for adhering to recommended follow-up care including future appointments with health care provider, activity level, medications prescribed, and wound care.

NURSING/COLLABORATIVE DIAGNOSES

Preoperative
1. Anxiety □ *828*
2. Pain: headache □ *829*
3. Sensory-perceptual alteration: visual □ *830*
Postoperative
1. Altered nutrition: less than body requirements □ *831*
2. Altered comfort:
    a. anterior thigh pain
    b. blockage of nasal passages
    c. headache □ *832*
3. Sensory-perceptual alteration: visual □ *832*
4. Altered oral mucous membrane: dryness □ *833*
5. Potential complications:
    a. meningitis
    b. diabetes insipidus
    c. adrenal crisis □ *833*
6. Knowledge deficit regarding follow-up care □ *835*

Preoperative

Use in conjunction with the Standardized Preoperative Care Plan.

1. NURSING DIAGNOSIS

Anxiety related to unfamiliar environment; lack of understanding of diagnostic tests and planned surgical procedure; effects of anesthesia; and anticipated postoperative discomfort and effects of surgery on appearance, vision, senses of smell and taste, hormone levels, and usual life style and roles.

DESIRED OUTCOMES	NURSING ACTIONS AND *SELECTED RATIONALES*

1. The client will experience a reduction in fear and anxiety (see Standardized Preoperative Care Plan, Nursing Diagnosis 1, for outcome criteria).	1.a. Refer to Standardized Preoperative Care Plan, Nursing Diagnosis 1, for measures related to assessment and reduction of fear and anxiety.
	 b. Implement additional measures *to reduce fear and anxiety:*
	 1. explain all diagnostic tests that may be performed:
	   a. magnetic resonance imaging (MRI) or computed tomography of the head
	   b. brain scan

   c. culture of nasopharyngeal secretions (transsphenoidal approach is contraindicated if reports indicate presence of infection)

   d. blood studies (e.g. electrolytes, hormone levels)

   e. visual field examinations

2. reinforce physician's explanations about the surgical procedure and assure client that there will be no external incision on head or removal of hair with a transsphenoidal approach

3. inform client that the periocular edema and ecchymosis that occur following the surgery usually diminish after 2 to 3 days

4. emphasize that visual disturbances that may occur after surgery are expected to resolve as inflammation subsides; if appropriate, reinforce the fact that existing visual disturbances are also expected to improve postoperatively

5. assure client that there is usually very little pain associated with the transsphenoidal approach

6. assure client that while nasal packing is in place after surgery, he/she will be able to breathe through mouth without difficulty

7. inform client that numbness of front teeth and gingiva is expected postoperatively and should subside over a few months

8. inform client that temporary loss of sense of smell and diminished sense of taste are expected postoperatively and should resolve within 2–3 weeks

9. reinforce physician's explanations regarding effects of surgery on hormone levels and replacement therapy:

   a. enough functioning pituitary usually remains following removal of a pituitary adenoma so that lifelong replacement therapy of thyroid, gonadotropic, adrenocorticotropic, and antidiuretic hormones is not necessary

   b. adrenocorticotropic hormone (ACTH) and corticosteroids will be given preoperatively and postoperatively on a temporary basis *to help the body adapt to the stress of surgery*

   c. hormone replacement therapy will be available if needed on a temporary or permanent basis; assure client that prior to discharge he/she will be well informed of signs and symptoms of hormone imbalances to watch for.

---

2. NURSING DIAGNOSIS

Pain: headache related to stretching or compression of the pain-sensitive dura and blood vessels associated with the expanding adenoma and inflammation of or around the pituitary gland.

DESIRED OUTCOMES	NURSING ACTIONS AND *SELECTED RATIONALES*

2. The client will obtain relief from headache as evidenced by:
a. verbalization of headache relief
b. relaxed facial expression and body positioning.
	2.a. Determine how client usually responds to pain.
	b. Assess for nonverbal signs of headache (e.g. reluctance to move head, wrinkled brow, clenched fists, squinting, rubbing head, avoidance of bright lights and noises).
	c. Assess verbal complaints of pain. Ask client to be specific about type, location, and severity of headache.
	d. Assess for factors that seem to aggravate and alleviate headache.
	e. Implement measures *to relieve headache:*
	  1. position client with head of bed elevated at least 30° *to improve venous return and relieve pressure on the dura*
	  2. perform actions *to minimize environmental stimuli* (e.g. provide a quiet environment, restrict visitors, dim lights)

3. avoid jarring bed or startling client *to minimize risk of sudden movements*
4. provide nonpharmacological measures for headache relief (e.g. cool cloth to forehead, backrub, distraction)
5. monitor for therapeutic and nontherapeutic effects of the following if administered:
   a. corticosteroids *to reduce inflammation*
   b. nonnarcotic analgesics or codeine (other narcotic analgesics are usually contraindicated *because they have a greater depressant effect on the central nervous system*).
   f. Consult physician if headache persists or worsens.

□ ▇▇▇▇▇▇▇▇▇▇▇▇▇▇▇▇▇▇▇▇▇▇▇▇▇▇▇▇▇▇▇▇

3. NURSING DIAGNOSIS

Sensory-perceptual alteration: visual related to pressure on the optic chiasm and optic nerve associated with the expanding adenoma and/or inflammation.

□ ▇▇▇▇▇▇▇▇▇▇▇▇▇▇▇▇▇▇▇▇▇▇▇▇▇▇▇▇▇▇▇▇

DESIRED OUTCOMES	NURSING ACTIONS AND *SELECTED RATIONALES*

3.a. The client will not experience falls as a result of visual impairment.	3.a.1. Assess for visual disturbances (e.g. partial or total blindness [usually of just one eye], bitemporal hemianopsia).
	2. Implement measures *to prevent falls associated with visual impairment:*
	  a. orient client to surroundings, room, and arrangement of furniture
	  b. keep bed in low position with side rails up when client is in bed
	  c. place call signal and desired personal articles within easy reach and assist client to identify their location
	  d. instruct client to ask for assistance as needed
	  e. instruct client to scan the environment *in order to compensate for visual field cuts or decreased vision in one eye*
	  f. assist with ambulation by walking a half step ahead of client and describing approaching objects or obstacles; instruct client to grasp back of nurse's arm during ambulation
	  g. avoid unnecessary clutter in room
	  h. provide adequate lighting in room.

3.b. The client will have basic needs met.	3.b.1. Assist client with personal hygiene he/she is unable to perform independently. 2. Identify where items are placed on his/her plate or tray, cut food, open packages, or feed client if necessary. 3. Assist with activities that require reading (e.g. menu selection, mail, legal documents). 4. Provide auditory rather than visual diversionary activities.

Postoperative

Use in conjunction with the Standardized Postoperative Care Plan.

1. NURSING DIAGNOSIS

Altered nutrition: less than body requirements related to:

a. decreased oral intake associated with:
1. anorexia resulting from discomfort, fatigue, loss of sense of smell, diminished sense of taste, and decreased activity
2. fear of disrupting oral cavity incision
3. dysphagia resulting from dry mouth
4. prescribed dietary modifications;
b. inadequate nutritional replacement therapy;
c. increased nutritional needs associated with increased metabolic rate that occurs during wound healing.

DESIRED OUTCOMES	NURSING ACTIONS AND *SELECTED RATIONALES*

1. The client will maintain an adequate nutritional status (see Standardized Postoperative Care Plan, Nursing Diagnosis 6, for outcome criteria).	1.a. Refer to Standardized Postoperative Care Plan, Nursing Diagnosis 6, for measures related to assessment and maintenance of an adequate nutritional status.
	 b. Implement additional measures *to improve oral intake and maintain an adequate nutritional status:*
	  1. perform actions to relieve headache and blockage of nasal passages (see Preoperative Nursing Diagnosis 2, action e and Postoperative Nursing Diagnosis 2, action b.1)
	  2. assure client that adherence to prescribed diet (will advance to soft diet as tolerated) will not disrupt the oral cavity incision
	  3. perform actions *to reduce dysphagia:*
	   a. implement measures to reduce dryness of oral mucous membrane (see Postoperative Nursing Diagnosis 4, actions a and b)
	   b. if dryness of oral mucous membrane persists:
	    1. avoid serving foods/fluids that are sticky (e.g. peanut butter, soft bread, bananas)
	    2. moisten dry foods with gravy or sauces (e.g. catsup, salad dressing, sour cream)
	  4. provide meals that are visually appealing *to help stimulate appetite*
	  5. experiment with different flavorings, seasonings, and textures
	  6. serve food warm *to stimulate sense of smell following removal of nasal packing.*

☐ ▊▊▊▊▊▊▊▊▊▊▊▊▊▊▊▊▊▊▊▊▊▊▊▊▊▊▊▊▊▊

2. NURSING DIAGNOSIS

Altered comfort:*

a. **anterior thigh pain** related to tissue trauma associated with removal of a small portion of muscle for repair of the surgical site;
b. **blockage of nasal passages** related to inflammation of the sphenoid sinuses and presence of nasal packing;
c. **headache** related to inflammation of and around the remaining pituitary gland.

---

* In this care plan, the nursing diagnosis "pain" is included under the diagnostic label of altered comfort.

☐ ▊▊▊▊▊▊▊▊▊▊▊▊▊▊▊▊▊▊▊▊▊▊▊▊▊▊▊▊▊▊

DESIRED OUTCOMES	NURSING ACTIONS AND *SELECTED RATIONALES*

2. The client will experience diminished discomfort as evidenced by:
  a. verbalization of diminished discomfort
  b. relaxed facial expression and body positioning
  c. increased participation in activities.
	2.a. Refer to Standardized Postoperative Care Plan, Nursing Diagnosis 7.A, for measures related to assessment and reduction of pain.
	  b. Implement additional measures *to reduce discomfort:*
	    1. perform actions *to relieve blockage of nasal passages:*
	      a. keep head of bed elevated at least 30° *to promote nasal drainage*
	      b. remove nasal packing as soon as allowed (usually 2–4 days after surgery)
	      c. monitor for therapeutic and nontherapeutic effects of decongestants if administered
	    2. perform actions to relieve headache (see Preoperative Nursing Diagnosis 2, action e).

☐ ▊▊▊▊▊▊▊▊▊▊▊▊▊▊▊▊▊▊▊▊▊▊▊▊▊▊▊▊▊▊

3. NURSING DIAGNOSIS

Sensory-perceptual alteration: visual related to:

a. periocular edema associated with pressure from head stabilization device used during surgery and inflammation of the surgical area;
b. pressure on the optic chiasm and optic nerve associated with inflammation of the surgical area.

☐ ▊▊▊▊▊▊▊▊▊▊▊▊▊▊▊▊▊▊▊▊▊▊▊▊▊▊▊▊▊▊

DESIRED OUTCOMES	NURSING ACTIONS AND *SELECTED RATIONALES*

3. The client will have gradual improvement of any visual disturbance as evidenced by:
  a. increased participation in activities
  b. verbalization of improved vision.
	3.a. Assess for visual disturbances (e.g. decreased ability to see due to edema of and around eyelids, partial or total blindness [usually in just one eye], bitemporal hemianopsia).
	  b. Implement measures *to improve vision:*
	    1. position client with head of bed elevated at least 30° *to reduce inflammation in the surgical area and periocular edema*
	    2. apply cold packs to periocular area for first 24–48 hours after surgery *in order to reduce periocular edema*
	    3. monitor for therapeutic and nontherapeutic effects of corticosteroids if administered *to reduce inflammation around the optic chiasm and optic nerve.*

c. If vision is impaired:
1. refer to Preoperative Nursing Diagnosis 3 for measures related to preventing falls and meeting client's self-care needs
2. consult physician if visual disturbances worsen or there is no improvement in vision as periocular edema subsides.

4. NURSING DIAGNOSIS

Altered oral mucous membrane: dryness related to:

a. mouth breathing associated with presence of nasal packing;
b. decreased salivation associated with food and oral fluid restrictions and some medications (e.g. anesthetic agents, narcotic analgesics).

DESIRED OUTCOMES	NURSING ACTIONS AND *SELECTED RATIONALES*
4. The client will maintain a moist, intact oral mucous membrane.	4.a. Refer to Standardized Postoperative Care Plan, Nursing Diagnosis 8, for measures related to assessment and reduction of dryness of the oral mucous membrane. b. Provide client with a mist mask or room humidifier if indicated *to further relieve dryness of the oral mucous membrane.* c. Consult physician if signs and symptoms of parotitis (e.g. swelling of the parotid glands, ear pain, difficulty swallowing, fever) occur.

5. COLLABORATIVE DIAGNOSIS

Potential complications:

a. **meningitis** related to infection associated with intraoperative or postoperative wound contamination;
b. **diabetes insipidus** related to decreased secretion of antidiuretic hormone (ADH) associated with inflammation of or trauma to the posterior pituitary gland;
c. **adrenal crisis** related to lack of adrenocorticotropic hormone (ACTH) associated with inflammation of or trauma to the anterior portion of the pituitary gland.

DESIRED OUTCOMES	NURSING ACTIONS AND *SELECTED RATIONALES*
5.a. The client will not develop meningitis as evidenced by: 1. absence of fever and chills 2. absence of nuchal rigidity and photophobia 3. gradual resolution of headache 4. negative Kernig's and Brudzinski's signs	5.a.1. Assess for and report signs and symptoms of a CSF leak: a. presence of glucose in nasal drainage as shown by positive Tes-Tape or Dextrostix results; be aware that any drainage containing blood will also test positive for glucose b. clear halo or watery, pale ring around bloody or serosanguineous drainage on nasal drip pad or pillowcase c. complaints of postnasal drip d. complaints of severe supraorbital headache *(may indicate CSF in sinuses)* e. constant swallowing.

UNIT
XIV

5. normal cerebral spinal fluid (CSF) analysis.

2. Assess for and report signs and symptoms of meningitis:
   a. fever, chills
   b. nuchal rigidity
   c. photophobia
   d. increasing or persistent headache
   e. positive Kernig's sign (inability to straighten knee when hip is flexed)
   f. positive Brudzinski's sign (flexion of hip and knee in response to forward flexion of the neck).
3. Assist with lumbar puncture if indicated. Document appearance of CSF (a milky appearance indicates elevated WBC levels) and CSF pressure (pressure is usually elevated with meningitis).
4. Monitor results of CSF analysis and report increased WBC and protein levels.
5. Implement measures *to prevent meningitis:*
   a. perform actions *to prevent disruption of the graft site in order to reduce risk of wound contamination:*
      1. implement measures *to reduce pressure on the graft site:*
         a. instruct client to avoid coughing, sneezing, blowing nose, and straining to have a bowel movement; consult physician regarding an order for antitussives, decongestants, stool softeners, and laxatives if indicated
         b. if client feels the urge to sneeze, instruct him/her to put gentle pressure on both sides of nose *in order to prevent sneezing*
         c. instruct client to avoid bending at the waist or tilting head forward
         d. assist with lumbar puncture to remove some CSF if indicated
      2. do not perform nasal suctioning or irrigations
   b. perform actions *to prevent wound contamination:*
      1. utilize good handwashing technique and encourage client to do the same
      2. instruct client to avoid touching nasal packing and dressings and putting fingers in his/her nose; use restraints or mittens if necessary
      3. provide good oral hygiene (e.g. mouth rinses, gentle brushing) as ordered
      4. use aseptic technique when changing nasal drip pad; change pad as soon as it becomes damp
      5. do not reinsert packing if it begins to come out of nares; cover it with a sterile drip pad and consult physician about cutting off the external packing
      6. following removal of nasal packing, do not attempt to clean nose unless ordered by physician; if cleansing is ordered, perform it using aseptic technique
   c. elevate head of bed at least 30° *to allow free drainage of fluid*
   d. if graft site is disrupted, prepare client for surgical repair if planned
   e. monitor for therapeutic and nontherapeutic effects of anti-infectives if administered prophylactically.
6. If signs and symptoms of meningitis occur:
   a. continue with above measures
   b. initiate seizure precautions *(cerebral irritation can cause seizures)*
   c. maintain activity restrictions as ordered (bedrest is usually ordered *to promote healing of area of leakage)*
   d. provide a quiet environment with dim lighting *to reduce discomfort associated with headache and photophobia*
   e. monitor for therapeutic and nontherapeutic effects of the following medications if administered:
      1. corticosteroids *to reduce inflammation*
      2. anti-infectives
   f. assess for and report signs and symptoms of increased intracranial pressure (e.g. restlessness; decreasing level of consciousness; loss of motor and sensory function; sluggish pupillary response to light; papilledema; slow, bounding pulse; rise in systolic B/P with widening pulse pressure)
   g. provide emotional support to client and significant others.

5.b. The client will experience gradual resolution of

5.b.1. Assess for and report signs and symptoms of diabetes insipidus:
   a. polyuria (urine output can range from 4–10 or more liters/day)

diabetes insipidus if it occurs as evidenced by:
1. decreasing polyuria and polydipsia
2. urine specific gravity returning toward normal range.

b. polydipsia (if the client is able to tolerate oral liquids, he/she may drink 4–10 or more liters of fluid/day)
c. urine specific gravity less than 1.005.
2. If signs and symptoms of diabetes insipidus are present:
a. maintain fluid intake equal to output *in order to prevent dehydration*
b. monitor for therapeutic and nontherapeutic effects of the following if administered:
1. ADH replacements (e.g. vasopressin, lypressin, desmopressin acetate [DDAVP])
2. medications that enhance the action of available ADH (e.g. chlorpropamide, clofibrate, carbamazepine)
c. assess closely for and report signs and symptoms of dehydration (e.g. decreased skin turgor, significant weight loss, dry mucous membranes, decreased B/P, increased pulse, elevated serum sodium and osmolality).

5.c. The client will not develop adrenal crisis as evidenced by:
1. stable vital signs
2. usual mental status
3. absence of abdominal pain, nausea, vomiting, diarrhea
4. normal skin turgor
5. serum sodium and potassium within normal range.

5.c.1. Assess for and report signs and symptoms of adrenal crisis:
a. temperature above 38°C
b. drop of 20 mm Hg in systolic B/P, a systolic pressure below 80 mm Hg, or a continual drop of 5–10 mm Hg in systolic pressure with each reading
c. pattern of increasing pulse or pulse rate above 100 beats/minute
d. confusion, lethargy, unresponsiveness
e. nausea, vomiting, abdominal pain, diarrhea
f. poor skin turgor
g. decline in serum sodium and/or increase in serum potassium levels.
2. Assess for and report significant changes in cardiac rhythm *(may be an early indication of potassium imbalance)*.
3. Implement measures *to prevent adrenal crisis:*
a. administer corticosteroids on a regularly scheduled basis as ordered *to maintain therapeutic blood levels* (this is usually started preoperatively)
b. administer analgesics at scheduled intervals if indicated *(pain is a stressor that may precipitate crisis)*
c. minimize exposure to factors that can precipitate adrenal insufficiency (e.g. psychological stress, trauma, extremes in temperature).
4. If adrenal crisis occurs:
a. maintain client on strict bedrest
b. maintain oxygen therapy as ordered
c. perform actions *to reduce fever* (e.g. antipyretics, hypothermia blanket, tepid water bath)
d. maintain intravenous fluid and electrolyte therapy as ordered
e. monitor for therapeutic and nontherapeutic effects of the following medications if administered:
1. intravenous corticosteroids (glucocorticoids and mineralocorticoids may both be given)
2. vasopressors *to maintain adequate mean arterial pressure*
f. institute appropriate safety measures if client is irrational or comatose
g. provide emotional support to client and significant others.

☐ ▬▬▬▬▬▬▬▬▬▬▬▬▬▬▬▬▬▬▬▬

6. NURSING DIAGNOSIS

Knowledge deficit regarding follow-up care.

☐ ▬▬▬▬▬▬▬▬▬▬▬▬▬▬▬▬▬▬▬▬

DESIRED OUTCOMES	NURSING ACTIONS AND *SELECTED RATIONALES*

6.a. The client will identify ways to promote healing of the operative site.

6.a. Instruct client in ways *to promote healing of the operative site* (he/she will be expected to continue with these actions for 1–2 months after surgery):
1. avoid bending at the waist

UNIT XIV

2. avoid tilting head forward (client should wash hair in the shower with head tilted back rather than forward)
3. avoid vigorous coughing and nose blowing
4. avoid sneezing (instruct client to place gentle pressure on both sides of nose when he/she feels the urge to sneeze)
5. keep fingers out of nose
6. prevent constipation (e.g. drink at least 10 glasses of liquid/day, eat foods high in fiber, progressively increase activity) *in order to reduce straining and subsequent increased pressure on operative site*
7. practice good oral hygiene (e.g. gentle brushing, mouth rinses) as ordered
8. avoid trauma to oral cavity incision line:
   a. adhere to soft diet as prescribed
   b. avoid putting sharp or hard objects (e.g. toothpick, end of pen) in mouth
   c. when allowed to brush, use a soft bristle brush and brush gently.

6.b. The client will state signs and symptoms to report to the health care provider.

6.b.1. Refer to Standardized Postoperative Care Plan, Nursing Diagnosis 20, action c, for signs and symptoms to report to the health care provider.
  2. Instruct client to also report:
     a. bloody or clear discharge from nose
     b. constant swallowing
     c. increased postnasal drip or nasal congestion
     d. persistent headache
     e. stiff neck
     f. changes in vision (e.g. double vision, blurred vision, visual field cut)
     g. continued loss of senses of smell and taste (these are expected to have returned to normal about 2–3 weeks after surgery)
     h. excessive thirst or urine output (*could indicate that ADH replacement therapy is needed*)
     i. increasing fatigue and muscle weakness, loss of appetite, nausea, vomiting (*could indicate that corticosteroid replacement therapy is needed*)
     j. apathy, fatigue, mental sluggishness, weight gain, sensitivity to cold, menstrual irregularities, decreased sex drive (*could indicate that thyroid replacement therapy is needed*)
     k. impotence or decreased vaginal lubrication (*could indicate that gonadotropin replacement therapy is needed*).

6.c. The client will verbalize an understanding of and a plan for adhering to recommended follow-up care including future appointments with health care provider, activity level, medications prescribed, and wound care.

6.c.1. Refer to Standardized Postoperative Care Plan, Nursing Diagnosis 20, for routine postoperative instructions and measures to improve client compliance.
  2. Explain the rationale for, side effects of, methods of administering, schedule for taking, and importance of taking medications prescribed (e.g. ADH replacement therapy, corticosteroids).

Hypothyroidism

Hypothyroidism is a condition resulting from a deficiency of circulating thyroid hormone. When it occurs in infants, it is called cretinism. Hypothyroidism that develops in an adult is often referred to as myxedema.* The term myxedema denotes the presence of nonpitting edema associated with accumulation of hydrophilic mucinous substances (protein coupled with hyaluronic acid, chondroitin sulfate B, and mucopolysaccharides) in subcutaneous, connective, and/or muscle tissue. This edema is a typical manifestation of hypothyroidism.

Hypothyroidism is classified as primary, secondary, or tertiary depending on the origin of thyroid dysfunction. Primary hypothyroidism accounts for approximately 95% of all cases of hypothyroidism and is due to failure of the thyroid gland itself. It may be caused by autoim-

mune disease, radioiodine therapy, external radiation, thyroidectomy, idiopathic atrophy, hereditary biochemical defects, iodine deficiency, and certain drugs (e.g. iodine, antithyroid drugs, lithium, para-aminosalicylic acid, thiocyanates, phenylbutazone). Secondary hypothyroidism is caused by pituitary dysfunction and tertiary hypothyroidism is a result of hypothalamic dysfunction. Some sources classify both pituitary and hypothalamic dysfunction as secondary or trophoprivic. The clinical manifestations of hypothyroidism are the same regardless of the etiology, with the severity of signs and symptoms being dependent on the degree of thyroid hormone deficiency.

This care plan focuses on the adult client hospitalized for diagnosis and initiation of treatment of hypothyroidism. Goals of care are to restore adequate circulating thyroid hormone levels, maintain comfort, prevent complications, and educate the client regarding follow-up care.

---

* In this care plan, the terms hypothyroidism and myxedema will be used interchangeably.

DISCHARGE CRITERIA

Prior to discharge, the client will:

- identify ways to prevent constipation until usual bowel habits are regained
- identify appropriate safety precautions to follow if alterations in coagulation, sensory-perceptual function, and thought processes are present
- demonstrate accuracy in counting pulse
- verbalize an understanding of medication therapy including rationale for, side effects of, schedule for taking, and importance of taking as prescribed
- identify ways to maintain an adequate nutritional status
- state signs and symptoms to report to the health care provider
- verbalize an understanding of and a plan for adhering to recommended follow-up care including future appointments with health care provider and activity level.

Use in conjunction with the Care Plan on Immobility.

NURSING/COLLABORATIVE DIAGNOSES

1. Anxiety □ *838*
2. Decreased cardiac output □ *839*

□ ▬▬▬▬▬▬▬▬▬▬▬▬▬▬▬▬▬▬▬▬▬▬▬▬▬

1. NURSING DIAGNOSIS

Anxiety related to unfamiliar environment, current symptoms, unknown diagnosis, and lack of understanding of diagnostic tests and treatments.

□ ▬▬▬▬▬▬▬▬▬▬▬▬▬▬▬▬▬▬▬▬▬▬▬▬▬

DESIRED OUTCOMES	NURSING ACTIONS AND *SELECTED RATIONALES*
1. The client will experience a reduction in fear and anxiety (see Care Plan on Immobility, Nursing Diagnosis 1, for outcome criteria).	1.a. Assess client for signs and symptoms of fear and anxiety (e.g. verbalization of fears and concerns; tenseness; tremors; irritability; restlessness; diaphoresis; tachypnea; tachycardia; elevated blood pressure; facial tension, pallor, or flushing; noncompliance with treatment plan). Validate perceptions carefully, remembering that some of these responses may be

less apparent *because of the altered thought processes and decreased sympathetic-type responses that occur with a lack of thyroid hormone.*
   b. Ascertain effectiveness of current coping skills.
   c. Refer to Care Plan on Immobility, Nursing Diagnosis 1, action c, for measures to reduce fear and anxiety.
   d. Implement additional measures *to reduce fear and anxiety:*
      1. explain all diagnostic tests:
         a. blood studies (e.g. total T_3 and T_4, free T_4 index, resin T_3 uptake, protein-bound iodine [PBI], TSH level, TRH stimulation test, thyroid antibodies, cholesterol level)
         b. radioactive iodine uptake test (RAIU)
         c. thyroid scan
         d. basal metabolic rate (BMR)
         e. deep tendon reflex contraction and relaxation times
         f. needle biopsy or aspiration of thyroid gland
      2. assure client that current symptoms should resolve with treatment, but caution him/her that it may take from 2 weeks to several months.

2. NURSING DIAGNOSIS

Decreased cardiac output related to:

a. decreased stroke volume and heart rate associated with diminished thyroid hormone levels (thyroid hormone has positive inotropic and chronotropic effects on the heart);
b. increased peripheral resistance associated with atherosclerosis (may be present due to reduced lipid metabolism when thyroid hormone levels are diminished) and the vasoconstriction that occurs to compensate for decreased cardiac output;
c. lower demand for oxygen asssociated with a decreased metabolic rate;
d. weakened myocardium (can occur because of myxedematous changes in myocardium);
e. restricted contractility associated with pericardial effusion (can occur as a result of the increased capillary permeability present in hypothyroidism and accumulation of hydrophilic mucinous substances in the pericardial space).

DESIRED OUTCOMES	NURSING ACTIONS AND *SELECTED RATIONALES*

2. The client will maintain adequate cardiac output as evidenced by:
  a. B/P within normal range for client
  b. apical pulse audible, regular, and at least 60 beats/minute
  c. absence of gallop rhythms
  d. B/P and pulse stable with position change
  e. unlabored respirations at 16–20/minute
  f. normal breath sounds
  g. usual mental status
  h. absence of lightheadedness and syncope
	2.a. Assess for and report signs and symptoms of decreased cardiac output:
	  1. drop of 20 mm Hg in systolic B/P, systolic pressure below 80 mm Hg, or continual drop of 5–10 mm Hg in systolic pressure with each reading
	  2. narrowed pulse pressure
	  3. irregular pulse
	  4. pulse rate less than 60 beats/minute
	  5. muffled heart sounds
	  6. presence of an S_3 and/or S_4 gallop rhythm
	  7. decline in systolic BP of at least 15 mm Hg with a concurrent rise in pulse when client sits up
	  8. rapid, labored, or irregular respirations
	  9. crackles and diminished or absent breath sounds
	  10. restlessness, confusion
	  11. lightheadedness, syncope
	  12. diminished or absent peripheral pulses
	  13. decreased amplitude of carotid pulse
	  14. cool, pale, mottled, or cyanotic skin

UNIT XIV

i. palpable peripheral pulses
j. normal amplitude of carotid pulse
k. skin warm and usual color
l. capillary refill time less than 3 seconds
m. urine output at least 30 cc/hour
n. hemodynamic measurements such as pulmonary artery pressure (PAP), pulmonary capillary wedge pressure (PCWP), cardiac output (CO), and central venous pressure (CVP) within normal range
o. BUN and serum creatinine and alkaline phosphatase levels within normal range.

15. capillary refill time greater than 3 seconds
16. urine output less than 30 cc/hour
17. decreased CO; increased PAP, PCWP, and CVP (use internal jugular vein pulsation method to estimate CVP if monitoring device not present)
18. elevated BUN and serum creatinine and alkaline phosphatase levels.

b. Monitor EKG readings and report any abnormalities.
c. Monitor chest x-ray results. Report findings of cardiomegaly, pleural effusion, or pulmonary edema.
d. Implement measures *to improve cardiac output:*
  1. perform actions *to reduce cardiac workload:*
    a. place client in a semi- to high Fowler's position
    b. instruct client to avoid activities that create a Valsalva response (e.g. straining to have a bowel movement, bending at the waist, holding breath while moving)
    c. promote physical and emotional rest
    d. implement measures to improve breathing pattern (see Nursing Diagnosis 3, actions d and e)
    e. discourage smoking *(smoking has a cardiostimulatory effect, causes vasoconstriction, and reduces oxygen availability)*
    f. provide frequent, small meals rather than 3 large ones *(large meals require an increase in blood supply to gastrointestinal tract for digestion)*
    g. discourage intake of foods/fluids high in caffeine such as coffee, tea, chocolate, and colas *(caffeine is a myocardial stimulant and increases myocardial oxygen consumption)*
    h. increase activity gradually
    i. implement measures as ordered to treat anemia, hypertension, and chronic obstructive pulmonary disease *(these conditions increase cardiac workload)*
  2. monitor for therapeutic and nontherapeutic effects of the following medications if administered:
    a. positive inotropic agents (e.g. digitalis preparations, dobutamine, amrinone) *to improve myocardial contractility*
    b. sympathomimetics (e.g. ephedrine, isoproterenol) *to increase heart rate*
    c. thyroid hormone (e.g. levothyroxine, liothyronine, liotrix) *to improve myocardial contractility and increase heart rate.*
e. Consult physician if signs and symptoms of decreased cardiac output persist or worsen.

3. NURSING DIAGNOSIS

Ineffective breathing pattern: shallow respirations related to restricted lung expansion associated with:

a. weakness, fatigue, and positioning;
b. transudative pleural effusion resulting from the increased capillary permeability present in hypothyroidism, accumulation of hydrophilic mucinous substances in the pleural space, and congestive heart failure (CHF) if it occurs;
c. pressure on the diaphragm as a result of abdominal distention;
d. weakness of the diaphragm and muscles of the chest wall resulting from diminished levels of thyroid hormone.

DESIRED OUTCOMES	NURSING ACTIONS AND *SELECTED RATIONALES*
3. The client will maintain an effective breathing pattern	3.a. Assess for and report: 1. shallow respirations

(see Care Plan on Immobility, Nursing Diagnosis 3, for outcome criteria).

2. signs and symptoms of pleural effusion:
  a. dyspnea
  b. diminished or absent breath sounds
  c. dull percussion note over area of diminished breath sounds
  d. chest x-ray showing pleural effusion.
  b. Monitor blood gases. Report abnormal results.
  c. Monitor for and report significant changes in ear oximetry and capnograph results.
  d. Refer to Care Plan on Immobility, Nursing Diagnosis 3, action d, for measures to improve breathing pattern.
  e. Implement additional measures *to improve breathing pattern:*
    1. question any order for a normal adult dose of a central nervous system depressant such as a narcotic analgesic, sedative, or hypnotic (regular doses of these agents may depress respirations *because these clients metabolize medications slowly)*
    2. perform actions to reduce abdominal distention (see Nursing Diagnosis 7.B, action 3)
    3. perform actions *to prevent and treat pleural effusion:*
      a. implement measures to promote resolution of interstitial edema and prevent further accumulation of fluid in the interstitial spaces (see Nursing Diagnosis 4, action c)
      b. prepare client for and assist with thoracentesis if planned.
  f. Consult physician if:
    1. ineffective breathing pattern continues
    2. signs and symptoms of impaired gas exchange (e.g. confusion, restlessness, irritability, cyanosis, decreased PaO_2 and increased $PaCO_2$ levels) are present.

□ ▬▬▬▬▬▬▬▬▬▬▬▬▬▬▬▬

4. NURSING DIAGNOSIS

Altered fluid balance: interstitial edema related to:

a. increased capillary permeability present in hypothyroidism;
b. accumulation of hydrophilic mucinous substances in the interstitial spaces (these substances then draw additional fluid into the interstitial spaces);
c. decreased excretion of water associated with reduced renal blood flow and glomerular filtration.

□ ▬▬▬▬▬▬▬▬▬▬▬▬▬▬▬▬

DESIRED OUTCOMES	NURSING ACTIONS AND *SELECTED RATIONALES*

4. The client will experience resolution of interstitial edema as evidenced by:
  a. gradual resolution of generalized and localized edema
  b. unlabored respirations
  c. normal breath sounds.

4.a. Assess for and report signs and symptoms of interstitial edema:
  1. generalized or localized nonpitting edema (most noticeable in the periorbital area, hands, and lower extremities)
  2. dyspnea
  3. diminished or absent breath sounds.
  b. Monitor chest x-ray results. Report findings of pleural effusion.
  c. Implement measures *to promote resolution of interstitial edema and prevent further accumulation of fluid in the interstitial spaces:*
    1. perform actions to improve cardiac output (see Nursing Diagnosis 2, action d) *in order to maintain an adequate renal blood flow and promote normal fluid excretion*
    2. perform actions to treat CHF (see Collaborative Diagnosis 18, action b.4) if it occurs *in order to reduce edema and promote optimal renal blood flow*
    3. monitor for therapeutic and nontherapeutic effects of the following medications if administered:

     a. thyroid hormone (e.g. levothyroxine, liothyronine, liotrix) *to decrease capillary permeability, reduce accumulation of hydrophilic mucinous substances in the interstitium, and improve glomerular filtration*

     b. diuretics *to promote excretion of water* (used primarily if urine output is inadequate).

   d. Consult physician if signs and symptoms of interstitial edema persist or worsen.

5.A. NURSING DIAGNOSIS

Altered nutrition: less than body requirements related to:

1. decreased oral intake associated with:
   a. anorexia resulting from general apathy, a reduced metabolic rate, and early satiety associated with decreased gastrointestinal motility (a result of thyroid hormone deficiency and decreased activity)
   b. dyspepsia resulting from gastrointestinal gas accumulation
   c. weakness and fatigue
   d. dysphagia resulting from pressure on the esophagus if the thyroid gland is enlarged;
2. impaired digestion and absorption of nutrients associated with:
   a. decreased production of hydrochloric acid and intrinsic factor (some clients with autoimmune hypothyroidism have circulating antibodies against gastric parietal cells)
   b. atrophy and/or myxedematous infiltration of the gastric and intestinal mucosa
   c. slowed absorption due to a reduced metabolic rate.

DESIRED OUTCOMES	NURSING ACTIONS AND *SELECTED RATIONALES*

5.A. The client will maintain an adequate nutritional status as evidenced by:
1. weight returning toward normal range for client's age, height, and build
2. normal BUN and serum albumin, protein, Hct., Hgb., cholesterol, and lymphocyte levels
3. increased strength and activity tolerance
4. healthy oral mucous membrane.
	5.A.1. Assess the client for signs and symptoms of malnutrition:
	  a. abnormal weight for client's age, height, and build (many of these clients are overweight)
	  b. abnormal BUN and low serum albumin, protein, Hct., Hgb., cholesterol, and lymphocyte levels
	  c. weakness and fatigue
	  d. stomatitis.
	2. Reassess nutritional status on a regular basis and report decline.
	3. Monitor percentage of meals eaten.
	4. Assess the client to determine causes of inadequate intake (e.g. anorexia, dyspepsia, weakness, fatigue, dysphagia).
	5. Implement measures *to improve nutritional status:*
	  a. perform actions *to improve oral intake:*
	    1. implement measures to reduce dyspepsia (see Nursing Diagnosis 7.B, action 3)
	    2. provide oral care before meals
	    3. eliminate noxious stimuli from the environment
	    4. serve small portions of nutritious foods/fluids that are appealing to the client
	    5. provide a clean, relaxed, pleasant atmosphere
	    6. obtain a dietary consult if necessary to assist client in selecting foods/fluids that meet nutritional needs as well as preferences
	    7. encourage significant others to bring in client's favorite foods
	    8. implement measures to improve swallowing (see Nursing Diagnosis 6, action b)
	    9. encourage a rest period before meals *to minimize fatigue*

10. allow adequate time for meals; reheat food if necessary
11. increase activity as tolerated *(activity stimulates appetite)*
    b. instruct and assist client to select foods and fluids that are high in the following nutrients yet do not contribute to atherogenesis:
       1. protein (e.g. lean meats, fish, poultry)
       2. vitamin B$_{12}$ (e.g. lean meats, chicken)
       3. folic acid (e.g. green leafy vegetables, asparagus, lima beans, fruit, yeast)
       4. iron (e.g. apricots, figs, green leafy vegetables, whole-grain and enriched breads and cereals)
       5. vitamin C (e.g. citrus fruits and juices) *to increase iron absorption*
    c. monitor for therapeutic and nontherapeutic effects of the following medications if administered:
       1. gastrointestinal stimulants (e.g. metoclopramide) *to increase gastrointestinal motility in order to reduce early satiety*
       2. iron preparations (e.g. ferrous sulfate, ferrous gluconate)
       3. vitamin B$_{12}$ (e.g. cyanocobalamin) injections or vitamin B$_{12}$ with intrinsic factor
       4. folic acid (e.g. Folvite, sodium folate)
       5. vitamin C (ascorbic acid) *to increase absorption of iron*
       6. glutamic acid hydrochloride *to aid digestion and increase iron absorption*
       7. thyroid hormone (e.g. levothyroxine, liothyronine, liotrix) *to resolve the multiple causes of decreased oral intake and impaired absorption.*
6. Perform a 72-hour calorie count if nutritional status declines or fails to improve.
7. Consult physician regarding alternative methods of providing nutrition (e.g. parenteral nutrition, tube feeding) if client does not consume enough food or fluid to meet nutritional needs.

5.B. NURSING DIAGNOSIS

Altered nutrition: more than body requirements related to decreased metabolism of nutrients associated with a reduced metabolic rate.

DESIRED OUTCOMES	NURSING ACTIONS AND *SELECTED RATIONALES*
5.B. The client will experience a gradual reduction in weight as evidenced by: 1. weight declining toward normal range for client's age, height, and build 2. decrease in size of triceps skinfold measurements.	5.B.1. Assess the client for signs of weight excess: a. weight at least 10–20% over ideal weight for age, height, and build (frank obesity is often not present despite the reduced metabolic rate *because of the concomitant decrease in oral intake*) b. triceps skinfold measurement greater than normal for build. 2. Reassess nutritional status on a regular basis (every 3–5 days) and report an increase in weight and size of triceps skinfold. 3. Monitor the amount of foods/fluids consumed *to determine if intake appears excessive.* 4. Implement measures *to promote a gradual reduction of weight:* a. maintain caloric restrictions as ordered b. obtain a dietary consult to assist client to select foods/fluids that meet caloric restrictions, nutritional needs, and personal preferences c. increase activity as allowed and tolerated d. monitor for therapeutic and nontherapeutic effects of thyroid hormone (e.g. levothyroxine, liothyronine, liotrix) if administered *to increase metabolic rate.* 5. Consult physician if client continues to gain weight despite implementation of the above measures.

UNIT XIV

6. NURSING DIAGNOSIS

Impaired swallowing related to pressure on the esophagus associated with enlargement of the thyroid gland (goiter) if present.

DESIRED OUTCOMES	NURSING ACTIONS AND *SELECTED RATIONALES*

6. The client will experience an improvement in swallowing as evidenced by:
a. verbalization of same
b. absence of coughing and choking when eating and drinking.
	6.a. Assess for and report signs and symptoms of impaired swallowing (e.g. coughing or choking when eating or drinking, stasis of food in oral cavity).
	b. Implement measures *to improve ability to swallow:*
	  1. place client in a high Fowler's position for meals and snacks *to increase the gravity flow of food*
	  2. assist client to select foods that are easy to swallow (e.g. custards, applesauce, pureed foods)
	  3. encourage client to chew food thoroughly and concentrate on the act of swallowing
	  4. moisten dry foods with gravy or sauces (e.g. catsup, salad dressing, sour cream).
	c. Consult physician if difficulty swallowing persists or worsens.

7.A. NURSING DIAGNOSIS

Altered comfort:*

1. **muscle stiffness and aching** related to separation of muscle fibers by hydrophilic mucinous substances;
2. **joint stiffness and aching** related to joint effusions associated with increased capillary permeability and accumulations of hydrophilic mucinous substances.

---

* In this care plan, the nursing diagnosis "pain" is included under the diagnostic label of altered comfort.

DESIRED OUTCOMES	NURSING ACTIONS AND *SELECTED RATIONALES*

7.A. The client will experience diminished muscle and joint discomfort as evidenced by:
1. verbalization of same
2. relaxed facial expression and body positioning
3. increased participation in activities.
	7.A.1. Determine how the client usually responds to discomfort.
	2. Assess for nonverbal signs of discomfort (e.g. wrinkled brow, clenched fists, reluctance to move, guarding of a particular extremity, restlessness).
	3. Assess verbal complaints of discomfort. Ask client to be specific about location, severity, and type of discomfort.
	4. Assess for factors that seem to aggravate and alleviate discomfort.
	5. Implement measures *to reduce discomfort:*
	  a. consult physician about application of heat or cold to areas of discomfort
	  b. perform actions *to protect affected extremities from trauma, pressure, or excessive movement:*
	    1. avoid jarring the bed

    2. use a bed cradle or footboard *to relieve pressure from bedding*

    3. instruct and assist client to support affected extremities with hands or pillows when changing positions

    4. remind client to move affected extremities slowly and cautiously

    5. apply a splint to the affected joint(s) if ordered

  c. provide or assist with nonpharmacological measures for relief of discomfort (e.g. back rub, position change, relaxation techniques, guided imagery, quiet conversation, restful environment, diversional activity)

  d. monitor for therapeutic and nontherapeutic effects of analgesics if administered.

6. Consult physician if above measures fail to provide adequate relief of muscle and/or joint discomfort.

7.B. NURSING DIAGNOSIS

Altered comfort: dyspepsia, gas pain, and abdominal distention related to accumulation of gas and fluid in gastrointestinal tract associated with impaired digestion (results from a lack of hydrochloric acid) and decreased gastrointestinal motility.

DESIRED OUTCOMES	NURSING ACTIONS AND *SELECTED RATIONALES*

7.B. The client will experience a reduction in dyspepsia, gas pain, and abdominal distention as evidenced by:
1. verbalization of same
2. relaxed facial expression and body positioning
3. diminished eructation
4. decrease in abdominal girth.
	7.B.1. Assess for nonverbal signs of dyspepsia, gas pain, and abdominal distention (e.g. clutching and guarding of abdomen, restlessness, reluctance to move, grimacing, frequent eructation, increase in abdominal girth, dyspnea).
	2. Assess for verbal complaints of indigestion, gas pain, and abdominal fullness.
	3. Implement measures *to reduce accumulation of gas and fluid in gastrointestinal tract in order to prevent dyspepsia, gas pain, and abdominal distention:*
	  a. encourage and assist client with frequent position change and ambulation as soon as allowed and tolerated *(activity stimulates peristalsis)*
	  b. instruct client to avoid activities such as gum chewing, sucking on hard candy, and smoking *in order to reduce air swallowing*
	  c. encourage client to drink warm liquids *in order to stimulate peristalsis*
	  d. instruct client to avoid gas-producing foods/fluids (e.g. cabbage, onions, popcorn, baked beans, carbonated beverages)
	  e. encourage client to eructate and expel flatus whenever he/she feels the urge
	  f. monitor for therapeutic and nontherapeutic effects of the following medications if administered:
	    1. antiflatulents *to reduce gas accumulation*
	    2. gastrointestinal stimulants (e.g. bisacodyl, metoclopramide) *to increase gastrointestinal motility*
	    3. glutamic acid hydrochloride *to aid digestion*
	    4. thyroid hormone (e.g. levothyroxine, liothyronine, liotrix) *to increase gastrointestinal motility.*
	4. Consult physician if signs and symptoms of dyspepsia, gas pain, and abdominal distention persist or worsen.

UNIT
XIV

□ ▬▬▬▬▬▬▬▬▬▬▬▬▬▬▬▬▬▬

7.C. NURSING DIAGNOSIS

Altered comfort: chills and feeling of coldness related to hypothermia and a compensatory peripheral vasoconstriction that occurs as a result of decreased cardiac output.

□ ▬▬▬▬▬▬▬▬▬▬▬▬▬▬▬▬▬▬

DESIRED OUTCOMES	NURSING ACTIONS AND *SELECTED RATIONALES*

7.C. The client will not experience chills and a feeling of being cold.	7.C.1. Assess client for chills and statements of feeling cold.
	2. Implement measures *to prevent chills and feeling of being cold:*
	  a. perform actions to prevent and treat hypothermia (see Nursing Diagnosis 8, action b)
	  b. perform actions to improve cardiac output (see Nursing Diagnosis 2, action d) *in order to reduce compensatory vasoconstriction.*
	3. Implement measures *to promote comfort if chills and a feeling of being cold occur:*
	  a. eliminate drafts in room as possible
	  b. maintain a room temperature that is comfortable for client
	  c. provide client with extra blankets and clothing as needed
	  d. provide warm liquids to drink.
	4. Consult physician if client continues to have chills or complains of being cold.

□ ▬▬▬▬▬▬▬▬▬▬▬▬▬▬▬▬▬▬

8. NURSING DIAGNOSIS

Hypothermia related to a decreased basal metabolic rate associated with thyroid hormone deficiency.

□ ▬▬▬▬▬▬▬▬▬▬▬▬▬▬▬▬▬▬

DESIRED OUTCOMES	NURSING ACTIONS AND *SELECTED RATIONALES*

8. The client will have a normal body temperature.	8.a. Monitor for signs and symptoms of hypothermia (e.g. cool skin, pallor, slow capillary refill, complaints of feeling cold, body temperature below normal).
	b. Implement measures *to prevent and treat hypothermia:*
	  1. maintain a room temperature of at least 70°F
	  2. provide client with extra blankets and clothing
	  3. monitor for therapeutic and nontherapeutic effects of thyroid hormone (e.g. levothyroxine, liothyronine, liotrix) if administered.
	c. Consult physician if signs and symptoms of hypothermia persist.

□ ▬▬▬▬▬▬▬▬▬▬▬▬▬▬▬▬▬▬

9. NURSING DIAGNOSIS

Sensory-perceptual alteration: auditory: decreased hearing ability related to accumulation of hydrophilic mucinous substances on cranial nerve VIII.

□ ▬▬▬▬▬▬▬▬▬▬▬▬▬▬▬▬▬▬

DESIRED OUTCOMES	**NURSING ACTIONS AND *SELECTED RATIONALES***

9. The client will be able to comprehend others as evidenced by:
   a. appropriate responses
   b. cooperation with treatment regimen.

9.a. Assess client's ability to hear by:
    1. observing for cues indicative of decreased hearing ability (e.g. speaking loudly, staring at other person's lips during conversation, moving closer to others when they speak, acts of frustration, nodding yes with subsequent inappropriate responses)
    2. noting client's verbal complaints of not being able to hear or understand what others are saying.
  b. If client's hearing ability is diminished:
    1. determine from significant others what techniques have been effective in communicating with client
    2. implement measures *to facilitate communication:*
      a. provide adequate lighting in room *so client can read lips*
      b. reduce environmental noise
      c. speak slightly louder and more slowly than usual; avoid lowering voice at end of sentences
      d. use simple sentences
      e. avoid overenunciation of words
      f. face client while speaking
      g. avoid chewing gum or eating while talking to client
      h. talk into the less impaired ear
      i. rephrase sentences when client does not understand
      j. employ related nonverbal cues such as facial expressions or pointing when appropriate
      k. use alternative forms of communication (e.g. flash cards, paper and pencil, magic slate) if indicated
      l. respond to client's call signal in person rather than over intercommunication system
      m. remind client to use his/her hearing aid
    3. instruct significant others regarding communication techniques that are effective with client
    4. reinforce physician's explanation about permanency of hearing loss (hearing usually improves as thyroid hormone levels are restored)
    5. consult physician if hearing loss worsens.

☐ ▬▬▬▬▬▬▬▬▬▬▬▬▬▬▬▬▬▬▬▬▬▬▬▬▬▬▬▬▬

10. NURSING DIAGNOSIS

Impaired verbal communication related to accumulation of hydrophilic mucinous substances in the tongue or larynx and pressure on the larynx if thyroid is enlarged.

☐ ▬▬▬▬▬▬▬▬▬▬▬▬▬▬▬▬▬▬▬▬▬▬▬▬▬▬▬▬▬

DESIRED OUTCOMES	**NURSING ACTIONS AND *SELECTED RATIONALES***

10. The client will communicate needs and desires effectively.

10.a. Assess for difficulties in verbal communication (e.g. hoarseness; thick, slurred speech).
  b. If client has difficulty communicating verbally:
    1. implement measures *to facilitate communication:*
      a. maintain a patient, calm approach; avoid interrupting client and allow ample time for communication
      b. maintain a quiet environmment *so that client does not have to raise voice to be heard*
      c. ask questions that require short answers or nod of head
      d. provide materials necessary for communication (e.g. magic slate, pad and pencil, flash cards)

UNIT XIV

    e. answer call signal promptly and in person rather than using the
   intercommunication system

    f. make frequent rounds to ascertain needs

    g. if client is frustrated or fatigued, try to anticipate needs *in order to
   minimize necessity of verbal communication*

2. inform significant others and health care personnel of approaches being
   used to maximize client's ability to communicate; encourage significant
   others and staff to talk to client even if he/she has difficulty speaking

3. assure client that hoarseness and/or thick, slurred speech should subside
   when thyroid hormone levels are restored

4. consult physician if client experiences increasing impairment of verbal
   communication.

□ ▬▬▬▬▬▬▬▬▬▬▬▬▬▬▬▬▬▬▬▬▬▬▬

11. NURSING DIAGNOSIS

Impaired skin integrity: irritation or breakdown related to:

a. prolonged pressure on tissues associated with decreased mobility;
b. increased fragility of the skin associated with dryness and interstitial edema.

□ ▬▬▬▬▬▬▬▬▬▬▬▬▬▬▬▬▬▬▬▬▬▬▬

DESIRED OUTCOMES	NURSING ACTIONS AND *SELECTED RATIONALES*

11. The client will maintain skin integrity (see Care Plan on Immobility, Nursing Diagnosis 7, for outcome criteria).	11.a. Inspect the skin (especially bone prominences, dependent areas, and areas that are dry or edematous) for pallor, redness, and breakdown.
	b. Refer to Care Plan on Immobility, Nursing Diagnosis 7, action b, for measures related to prevention of skin breakdown associated with decreased mobility.
	c. Implement measures *to reduce dryness of skin:*
	  1. avoid use of harsh soaps and hot water
	  2. gently pat the skin dry
	  3. apply moisturizers or emollient creams to skin at least once/day.
	d. Implement measures *to reduce skin breakdown associated with edema:*
	  1. perform actions to promote resolution of interstitial edema and prevent further accumulation of fluid in the interstitial spaces (see Nursing Diagnosis 4, action c)
	  2. place a bed cradle over affected areas *to relieve pressure from bedding*
	  3. handle edematous areas gently.
	e. If skin breakdown occurs:
	  1. notify physician
	  2. continue with above measures to prevent further irritation and breakdown
	  3. perform decubitus care as ordered or per standard hospital policy
	  4. monitor client closely and report signs and symptoms of infection (e.g. elevated temperature; redness, warmth, and edema around area of breakdown; unusual drainage from site).

□ ▬▬▬▬▬▬▬▬▬▬▬▬▬▬▬▬▬▬▬▬▬▬▬

12. NURSING DIAGNOSIS

Activity intolerance related to:

a. tissue hypoxia associated with:
    1. anemia resulting from:
        a. decreased iron, vitamin B_{12}, and folic acid levels associated with decreased
           oral intake and impaired absorption

b. blood loss associated with menorrhagia (can result from imbalances of progesterone and estradiol) if it occurs
c. atrophy of erythropoietin-producing tissue as a result of the decreased need for oxygen associated with a lower metabolic rate
2. decreased tissue perfusion resulting from decreased cardiac output;
b. low energy levels associated with decreased metabolic rate;
c. inadequate nutritional status.

□ ▬▬▬▬▬▬▬▬▬▬▬▬▬▬▬▬▬▬▬▬▬▬

DESIRED OUTCOMES	NURSING ACTIONS AND *SELECTED RATIONALES*

12. The client will demonstrate an increased tolerance for activity (see Care Plan on Immobility, Nursing Diagnosis 8, for outcome criteria).	12.a. Refer to Care Plan on Immobility, Nursing Diagnosis 8, for measures related to assessment and improvement of activity tolerance.
	b. Implement additional measures *to promote rest and improve activity tolerance:*
	  1. maintain activity restrictions as ordered
	  2. perform actions to reduce fear and anxiety (see Nursing Diagnosis 1, actions c and d)
	  3. perform actions to increase cardiac output (see Nursing Diagnosis 2, action d)
	  4. perform actions to improve breathing pattern (see Nursing Diagnosis 3, actions d and e) *in order to maintain adequate alveolar gas exchange*
	  5. maintain an optimal nutritional status (see Nursing Diagnosis 5.A, action 5)
	  6. monitor for therapeutic and nontherapeutic effects of thyroid hormone (e.g. levothyroxine, liothyronine, liotrix) if administered.

□ ▬▬▬▬▬▬▬▬▬▬▬▬▬▬▬▬▬▬▬▬▬▬

13. NURSING DIAGNOSIS

Impaired physical mobility related to:

a. activity intolerance;
b. delayed muscle contraction and relaxation (results in slowed movements);
c. joint and muscle discomfort;
d. impaired coordination and unsteady gait associated with deposits of hydrophilic mucinous substances in the cerebellum.

□ ▬▬▬▬▬▬▬▬▬▬▬▬▬▬▬▬▬▬▬▬▬▬

DESIRED OUTCOMES	NURSING ACTIONS AND *SELECTED RATIONALES*

13.a. The client will achieve maximum physical mobility within limitations imposed by the disease process.	13.a.1. Assess for factors that impair physical mobility (e.g. weakness, fatigue, joint or muscle discomfort, uncoordinated movements).
	2. Implement measures *to increase mobility:*
	  a. perform actions to improve activity tolerance (see Nursing Diagnosis 12)
	  b. instruct client in and assist with range of motion exercises every 4 hours
	  c. monitor for therapeutic and nontherapeutic effects of thyroid hormone (e.g. levothyroxine, liothyronine, liotrix) if administered *to reduce accumulation of hydrophilic mucinous substances in muscles, joints, and cerebellum*
	  d. perform actions to reduce muscle and joint discomfort (see Nursing Diagnosis 7.A, action 5)

UNIT XIV

e. instruct client in and assist with correct use of mobility aids (e.g. cane, walker).
3. Increase activity and participation in self-care activities as tolerated.
4. Provide praise and encouragement for all efforts to increase physical mobility.
5. Encourage the support of significant others. Allow them to assist with range of motion exercises and activity if desired.
6. Consult physician if physical mobility does not improve after thyroid hormone replacement has been initiated.

13.b. The client will not experience problems associated with immobility.

13.b. Refer to Care Plan on Immobility for actions to prevent problems associated with immobility if client remains on bedrest for longer than 48 hours.

14. NURSING DIAGNOSIS

Self-care deficit related to altered thought processes and impaired physical mobility.

DESIRED OUTCOMES	NURSING ACTIONS AND *SELECTED RATIONALES*

14. The client will demonstrate increased participation in self-care activities.	14.a. Refer to Care Plan on Immobility, Nursing Diagnosis 9, for measures related to assessment of, planning for, and meeting client's self-care needs.
	b. Implement additional measures *to facilitate the client's ability to perform self-care activities:*
	  1. perform actions to increase mobility (see Nursing Diagnosis 13, action a.2)
	  2. perform actions to improve thought processes (see Nursing Diagnosis 16, action c).

15. NURSING DIAGNOSIS

Constipation related to decreased gastrointestinal motility (a result of thyroid hormone deficiency, anxiety, and decreased activity) and diminished intake of fluid and foods high in fiber.

DESIRED OUTCOMES	NURSING ACTIONS AND *SELECTED RATIONALES*
15. The client will have a gradual return of usual bowel elimination pattern.	15.a. Refer to Care Plan on Immobility, Nursing Diagnosis 11, actions a–e, for measures related to assessment and prevention of constipation. b. Avoid enemas and manual removal of stool if possible *(both cause vagal stimulation, which can further slow client's pulse)*. c. Consult physician if constipation persists once thyroid hormone replacement therapy is initiated.

16. NURSING DIAGNOSIS

Altered thought processes: slowed verbal responses, impaired memory, and apathy related to:

a. cerebral hypoxia associated with anemia and diminished cerebral blood flow (a result of decreased cardiac output);
b. decreased central nervous system stimulation associated with lack of thyroid hormone.

DESIRED OUTCOMES	NURSING ACTIONS AND *SELECTED RATIONALES*
16. The client will regain usual thought processes as evidenced by: a. improved verbal response time b. improved memory c. increased interest in surroundings and activities.	16.a. Assess client for alterations in thought processes (e.g. slowed verbal responses, inability to remember things, lack of interest in environment). b. Ascertain from significant others client's usual level of intellectual functioning. c. Implement measures *to improve thought processes:* 1. perform actions to improve cardiac output (see Nursing Diagnosis 2, action d) *in order to increase cerebral blood flow* 2. perform actions to improve nutritional status (see Nursing Diagnosis 5.A, action 5) *in order to prevent or treat anemia* 3. monitor for therapeutic and nontherapeutic effects of thyroid hormone (e.g. levothyroxine, liothyronine, liotrix) if administered. d. If client shows evidence of altered thought processes: 1. allow adequate time for communication and performance of activities 2. repeat instructions as necessary using clear, simple language 3. write out a schedule of activities for client to refer to if desired 4. encourage significant others to be supportive of and patient with client 5. inform client and significant others that intellectual functioning will improve once thyroid hormone levels have been restored 6. consult physician if client does not demonstrate a gradual improvement in thought processes once thyroid hormone replacement therapy has been initiated.

17. NURSING DIAGNOSIS

Potential for trauma related to:

a. falls associated with unsteady gait, joint and muscle stiffness, fatigue and weakness, oversedation (may occur if client receives usual adult dose of central nervous system depressants), and night blindness (can develop as a result of decreased conversion of carotene to vitamin A due to deficiency of thyroid hormone);
b. burns and cuts associated with:
1. paresthesias resulting from compression of nerves by hydrophilic mucinous substances (most often affects the median nerve)
2. altered thought processes
3. impaired coordination.

DESIRED OUTCOMES	NURSING ACTIONS AND *SELECTED RATIONALES*

17. The client will not experience falls, burns, or cuts.

17.a. Determine whether factors predisposing the client to falls, burns, or cuts exist:
    1. weakness and fatigue
    2. joint stiffness
    3. uncoordinated movements
    4. altered thought processes
    5. decreased sensation in extremities
    6. unsteady gait
    7. night blindness
    8. receiving central nervous system depressants.

  b. Implement measures *to prevent falls:*
    1. keep bed in low position with side rails up when client is in bed
    2. keep needed items within easy reach
    3. encourage client to request assistance whenever needed; have call signal within easy reach
    4. use lap belt when client is in chair if indicated
    5. instruct client to wear shoes with nonskid soles and low heels when ambulating
    6. avoid unnecessary clutter in room
    7. accompany client during ambulation utilizing a transfer safety belt
    8. provide ambulatory aids (e.g. walker, cane) if the client is weak or unsteady on feet
    9. instruct client to ambulate in well-lit areas and to utilize handrails if needed
    10. do not rush client; allow adequate time for trips to the bathroom and ambulation in hallway
    11. perform actions to increase strength and activity tolerance (see Nursing Diagnosis 12)
    12. if client has night blindness, provide low lighting in room at night
    13. administer central nervous system depressants such as narcotics, sedatives, and hypnotics judiciously; question any order for a usual adult dose of these medications *because the client is unable to metabolize them at a normal rate.*

  c. Implement measures *to prevent burns:*
    1. let hot foods and fluids cool slightly before serving *to reduce risk of burns if spills occur*
    2. supervise client while smoking if indicated
    3. assess temperature of bath water and heating pad before and during use.

  d. Assist client with tasks that require fine motor skills (e.g. shaving) *in order to prevent cuts.*

  e. Include client and significant others in planning and implementing measures to prevent injury.

  f. If injury does occur, initiate appropriate first aid and notify physician.

18. COLLABORATIVE DIAGNOSIS

Potential complications:

a. **myxedema coma (exacerbation of all the manifestations of hypothyroidism)** precipitated by:
    1. an increased need for thyroid hormone resulting from conditions such as stress, infection, and trauma
    2. central nervous system (CNS) depression as a result of certain medications (e.g. narcotics, sedatives) and CO_2 narcosis;

b. **congestive heart failure (CHF)** related to increasing weakness of the myocardium and restricted contractility if pericardial effusion is present;

c. **myxedema ileus (myxedema megacolon)** related to diminished or absent gastrointestinal motility associated with thyroid hormone deficiency;

d. **bleeding** related to increased capillary fragility and deficiency of certain clotting factors associated with thyroid hormone deficiency.

□ ▬▬▬▬▬▬▬▬▬▬▬▬▬▬▬▬

DESIRED OUTCOMES	NURSING ACTIONS AND *SELECTED RATIONALES*

18.a. The client will not experience myxedema coma as evidenced by:
1. vital signs within normal range for client
2. usual or improved mental status
3. stable or improved reflexes
4. blood gases within normal range.

18.a.1. Assess for and immediately report signs and symptoms of myxedema coma (e.g. further decline in temperature, further slowing of pulse rate, decreased B/P, hypoventilation, marked lethargy, confusion, further slowing or absence of reflexes, elevated $PaCO_2$).

2. Implement measures *to prevent myxedema coma:*
   a. minimize exposure to factors that may precipitate myxedema coma (e.g. infection, trauma, psychological stress)
   b. perform actions *to prevent CNS depression:*
      1. implement measures to improve breathing pattern (see Nursing Diagnosis 3, actions d and e) *in order to prevent CO_2 narcosis*
      2. administer any CNS depressant (e.g. narcotics, sedatives) judiciously; question any order for a normal adult dose of these agents
   c. monitor for therapeutic and nontherapeutic effects of thyroid hormone (e.g. levothyroxine, liothyronine, liotrix) if administered.

3. If signs and symptoms of myxedema coma occur:
   a. continue with above actions
   b. maintain oxygen therapy as ordered
   c. warm client gradually with extra blankets *(rapid warming may cause vasodilation and a further decline in B/P)*
   d. maintain intravenous fluid and electrolyte therapy as ordered; hypertonic saline and dextrose solutions may be given *to treat the hyponatremia and hypoglycemia that can occur as a result of water intoxication and decreased metabolism of insulin*
   e. maintain fluid restrictions if ordered *to correct hyponatremia*
   f. monitor for therapeutic and nontherapeutic effects of the following medications if administered:
      1. intravenous thyroid hormone
      2. positive inotropic agents and sympathomimetics *to improve cardiac output*
      3. vasopressors *to maintain an adequate mean arterial pressure*
   g. assist with intubation and mechanical ventilation if indicated
   h. provide emotional support to client and significant others.

18.b. The client will not develop CHF as evidenced by:
1. vital signs within normal range for client
2. audible heart sounds without an S_3 or S_4 or softening of pre-existing murmurs
3. normal breath sounds
4. absence of or no increase in dyspnea and orthopnea
5. palpable peripheral pulses and normal carotid pulse amplitude
6. balanced intake and output
7. stable weight
8. CVP within normal range

18.b.1. Assess for and report signs and symptoms of CHF:
   a. further narrowing of pulse pressure and slowing of pulse rate
   b. softened or muffled heart sounds
   c. development of or intensified S_3 and/or S_4 gallop rhythm
   d. crackles and diminished or absent breath sounds
   e. dyspnea, orthopnea
   f. displaced apical impulse
   g. diminished or absent peripheral pulses
   h. decreased amplitude of carotid pulse
   i. intake greater than output
   j. weight gain
   k. elevated CVP
   l. peripheral edema
   m. distended neck veins
   n. enlarged, tender liver
   o. elevated BUN and serum creatinine and alkaline phosphatase levels.

2. Monitor chest x-ray results. Report findings of cardiomegaly, pleural effusion, or pulmonary edema.

3. Implement measures to improve cardiac output (see Nursing Diagnosis 2, action d) *in order to prevent CHF.*

UNIT XIV

9. absence of peripheral edema; distended neck veins; enlarged, tender liver
10. BUN and serum creatinine and alkaline phosphatase levels within normal range.

4. If signs and symptoms of CHF occur:
   a. continue with above actions to improve cardiac output
   b. monitor for therapeutic and nontherapeutic effects of medications that may be administered *to reduce vascular congestion and/or cardiac workload* (e.g. diuretics, cardiotonics, vasodilators, morphine sulfate)
   c. apply rotating tourniquets according to hospital policy if ordered *to reduce pulmonary vascular congestion*
   d. refer to Care Plan on Congestive Heart Failure for additional care measures.

18.c. The client will not develop myxedema ileus as evidenced by:
1. active bowel sounds
2. gradual return of usual bowel elimination pattern
3. absence of nausea and vomiting
4. no increase in abdominal distention and discomfort.

18.c.1. Assess for and report signs and symptoms of myxedema ileus (e.g. diminished or absent bowel sounds, decrease in frequency of bowel movements, nausea and vomiting, increased abdominal distention and discomfort).
2. Monitor abdominal x-ray results. Report findings of colonic distention or obstruction.
3. Implement measures *to prevent an ileus*:
   a. perform actions to prevent constipation (see Care Plan on Immobility, Nursing Diagnosis 11, action e)
   b. monitor for therapeutic and nontherapeutic effects of the following medications if administered *to increase gastrointestinal motility*:
      1. thyroid hormone (e.g. levothyroxine, liothyronine, liotrix)
      2. gastrointestinal stimulants (e.g. bisacodyl, metoclopramide).
4. If signs and symptoms of an ileus occur:
   a. maintain food and fluid restrictions as ordered
   b. insert a nasogastric or intestinal tube and maintain suction as ordered
   c. maintain intravenous fluid and electrolyte therapy as ordered.

18.d. The client will not experience unusual bleeding as evidenced by:
1. skin and mucous membranes free of bleeding, petechiae, and ecchymosis
2. absence of unusual joint pain and swelling
3. no increase in abdominal girth
4. absence of frank or occult blood in stool, urine, and vomitus
5. usual menstrual flow
6. vital signs within normal range for client
7. stable or improved Hct. and Hgb.
8. usual mental status.

18.d.1. Assess client for and report signs and symptoms of unusual bleeding:
   a. petechiae
   b. multiple ecchymotic areas
   c. bleeding gums
   d. frequent or uncontrollable episodes of epistaxis
   e. unusual oozing from injection sites
   f. unusual joint pain or swelling
   g. increase in abdominal girth
   h. hematemesis, melena, red or smoke-colored urine
   i. hypermenorrhea
   j. significant drop in B/P accompanied by an increased pulse rate
   k. decline in Hct. and Hgb. levels
   l. restlessness, confusion.
2. Monitor coagulation test results (e.g. tourniquet or Rumpel-Leede test, activated partial thromboplastin time, bleeding time). Report abnormal values.
3. If coagulation test results are abnormal or Hct. and Hgb. levels decline, test all stools, urine, and vomitus for occult blood. Report positive results.
4. Implement measures *to prevent bleeding*:
   a. use the smallest gauge needle possible when giving injections and performing venous or arterial punctures
   b. apply gentle, prolonged pressure after injections and venous or arterial punctures
   c. take B/P only when necessary and avoid overinflating the cuff
   d. caution client to avoid activities that increase potential for trauma (e.g. shaving with a straight-edge razor, cutting nails, using stiff bristle toothbrush or dental floss)
   e. pad side rails if client is confused or restless
   f. perform actions to prevent falls (see Nursing Diagnosis 17, action b)
   g. instruct client to avoid blowing nose forcefully or straining to have a bowel movement; consult physician about an order for decongestants, stool softeners, and/or laxatives if indicated
   h. monitor for therapeutic and nontherapeutic effects of the following medications and blood products if administered:
      1. estrogen-progestin preparations *to suppress menses*
      2. platelets
      3. plasma or whole blood.

5. If bleeding occurs and does not subside spontaneously:
   a. apply firm, prolonged pressure to bleeding area if possible
   b. if epistaxis occurs, place client in a high Fowler's position and apply pressure and ice packs to nasal area
   c. maintain oxygen therapy as ordered
   d. perform iced water or saline lavage as ordered *to control gastric bleeding*
   e. administer whole blood, fresh frozen plasma, or clotting factors as ordered
   f. prepare client for surgical repair of bleeding vessels if planned
   g. provide emotional support to client and significant others.

19. NURSING DIAGNOSIS

Sexual dysfunction:

a. **decreased libido** related to general apathy, weakness, fatigue, altered self-concept, and hormone imbalances (altered secretion and metabolism of androgens, progesterone, and estradiol);
b. **impotence** related to altered self-concept and altered secretion and metabolism of androgens.

DESIRED OUTCOMES	NURSING ACTIONS AND *SELECTED RATIONALES*

19. The client will demonstrate beginning acceptance of changes in sexual functioning (see Care Plan on Immobility, Nursing Diagnosis 15, for outcome criteria).	19.a. Refer to Care Plan on Immobility, Nursing Diagnosis 15, for measures related to assessment and management of sexual dysfunction.
	b. Implement additional measures *to promote optimal sexual functioning:*
	  1. reassure client and partner that hormone imbalances causing sexual dysfunction often resolve once thyroid hormone levels are restored to normal
	  2. perform actions to improve the client's self-concept (see Nursing Diagnosis 20)
	  3. instruct client to allow adequate rest periods before and after sexual activity.

20. NURSING DIAGNOSIS

Disturbance in self-concept* related to:

a. changes in appearance (e.g. yellow, dry skin; hair breakage and loss; broken nails; weight gain; edema of face, hands, and feet);
b. difficulty communicating verbally associated with slurred speech and hoarseness;
c. alterations in sexual functioning;
d. infertility associated with oligospermia and failure to ovulate as a result of hormone imbalances (particularly in secondary hypothyroidism);
e. altered thought processes;
f. dependence on others to meet self-care needs.

---

* This diagnostic label includes the nursing diagnoses of body image disturbance and self-esteem disturbance.

DESIRED OUTCOMES	NURSING ACTIONS AND *SELECTED RATIONALES*

20. The client will demonstrate beginning adaptation to changes in appearance, level of independence, and body functioning (see Care Plan on Immobility, Nursing Diagnosis 16, for outcome criteria).	20.a. Refer to Care Plan on Immobility, Nursing Diagnosis 16, for measures related to assessment and promotion of a positive self-concept.
	b. Implement additional measures *to promote a positive self-concept:*
	  1. assure client that most of the changes in appearance and body functioning should gradually resolve as thyroid hormone levels are restored
	  2. perform actions to promote optimal sexual functioning (see Nursing Diagnosis 19)
	  3. encourage maximum participation in self-care within the prescribed activity restrictions and encourage significant others to allow client to do what he/she is able *so that independence can be re-established and self-esteem redeveloped*
	  4. perform actions *to assist client to adapt to changes in appearance:*
	    a. instruct and assist client in ways *to minimize breakage and/or loss of hair:*
	      1. brush and comb hair gently
	      2. avoid frequent shampooing and use of harsh hair products
	      3. avoid using hair dryer and curling irons
	      4. do not use elastic bands to contain hair
	      5. avoid coloring and permanenting hair
	    b. assist client with usual grooming and makeup habits
	    c. assist and instruct client to apply moisturizers and emollients to skin as necessary *to reduce dryness*
	    d. assist and instruct client about ways *to reduce nail breakage* (e.g. keep nails short and filed smoothly, use polish specifically designed to strengthen nails).

□ ▬▬▬▬▬▬▬▬▬▬▬▬▬▬▬▬▬▬▬▬▬▬▬▬▬▬

21. NURSING DIAGNOSIS

Knowledge deficit regarding follow-up care.

□ ▬▬▬▬▬▬▬▬▬▬▬▬▬▬▬▬▬▬▬▬▬▬▬▬▬▬

DESIRED OUTCOMES	NURSING ACTIONS AND *SELECTED RATIONALES*

21.a. The client will identify ways to prevent constipation until usual bowel habits are regained.	21.a. Provide the following instructions regarding ways *to prevent constipation:*
	  1. drink at least 10 glasses of liquid/day unless physician has prescribed a fluid restriction
	  2. increase intake of foods high in fiber (e.g. bran, whole grains, raw fruits and vegetables, dried fruits)
	  3. increase activity as tolerated
	  4. take stool softeners as prescribed.

21.b. The client will identify appropriate safety precautions to follow if alterations in coagulation, sensory-perceptual function, and thought processes are present.	21.b. Instruct client regarding appropriate safety precautions to follow if alterations in coagulation, sensory-perceptual function, and thought processes are present:
	  1. reduce risk of bleeding by:
	    a. avoiding taking aspirin, aspirin-containing products, and ibuprofen
	    b. using an electric rather than a straight-edge razor
	    c. flossing and brushing teeth gently
	    d. cutting nails carefully
	    e. avoiding situations that could result in injury (e.g. contact sports)
	    f. avoiding blowing nose forcefully
	    g. avoiding straining to have a bowel movement

2. if night blindness is present:
   a. keep sleeping room dimly lit at night
   b. remove unnecessary furnishings in room
   c. do not drive at night
3. if hearing loss has occurred:
   a. have devices for the hearing-impaired installed on phone and alarm systems
   b. do not drive if hearing remains severely impaired
4. if paresthesias are present:
   a. use care in application of heat and cold to involved area(s)
   b. wear slippers or shoes whenever ambulating if paresthesias involve feet
5. if altered intellectual function or impaired coordination are present:
   a. do not drive
   b. avoid operating any hazardous equipment.

21.c. The client will demonstrate accuracy in counting pulse.	21.c.1. Teach client how to count his/her pulse, being alert to regularity of the rhythm. 2. Allow time for return demonstration and accuracy check.
21.d. The client will verbalize an understanding of medication therapy including rationale for, side effects of, schedule for taking, and importance of taking as prescribed.	21.d.1. Explain the rationale for, side effects of, and importance of taking medications prescribed. 2. If client is discharged on thyroid hormone, instruct to: a. take medication in the morning *(thyroid hormone has a stimulating effect that disrupts sleep if taken in the evening)* b. avoid altering the prescribed medication regimen c. take pulse before taking medication; hold medication and consult physician if pulse is over 100 beats/minute d. expect changes such as weight loss, reduction in swelling or puffiness, return of usual bowel habits, increased appetite, and increased strength and energy within 1–4 weeks after medication therapy is started e. store thyroid medication in an airtight, light-resistant container away from heat f. monitor blood and/or urine sugar closely if a diabetic *(thyroid hormone elevates blood sugar)* and inform physician of changes in usual pattern of results g. wear a Medic-Alert tag and inform all health care providers of thyroid hormone regimen h. report signs and symptoms of excessive thyroid hormone replacement (e.g. restlessness, sleeplessness, weight loss of more than 5 pounds in a week, persistent diarrhea, palpitations, chest pain, shortness of breath, excessive sweating, frequent or unusual mood swings, irregular pulse or pulse over 100 beats/minute). 3. Instruct client to consult health care provider before taking other prescription and nonprescription medications.
21.e. The client will identify ways to maintain an adequate nutritional status.	21.e.1. Reinforce instructions about foods/fluids high in vitamins and nutrients that should be included in diet (see Nursing Diagnosis 5.A, action 5.b). 2. Instruct client to take nutritional supplements (e.g. vitamins, hematinics) as prescribed. 3. Reinforce physician's instructions on weight loss. Provide information about weight loss programs if indicated.
21.f. The client will state signs and symptoms to report to the health care provider.	21.f. Instruct client to report signs and symptoms of: 1. inadequate thyroid hormone replacement (e.g. persistent or recurrent fatigue, weakness, muscle and joint aching, cold intolerance, weight gain, constipation, abdominal distention, impaired memory, apathy, hair breakage or loss , shortness of breath, swelling of feet and ankles) 2. excessive thyroid hormone replacement (see action d.2.h in this diagnosis).
21.g. The client will verbalize an understanding of and a plan for adhering to	21.g.1. Reinforce the importance of keeping follow-up appointments with health care provider and continuing lifelong thyroid hormone replacement and health supervision.

UNIT
XIV

recommended follow-up care including future appointments with health care provider and activity level.

2. Reinforce the physician's instructions regarding activity level.
3. Implement measures *to improve client compliance:*
   a. include significant others in teaching sessions if possible
   b. encourage questions and allow time for reinforcement and clarification of information provided
   c. provide written instructions regarding future appointments with health care provider, dietary modifications, activity progression, medications prescribed, and signs and symptoms to report.

■ ■

Thyroidectomy

Thyroidectomy is the surgical removal of the thyroid gland. It may be performed to treat neoplasms of the thyroid, unusually large goiters, or hyperthyroidism that has been refractory to conservative treatment. A subtotal thyroidectomy (removal of up to 90% of the thyroid gland) is the preferred procedure unless the surgery is being done to treat a malignancy, in which case a total thyroidectomy will be performed. Following a subtotal thyroidectomy, the remaining gland tissue usually hypertrophies enough to supply adequate amounts of thyroid hormone. Prior to hospitalization for surgery, the client is treated with antithyroid agents and iodine to achieve a euthyroid state in order to minimize the risk of thyroid crisis and hemorrhage intraoperatively and postoperatively.

This care plan focuses on the adult client with hyperthyroidism whose condition has been medically stabilized and who is being hospitalized for a subtotal thyroidectomy. Preoperative goals of care are to reduce fear and anxiety and educate the client regarding postoperative care and management. Postoperatively, the goals of care are to maintain comfort, prevent complications, and educate the client regarding follow-up care.

DISCHARGE CRITERIA

Prior to discharge, the client will:

- demonstrate the ability to correctly perform range of motion exercises of the neck
- identify ways to maintain function of the remaining thyroid tissue
- state signs and symptoms to report to the health care provider
- verbalize an understanding of and a plan for adhering to recommended follow-up care including future appointments with health care provider, medications prescribed, activity level, and wound care.

□

NURSING/COLLABORATIVE DIAGNOSES

Preoperative
1. Knowledge deficit □ *859*
Postoperative
1. Impaired skin integrity:
   a. surgical incision
   b. impaired wound healing □ *860*

2. Impaired verbal communication □ *860*
3. Potential complications:
   a. hypovolemic shock
   b. respiratory distress
   c. hypocalcemia
   d. thyroid storm (excessive output of thyroid hormone)
   e. vocal cord paralysis □ *861*
4. Knowledge deficit regarding follow-up care □ *863*

Preoperative

Use in conjunction with the Standardized Preoperative Care Plan.

1. NURSING DIAGNOSIS

Knowledge deficit regarding hospital routines associated with surgery, physical preparation for a thyroidectomy, and postoperative care and management.

DESIRED OUTCOMES	NURSING ACTIONS AND *SELECTED RATIONALES*
1.a. The client will verbalize an understanding of usual preoperative and postoperative care and routines.	1.a. Refer to Standardized Preoperative Care Plan, Nursing Diagnosis 4, action a, for information to include in preoperative teaching.

1.b. The client will demonstrate the ability to perform techniques designed to prevent postoperative complications.	1.b.1. Refer to Standardized Preoperative Care Plan, Nursing Diagnosis 4, action b.1, for instructions on ways to prevent postoperative complications.
	2. Provide additional instructions on ways *to prevent complications after a thyroidectomy:*
	  a. instruct client on ways *to minimize stress on the suture line:*
	    1. support head and neck with hands when turning head and moving in bed for first few days after surgery
	    2. avoid turning head abruptly and hyperextending neck
	  b. instruct client regarding the need to do neck range of motion exercises beginning 2–4 days after surgery *in order to prevent neck contractures;* demonstrate flexion, extension, rotation, and lateral movements of head and neck.
	3. Allow time for questions, clarification, and return demonstration.

UNIT
XIV

Postoperative

Use in conjunction with the Standardized Postoperative Care Plan.

1. NURSING DIAGNOSIS

Impaired skin integrity:

a. **surgical incision;**
b. **impaired wound healing** related to inadequate nutritional status, inadequate blood supply to wound area, stress on wound area, infection, and increased levels of glucocorticoids (levels usually rise with stress).

DESIRED OUTCOMES	NURSING ACTIONS AND *SELECTED RATIONALES*

1. The client will experience normal healing of surgical wound (see Standardized Postoperative Care Plan, Nursing Diagnosis 9, outcome a, for outcome criteria).	1.a. Refer to Standardized Postoperative Care Plan, Nursing Diagnosis 9, action a, for measures related to assessment and promotion of normal wound healing.
	  b. Implement additional measures *to reduce stress on the incision:*
	  1. place client in a semi-Fowler's position with small pillow under head
	  2. maintain client's head and neck in proper alignment using pillows or sandbags
	  3. support client's head and neck during position change until client is able to do so
	  4. reinforce preoperative instructions on need to support head and neck with hands when moving and to avoid turning head abruptly and hyperextending neck
	  5. place personal articles and call signal within easy reach *so client does not have to turn or strain to reach them*
	  6. focus on deep breathing and use of inspiratory exerciser rather than vigorous coughing to promote an effective breathing pattern and airway clearance (some physicians prefer that client not cough *because it increases stress on suture line)*
	  7. stress importance of doing neck range of motion exercises gently (exercises are usually started 2–4 days postoperatively).

2. NURSING DIAGNOSIS

Impaired verbal communication related to surgical trauma to or edema surrounding the recurrent laryngeal nerve(s).

DESIRED OUTCOMES	NURSING ACTIONS AND *SELECTED RATIONALES*

2. The client will communicate needs and desires effectively.	2.a. Assess for difficulties in verbal communication (e.g. hoarseness, change in pitch of voice, complete loss of voice).
	   b. Implement measures *to facilitate communication:*
	     1. maintain a quiet environment *so that client does not have to raise voice to be heard*
	     2. ask questions that require short answers or nod of head
	     3. provide materials necessary for communication (e.g. magic slate, pad and pencil)
	     4. ensure that intravenous therapy does not interfere with client's ability to write
	     5. answer call signal promptly and in person rather than using the intercommunication system
	     6. make frequent rounds to ascertain needs
	     7. allow ample time for communication.
	   c. Inform significant others and health care personnel of approaches being used to maximize client's ability to communicate.
	   d. Assess for voice changes routinely. Report increasing hoarseness or voice loss (hoarseness is expected but should not persist for longer than 4 days).

□ ▬▬▬▬▬▬▬▬▬▬▬▬▬▬▬▬▬▬▬▬▬▬

3. COLLABORATIVE DIAGNOSIS

Potential complications:

a. **hypovolemic shock** related to hemorrhage (the thyroid gland is a very vascular organ) and fluid volume deficit (results from excessive fluid loss and inadequate fluid replacement);

b. **respiratory distress** related to airway obstruction associated with:
   1. tracheal compression resulting from edema and bleeding in the surgical area
   2. laryngeal spasm resulting from bilateral recurrent laryngeal nerve damage and tetany (occurs with marked reduction in serum calcium)
   3. aspiration;

c. **hypocalcemia** related to damage to or inadvertent removal of the parathyroid gland(s) during surgery;

d. **thyroid storm (excessive output of thyroid hormone)** related to the stress of surgery and trauma to the thyroid gland during surgery;

e. **vocal cord paralysis** related to damage to the recurrent laryngeal nerve(s) during surgery.

□ ▬▬▬▬▬▬▬▬▬▬▬▬▬▬▬▬▬▬▬▬▬▬

DESIRED OUTCOMES	NURSING ACTIONS AND *SELECTED RATIONALES*

3.a. The client will not develop hypovolemic shock (see Standardized Postoperative Care Plan, Collaborative Diagnosis 19, outcome a, for outcome criteria).	3.a.1. Assess for and report the following:
	   a. signs and symptoms of hemorrhage (e.g. increased tightness of neck dressing; complaints of fullness or pressure in neck; excessive bloody drainage on pillow, back of neck, or shoulders; decline in B/P; tachycardia; difficulty breathing; decline in RBCs, Hct., and Hgb.)
	   b. persistent vomiting
	   c. difficulty maintaining intravenous or oral fluid intake
	   d. signs and symptoms of hypovolemic shock (see Standardized Postoperative Care Plan, Collaborative Diagnosis 19, action a.3, for signs and symptoms).

2. Implement measures *to prevent hypovolemic shock:*
   a. administer fluid volume replacements as ordered
   b. perform actions to prevent nausea and vomiting (see Standardized Postoperative Care Plan, Nursing Diagnosis 7.C, action 2)
   c. perform actions to reduce stress on the surgical site (see Postoperative Nursing Diagnosis 1, action b) *in order to reduce risk of hemorrhage*
   d. when oral intake is allowed, maintain a fluid intake of 2500 cc/day unless contraindicated
   e. if signs and symptoms of bleeding occur:
      1. apply ice bag to neck
      2. prepare client for surgical intervention (e.g. ligation of bleeding vessels) if planned.
3. Implement measures to treat hypovolemic shock if it occurs (see Standardized Postoperative Care Plan, Collaborative Diagnosis 19, action a.5).

3.b. The client will not experience respiratory distress as evidenced by:
1. unlabored respirations at 16–20/minute
2. absence of stridor and sternocleidomastoid muscle retraction
3. usual skin color
4. usual mental status
5. blood gases within normal range.

3.b.1. Assess for and immediately report:
   a. increased edema or expanding hematoma in surgical area
   b. deviation of trachea from midline
   c. persistent or increased difficulty swallowing
   d. signs and symptoms of respiratory distress (e.g. rapid and/or labored respirations, stridor, sternocleidomastoid muscle retraction, cyanosis, restlessness, agitation)
   e. abnormal blood gases
   f. significant changes in ear oximetry and capnograph results.
2. Have skin clip or suture removal, tracheostomy, and suction equipment readily available.
3. Implement measures *to prevent respiratory distress:*
   a. perform actions *to minimize edema of surgical site:*
      1. keep head of bed elevated 30°
      2. apply ice bag to neck as ordered
   b. perform actions to reduce stress on incision (see Postoperative Nursing Diagnosis 1, action b) *in order to reduce risk of bleeding*
   c. if signs and symptoms of bleeding occur, loosen dressing *to promote drainage of blood and reduce the risk of respiratory distress*
   d. assess for and immediately report signs and symptoms of hypocalcemia (see action c.1 in this diagnosis) *so that treatment can be initiated and risk of laryngeal spasm reduced*
   e. perform actions to prevent aspiration (see Standardized Postoperative Care Plan, Nursing Diagnosis 18, actions d.2–6).
4. If signs and symptoms of respiratory distress occur:
   a. place client in a high Fowler's position unless he/she is hypotensive
   b. loosen dressings on neck *to prevent further compression of trachea*
   c. maintain oxygen therapy as ordered
   d. suction client if indicated
   e. assist with emergency tracheostomy if performed
   f. provide emotional support to client and significant others.

3.c. The client will experience resolution of hypocalcemia if it occurs as evidenced by:
1. usual mental status
2. regular pulse at 60–100 beats/minute
3. negative Chvostek's and Trousseau's signs
4. absence of paresthesias, muscle cramps, tetany, seizure activity
5. serum calcium level within normal range.

3.c.1. Assess for and report signs and symptoms of hypocalcemia (e.g. change in mental status; cardiac arrhythmias; positive Chvostek's and Trousseau's signs; numbness and tingling of fingers, toes, and circumoral area; muscle cramps; tetany; seizures; low serum calcium level).
2. If signs and symptoms of hypocalcemia occur:
   a. institute seizure precautions
   b. perform actions to treat respiratory distress if it occurs (see action b.4 in this diagnosis)
   c. monitor for therapeutic and nontherapeutic effects of intravenous calcium gluconate or calcium chloride if administered
   d. provide emotional support to client and significant others.
3. Once signs and symptoms of hypocalcemia have resolved, implement measures *to maintain serum calcium and phosphorus levels within a safe range:*
   a. encourage client to increase intake of foods/fluids high in calcium (e.g. dairy products) and vitamin D (e.g. fortified dairy products, egg yolk, liver)
   b. monitor for therapeutic and nontherapeutic effects of the following medications if administered:

1. oral calcium supplements and vitamin D preparations
2. phosphate-binding preparations such as aluminum hydroxide gel and aluminum carbonate *to lower elevated phosphorus level that can occur in hypoparathyroidism.*

3.d. The client will not develop thyroid storm as evidenced by:
1. stable vital signs
2. usual mental status
3. absence of nausea, vomiting, tremors.

3.d.1. Assess for and report signs and symptoms of thyroid storm:
   a. significant temperature elevation (usually above 39°C)
   b. marked increase in client's usual pulse rate and B/P
   c. increasing restlessness, agitation, irritability, and tremors
   d. nausea and vomiting
   e. delirium, unresponsiveness.
2. Minimize exposure to factors that may precipitate thyroid storm (e.g. infection, sudden increase in activity, trauma, psychological stress).
3. If signs and symptoms of thyroid storm occur:
   a. utilize hypothermia techniques (e.g. cooling blanket, tepid water bath) *to reduce fever*
   b. maintain intravenous fluid and electrolyte therapy as ordered *to correct insensible losses associated with vomiting and hyperthermia-induced diaphoresis*
   c. maintain oxygen therapy as ordered
   d. institute appropriate safety measures if client is irrational, delirious, or comatose
   e. monitor for therapeutic and nontherapeutic effects of the following medications if administered:
      1. antipyretics *to reduce fever* (avoid aspirin *because it increases free T_3 and T_4 levels*)
      2. antithyroid agents (e.g. propylthiouracil, methimazole) and iodine preparations (e.g. sodium iodide) *to suppress activity of the remaining thyroid tissue; propylthiouracil also blocks the peripheral conversion of T_4 to the more potent T_3*
      3. glucocorticoids *to aid the body in handling stress and replenish endogenous glucocorticoids that have probably been depleted by the increased metabolism (dexamethasone has also been found to inhibit thyroid gland secretions and peripheral conversion of T_4 to T_3)*
      4. adrenergic inhibiting agents (e.g. propranolol, reserpine) *to reduce the peripheral and cardiac manifestations of thyroid hormone excess*
      5. cardiac glycosides (e.g. digitalis preparations) *to strengthen myocardial contractions in order to meet the demand for increased cardiac output*
      6. vitamin supplements *to replace vitamins utilized during increased metabolism*
   f. provide emotional support to client and significant others.

3.e. The client will experience resolution of vocal cord paralysis if it occurs as evidenced by return of usual voice tone and quality by 4th postoperative day.

3.e.1. Have client speak periodically. Assess for signs of vocal cord paralysis (e.g. hoarseness, high pitch or complete absence of voice).
2. If voice changes occur:
   a. encourage client to limit verbal communication *in order to rest the vocal cords*
   b. implement measures to facilitate communication (see Postoperative Nursing Diagnosis 2, action b)
   c. reinforce physician's explanation about permanence of voice changes (voice changes are usually temporary)
   d. consult physician if signs and symptoms of vocal cord paralysis persist or worsen (hoarseness is expected but should not persist for longer than 4 days).

4. NURSING DIAGNOSIS

Knowledge deficit regarding follow-up care.

UNIT XIV

DESIRED OUTCOMES	NURSING ACTIONS AND *SELECTED RATIONALES*

4.a. The client will demonstrate the ability to correctly perform range of motion exercises of the neck.

4.a.1. Reinforce preoperative teaching about range of motion exercises of the neck. Instruct client to do the exercises 3–4 times/day for first few weeks after discharge.
    2. Allow time for questions, clarification, practice, and return demonstration.

4.b. The client will identify ways to maintain function of the remaining thyroid tissue.

4.b. Provide the following instructions on ways *to maintain function of the remaining thyroid tissue:*
    1. maintain an adequate iodine intake (use of iodized salt is usually sufficient)
    2. avoid intake of substances that inhibit thyroid activity (goitrogens) such as turnips, rutabagas, peanut skins, soybeans, and large amounts of seafood
    3. maintain a regular exercise program *(exercise stimulates the thyroid gland).*

4.c. The client will state signs and symptoms to report to the health care provider.

4.c.1. Refer to Standardized Postoperative Care Plan, Nursing Diagnosis 20, action c, for signs and symptoms to report to the health care provider.
    2. Instruct client to also report signs and symptoms of:
      a. recurrent hyperthyroidism (e.g. insomnia, heat intolerance, diarrhea, restlessness, unexplained weight loss)
      b. hypothyroidism (e.g. unexplained weight gain, persistent fatigue and weakness, drowsiness, cold intolerance, constipation)
      c. hypoparathyroidism (e.g. numbness and tingling of toes or fingers or around mouth, muscle cramping, tremors).

4.d. The client will verbalize an understanding of and a plan for adhering to recommended follow-up care including future appointments with health care provider, medications prescribed, activity level, and wound care.

4.d. Refer to Standardized Postoperative Care Plan, Nursing Diagnosis 20, for routine postoperative instructions and measures to improve client compliance.

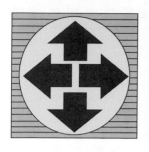

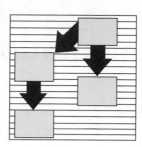
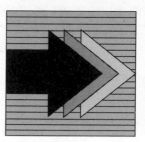
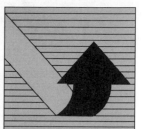

Unit XV

Nursing Care of the Client with Disturbances of Musculoskeletal Function

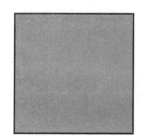
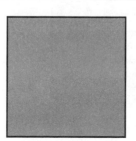

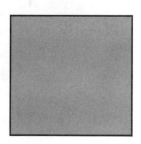

Amputation

An amputation is the removal of all or part of a limb. Amputation of the upper extremities is usually the result of trauma and tends to occur in younger people. The majority of amputations, however, are surgically performed and involve the lower extremities of persons with inadequate peripheral circulation resulting from atherosclerosis or diabetes mellitus. In these instances, amputation is considered to be a reconstructive surgery performed to improve quality of life by relieving severe, persistent discomfort. Amputation may also be indicated in the treatment of clients who have experienced severe tissue destruction as a result of mechanical or thermal trauma, cancer, uncontrollable infection, gangrene, or congenital anomalies. The two types of surgical amputations are open and closed. The open or guillotine type is used for the client with an infected limb. The wound is left open, treated until infection resolves, and then closed during a second surgical procedure. A closed amputation, which consists of soft tissue flaps sutured over the bone, is performed on the client with no evidence of infection. A disarticulation is a closed amputation of a limb through a joint.

The three basic techniques for postoperative residual limb management are the use of a soft compression dressing with delayed prosthetic fitting, casting with early prosthetic fitting, and casting with immediate prosthetic fitting. The technique selected depends on the underlying pathological condition, physiological and psychological status of the client, and his/her age.

This care plan focuses on the adult client hospitalized for a planned above the knee, closed amputation. Preoperatively, goals of care are to reduce fear and anxiety and educate the client regarding postoperative care and expectations. Goals of postoperative care are to maintain comfort, prevent complications, assist the client to adjust to the change in body image and effects of the amputation on mobility, assist with rehabilitative efforts, and educate the client regarding follow-up care.

DISCHARGE CRITERIA

Prior to discharge, the client will:

- identify ways to assess and maintain health of the remaining extremities
- demonstrate the ability to appropriately care for the residual limb
- verbalize how to appropriately care for the prosthesis
- identify ways to manage phantom limb pain
- state signs and symptoms of complications to report to the health care provider
- share feelings and thoughts about the change in body image and effects of the amputation on life style and roles
- identify community resources that can assist with home management and adjustment to changes resulting from the amputation
- verbalize an understanding of and a plan for adhering to recommended follow-up care including future appointments with health care provider, prosthetist, and physical therapist; medications prescribed; and activity level.

NURSING/COLLABORATIVE DIAGNOSES

Preoperative
1. Anxiety □ *867*
2. Knowledge deficit □ *868*
Postoperative
1. Pain:
   a. surgical pain
   b. phantom limb pain □ *869*

2. Impaired skin integrity:
   a. surgical incision
   b. impaired wound healing
   c. irritation or breakdown ☐ *870*
3. Impaired physical mobility ☐ *871*
4. Self-care deficit ☐ *872*
5. Potential for trauma ☐ *872*
6. Potential complications:
   a. hematoma formation
   b. residual limb edema
   c. necrosis of skin flap
   d. hip contractures on the operative side ☐ *873*
7. Disturbance in self-concept ☐ *874*
8. Grieving ☐ *875*
9. Knowledge deficit regarding follow-up care ☐ *876*

Preoperative

Use in conjunction with the Standardized Preoperative Care Plan.

1. NURSING DIAGNOSIS

Anxiety related to unfamiliar environment, lack of understanding of diagnostic tests, impending mutilating surgery, effects of anesthesia, and anticipated postoperative pain and effects of the amputation on usual life style and roles.

DESIRED OUTCOMES	NURSING ACTIONS AND *SELECTED RATIONALES*

1. The client will experience a reduction in fear and anxiety (see Standardized Preoperative Care Plan, Nursing Diagnosis 1, for outcome criteria).	1.a. Refer to Standardized Preoperative Care Plan, Nursing Diagnosis 1, for measures related to assessment and reduction of fear and anxiety.
	b. Implement additional measures *to reduce fear and anxiety:*
	  1. explain all diagnostic studies performed to determine adequacy of circulation in the affected leg (e.g. oscillometry, skin temperature studies, arteriography, treadmill exercise test, Doppler ultrasound, segmental blood pressure measurements, muscle perfusion studies, ^{133}xenon clearance)
	  2. reinforce physician's explanation about the level of amputation planned (level is determined by adequacy of limb circulation, requirements of planned prosthesis, and muscle balance)
	  3. encourage client to discuss feelings about the amputation and how it will change his/her life style and roles
	  4. if desired by client, arrange for a visit with an amputee who has successfully adjusted to the loss of a lower limb.

UNIT XV

2. NURSING DIAGNOSIS

Knowledge deficit regarding:

a. hospital routines associated with surgery;
b. physical preparation for the amputation;
c. postoperative care and management of the residual limb;
d. activity and exercise schedule postoperatively;
e. phantom limb phenomena.

DESIRED OUTCOMES	NURSING ACTIONS AND *SELECTED RATIONALES*
2.a. The client will verbalize an understanding of usual preoperative and postoperative care and routines.	2.a.1. Refer to Standardized Preoperative Care Plan, Nursing Diagnosis 4, actions a.1–4, for information to include in preoperative teaching. 2. Explain that limited ambulation will be encouraged within 48 hours postoperatively if a temporary prosthesis is in place. 3. Explain that turning in bed may be difficult at first until he/she adapts to the change in the body's center of gravity. 4. Allow time for questions and clarification of information provided.
2.b. The client will demonstrate the ability to perform recommended techniques to prevent postoperative complications.	2.b.1. Refer to Standardized Preoperative Care Plan, Nursing Diagnosis 4, action b.1, for instructions on ways to prevent postoperative complications. 2. Provide additional instructions on ways *to prevent postoperative complications:* a. inform client that the following precautions will need to be adhered to postoperatively *in order to prevent flexion, abduction, and/or external rotation of the hip:* 1. avoid sitting for long periods 2. avoid placing pillows under residual limb 3. maintain residual limb in proper alignment 4. lie prone for several periods during the day *to promote hip extension* b. instruct in active and isometric limb exercises *to prevent hip joint contractures.* 3. Allow time for clarification, practice, and return demonstration.
2.c. The client will demonstrate ways to improve strength and facilitate mobility postoperatively.	2.c.1. Instruct client in the following exercises performed *to improve strength and facilitate mobility postoperatively:* a. hip extension, adduction, and abduction b. range of motion and strengthening exercises for the upper extremities, chest, and abdominal muscles *to facilitate crutch walking and transfer activities.* 2. Provide instructions related to: a. use of trapeze b. transfer techniques c. use of mobility aids (e.g. crutches, walker) d. weight-bearing modifications for the affected side; emphasize that full weight-bearing will not be done until the permanent prosthesis is in place. 3. Allow time for practice and return demonstration of exercises and transfer techniques.
2.d. The client will verbalize an understanding of the prosthesis and dressings planned.	2.d.1. Reinforce the physician's explanation about the type of prosthesis and dressings planned. 2. If an immediate or early prosthetic fitting will be done: a. show client what the prosthesis will look like and how it will be held in place b. inform client that:

1. the residual limb will be wrapped with a soft material or "sock" and casted
2. the purpose of casting the residual limb *is to facilitate shaping, provide controlled pressure in order to reduce edema and support tissue, minimize pain on movement, and allow attachment of a pylon (foot and pipe)*
3. the cast will be changed as the residual limb shrinks (the first cast is usually replaced about 2 weeks after surgery).

3. If prosthesis fitting is delayed or not planned:
    a. explain that a cast or compression dressing will be applied *to support tissue, reduce edema, and promote residual limb maturation*
    b. inform client of the type and frequency of wound care.
4. Allow time for questions and clarification of information provided.

DESIRED OUTCOMES	NURSING ACTIONS AND *SELECTED RATIONALES*

2.e. The client will verbalize an awareness of phantom limb sensation versus phantom limb pain.	2.e.1. Explain the normal phantom limb sensation that is experienced by all clients after an amputation. Assure client that this sensation will serve as a proprioceptive aid when ambulating with his/her prosthesis.
	2. Reinforce the physician's explanation about the phantom limb pain that may also be experienced postoperatively. Explanation may include that:
	  a. it does not occur in all clients
	  b. it usually starts several weeks postoperatively and disappears gradually over several months to years
	  c. the type of pain experienced varies from client to client and can be very similar to pain experienced before the amputation (e.g. burning, cramping, electric shock–like, tingling)
	  d. it may be triggered by pressure on other body areas.

Postoperative

Use in conjunction with the Standardized Postoperative Care Plan.

1. NURSING DIAGNOSIS

Pain:

a. **surgical pain** related to tissue trauma and reflex muscle spasm associated with the amputation;

b. **phantom limb pain** possibly related to an interruption of the neural reflex pathways (occurs in approximately 10% of clients and may begin early in the postoperative period or several weeks later).

DESIRED OUTCOMES	NURSING ACTIONS AND *SELECTED RATIONALES*
1. The client will experience diminished pain (see Standardized Postoperative Care Plan, Nursing Diagnosis 7.A, for outcome criteria).	1.a. Refer to Standardized Postoperative Care Plan, Nursing Diagnosis 7.A, for measures related to assessment and management of postoperative pain. b. Encourage client to report phantom limb pain. c. Implement additional measures *to reduce phantom limb pain if it occurs:* 1. instruct client to apply pressure on residual limb by walking on pylon or pressing limb against a firm surface

2. consult physician about application of heat to residual limb
3. instruct client to mentally put absent limb through range of motion exercises
4. assist with a nerve block if performed.

☐ ▬▬▬▬▬▬▬▬▬▬▬▬▬▬▬▬▬▬▬▬▬▬▬▬▬▬

2. NURSING DIAGNOSIS

Impaired skin integrity:

a. **surgical incision;**
b. **impaired wound healing** related to:
1. decreased circulation to wound area associated with inadequate peripheral vascular circulation resulting from the underlying disease process, edema of residual limb, and/or excessive pressure on operative site (may be due to non-compliance with weight-bearing limitations, improper residual limb wrapping, and/or slippage of cast or compression dressing)
2. inadequate nutritional status, infection, and increased levels of glucocorticoids (levels usually rise with stress);
c. **irritation or breakdown** related to:
1. contact of skin with wound drainage, pressure from drainage tube, and use of tape
2. prolonged pressure on tissues associated with decreased mobility.

☐ ▬▬▬▬▬▬▬▬▬▬▬▬▬▬▬▬▬▬▬▬▬▬▬▬▬▬

DESIRED OUTCOMES	NURSING ACTIONS AND *SELECTED RATIONALES*

2.a. The client will experience normal healing of surgical wound (see Standardized Postoperative Care Plan, Nursing Diagnosis 9, outcome a, for outcome criteria).	2.a.1. Refer to Standardized Postoperative Care Plan, Nursing Diagnosis 9, actions a.1 and 2, for measures related to assessment and promotion of normal wound healing.
	2. Implement additional measures *to promote normal wound healing:*
	  a. perform actions to prevent residual limb edema (see Postoperative Collaborative Diagnosis 6, action b.2)
	  b. monitor for and report slippage of cast or compression dressing *(can act as a tourniquet and impede circulation)*
	  c. caution client to comply with weight-bearing limitations *in order to prevent excessive pressure on wound site and wound disruption.*
	3. If signs and symptoms of impaired wound healing occur:
	  a. prepare client for surgical revision of residual limb or wound debridement if indicated
	  b. provide emotional support to client and significant others.

2.b. The client will maintain skin integrity (see Standardized Postoperative Care Plan, Nursing Diagnosis 9, outcome b, for outcome criteria).	2.b.1. Refer to Standardized Postoperative Care Plan, Nursing Diagnosis 9, actions b.1 and 2, for measures related to assessment and prevention of skin irritation or breakdown resulting from wound drainage, drainage tubing, and tape.
	2. Implement measures *to prevent skin breakdown due to decreased mobility:*
	  a. turn client and gently massage over bone prominences and around reddened areas at least every 2 hours
	  b. lift and move client carefully using a turn sheet and adequate assistance *to prevent linen from shearing skin*
	  c. instruct or assist client to shift weight every 30 minutes
	  d. if fade time (length of time it takes for reddened area to fade after pressure is removed) is greater than 15 minutes, increase frequency of position changes and/or provide more effective methods of cushioning, padding, and positioning

e. keep skin lubricated, clean, and dry
f. keep bed linens wrinkle-free
g. provide alternating pressure or eggcrate mattress, floatation pad, sheepskin, and elbow and heel protectors if indicated
h. perform actions to increase mobility (see Postoperative Nursing Diagnosis 3, action a).
3. If skin breakdown occurs:
a. notify physician
b. continue with above measures to prevent further irritation and breakdown
c. perform wound and decubitus care as ordered or per standard hospital policy
d. monitor client closely and report signs and symptoms of infection (e.g. elevated temperature; redness, warmth, and edema around area of breakdown; unusual drainage from site).

☐ ▬▬▬▬▬▬▬▬▬▬▬▬▬▬▬▬▬▬▬▬▬▬▬▬▬▬▬▬▬

3. NURSING DIAGNOSIS

Impaired physical mobility related to:

a. pain, weakness, and fatigue;
b. depressant effects of anesthesia and some medications (e.g. narcotic analgesics, muscle relaxants, antiemetics);
c. balance difficulties associated with change in the body's center of gravity as a result of loss of a lower limb;
d. inability to control prosthesis;
e. activity restrictions imposed by the treatment plan;
f. reluctance to move associated with fear of falling.

☐ ▬▬▬▬▬▬▬▬▬▬▬▬▬▬▬▬▬▬▬▬▬▬▬▬▬▬▬▬▬

DESIRED OUTCOMES	NURSING ACTIONS AND *SELECTED RATIONALES*

3.a. The client will achieve maximum physical mobility within limitations imposed by the amputation and prescribed activity restrictions.	3.a.1. Refer to Standardized Postoperative Care Plan, Nursing Diagnosis 11, for measures related to assessing and increasing client's mobility.
	2. Implement additional measures *to increase mobility:*
	  a. perform actions to reduce pain (see Postoperative Nursing Diagnosis 1)
	  b. reinforce physical therapist's instructions on ways to adapt to the body's new center of gravity (e.g. ambulate with residual limb extended and adducted)
	  c. reinforce preoperative instructions and assist client with exercises, transfer activities, and ambulation techniques
	  d. assure client that pylon will provide adequate support during ambulation
	  e. reinforce prosthetist's instructions about control and use of prosthesis and correct gait technique
	  f. if application of a prosthesis is delayed or not planned, assist client in exercises to:
	    1. develop standing balance and strength (e.g. knee bends, standing on toes, hopping on the remaining foot while holding on to a chair, balancing on the unoperative leg without support, quadriceps- and gluteal-setting exercises)
	    2. increase strength of arm extensor and shoulder depressor muscles (e.g. pushups, use of trapeze to lift body off bed, flexion and extension of arms holding traction weights or a weighted wand, arm pulley exercises) *to facilitate crutch walking*
	    3. prevent contractures (e.g. range of motion of residual limb and unaffected extremities)

UNIT XV

g. provide support and encouragement if frustration and discouragement with lack of progress are evident.

3.b. The client will not experience problems associated with immobility.

3.b. Refer to Care Plan on Immobility for actions to prevent problems associated with immobility if client remains on bedrest for longer than 48 hours.

4. NURSING DIAGNOSIS

Self-care deficit related to impaired physical mobility associated with pain, weakness, fatigue, balance difficulties, and restrictions imposed by the treatment plan.

DESIRED OUTCOMES	NURSING ACTIONS AND *SELECTED RATIONALES*
4. The client will perform self-care activities within physical limitations and prescribed activity restrictions.	4.a. Refer to Standardized Postoperative Care Plan, Nursing Diagnosis 12, for measures related to assessment of, planning for, and meeting client's self-care needs. b. Implement measures to increase mobility (see Postoperative Nursing Diagnosis 3, action a) *in order to further facilitate the client's ability to perform self-care activities.*

5. NURSING DIAGNOSIS

Potential for trauma related to falls associated with:

a. weakness and fatigue;
b. orthostatic hypotension resulting from peripheral pooling of blood and blood loss during surgery;
c. depressant effects of some medications (e.g. narcotic analgesics, muscle relaxants) on central nervous system;
d. change in body's center of gravity resulting from loss of a lower limb;
e. difficulty with prosthesis control and transfer and ambulation techniques.

DESIRED OUTCOMES	NURSING ACTIONS AND *SELECTED RATIONALES*
5. The client will not experience falls.	5.a. Refer to Standardized Postoperative Care Plan, Nursing Diagnosis 17, for measures related to assessment and prevention of falls. b. Implement additional measures *to prevent falls:* 1. perform actions to increase client's mobility and stability (see Postoperative Nursing Diagnosis 3, action a) 2. encourage client to ask for assistance when he/she wishes to ambulate; accompany client until control of the prosthesis and transfer and ambulation techniques are mastered.

6. COLLABORATIVE DIAGNOSIS

Potential complications:

a. **hematoma formation** related to oozing from small blood vessels at surgical site;

b. **residual limb edema** related to slippage of the cast or compression dressing, inadequate residual limb bandaging, and/or prolonged dependent positioning;

c. **necrosis of skin flap** related to impaired wound healing and infection;

d. **hip contractures on the operative side** (particularly with delayed prosthesis fitting) related to poor positioning and failure to perform prescribed exercises.

DESIRED OUTCOMES	NURSING ACTIONS AND *SELECTED RATIONALES*
6.a. The client will not develop a hematoma at the operative site as evidenced by: 1. expected amount of drainage from incision and drain 2. no unusual increase in swelling and pain in operative area 3. no increase in skin discoloration at surgical site.	6.a.1. Assess for and report signs and symptoms of hematoma formation (e.g. less than expected amount of drainage from incision and drain; increased pain, swelling, and/or discoloration in surgical area). 2. Implement measures *to prevent hematoma formation:* a. maintain patency of drain (e.g. keep tubing free of kinks, empty collection device as often as necessary, maintain suction if ordered) if present b. wrap residual limb properly *so that adequate pressure is maintained to site* c. protect the residual limb from trauma. 3. If a hematoma develops, prepare client for aspiration of blood and reapplication of a pressure dressing.
6.b. The client will experience limited residual limb edema.	6.b.1. Assess for and report increasing edema of residual limb. 2. Implement measures *to prevent residual limb edema:* a. use proper residual limb wrapping technique b. maintain elevation of foot of bed as ordered c. caution client to avoid placing residual limb in a dependent position (e.g. over side of bed) for long periods d. if cast slippage occurs, immediately wrap residual limb firmly with elastic bandages and notify physician. 3. If residual limb edema becomes excessive, prepare client for and assist with recasting or reapplication of a soft compression dressing.
6.c. The client will not experience necrosis of the skin flap as evidenced by: 1. skin warm and usual color 2. no skin breakdown 3. absence of a foul odor.	6.c.1. Assess for and report signs and symptoms of necrosis of skin flap (e.g. pale, cool, darkened skin; skin breakdown; foul odor). 2. Implement measures *to prevent necrosis of the skin flap:* a. perform actions to promote wound healing (see Postoperative Nursing Diagnosis 2, actions a.1 and 2) b. perform actions to prevent and treat wound infection (see Standardized Postoperative Care Plan, Nursing Diagnosis 16, actions b.4 and 5). 3. If necrosis occurs: a. prepare client for surgical revision of the residual limb b. provide emotional support to client and significant others.
6.d. The client will not develop hip contractures on the operative side as evidenced by the ability to move the joint through its full range of motion.	6.d.1. Assess client frequently for beginning development of contractures (e.g. inability to fully extend, adduct, and/or internally rotate residual limb). 2. Implement measures *to prevent hip contractures:* a. if residual limb elevation is ordered postoperatively, place bed in Trendelenburg position rather than placing limb on pillows b. turn client to prone position at least once the 1st postoperative day, then several times daily *in order to promote hip extension;* place a pillow under abdomen and residual limb *to maintain hip extension and stretch flexor muscles*

    c. position legs close to one another in good alignment *in order to prevent hip abduction*

    d. caution client not to raise head of the bed or sit for extended periods

    e. place trochanter roll or sandbags along outer aspect of thigh when client is supine *to prevent external rotation of hip*

    f. assist client with range of motion and prescribed exercise program at least 3–4 times/day

    g. encourage crutch walking as soon as allowed and tolerated

    h. perform actions to reduce pain (see Postoperative Nursing Diagnosis 1) *in order to reduce the risk of client's flexing residual limb in response to pain.*

3. If contractures develop:

    a. assist with rehabilitative efforts to improve range of motion of hip

    b. provide emotional support to client and significant others.

☐ ▇▇▇▇▇▇▇▇▇▇▇▇▇▇▇▇▇▇▇▇▇▇▇▇▇▇▇▇

7. NURSING DIAGNOSIS

Disturbance in self-concept* related to:

a. change in appearance and perceived loss of physical attractiveness and mobility associated with loss of a limb;

b. inability to participate in usual life style and roles associated with physical limitations imposed by loss of a leg;

c. dependence on others to meet self-care needs.

---

  * This diagnostic label includes the nursing diagnoses of body image disturbance and self-esteem disturbance.

☐ ▇▇▇▇▇▇▇▇▇▇▇▇▇▇▇▇▇▇▇▇▇▇▇▇▇▇▇▇

DESIRED OUTCOMES	NURSING ACTIONS AND *SELECTED RATIONALES*

7. The client will demonstrate beginning adaptation to the loss of a lower limb and resulting changes in body functioning, life style, and roles as evidenced by:

  a. verbalization of feelings of self-worth

  b. maintenance of relationships with significant others

  c. active participation in activities of daily living

  d. active interest in personal appearance

  e. willingness to participate in social activities

  f. verbalization of a beginning plan for adapting life style to meet restrictions imposed by the loss of a lower limb.

7.a. Determine the meaning of changes in body image and functioning, life style, and roles to the client by encouraging him/her to verbalize feelings and by noting nonverbal responses to changes experienced.

b. Assess for signs and symptoms of a disturbance in self-concept (e.g. verbal or nonverbal cues denoting a negative response to changes in body functioning and appearance such as denial of or preoccupation with changes that have occurred, refusal to look at or touch residual limb, or withdrawal from significant others).

c. Implement measures to facilitate the grieving process (see Postoperative Nursing Diagnosis 8, action d).

d. Stay with the client during first dressing change *to provide support as he/she views the residual limb for the first time.*

e. Assist client to identify strengths and qualities that have a positive effect on self-concept.

f. Implement measures to assist client *to increase self-esteem* (e.g. limit negative self-criticism, encourage positive comments about self, give positive feedback about accomplishments).

g. Assist client to identify and utilize coping techniques that have been helpful in the past.

h. Clarify misconceptions about future limitations on physical activity. If appropriate, emphasize that a high degree of mobility can be achieved with a prosthesis in place.

i. Assist client with usual grooming and makeup habits if necessary.

j. Demonstrate acceptance of client using techniques such as therapeutic touch and frequent visits. Encourage significant others to do the same.

k. Assess for and support behaviors suggesting positive adaptation to changes experienced (e.g. willingness to care for residual limb, compliance with treatment plan).

l. Encourage significant others to allow client to do what he/she is able *so that independence can be re-established and/or self-esteem redeveloped.*

m. Encourage client contact with others *so that he/she can test and establish a new self-image.*

n. Assist client's and significant others' adjustment by listening, facilitating communication, and providing information.

o. Provide opportunity for client to discuss life-style changes he/she feels might be necessary as a result of the amputation. Assist him/her to explore available options.

p. Ensure that client and significant others have similar expectations and understanding of future life style.

q. Assist the client and significant others to identify ways that personal and family goals can be adjusted rather than abandoned.

r. Teach client the rationale for treatments and encourage maximum participation in treatment regimen *to enable him/her to maintain a sense of control over life.*

s. Encourage visits and support from significant others.

t. Encourage client to continue involvement in social activities and to pursue interests. If previous interests and hobbies cannot be pursued, encourage development of new ones.

u. Arrange for a visit with an amputee who has successfully adjusted to loss of a limb.

v. Provide information about and encourage utilization of community agencies or support groups (e.g. Mutual Amputee Aid Foundation; vocational rehabilitation; family, individual, and/or financial counseling).

w. Consult physician about psychological counseling if client desires or if he/she seems unwilling or unable to adapt to changes that have occurred as a result of the amputation.

8. NURSING DIAGNOSIS

Grieving* related to the loss of a limb and resulting changes in body image and usual life style and roles.

---

* This diagnostic label includes anticipatory grieving and grieving following the actual losses/changes.

DESIRED OUTCOMES	NURSING ACTIONS AND *SELECTED RATIONALES*

8. The client will demonstrate beginning progression through the grieving process as evidenced by:
a. verbalization of feelings about the loss of his/her leg
b. expression of grief
c. participation in treatment plan and self-care activities
d. utilization of available support systems
e. verbalization of a plan for integrating prescribed follow-up care into life style.
	8.a. Determine client's perception of the impact of the amputation on his/her future.
	b. Determine how client usually expresses grief.
	c. Observe for signs of grieving (e.g. changes in eating habits, insomnia, anger, noncompliance, denial).
	d. Implement measures *to facilitate the grieving process:*
	  1. assist client to acknowledge the losses and changes experienced *so grief work can begin;* assess for factors that may hinder or facilitate acknowledgment
	  2. discuss the grieving process and assist client to accept the stages of grieving as an expected response to the loss of his/her limb and anticipated life changes; support the realization that grief may recur *because of the long rehabilitation process*
	  3. allow time for client to progress through the stages of grieving (denial, anger, bargaining, depression, acceptance [Kübler-Ross, 1969]); be aware that not every stage is experienced or expressed by all individuals

4. provide an atmosphere of care and concern (e.g. provide privacy, be available and nonjudgmental, display empathy and respect) *so that client will feel free to verbalize both positive and negative feelings and concerns*
5. perform actions *to promote trust* (e.g. answer questions honestly, provide requested information)
6. encourage the expression of anger and sadness about the losses/changes experienced; recognize displacement of anger and assist client to see actual cause of angry feelings and resentment; establish limits on abusive behavior
7. encourage client to express his/her feelings in whatever ways are comfortable (e.g. writing, drawing, conversation)
8. assist client to identify personal strengths that have helped him/her to cope in previous situations of loss
9. support realistic hope about his/her ability to be successfully rehabilitated.

e. Assess for and support behaviors suggesting successful resolution of grief (e.g. verbalizing feelings about loss of the leg, expressing sorrow, focusing on ways to adapt to changes that might occur).

f. Explain the stages of the grieving process to significant others. Encourage their support and understanding.

g. Provide information regarding counseling services and support groups that might be of assistance to client in working through grief.

h. Arrange for visit from clergy if desired by client.

i. Monitor for therapeutic and nontherapeutic effects of antidepressants if administered.

j. Consult physician regarding referral for counseling if signs of dysfunctional grieving (e.g. persistent denial of loss and necessary changes in activities, excessive anger or sadness, hysteria, suicidal behaviors, phobias) occur.

☐ ▮▮▮▮▮▮▮▮▮▮▮▮▮▮▮▮▮▮▮▮▮▮▮▮▮▮▮▮▮▮▮▮

9. NURSING DIAGNOSIS

Knowledge deficit regarding follow-up care.

☐ ▮▮▮▮▮▮▮▮▮▮▮▮▮▮▮▮▮▮▮▮▮▮▮▮▮▮▮▮▮▮▮▮

DESIRED OUTCOMES	NURSING ACTIONS AND *SELECTED RATIONALES*

9.a. The client will identify ways to assess and maintain health of the remaining extremities.	9.a.1. Instruct client in ways *to maintain health of the remaining extremities:*
	  a. wear a well-fitting shoe *to protect remaining foot from pressure and trauma*
	  b. perform nail care using appropriate technique
	  c. avoid breaks in the skin *to reduce risk of infection*
	  d. stop smoking
	  e. adhere to regular follow-up care if diabetes or peripheral vascular disease was a factor leading to the need for amputation.
	2. Instruct client to report signs and symptoms of altered circulation in extremities (e.g. tingling, color changes, numbness, swelling, pallor, absent peripheral pulses).
	3. Instruct client in how to check peripheral pulses.
	4. Allow time for questions, clarification, and return demonstration.

9.b. The client will demonstrate the ability to appropriately care for the residual limb.	9.b.1. Instruct client *in ways to care for residual limb:*
	  a. inspect all aspects of residual limb daily using a hand mirror if necessary to check for redness, skin irritation, and breakdown
	  b. if the residual limb is bandaged:
	    1. reinforce preoperative teaching about the purpose of bandaging residual limb

2. instruct client and significant others in appropriate wrapping technique; stress importance of using the proper width and length of elastic wraps (usually an above the knee amputee needs three 6-inch bandages sewn together)
3. instruct client to use a clean bandage each day and rewrap the residual limb at least 4 times/day (wrap should be worn 24 hours/day until prosthetic fitting is completed and/or residual limb size has stabilized)
  c. if client has a prosthesis, instruct him/her to:
  1. wash residual limb daily using a mild soap, rinse thoroughly, and pat dry; allow the limb to air dry for at least an hour before applying prosthesis
  2. avoid use of emollients and powders on residual limb
  3. toughen residual limb once healing has taken place by massaging it, pushing it against a firm surface, or pulling on it with a hand-held towel
  4. use only residual limb socks supplied by the prosthetist; socks should be changed daily, laundered gently in cool water with a mild soap, and laid flat to dry
  5. replace worn or damaged residual limb socks; never mend them
  6. emphasize the need to monitor fit of the socket; inform client that the residual limb will continue to shrink for up to 2 years and adjustments of socket will need to be done by prosthetist as this occurs; caution client not to make even minor adjustments on his/her own
  7. caution client to follow weight-bearing limitations until healing is complete
  8. if skin breakdown occurs, avoid use of prosthesis until area has been checked by physician and/or prosthetist
  9. apply prosthesis on arising and wear for prescribed length of time *to prevent residual limb edema.*
2. Allow time for questions, clarification, and return demonstration.

9.c. The client will verbalize how to appropriately care for the prosthesis.	9.c. Instruct client in ways *to care for the prosthesis:* 1. cleanse socket daily with a damp, soapy cloth; rinse and dry thoroughly 2. do not allow leather or metal components of prosthesis to get wet 3. have prosthesis examined on a regular basis for general maintenance 4. have prosthesis readjusted if a weight loss or gain of 10 pounds occurs 5. make sure that shoes worn with prosthesis are in good repair *to avoid damage to prosthesis and gait alteration.*
9.d. The client will identify ways to manage phantom limb pain.	9.d.1. Instruct client in ways *to manage phantom limb pain:* a. apply intermittent pressure to residual limb by walking on pylon or pressing the limb against a firm surface b. mentally put absent limb through range of motion exercises c. apply moist or dry heat to residual limb d. participate in diversional activities. 2. Reassure client that phantom pain (if it occurs) should gradually disappear.
9.e. The client will state signs and symptoms of complications to report to the health care provider.	9.e.1. Refer to Standardized Postoperative Care Plan, Nursing Diagnosis 20, action c, for signs and symptoms to report to the health care provider. 2. Instruct client to report these additional signs and symptoms: a. occurrence of and/or persistent phantom limb pain b. persistent residual limb swelling c. inability to maintain balance d. difficulty controlling prosthesis e. numbness, tingling, color changes, and swelling of residual limb and/or remaining extremities f. absent peripheral pulses.
9.f. The client will identify community resources that can assist with home management and adjustment to changes resulting from the amputation.	9.f.1. Provide information about community resources that can assist the client and significant others with home management and adjustment to changes resulting from the amputation (e.g. Visiting Nurse Association; homemakers service; social services; individual, family, and occupational counseling; amputee support groups). 2. Initiate a referral if indicated.

UNIT XV

9.g. The client will verbalize an understanding of and a plan for adhering to recommended follow-up care including future appointments with health care provider, prosthetist, and physical therapist; medications prescribed; and activity level.	9.g.1. Refer to Standardized Postoperative Care Plan, Nursing Diagnosis 20, for routine postoperative instructions and measures to improve client compliance.
	2. Emphasize the importance of adhering to recommended progression of weight-bearing on residual limb.

Reference

Kübler-Ross, E. On death and dying. New York: Macmillan, 1969.

Fractured Femur with Skeletal Traction

Femoral fractures are usually a result of accidents involving severe trauma with considerable force to the femur. Reduction of the fracture may be accomplished surgically by fixation with an intramedullary nail or heavy plate (internal fixation) or nonsurgically. Following nonsurgical reduction, skin traction or, more commonly, skeletal traction is applied to immobilize the fracture segments. Fixation of the fracture segments by skeletal traction (external fixation) is accomplished by inserting a pin or wire through the proximal tibia or distal femur and attaching it to a suspension device (e.g. Thomas or Harris splint with a Pearson attachment, Neufield roller traction). Skeletal traction is often used as preliminary treatment for a fracture of the shaft of the femur until the client is able to undergo internal fixation (usually 7–10 days) or until the fracture is stable and a cast brace can be applied (usually 2–4 weeks). In persons who have complicated fractures or who are not good surgical candidates, skeletal traction may be utilized until bone healing is complete (about 8–12 weeks). The method of fracture reduction and immobilization depends on the area of the femoral shaft that is fractured, the type of fracture, the client's overall health status, and physician and client preferences.

This care plan focuses on the adult client who has sustained a fracture of the distal shaft of the femur and has been hospitalized for initial reduction and fixation of the fracture by means of skeletal traction with plans for subsequent application of a cast brace. The goals of care are to maintain comfort; prevent complications associated with the fracture, skeletal traction, and prolonged immobility; and educate the client regarding follow-up care.

DISCHARGE CRITERIA

Prior to discharge, the client will:

- demonstrate correct transfer and ambulation techniques and proper use of ambulatory aids
- demonstrate the ability to correctly perform the prescribed exercises
- identify appropriate skin care measures and ways to care for a cast brace
- state signs and symptoms to report to the health care provider

- verbalize an understanding of and a plan for adhering to recommended follow-up care including future appointments with health care provider and physical therapist, activity limitations, medications prescribed, and dietary needs.

Use in conjunction with the Care Plan on Immobility.

NURSING/COLLABORATIVE DIAGNOSES

1. Anxiety □ *879*
2. Altered nutrition: less than body requirements □ *880*
3. Pain: leg □ *880*
4. Impaired skin integrity:
   a. irritation and breakdown
   b. tearing of skin at pin or wire sites □ *881*
5. Impaired physical mobility □ *882*
6. Constipation □ *883*
7. Sleep pattern disturbance □ *883*
8. Potential for infection: injured extremity:
   a. pin site infection
   b. osteomyelitis
   c. gas gangrene
   d. tetanus □ *883*
9. Potential for trauma □ *885*
10. Potential complications:
    a. shock
    b. neurovascular damage in the injured extremity
    c. fat embolism syndrome
    d. contractures of the hips, knees, or feet
    e. delayed union or nonunion of the fractured bone
    f. malunion
    g. thromboembolism □ *886*
11. Knowledge deficit regarding follow-up care □ *889*

UNIT XV

1. NURSING DIAGNOSIS

Anxiety related to unfamiliar environment; severe pain; insertion of skeletal pin or wire; feeling of confinement; lack of understanding of diagnostic tests, treatment plan, and traction device; and fear of future disability.

DESIRED OUTCOMES	NURSING ACTIONS AND *SELECTED RATIONALES*

1. The client will experience a reduction in fear and anxiety (see Care Plan on Immobility, Nursing Diagnosis 1, for outcome criteria).	1.a. Refer to Care Plan on Immobility, Nursing Diagnosis 1, for measures related to assessment and reduction of fear and anxiety.
	b. Implement additional measures *to reduce fear and anxiety:*
	  1. perform actions to reduce pain (see Nursing Diagnosis 3, action e)
	  2. explain the skeletal pin or wire insertion procedure; assure client that adequate pain medication will be provided and that a local anesthetic will be used
	  3. explain the purpose for the traction and how it works; inform client that he/she can move freely in a balanced suspension device as long as the injured leg is kept in proper alignment
	  4. assure client that staff are knowledgeable about traction equipment
	  5. reinforce physician's explanation about the plan of treatment (e.g. skeletal traction followed by application of cast) and its effectiveness with regard to future mobility.

2. NURSING DIAGNOSIS

Altered nutrition: less than body requirements related to:

a. decreased oral intake associated with anorexia resulting from boredom, depression, constipation, pain, and early satiety (results from decreased gastrointestinal motility [slowed motility is due to decreased activity, use of narcotic analgesics, and the hypercalcemia that can develop from disuse osteoporosis]);
b. increased utilization of nutrients associated with the increased metabolic rate that occurs with healing of the fracture.

DESIRED OUTCOMES	NURSING ACTIONS AND *SELECTED RATIONALES*

2. The client will maintain an adequate nutritional status (see Care Plan on Immobility, Nursing Diagnosis 6, for outcome criteria).	2.a. Refer to Care Plan on Immobility, Nursing Diagnosis 6, for measures related to assessment and maintenance of an optimal nutritional status.
	b. Implement additional measures *to provide the nutrients and calories necessary for optimal bone healing:*
	  1. assist and instruct client to maintain a caloric intake of 3000–4000 calories/day and to increase intake of foods/fluids high in protein (e.g. meat, legumes, poultry, fish, eggs) and vitamin C (e.g. citrus fruits and juices, potatoes)
	  2. instruct client to maintain an adequate intake of calcium and vitamin D (e.g. 3 servings of fortified milk/day) but caution him/her to avoid excessive calcium and vitamin D intake *(hypercalcemia can develop as a result of disuse osteoporosis while client is immobile)*
	  3. consult physician about protein or vitamin supplements if client's dietary intake is insufficient.

3. NURSING DIAGNOSIS

Pain: leg related to fracture of the bone, soft tissue injury, and muscle spasms.

DESIRED OUTCOMES	**NURSING ACTIONS AND *SELECTED RATIONALES***

3. The client will experience diminished leg pain as evidenced by:
   a. verbalization of a reduction of pain
   b. relaxed facial expression and body positioning
   c. increased participation in activities
   d. stable vital signs.

3.a. Determine how client usually responds to pain.
   b. Assess for nonverbal signs of pain (e.g. wrinkled brow, clenched fists, reluctance to move, clutching leg, restlessness, diaphoresis, facial pallor or flushing, change in B/P, tachycardia).
   c. Assess verbal complaints of pain. Ask client to be specific about location, severity, and type of pain.
   d. Assess for factors that seem to aggravate or alleviate pain.
   e. Implement measures *to reduce pain:*
      1. maintain traction and proper alignment of extremity
      2. instruct and assist client to move carefully; obtain adequate assistance when lifting client
      3. do not remove or lift weights to facilitate lifting or other care *(a sudden reduction of traction can cause severe muscle spasm and misalignment of the fracture)*
      4. avoid bumping the skeletal pin or wire, traction device, and weights
      5. medicate prior to any painful treatments or procedures (e.g. linen changes) and before pain is severe; if client has patient-controlled analgesia (PCA) device, encourage him/her to use it as instructed
      6. provide or assist with nonpharmacological measures for pain relief (e.g. realignment, position change, relaxation techniques, transcutaneous electrical nerve stimulation, guided imagery, quiet conversation, diversional activities)
      7. monitor for therapeutic and nontherapeutic effects of analgesics and muscle relaxants if administered.
   f. Consult physician if above measures fail to provide adequate pain relief.

4. NURSING DIAGNOSIS

Impaired skin integrity:

a. **irritation and breakdown** related to:
   1. prolonged pressure on tissues associated with decreased mobility
   2. increased fragility of skin associated with dependent edema and decreased tissue perfusion resulting from decreased mobility
   3. excessive or prolonged pressure on the injured extremity from the splint device
   4. friction on elbows and unaffected heel (can occur when client pushes self up or moves around in bed);
b. **tearing of skin at pin or wire sites** related to excessive or forceful movement of the pin or wire.

DESIRED OUTCOMES	**NURSING ACTIONS AND *SELECTED RATIONALES***

4. The client will maintain skin integrity (see Care Plan on Immobility, Nursing Diagnosis 7, for outcome criteria).

4.a. Inspect the following areas for pallor, redness, and breakdown:
      1. back, coccyx, and buttocks
      2. elbows and heels
      3. groin, gluteal fold, and ischial area
      4. lateral and medial aspects of knee and ankle
      5. pin or wire sites.
   b. Use a long-handled mirror to inspect areas that may be difficult to fully visualize (e.g. buttocks, gluteal fold or groin area under ring on splint device).
   c. Refer to Care Plan on Immobility, Nursing Diagnosis 7, action b, for measures to prevent skin breakdown associated with decreased mobility.

UNIT
XV

d. Implement measures *to prevent skin irritation and breakdown underneath the splint device:*
   1. maintain proper position of the ring on the splint device *in order to keep it from slipping or causing undue pressure on any area in the groin, gluteal fold, or ischial area*
   2. perform meticulous skin care to area under ring
   3. consult physician if ring is too tight
   4. do not pad ring *(the padding often becomes wrinkled and wet, causing increased skin irritation)*
   5. maintain proper alignment of the injured extremity in the splint *in order to keep splint from putting pressure on the medial or lateral aspects of knee or ankle*
   6. keep slings on the splint and Pearson attachment dry and wrinkle-free.
e. Implement measures *to prevent skin irritation and breakdown on elbows and unaffected heel:*
   1. massage elbows and heels with lotion frequently
   2. encourage client to use trapeze to move self rather than pushing with elbows and heel
   3. reduce pressure on the unaffected heel by placing heel on a rubber glove filled with water or placing a rolled towel under ankle
   4. provide elbow and heel pads if indicated.
f. Implement measures *to prevent tearing of skin at the pin or wire sites:*
   1. consult physician if skin around pin or wire is taut *(physician may choose to incise the area because taut skin is likely to tear)*
   2. place a cork or adhesive tape over pin or wire ends *to reduce risk of having bedclothes and linens catch and pull on them.*
g. If skin breakdown occurs:
   1. notify physician
   2. continue with above measures to prevent further irritation and breakdown
   3. perform wound or decubitus care as ordered or per standard hospital policy
   4. monitor client closely and report signs and symptoms of infection (e.g. elevated temperature; redness, warmth, and edema around area of breakdown; unusual drainage from site).

□ ▬▬▬▬▬▬▬▬▬▬▬▬▬▬▬▬▬▬▬▬▬▬

5. NURSING DIAGNOSIS

Impaired physical mobility related to immobilization in traction and reluctance to move associated with pain and fear of disturbing traction and alignment.

□ ▬▬▬▬▬▬▬▬▬▬▬▬▬▬▬▬▬▬▬▬▬▬

DESIRED OUTCOMES	NURSING ACTIONS AND *SELECTED RATIONALES*

5.a. The client will achieve maximum physical mobility within limitations imposed by physical condition and treatment plan.	5.a.1. Assess for factors that impair physical mobility (e.g. traction, pain, fear of disturbing traction).
	2. Implement measures *to increase mobility:*
	  a. perform actions to reduce pain (see Nursing Diagnosis 3, action e)
	  b. reassure client that purpose of balanced suspension is to allow increased mobility while in traction
	  c. assist client with range of motion exercises to unaffected extremities at least 4 times/day.
	3. Increase activity and participation in self-care as allowed and tolerated.

5.b. The client will not experience problems associated with immobility.	5.b. Refer to Care Plan on Immobility for actions to prevent problems associated with immobility.

6. NURSING DIAGNOSIS

Constipation related to:

a. decreased intake of fluid and foods high in fiber;
b. reluctance to use a bedpan;
c. weakened abdominal and perineal muscles associated with generalized loss of muscle tone resulting from prolonged immobility;
d. decreased gastrointestinal motility (results from decreased activity, use of narcotic analgesics, anxiety, and neuromuscular depressant effects of hypercalcemia if present).

DESIRED OUTCOMES	NURSING ACTIONS AND *SELECTED RATIONALES*
6. The client will maintain usual bowel elimination pattern.	6.a. Refer to Care Plan on Immobility, Nursing Diagnosis 11, for measures related to assessment and prevention of constipation. b. Once severe pain subsides, encourage client to use nonnarcotic analgesics.

7. NURSING DIAGNOSIS

Sleep pattern disturbance related to decreased physical activity, fear, anxiety, inability to assume usual sleep position, pain, frequent assessments and treatments, and unfamiliar environment.

DESIRED OUTCOMES	NURSING ACTIONS AND *SELECTED RATIONALES*

7. The client will attain optimal amounts of sleep within the parameters of the treatment regimen (see Care Plan on Immobility, Nursing Diagnosis 12, for outcome criteria).	7.a. Refer to Care Plan on Immobility, Nursing Diagnosis 12, for measures related to assessment and promotion of sleep.
	  b. Implement additional measures *to promote sleep:*
	    1. perform actions to reduce pain (see Nursing Diagnosis 3, action e)
	    2. encourage client to be as active as possible within limitations imposed by traction:
	      a. have client perform as much of self-care as possible
	      b. consult occupational therapist regarding diversional activities that provide physical and mental stimulation.

8. NURSING DIAGNOSIS

Potential for infection: injured extremity:

a. **pin site infection** related to a break in skin integrity associated with the presence of a pin or wire;
b. **osteomyelitis** related to organisms reaching the bone through an open wound or the pin or wire sites;

UNIT
XV

c. **gas gangrene** related to growth of clostridia in a deep wound (can occur with a compound fracture);
d. **tetanus** related to growth of *Clostridium tetani* in a deep wound (can occur with a compound fracture).

☐ ███

DESIRED OUTCOMES	NURSING ACTIONS AND *SELECTED RATIONALES*

8. The client will remain free of infection in the injured extremity as evidenced by:
   a. absence of chills and fever
   b. pulse rate within normal limits
   c. absence of discoloration, swelling, and unusual odor and drainage at pin or wire sites and open wound(s)
   d. usual mental status
   e. absence of twitching or spasms
   f. WBC and differential counts returning toward normal range within 3–5 days after the injury
   g. negative cultures of pin or wire sites and wound drainage.

8.a. Assess for and report signs and symptoms of the following:
   1. infection in injured extremity:
      a. elevated temperature
      b. chills
      c. pattern of increased pulse or pulse rate greater than 100 beats/minute
      d. redness, swelling, or unusual odor or drainage at pin or wire sites or open wound(s)
      e. complaints of increased pain and tenderness in extremity
   2. gas gangrene:
      a. severe localized pain and increased swelling in injured leg
      b. change in mental status
      c. crepitation around wound site *(created by gas bubbles)*
      d. formation of bullae around wound site
      e. frothy, sweet, or foul-smelling wound drainage
      f. bronze discoloration of skin
      g. dehiscence of wound revealing dark red or black muscle tissue
      h. significant decline in B/P
   3. tetanus:
      a. muscle rigidity
      b. tonic spasms of the jaw muscles
      c. dysphagia.
   b. Monitor WBC and differential counts. Report persistent elevation or increasing values of WBC count and/or significant change in differential.
   c. Obtain culture specimens as ordered. Report positive results.
   d. Implement measures *to reduce risk of wound and/or pin/wire site infection:*
      1. instruct client and significant others to avoid touching wound and pin/wire sites
      2. place a cork or adhesive tape over pin or wire ends *in order to reduce risk of catching bedclothes and linen on the pin or wire and further traumatizing skin and underlying tissue*
      3. perform pin/wire site care according to physician's orders using sterile technique (care usually includes cleaning sites with hydrogen peroxide and applying a povidone-iodine preparation or anti-infective ointment and a sterile dressing)
      4. if client has open wounds associated with a compound fracture, perform wound care as ordered or per hospital policy using sterile technique
      5. administer tetanus toxoid and/or tetanus immune globulin as ordered (this will usually be administered in emergency room)
      6. monitor for therapeutic and nontherapeutic effects of anti-infectives if administered prophylactically.
   e. If signs and symptoms of infection occur:
      1. perform wound irrigations as ordered
      2. apply warm moist packs to infected areas as ordered
      3. prepare client for hyperbaric oxygen therapy (used in some institutions where available to treat gas gangrene and persistent osteomyelitis)
      4. prepare client for incision, drainage, and debridement of infected area if planned
      5. monitor for therapeutic and nontherapeutic effects of anti-infectives if administered
      6. if tetanus is diagnosed:

a. monitor for therapeutic and nontherapeutic effects of sedatives and muscle relaxants if administered *to control muscle rigidity*
b. monitor client closely for respiratory distress
7. provide emotional support to client and significant others.

□ ▉▉

9. NURSING DIAGNOSIS

Potential for trauma related to falls (once allowed out of bed) associated with:

a. generalized weakness and decreased muscle strength resulting from prolonged immobility;
b. pain, weakness, and decreased joint mobility in a weight-bearing extremity as a result of the bone fracture and prolonged immobilization of extremity;
c. heaviness of cast brace if present and improper transfer and ambulation techniques.

□ ▉▉

DESIRED OUTCOMES	NURSING ACTIONS AND *SELECTED RATIONALES*

9. The client will not experience falls.	9.a. Determine whether conditions predisposing the client to falls (e.g. prolonged immobility, generalized weakness, pain or limited joint mobility in the injured extremity) exist.
	b. Implement measures *to assist client to maintain muscle strength and joint mobility while in traction in order to reduce risk of falls once he/she is allowed out of bed:*
	  1. perform actions to prevent contractures (see Collaborative Diagnosis 10, actions d.2–6)
	  2. instruct client to do quadriceps- and gluteal-setting exercises as soon as allowed (usually 3–4 days after injury)
	  3. encourage client to use trapeze to lift self *(builds arm strength, which will be beneficial for crutch walking).*
	c. When traction is discontinued and client is allowed to increase activity, implement the following measures *to prevent falls:*
	  1. encourage client to request assistance whenever getting out of bed; have call signal within easy reach
	  2. reinforce physical therapist's instructions and assist with correct transfer and ambulation techniques and use of crutches or walker
	  3. instruct client to wear shoes with nonskid soles and low heels when ambulating
	  4. avoid unnecessary clutter in room
	  5. accompany client during ambulation utilizing a transfer safety belt
	  6. instruct client to ambulate in well-lit areas
	  7. do not rush client; allow adequate time for trips to the bathroom and ambulation in hallway
	  8. perform actions *to maintain strength and increase activity tolerance:*
	    a. maintain an optimal nutritional status (see Nursing Diagnosis 2)
	    b. provide adequate rest periods between periods of activity
	    c. increase activity gradually
	  9. administer prescribed analgesics at least 30–60 minutes before exercise and ambulation sessions *in order to maximize client's ability to utilize proper transfer and ambulation techniques.*
	d. Include client and significant others in planning and implementing measures to prevent falls.
	e. If falls occur, initiate appropriate first aid measures and notify physician.

UNIT
XV

10. COLLABORATIVE DIAGNOSIS

Potential complications:

a. **shock** related to severe pain and excessive blood loss (may occur because the femoral shaft is very vascular);

b. **neurovascular damage in the injured extremity** related to trauma to the nerves or blood vessels as a result of the fracture, insertion of pin or wire, and improper traction on or alignment of the injured extremity;

c. **fat embolism syndrome** related to release of bone marrow fat into the bloodstream (can occur with a fracture of a long bone) and an alteration in fat metabolism associated with trauma and stress;

d. **contractures of the hips, knees, or feet** related to improper positioning, prolonged immobility, and pressure exerted on the nerves by the traction device;

e. **delayed union or nonunion of the fractured bone** related to inadequate reduction and/or immobilization of the fracture, inadequate nutritional status, inadequate blood supply to the fracture site, or infection of the fractured bone or surrounding tissue;

f. **malunion** related to inadequate reduction or improper immobilization of the fracture;

g. **thromboembolism** related to:
   1. venous stasis associated with prolonged immobility, the inability to perform active exercises of the injured leg, and pressure exerted on blood vessels by traction device
   2. trauma to blood vessels associated with fracture.

DESIRED OUTCOMES	NURSING ACTIONS AND *SELECTED RATIONALES*

10.a. The client will not develop shock as evidenced by:
1. usual mental status
2. stable vital signs
3. skin warm and usual color
4. palpable peripheral pulses
5. capillary refill time less than 3 seconds
6. urine output at least 30 cc/hour.

10.a.1. Assess for and report conditions that may precipitate shock:
   a. severe pain
   b. bleeding (signs and symptoms include excessive blood loss from open wound; extreme swelling and/or discoloration of injured extremity; decline in B/P; increased pulse; and declining RBC, Hct., and Hgb. levels).

2. Assess for and report signs and symptoms of shock:
   a. restlessness, agitation, confusion
   b. significant decrease in B/P
   c. decline in B/P of at least 15 mm Hg with concurrent rise in pulse when client changes from lying to sitting or standing position
   d. resting pulse rate greater than 100 beats/minute
   e. rapid or labored respirations
   f. cool, pale, or cyanotic skin
   g. diminished or absent peripheral pulses
   h. capillary refill time greater than 3 seconds
   i. urine output less than 30 cc/hour.

3. Implement measures *to prevent shock:*
   a. assist with measures *to control bleeding at the fracture site* (e.g. firm pressure, tourniquet proximal to fracture site, surgical ligation of bleeding vessels)
   b. assist with measures to stabilize and immobilize fracture as soon as possible *in order to decrease pain and bleeding*
   c. perform actions to reduce pain (see Nursing Diagnosis 3, action e)
   d. maintain fluid and blood replacement therapy as ordered.

4. If signs and symptoms of shock occur:
   a. continue with above measures
   b. place client flat in bed with legs elevated unless contraindicated
   c. monitor vital signs frequently

      d. administer oxygen as ordered
      e. monitor for therapeutic and nontherapeutic effects of the following if administered:
        1. blood products and/or volume expanders
        2. vasoconstrictors (may be given for a short period *to maintain mean arterial pressure*)
      f. provide emotional support to client and significant others.

10.b. The client will maintain normal circulatory, motor, and sensory function in the injured extremity as evidenced by:
1. palpable pedal pulses
2. capillary refill time in toes less than 3 seconds
3. extremity warm and usual color
4. ability to flex and extend foot and toes
5. absence of numbness and tingling in leg and foot
6. absence of foot pain during passive movement of toes or foot
7. ability to maintain foot in proper alignment.

10.b.1. Frequently assess neurovascular status in injured extremity. Compare assessments to unaffected limb and previous assessments.
    2. Assess for and report signs and symptoms of neurovascular damage in injured extremity:
      a. diminished or absent pedal pulses
      b. capillary refill time in toes greater than 3 seconds
      c. pallor, blanching, cyanosis, or coolness of extremity
      d. inability to flex or extend foot or toes
      e. numbness or tingling in leg or foot
      f. pain in foot during passive motion of toes or foot
      g. unusual external or internal rotation of lower leg and foot.
    3. Implement measures *to prevent neurovascular damage in injured extremity:*
      a. maintain traction as ordered
      b. maintain proper alignment of injured extremity (slight external rotation is normal) in splint; if appropriate, instruct client to reposition splint by grasping both sides of the ring and shifting it into place
      c. do not allow the sling or metal parts of the splint to exert uneven or excessive pressure on any area of the leg (be especially alert to pressure on the groin, ischial area, greater trochanteric area of thigh, popliteal space, Achilles tendon, heel, and lateral and medial aspects of knee and ankle).
    4. If signs and symptoms of neurovascular damage occur:
      a. assess for and correct improper positioning of extremity, sling, or splint device
      b. notify physician if the signs and symptoms persist or worsen
      c. prepare client for surgical intervention if planned.

10.c. The client will not experience fat embolism syndrome as evidenced by:
1. usual mental status
2. absence of sudden chest pain
3. unlabored respirations at 16–20/minute
4. usual skin color
5. absence of petechiae
6. PaO_2 within normal limits.

10.c.1. Assess for and report signs and symptoms of fat embolism syndrome (usually occurs within first 72 hours after the injury):
      a. restlessness, apprehension, confusion
      b. sudden onset of chest pain, dyspnea, tachypnea
      c. pallor with subsequent cyanosis
      d. elevated temperature and pulse
      e. petechiae on the buccal membranes, conjunctival sac, face, neck, or chest (petechiae are a late sign)
      f. low PaO_2 level.
    2. Minimize movement of the fractured extremity during first few days after the injury *in order to reduce risk of fat emboli.*
    3. If signs and symptoms of fat embolism syndrome occur:
      a. prepare client for an immediate chest x-ray or lung scan
      b. obtain urine and blood specimens as ordered (*the presence of free fat globules in urine and blood helps confirm a diagnosis of fat emboli*)
      c. move client as little as possible *to prevent further embolization*
      d. implement measures *to treat the hypoxia that results with fat embolism syndrome:*
        1. administer high-flow oxygen unless contraindicated
        2. instruct client to deep breathe or use inspiratory exerciser at least every hour
      e. monitor for therapeutic and nontherapeutic effects of corticosteroids if administered *to reduce pulmonary inflammation*
      f. provide emotional support to client and significant others.

10.d. The client will maintain normal range of motion.

10.d.1. Assess for and report limitations in range of motion.
    2. Implement general measures *to prevent contractures:*
      a. maintain proper body alignment at all times

UNIT XV

b. instruct client in and assist with range of motion exercises to unaffected joints at least every 4 hours

c. encourage client to perform as much of self-care as possible

d. progress activity as allowed.

3. Place client in a flat, supine position for 30 minutes at least every 4 hours (unless physician has ordered head of bed to be elevated at all times) *in order to reduce risk of hip flexion contractures.*

4. Place trochanter roll or sandbag along outer aspect of each thigh *to prevent external rotation of the hips.*

5. Implement measures *to prevent stiffening and/or contractures of the affected knee:*
   a. maintain knee in a slightly flexed position (approximately 15°) throughout the period of immobilization
   b. begin passive and active knee exercises as soon as allowed.

6. Implement measures *to prevent footdrop:*
   a. attach a footplate to the splint device
   b. instruct and assist client to flex, extend, and rotate feet for 5–10 minutes every 1–2 hours
   c. do not allow metal frame of splint to press against lateral aspect of the knee *(exerts pressure on the peroneal nerve, which may cause footdrop).*

7. Consult physician if range of motion of any extremity becomes restricted.

10.e. The client will have normal healing of the fracture as evidenced by:
1. stability of the fracture site
2. freedom from pain when angulatory strain is applied
3. x-rays showing beginning evidence of union of the fracture.

10.e.1. Assess for and report signs and symptoms of delayed healing or nonunion of the fracture (not significant until about 4–7 weeks after the injury, when the fracture union should begin to firm up):
   a. mobility at the fracture site (indicates that union has not begun to firm up)
   b. pain upon angulatory movement of the injured leg
   c. inability to move knee.

2. Monitor x-ray results. Report findings indicating delayed healing or nonunion.

3. Implement measures *to promote healing of the fracture:*
   a. maintain alignment of extremity as ordered (leg should be in a neutral position with patella straight up or in slight external rotation *to prevent rotational deformities)*
   b. perform actions *to maintain effective traction:*
      1. keep weights hanging freely and knots away from pulley device
      2. do not allow end of splint to rest on the bed
      3. do not remove traction unless specifically ordered
      4. consult physician about a reduction of traction weight if more than 20 pounds is present after the first 24 hours (heavy traction is ordered for the first few hours to reduce overriding and is then usually reduced)
      5. encourage client to limit head of bed elevation to 20–25° when resting *in order to maintain prescribed traction force*
   c. maintain activity restrictions and reinforce importance of adhering to weight-bearing restrictions (usually full weight-bearing is not allowed until union of fracture has been confirmed)
   d. maintain an optimal nutritional status (see Nursing Diagnosis 2)
   e. perform actions to prevent and treat wound and pin/wire site infection (see Nursing Diagnosis 8, actions d and e).

4. If signs and symptoms of delayed healing and nonunion occur:
   a. continue with above measures to promote healing
   b. assist with partial weight-bearing activities as ordered *(weight-bearing stimulates osteoblastic activity and may increase circulation to fracture site)*
   c. assist with recasting if performed *(would be necessary if cast brace is not providing adequate immobilization)*
   d. assist with electrical stimulation (e.g. percutaneous stimulation, noninvasive pulsing electromagnetic fields) to fracture site if performed *to promote bone healing*
   e. prepare client for internal fixation and/or bone grafting if planned
   f. provide emotional support to client and significant others.

10.f. The client will not experience malunion as evidenced by:
1. expected alignment and movement of injured extremity
2. length of injured extremity equal to unaffected extremity
3. resolution of thigh pain.

10.f.1. Assess for and report signs and symptoms of malunion:
  a. significant (greater than 10°) internal or external rotation of the injured extremity
  b. limitation in expected range of motion of injured extremity
  c. injured extremity more than 2.5 cm (1 inch) shorter than unaffected extremity
  d. persistent pain in injured thigh.
  2. Implement measures *to prevent malunion:*
    a. perform actions to promote healing of the fracture (see action e.3 in this diagnosis)
    b. once cast brace is applied, monitor for and report poor alignment of extremity in cast.
  3. If signs and symptoms of malunion occur:
    a. prepare client for wedging of cast, recasting, or surgical realignment
    b. provide emotional support to client and significant others.

10.g. The client will not develop a venous thrombus or pulmonary embolism (see Care Plan on Immobility, Collaborative Diagnosis 14, outcomes a.1 and 2, for outcome criteria).

10.g.1. Refer to Care Plan on Immobility, Collaborative Diagnosis 14, actions a.1 and 2, for measures related to assessment, prevention, and treatment of a venous thrombus and pulmonary embolism.
  2. Implement additional measures *to prevent thrombus formation:*
    a. encourage client to be as mobile as possible within restraints imposed by traction
    b. perform actions *to reduce risk of compromising venous return:*
      1. make sure that sling and splint device are not exerting uneven or excessive pressure on any one area (be especially alert for pressure on popliteal space)
      2. do not place pillow under unaffected leg or elevate knee gatch
    c. begin active leg exercises of injured leg as soon as allowed.

11. NURSING DIAGNOSIS

Knowledge deficit regarding follow-up care.

DESIRED OUTCOMES	**NURSING ACTIONS AND *SELECTED RATIONALES***

11.a. The client will demonstrate correct transfer and ambulation techniques and proper use of ambulatory aids.

11.a.1. Reinforce instructions about correct transfer and ambulation techniques and proper use of crutches or walker.
  2. Reinforce physician's instructions about weight-bearing on injured extremity.
  3. Allow time for client to practice transfer and ambulation techniques. Reinforce teaching as necessary.

11.b. The client will demonstrate the ability to correctly perform the prescribed exercises.

11.b.1. Reinforce importance of exercise in rehabilitation process.
  2. Reinforce physical therapist's instructions regarding the prescribed exercise program.
  3. Allow time for questions, clarification, and return demonstration of prescribed exercises.

11.c. The client will identify appropriate skin care measures and ways to care for a cast brace.

11.c. Instruct client regarding ways *to care for skin and cast brace:*
  1. caution client to avoid:
    a. inserting any foreign object under cast
    b. covering cast with plastic for prolonged time
    c. removing padding from inside cast

UNIT
XV

2. encourage client to:
   a. keep cast dry; if cast becomes damp or wet, dry with a blow dryer set at a cool temperature
   b. remove easy to reach loose pieces of cast material from inside the cast
   c. keep skin around edges of cast clean and dry; apply alcohol to area daily (unless skin dryness is a problem)
   d. cover rough edges of cast with adhesive tape or stockinette.

11.d. The client will state signs and symptoms to report to the health care provider.	11.d. Stress the importance of reporting the following signs and symptoms: 1. persistent or increased pain or spasms in injured extremity 2. loss of sensation or movement in injured extremity 3. inability to maintain injured extremity in a neutral position 4. shortening of injured extremity (may be noticed as a limp once full weight-bearing is resumed) 5. excessive or unusual drainage on cast 6. foul smell from cast 7. burning or tingling sensation underneath cast 8. elevated temperature 9. areas of skin breakdown.

11.e. The client will verbalize an understanding of and a plan for adhering to recommended follow-up care including future appointments with health care provider and physical therapist, activity limitations, medications prescribed, and dietary needs.	11.e.1. Reinforce the importance of keeping follow-up appointments with health care provider and physical therapist.
	2. Reinforce physician's instructions regarding activity limitations.
	3. Encourage client to schedule periods during the day when he/she can rest with injured extremity elevated.
	4. Reinforce the need to increase intake of foods high in protein and vitamins (especially C) and maintain a sufficient calcium and vitamin D intake.
	5. Explain the rationale for, side effects of, and importance of taking medications prescribed.
	6. Implement measures *to improve client compliance:*
	  a. include significant others in teaching sessions if possible
	  b. encourage questions and allow time for reinforcement and clarification of information provided
	  c. provide written instructions regarding scheduled appointments with health care provider and physical therapist, exercise regimen, medications prescribed, and signs and symptoms to report.

Fractured Hip with Internal Fixation or Prosthesis Insertion

A fractured hip is the term used to describe a fracture of the proximal end of the femur that includes the head, neck, and trochanteric area of the femur. A fractured hip is classified according to the specific location of the fracture. An intracapsular fracture occurs in the femoral neck and may be specifically identified as a subcapital, transcervical, or basilar neck fracture. An extracapsular fracture occurs distal to the hip joint and may be classified as intertrochanteric or subtrochanteric.

A fractured hip is a leading orthopedic injury in the elderly because of the increased incidence of osteoporosis and falls in the elderly population. Although a fractured hip can be treated by traction for 8–12 weeks, the preferred treatment is surgery because it allows earlier mobility. Surgery involves internal fixation of the fracture or insertion of a femoral head prosthesis. Prosthetic devices such as an Austin-Moore or Thompson prosthesis are used to replace the femoral head and neck if the fracture occurred in the intracapsular region. If the fracture occurred in the extracapsular region, internal fixation of the fracture with pins, nails, a nail and plate device, or a compression screw device will be performed. Ideally, surgery is performed within 12–24 hours after the injury, especially if the client has a displaced femoral neck. If the client's condition is less than optimal, surgery may be delayed for 24–72 hours in order to stabilize the client's condition. During the preoperative period, traction is usually applied to stabilize and reduce the fracture.

This care plan focuses on the elderly adult client who is hospitalized for surgical repair of a hip fracture. The goals of preoperative care are to reduce fear and anxiety, maintain comfort, and prevent complications associated with the fracture and immobility. Postoperatively, the goals of care are to maintain comfort, prevent complications, assist the client to regain maximum mobility and independence, and educate the client regarding follow-up care.

DISCHARGE CRITERIA

Prior to discharge, the client will:

- verbalize an understanding of activity and position restrictions
- demonstrate correct transfer and ambulation techniques and proper use of ambulatory aids
- demonstrate the ability to correctly perform the prescribed exercises
- identify ways to reduce the risk of falls in the home environment
- share thoughts and feelings about the need to transfer to an extended care facility if planned
- state signs and symptoms of complications to report to the health care provider
- identify community resources that can assist with home management and provide transportation
- verbalize an understanding of and a plan for adhering to recommended follow-up care including future appointments with health care provider and physical therapist, medications prescribed, activity level, and wound care.

NURSING/COLLABORATIVE DIAGNOSES

Preoperative
1. Anxiety □ *892*
2. Pain: hip □ *892*
3. Impaired physical mobility □ *893*
4. Potential complications:
   a. neurovascular damage
   b. fat embolism syndrome □ *893*
Postoperative
1. Pain: hip and leg □ *895*
2. Potential for trauma □ *895*
3. Potential complications:
   a. dislocation of prosthesis or internal fixation device
   b. neurovascular damage in the operative extremity
   c. fat embolism syndrome
   d. contractures of the hips, knees, or feet
   e. delayed healing or nonunion of the fractured bone
   f. avascular necrosis
   g. malposition of the operative extremity □ *896*
4. Powerlessness □ *899*
5. Knowledge deficit regarding follow-up care □ *899*

UNIT
XV

Preoperative

Use in conjunction with the Standardized Preoperative Care Plan.

1. NURSING DIAGNOSIS

Anxiety related to unfamiliar environment; severe pain; lack of understanding of diagnostic tests, traction device, and planned surgery; anticipated postoperative discomfort and changes in life style; and possible permanent disability or death.

DESIRED OUTCOMES	NURSING ACTIONS AND *SELECTED RATIONALES*
1. The client will experience a reduction in fear and anxiety (see Standardized Preoperative Care Plan, Nursing Diagnosis 1, for outcome criteria).	1.a. Refer to Standardized Preoperative Care Plan, Nursing Diagnosis 1, for measures related to assessment and reduction of fear and anxiety. b. Implement additional measures *to reduce fear and anxiety*: 1. perform actions to reduce pain (see Preoperative Nursing Diagnosis 2, action e) 2. explain the purpose of the traction and how it works 3. assure client that staff are knowledgeable about traction equipment 4. reassure client that modern treatment methods for a fractured hip have significantly reduced permanent disability and death rates; inform client that he/she will probably begin ambulation on 3rd postoperative day.

2. NURSING DIAGNOSIS

Pain: hip related to fracture of the bone, soft tissue injury, and muscle spasms.

DESIRED OUTCOMES	NURSING ACTIONS AND *SELECTED RATIONALES*
2. The client will experience diminished hip pain as evidenced by: a. verbalization of a reduction of pain b. relaxed facial expression and body positioning c. stable vital signs.	2.a. Determine how the client usually responds to pain. b. Assess for nonverbal signs of pain (e.g. wrinkled brow, clenched fists, reluctance to move, clutching hip or thigh, restlessness, diaphoresis, facial pallor or flushing, change in B/P, tachycardia). c. Assess verbal complaints of pain. Ask client to be specific regarding location, severity, and type of pain. d. Assess for factors that seem to aggravate or alleviate pain. e. Implement measures *to reduce pain*: 1. perform actions *to maintain effective traction on the injured extremity*: a. ensure that weights are hanging freely b. do not allow footplate or ropes to rest on end of bed c. keep affected heel off bed d. keep knots away from pulley device e. do not remove traction unless specifically ordered

f. do not lift the weights in order to facilitate lifting and other care *(this reduces traction pull and can cause severe muscle spasm)*

g. limit head of bed elevation to 20–25° except for meals and toileting *in order to maintain the prescribed traction force*

2. avoid bumping the traction device
3. place a trochanter roll or sandbag firmly against the lateral aspect of injured hip and upper thigh (should extend from iliac crest to midthigh) *in order to maintain leg in proper alignment*
4. consult physician if extremity appears out of alignment; do not attempt to realign extremity *(an attempt to realign the extremity may cause further tissue injury)*
5. move client carefully, keeping injured extremity well supported
6. if turning is allowed, place pillow between legs before turning *in order to prevent adduction and further strain on the fracture site*
7. provide or assist with nonpharmacological measures for pain relief (e.g. position change, relaxation techniques, quiet conversation, diversional activities)
8. monitor for therapeutic and nontherapeutic effects of analgesics and muscle relaxants if administered.

f. Consult physician if above measures fail to provide adequate pain relief.

3. NURSING DIAGNOSIS

Impaired physical mobility related to prescribed activity restrictions, traction, and reluctance to move associated with pain and fear of disturbing the traction and alignment.

DESIRED OUTCOMES	NURSING ACTIONS AND *SELECTED RATIONALES*
3.a. The client will achieve maximum physical mobility within limitations imposed by physical condition and treatment plan.	3.a.1. Assess for factors that impair physical mobility (e.g. traction, pain, fear of disturbing traction). 2. Implement measures *to increase mobility:* 　a. perform actions to reduce pain (see Preoperative Nursing Diagnosis 2, action e) 　b. assure client that he/she can move unaffected extremities freely as long as injured hip is kept in proper alignment. 3. Increase participation in self-care activities as allowed and tolerated.
3.b. The client will not experience problems associated with immobility.	3.b. Refer to Care Plan on Immobility for actions to prevent problems associated with immobility if client remains on bedrest for longer than 24 hours.

4. COLLABORATIVE DIAGNOSIS

Potential complications:

a. **neurovascular damage** related to trauma to the nerves or blood vessels as a result of the injury; displaced bone fragments; and improper wrapping, alignment, or traction of the injured extremity;

b. **fat embolism syndrome** related to a release of bone marrow fat into the bloodstream (may occur when a long bone is fractured) and an alteration in fat metabolism associated with trauma or stress.

UNIT
XV

DESIRED OUTCOMES	NURSING ACTIONS AND *SELECTED RATIONALES*

4.a. The client will maintain normal circulatory, motor, and sensory function in the injured extremity as evidenced by:
1. palpable pedal pulses
2. capillary refill time in toes less than 3 seconds
3. extremity warm and usual color
4. ability to flex and extend foot and toes
5. absence of numbness and tingling in leg and foot
6. absence of foot pain during passive movement of toes or foot.

4.a.1. Frequently assess neurovascular status in the injured extremity. Compare assessments to the unaffected limb and previous assessments.
2. Assess for and report signs and symptoms of neurovascular damage in the injured extremity:
  a. diminished or absent pedal pulses
  b. capillary refill time in toes greater than 3 seconds
  c. pallor, blanching, cyanosis, or coolness of the extremity
  d. inability to flex or extend foot or toes
  e. numbness or tingling in leg or foot
  f. pain in foot during passive motion of toes or foot.
3. Implement measures *to prevent neurovascular damage in injured extremity:*
  a. maintain traction as ordered
  b. place a trochanter roll or sandbag firmly against lateral aspect of injured hip and upper thigh (should extend from the iliac crest to midthigh) *in order to help maintain proper alignment*
  c. do not attempt to realign injured leg unless specifically ordered *(an attempt to align extremity may cause further trauma to the nerves)*
  d. make sure elastic wraps are applied properly (if necessary to reapply elastic wraps, obtain assistance *so that one person can maintain traction on the leg during the reapplication process)*
  e. make sure that excessive or prolonged pressure is not exerted on heel and medial and lateral aspects of knee and ankle
  f. do not turn client on injured side unless specifically ordered *(may cause further displacement of fracture and decrease tissue perfusion to area).*
4. If signs and symptoms of neurovascular damage occur:
  a. assess for and correct improper positioning of the injured extremity or traction device and external causes of uneven or excessive pressure
  b. notify physician if the signs and symptoms persist or worsen
  c. prepare client for surgical intervention (e.g. internal fixation, insertion of hip prosthesis) if planned.

4.b. The client will not experience fat embolism syndrome as evidenced by:
1. usual mental status
2. absence of sudden chest pain
3. unlabored respirations at 16–20/minute
4. usual skin color
5. absence of petechiae
6. PaO$_2$ within normal limits.

4.b.1. Assess for and report signs and symptoms of fat embolism syndrome (usually occurs within first 72 hours after the injury):
  a. restlessness, apprehension, confusion
  b. sudden onset of chest pain, dyspnea, tachypnea
  c. pallor with subsequent cyanosis
  d. elevated temperature and pulse
  e. petechiae on buccal membranes, conjunctival sac, face, neck, or chest (petechiae are a late sign)
  f. low PaO$_2$ level.
2. Minimize movement of injured extremity for the first few days after injury *in order to reduce risk of fat emboli.*
3. If signs and symptoms of fat embolism syndrome occur:
  a. prepare client for immediate chest x-ray or lung scan
  b. obtain urine and blood specimens as ordered *(the presence of free fat globules in urine and blood helps confirm the diagnosis of fat emboli)*
  c. move client as little as possible *to prevent further embolization*
  d. implement measures *to treat the hypoxia that results with fat embolism syndrome:*
    1. administer high-flow oxygen unless contraindicated
    2. instruct client to deep breathe or use inspiratory exerciser at least every hour
  e. monitor for therapeutic and nontherapeutic effects of corticosteroids if administered *to reduce pulmonary inflammation*
  f. provide emotional support to client and significant others.

Postoperative

Use in conjunction with the Standardized Postoperative Care Plan.

1. NURSING DIAGNOSIS

Pain: hip and leg related to tissue trauma and reflex muscle spasm associated with the surgery and poor alignment of the extremity postoperatively.

DESIRED OUTCOMES	NURSING ACTIONS AND *SELECTED RATIONALES*

1. The client will experience diminished hip and leg pain (see Standardized Postoperative Care Plan, Nursing Diagnosis 7.A, for outcome criteria).	1.a. Refer to Standardized Postoperative Care Plan, Nursing Diagnosis 7.A, for measures related to assessment and reduction of pain.
	 b. Implement additional measures *to reduce pain in operative extremity:*
	   1. maintain extremity in proper alignment by placing trochanter roll or sandbag along lateral and medial aspects of thigh and lower leg (make sure excessive pressure is not exerted on medial and lateral aspects of knee and ankle)
	   2. keep pillows between legs while in a side-lying position *in order to prevent adduction and the resultant strain on surgical site*
	   3. move the operative extremity gently.

2. NURSING DIAGNOSIS

Potential for trauma related to falls associated with:

a. weakness, fatigue, and orthostatic hypotension resulting from the effects of major surgery and physiological changes that occur with aging;
b. central nervous system depressant effects of some medications (e.g. narcotic analgesics, muscle relaxants);
c. weakness and pain in weight-bearing extremity as a result of the surgery;
d. improper transfer and ambulation techniques.

DESIRED OUTCOMES	NURSING ACTIONS AND *SELECTED RATIONALES*
2. The client will not experience falls.	2.a. Determine whether conditions predisposing client to falls (e.g. weakness, fatigue, advanced age, orthostatic hypotension, use of narcotic analgesics or muscle relaxants) exist. b. Refer to Standardized Postoperative Care Plan, Nursing Diagnosis 17, action b, for measures to prevent falls.

UNIT
XV

    c. Implement additional measures *to reduce risk of falls:*
      1. perform actions *to assist client to increase muscle strength:*
        a. instruct and encourage client to perform isometric quadriceps, gluteal, and abdominal exercises
        b. reinforce physical therapist's instructions and assist client with muscle strengthening exercises (usually started 2–3 days after surgery)
        c. encourage client to use the trapeze to lift self *(strengthens arm muscles, which will facilitate use of crutches or walker)*
      2. reinforce physical therapist's instructions regarding correct transfer and ambulation techniques and proper use of ambulatory aids (e.g. crutches, walker)
      3. administer prescribed analgesics at least 30–60 minutes before exercise and ambulation sessions *in order to maximize client's ability to utilize proper transfer and ambulation techniques.*
    d. Include client and significant others in planning and implementing measures to prevent falls.
    e. If falls occur, initiate appropriate first aid measures and notify physician.

3. COLLABORATIVE DIAGNOSIS

Potential complications:

a. **dislocation of prosthesis or internal fixation device** related to improper positioning of operative extremity or early weight-bearing;
b. **neurovascular damage in the operative extremity** related to trauma to the nerves or blood vessels as a result of the surgery, blood accumulation and edema in surgical area, improper alignment of operative extremity, and dislocation of the prosthesis or internal fixation device postoperatively;
c. **fat embolism syndrome** related to a release of bone marrow fat into the bloodstream (may occur when a long bone is fractured) and an alteration in fat metabolism associated with trauma and stress;
d. **contractures of the hips, knees, or feet** related to improper positioning and decreased mobility;
e. **delayed healing or nonunion of the fractured bone** related to an inadequate blood supply to the fracture site, inadequate nutritional status, and wound infection;
f. **avascular necrosis** related to an inadequate blood supply to the bone (occurs primarily following intracapsular fractures);
g. **malposition of the operative extremity** related to improper alignment.

DESIRED OUTCOMES	NURSING ACTIONS AND *SELECTED RATIONALES*

3.a. The client will not experience dislocation of the prosthesis or internal fixation device as evidenced by:
1. continued resolution of hip pain
2. ability to maintain operative leg in proper alignment
	3.a.1. Assess for and report signs and symptoms of dislocation of the hip prosthesis or internal fixation device:
	  a. sudden, severe pain in operative hip
	  b. significant (greater than 10°) external or internal rotation of the operative leg
	  c. sudden inability to participate in usual exercise and ambulation regimen
	  d. decline in neurovascular status in operative leg.
	  2. If a prosthesis was inserted, implement measures *to prevent its dislocation:*
	    a. perform actions *to maintain operative extremity in proper alignment:*

3. ability to adhere to exercise and ambulation regimen

4. normal neurovascular status in operative leg.

1. place a trochanter roll or sandbag on lateral side of thigh and calf (should not press on the lateral calf immediately below the knee and on the lateral malleolus) *in order to prevent external rotation* (important when anterolateral approach used)

2. place a pillow, sandbag, or trochanter roll along medial side of the operative leg (should not press on medial aspect of knee and ankle) *in order to prevent internal rotation*

3. instruct client not to rotate leg internally or externally

b. maintain restrictions on head of bed elevation as ordered (some physicians order a 45–60° maximum elevation for first 2–3 days after surgery) *in order to prevent excessive hip flexion*

c. perform actions *to prevent extreme (beyond 90°) hip flexion:*
   1. instruct client not to lean forward to reach objects on end of bed or on floor or to put on slippers, socks, or shoes
   2. raise the entire bed to client's midthigh level before he/she gets in or out of bed *in order to reduce the degree of hip flexion that occurs when client sits on edge of bed*
   3. provide a high, firm chair (or elevate sitting surface with pillows) and raised toilet seat for client's use *in order to reduce degree of hip flexion when client sits down*
   4. do not elevate operative leg when sitting in chair

d. perform actions *to prevent adduction of the operative extremity:*
   1. keep 2–3 pillows or abductor device between legs at all times
   2. remind client not to cross legs
   3. do not move operative extremity past midline

e. do not turn client on operative side unless orders specify to do so

f. reinforce importance of adhering to recommended weight-bearing restrictions (partial weight-bearing is usually allowed as soon as ambulation is started).

3. If internal fixation of the fracture was performed, implement measures *to prevent dislocation of the internal fixation device:*

a. perform actions to prevent extreme hip flexion and adduction (see actions a.2.c and d in this diagnosis)

b. place pillow, sandbag, or trochanter roll along medial thigh and calf of operative extremity *to prevent internal rotation*

c. reinforce weight-bearing limitations as ordered (weight-bearing restrictions following internal fixation vary but often progress from no weight-bearing initially to partial weight-bearing before discharge and resumption of full weight-bearing after about 10 weeks)

d. turn client only as ordered (usually allowed to turn on unoperative side only) and always with pillows between legs

e. perform actions to promote healing of fracture (see action e.2 in this diagnosis).

4. If signs and symptoms of dislocation of prosthesis or internal fixation device occur:

a. maintain client on bedrest

b. prepare client for x-rays of surgical area

c. prepare client for closed reduction or surgical repair of the dislocation if planned

d. provide emotional support to client and significant others.

3.b. The client will maintain normal circulatory, motor, and sensory function in the operative extremity (see Preoperative Collaborative Diagnosis 4, outcome a, for outcome criteria).

3.b.1. Refer to Preoperative Collaborative Diagnosis 4, actions a.1 and 2, for measures related to assessment of neurovascular status in operative extremity.

2. Implement measures *to prevent neurovascular damage in operative extremity:*
   a. maintain extremity in proper alignment
   b. perform actions to prevent dislocation of prosthesis or internal fixation device (see actions a.2 and 3 in this diagnosis)
   c. consult physician about application of ice to surgical site if edema develops.

3. If signs and symptoms of neurovascular damage occur:
   a. assess for and correct improper positioning of operative extremity; do not attempt realignment if extreme rotation has occurred
   b. notify physician if the signs and symptoms persist or worsen
   c. prepare client for closed reduction or return to surgery if planned.

UNIT XV

3.c. The client will not experience fat embolism syndrome (see Preoperative Collaborative Diagnosis 4, outcome b, for outcome criteria).

3.c. Refer to Preoperative Collaborative Diagnosis 4, action b, for measures related to assessment, prevention, and treatment of fat embolism syndrome.

3.d. The client will maintain normal range of motion.

3.d.1. Assess for and report limitations in range of motion.
   2. Implement general measures *to prevent contractures:*
      a. maintain proper body alignment at all times
      b. instruct client in and assist with range of motion and muscle strengthening exercises of unaffected extremities at least every 4 hours
      c. encourage client to perform as much of self-care as possible
      d. progress activity as allowed.
   3. Implement measures *to reduce risk of hip and knee contractures:*
      a. place client in a flat, supine position for 30 minutes at least every 4 hours
      b. as activity progresses, limit the length of time client is in a high Fowler's position or chair (usually no longer than an hour at a time)
      c. avoid use of the knee gatch or pillows under knees
      d. assist with ambulation training as soon as allowed (usually 3–5 days after surgery)
      e. when client is in a supine position, place trochanter roll or sandbag along outer aspect of each thigh *to prevent external rotation of the hips.*
   4. Implement measures *to prevent footdrop:*
      a. instruct and assist client to flex, extend, and rotate feet for 5–10 minutes every 1–2 hours
      b. perform actions to prevent neurovascular damage in the operative extremity (see action b.2 in this diagnosis)
      c. use a footboard, sandbags, pillows, high-topped tennis shoes, foam boots, or foot positioners if necessary *to keep feet in a neutral or slightly dorsiflexed position*
      d. keep bed linen from exerting excessive pressure on toes and feet.
   5. Consult physician if range of motion of any extremity becomes more restricted.

3.e. The client will not experience avascular necrosis or delayed healing or nonunion of the fracture as evidenced by:
   1. resolution of hip pain and muscle spasms
   2. proper alignment of operative extremity
   3. expected progression in prescribed physiotherapy program
   4. x-rays showing evidence of union of fracture.

3.e.1. Assess for and report signs and symptoms of avascular necrosis and delayed healing or nonunion of the fracture:
      a. persistent hip pain and muscle spasms
      b. inability to maintain operative leg in proper alignment
      c. inability to make expected progress in physical therapy program
      d. x-rays showing delayed healing or nonunion of fracture.
   2. Implement measures *to promote healing of the fracture:*
      a. maintain operative leg in proper alignment
      b. maintain restrictions on weight-bearing as ordered
      c. maintain an optimal nutritional status (see Standardized Postoperative Care Plan, Nursing Diagnosis 6, action f)
      d. encourage client to consume foods/fluids high in calcium and vitamin D (e.g. fortified dairy products)
      e. perform actions to prevent and treat wound infection (see Standardized Postoperative Care Plan, Collaborative Diagnosis 16, actions b.4 and 5)
      f. monitor for therapeutic and nontherapeutic effects of supplemental calcium and vitamin D if administered.
   3. If signs and symptoms of avascular necrosis or delayed healing or nonunion of the fracture occur:
      a. continue with above measures to promote healing
      b. assist with electrical stimulation (e.g. percutaneous stimulation, noninvasive pulsing electromagnetic fields) to fracture site if performed *to promote healing*
      c. prepare client for surgical intervention (e.g. bone grafting, prosthesis insertion or replacement) if indicated
      d. provide emotional support to client and significant others.

3.f. The client will not experience malposition of

3.f.1. Assess for and report signs and symptoms of malposition of the operative extremity:

the operative extremity as evidenced by:
1. normal alignment and movement of the extremity
2. length of operative extremity equal to unoperative extremity
3. resolution of hip pain.

   a. significant (greater than 10°) internal or external rotation of the extremity
   b. limitation in expected range of motion of hip
   c. operative extremity more than 2.5 cm (1 inch) shorter than unoperative extremity
   d. persistent hip pain.
2. Implement measures *to prevent malposition of operative extremity:*
   a. maintain proper alignment of extremity
   b. reinforce the importance of not bearing weight on extremity until allowed (particularly important after internal fixation)
   c. perform additional actions to promote healing (see actions e.2.c–f in this diagnosis).
3. If signs and symptoms of malposition of the operative extremity occur:
   a. prepare client for closed reduction or surgical realignment
   b. provide emotional support to client and significant others.

4. NURSING DIAGNOSIS

Powerlessness related to temporary physical limitations, dependence on others to meet basic needs, and possible change in roles and future living situation.

DESIRED OUTCOMES	NURSING ACTIONS AND *SELECTED RATIONALES*
4. The client will demonstrate increasing feelings of control over his/her situation as evidenced by: a. verbalization of same b. active participation in planning of care and decision making regarding future living situation c. participation in self-care activities within physical limitations.	4.a. Assess for feelings of powerlessness (e.g. verbalization of lack of control, anger, apathy, hostility, lack of participation in self-care or discharge planning). b. Obtain information from client and significant others regarding client's usual response to situations in which client has had limited control (e.g. loss of job, financial stress). c. Encourage client to verbalize feelings about self, current situation, and possible changes in roles and living situation (e.g. transfer to an extended care facility, need for a live-in attendant, move to another person's home). Focus on the positive aspects of the planned living arrangement changes. d. Reinforce physician's explanations about the hip surgery and rehabilitation plan. e. Support realistic hope about effects of rehabilitation and probability of future independence. f. Remind client of his/her right to ask questions about condition and treatment regimen. g. Include client in planning of care, encourage maximum participation in the treatment plan, and allow choices whenever possible *to enable him/her to maintain a sense of control.* h. Encourage significant others to allow client to do as much as he/she is able *so that a feeling of independence can be maintained.* i. Assist client to establish realistic short- and long-term goals. j. Provide continuity of care through written care plans *to ensure that client can maintain control over his/her situation.*

UNIT
XV

5. NURSING DIAGNOSIS

Knowledge deficit regarding follow-up care.

DESIRED OUTCOMES	NURSING ACTIONS AND *SELECTED RATIONALES*

5.a. The client will verbalize an understanding of activity and position restrictions.	5.a. Provide instructions about restrictions on activities and positioning (restrictions are necessary for 2 months to a year depending on client condition, surgical procedure, and physician preference):
	  1. turn only as directed by physician (many physicians allow turning to unoperative side only and instruct client to keep pillows between legs while on side)
	  2. never cross legs
	  3. do not sit on low chairs, stools, or toilets; place a cushion on low chairs, rent or purchase a raised toilet seat for home use, and use the high toilets designed for the handicapped when in public facilities
	  4. do not elevate operative leg when sitting
	  5. sit in chairs with arms and utilize the arms to raise self off chair
	  6. support weight on unoperative leg when raising self from a sitting position
	  7. do not sit for more than 1 hour at a time
	  8. do not bend down to reach objects on the floor or in low cupboards or drawers
	  9. do not reach to end of bed to pull covers up
	  10. do not put on shoes or socks without using an adaptive device (e.g. long-handled shoehorn)
	  11. keep operative leg in proper alignment and avoid turning the hip and knee inward or outward
	  12. when riding in a car:
	    a. sit on a firm pillow or cushion *to prevent hip flexion of more than 90°*
	    b. keep operative leg extended *(a sudden impact of the knee against the dashboard can dislodge the prosthesis)*
	  13. do not resume sexual activity until approved by physician
	  14. when sexual activity is resumed, avoid positions that involve turning knee and hip inward, flexing hip beyond 90°, and moving operative leg past the midline
	  15. avoid lifting heavy objects, excessive twisting and turning of body, and activities that place excessive strain on hip (e.g. jogging).

5.b. The client will demonstrate correct transfer and ambulation techniques and proper use of ambulatory aids.	5.b.1. Reinforce instructions about correct transfer and ambulation techniques, amount of weight-bearing allowed, and proper use of ambulatory aids (a walker is preferable for most of these clients *because it provides the greatest stability*). 2. Allow time for questions, clarification, and practice of transfer and ambulation techniques.

5.c. The client will demonstrate the ability to correctly perform the prescribed exercises.	5.c.1. Reinforce instructions on muscle strengthening and range of motion exercises.
	  2. Explain importance of continuing muscle strengthening and range of motion exercises 3–4 times/day.
	  3. Allow time for questions, clarification, and return demonstration of prescribed exercises.

5.d. The client will identify ways to reduce the risk of falls in the home environment.	5.d. If client is to return home, provide the following instructions on how to reduce risk of falls at home:
	  1. keep electrical cords out of pathways
	  2. remove unnecessary furniture and provide wide pathways for ambulation
	  3. remove scatter rugs
	  4. provide adequate lighting at all times
	  5. do not climb stairs until permission is given by physician
	  6. allow ample time for activities.

5.e. The client will state signs and symptoms of complications to report to the health care provider.	5.e.1. Refer to Standardized Postoperative Care Plan, Nursing Diagnosis 20, action c, for signs and symptoms to report to the health care provider.
	  2. Instruct client to report these additional signs and symptoms:
	    a. persistent or increased pain or spasms in operative extremity

b. loss of sensation or movement in operative extremity
c. inability to maintain operative extremity in a neutral position
d. inability to bear weight on operative extremity once weight-bearing is allowed
e. shortening of operative extremity (will probably be noticed as a limp once full weight-bearing is resumed).

5.f. The client will identify community resources that can assist with home management and provide transportation.	5.f.1. Provide information about community resources that can assist the client and significant others with home management and provide transportation (e.g. Visiting Nurse Association, home health agencies, Meals on Wheels, church groups, transportation services). 2. Initiate a referral if indicated.
5.g. The client will verbalize an understanding of and a plan for adhering to recommended follow-up care including future appointments with health care provider and physical therapist, medications prescribed, activity level, and wound care.	5.g.1. Refer to Standardized Postoperative Care Plan, Nursing Diagnosis 20, for routine postoperative instructions and measures to improve client compliance. 2. Reinforce the importance of keeping appointments with physical therapist.

■ ■

Laminectomy/Discectomy with or without Fusion

A laminectomy is the surgical removal of the lamina of a vertebra. It may be performed to allow the removal of a neoplasm or bone fragments that are putting pressure on spinal nerve roots or the spinal cord or to enable a rhizotomy or cordotomy to be performed to treat intractable pain. Most commonly, a laminectomy or a laminotomy (the surgical division of the lamina of a vertebra) is performed to gain access to a herniated nucleus pulposus ("ruptured disc") so that a discectomy (removal of the herniated portion of the disc) can be accomplished. A disc herniation is usually the result of degenerative changes in the vertebrae and supporting ligaments or trauma to the vertebrae due to falls, motor vehicle accidents, or continued use of poor body mechanics. It occurs most frequently in the cervical interspaces (particularly C5–6 and C6–7) and lumbar interspaces (particularly L4–5 and L5–S1). A discectomy is usually indicated if conservative measures fail to control discomfort, neurological impairments persist or worsen, and/or chemonucleolysis (injection of chymopapain into the nucleus pulposus of the herniated disc) is contrain-

dicated or unsuccessful in reducing the size of the protruding disc. The disc removal can be accomplished in conjunction with a laminotomy or laminectomy as noted previously or, in some instances, microdiscectomy is possible. If more than two herniated discs are removed or if the spinal column is unstable, a fusion may be performed using metal rods or wires or, more commonly, a bone graft from the iliac crest.

This care plan focuses on the adult client hospitalized for a laminectomy* that is being performed to remove a herniated nucleus pulposus that has not responded to conservative management. Preoperatively, goals of care are to reduce discomfort and educate the client regarding postoperative management. Postoperative goals of care are to maintain comfort, prevent complications, and educate the client regarding follow-up care.

---

* The care of a client hospitalized for a laminectomy/discectomy with fusion is also discussed. If a fusion is performed and activity is limited for longer than 48 hours, refer to the Care Plan on Immobility.

UNIT
XV

DISCHARGE CRITERIA

Prior to discharge, the client will:

- identify ways to prevent recurrent disc herniation
- demonstrate the ability to correctly apply and remove a brace, cast, or collar if one is required
- verbalize an understanding of ways to maintain skin integrity when wearing a brace, cast, or collar
- state signs and symptoms of complications to report to the health care provider
- verbalize an understanding of and a plan for adhering to recommended follow-up care including future appointments with health care provider, medications prescribed, activity level, and wound care.

NURSING/COLLABORATIVE DIAGNOSES

Preoperative
1. Altered comfort:
   a. pain
   b. paresthesias (burning, numbness, and tingling) □ *903*
2. Knowledge deficit □ *904*
Postoperative
1. Altered comfort:
   a. pain
   b. paresthesias (burning, numbness, and tingling) □ *905*
2. Impaired skin integrity:
   a. surgical incision
   b. impaired wound healing
   c. irritation and breakdown □ *906*
3. Urinary retention □ *907*
4. Potential complications:
   a. respiratory distress
   b. neurovascular damage
   c. development of cerebrospinal fistula
   d. vocal cord paralysis
   e. paralytic ileus □ *907*
5. Knowledge deficit regarding follow-up care □ *910*

Preoperative

Use in conjunction with the Standardized Preoperative Care Plan.

1. NURSING DIAGNOSIS

Altered comfort:*

a. **pain** related to muscle spasm and irritation of the spinal nerve roots associated with pressure from the herniated nucleus pulposus and inflammation;

b. **paresthesias (burning, numbness, and tingling)** related to irritation of the spinal nerve roots associated with pressure from the herniated nucleus pulposus and inflammation.

---

* In this care plan, the nursing diagnosis "pain" is included under the diagnostic label of altered comfort.

DESIRED OUTCOMES	NURSING ACTIONS AND *SELECTED RATIONALES*

1. The client will experience diminished pain, burning, numbness, and tingling as evidenced by:
a. verbalization of same
b. relaxed facial expression and body positioning
c. stable vital signs.
	1.a. Determine how client usually responds to pain.
	b. Assess for nonverbal signs of discomfort (e.g. wrinkled brow, rubbing lower back and hips or neck and shoulders, clenched fists, guarding of affected extremity, reluctance to move, restlessness, diaphoresis, facial pallor or flushing, change in B/P, tachycardia).
	c. Assess verbal complaints of discomfort. Ask client to be specific about location, severity, and type of discomfort (clients with lumbar disc herniation usually complain of muscle spasm and pain in lower back and hips and pain, numbness, or tingling in the affected lower extremity; clients with cervical disc herniation usually complain of pain and muscle spasm in back of neck and shoulders and pain, numbness, or tingling in the affected arm and fingers).
	d. Assess for factors that seem to aggravate and alleviate discomfort.
	e. Implement measures *to reduce discomfort:*
	  1. perform actions *to reduce stress on the affected area:*
	    a. provide a firm mattress or place a bed board under mattress for added support
	    b. maintain activity restrictions (activity is usually limited to bedrest with bathroom privileges)
	    c. instruct client to avoid lying in prone position
	    d. if client has cervical disc herniation, instruct him/her to:
	      1. keep head of bed flat or just slightly elevated except for meals and snacks
	      2. use a flat rather than thick pillow under head *in order to prevent flexion of the neck*
	      3. avoid flexing or hyperextending neck
	      4. move entire upper body rather than just neck when turning head
	    e. if client has lumbar disc herniation:
	      1. elevate head of bed about 30–45° and use knee gatch to maintain knees in a slightly flexed position *in order to reduce tension on lumbar area by flattening the lumbosacral curve*
	      2. instruct client to avoid twisting or sudden turning
	    f. provide client with a firm, straight-backed arm chair to sit on

UNIT XV

g. maintain pelvic or cervical traction if ordered *to keep the affected area in proper alignment and reduce pressure on spinal nerve roots*

h. assist client to apply a corset, brace, or cervical collar if ordered *to maintain proper alignment of and provide additional support to the affected area of the spine*

i. implement measures *to keep client from bending, twisting, and turning* (e.g. keep personal articles within easy reach, assist him/her to put on shoes or slippers)

j. instruct client to avoid coughing, sneezing, or straining to have a bowel movement; consult physician about an order for an antitussive, decongestant, laxative, or stool softener if indicated

2. consult physician about application of a heating pad, moist hot pack, or ice pack to lumbar or cervical spine area

3. consult physician regarding an order for ultrasonic heat treatment, diathermy, and/or massage

4. use a bed cradle *to keep weight of the covers off any areas of paresthesia*

5. provide or assist with nonpharmacological measures for relief of discomfort (e.g. back rub, position change, relaxation techniques, transcutaneous electrical nerve stimulation, guided imagery, quiet conversation, restful environment, diversional activities)

6. monitor for therapeutic and nontherapeutic effects of the following medications if administered:
   a. analgesics
   b. muscle relaxants
   c. anti-inflammatory agents *to reduce inflammation of and around the nerve root.*

f. Consult physician if above measures fail to provide adequate pain relief.

---

2. NURSING DIAGNOSIS

Knowledge deficit regarding hospital routines associated with surgery, physical preparation for laminectomy/discectomy and/or spinal fusion, and postoperative care and management.

DESIRED OUTCOMES	NURSING ACTIONS AND *SELECTED RATIONALES*

2.a. The client will verbalize an understanding of usual preoperative and postoperative care and routines.

2.a.1. Refer to Standardized Preoperative Care Plan, Nursing Diagnosis 4, actions a.1–4, for information to include in preoperative teaching.

2. Provide additional information regarding preoperative and postoperative care for clients having a laminectomy/discectomy:

a. explain that client may begin progressive activity the evening of or morning after surgery (depending on physician preference)

b. if a laminectomy with fusion is planned, inform client that:
   1. progressive activity will usually begin between 3–7 days after surgery depending on physician preference and extensiveness of surgery
   2. after surgery a brace or cast must be worn *to provide additional stability to the spine* (the stabilizing device may need to be worn during activity for up to 6 months)
   3. there will be an incision in the hip area (if bone graft is taken from the iliac crest) in addition to the lower back or neck incision

c. explain to client that the pain he/she is experiencing preoperatively will probably still be present postoperatively due to nerve irritation and edema resulting from the surgery; assure him/her that the presence of pain does not indicate that the surgery was unsuccessful

d. explain that a physical therapist may come to instruct the client about the postoperative exercise plan.

3. Allow time for questions and clarification of information provided.

2.b. The client will demonstrate the ability to perform techniques designed to prevent postoperative complications.

2.b.1. Refer to Standardized Preoperative Care Plan, Nursing Diagnosis 4, action b.1, for instructions on ways to prevent postoperative complications.

2. Provide additional instructions about ways *to prevent postoperative complications:*

a. instruct client how to logroll and stress the importance of turning in this manner for at least 48 hours after surgery (the length of time increases if a fusion was performed)

b. instruct client to avoid flexing, hyperextending, turning, and twisting the cervical or lumbar spine postoperatively

c. demonstrate the correct way to change from a lying to standing position (e.g. keep spine in proper alignment, utilize arm and leg muscles)

d. reinforce physician's or physical therapist's instructions about exercises to strengthen arms, legs, and abdomen *(increased strength of these areas decreases strain on the spine)*

e. if client is expected to have a brace or cast postoperatively, obtain it preoperatively *in order to check for proper fit and allow time for client to practice putting it on, taking it off, and moving around in it* (the cast is made in 2 sections and client will "sandwich" self between the sections and fasten them together with straps).

3. Allow time for questions, clarification, and return demonstration.

Postoperative

Use in conjunction with the Standardized Postoperative Care Plan.

1. NURSING DIAGNOSIS

Altered comfort:*

a. **pain** related to tissue trauma, reflex muscle spasm, and irritation of and pressure on the spinal nerve roots associated with surgical trauma and inflammation;

b. **paresthesias (burning, numbness, and tingling)** related to irritation of and pressure on the spinal nerve roots associated with surgical trauma and inflammation.

---

* In this care plan, the nursing diagnosis "pain" is included under the diagnostic label of altered comfort.

UNIT XV

DESIRED OUTCOMES	NURSING ACTIONS AND *SELECTED RATIONALES*
1. The client will experience diminished pain, burning, numbness, and tingling as evidenced by:	1.a. Refer to Standardized Postoperative Care Plan, Nursing Diagnosis 7.A, for measures related to assessment and management of pain. b. Implement additional measures *to reduce discomfort:* 1. perform actions *to reduce strain on the surgical area:*

a. verbalization of same
b. relaxed facial expression and body positioning
c. increased participation in activities when allowed
d. stable vital signs.

a. logroll client for first 48 hours postoperatively and then instruct him/her to continue to logroll when turning self
b. ensure that client is always positioned with spine in proper alignment
c. apply stabilizing device (brace, cervical collar, or cast) as ordered *to provide additional support to surgical area*
d. reinforce preoperative teaching about the need to avoid twisting, flexing, and hyperextending spine
e. instruct client to avoid prolonged sitting (some physicians allow clients to sit only for meals for first few postoperative days)
f. instruct client to avoid straining to have a bowel movement (especially after lumbar laminectomy); consult physician about an order for a laxative or stool softener if indicated
2. use bed cradle to keep covers off any area of paresthesia
3. monitor for therapeutic and nontherapeutic effects of corticosteroids if administered *to reduce inflammation in the surgical area.*

☐ ▆▆▆▆▆▆▆▆▆▆▆▆▆▆▆▆▆▆▆▆▆▆▆▆▆▆▆▆▆

2. NURSING DIAGNOSIS

Impaired skin integrity:

a. **surgical incision;**
b. **impaired wound healing** related to inadequate blood supply to wound area, stress on wound area, infection, and increased levels of glucocorticoids (levels usually rise with stress);
c. **irritation and breakdown** related to contact of the skin with wound drainage; pressure from drainage tube (may be present if fusion was performed); use of tape; and pressure from a cast, brace, or collar if used to stabilize the spine following fusion.

☐ ▆▆▆▆▆▆▆▆▆▆▆▆▆▆▆▆▆▆▆▆▆▆▆▆▆▆▆▆▆

DESIRED OUTCOMES	NURSING ACTIONS AND *SELECTED RATIONALES*
2.a. The client will experience normal healing of the surgical wound (see Standardized Postoperative Care Plan, Nursing Diagnosis 9, outcome a, for outcome criteria).	2.a. Refer to Standardized Postoperative Care Plan, Nursing Diagnosis 9, action a, for measures related to assessment and promotion of normal wound healing.

2.b. The client will maintain skin integrity as evidenced by:
1. absence of redness and irritation
2. no skin breakdown.
	2.b.1. Inspect the following skin areas for signs and symptoms of irritation and breakdown:
	  a. areas in contact with wound drainage, tape, and drainage tubing
	  b. area under stabilizing device (brace, cast, or collar).
	2. Refer to Standardized Postoperative Care Plan, Nursing Diagnosis 9, action b.2, for measures related to prevention of skin irritation and breakdown resulting from wound drainage, drainage tubing, and tape.
	3. Implement measures *to prevent skin irritation and breakdown under stabilizing device:*
	  a. apply stabilizing device securely enough to keep it from rubbing and irritating the skin but not too tightly
	  b. position client so that the stabilizing device is not causing uneven pressure on any one area
	  c. if client is wearing a cotton T-shirt under the brace or cast, ensure that it is dry and wrinkle-free
	  d. apply cornstarch to skin under collar, brace, or cast *in order to keep skin dry and reduce irritation*

   e. keep stabilizing device dry
   f. keep skin around edges of stabilizing device clean and dry
   g. instruct client to refrain from poking anything under the collar, brace, or cast
   h. if the client has a brace or removable cast, pad areas over bone prominences
   i. if client has a cast:
      1. petal the cast edges or secure stockinette over the edges *to reduce irritation from rough edges and decrease the number of cast pieces falling inside the cast*
      2. if client complains of irritation under the cast, assist him/her to remove cast *in order to remove loose cast pieces*
   j. consult physician, physical therapist, or orthotist if cast, brace, or collar is putting excessive pressure on the skin.
   4. If skin breakdown occurs:
      a. notify physician
      b. continue with above measures to prevent further irritation and breakdown
      c. perform wound and decubitus care as ordered or per standard hospital policy
      d. monitor client closely and report signs and symptoms of infection (e.g. elevated temperature; redness, warmth, and edema around incision or area of breakdown; unusual drainage or odor from site).

3. NURSING DIAGNOSIS

Urinary retention related to:

a. pooling of urine in kidney and bladder associated with horizontal positioning;
b. stimulation of the sympathetic nervous system associated with pain, fear, and anxiety;
c. direct stimulation of the sympathetic fibers that innervate the bladder (may occur with a lumbar laminectomy);
d. depressant effects of some medications (e.g. anesthetic agents, narcotic analgesics) on bladder muscle tone.

DESIRED OUTCOMES	NURSING ACTIONS AND *SELECTED RATIONALES*
3. The client will not experience urinary retention (see Standardized Postoperative Care Plan, Nursing Diagnosis 13, for outcome criteria).	3. Refer to Standardized Postoperative Care Plan, Nursing Diagnosis 13, for measures related to assessment and management of urinary retention.

4. COLLABORATIVE DIAGNOSIS

Potential complications:

a. **respiratory distress** related to:
   1. damage to the phrenic nerve during surgery or compression of the nerve associated with inflammation (this is a possibility in clients who have had a cer-

vical laminectomy with or without fusion because the phrenic nerve arises at the C3–5 level)
   2. tracheal compression associated with a hematoma or inflammation following a cervical laminectomy (particularly when the anterior approach was utilized);
b. **neurovascular damage** related to:
   1. spinal nerve root and/or spinal cord trauma during surgery
   2. pressure on the spinal cord or nerve roots associated with a hematoma in the surgical area, inflammation, and/or dislodgment of the bone graft at the fusion site
   3. excessive or uneven pressure exerted by stabilizing device;
c. **development of a cerebrospinal fistula** related to inadvertent damage to and/or incomplete closure of the dura (care is taken during surgery to keep the dura intact; however, it is sometimes necessary to incise dura that extends along the involved nerve root);
d. **vocal cord paralysis** related to damage to the recurrent laryngeal nerve(s) during an anterior cervical laminectomy;
e. **paralytic ileus** related to stimulation of the sympathetic fibers that innervate the gastrointestinal tract (may occur with a lumbar laminectomy) and effects of anesthesia and some medications (e.g. muscle relaxants, narcotic analgesics).

DESIRED OUTCOMES	NURSING ACTIONS AND *SELECTED RATIONALES*
4.a. The client will not experience respiratory distress as evidenced by: 1. unlabored respirations at 16–20/minute 2. absence of stridor or sternocleidomastoid muscle retraction 3. usual skin color 4. usual mental status 5. blood gases within normal range.	4.a.1. Following a cervical laminectomy, assess for and immediately report: a. increased edema or an expanding hematoma in surgical area b. deviation of trachea from midline c. persistent or increased difficulty swallowing d. signs and symptoms of respiratory distress (e.g. rapid and/or labored respirations, stridor, sternocleidomastoid muscle retractions, cyanosis, restlessness, agitation) e. abnormal blood gases f. significant changes in ear oximetry and capnograph results. 2. Have tracheostomy tray and suction equipment readily available following a cervical laminectomy. 3. Implement measures *to prevent respiratory distress following a cervical laminectomy:* a. perform actions to reduce strain on the surgical area (see Postoperative Nursing Diagnosis 1, actions b.1.a–d) *in order to decrease risk of bleeding and increased inflammation* b. maintain patency of wound drainage system *in order to prevent development of a hematoma* c. monitor for therapeutic and nontherapeutic effects of corticosteroids if administered *to reduce inflammation in the surgical area.* 4. If signs and symptoms of respiratory distress occur: a. place client in a high Fowler's position unless contraindicated b. loosen neck dressing or cervical brace or collar if it appears tight c. administer oxygen as ordered d. assist with intubation or emergency tracheostomy if indicated e. prepare client for surgical evacuation of hematoma or repair of the bleeding vessel(s) if indicated f. provide emotional support to client and significant others.
4.b. The client will maintain normal circulatory, motor, and sensory function in the extremities as evidenced by: 1. palpable peripheral pulses 2. capillary refill time less than 3 seconds	4.b.1. Assess neurovascular status frequently (check upper extremities after surgery on the cervical area and lower extremities after surgery on the lumbar area). Compare findings to previous assessments. 2. Assess for and report signs and symptoms of neurovascular damage: a. diminished or absent peripheral pulses b. capillary refill time greater than 3 seconds c. pallor, blanching, cyanosis, and coolness of extremities d. inability to flex or extend foot and toes or hands and fingers

3. skin warm and usual color
4. ability to flex and extend foot and toes and/or hands and fingers
5. usual tone and strength in biceps, triceps, and quadriceps muscles
6. expected resolution of numbness and tingling in extremities
7. absence of pain during passive range of motion of feet and/or hands.

e. decreased tone or strength in biceps, triceps, or quadriceps muscles
f. increased numbness or tingling in extremities
g. pain in foot during passive range of motion of foot or toes; pain in hand during passive range of motion of hand or fingers.
3. Implement measures *to prevent neurovascular damage in the extremities:*
   a. perform actions to reduce strain on surgical area (see Postoperative Nursing Diagnosis 1, action b.1) *in order to decrease risk of bleeding and increased inflammation and prevent dislodgment of the bone graft if fusion was performed*
   b. maintain patency of the wound drainage system *in order to prevent development of a hematoma*
   c. apply stabilizing device properly; notify physician, physical therapist, or orthotist if brace, cast, or collar appears to cause pressure on any area
   d. monitor for therapeutic and nontherapeutic effects of corticosteroids if administered *to reduce inflammation in surgical area.*
4. If signs and symptoms of neurovascular damage occur:
   a. assess for and correct improper alignment and causes of uneven or excessive pressure (e.g. tight or improperly applied stabilizing device)
   b. notify physician if signs and symptoms persist
   c. if footdrop occurs:
      1. flex, extend, and rotate client's feet for 5–10 minutes every 1–2 hours
      2. use a footboard, sandbags, pillows, foam boots, or foot positioners *to keep feet in a neutral or slightly dorsiflexed position*
   d. if wristdrop occurs:
      1. use wrist splint *to maintain wrist in a neutral or slightly extended position*
      2. flex, extend, and rotate client's wrist for 5–10 minutes every 1–2 hours
   e. prepare client for surgical intervention (e.g. evacuation of hematoma, repositioning of dislodged bone graft) if planned.

4.c. The client will not develop a cerebrospinal fistula as evidenced by:
1. absence of cerebrospinal fluid drainage from lower back or neck incision
2. no complaints of headache.

4.c.1. Assess for and report signs and symptoms of a cerebrospinal fistula:
   a. presence of glucose in wound drainage as shown by positive Tes-Tape or Dextrostix results; be aware that any drainage containing blood will also test positive for glucose
   b. clear halo or watery, pale ring around bloody or serosanguineous drainage on lower back or neck dressing, sheet, or pillowcase
   c. complaints of a headache.
2. Implement measures to reduce strain on surgical area (see Postoperative Nursing Diagnosis 1, action b.1) *in order to promote healing of the dura if it was incised during surgery.*
3. If signs and symptoms of cerebrospinal fistula occur:
   a. maintain activity restrictions as ordered
   b. maintain meticulous sterile technique when changing dressings
   c. change dressings as soon as they become damp
   d. monitor for therapeutic and nontherapeutic effects of anti-infectives if administered
   e. assess for and report signs and symptoms of meningitis (e.g. fever, chills, increasing or persistent headache, nuchal rigidity, photophobia, positive Kernig's and Brudzinski's signs)
   f. prepare client for surgical repair of the torn dura if it does not heal spontaneously
   g. provide emotional support to the client and significant others.

4.d. The client will experience resolution of vocal cord paralysis if it occurs as evidenced by gradual return of usual voice tone and quality.

4.d.1. Have client speak periodically. Assess for signs of vocal cord paralysis (e.g. hoarseness, high pitched voice, complete absence of voice).
2. If voice changes occur:
   a. encourage client to limit verbal communication *in order to rest the vocal cords*
   b. implement measures to facilitate communication (e.g. provide pen and pencil, flash cards, or magic slate; maintain quiet environment *so client does not have to raise voice to be heard)*
   c. reinforce physician's explanation regarding the permanence of voice changes (voice tone and quality usually return to normal once inflammation subsides)

d. consult physician if signs and symptoms of vocal cord paralysis persist or worsen.

4.e. The client will not develop a paralytic ileus (see Standardized Postoperative Care Plan, Collaborative Diagnosis 19, outcome d, for outcome criteria).

4.e. Refer to Standardized Postoperative Care Plan, Collaborative Diagnosis 19, action d, for measures related to assessment and management of a paralytic ileus.

5. NURSING DIAGNOSIS

Knowledge deficit regarding follow-up care.

DESIRED OUTCOMES	NURSING ACTIONS AND *SELECTED RATIONALES*

5.a. The client will identify ways to prevent recurrent disc herniation.

5.a.1. Provide instructions regarding ways *to reduce back and/or neck strain and reduce risk of recurrent disc herniation:*
- a. maintain an optimal weight
- b. provide adequate support for spine (e.g. sleep on a firm mattress; sit on firm, straight-backed or contoured chairs; wear stabilization device during activity if prescribed)
- c. always use proper body mechanics (e.g. bend at the knees rather than waist, carry items close to body)
- d. always maintain good posture
- e. begin prescribed, progressive exercise program to strengthen back, neck, arms, legs, and abdominal muscles when allowed.

2. Provide a dietary consult regarding a weight reduction program if indicated.
3. Allow time for client to practice good posture when sitting, standing, and walking; proper positioning when resting; and any exercises allowed in immediate postoperative period. Encourage client to think about and plan movements before doing them.
4. Allow time for questions, clarification, and return demonstration of proper body mechanics, positioning, and exercises allowed.

5.b. The client will demonstrate the ability to correctly apply and remove a brace, cast, or collar if one is required.

5.b.1. Reinforce instructions on the correct way to apply and remove brace, cast, or collar if client needs to wear one after discharge.
2. Allow time for questions, clarification, and return demonstration.

5.c. The client will verbalize an understanding of ways to maintain skin integrity when wearing a brace, cast, or collar.

5.c.1. If client is to be discharged with a stabilization device, instruct him/her to examine skin under brace, cast, or collar daily when device is off during personal hygiene (if device should not be removed, demonstrate how to examine under device using a mirror and flashlight).
2. Instruct client in ways *to maintain skin integrity if he/she needs to wear a stabilizing device:*
- a. apply device properly and maintain spine in good alignment *to avoid undue pressure in any area*
- b. wear a cotton T-shirt under brace or cast and keep shirt dry and wrinkle-free
- c. apply cornstarch to skin *to keep it dry and reduce irritation from the stabilizing device*
- d. avoid poking anything under the device
- e. petal cast edges or secure stockinette over edges if cast is rough or cracking
- f. if pieces of cast material fall between cast and skin, remove easy to reach pieces, take off cast if allowed and carefully clean skin, or call

health care provider if cast cannot be removed and debris is irritating skin
g. pad areas of brace or cast that put excessive or uneven pressure on a particular body area.

5.d. The client will state signs and symptoms of complications to report to the health care provider.	5.d.1. Refer to Standardized Postoperative Care Plan, Nursing Diagnosis 20, action c, for signs and symptoms to report to the health care provider. 2. Instruct client to report these additional signs and symptoms: a. decreased movement or sensation in extremities b. coolness or bluish color of extremities c. increasing pain in surgical area or extremity d. difficulty standing up straight (with lumbar surgery) or keeping neck straight (with cervical surgery) e. persistent and/or severe headache f. drainage of clear or bloody fluid from incision on spine g. persistent or increasing hoarseness or difficulty swallowing (may occur following cervical laminectomy) h. reddened or irritated pressure area on skin underneath cast, brace, or collar.
5.e. The client will verbalize an understanding of and a plan for adhering to recommended follow-up care including future appointments with health care provider, medications prescribed, activity level, and wound care.	5.e.1. Refer to Standardized Postoperative Care Plan, Nursing Diagnosis 20, for routine postoperative instructions and measures to improve client compliance. 2. Reinforce physician's instructions regarding activity (the restrictions will vary depending on extensiveness of surgery, client condition, and physician preference): a. avoid lifting heavy objects b. progress through exercise program at the rate prescribed c. avoid sitting or standing for prolonged periods (especially after surgery on lumbar area) d. schedule adequate rest periods e. avoid driving a car *(causes increased flexion of the spine)* and taking long car rides *(the vibrations can jar the spine and long periods without significant changes in position can increase stiffness and discomfort)* until allowed.

■ ■

Total Hip Replacement

A total hip replacement is a surgical procedure in which the ball and socket components of the hip joint are replaced with prosthetic devices. To date, the most commonly used prosthetic devices are a polyethylene cup to replace the acetabulum and a stainless steel or Vitallium ball to replace the femoral component of the hip. The prostheses are secured in place by a cement-like agent called methylmethacrylate. Other prosthetic devices being used are bipolar (consists of a femoral component and a metallic acetabular cup with a poly-ethylene liner) and uncemented prostheses, particularly the acetabular component. Uncemented prostheses are secured in place by a bone-prosthesis interlock provided by flanged pegs or a porous surface, which allows bone

ingrowth. A total hip replacement is performed to relieve joint pain that has been resistant to conservative management and/or improve joint mobility in persons with severe degenerative or rheumatoid arthritis, septic arthritis, necrosis of the femoral head, or congenital hip deformity. It may also be performed following failure of previous reconstructive surgery.

This care plan focuses on the adult client hospitalized for a total hip replacement. Preoperative goals of care are to reduce fear and anxiety, reduce discomfort, and educate the client regarding ways to prevent postoperative complications and facilitate rehabilitation. Postoperatively, the goals of care are to maintain comfort, prevent complications, assist the client to regain maximum mobility, and educate the client regarding follow-up care. Prevention of infection is of major importance in caring for the client who has had a total hip replace-ment since infection of the operative hip usually neces-sitates surgical debridement and/or removal of the prostheses.

DISCHARGE CRITERIA

Prior to discharge, the client will:

- verbalize an understanding of activity and position restrictions
- demonstrate correct transfer and ambulation techniques and proper use of am-bulatory aids
- demonstrate the ability to correctly perform the prescribed exercises
- identify ways to reduce the risk of falls in the home environment
- state signs and symptoms of complications to report to the health care provider
- identify community resources that can assist with home management and provide transportation
- verbalize an understanding of and a plan for adhering to recommended follow-up care including future appointments with health care provider and physical ther-apist, medications prescribed, activity level, and wound care.

NURSING/COLLABORATIVE DIAGNOSES

Preoperative
1. Pain: hip □ *913*
2. Knowledge deficit □ *913*
Postoperative
1. Pain:
   a. hip pain
   b. low back pain □ *915*
2. Impaired skin integrity:
   a. surgical incision
   b. impaired wound healing
   c. irritation and breakdown □ *916*
3. Potential for infection: operative hip □ *917*
4. Potential for trauma □ *918*
5. Potential complications:
   a. shock
   b. neurovascular damage in the operative extremity
   c. dislocation of hip prosthesis(es)
   d. fat embolism syndrome
   e. thromboembolism
   f. contractures of hips, knees, or feet □ *918*
6. Knowledge deficit regarding follow-up care □ *922*

Preoperative

Use in conjunction with the Standardized Preoperative Care Plan.

1. NURSING DIAGNOSIS

Pain: hip related to irritation of or pressure on the nerves associated with processes such as inflammation and degeneration of protective surfaces and support structures that result from the joint disorder necessitating the surgery.

DESIRED OUTCOMES	NURSING ACTIONS AND *SELECTED RATIONALES*

1. The client will experience diminished hip pain as evidenced by:
  a. verbalization of a reduction of pain
  b. relaxed facial expression and body positioning
  c. increased participation in activities
  d. stable vital signs.
	1.a. Determine how the client usually responds to pain.
	  b. Assess for nonverbal signs of pain (e.g. wrinkled brow, clenched fists, reluctance to move, difficulty walking, guarding of affected hip, restlessness, diaphoresis, facial pallor or flushing, change in B/P, tachycardia).
	  c. Assess verbal complaints of pain. Ask client to be specific about location, severity, and type of pain.
	  d. Assess for factors that seem to aggravate or alleviate pain.
	  e. Implement measures *to reduce hip pain:*
	    1. apply heat or cold (e.g. heating pad, ice packs) to hip as ordered
	    2. provide or assist with nonpharmacological measures for pain relief (e.g. position change, transcutaneous electrical nerve stimulation, relaxation techniques, guided imagery, quiet conversation, restful environment, diversional activities)
	    3. monitor for therapeutic and nontherapeutic effects of analgesics and anti-inflammatory agents if administered.
	  f. Consult physician if above measures fail to provide adequate pain relief.

2. NURSING DIAGNOSIS

Knowledge deficit regarding hospital routines associated with surgery, physical preparation for total hip replacement, and postoperative care and management.

DESIRED OUTCOMES	NURSING ACTIONS AND *SELECTED RATIONALES*

2.a. The client will verbalize an understanding of usual preoperative and postoperative care and routines.	2.a.1. Refer to Standardized Preoperative Care Plan, Nursing Diagnosis 4, actions a.1–4, for information to include in preoperative teaching.
	  2. Provide additional information on specific preoperative care for clients having a total hip replacement:
	    a. explain that the following measures will be performed *to reduce risk of a postoperative hip infection:*

UNIT
XV

1. the operative hip and thigh will be scrubbed with an antiseptic solution at least twice before surgery (some institutions require a sterile prep of the area followed by application of a sterile wrap)
2. injections will not be given in the operative extremity
3. existing infections will be treated before surgery; instruct client to report any symptoms of infection (e.g. cough, runny nose, burning on urination)
4. anti-infectives will probably be administered prophylactically before and after surgery

b. explain that anticoagulants (e.g. heparin, Embolex, warfarin) and/or antiplatelet agents (e.g. low-weight dextran, aspirin) may be administered before surgery *to reduce risk of postoperative thrombus formation*; inform client that coagulation studies are usually done before starting these medications, especially if he/she has been taking aspirin, aspirin-containing compounds, or ibuprofen

c. explain that a physical therapist will fit crutches or walker and provide instructions about the postoperative physical therapy regimen.

3. Allow time for questions and clarification of information provided.

2.b. The client will demonstrate the ability to perform techniques designed to prevent postoperative complications.	2.b.1. Refer to Standardized Preoperative Care Plan, Nursing Diagnosis 4, action b.1, for instructions on ways to prevent postoperative complications.

2. Provide additional instructions about ways *to prevent postoperative complications:*
   a. reinforce physician's or physical therapist's instructions on:
      1. transfer techniques that can be performed without flexing hip beyond the prescribed limit
      2. exercises *to improve strength and facilitate mobility:*
         a. quadriceps- and gluteal-setting
         b. upper extremity strengthening
         c. sling-assisted hip and knee flexion and extension
         d. isometric hip extension and abduction exercises (spreading legs apart and pushing knee backward into bed)
      3. ambulation techniques and proper use of ambulatory aids (weight-bearing limitations are determined by the physician and vary depending on the type of prostheses utilized; weight-bearing is allowed earlier with cemented prostheses)
   b. instruct client in the correct way to use trapeze and unoperative extremity to move self
   c. explain the following activity and positioning limitations that need to be adhered to postoperatively *to prevent dislocation of prosthesis(es):*
      1. bedrest will be maintained for first 1–3 days with head of bed elevated no more than 45° for short periods
      2. operative extremity should be maintained in an abducted position by a splint, traction, abduction wedge, or 2–3 pillows for first few days after surgery
      3. legs should not be brought toward the midline, crossed, or rotated inwardly
      4. if turning is allowed, it should be done only with assistance of trained personnel
      5. hip flexion of 45–60° will be permitted initially and should not exceed 90° during the rehabilitation phase.
3. Allow time for questions, clarification, and return demonstration.

Postoperative

Use in conjunction with the Standardized Postoperative Care Plan.

1. NURSING DIAGNOSIS

Pain:

a. **hip pain** related to tissue trauma and reflex muscle spasms associated with the surgery, blood accumulation and edema in surgical area, and improper positioning of the operative extremity;
b. **low back pain** related to body positioning (client usually has to remain in a supine position when in bed).

DESIRED OUTCOMES	NURSING ACTIONS AND *SELECTED RATIONALES*

1. The client will experience diminished hip and back pain (see Standardized Postoperative Care Plan, Nursing Diagnosis 7.A, for outcome criteria).	1.a. Refer to Standardized Postoperative Care Plan, Nursing Diagnosis 7.A, for measures related to assessment and reduction of pain.
	b. Implement additional measures *to reduce pain:*
	  1. perform actions *to reduce pain in the operative extremity:*
	    a. keep operative extremity in an abducted position (certain physicians ensure this position by placing the extremity in a splint for 24–72 hours after surgery; others order placement of an abduction wedge or 2–3 pillows between legs at all times)
	    b. maintain restrictions on the degree of hip flexion as ordered (usually a 45–60° maximum is allowed for first 2–3 days with a maximum of 90° during rehabilitation period)
	    c. place trochanter or hip roll at the operative site for first 24 hours after surgery *(pressure on the operative area helps maintain alignment and prevent hematoma formation)*
	    d. apply ice packs to the operative hip for the first 24–48 hours after surgery *in order to reduce bleeding and edema in the surgical area*
	    e. maintain patency of wound drainage system (e.g. prevent kinking of tubing, empty collection device as needed, keep collection device below surgical wound, maintain suction as ordered) *to reduce accumulation of fluid in surgical area*
	    f. maintain traction as ordered (light traction may be ordered for first 24–48 hours *to reduce muscle spasms and maintain abduction)*
	    g. move operative extremity gently
	    h. if turning is allowed, keep pillows between legs while in side-lying position *in order to prevent adduction and resultant strain on surgical site*
	    i. maintain proper placement and function of transcutaneous electrical nerve stimulator if ordered
	    j. administer prescribed analgesics at least 30–60 minutes before exercise and ambulation sessions
	  2. perform actions *to help relieve low back discomfort:*
	    a. place alternating pressure or eggcrate mattress or floatation pad on bed
	    b. massage client's back at least every 3–4 hours
	    c. if turning is allowed, turn client every 2 hours (certain physicians allow turning to unoperative side; others allow no turning at all).

UNIT XV

2. NURSING DIAGNOSIS

Impaired skin integrity:

a. **surgical incision;**
b. **impaired wound healing** related to inadequate nutritional status, inadequate blood supply to wound area, stress on wound area, infection, and increased levels of glucocorticoids (levels usually rise with stress);
c. **irritation and breakdown** related to:
1. contact of skin with wound drainage, pressure from drainage tubes, and use of tape
2. prolonged pressure on tissues associated with decreased mobility
3. excessive or prolonged pressure on tissues from immobilizing device (e.g. splint, traction) and elastic wraps or hose.

DESIRED OUTCOMES	NURSING ACTIONS AND *SELECTED RATIONALES*
2.a. The client will experience normal healing of the surgical wound (see Standardized Postoperative Care Plan, Nursing Diagnosis 9, outcome a, for outcome criteria).	2.a. Refer to Standardized Postoperative Care Plan, Nursing Diagnosis 9, action a, for measures related to assessment and promotion of normal wound healing.
2.b. The client will maintain skin integrity as evidenced by: 1. absence of redness and irritation 2. no skin breakdown.	2.b.1. Frequently inspect the following sites for pallor, redness, and breakdown: 　a. skin areas in contact with wound drainage, tape, and drainage tubings 　b. back, coccyx, and buttocks 　c. elbows and heels 　d. pressure points on operative extremity if traction or splint is present 　e. areas under elastic wraps or hose. 2. Refer to Standardized Postoperative Care Plan, Nursing Diagnosis 9, action b.2, for measures related to prevention of skin irritation and breakdown resulting from wound drainage, drainage tubings, and tape. 3. Implement measures *to prevent skin breakdown associated with decreased mobility*: 　a. instruct client to use trapeze to lift self and shift weight every 30 minutes 　b. gently massage back, coccyx, buttocks, elbows, and heels every 2 hours 　c. lift and move client carefully using a turn sheet and adequate assistance *to prevent linen from shearing skin* 　d. turn client every 2 hours if allowed (may be allowed to turn on unoperative side) 　e. if fade time (length of time it takes for reddened area to fade after pressure is removed) is greater than 15 minutes, increase the frequency of position changes and massages 　f. keep skin lubricated, clean, and dry 　g. keep bed linens wrinkle-free 　h. provide alternating pressure or eggcrate mattress, floatation pad, or sheepskin if indicated 　i. increase activity as allowed and tolerated. 4. If operative extremity is immobilized by traction or a splint, implement measures *to reduce risk of skin breakdown associated with excessive or uneven pressure*: 　a. if elastic wraps are used to maintain skin traction, make sure they are wrinkle-free and exerting even pressure 　b. make sure traction boot is not too tight (should be able to slip index finger under straps) and does not extend into the popliteal space

      c. make sure metal parts on suspension device are not resting on any area of extremity

      d. maintain proper alignment of extremity in traction or splint device.

5. Implement measures *to prevent irritation and breakdown on elbows and heels:*

      a. massage elbows and heels with lotion frequently

      b. encourage client to use trapeze to move self rather than pushing up with heel and elbows

      c. reduce pressure on heels by placing them on rubber gloves filled with water or placing rolled towel under ankles

      d. provide elbow and heel protectors if indicated.

6. Implement measures *to prevent skin breakdown under elastic wraps or hose:*

      a. remove elastic wraps or hose once a shift, bathe and thoroughly dry skin, and reapply wraps or hose smoothly

      b. check wraps or hose frequently and reapply if they have loosened, slipped, or become wrinkled

      c. if areas of redness develop under wraps or hose, consult physician before reapplying.

7. If skin breakdown occurs:

      a. notify physician

      b. continue with above measures to prevent further irritation and breakdown

      c. perform wound and decubitus care as ordered or per standard hospital policy

      d. monitor client closely and report signs and symptoms of infection (e.g. elevated temperature; redness, warmth, and edema around area of breakdown; unusual drainage from site).

---

3. NURSING DIAGNOSIS

Potential for infection: operative hip related to:

a. introduction of organisms into the wound during or after surgery;

b. tissue necrosis associated with heat given off during solidification of methyl-methacrylate (the necrotic area and presence of heat provide an environment conducive to bacterial growth);

c. hematoma formation (increases the likelihood of infection by providing a good medium for bacterial growth and compromising blood flow to the area).

DESIRED OUTCOMES	NURSING ACTIONS AND *SELECTED RATIONALES*

3. The client will remain free of infection in the operative hip (see Standardized Postoperative Care Plan, Nursing Diagnosis 16, outcome b, for outcome criteria).	3.a. Assess for and report the following:
	  1. continuous drainage of fluid from incision *(may be indicative of a sinus tract, which provides a good pathway for infection)*
	  2. sloughing or necrosis of skin in the operative area
	  3. signs and symptoms of wound infection (e.g. chills; fever; redness, warmth, and swelling of wound area; unusual wound drainage; foul odor from wound area).
	b. Refer to Standardized Postoperative Care Plan, Nursing Diagnosis 16, actions b.4 and 5, for measures related to prevention and treatment of wound infection.
	c. Implement additional measures *to reduce risk of infection in the operative hip:*

1. use strict aseptic technique when emptying wound drainage device (some physicians do not allow other health care personnel to empty drainage device *because of risk of contamination*)
2. maintain patency of wound drainage device *in order to reduce risk of hematoma formation*
3. do not administer injections in operative extremity
4. prepare client for surgical repair of sinus tract or grafting of any area of skin sloughing or necrosis if indicated.

4. NURSING DIAGNOSIS

Potential for trauma related to falls associated with:

a. weakness, fatigue, and orthostatic hypotension resulting from the effects of major surgery;
b. central nervous system depressant effects of some medications (e.g. narcotic analgesics, muscle relaxants);
c. weakness and pain in weight-bearing extremity as a result of the surgery;
d. improper transfer and ambulation techniques.

DESIRED OUTCOMES	NURSING ACTIONS AND *SELECTED RATIONALES*

4. The client will not experience falls.	4.a. Determine whether conditions predisposing client to falls (e.g. weakness, fatigue, advanced age, orthostatic hypotension, use of narcotic analgesics or muscle relaxants) exist.
	b. Refer to Standardized Postoperative Care Plan, Nursing Diagnosis 17, action b, for measures to prevent falls.
	c. Implement additional measures *to reduce risk of falls:*
	  1. reinforce preoperative instructions and assist client with exercises to improve muscle strength, transfer and ambulation techniques, and use of ambulatory aids
	  2. administer prescribed analgesics 30–60 minutes before exercise and ambulation sessions *in order to maximize client's ability to utilize proper transfer and ambulation techniques*
	  3. monitor for therapeutic and nontherapeutic effects of blood products if administered *to treat weakness associated with anemia (these clients usually lose a large amount of blood during surgery because the hip is a highly vascular area).*
	d. Include client and significant others in planning and implementing measures to prevent falls.
	e. If falls occur, initiate appropriate first aid and notify physician.

5. COLLABORATIVE DIAGNOSIS

Potential complications:

a. **shock** related to hypovolemia associated with hemorrhage during or after surgery (client is very prone to bleeding because of the high vascularity of the area and treatment with anticoagulants and/or antiplatelet agents) and fluid volume deficit (results from excessive fluid loss and inadequate fluid replacement);

b. **neurovascular damage in the operative extremity** related to trauma to the nerves or blood vessels as a result of the surgery, blood accumulation and edema in surgical area, improper alignment of operative extremity, excessive pressure exerted by traction or abductor splint, and dislocation of the prosthesis;

c. **dislocation of hip prosthesis(es)** related to weakness of the hip muscles, improper positioning of the operative extremity, and/or noncompliance with weight-bearing limitations;

d. **fat embolism syndrome** related to a release of bone marrow fat into the bloodstream (may occur as a result of surgical trauma to pelvis and/or long bone) and an alteration in fat metabolism associated with trauma and stress;

e. **thromboembolism** related to:
   1. trauma to vein walls during surgery
   2. venous stasis associated with decreased mobility and pressure exerted by abductor device (e.g. splint, traction, wedge)
   3. hypercoagulability associated with fluid volume deficit;

f. **contractures of hips, knees, or feet** related to decreased mobility preoperatively and improper positioning and decreased mobility postoperatively.

DESIRED OUTCOMES	NURSING ACTIONS AND *SELECTED RATIONALES*
5.a. The client will not develop shock (see Standardized Postoperative Care Plan, Collaborative Diagnosis 19, outcome a, for outcome criteria).	5.a.1. Assess for and report the following: a. excessive wound drainage (expected loss is 200–500 cc in the first 24 hours, diminishing to 30 cc/shift by 48 hours after surgery) b. persistent vomiting c. difficulty maintaining intravenous or oral fluid intake d. significant decline in RBC, Hct., and Hgb. levels e. prothrombin time (PT) and activated partial thromboplastin time (APTT) more than 2½ times the control *(indicates a high risk for hemorrhage)* f. signs and symptoms of shock (see Standardized Postoperative Care Plan, Collaborative Diagnosis 19, action a.3). 2. Refer to Standardized Postoperative Care Plan, Collaborative Diagnosis 19, actions a.4 and 5, for measures related to prevention and treatment of shock. 3. Implement additional measures *to reduce risk of shock:* a. apply ice packs to operative hip for first 24–48 hours after surgery *in order to promote vasoconstriction and reduce blood loss* b. take additional precautions *to prevent bleeding if client is taking an anticoagulant:* 1. use the smallest gauge needle possible when giving injections and performing venous or arterial punctures 2. apply gentle, prolonged pressure after injections and venous or arterial punctures 3. take B/P only when necessary and avoid overinflating the cuff 4. caution client to avoid activities that increase the potential for trauma (e.g. shaving with a straight-edge razor, cutting nails, using stiff bristle toothbrush or dental floss) 5. pad side rails if client is confused or restless 6. remove hazardous objects from pathway *to prevent bumps or falls* 7. instruct client to avoid blowing nose forcefully or straining to have a bowel movement; consult physician about an order for decongestants, stool softeners, and/or laxatives if indicated.
5.b. The client will maintain normal circulatory, motor, and sensory function in the operative extremity as evidenced by: 1. palpable pedal pulses	5.b.1. Frequently assess neurovascular status in operative extremity. Compare assessments to the unaffected limb and previous assessments. 2. Assess for and report signs and symptoms of neurovascular damage in the operative extremity: a. diminished or absent pedal pulses b. capillary refill time in toes greater than 3 seconds

2. capillary refill time in toes less than 3 seconds
3. extremity warm and usual color
4. ability to flex and extend foot and toes
5. absence of numbness and tingling in foot and toes
6. absence of foot pain during passive movement of toes or foot
7. ability to maintain extremity in proper alignment.

    c. pallor, blanching, cyanosis, or coolness of the extremity
    d. inability to flex or extend foot or toes
    e. numbness or tingling in foot or toes
    f. pain in foot during passive motion of the toes or foot
    g. significant (greater than 10°) internal or external rotation of extremity.
3. Implement measures *to prevent neurovascular damage in operative extremity:*
    a. apply ice packs to operative hip for first 24–48 hours after surgery *in order to reduce bleeding and edema in surgical area*
    b. maintain patency of the wound drainage system *in order to reduce accumulation of fluid in surgical area*
    c. make sure that elastic wraps, trochanter roll, traction, or sling is not exerting pressure on the popliteal space, Achilles tendon, and lateral and medial aspects of the knee and ankle
    d. perform actions to prevent dislocation of the prosthesis (see action c.2 in this diagnosis).
4. If signs and symptoms of neurovascular damage occur:
    a. assess for and correct causes of uneven pressure (e.g. tight elastic wraps, improper positioning of abductor device)
    b. notify physician if the signs and symptoms persist
    c. prepare client for closed reduction or surgical intervention (e.g. relocation of prosthesis, hematoma evacuation) if planned.

5.c. The client will not experience dislocation of the hip prosthesis(es) as evidenced by:
1. continued resolution of hip pain
2. ability to maintain operative leg in proper alignment
3. ability to adhere to expected exercise and ambulation regimen
4. usual length of operative extremity
5. normal neurovascular status in operative leg.

5.c.1. Assess for and report signs and symptoms of dislocation of hip prosthesis(es):
    a. sudden, severe hip pain followed by continued pain and muscle spasms during hip movement
    b. palpable bulge over femur head
    c. abnormal rotation of operative leg
    d. inability to move or bear weight on operative leg
    e. shortening of operative leg
    f. decline in neurovascular status in operative leg.
2. Implement measures *to prevent dislocation of the prosthesis(es):*
    a. maintain bedrest as ordered (usually on bedrest for first 1–3 days after surgery)
    b. perform actions *to prevent adduction:*
       1. keep an abduction wedge or 2–3 pillows between legs while in bed
       2. remind client to avoid crossing legs
       3. do not move operative extremity past midline
       4. turn client only as ordered and always with pillows between legs
    c. perform actions *to maintain operative extremity in proper alignment:*
       1. place a trochanter roll on lateral side of thigh and calf (should not press on the lateral calf immediately below the knee and on the lateral malleolus) *in order to prevent external rotation* (especially important following anterolateral surgical approach)
       2. position pillow or trochanter roll along medial side of operative leg (should not press on medial aspect of knee and ankle) *in order to prevent internal rotation*
       3. instruct client not to rotate leg internally or externally
    d. maintain restrictions on head of bed elevation as ordered (some physicians order a 45–60° maximum for first 2–3 days after surgery) *in order to prevent excessive hip flexion*
    e. perform actions *to prevent extreme (beyond 90°) hip flexion:*
       1. instruct client not to lean forward to reach objects on end of bed or on floor or to put on slippers, socks, or shoes
       2. raise the entire bed to client's midthigh level before he/she gets in or out of bed *in order to reduce the degree of hip flexion that occurs when client sits on edge of bed*
       3. provide a high, firm chair (or elevate sitting surface with pillows) and a raised toilet seat for client's use *in order to reduce degree of hip flexion when client sits down*
       4. do not elevate operative leg when client is sitting in chair
    f. reinforce importance of adhering to recommended weight-bearing restrictions (the amount of weight-bearing allowed is based on the type of prostheses inserted; with cemented prostheses, partial weight-bearing is usually allowed as soon as ambulation is started).

3. If signs and symptoms of dislocation of the prosthesis(es) occur:
   a. maintain client on bedrest
   b. prepare client for x-rays of the surgical area
   c. prepare client for closed reduction (e.g. traction) or surgical relocation of the prosthesis if planned
   d. provide emotional support to client and significant others.

5.d. The client will not experience fat embolism syndrome as evidenced by:
1. usual mental status
2. absence of sudden chest pain
3. unlabored respirations at 16–20/minute
4. usual skin color
5. absence of petechiae
6. PaO₂ within normal limits.

5.d.1. Assess for and report signs and symptoms of fat embolism syndrome (usually occurs within first 72 hours after surgery):
   a. restlessness, apprehension, confusion
   b. sudden onset of chest pain, dyspnea, tachypnea
   c. pallor with subsequent cyanosis
   d. elevated temperature and pulse
   e. petechiae on buccal membranes, conjunctival sac, face, neck, or chest (petechiae are a late sign)
   f. low PaO_2 level.
2. Minimize movement of operative extremity during first few days after surgery *in order to reduce risk of fat emboli.*
3. If signs and symptoms of fat embolism syndrome occur:
   a. prepare client for immediate chest x-ray or lung scan
   b. obtain urine and blood specimens as ordered *(the presence of free fat globules in urine and blood helps confirm a diagnosis of fat emboli)*
   c. move client as little as possible *to prevent further embolization*
   d. implement measures *to treat the hypoxia that results with fat embolism syndrome:*
      1. administer high-flow oxygen unless contraindicated
      2. instruct client to deep breathe or use inspiratory exerciser at least every hour
   e. monitor for therapeutic and nontherapeutic effects of corticosteroids if administered *to reduce pulmonary inflammation*
   f. provide emotional support to client and significant others.

5.e. The client will not develop a venous thrombus or pulmonary embolism (see Standardized Postoperative Care Plan, Collaborative Diagnosis 19, outcomes c.1 and 2, for outcome criteria).

5.e.1. Refer to Standardized Postoperative Care Plan, Collaborative Diagnosis 19, actions c.1 and 2, for measures related to assessment, prevention, and treatment of a venous thrombus and pulmonary embolism.
2. Implement additional measures *to improve venous return and prevent thrombus formation:*
   a. keep head of bed flat as much as possible during first few days after surgery
   b. assist client with exercises and ambulation as allowed
   c. promote active foot and leg exercises by having client rock in a rocking chair once activity is progressed
   d. perform actions *to reduce risk of compromising venous return:*
      1. make sure elastic wraps or traction boot is not too tight
      2. make sure that sling on splint device, elastic wraps, or traction boot is not exerting pressure on popliteal space
      3. avoid use of knee gatch or pillows under knees
      4. discourage prolonged sitting or standing.

5.f. The client will maintain or regain normal range of motion.

5.f.1. Assess for and report limitations in range of motion (range of motion of operative extremity cannot be fully assessed for first 2–3 days because of position and movement restrictions).
2. Implement general measures *to prevent contractures:*
   a. maintain proper body alignment at all times
   b. instruct and assist client with range of motion exercises to unaffected joints at least every 4 hours
   c. encourage client to perform as much of self-care as possible
   d. progress activity as allowed.
3. Implement measures *to reduce risk of hip and knee contractures:*
   a. place client in a flat, supine position at least every 4 hours
   b. limit length of time client is in a high Fowler's position (usually no longer than an hour at a time)
   c. avoid use of the knee gatch or pillows under knees
   d. reinforce instructions and assist with hip and knee flexion-extension exercises as allowed (usually started 4–5 days after surgery)

UNIT XV

e. when client is in a supine position, place trochanter roll or sandbag along outer aspect of each thigh *to prevent external rotation of the hips.*
4. Implement measures *to prevent footdrop:*
   a. instruct client to flex, extend, and rotate feet for 5–10 minutes every 1–2 hours
   b. perform actions to prevent neurovascular damage in the operative extremity (see action b.3 in this diagnosis)
   c. use a footboard, sandbags, pillows, high-topped tennis shoes, foam boots, or foot positioners if necessary *to keep feet in a neutral or slightly dorsiflexed position*
   d. keep bed linen from exerting excessive pressure on toes and feet.
5. Consult physician if client is unable to make expected progress with flexion-extension exercises or if any other joint range of motion becomes restricted.

----

6. NURSING DIAGNOSIS

Knowledge deficit regarding follow-up care.

DESIRED OUTCOMES	NURSING ACTIONS AND *SELECTED RATIONALES*

6.a. The client will verbalize an understanding of activity and position restrictions.	6.a. Provide instructions about restrictions on activities and positioning (length of time the restrictions are necessary varies but ranges from 2 months to a year):
	1. turn only as directed by physician (many physicians allow turning to unoperative side only and instruct client to keep pillow between legs while on side)
	2. never cross legs
	3. do not sit on low chairs, stools, or toilets; place a cushion on low chairs, rent or purchase a raised toilet seat for home use, and use the high toilets designated for the handicapped when in public facilities
	4. do not elevate operative leg when sitting
	5. sit in chairs with arms and utilize the arms to raise self off chair
	6. support weight on unoperative leg when raising self from a sitting position
	7. do not sit for more than 1 hour at a time
	8. do not bend down to reach objects on the floor or in low cupboards or drawers
	9. do not reach to the end of bed to pull covers up
	10. do not put on shoes or socks without using an adaptive device
	11. keep operative leg in proper alignment and avoid rotating hip and knee
	12. when riding in a car:
	  a. sit on a firm pillow or cushion *to prevent hip flexion of more than 90°*
	  b. keep operative leg extended *(a sudden impact of the knee against the dashboard can dislodge the prosthesis)*
	13. do not resume sexual activity until approved by physician (usually about 6 weeks postoperatively)
	14. when sexual activity is resumed, avoid positions that involve turning knee or hip inward, flexing hip beyond 90°, and moving operative leg past the midline
	15. avoid lifting heavy objects, excessive twisting and turning of body, and activities that place excessive strain on hip (e.g. jogging, jumping).

6.b. The client will demonstrate correct transfer and	6.b.1. Reinforce instructions about correct transfer and ambulation techniques and proper use of walker, quad cane, or crutches.

ambulation techniques and proper use of ambulatory aids.

2. Reinforce physician's instructions about amount of weight-bearing on operative extremity (full weight-bearing may be allowed by the time of discharge if cemented prostheses were inserted).
3. Allow time for questions, clarification, and practice of transfer techniques and ambulation.

6.c. The client will demonstrate the ability to correctly perform the prescribed exercises.

6.c.1. Reinforce the physical therapist's instructions on prescribed exercises.
2. Reinforce importance of continuing the prescribed exercises for at least a year after surgery.
3. Allow time for questions, clarification, and return demonstration of prescribed exercises.

6.d. The client will identify ways to reduce the risk of falls in the home environment.

6.d. Provide the following instructions on ways *to reduce risk of falls at home:*
1. keep electrical cords out of pathways
2. remove unnecessary furniture and provide wide pathways for ambulation
3. remove scatter rugs
4. provide adequate lighting at all times
5. avoid unnecessary stair climbing
6. allow ample time for activities.

6.e. The client will state signs and symptoms of complications to report to the health care provider.

6.e.1. Refer to Standardized Postoperative Care Plan, Nursing Diagnosis 20, action c, for signs and symptoms to report to the health care provider.
2. Instruct client to report these additional signs and symptoms:
a. persistent or increased pain or spasms in operative extremity
b. loss of sensation or movement in operative extremity
c. inability to bear weight on operative extremity
d. inability to maintain operative extremity in a neutral position
e. shortening of operative extremity (will probably be noticed as a limp)
f. unusual or excessive bleeding.

6.f. The client will identify community resources that can assist with home management and provide transportation.

6.f.1. Provide information about community resources that can assist the client and significant others with home management and provide transportation (e.g. Visiting Nurse Association, home health agencies, Meals on Wheels, church groups, transportation services).
2. Initiate a referral if indicated.

6.g. The client will verbalize an understanding of and a plan for adhering to recommended follow-up care including future appointments with health care provider and physical therapist, medications prescribed, activity level, and wound care.

6.g.1. Refer to Standardized Postoperative Care Plan, Nursing Diagnosis 20, for routine postoperative instructions and measures to improve client compliance.
2. Reinforce importance of keeping appointments with physical therapist.
3. If client is discharged on a coumarin derivative (e.g. dicumarol, warfarin, phenprocoumon), instruct to:
a. keep scheduled appointments for periodic blood studies to monitor coagulation times
b. take medication at same time each day *in order to maintain a therapeutic blood level*
c. avoid regular and/or excessive intake of alcohol *(may alter responsiveness to coumarins)*
d. take the following precautions *to minimize risk of bleeding:*
1. avoid taking aspirin, aspirin-containing compounds, and ibuprofen
2. use an electric rather than a straight-edge razor
3. floss and brush teeth gently
4. cut nails carefully
5. avoid situations that could result in injury (e.g. contact sports)
6. avoid blowing nose forcefully
7. avoid straining to have a bowel movement
e. report prolonged or excessive bleeding from skin, nose, or mouth; blood in urine, vomitus, sputum, or stools; prolonged or excessive menses; excessive bruising; severe headache; or sudden abdominal or back pain
f. apply firm, prolonged pressure to any bleeding area if possible
g. wear a Medic-Alert band identifying self as being on anticoagulant therapy.
4. Instruct client to inform other health care providers of history of total hip replacement so prophylactic anti-infectives may be started before any dental work, invasive diagnostic procedures, or surgery.

UNIT XV

Total Knee Replacement

A total knee replacement is a surgical procedure in which the articular surfaces of the tibia and femur and sometimes the patella are replaced with prosthetic devices. It is performed to relieve joint pain that has not been controlled by conservative management and/or improve joint mobility in persons with severe degenerative, rheumatoid, or traumatic arthritis; congenital knee deformity; or severe intra-articular injury.

The two major types of prosthetic devices currently being used to replace the knee joint are the condylar and the hinge prostheses. The condylar prostheses consist of a metal femoral implant and a polyethylene tibial implant that are secured in place with a cement-like agent called methylmethacrylate. The hinge prosthesis is a one-piece metal device that has either long intramedullary portions on both ends to secure it in place or shorter ends that can be secured in place with methylmethac-rylate. Increasingly popular is the use of uncemented tibial, femoral, and/or patellar components. These are secured in place by bone growth or, more frequently, by a bone-prosthesis interlock provided by flanged pegs.

This care plan focuses on the adult client hospitalized for a total knee replacement. Preoperative goals of care are to reduce fear and anxiety, reduce discomfort, and educate the client regarding ways to prevent postoperative complications and facilitate rehabilitation. Postoperatively, the goals of care are to maintain comfort, prevent complications, assist the client to regain maximum mobility, and educate the client regarding follow-up care. Prevention of infection is of major importance in caring for the client who has had a total knee replacement since infection of the operative knee usually necessitates surgical debridement and/or removal of the prosthesis(es).

DISCHARGE CRITERIA

Prior to discharge, the client will:

- demonstrate correct transfer and ambulation techniques and proper use of ambulatory aids
- demonstrate the ability to correctly perform the prescribed exercises
- identify ways to reduce the risk of loosening of the prosthesis(es)
- identify ways to reduce the risk of falls in the home environment
- state signs and symptoms of complications to report to the health care provider
- identify community resources that can assist with home management and provide transportation
- verbalize an understanding of and a plan for adhering to recommended follow-up care including future appointments with health care provider and physical therapist, medications prescribed, activity level, and wound care.

NURSING/COLLABORATIVE DIAGNOSES

Preoperative
1. Pain: knee □ 925
2. Knowledge deficit □ 926
Postoperative
1. Pain:
   a. knee pain
   b. low back pain □ 927
2. Impaired skin integrity:
   a. surgical incision
   b. impaired wound healing
   c. irritation and breakdown □ 928

3. Potential for infection: operative knee □ *929*
4. Potential for trauma □ *930*
5. Potential complications:
   a. shock
   b. neurovascular damage in the operative extremity
   c. dislocation of knee prosthesis(es) or stress fracture of tibia or femur
   d. fat embolism syndrome
   e. thromboembolism
   f. contractures of the hips, knees, or feet □ *931*
6. Knowledge deficit regarding follow-up care □ *934*

Preoperative

Use in conjunction with the Standardized Preoperative Care Plan.

1. NURSING DIAGNOSIS

Pain: knee related to irritation of or pressure on the nerves associated with processes such as inflammation and degeneration of protective surfaces and support structures and/or dislocation of bone fragments that occur with the joint disorder necessitating the surgery.

DESIRED OUTCOMES	NURSING ACTIONS AND *SELECTED RATIONALES*

1. The client will experience diminished knee pain as evidenced by:
   a. verbalization of a reduction of pain
   b. relaxed facial expression and body positioning
   c. increased participation in activities
   d. stable vital signs.
	1.a. Determine how the client usually responds to pain.
	   b. Assess for nonverbal signs of pain (e.g. wrinkled brow, clenched fists, reluctance to move, difficulty walking, guarding of affected knee, restlessness, diaphoresis, facial pallor or flushing, change in B/P, tachycardia).
	   c. Assess verbal complaints of pain. Ask client to be specific about location, severity, and type of pain.
	   d. Assess for factors that seem to aggravate or alleviate pain.
	   e. Implement measures *to reduce pain:*
	      1. apply heat or cold (e.g. heating pad, ice packs) to knee as ordered
	      2. provide or assist with nonpharmacological measures for pain relief (e.g. position change, transcutaneous electrical nerve stimulation, relaxation techniques, guided imagery, quiet conversation, restful environment, diversional activities)
	      3. monitor for therapeutic and nontherapeutic effects of analgesics and anti-inflammatory agents if administered.
	   f. Consult physician if above measures fail to provide adequate pain relief.

UNIT
XV

2. NURSING DIAGNOSIS

Knowledge deficit regarding hospital routines associated with surgery, physical preparation for total knee replacement, and postoperative care and management.

DESIRED OUTCOMES	NURSING ACTIONS AND *SELECTED RATIONALES*

2.a. The client will verbalize an understanding of usual preoperative and postoperative care and routines.	2.a.1. Refer to Standardized Preoperative Care Plan, Nursing Diagnosis 4, actions a.1-4, for information to include in preoperative teaching.
	2. Provide additional information about specific preoperative care for clients having a total knee replacement:
	 a. explain that the following measures will be performed *to reduce risk of a postoperative knee infection:*
	  1. the operative leg will be scrubbed with an antiseptic solution at least twice before surgery (some institutions require a sterile prep of the area followed by application of a sterile wrap)
	  2. injections will not be given in the operative extremity
	  3. existing infections will be treated before surgery; instruct client to report any symptoms of infection (e.g. cough, runny nose, burning on urination)
	  4. anti-infectives will probably be administered prophylactically before and after surgery
	 b. explain that anticoagulants (e.g. heparin, Embolex, warfarin) and/or antiplatelet agents (e.g. low-weight dextran, aspirin) may be administered before surgery *to reduce risk of postoperative thrombus formation;* inform client that coagulation studies are usually done before starting these medications, especially if he/she has been taking aspirin, aspirin-containing compounds, or ibuprofen
	 c. explain that a physical therapist will fit crutches or walker and provide instructions on postoperative physical therapy regimen.
	3. Allow time for questions and clarification of information provided.

2.b. The client will demonstrate the ability to perform techniques designed to prevent postoperative complications.	2.b.1. Refer to Standardized Preoperative Care Plan, Nursing Diagnosis 4, action b.1, for instructions on ways to prevent postoperative complications.
	2. Provide additional instructions about ways *to prevent postoperative complications:*
	 a. reinforce physician's or physical therapist's instructions on:
	  1. exercises *to improve strength and facilitate mobility:*
	   a. hamstring, quadriceps-, and gluteal-setting
	   b. upper extremity strengthening
	   c. knee flexion
	   d. sling-assisted and independent straight leg raising
	  2. transfer and ambulation techniques and proper use of ambulatory aids (weight-bearing limitations are determined by the physician and vary depending on the type of prostheses inserted; less weight-bearing is allowed initially with uncemented prostheses)
	 b. instruct client in the correct way to use trapeze and unoperative extremity to move self
	 c. inform client that he/she will need to avoid abrupt flexion of the knee for first few weeks after surgery *in order to prevent displacement of the prosthesis(es)*
	 d. explain the need to leave operative extremity in the continuous passive motion (CPM) machine if ordered.
	3. Allow time for questions, clarification, and return demonstration.

Postoperative

Use in conjunction with the Standardized Postoperative Care Plan.

1. NURSING DIAGNOSIS

Pain:

a. **knee pain** related to tissue trauma and reflex muscle spasms associated with the surgery, blood accumulation and edema in surgical area, and improper positioning of the operative extremity;

b. **low back pain** related to body positioning (for at least 48 hours after surgery, client usually must remain in a supine position when in bed).

DESIRED OUTCOMES	NURSING ACTIONS AND *SELECTED RATIONALES*

1. The client will experience diminished knee and back pain (see Standardized Postoperative Care Plan, Nursing Diagnosis 7.A, for outcome criteria).	1.a. Refer to Standardized Postoperative Care Plan, Nursing Diagnosis 7.A, for measures related to assessment and reduction of pain.
	b. Implement additional measures *to reduce pain:*
	  1. perform actions *to alleviate pain in the operative extremity:*
	    a. maintain operative extremity in proper alignment
	    b. move the operative extremity carefully
	    c. implement measures *to reduce bleeding and edema in the surgical area:*
	      1. apply ice packs to the operative knee for first 24–48 hours after surgery (if client has a cast, do not place ice packs directly on top of it *because the weight will dent a damp cast*)
	      2. elevate the operative extremity above heart level for first 48 hours after surgery
	    d. maintain patency of the wound drainage system (e.g. prevent kinking of tubing, empty collection device as needed, keep collection device below wound level, maintain suction as ordered) *to prevent accumulation of fluid in the surgical area*
	    e. remind client to avoid abrupt flexion of operative knee
	    f. maintain proper placement and function of transcutaneous electrical nerve stimulator if ordered
	    g. administer prescribed analgesics at least 30–60 minutes before exercise and ambulation sessions
	    h. apply ice packs to operative knee for 20–30 minutes before and after exercise and ambulation sessions as ordered
	  2. perform actions *to help relieve low back discomfort:*
	    a. lower the foot of bed for 30- to 60-minute periods as allowed if leg elevation is being maintained
	    b. place alternating pressure or eggcrate mattress or floatation pad on bed
	    c. massage client's back at least every 3–4 hours
	    d. if turning is allowed (many physicians allow turning after the first 48 hours), routinely position client on side with pillows between legs and operative leg in an extended position.

UNIT XV

2. NURSING DIAGNOSIS

Impaired skin integrity:

a. **surgical incision;**
b. **impaired wound healing** related to inadequate nutritional status, inadequate blood supply to wound area, stress on wound area, infection, and increased levels of glucocorticoids (levels usually rise with stress);
c. **irritation and breakdown** related to:
   1. contact of skin with wound drainage, pressure from drainage tubes, and use of tape
   2. prolonged pressure on tissues associated with decreased mobility
   3. excessive or prolonged pressure on tissues from immobilizing device (e.g. compression dressing, knee immobilizer, cast) and elastic wraps or hose.

DESIRED OUTCOMES	NURSING ACTIONS AND *SELECTED RATIONALES*
2.a. The client will experience normal healing of the surgical wound (see Standardized Postoperative Care Plan, Nursing Diagnosis 9, outcome a, for outcome criteria).	2.a. Refer to Standardized Postoperative Care Plan, Nursing Diagnosis 9, action a, for measures related to assessment and promotion of normal wound healing.
2.b. The client will maintain skin integrity as evidenced by: 1. absence of redness and irritation 2. no skin breakdown.	2.b.1. Frequently inspect the following sites for pallor, redness, and breakdown: a. skin areas in contact with wound drainage, tape, and drainage tubings b. back, coccyx, and buttocks c. elbows and heels d. edges of compression dressing, cast, or knee immobilizer e. areas under elastic wraps or hose. 2. Refer to Standardized Postoperative Care Plan, Nursing Diagnosis 9, action b.2, for measures related to prevention of skin irritation and breakdown resulting from wound drainage, drainage tubings, and tape. 3. Implement measures *to prevent skin breakdown associated with decreased mobility:* a. instruct client to use trapeze to lift self and shift weight every 30 minutes b. gently massage back, coccyx, buttocks, elbows, and heels every 2 hours c. lift and move client carefully using a turn sheet and adequate assistance *to prevent linen from shearing skin* d. if turning is allowed (some physicians may not allow turning for first 48 hours), turn client every 2 hours keeping pillows between legs and operative knee extended e. if fade time (length of time it takes for reddened area to fade after pressure is removed) is greater than 15 minutes, increase the frequency of position changes and massages f. keep skin lubricated, clean, and dry g. keep bed linens wrinkle-free h. provide alternating pressure or eggcrate mattress, floatation pad, or sheepskin if indicated i. increase activity as allowed and tolerated. 4. Implement measures *to prevent irritation and breakdown on elbows and heels:* a. massage elbows and heels with lotion frequently b. encourage client to use trapeze to move self rather than pushing up with heel and elbows

      c. reduce pressure on heels by placing them on rubber gloves filled with water or placing rolled towel under ankles

      d. provide elbow and heel protectors if indicated.

5. Implement measures *to prevent skin breakdown under the compression dressing, knee immobilizer, or cast:*

      a. assess for and report tightness of the cast or dressing and complaints of burning under the immobilizing device

      b. loosen straps on knee immobilizer if it appears too tight

      c. apply cornstarch to skin under immobilizer *in order to keep skin dry and reduce irritation*

      d. keep dressing or cast dry

      e. position the operative extremity so that immobilizing device is not causing uneven pressure on any one area

      f. keep skin around edges of immobilizing device clean and dry (alcohol is often used unless skin is overly dry)

      g. instruct client to refrain from poking anything inside the immobilizing device

      h. if the client has a cast:

         1. petal the cast edges or secure the stockinette over the edges *to reduce irritation from rough edges and decrease the amount of cast debris falling inside the cast*

         2. remove easy to reach loose pieces of cast material from inside the cast.

6. Implement measures *to prevent skin breakdown under elastic wraps or hose:*

      a. remove elastic wraps or hose once a shift, bathe and thoroughly dry skin, and reapply wraps or hose smoothly

      b. check wraps or hose frequently and reapply if they have slipped, loosened, or become wrinkled

      c. if areas of redness develop under wraps or hose, consult physician before reapplying.

7. If skin breakdown occurs:

      a. notify physician

      b. continue with above measures to prevent further irritation and breakdown

      c. perform wound and decubitus care as ordered or per standard hospital policy

      d. monitor client closely and report signs and symptoms of infection (e.g. elevated temperature; redness, warmth, and edema around area of breakdown; unusual drainage from site; foul odor from cast or dressing).

3. NURSING DIAGNOSIS

Potential for infection: operative knee related to:

a. introduction of organisms into the wound during or following surgery;

b. tissue necrosis associated with heat given off during solidification of methyl-methacrylate (the necrotic area and presence of heat provide an environment conducive to bacterial growth);

c. hematoma formation (increases the likelihood of infection by providing a good medium for bacterial growth and compromising blood flow to the area).

DESIRED OUTCOMES	NURSING ACTIONS AND *SELECTED RATIONALES*
3. The client will remain free of infection in the operative knee (see Standardized	3.a. Assess for and report the following: 1. continuous drainage of fluid from incision *(may indicate a sinus tract, which provides a good pathway for infection)*

Postoperative Care Plan, Nursing Diagnosis 16, outcome b, for outcome criteria).

2. sloughing or necrosis of skin in operative area
3. signs and symptoms of wound infection (e.g. chills; fever; redness, warmth, and swelling of wound area; unusual wound drainage; foul odor from wound area).

b. Refer to Standardized Postoperative Care Plan, Nursing Diagnosis 16, actions b.4 and 5, for measures related to prevention and treatment of wound infection.

c. Implement additional measures *to reduce risk of infection in the operative knee:*
   1. use strict aseptic technique when emptying wound drainage device (some physicians do not want other health care personnel to empty drainage device *because of risk of contamination)*
   2. maintain patency of the wound drainage device *in order to reduce risk of hematoma formation*
   3. do not administer injections in operative extremity
   4. keep continuous passive motion (CPM) machine off the floor when not in use
   5. prepare client for surgical repair of a sinus tract or grafting of any area of skin sloughing or necrosis if indicated.

---

4. NURSING DIAGNOSIS

Potential for trauma related to falls associated with:

a. weakness, fatigue, and orthostatic hypotension resulting from the effects of major surgery;
b. central nervous system depressant effects of some medications (e.g. narcotic analgesics, muscle relaxants);
c. weakness and pain in weight-bearing extremity as a result of the surgery;
d. improper transfer and ambulation techniques.

DESIRED OUTCOMES	NURSING ACTIONS AND *SELECTED RATIONALES*

4. The client will not experience falls.

4.a. Determine whether conditions predisposing client to falls (e.g. weakness, fatigue, advanced age, orthostatic hypotension, use of narcotic analgesics or muscle relaxants) exist.

b. Refer to Standardized Postoperative Care Plan, Nursing Diagnosis 17, action b, for measures to prevent falls.

c. Implement additional measures *to reduce risk of falls:*
   1. reinforce preoperative instructions and assist client with transfer and ambulation techniques, use of ambulatory aids, and exercises to improve muscle strength
   2. administer prescribed analgesics and/or cold applications 30–60 minutes before exercise and ambulation sessions *in order to maximize the client's ability to utilize proper transfer and ambulation techniques*
   3. ensure that client has knee splint (immobilizer) on for ambulation sessions *to provide additional stabilization of operative leg.*

d. Include client and significant others in planning and implementing measures to prevent falls.

e. If falls occur, initiate appropriate first aid and notify physician.

5. COLLABORATIVE DIAGNOSIS

Potential complications:

a. **shock** related to hypovolemia associated with hemorrhage during or after surgery (client is more prone to bleeding if on anticoagulant therapy) and fluid volume deficit (results from excessive fluid loss and inadequate fluid replacement);
b. **neurovascular damage in the operative extremity** related to trauma to the nerves or blood vessels as a result of surgery, blood accumulation and edema in surgical area, improper alignment of operative extremity, excessive pressure exerted by the immobilizing device, dislocation of the prosthesis, and stress fracture of tibia or femur;
c. **dislocation of knee prosthesis(es) or stress fracture of tibia or femur** related to rotation of or excessive pressure on the knee;
d. **fat embolism syndrome** related to release of bone marrow fat into the bloodstream (may occur as a result of surgical trauma to a long bone) and an alteration in fat metabolism that occurs with trauma and stress;
e. **thromboembolism** related to:
   1. trauma to vein walls during surgery
   2. venous stasis associated with use of a tourniquet on operative leg during surgery, pressure created by the immobilizing device, and decreased mobility
   3. hypercoagulability associated with fluid volume deficit;
f. **contractures of the hips, knees, or feet** related to decreased mobility preoperatively and improper positioning and decreased mobility postoperatively.

DESIRED OUTCOMES	NURSING ACTIONS AND *SELECTED RATIONALES*
5.a. The client will not develop shock (refer to Standardized Postoperative Care Plan, Collaborative Diagnosis 19, outcome a, for outcome criteria).	5.a.1. Assess for and report the following: a. excessive wound drainage (expected loss is 300–500 cc in first 24 hours, diminishing to 30 cc/shift by 48 hours after surgery) b. persistent vomiting c. difficulty maintaining intravenous or oral fluid intake d. significant decline in RBC, Hct., and Hgb. levels e. prothrombin time (PT) and activated partial thromboplastin time (APTT) more than 2½ times the control *(indicates a high risk for hemorrhage)* f. signs and symptoms of shock (see Standardized Postoperative Care Plan, Collaborative Diagnosis 19, action a.3). 2. Refer to Standardized Postoperative Care Plan, Collaborative Diagnosis 19, actions a.4 and 5, for measures related to prevention and treatment of shock. 3. Implement additional measures *to reduce risk of shock:* a. apply ice packs to operative knee for first 24–48 hours after surgery *in order to promote vasoconstriction and reduce blood loss* b. take additional precautions *to prevent bleeding if client is taking an anticoagulant:* 1. use smallest gauge needle possible when giving injections and performing venous or arterial punctures 2. apply gentle, prolonged pressure following injections and venous or arterial punctures 3. take B/P only when necessary and avoid overinflating the cuff 4. caution client to avoid activities that increase the potential for trauma (e.g. shaving with a straight-edge razor, cutting nails, using stiff bristle toothbrush or dental floss) 5. pad side rails if client is confused or restless 6. remove hazardous objects from pathway *to prevent bumps or falls*

7. instruct client to avoid blowing nose forcefully or straining to have a bowel movement; consult physician regarding order for decongestants, stool softeners, and/or laxatives if indicated.

5.b. The client will maintain normal circulatory, motor, and sensory function in the operative extremity as evidenced by:
1. palpable pedal pulses
2. capillary refill time in toes less than 3 seconds
3. extremity warm and usual color
4. ability to flex and extend foot and toes
5. absence of numbness and tingling in foot and toes
6. absence of foot pain during passive movement of toes or foot.

5.b.1. Frequently assess neurovascular status in the operative extremity. Compare assessments to the unaffected limb and previous assessments.
2. Assess for and report signs and symptoms of neurovascular damage in operative extremity:
   a. diminished or absent pedal pulses
   b. capillary refill time in toes greater than 3 seconds
   c. pallor, blanching, cyanosis, or coolness of the extremity
   d. inability to flex or extend foot or toes
   e. numbness or tingling in foot or toes
   f. pain in foot during passive motion of toes or foot.
3. Implement measures *to prevent neurovascular damage in the operative extremity:*
   a. perform actions *to reduce bleeding and edema in surgical area:*
      1. elevate operative extremity above heart level for the first 48 hours after surgery
      2. apply ice packs to both sides of the operative knee for the first 24–48 hours after surgery (if client has a cast, do not place ice packs directly on top of it *because the weight will dent the damp cast)*
   b. maintain patency of the wound drainage system *in order to reduce accumulation of fluid in surgical area*
   c. maintain extremity in proper alignment
   d. perform actions *to relieve pressure from the immobilizing device:*
      1. position leg so that immobilizing device is not causing uneven pressure on any one area
      2. if client has a knee immobilizer, loosen straps if it appears to be too tight
      3. if client has a cast, "fishtail" (make several longitudinal cuts in the edges and bend the edges back) the edges if cast appears tight
   e. notify physician if cast or dressing appears to be too tight
   f. perform actions to prevent dislocation of the prosthesis(es) and a stress fracture of the tibia and femur (see action c.2 in this diagnosis).
4. If signs and symptoms of neurovascular damage occur:
   a. assess for and correct causes of uneven or excessive pressure (e.g. tight or improper positioning of immobilizing device, increased swelling)
   b. notify physician if the signs and symptoms persist
   c. prepare client for closed reduction or surgical intervention (e.g. relocation of the prosthesis, hematoma evacuation) if planned.

5.c. The client will not experience dislocation of the knee prosthesis(es) or stress fracture of tibia or femur as evidenced by:
1. continued resolution of knee pain
2. ability to maintain operative leg in proper alignment
3. ability to adhere to expected exercise and ambulation regimen
4. normal neurovascular status in operative leg.

5.c.1. Assess for and report signs and symptoms of dislocation of the knee prosthesis(es) and stress fracture of tibia or femur:
   a. sudden, severe knee pain followed by continued pain and muscle spasms during knee movement
   b. abnormal rotation of the lower portion of operative leg
   c. inability to move or bear weight on operative leg
   d. decline in neurovascular status in operative leg.
2. Implement measures *to prevent dislocation of the prosthesis(es) and stress fracture of the tibia and femur:*
   a. instruct client to avoid acute flexion, rotation, and twisting of knee
   b. reinforce physician's instructions regarding the amount of weight-bearing allowed (with uncemented prostheses, less weight-bearing is allowed) and the importance of only partial weight-bearing for about 6 weeks
   c. reinforce instructions and assist client with gait training and proper use of ambulatory aids
   d. reinforce the importance of wearing knee splint (immobilizer) when ambulating.
3. If signs and symptoms of prosthesis(es) dislocation or stress fracture occur:
   a. maintain client on bedrest
   b. prepare client for x-rays of operative leg
   c. prepare client for closed reduction or surgical intervention if planned
   d. provide emotional support to client and significant others.

5.d. The client will not experience fat embolism syndrome as evidenced by:
1. usual mental status
2. absence of sudden chest pain
3. unlabored respirations at 16–20/minute
4. usual skin color
5. absence of petechiae
6. PaO₂ within normal limits.

5.d.1. Assess for and report signs and symptoms of fat embolism syndrome (usually occurs within first 72 hours after surgery):
 a. restlessness, apprehension, confusion
 b. sudden onset of chest pain, dyspnea, tachypnea
 c. pallor with subsequent cyanosis
 d. elevated temperature and pulse
 e. petechiae on the buccal membranes, conjunctival sac, face, neck, or chest (petechiae are a late sign)
 f. low PaO₂ level.
 2. Minimize movement of operative extremity during first few days after surgery *in order to reduce risk of fat emboli* (a constant passive motion [CPM] machine may be used immediately after surgery *to limit movement yet still provide gentle range of motion*).
 3. If signs and symptoms of fat embolism syndrome occur:
 a. prepare client for an immediate chest x-ray or lung scan
 b. obtain urine and blood specimens as ordered (*the presence of free fat globules in urine and blood helps confirm a diagnosis of fat emboli*)
 c. move client as little as possible *to prevent further embolization*
 d. implement measures *to treat the hypoxia that results with fat embolism syndrome:*
  1. administer high-flow oxygen unless contraindicated
  2. instruct client to deep breathe or use inspiratory exerciser at least every hour
 e. monitor for therapeutic and nontherapeutic effects of corticosteroids if administered *to reduce pulmonary inflammation*
 f. provide emotional support to client and significant others.

5.e. The client will not develop a venous thrombus or pulmonary embolism (see Standardized Postoperative Care Plan, Collaborative Diagnosis 19, outcomes c.1 and 2 for outcome criteria).

5.e.1. Refer to Standardized Postoperative Care Plan, Collaborative Diagnosis 19, actions c.1 and 2 for measures related to assessment, prevention, and treatment of a venous thrombus and pulmonary embolism.
 2. Implement additional measures *to improve venous return and prevent thrombus formation following total knee replacement:*
 a. elevate operative extremity above heart level for the first 48 hours after surgery
 b. assist client with leg exercises and ambulation as allowed
 c. perform actions *to reduce risk of compromising venous return:*
  1. consult physician if dressing or cast appears too tight
  2. loosen knee immobilizer if it appears to be too tight
  3. make sure exercise sling is not exerting pressure on the popliteal space
  4. avoid use of the knee gatch or pillows under knees
  5. discourage prolonged sitting or standing.

5.f. The client will maintain or regain normal range of motion.

5.f.1. Assess for and report limitations in range of motion (range of motion of the operative knee and hip cannot be fully assessed until the bulky dressing has been removed and the client can begin sling-assisted or active exercises).
 2. Implement general measures *to prevent contractures:*
 a. maintain proper body alignment at all times
 b. instruct and assist client with range of motion exercises to unaffected joints at least every 4 hours
 c. encourage client to perform as much of self-care as possible
 d. gradually progress activity as allowed.
 3. Implement measures *to reduce risk of hip contractures:*
 a. place client in a flat, supine position at least every 4 hours
 b. limit the length of time client is in a high Fowler's position (usually no longer than an hour at a time)
 c. avoid use of the knee gatch or pillows under knees
 d. assist client with straight leg raising exercises (usually started 2–3 days after surgery)
 e. when client is in a supine position, place trochanter roll or sandbag along outer aspect of each thigh *to prevent external rotation of the hips.*
 4. Implement measures *to prevent or reduce flexion and extension contractures of the operative knee:*
 a. avoid use of the knee gatch or pillows under knees

UNIT XV

b. assist client with knee flexion-extension exercises as soon as allowed (usually started 2–4 days postoperatively)

c. ensure that continuous passive motion (CPM) machine is set at and maintains the degree of flexion and extension ordered (flexion is set at 30–50° initially, progressing to 90° by discharge).

5. Implement measures *to prevent footdrop:*
   a. instruct the client to flex, extend, and rotate feet for 5–10 minutes every 1–2 hours while awake
   b. perform actions to prevent neurovascular damage in the operative extremity (see action b.3 in this diagnosis)
   c. use a footboard, sandbags, pillows, high-topped tennis shoes, foam boots, or foot positioners if necessary *to keep feet in a neutral or slightly dorsiflexed position*
   d. keep bed linen from exerting excessive pressure on toes and feet.

6. Consult physician if client is unable to make expected progress with knee flexion (90° flexion is expected within 12–14 days) or if any other joint range of motion becomes restricted.

□ ▬▬▬▬▬▬▬▬▬▬▬▬▬▬▬▬▬▬

6. NURSING DIAGNOSIS

Knowledge deficit regarding follow-up care.

□ ▬▬▬▬▬▬▬▬▬▬▬▬▬▬▬▬▬▬

DESIRED OUTCOMES	NURSING ACTIONS AND *SELECTED RATIONALES*
6.a. The client will demonstrate correct transfer and ambulation techniques and proper use of ambulatory aids.	6.a.1. Reinforce instructions about correct transfer and ambulation techniques and proper use of crutches, cane, or walker. 2. Reinforce the importance of not bearing full weight on the operative extremity until instructed (usually about 6 weeks postoperatively). 3. Allow time for questions, clarification, and practice of transfer techniques and ambulation.
6.b. The client will demonstrate the ability to correctly perform the prescribed exercises.	6.b.1. Reinforce the physical therapist's instructions about prescribed exercises. 2. Reinforce the importance of continuing prescribed exercises for at least a year after surgery. 3. Allow time for questions, clarification, and return demonstration of prescribed exercises.
6.c. The client will identify ways to reduce the risk of loosening of the prosthesis(es).	6.c.1. Inform client of the possibility of loosening of the prosthesis (usually does not occur until 2–3 years after surgery). 2. Instruct client to report increasing pain or instability of operative knee (may indicate loosening of the prosthesis). 3. Instruct client regarding ways *to minimize risk of loosening of the prosthesis(es):* a. avoid full weight-bearing for at least 6 weeks b. avoid unusual twisting or rotation of knee c. avoid contact sports d. do not force knee beyond comfortable degree of flexion e. avoid placing undue stress on knees (e.g. do not lift and carry heavy objects, maintain a desirable body weight, avoid activities such as jogging).
6.d. The client will identify ways to reduce the risk of falls in the home environment.	6.d. Provide the following instructions on ways *to reduce risk of falls at home:* 1. keep electrical cords out of pathways 2. remove unnecessary furniture and provide wide pathways for ambulation 3. remove scatter rugs 4. provide adequate lighting at all times

5. avoid unnecessary stair climbing
6. allow ample time for activities.

6.e. The client will state signs and symptoms of complications to report to the health care provider.

6.e.1. Refer to Standardized Postoperative Care Plan, Nursing Diagnosis 20, action c, for signs and symptoms to report to the health care provider.
2. Instruct client to report these additional signs and symptoms:
    a. persistent or increased pain or spasms in operative extremity
    b. loss of sensation or movement in operative extremity
    c. inability to bear expected amount of weight on operative extremity
    d. inability to maintain operative extremity in a neutral position
    e. instability of operative extremity (knee "giving out")
    f. unusual or excessive bleeding.

6.f. The client will identify community resources that can assist with home management and provide transportation.

6.f.1. Provide information about community resources that can assist client and significant others with home management and provide transportation (e.g. Visiting Nurse Association, home health agencies, Meals on Wheels, church groups, transportation services).
2. Initiate a referral if indicated.

6.g. The client will verbalize an understanding of and a plan for adhering to recommended follow-up care including future appointments with health care provider and physical therapist, medications prescribed, activity level, and wound care.

6.g.1. Refer to Standardized Postoperative Care Plan, Nursing Diagnosis 20, for routine postoperative instructions and measures to improve client compliance.
2. Reinforce the importance of keeping appointments with physical therapist.
3. Instruct client to inform other health care providers of history of total knee replacement so prophylactic anti-infectives may be started before any dental work, invasive diagnostic procedures, or surgery.

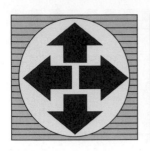
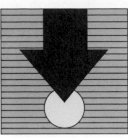
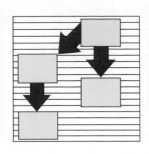
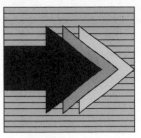
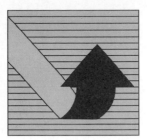

Unit XVI

Nursing Care of the Client with Disturbances of the Integumentary System

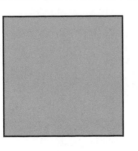
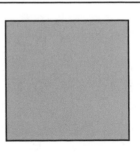
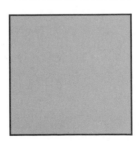

Burns

Burn injuries are one of the major causes of accidental death in the United States. Types of burn injury include thermal burns caused by contact with flames or hot surfaces, steam, and/or liquids; chemical burns resulting from contact with necrotizing substances such as acid and alkalies; and electrical burns due to contact with electrical currents. Burns can also occur as a result of exposure to radiation. Smoke inhalation injury occurs in approximately one third of persons who experience a major burn. Burns are categorized according to the depth of damage to the integument and are labeled as partial-thickness or full-thickness burns. Partial-thickness burns involve the epidermis and, to some degree, the dermis. Regeneration of tissue is possible with a partial-thickness burn because some of the remaining dermal tissue is viable. A full-thickness burn involves destruction of all skin layers and nerve endings, thus making spontaneous regeneration impossible.

There are three periods or phases that a client with a major burn injury experiences. These are the emergent phase (fluid accumulation or shock), acute phase (fluid remobilization or stage of diuresis), and rehabilitation phase. The emergent phase begins with the burn injury, usually lasts from 24 to 48 hours, and if the burn is severe, may persist for as long as 2 weeks. During this phase, increased capillary permeability leads to a fluid shift from the intravascular to the interstitial spaces resulting in a major risk of hypovolemic shock. The acute phase begins when the initial fluid replacement or resuscitation is complete, the fluid reshifts into the vascular space, and the client begins to diurese. This period ends when all of the full-thickness burns are covered with autografts. The rehabilitation phase begins on admission to the hospital and continues until the client is able to resume a functional role in society.

This care plan focuses on the adult client hospitalized with a major burn injury. The treatment plan is based on the depth of the burn, extensiveness of the burn (calculated according to percentage of body surface area [BSA] involved), body parts affected, age of the client, pre-existing medical conditions (e.g. lung or heart disease, diabetes), and concurrent injuries. The goals of nursing care are to participate in the team effort to resuscitate the client; prevent infection and other complications; maintain comfort, an adequate nutritional status, and joint mobility and function; support the client as he/she begins to cope with the effects of the burn injury; and educate the client regarding follow-up care.

DISCHARGE CRITERIA

Prior to discharge, the client will:

- identify ways to reduce the risk of recurrent burn injury
- demonstrate the ability to care for wounds appropriately
- demonstrate ways to maintain joint mobility and function
- demonstrate the ability to correctly use adaptive devices
- state signs and symptoms to report to the health care providers
- share thoughts and feelings about the effects of the burn injury on his/her future
- identify community resources that can assist with home management and adjustment to changes and losses resulting from the burn injury
- verbalize an understanding of and a plan for adhering to recommended follow-up care including future appointments with health care providers and physical and occupational therapists, medications prescribed, activity level, exercise regimen, dietary recommendations, and future reconstructive procedures.

Use in conjunction with the Care Plan on Immobility.

NURSING/COLLABORATIVE DIAGNOSES

1. Anxiety ☐ *940*
2. Altered systemic tissue perfusion ☐ *941*
3. Altered respiratory function:
   a. ineffective airway clearance
   b. ineffective breathing patterns:
      1. hyperventilation
      2. hypoventilation
   c. impaired gas exchange ☐ *942*
4A. Altered fluid and electrolyte balance in the emergent (fluid accumulation or shock) phase:
   1. hypovolemia
   2. hyperkalemia
   3. hyponatremia
   4. metabolic acidosis ☐ *944*
4B. Altered fluid and electrolyte balance during the acute phase (fluid remobilization or stage of diuresis):
   1. fluid volume excess
   2. hyponatremia
   3. hypernatremia
   4. hypokalemia
   5. hypochloremia
   6. hypophosphatemia
   7. metabolic alkalosis ☐ *946*
5. Altered nutrition: less than body requirements ☐ *949*
6A. Altered comfort: pain ☐ *951*
6B. Altered comfort: nausea and vomiting ☐ *952*
6C. Altered comfort: chills ☐ *952*
7. Hypothermia ☐ *953*
8. Impaired skin integrity:
   a. burn injury, extensive debridement of damaged tissue, and grafting procedures
   b. impaired healing of burn or graft sites
   c. irritation or breakdown ☐ *953*
9. Activity intolerance ☐ *955*
10. Impaired physical mobility ☐ *956*
11. Self-care deficit ☐ *956*
12. Constipation ☐ *957*
13. Diarrhea ☐ *957*
14. Sleep pattern disturbance ☐ *958*
15. Potential for infection:
   a. wound infection
   b. pneumonia ☐ *959*
16. Potential for trauma ☐ *960*
17. Potential complications:
   a. gastrointestinal (GI) bleeding
   b. thromboembolism
   c. impaired renal function
   d. shock

UNIT
XVI

---

e. paralytic ileus
  f. contractures □ *961*
18. Sexual dysfunction □ *964*
19. Disturbance in self-concept □ *965*
20. Ineffective individual coping □ *966*
21. Grieving □ *967*
22. Diversional activity deficit □ *968*
23. Social isolation □ *968*
24. Knowledge deficit regarding follow-up care □ *969*

---

1. NURSING DIAGNOSIS

Anxiety related to:

a. sudden extensive injury;
b. unfamiliar environment;
c. pain;
d. difficulty breathing;
e. effects of burns on appearance and usual life style and roles;
f. loss of control over environment and body functions;
g. treatments to debride wounds;
h. possible death.

DESIRED OUTCOMES	NURSING ACTIONS AND *SELECTED RATIONALES*

1. The client will experience a reduction in fear and anxiety as evidenced by:
a. verbalization of feeling less anxious or fearful
b. relaxed facial expression and body movements
c. stable vital signs
d. usual skin color in unburned areas
e. verbalization of an understanding of hospital routines, extensiveness of the injury, treatments, and prognosis.
	1.a. Assess client for signs and symptoms of fear and anxiety (e.g. verbalization of fears and concerns; tenseness; tremors; irritability; restlessness; increased dyspnea; diaphoresis; tachycardia; elevated blood pressure; facial tension, pallor, or flushing; noncompliance with treatment plan). Validate perceptions carefully, remembering that some behavior may result from hypoxia and fluid and electrolyte imbalances.
	b. Ascertain effectiveness of current coping skills.
	c. Implement measures *to reduce fear and anxiety:*
	  1. maintain a calm, confident manner when interacting with client
	  2. perform actions to reduce pain (see Nursing Diagnosis 6.A, action 5)
	  3. perform actions to improve respiratory status (see Nursing Diagnosis 3, action f)
	  4. assure client that staff members are nearby; respond to call signal as soon as possible
	  5. following period of acute distress:
	    a. orient to hospital environment, equipment, and routines
	    b. keep monitoring equipment out of client's direct view whenever possible
	    c. introduce staff who will be participating in his/her care; if possible, maintain consistency in staff assigned to his/her care *to provide feelings of stability and comfort with the environment*

    d. encourage verbalization of fear and anxiety; provide feedback
    e. reinforce physician's explanations and clarify any misconceptions client may have about extensiveness of burn injury and prognosis
    f. explain all diagnostic tests (e.g. blood and urine studies, chest x-ray, EKG, pulmonary artery catheterization and pressure measurements)
    g. explain planned or expected treatments using visual aids if necessary for clarification
    h. provide a calm, restful environment
    i. instruct in relaxation techniques and encourage participation in diversional activities
    j. perform actions to assist the client to cope with the diagnosis and its implications (see Nursing Diagnosis 20, action e)
    k. arrange for a visit from clergy if client desires
    l. encourage significant others to project a caring, concerned attitude without obvious anxiousness
    m. if surgical intervention is indicated, begin preoperative teaching
    n. monitor for therapeutic and nontherapeutic effects of anti-anxiety agents if administered.
  d. Prepare significant others for changes in client's appearance *so that they are better able to be supportive.*
  e. Include significant others in orientation and teaching sessions and encourage their continued support of client.
  f. Provide information based on current needs of client and significant others at a level they can understand. Encourage questions and clarification of information provided.
  g. Consult physician if above actions fail to control fear and anxiety.

□ ▬▬▬▬▬▬▬▬▬▬▬▬▬▬▬▬▬▬▬▬▬▬▬▬▬▬▬▬

2. NURSING DIAGNOSIS

Altered systemic tissue perfusion related to:

a. hypovolemia in the emergent phase associated with third-spacing and fluid loss;
b. restricted blood flow in extremities associated with increasing edema under eschar of circumferential burns;
c. vasoconstriction associated with hypothermia resulting from excessive heat loss through denuded skin areas;
d. peripheral pooling of blood associated with venous stasis resulting from decreased mobility and loss of muscle tone.

□ ▬▬▬▬▬▬▬▬▬▬▬▬▬▬▬▬▬▬▬▬▬▬▬▬▬▬▬▬

DESIRED OUTCOMES	NURSING ACTIONS AND *SELECTED RATIONALES*
2. The client will maintain adequate systemic tissue perfusion as evidenced by: a. B/P and pulse within normal range for client and stable with position change b. unlabored respirations at 16–20/minute c. usual mental status d. skin in unburned areas warm and usual color (may be cool and pale early postburn) e. palpable peripheral pulses	2.a. Assess for and report signs and symptoms of diminished systemic tissue perfusion: 1. significant decrease in B/P 2. resting pulse rate greater than 100 beats/minute 3. decline in systolic B/P of at least 15 mm Hg with a concurrent rise in pulse when client changes from lying to sitting or standing position 4. rapid or labored respirations 5. restlessness, slow responses, confusion 6. cool, pale, mottled, or cyanotic skin in unburned areas (areas, particularly those distal to burn, may be cool and pale early in postburn period) 7. diminished or absent peripheral pulses (pulses should be checked with a Doppler flowmeter every hour for at least 48 hours postburn or until edema subsides) 8. capillary refill time greater than 3 seconds

f. capillary refill time less than 3 seconds

g. urine output at least 30 cc/hour.

9. urine output less than 30 cc/hour (an indwelling catheter is usually ordered during the emergent phase *to provide a way to accurately assess hourly urine output*).

b. Implement measures *to maintain adequate systemic tissue perfusion:*

1. perform actions to prevent and treat hypovolemia (see Nursing Diagnosis 4.A, action 1.b)
2. maintain client in a horizontal position for first 48–72 hours postburn or as long as signs and symptoms of inadequate tissue perfusion are present *in order to maintain adequate cerebral blood flow and prevent orthostatic hypotension associated with hypovolemia*
3. change client's position slowly *to allow time for autoregulatory mechanisms to adjust to position changes*
4. perform actions to prevent peripheral pooling of blood and increase venous return (see Care Plan on Immobility, Nursing Diagnosis 2, action b.2)
5. maintain slight elevation of extremities with circumferential burns as ordered *to increase venous return without compromising arterial flow*
6. assist with escharotomy or fasciotomy of circumferential burns if edema is impairing circulation
7. perform actions to prevent hypothermia (see Nursing Diagnosis 7, action b) *in order to minimize generalized vasoconstriction.*

c. Consult physician if signs and symptoms of decreased systemic tissue perfusion persist or worsen.

3. NURSING DIAGNOSIS

Altered respiratory function:*

a. **ineffective airway clearance** related to:
  1. airway obstruction associated with upper airway edema (results from inhalation of heat and smoke; burn injury to head, neck, or upper thorax; and/or trauma occurring with intubation during resuscitation efforts), interstitial edema of lower airways (due to chemical injury resulting from inhalation of noxious gases), bronchospasm (results from airway or neural reflex irritation), and formation of pseudomembranous casts by damaged epithelial cells
  2. stasis of secretions associated with poor cough effort, decreased mobility, and impaired ciliary movement;
b. **ineffective breathing patterns:**
  1. **hyperventilation** related to fear, anxiety, and pain
  2. **hypoventilation** related to the depressant effects of certain medications (e.g. narcotic analgesics) and inability to fully expand chest wall associated with burn injury of the thorax, body positioning, and gastric distention;
c. **impaired gas exchange** related to:
  1. ineffective breathing patterns and/or airway clearance
  2. carbon monoxide (CO) poisoning (the high affinity of CO for hemoglobin results in displacement of oxygen, formation of carboxyhemoglobin, and hypoxia)
  3. decrease in effective lung surface associated with atelectasis (due to stasis of secretions and ineffective breathing patterns) and formation of hyaline membrane which occurs with necrosis of type 1 alveolar cells
  4. a thickened alveolar-capillary membrane associated with pulmonary edema (results from fluid overload, interstitial edema of lower airway if smoke inhalation has occurred, and an increase in pulmonary capillary perfusion due to an increased basal metabolic rate and cardiac output following resuscitation).

---

* This diagnostic label includes the following nursing diagnoses: ineffective breathing pattern, ineffective airway clearance, and impaired gas exchange (Carpenito, 1989).

DESIRED OUTCOMES	NURSING ACTIONS AND *SELECTED RATIONALES*

3. The client will maintain adequate respiratory function as evidenced by:
   a. normal rate, rhythm, and depth of respirations
   b. decreased dyspnea
   c. usual or improved breath sounds
   d. usual mental status
   e. usual skin color in unburned areas
   f. blood gases and carboxyhemoglobin (COHb) levels within a safe range for client.

3.a. Assess for and report signs and symptoms of the following:
   1. smoke or heat inhalation injury (closely monitor clients who have sustained burns of head and neck or whose burn occurred in a closed or poorly ventilated space):
      a. singed nasal hairs
      b. persistent cough
      c. soot or carbon particles in sputum (usually does not occur until 24–48 hours following injury)
      d. hoarseness, stridor
      e. choking
      f. dyspnea, tachypnea
      g. wheezing (indicative of severe inhalation injury if occurs earlier than 24–48 hours following injury)
   2. toxic chemical inhalation (e.g. shortness of breath, tenacious sputum with or without carbon particles, cough, rhinorrhea)
   3. carbon monoxide poisoning (e.g. headache, irritability, flushed appearance, nausea, vomiting, visual disturbances, dyspnea, dizziness, confusion, seizures)
   4. burn injury to upper airway without smoke inhalation (e.g. increasing edema above glottis, stridor, dyspnea, decreasing level of consciousness).

b. Assess for and report signs and symptoms of altered respiratory function:
   1. rapid, shallow, slow, or irregular respirations
   2. dyspnea
   3. use of accessory muscles when breathing
   4. adventitious and/or diminished or absent breath sounds
   5. restlessness, irritability
   6. confusion, somnolence
   7. dusky or cyanotic skin color in unburned areas.

c. Monitor blood gas and carboxyhemoglobin values. Report abnormal results.

d. Monitor for and report significant changes in ear oximetry and capnograph results.

e. Prepare client for the following if indicated:
   1. fiberoptic bronchoscopy and/or laryngoscopy *to determine if inhalation injury has occurred* (may be performed serially during the first 24–48 hours postburn *because of edema progression during that time*)
   2. xenon perfusion-ventilation lung scan *to aid in early diagnosis of smoke inhalation and identify small airway obstruction*
   3. pulmonary function studies *to evaluate lower respiratory tract injury and effectiveness of treatment.*

f. Implement measures *to improve respiratory status:*
   1. assist with intubation, mechanical ventilation, and/or tracheostomy if indicated
   2. if signs and symptoms of carbon monoxide poisoning exist, be prepared to assist with the following treatments:
      a. administration of 100% O_2 (*reduces half-life of COHb to less than 1 hour and facilitates return of normal oxyhemoglobin levels*)
      b. use of hyperbaric oxygen chamber
      c. ventilator assistance
   3. place client in a semi- to high Fowler's position unless contraindicated
   4. administer oxygen as ordered
   5. perform actions to reduce fear and anxiety (see Nursing Diagnosis 1, action c)
   6. instruct client to breathe slowly if he/she is hyperventilating
   7. perform actions to relieve pain (see Nursing Diagnosis 6.A, action 5)
   8. instruct client to turn and deep breathe or use inspiratory exerciser at least every 2 hours
   9. perform actions *to facilitate removal of pulmonary secretions and debris:*
      a. prepare client for laryngoscopy, bronchoscopy, and lung lavage if indicated
      b. instruct and assist client to cough every 1–2 hours

UNIT
XVI

   c. implement measures *to liquefy tenacious secretions:*
    1. continue with intravenous fluid resuscitation as ordered
    2. humidify inspired air as ordered
    3. assist with administration of mucolytic agents via nebulizer or IPPB treatment
   d. assist with or perform postural drainage, percussion, and vibration if ordered
   e. perform tracheal suctioning if client is unable to cough up secretions
   f. monitor for therapeutic and nontherapeutic effects of expectorants if administered
  10. perform actions to prevent and treat fluid volume excess (see Nursing Diagnosis 4.B, action 1.c) *in order to prevent pulmonary edema*
  11. monitor for therapeutic and nontherapeutic effects of bronchodilators if administered *to decrease bronchospasm*
  12. increase activity as allowed and tolerated
  13. administer central nervous system depressants (e.g. narcotic analgesics, sedatives) judiciously *to prevent further respiratory depression*; hold medication and consult physician if respiratory rate is less than 12/minute
  14. assist with escharotomy if burns of chest wall are circumferential and are inhibiting chest expansion
  15. when oral intake is allowed, instruct client to avoid gas-producing foods/fluids (e.g. beans, cauliflower, cabbage, onions, carbonated beverages) and large meals *to prevent gastric distention and increased pressure on diaphragm*
  16. discourage smoking.
 g. Consult physician if:
  1. signs and symptoms of altered respiratory function worsen or fail to improve
  2. signs and symptoms of respiratory acidosis (e.g. change in mental status, increased pulse, dizziness, headache, feeling of fullness in head, muscle twitching, seizures, increase in $PaCO_2$ and decline in pH) are present
  3. signs and symptoms of respiratory alkalosis (e.g. inability to concentrate, lightheadedness, palpitations, circumoral paresthesias, numbness and tingling of extremities, diaphoresis, tinnitus, blurred vision, low $PaCO_2$ and elevated pH) are present.

□ ▬▬▬▬▬▬▬▬▬▬▬▬▬▬▬▬▬▬▬▬▬▬▬▬▬▬

4.A. NURSING/COLLABORATIVE DIAGNOSIS

Altered fluid and electrolyte balance in the emergent (fluid accumulation or shock) phase:

1. **hypovolemia** related to:
 a. third-spacing associated with increased capillary permeability resulting from trauma
 b. blood loss associated with leakage from damaged capillaries
 c. excessive loss of fluid associated with evaporation and exudation from denuded body surfaces, vomiting, nasogastric tube drainage, and diarrhea
 d. delayed or inadequate fluid replacement;
2. **hyperkalemia** related to:
 a. release of potassium from damaged cells
 b. metabolic acidosis (results in cellular release of potassium)
 c. impaired renal function (may result from hemoglobinuria, myoglobinuria, and decreased renal blood flow);
3. **hyponatremia** related to excessive loss from denuded skin areas, shift of sodium into interstitial space (associated with increased capillary permeability), vomiting, nasogastric tube drainage, diarrhea, and excessive administration of electrolyte-free water;

4. **metabolic acidosis** related to:
  a. release of fixed acids from damaged cells
  b. hyperkalemia and hyponatremia
  c. excessive lactic acid production associated with cellular hypoxia resulting from inadequate tissue perfusion
  d. ketosis associated with an increased metabolism of fats resulting from an inadequate carbohydrate intake
  e. excessive loss of bicarbonate associated with diarrhea and impaired renal reabsorptive function
  f. use of mafenide acetate as a topical anti-infective agent on extensive burn areas (mafenide is a carbonic anhydrase inhibitor and results in a rapid alkaline diuresis).

DESIRED OUTCOMES	NURSING ACTIONS AND *SELECTED RATIONALES*

4.A.1. The client will not experience hypovolemia as evidenced by:
a. usual mental status
b. stable vital signs
c. balanced intake and output within 48 hours following burn injury
d. palpable peripheral pulses
e. capillary refill time less than 3 seconds.
	4.A.1.a. Assess for and report signs and symptoms of:
	1. hypovolemia:
	  a. restlessness, agitation
	  b. significant decrease in B/P
	  c. significant increase in resting pulse rate
	  d. decline in B/P of at least 15 mm Hg with concurrent rise in pulse when client changes from lying to sitting or standing position
	  e. rapid or labored respirations
	  f. decline in urine output
	  g. diminished or absent peripheral pulses
	  h. capillary refill time greater than 3 seconds
	2. third-spacing (e.g. peripheral edema, ascites, dyspnea, crackles and/or diminished breath sounds).
	b. Implement measures *to prevent and treat hypovolemia:*
	1. maintain intravenous fluid therapy as ordered (a variety of formulas and protocols using colloids, crystalloids [e.g. lactated Ringer's solution], and glucose in water may be utilized depending on physician preference and extent of burn injury)
	2. monitor for therapeutic and nontherapeutic effects of blood replacements if administered (blood replacement is usually delayed until fluid resuscitation is complete *because of the increased capillary permeability during emergent phase*; it is given as part of the resuscitation effort if blood loss is due to associated injuries or if there is pre-existing anemia)
	3. assist with application of occlusive or biological dressings *to reduce evaporative fluid loss*
	4. perform actions to control diarrhea (see Nursing Diagnosis 13, action d)
	5. perform actions to prevent nausea and vomiting (see Nursing Diagnosis 6.B, action 2).
	c. If signs and symptoms of hypovolemia persist:
	1. continue with above measures
	2. consult physician if signs and symptoms of hypovolemic shock (see Collaborative Diagnosis 17, action d.1.c) occur.

4.A.2. The client will maintain a safe serum potassium level as evidenced by: a. regular pulse at 60–100 beats/minute b. usual muscle tone and strength c. normal bowel sounds d. serum potassium within normal range.	4.A.2.a. Assess for and report signs and symptoms of hyperkalemia (e.g. slow or irregular pulse; paresthesias; muscle weakness and flaccidity; hyperactive bowel sounds with diarrhea and intestinal colic; EKG reading showing peaked T wave, prolonged PR interval, and/or widened QRS; elevated serum potassium level). b. Implement measures *to prevent or treat hyperkalemia:* 1. perform actions to prevent or treat acidosis (see action 4.b in this diagnosis) *in order to decrease cellular release of potassium* 2. if oral intake is allowed, maintain dietary restrictions of potassium as ordered

3. if signs and symptoms of hyperkalemia are present, consult physician before administering prescribed potassium supplements
4. monitor for therapeutic and nontherapeutic effects of the following if administered:
   a. cation-exchange resins (e.g. Kayexalate) *to increase potassium excretion via the intestines (act by exchanging sodium for potassium)*
   b. intravenous insulin and hypertonic glucose solutions *to enhance transport of potassium back into cells*
5. prepare client for dialysis if planned.
c. Consult physician if signs and symptoms of hyperkalemia persist or worsen.

4.A.3. The client will maintain a safe serum sodium level as evidenced by:
a. usual mental status
b. usual strength and muscle tone
c. absence of nausea, vomiting, abdominal cramps, twitching, seizure activity
d. serum sodium within normal range.

4.A.3.a. Assess for and report signs and symptoms of hyponatremia (e.g. lethargy, confusion, weakness, nausea, vomiting, abdominal cramps, twitching, seizures, low serum sodium level).
b. Implement measures *to prevent or treat hyponatremia:*
   1. maintain fluid and electrolyte replacement therapy as ordered
   2. perform actions to reduce nausea and vomiting (see Nursing Diagnosis 6.B, action 2)
   3. perform actions to prevent or control diarrhea (see Nursing Diagnosis 13, action d)
   4. if irrigation of nasogastric tube is indicated, use normal saline rather than water
   5. if oral intake is allowed during this phase:
      a. encourage intake of foods/fluids high in sodium (e.g. soups, bouillon)
      b. limit intake of water as ordered *to prevent dilutional hyponatremia (oral electrolyte solutions may be allowed to replenish sodium levels and ease thirst).*
c. Consult physician if signs and symptoms of hyponatremia persist or worsen.

4.A.4. The client will maintain acid-base balance as evidenced by:
a. usual mental status
b. unlabored respirations at 16–20/minute
c. absence of headache, nausea, vomiting
d. blood gases within normal range for client
e. anion gap less than 16 mEq/liter.

4.A.4.a. Assess for and report signs and symptoms of metabolic acidosis (e.g. drowsiness; disorientation; stupor; rapid, deep respirations; headache; nausea; vomiting; low pH and CO_2 content and negative base excess; anion gap greater than 16 mEq/liter).
b. Implement measures *to prevent or treat metabolic acidosis:*
   1. perform actions to promote adequate tissue perfusion (see Nursing Diagnosis 2, action b) *in order to prevent tissue hypoxia and subsequent lactic acid release*
   2. perform actions to control diarrhea (see Nursing Diagnosis 13, action d)
   3. perform actions to maintain serum potassium within normal range (see action 2.b in this diagnosis)
   4. perform actions to maintain an adequate nutritional status (see Nursing Diagnosis 5, action c) *in order to reduce ketosis*
   5. perform actions to prevent or treat hyponatremia (see action 3.b in this diagnosis)
   6. monitor for therapeutic and nontherapeutic effects of sodium bicarbonate if administered (reserved for use in severe acidosis when pH is less than 7.1).
c. Consult physician if signs and symptoms of acidosis persist or worsen.

4.B. NURSING/COLLABORATIVE DIAGNOSIS

Altered fluid and electrolyte balance during the acute phase (fluid remobilization or stage of diuresis):

1. fluid volume excess related to:
a. reabsorption of third-space fluid

    b. excessive fluid replacement

    c. decreased fluid excretion associated with impaired renal function (may result from hemoglobinuria, myoglobinuria, and decreased renal blood flow) and high levels of antidiuretic hormone resulting from pain and stress;

2. **hyponatremia** related to:

    a. hemodilution associated with disproportionate fluid and sodium replacements in relation to evaporative losses

    b. increased sodium loss associated with:

        1. topical wound treatment with silver nitrate (increases transeschar loss)

        2. extensive denuded skin areas and lengthy hydrotherapy sessions (increase electrolyte loss through large open wounds)

        3. excessive diuresis (may occur when fluid shifts back into intravascular space if renal function is adequate)

        4. vomiting, nasogastric tube drainage, and diarrhea;

3. **hypernatremia** related to:

    a. inadequate fluid replacement in proportion to fluid loss (fluid is lost as a result of evaporation from denuded areas and diaphoresis and rapid respirations if sepsis is present)

    b. excessive saline administration

    c. osmotic diuresis associated with glucosuria (resulting from stress-related glucose elevation) or increased urinary urea nitrogen excretion resulting from excessive protein catabolism;

4. **hypokalemia** related to:

    a. hemodilution associated with fluid volume excess

    b. inadequate potassium replacement

    c. loss of potassium associated with diuresis, diarrhea, vomiting, nasogastric tube drainage, application of silver nitrate (increases transeschar loss) or mafenide acetate (increases renal loss) to burn areas, and lengthy hydrotherapy sessions (increases electrolyte loss through large open wounds)

    d. shift of potassium from the intravascular space back into the cells once acidosis is corrected;

5. **hypochloremia** related to hemodilution and excessive loss of chloride associated with vomiting, nasogastric tube drainage, and diarrhea;

6. **hypophosphatemia** related to:

    a. hemodilution associated with fluid volume excess

    b. phosphate-free fluid replacements

    c. shift of phosphate into the cells associated with intravenous glucose infusions

    d. loss of phosphate associated with diarrhea

    e. excessive administration of phosphate-binding antacids;

7. **metabolic alkalosis** related to hypochloremia, hypokalemia, and loss of hydrochloric acid associated with vomiting and nasogastric tube drainage.

DESIRED OUTCOMES	NURSING ACTIONS AND *SELECTED RATIONALES*
4.B.1. The client will not experience fluid volume excess as evidenced by: a. return to preburn weight b. stable B/P and pulse c. absence of gallop rhythms d. balanced intake and output e. usual mental status f. normal breath sounds	4.B.1.a. Assess for and report signs and symptoms of fluid volume excess: 1. significant weight gain (client should be weighed daily, gain no more than 15–20% of his/her normal body weight with fluid replacement therapy, and return to preburn weight by 10th postburn day) 2. elevated B/P and pulse 3. development or worsening of an S_3 and/or S_4 gallop rhythm 4. intake greater than output 5. change in mental status 6. crackles and diminished or absent breath sounds 7. decreased Hct. level (may also be decreased due to capillary leakage) 8. dyspnea, orthopnea

g. Hct. within normal range
h. absence of dyspnea, peripheral edema, distended neck veins
i. CVP within normal range.

9. peripheral edema
10. distended neck veins
11. elevated CVP (use internal jugular vein pulsation method to estimate CVP if monitoring device not present).

b. Monitor chest x-ray results. Report findings of vascular congestion, pleural effusion, or pulmonary edema.

c. Implement measures *to prevent or treat fluid volume excess:*
1. maintain intravenous infusion rates and oral fluid restrictions as ordered
2. monitor for therapeutic and nontherapeutic effects of the following medications if administered:
   a. diuretics *to increase excretion of water*
   b. positive inotropic agents and arterial vasodilators *to increase cardiac output and subsequently improve renal blood flow.*

d. Consult physician if signs and symptoms of fluid volume excess persist or worsen.

4.B.2. The client will maintain a safe serum sodium level as evidenced by:
a. moist mucous membranes
b. absence of fever
c. usual mental status
d. usual strength and muscle tone
e. absence of nausea, vomiting, twitching, seizure activity
f. serum sodium level within normal range.

4.B.2.a. Assess for and report signs and symptoms of the following:
1. hyponatremia (e.g. lethargy, confusion, weakness, nausea, vomiting, abdominal cramps, twitching, seizures, low serum sodium level)
2. hypernatremia (e.g. thirst; dry, sticky mucous membranes; elevated temperature; restlessness; lethargy; weakness; seizures; elevated serum sodium level).

b. Implement measures *to prevent or treat hyponatremia:*
1. refer to Nursing Diagnosis 4.A, action 3.b, for measures related to prevention and treatment of hyponatremia
2. limit hydrotherapy sessions to no longer than 20 minutes *in order to prevent further sodium loss*
3. perform actions to prevent or treat fluid volume excess (see action 1.c in this diagnosis).

c. Implement measures *to prevent or treat hypernatremia:*
1. maintain intravenous fluid therapy as ordered
2. maintain dietary sodium restrictions as ordered
3. monitor blood and urine glucose levels and report increased levels *(glucosuria causes osmotic diuresis)*
4. monitor for therapeutic and nontherapeutic effects of insulin if administered *to reduce hyperglycemia and prevent osmotic diuresis*
5. perform actions to prevent and/or treat wound infection (see Nursing Diagnosis 15, actions a.4 and 5) *in order to reduce risk of diaphoresis and rapid respirations associated with sepsis.*

d. Consult physician if signs and symptoms of sodium imbalance persist or worsen.

4.B.3. The client will maintain safe serum potassium and chloride levels as evidenced by:
a. regular pulse at 60–100 beats/minute
b. respiratory rate at 16–20/minute
c. usual muscle tone and strength
d. normal bowel sounds
e. serum potassium and chloride within normal range.

4.B.3.a. Assess for and report signs and symptoms of:
1. hypokalemia (e.g. irregular pulse; muscle weakness and cramping; paresthesias; nausea and vomiting; hypoactive or absent bowel sounds; drowsiness; EKG reading showing ST depression, T wave inversion or flattening, and presence of U waves; low serum potassium level)
2. hypochloremia (e.g. twitching, tetany, depressed respirations, low serum chloride level).

b. Implement measures *to prevent or treat hypokalemia and/or hypochloremia:*
1. perform actions to reduce nausea and vomiting (see Nursing Diagnosis 6.B, action 2)
2. if irrigation of nasogastric tube is indicated, use normal saline rather than water
3. perform actions to reduce diarrhea (see Nursing Diagnosis 13, action d)
4. limit hydrotherapy sessions to no more than 20 minutes *to prevent excessive loss of potassium*
5. perform actions to prevent or treat fluid volume excess (see action 1.c in this diagnosis)
6. monitor for therapeutic and nontherapeutic effects of fluid and electrolyte replacements if administered

7. when oral intake is allowed, encourage intake of foods/fluids high in potassium (e.g. bananas, oranges, potatoes, raisins, figs, apricots, dates, tomatoes, Gatorade, fruit juices).
   c. Consult physician if signs and symptoms of hypokalemia and hypochloremia persist or worsen.

4.B.4. The client will maintain a safe serum phosphorus level as evidenced by:
   a. usual mental status
   b. usual strength and muscle tone
   c. absence of paresthesias, ataxia, seizure activity
   d. serum phosphorus within normal range.

4.B.4.a. Assess for and report signs and symptoms of hypophosphatemia (e.g. confusion, muscle weakness, paresthesias, ataxia, seizures, low serum phosphorus level).
   b. Implement measures *to prevent or treat hypophosphatemia:*
      1. perform actions to control diarrhea (see Nursing Diagnosis 13, action d)
      2. perform actions to prevent or treat fluid volume excess (see action 1.c in this diagnosis)
      3. if oral intake is allowed, encourage client to select foods/fluids high in phosphorus (e.g. fish, poultry, eggs, red meat, milk, peas, cheese, corn)
      4. monitor for therapeutic and nontherapeutic effects of phosphate supplements if administered
      5. if client is receiving phosphorus-binding antacids (e.g. Amphojel, ALternaGEL), consult physician about a change in antacids if serum phosphorus is low or if signs and symptoms of hypophosphatemia occur.
   c. Consult physician if signs and symptoms of hypophosphatemia persist or worsen.

4.B.5. The client will maintain acid-base balance as evidenced by:
   a. absence of dizziness and confusion
   b. respiratory rate at 16–20/minute
   c. usual sensation in unburned fingers, toes, and circumoral area
   d. absence of muscle twitching and seizure activity
   e. blood gases within normal range.

4.B.5.a. Assess for and report signs and symptoms of metabolic alkalosis (e.g. dizziness; confusion; bradypnea; tingling of unburned fingers, toes, and circumoral area; muscle twitching; seizures; elevated pH and CO_2 content and positive base excess).
   b. Implement measures to prevent or treat hypokalemia and hypochloremia (see action 3.b in this diagnosis) *in order to prevent or treat metabolic alkalosis.*
   c. Consult physician if signs and symptoms of metabolic alkalosis persist or worsen.

5. NURSING DIAGNOSIS

Altered nutrition: less than body requirements related to:

a. increased utilization of dietary proteins, fats, and carbohydrates associated with an increased metabolic rate (may be elevated 40%–100% depending on the amount of body surface area involved);
b. excessive albumin and protein losses from large draining wounds;
c. marked catabolic response associated with the stress of injury;
d. decreased oral intake associated with nausea, weakness, fatigue, prescribed dietary restrictions during emergent phase, and pain;
e. loss of nutrients associated with vomiting and diarrhea.

UNIT
XVI

DESIRED OUTCOMES	NURSING ACTIONS AND *SELECTED RATIONALES*

5. The client will maintain an adequate nutritional status as evidenced by:
   a. loss of no more than 10% of preburn weight
   b. BUN and serum albumin, protein, Hct., Hgb., cholesterol, and lymphocyte levels returning toward normal range
   c. triceps skinfold measurements within normal range
   d. usual strength and activity tolerance
   e. healthy oral mucous membrane.

5.a. Assess the client for signs and symptoms of malnutrition:
   1. loss of more than 10% of client's preburn weight
   2. abnormal BUN and low serum albumin, protein, Hct., Hgb., cholesterol, and lymphocyte levels
   3. triceps skinfold measurement less than normal for build
   4. weakness and fatigue
   5. stomatitis.
 b. When oral intake is allowed:
   1. monitor percentage of meals eaten
   2. assess the client to determine the causative factors of inadequate intake (e.g. nausea, weakness, fatigue).
 c. Implement measures *to maintain an optimal nutritional status:*
   1. monitor for therapeutic and nontherapeutic effects of tube feedings and total parenteral nutrition if administered
   2. perform actions to prevent or control diarrhea (see Nursing Diagnosis 13, action d)
   3. when foods/fluids are allowed, perform actions *to improve oral intake:*
      a. implement measures to reduce pain (see Nursing Diagnosis 6.A, action 5)
      b. implement measures to reduce nausea and vomiting (see Nursing Diagnosis 6.B, action 2)
      c. provide oral care before meals
      d. serve small portions of nutritious foods/fluids that are appealing to the client
      e. provide variety in commercial supplements if being used to augment caloric intake (e.g. puddings instead of liquids, different flavors)
      f. provide a clean, relaxed, pleasant atmosphere
      g. schedule wound care and other treatments at least an hour before meals
      h. encourage a rest period before meals *to minimize fatigue*
      i. encourage significant others to bring in client's favorite foods and eat with him/her *to make eating more of a familiar social experience*
      j. increase activity as allowed and tolerated *(activity stimulates appetite)*
   4. perform actions *to meet increased nutritional needs:*
      a. obtain a dietary consult if necessary to assist client in selecting foods/fluids that meet nutritional needs as well as preferences
      b. provide a diet high in calories (as much as 5000 calories daily depending on the amount of body surface area involved), protein, carbohydrate, vitamins, and minerals
      c. encourage client to drink or eat all of commercial supplements ordered
   5. perform actions *to reduce client's energy demands:*
      a. implement measures to reduce fear and anxiety (see Nursing Diagnosis 1, action c)
      b. implement measures to reduce pain (see Nursing Diagnosis 6.A, action 5)
      c. implement measures to prevent hypothermia and subsequent chilling (see Nursing Diagnosis 7, action b)
      d. implement measures to prevent or treat wound infection (see Nursing Diagnosis 15, actions a.4 and 5)
   6. monitor for therapeutic and nontherapeutic effects of vitamins, minerals, and hematinics if administered.
 d. Perform a 72-hour calorie count if nutritional status appears to be declining.
 e. Reassess nutritional status on a regular basis and report decline.

6.A. NURSING DIAGNOSIS

Altered comfort:* pain related to:

1. damaged or exposed nerve endings associated with a partial-thickness burn;
2. multiple donor sites for grafting;
3. exercising of burned limbs;
4. progressively tightening scar tissue;
5. extensive, frequent debridement of eschar;
6. wound care.

---

* In this care plan, the nursing diagnosis "pain" is included under the diagnostic label of altered comfort.

DESIRED OUTCOMES	NURSING ACTIONS AND *SELECTED RATIONALES*

6.A. The client will experience diminished pain as evidenced by:
1. verbalization of pain relief
2. relaxed facial expression and body positioning
3. increased participation in activities
4. stable vital signs.

6.A.1. Determine how the client usually responds to pain.
2. Assess for nonverbal signs of pain (e.g. guarding of affected body parts, wrinkled brow, clenched fists, reluctance to move, restlessness, diaphoresis, facial pallor or flushing, change in B/P, tachycardia).
3. Assess verbal complaints of pain. Ask client to be specific about location, severity, and type of pain.
4. Assess for factors that seem to aggravate and alleviate pain.
5. Implement measures *to reduce pain:*
    a. perform actions to reduce fear and anxiety about the pain experience (e.g. assure client that his/her needs for pain relief will be met, perform preoperative or preprocedure teaching)
    b. medicate before pain is severe; if client has patient-controlled analgesia (PCA) device, encourage him/her to use it as instructed
    c. perform actions *to reduce discomfort associated with wound care and exercise sessions:*
        1. administer analgesics 30 minutes before wound care and exercise sessions
        2. monitor for therapeutic and nontherapeutic effects of anesthetic agents (e.g. Penthrane, 50% nitrous oxide, ketamine) if administered in analgesic doses *to reduce pain during debridement sessions*
        3. moisten dressings with normal saline *to facilitate removal*
        4. provide emotional support during wound care and exercise sessions
    d. apply a light sterile covering to wounds or utilize a bed cradle *to relieve pain due to exposure of nerve endings to air currents*
    e. position burned parts in functional body alignment; instruct and assist client to perform range of motion exercises as ordered *to prevent progressively tightening scar tissue and contractures*
    f. obtain assistance when turning or transferring client *to provide adequate support to burn areas and donor sites*
    g. provide or assist with nonpharmacological measures for pain relief (e.g. back rub, position change, relaxation techniques, guided imagery, quiet conversation, restful environment, diversional activities)
    h. plan methods for achieving pain relief with client *in order to assist him/her to maintain a sense of control over the pain experience*
    i. monitor for therapeutic and nontherapeutic effects of analgesics if administered (in the early postburn period, small frequent intravenous doses of narcotics should be administered; intramuscular and subcutaneous routes are avoided *because of decreased absorption due to diminished tissue perfusion).*
6. Consult physician if above measures fail to provide adequate pain relief.

☐ ▆▆▆▆▆▆▆▆▆▆▆▆▆▆▆▆▆▆▆▆▆▆▆▆▆▆▆▆▆▆▆▆▆▆

6.B. NURSING DIAGNOSIS

Altered comfort: nausea and vomiting related to stimulation of the vomiting center associated with:

1. vagal and/or sympathetic stimulation resulting from visceral irritation associated with abdominal distention (may occur as a result of electrolyte imbalances and slowed gastrointestinal motility associated with stress response and decreased activity);
2. cortical stimulation due to pain and stress;
3. chemoreceptor trigger zone stimulation associated with electrolyte imbalance.

☐ ▆▆▆▆▆▆▆▆▆▆▆▆▆▆▆▆▆▆▆▆▆▆▆▆▆▆▆▆▆▆▆▆▆▆

DESIRED OUTCOMES	NURSING ACTIONS AND *SELECTED RATIONALES*

6.B. The client will experience relief of nausea and vomiting as evidenced by:
1. verbalization of relief of nausea
2. absence of vomiting.
	6.B.1. Assess client to determine factors that contribute to nausea and vomiting (e.g. electrolyte imbalances, fear, anxiety, abdominal distention, pain).
	2. Implement measures *to prevent nausea and vomiting:*
	  a. maintain patency of nasogastric tube (e.g. keep tubing free of kinks, irrigate and maintain suction as ordered) if present
	  b. perform actions to relieve pain (see Nursing Diagnosis 6.A, action 5)
	  c. perform actions to reduce fear and anxiety (see Nursing Diagnosis 1, action c)
	  d. perform actions to correct metabolic acidosis, hyponatremia, and hypokalemia (see Nursing Diagnoses 4.A, action 4.b and 4.B, actions 2.b and 3.b)
	  e. eliminate noxious sights and smells from the environment *(noxious stimuli cause cortical stimulation of the vomiting center)*
	  f. encourage client to change positions slowly *(movement stimulates the chemoreceptor trigger zone)*
	  g. encourage client to take deep, slow breaths when nauseated
	  h. provide oral hygiene after each emesis and before meals
	  i. maintain food and fluid restrictions as ordered
	  j. when oral intake is allowed:
	    1. progress diet from clear liquid to general as tolerated
	    2. avoid serving foods with an overpowering aroma; remove lids from hot foods before entering room
	    3. encourage client to eat dry foods (e.g. toast, crackers) and avoid drinking liquids with meals if nauseated
	    4. provide small, frequent meals rather than 3 large ones
	    5. instruct client to ingest foods and fluids slowly
	    6. instruct client to avoid foods/fluids that irritate the gastric mucosa (e.g. spicy foods; citrus fruits or juices; caffeine-containing items such as chocolate, coffee, tea, and colas)
	    7. instruct client to rest after eating with head of bed elevated
	  k. monitor for therapeutic and nontherapeutic effects of antiemetics and gastrointestinal stimulants (e.g. metoclopramide) if administered.
	3. Consult physician if above measures fail to control nausea and vomiting.

☐ ▆▆▆▆▆▆▆▆▆▆▆▆▆▆▆▆▆▆▆▆▆▆▆▆▆▆▆▆▆▆▆▆▆▆

6.C. NURSING DIAGNOSIS

Altered comfort: chills related to excessive heat loss associated with loss of skin integrity, body exposure if open method is used to treat burns, and tubbing procedures.

☐ ▆▆▆▆▆▆▆▆▆▆▆▆▆▆▆▆▆▆▆▆▆▆▆▆▆▆▆▆▆▆▆▆▆▆

DESIRED OUTCOMES	NURSING ACTIONS AND *SELECTED RATIONALES*
6.C. The client will not experience discomfort associated with chills as evidenced by: 1. verbalization of comfort 2. ability to rest.	6.C.1. Assess client frequently for chills. 2. Implement measures to prevent hypothermia (see Nursing Diagnosis 7, action b) *in order to prevent chilling.* 3. If chilling occurs, implement measures to increase comfort (e.g. provide additional blankets, increase room temperature, provide warm liquids to drink as tolerated). 4. Consult physician if above measures fail to prevent chilling.

☐ ████████████████████████████████████

7. NURSING DIAGNOSIS

Hypothermia related to:

a. inability to retain body heat associated with loss of microcirculation in burned areas;
b. loss of heat through extensive open wounds and during lengthy hydrotherapy sessions.

☐ ████████████████████████████████████

DESIRED OUTCOMES	NURSING ACTIONS AND *SELECTED RATIONALES*
7. The client will not experience hypothermia as evidenced by: a. body temperature within normal range b. warm skin in unburned areas c. usual mental status d. stable pulse and respirations.	7.a. Assess client for signs and symptoms of hypothermia (e.g. reduction in body temperature below normal, cool skin and piloerection in unburned areas, mental confusion, decreased pulse and respirations). b. Implement measures *to prevent hypothermia:* 1. perform actions to maintain adequate systemic tissue perfusion (see Nursing Diagnosis 2, action b) 2. limit hydrotherapy sessions to no longer than 20 minutes and maintain water temperature at 37.8°C (100°F) 3. maintain room temperature at 29.4°C (85°F) and utilize a bed cradle *to support additional blankets over client for warmth and to prevent drafts* 4. provide warm liquids to drink as tolerated 5. utilize heat lamps or heat shields with sensors as additional sources of heat if indicated 6. complete wound care quickly and efficiently *to prevent prolonged body exposure.* c. Consult physician if signs and symptoms of hypothermia persist or worsen.

☐ ████████████████████████████████████

8. NURSING DIAGNOSIS

Impaired skin integrity:

a. **burn injury, extensive debridement of damaged tissue, and grafting procedures;**
b. **impaired healing of burn or graft sites** related to malnutrition; inadequate tissue oxygenation associated with decreased tissue perfusion, anemia, and impaired alveolar gas exchange; infection; and high levels of glucocorticoids associated with pain and stress;
c. **irritation or breakdown** related to:
1. prolonged pressure on tissues associated with decreased mobility
2. increased tissue fragility associated with edema and tissue hypoxia resulting from decreased tissue perfusion, anemia, and a compromised respiratory status
3. dryness of unaffected and healed skin associated with frequent hydrotherapy.

☐ ████████████████████████████████████

UNIT
XVI

DESIRED OUTCOMES	NURSING ACTIONS AND *SELECTED RATIONALES*

8.a. The client will experience healing of burn, graft, and donor sites within expected period as evidenced by:
1. gradual reduction in redness and discomfort at burn, graft, and donor sites
2. presence of granulation tissue in healing wounds
3. intact graft edges.

8.a.1. Assess for and report signs and symptoms of impaired wound healing (e.g. increasing redness and edema at burn, graft, or donor sites; increasing pain in wound or donor areas; increase in necrotic tissue in burn areas; separation of graft edges).
2. Implement measures *to promote wound healing:*
   a. perform actions to maintain an optimal nutritional status (see Nursing Diagnosis 5, action c)
   b. perform actions to improve systemic tissue perfusion (see Nursing Diagnosis 2, action b) *in order to maintain adequate circulation to the wound areas*
   c. perform actions to improve respiratory status (see Nursing Diagnosis 3, action f) *in order to improve tissue oxygenation*
   d. perform actions to prevent and treat wound infection (see Nursing Diagnosis 15, actions a.4 and 5)
   e. perform appropriate wound care (i.e. open, semi-open, or closed method) as ordered
   f. perform actions *to prevent unnecessary trauma to wounds:*
      1. utilize bed cradle *to prevent linens from touching wounds open to air*
      2. moisten linens with saline before removal if they are adhering to burn areas
      3. if silver nitrate solution is being applied to wounds, thoroughly resaturate dressings as ordered *to maintain a safe concentration of silver nitrate (concentrations greater than 2–3% are caustic)*
   g. prepare client for grafting procedures when indicated *(allows earlier healing and minimizes excessive granulation tissue growth)*
   h. when grafting is done:
      1. perform actions *to prevent graft dislodgment* (e.g. avoid pressure on the graft site, use caution when performing wound care)
      2. perform actions to promote healing of donor site:
         a. use a bed cradle *to protect area from pressure of linens*
         b. if more than 30 cc of fluid collects under transparent occlusive dressing (e.g. Tegaderm) applied in surgery, aspirate it with a 25-gauge needle as ordered and patch needle hole with a small piece of occlusive dressing material rather than removing the dressing
         c. if a gauze dressing is used, expose to air or utilize a heat lamp as ordered *to facilitate drying*; when sufficient healing has occurred, dressing can be soaked off
      3. monitor for therapeutic and nontherapeutic effects of immunosuppressives if administered *to reduce risk of rejection of graft*.
3. Consult physician if:
   a. signs and symptoms of a wound infection (e.g. chills; fever; increased redness, warmth, and swelling of burn areas and/or donor site[s]; purulent, green, or gray, foul-smelling drainage from wounds) occur
   b. signs and symptoms of graft failure (e.g. sloughing, darkened edges) occur.
4. If signs and symptoms of impaired wound healing occur:
   a. assist with further wound debridement as indicated
   b. provide emotional support to client and significant others.

8.b. The client will maintain skin integrity in unaffected areas as evidenced by:
1. absence of redness and irritation
2. no skin breakdown.

8.b.1. Inspect the skin in unaffected areas (especially bone prominences and dependent and edematous areas) for redness, pallor, and breakdown.
2. Refer to Care Plan on Immobility, Nursing Diagnosis 7, action b, for measures related to prevention of skin breakdown associated with decreased mobility.
3. Implement measures *to prevent skin breakdown associated with increased tissue fragility:*
   a. perform actions to improve respiratory status (see Nursing Diagnosis 3, action f) *in order to improve tissue oxygenation*
   b. perform actions to improve systemic tissue perfusion (see Nursing Diagnosis 2, action b)

    c. perform actions to maintain an optimal nutritional status (see Nursing Diagnosis 5, action c)

    d. perform actions to prevent or treat fluid volume excess (see Nursing Diagnosis 4.B, action 1.c) *in order to reduce tissue edema.*

4. Implement measures *to prevent drying of unaffected and healed skin areas:*

    a. avoid use of harsh soaps and hot water

    b. apply skin moisturizers or emollient creams to unaffected and healed skin areas after each hydrotherapy session.

5. If skin breakdown occurs:

    a. notify physician

    b. continue with above measures to prevent further irritation and breakdown

    c. perform decubitus care as ordered or per standard hospital policy

    d. monitor client closely and report signs and symptoms of infection (e.g. elevated temperature; redness, warmth, and edema around area of breakdown; unusual drainage from site).

---

9. NURSING DIAGNOSIS

Activity intolerance related to:

a. inadequate tissue oxygenation associated with:
1. decreased tissue perfusion
2. impaired alveolar gas exchange resulting from ineffective airway clearance and/or breathing pattern, carbon monoxide poisoning, decrease in effective lung surface, and pulmonary edema
3. anemia resulting from thermal destruction of red cells, bleeding at the time of injury, blood loss during subsequent debridement of tissue, and malnutrition;

b. inadequate nutritional status;

c. difficulty resting and sleeping associated with discomfort, nightmares, inability to assume usual sleep position, fear, anxiety, and frequent assessments and treatments.

DESIRED OUTCOMES	NURSING ACTIONS AND *SELECTED RATIONALES*

9. The client will demonstrate an increased tolerance for activity (see Care Plan on Immobility, Nursing Diagnosis 8, for outcome criteria).	9.a. Refer to Care Plan on Immobility, Nursing Diagnosis 8, for measures related to assessment and improvement of activity tolerance.
	b. Implement additional measures *to promote rest and improve activity tolerance:*
	  1. perform actions to reduce fear and anxiety (see Nursing Diagnosis 1, action c)
	  2. perform actions to promote sleep (see Nursing Diagnosis 14)
	  3. perform actions to relieve discomfort (see Nursing Diagnoses 6.A, action 5; 6.B, action 2; and 6.C, actions 2 and 3)
	  4. perform actions to maintain adequate systemic tissue perfusion (see Nursing Diagnosis 2, action b)
	  5. perform actions to improve respiratory status (see Nursing Diagnosis 3, action f)
	  6. perform actions to maintain an optimal nutritional status (see Nursing Diagnosis 5, action c)
	  7. monitor for therapeutic and nontherapeutic effects of whole blood or packed red cells if administered.

UNIT
XVI

10. NURSING DIAGNOSIS

Impaired physical mobility related to:

a. pain;
b. activity restrictions associated with the treatment plan;
c. activity intolerance;
d. altered sensory and motor function associated with the burn injury and fluid and electrolyte imbalances;
e. decreased range of motion associated with contractures.

DESIRED OUTCOMES	NURSING ACTIONS AND *SELECTED RATIONALES*

10.a. The client will achieve maximum physical mobility within limitations imposed by the burn injury and prescribed activity restrictions.	10.a.1. Assess for factors that impair physical mobility (e.g. reluctance to move because of pain, activity restrictions, sensory or motor deficits, limitations in range of motion).
	2. Implement measures *to increase mobility:*
	  a. perform actions to control pain (see Nursing Diagnosis 6.A, action 5)
	  b. perform actions to maintain fluid and electrolyte balance (see appropriate actions in Nursing Diagnoses 4.A and 4.B)
	  c. perform actions to improve activity tolerance (see Nursing Diagnosis 9)
	  d. instruct and assist client in correct use of mobility aids (e.g. cane, walker, crutches) if appropriate
	  e. perform actions to reduce risk of contractures (see Collaborative Diagnosis 17, action f.2)
	  f. assist with prescribed exercise program to maintain muscle tone and joint mobility
	  g. encourage client to use unaffected extremities in performing activities of daily living
	  h. consult with physical and occupational therapists regarding adaptive devices for self-care activities if appropriate
	  i. reinforce need for increased activity and participation in physical therapy program.
	3. Increase activity and participation in self-care activities as allowed and tolerated.
	4. Provide praise and encouragement for all efforts to increase physical mobility.
	5. Encourage the support of significant others. Allow them to assist with range of motion exercises, positioning, and activity if desired.
	6. Consult physician if the client is unable to achieve an expected level of mobility or if range of motion becomes more restricted.

10.b. The client will not experience problems associated with immobility.	10.b. Refer to Care Plan on Immobility for actions to prevent problems associated with immobility.

11. NURSING DIAGNOSIS

Self-care deficit related to:

a. decreased activity tolerance associated with tissue hypoxia, nutritional deficits, and inability to rest and sleep;
b. impaired physical mobility associated with pain, sensory and motor deficits, contractures, and prescribed activity restrictions.

DESIRED OUTCOMES	NURSING ACTIONS AND *SELECTED RATIONALES*
11. The client will perform self-care activities within physical limitations and prescribed activity restrictions.	11.a. Refer to Care Plan on Immobility, Nursing Diagnosis 9, for measures related to assessment of, planning for, and meeting the client's self-care needs. b. Further facilitate the client's ability to meet self-care needs by performing actions to increase physical mobility (see Nursing Diagnosis 10, action a.2).

□ ▬▬▬▬▬▬▬▬▬▬▬▬▬▬▬▬▬▬▬

12. NURSING DIAGNOSIS

Constipation related to:

a. reluctance to use a bedpan;
b. inadequate intake of fluids and foods high in fiber;
c. use of antacids containing aluminum or calcium;
d. decreased gastrointestinal motility associated with sympathetic nervous system response to severe trauma, decreased activity, and use of narcotic analgesics;
e. weakened abdominal and perineal muscles associated with generalized loss of muscle tone resulting from prolonged immobility.

□ ▬▬▬▬▬▬▬▬▬▬▬▬▬▬▬▬▬▬▬

DESIRED OUTCOMES	NURSING ACTIONS AND *SELECTED RATIONALES*

12. The client will maintain usual bowel elimination pattern.	12.a. Refer to Care Plan on Immobility, Nursing Diagnosis 11, for measures related to assessment, prevention, and treatment of constipation.
	  b. Implement additional measures *to prevent constipation:*
	    1. if client is on antacid therapy, consult physician about alternating those containing aluminum or calcium with those containing a magnesium base
	    2. encourage use of nonnarcotic analgesics once the period of severe pain has subsided.

□ ▬▬▬▬▬▬▬▬▬▬▬▬▬▬▬▬▬▬▬

13. NURSING DIAGNOSIS

Diarrhea related to:

a. reduction in usual bowel flora associated with anti-infective therapy;
b. increased water in the bowel associated with the high osmolarity of commercial supplemental feedings;
c. rapid administration of tube feedings;
d. intestinal hypermotility associated with extreme stress;
e. use of antacids containing magnesium.

□ ▬▬▬▬▬▬▬▬▬▬▬▬▬▬▬▬▬▬▬

DESIRED OUTCOMES	NURSING ACTIONS AND *SELECTED RATIONALES*
13. The client will maintain usual bowel elimination pattern.	13.a. Ascertain client's usual bowel elimination habits. b. Assess for and report signs and symptoms of diarrhea (e.g. frequent, loose stools; abdominal pain and cramping).

    c. Assess bowel sounds regularly. Report an increase in frequency of and/or high-pitched bowel sounds.

    d. Implement measures *to prevent or control diarrhea:*

       1. instruct client to avoid foods/fluids that are poorly digested or act as irritants to the bowel:

         a. those high in fat (e.g. butter, cream, oils, whole milk, ice cream, pork, fried foods, gravies, nuts)

         b. those with high fiber content (e.g. whole-grain cereals, nuts, raw fruits and vegetables)

         c. those known to cause diarrhea or be gas-producers (e.g. cabbage, onions, popcorn, licorice, prunes, chili, baked beans, carbonated beverages)

         d. those high in caffeine (e.g. coffee, tea, chocolate, colas)

         e. spicy foods

         f. extremely hot or cold foods/fluids

       2. encourage consumption of low-residue foods (e.g. ripe bananas, cooked vegetables, chicken, fish, ground beef, white rice or bread, cooked cereals, pasta)

       3. provide small, frequent meals

       4. perform actions to reduce fear and anxiety (see Nursing Diagnosis 1, action c)

       5. discourage smoking *(nicotine has a stimulant effect on gastrointestinal tract)*

       6. if client is on antacid therapy, consult physician about alternating use of those containing magnesium with those containing aluminum or calcium

       7. initiate tube feedings at half-strength and at a slow rate; gradually increase concentration and rate as ordered until client is able to tolerate the feeding without diarrhea

       8. if client is receiving a commercial supplemental feeding, dilute it and administer or instruct the client to drink it slowly; consult physician about use of preparation with lower osmolarity if diarrhea persists

       9. monitor for therapeutic and nontherapeutic effects of the following medications if administered:

         a. opiate or opiate-like substances (e.g. loperamide, diphenoxylate hydrochloride) *to decrease gastrointestinal motility*

         b. bulk-forming agents (e.g. methylcellulose, psyllium hydrophylic mucilloid, calcium polycarbophil) *to absorb water in the bowel and produce a soft, formed stool.*

    e. Consult physician if diarrhea persists despite implementation of above actions.

14. NURSING DIAGNOSIS

Sleep pattern disturbance related to frequent assessments and treatments, decreased physical activity, fear, anxiety, nightmares, pain, inability to assume usual sleep position, and unfamiliar environment.

DESIRED OUTCOMES	NURSING ACTIONS AND *SELECTED RATIONALES*

14. The client will attain optimal amounts of sleep within the parameters of the treatment regimen (see Care Plan on Immobility, Nursing Diagnosis 12, for outcome criteria).	14.a. Refer to Care Plan on Immobility, Nursing Diagnosis 12, for measures related to assessment and promotion of sleep.
	b. Implement additional measures *to promote sleep:*
	  1. perform actions to reduce pain (see Nursing Diagnosis 6.A, action 5)
	  2. if client is experiencing frequent nightmares:
	    a. assure him/her that this is a temporary response to the injury

b. leave a dim light on in the room during rest and sleep periods if desired

c. allow significant others or a sitter to remain with client throughout the night *in order to provide constant reassurance*

3. perform actions to reduce fear and anxiety (see Nursing Diagnosis 1, action c).

---

15. NURSING DIAGNOSIS

Potential for infection:

a. **wound infection** related to:
  1. break in integrity of skin
  2. break in integrity of nasal, pharyngeal, and tracheal mucosa associated with inhalation injury
  3. colonization of microorganisms within the avascular eschar
  4. inability of systemic anti-infectives to penetrate eschar
  5. suppression of the normal immune response (occurs in proportion to the extent of the burn injury)
  6. repeated invasive procedures
  7. malnutrition
  8. wound contamination with both endogenous and environmental microorganisms
  9. compromised circulation to burn areas resulting in inadequate access of oxygen, antibodies, and phagocytes to wound
  10. administration of drugs with immunosuppressive properties (e.g. some anti-infectives);

b. **pneumonia** related to:
  1. stasis of pulmonary secretions associated with decreased activity, impaired ciliary movement, and ineffective cough effort
  2. suppression of the immune response associated with the burn injury and administration of some drugs with immunosuppressive properties (e.g. some anti-infectives).

DESIRED OUTCOMES	NURSING ACTIONS AND *SELECTED RATIONALES*

15.a. The client will remain free of infection in burn areas and donor sites as evidenced by:
1. absence of chills and fever
2. absence of redness, warmth, and swelling around donor sites and healing burn areas
3. absence of purulent, green, or gray foul-smelling exudate from wound(s)
4. WBC and differential counts returning to normal level
	15.a.1. Assess for and report signs and symptoms of wound infection (e.g. chills; fever; redness, warmth, and swelling of donor site or healing burn areas; rapid eschar separation; purulent, green, or gray foul-smelling drainage from wound[s]; increased subeschar suppuration; darkened areas around wound[s]).
	2. Monitor WBC count. Report persistent elevation, increasing values, and/or significant change in differential.
	3. Assist with wound biopsy for culture or obtain cultures of wound drainage as ordered. Report positive results.
	4. Implement measures *to prevent wound infection:*
	  a. maintain an optimal nutritional status (see Nursing Diagnosis 5, action c)
	  b. maintain a scrupulously clean or sterile environment depending on institution policy or physician preference
	  c. encourage and assist client with meticulous personal hygiene
	  d. wash hands thoroughly before any contact with client
	  e. utilize sterile technique during wound care whenever possible

UNIT
XVI

5. negative wound
   cultures.

    f. keep areas surrounding wound clean

    g. keep wound edges free of hair by shaving as often as necessary

    h. if burns involve the perineal area, wash with soap and water at least twice/day and after each bowel movement

    i. remove excessive debris and previously applied topical agents with each dressing change or as ordered (shower or hydrotherapy tub may be used)

    j. limit tub or bedside debridement sessions to no more than 20 minutes or 4 square inches of eschar *(extensive manipulation of wound during procedure allows bacteria to penetrate granulation tissue barrier)*

    k. apply enzyme debriding preparations correctly *to prevent damage to surrounding tissue and possible subsequent infection*

    l. monitor for therapeutic and nontherapeutic effects of topical anti-infectives (e.g. silver sulfadiazine, cerium nitrate solution, mafenide acetate, silver sulfadiazine–cerium nitrate cream) if applied

    m. apply physiological dressings (e.g. cutaneous allografts, porcine xenografts, amnion) or synthetic dressings (e.g. Hydron, Tegaderm) as ordered

    n. monitor for therapeutic and nontherapeutic effects of anti-infectives if administered prophylactically

    o. administer tetanus toxoid and/or tetanus immune globulin as ordered

    p. assist with subeschar anti-infective infusions as ordered.

5. If signs and symptoms of infection occur:
   a. continue with above measures
   b. monitor for therapeutic and nontherapeutic effects of anti-infectives if administered.

15.b. The client will not develop pneumonia (see Care Plan on Immobility, Nursing Diagnosis 13, outcome a, for outcome criteria).

15.b. Refer to Care Plan on Immobility, Nursing Diagnosis 13, action a, for measures related to the assessment, prevention, and management of pneumonia.

☐ ▄▄▄▄▄▄▄▄▄▄▄▄▄▄▄▄▄▄▄▄▄▄▄▄▄▄▄▄▄▄▄▄▄▄▄▄▄▄

16. NURSING DIAGNOSIS

Potential for trauma related to falls associated with:

a. weakness resulting from anemia, malnutrition, sleep deficit, fluid and electrolyte imbalances, and prolonged inactivity;
b. impaired physical mobility resulting from the burn injury.

☐ ▄▄▄▄▄▄▄▄▄▄▄▄▄▄▄▄▄▄▄▄▄▄▄▄▄▄▄▄▄▄▄▄▄▄▄▄▄▄

DESIRED OUTCOMES	**NURSING ACTIONS AND *SELECTED RATIONALES***

16. The client will not experience falls.

16.a. Determine whether conditions predisposing client to falls (e.g. weakness, fatigue, sensory or motor deficits, burn of a weight-bearing extremity) exist.

    b. Implement measures *to prevent falls:*

      1. keep bed in low position with side rails up when client is in bed

      2. keep needed items within easy reach

      3. encourage client to request assistance whenever needed; have call signal within easy reach

      4. use lap belt when client is in chair if indicated

      5. instruct client to wear shoes with nonskid soles and low heels when ambulating

      6. avoid unnecessary clutter in room

7. accompany client during ambulation utilizing a transfer safety belt
8. provide ambulatory aids (e.g. walker, cane) if client is weak or unsteady on feet
9. reinforce instructions from physical therapist regarding correct transfer and ambulation techniques
10. instruct client to ambulate in well-lit areas and to utilize handrails if needed
11. do not rush client; allow adequate time for trips to the bathroom and ambulation in hallway
12. perform actions to increase strength and activity tolerance (see Nursing Diagnosis 9)
13. perform actions to maintain fluid and electrolyte balance (see appropriate actions in Nursing Diagnoses 4.A and 4.B).

c. Include client and significant others in planning and implementing measures to prevent falls.

d. If falls occur, initiate appropriate first aid measures and notify physician.

□ ▬▬▬▬▬▬▬▬▬▬▬▬▬▬▬▬

17. COLLABORATIVE DIAGNOSIS

Potential complications:

a. **gastrointestinal (GI) bleeding** related to development of a stress (Curling's) ulcer associated with:
   1. ischemia of the gastric mucosa resulting from decreased tissue perfusion
   2. change in quantity or quality of mucus
   3. increased mucosal permeability resulting in an increase in the back diffusion of hydrogen ions
   4. increased gastric acid secretion resulting from a generalized stress response
   5. reflux of duodenal contents associated with paralytic ileus;

b. **thromboembolism** related to:
   1. hypercoagulability associated with increased blood viscosity due to hemoconcentration (may occur with hypovolemia)
   2. venous stasis associated with decreased mobility;

c. **impaired renal function** related to hemoglobinuria, myoglobinuria, and decreased renal blood flow (can result from hypovolemia);

d. **shock** related to:
   1. septicemia (septic shock) associated with invasion and proliferation of gram-negative and gram-positive organisms in open wounds, presence of a urinary catheter, and decreased resistance to infection resulting from general debilitation and suppression of the immune response associated with the burn injury
   2. hypovolemia associated with gastrointestinal bleeding and the massive fluid shift and loss of body fluid during the emergent phase of the burn injury;

e. **paralytic ileus** related to hypokalemia, the sympathetic nervous system response to severe trauma, and decreased tissue perfusion to the bowel associated with hypovolemia;

f. **contractures** related to poor positioning, prolonged immobility of joints, shortening of burn scar tissue, and hypertrophic scar tissue formation.

□ ▬▬▬▬▬▬▬▬▬▬▬▬▬▬▬▬

DESIRED OUTCOMES	NURSING ACTIONS AND *SELECTED RATIONALES*
17.a. The client will not experience GI bleeding as evidenced by: 1. no complaints of	17.a.1. Asssess for and report signs and symptoms of GI bleeding (e.g. complaints of epigastric discomfort and fullness, frank or occult blood in stool or gastric contents, decreased B/P, increased pulse). 2. Monitor RBC, Hct., and Hgb. levels. Report declining values.

epigastric discomfort
and fullness
2. absence of occult or
frank blood in stool and
gastric contents
3. B/P and pulse within
normal range for client
4. RBC, Hct., and Hgb.
levels within normal
range.

3. Implement measures *to prevent ulceration of the gastric mucosa:*
   a. perform actions to decrease fear and anxiety (see Nursing Diagnosis 1, action c)
   b. perform actions to maintain adequate systemic tissue perfusion (see Nursing Diagnosis 2, action b) *in order to prevent ischemia of gastric mucosa*
   c. encourage client to reduce intake of foods/fluids that are acidic, spicy, or high in caffeine (e.g. chocolate, colas, coffee, tea)
   d. monitor for therapeutic and nontherapeutic effects of antacids, histamine$_2$ receptor antagonists (e.g. cimetidine, ranitidine, famotidine), and mucosal barrier fortifiers (e.g. sucralfate) if administered.
4. If signs and symptoms of GI bleeding occur:
   a. insert nasogastric tube and maintain suction as ordered
   b. assist with iced water or saline gastric lavage, transendoscopic electrocoagulation, selective arterial embolization, endoscopic laser photocoagulation, and/or intra-arterial administration of vasopressors (e.g. vasopressin) if ordered
   c. monitor for therapeutic and/or nontherapeutic effects of blood products and/or volume expanders if administered
   d. prepare client for surgery if indicated
   e. provide emotional support to client and significant others
   f. refer to Care Plan on Peptic Ulcer for additional care measures.

17.b.1. The client will not develop a venous thrombus (see Care Plan on Immobility, Collaborative Diagnosis 14, outcome a.1, for outcome criteria).

17.b.1.a. Refer to Care Plan on Immobility, Collaborative Diagnosis 14, action a.1 for measures related to assessment, prevention, and treatment of a venous thrombus.
   b. Implement measures to prevent and treat hypovolemia (see Nursing Diagnosis 4.A, action 1.b) *in order to prevent increased blood viscosity, which leads to hypercoagulability.*

17.b.2. The client will not experience a pulmonary embolism (see Care Plan on Immobility, Collaborative Diagnosis 14, outcome a.2, for outcome criteria).

17.b.2. Refer to Care Plan on Immobility, Collaborative Diagnosis 14, action a.2, for measures related to assessment, prevention, and treatment of a pulmonary embolism.

17.c. The client will maintain adequate renal function as evidenced by:
1. urine output of at least 30 cc/hour
2. urine specific gravity between 1.010–1.030
3. BUN and serum creatinine within normal range
4. absence of protein in urine.

17.c.1. Assess for and report signs and symptoms of impaired renal function:
   a. urine output less than 30 cc/hour
   b. specific gravity fixed at or less than 1.010
   c. elevated BUN and serum creatinine
   d. presence of protein in the urine.
2. Collect a 24-hour urine specimen if ordered. Report decreased creatinine clearance.
3. Implement measures *to maintain adequate renal function:*
   a. perform actions to prevent and treat hypovolemia (see Nursing Diagnosis 4.A, action 1.b) *in order to reduce hemoconcentration and prevent precipitation of hemoglobin and myoglobin in the renal tubules (urine output should range from 50–100 cc/hour to speed the clearance of pigment from urine and blood)*
   b. perform actions to maintain adequate systemic tissue perfusion (see Nursing Diagnosis 2, action b) *in order to improve renal blood flow.*
4. If signs and symptoms of impaired renal function occur:
   a. continue with above actions
   b. administer diuretics as ordered
   c. assess for and report signs of acute renal failure (e.g. oliguria or anuria; weight gain; edema; elevated B/P; lethargy and confusion; increasing BUN and serum creatinine, phosphorus, and potassium levels)
   d. prepare client for dialysis if indicated
   e. refer to Care Plan on Renal Failure for additional care measures.

17.d. The client will not develop shock as evidenced by:

17.d.1. Assess for and report signs and symptoms of:
   a. GI bleeding (e.g. frank or occult blood in stools, vomitus, or

1. usual mental status
2. stable vital signs
3. skin warm and usual color in unburned areas
4. palpable peripheral pulses
5. capillary refill time less than 3 seconds
6. urine output at least 30 cc/hour.

nasogastric tube drainage; decline in Hct. and Hgb. levels; increase in pulse; decreased B/P)
   b. early or hyperdynamic stage of septic shock (e.g. confusion; chills and fever; warm, flushed skin; lower extremity mottling; tachycardia; tachypnea)
   c. shock:
      1. restlessness, agitation, confusion
      2. significant decrease in B/P
      3. decline in B/P of at least 15 mm Hg with concurrent rise in pulse when client changes from lying to sitting or standing position
      4. resting pulse rate greater than 100 beats/minute
      5. rapid or labored respirations
      6. cool, pale, or cyanotic skin
      7. diminished or absent peripheral pulses
      8. capillary refill time greater than 3 seconds
      9. urine output less than 30 cc/hour.
2. Implement measures *to prevent shock:*
   a. perform actions *to prevent septicemia:*
      1. implement measures to prevent and treat wound infection (see Nursing Diagnosis 15, actions a.4 and 5)
      2. consult physician about removal of urinary catheter as soon as client's condition stabilizes (*presence of a urinary catheter predisposes client to urinary tract infection, which is a common cause of septicemia)*
   b. perform actions to prevent ulceration and control bleeding of the gastric mucosa (see actions a.3 and 4 in this diagnosis)
   c. perform actions to prevent and treat hypovolemia (see Nursing Diagnosis 4.A, action 1.b).
3. If signs and symptoms of shock occur:
   a. continue with above measures to treat infection, control bleeding, and correct hypovolemia
   b. place client flat in bed with legs elevated unless contraindicated
   c. monitor vital signs frequently
   d. administer oxygen as ordered
   e. monitor for therapeutic and nontherapeutic effects of the following if administered:
      1. blood products and/or volume expanders
      2. vasopressors (may be given for a short time *to maintain mean arterial pressure)*
      3. positive inotropic agents (e.g. dopamine) *to increase cardiac output and improve blood flow to major organs*
      4. anti-infectives *to control the precipitating infection*
   f. provide emotional support to client and significant others.

17.e. The client will not develop a paralytic ileus as evidenced by:
1. absence of abdominal pain and cramping
2. soft, nondistended abdomen
3. normal bowel sounds
4. passage of flatus.

17.e.1. Assess for and report signs and symptoms of paralytic ileus (e.g. abdominal pain and cramping; firm, distended abdomen; absent bowel sounds; failure to pass flatus).
2. Implement measures *to prevent paralytic ileus:*
   a. perform actions to prevent and treat hypovolemia (see Nursing Diagnosis 4.A, action 1.b) *in order to help maintain adequate tissue perfusion to bowel*
   b. perform actions to prevent or treat hypokalemia (see Nursing Diagnosis 4.B, action 3.b)
   c. monitor for therapeutic and nontherapeutic effects of gastrointestinal stimulants (e.g. metoclopramide) if administered.
3. If signs and symptoms of paralytic ileus occur:
   a. continue with above measures to promote bowel activity
   b. withhold all oral intake
   c. insert nasogastric tube and maintain suction as ordered.

17.f. The client will maintain or regain normal range of motion.

17.f.1. Assess for and report limitations in range of motion.
2. Implement measures *to prevent contractures:*
   a. perform actions *to prevent contracture development associated with improper positioning and decreased mobility:*
      1. maintain affected joints in a neutral or extended position utilizing splints, pillows, or braces as necessary

2. if occlusive dressings are used, dress wound so that burned surfaces are not touching and body part is in functional or correct alignment
3. maintain traction devices if present
4. initiate or assist with a planned exercise program for all joints within 48–72 hours postburn and carry out on a regular schedule at least 4 times/day or with each dressing change
5. instruct and assist client with conditioning and strengthening exercises of major muscle groups as soon as feasible *to increase endurance and ability to participate in exercise program*
6. progress activity as allowed
7. encourage maximum participation in activities of daily living utilizing adaptive devices as necessary
8. encourage diversional activities that require use of involved joints

b. perform actions *to minimize scar formation:*
1. implement measures to prevent wound infection (see Nursing Diagnosis 15, action a.4) *in order to decrease the amount of scarring*
2. place dressing materials between digits during the healing process *to prevent scar band formation or webbing between digits*
3. utilize fine mesh gauze when dressing wounds *to flatten hypergranulation tissue (coarse mesh gauze can stimulate granulation tissue growth)*

c. if scar tissue is present, perform actions *to prevent hypertrophy and shortening:*
1. instruct client in and assist with sustained stretching exercises
2. position client to allow maximum stretch of scar tissue
3. apply elastic wraps or pressure garments as ordered *to prevent hypertrophic scar formation and flatten and soften formed scar tissue* (pressure garments are usually removed only for bathing and skin care)
4. lubricate healed areas with a nonirritating substance (e.g. mineral oil, cocoa butter) *to keep scar tissue soft and pliable*
5. assist with paraffin therapy as ordered *to facilitate sustained stretching in tight areas and increase softness and pliability of scar tissue*
6. massage scar tissue as ordered after paraffin therapy *to maintain pliability*
7. resume exercise to grafted areas as soon as allowed
8. implement measures *to facilitate compliance with the prescribed exercise program:*
   a. show client serial photographs of scar progression if preventive measures are not adhered to
   b. arrange for a visit with another who has successfully recovered from a similar burn injury.

3. If contractures develop, prepare client for serial splinting, sustained stretching with traction, or reconstructive surgery.

☐ ▇▇▇▇▇▇▇▇▇▇▇▇▇▇▇▇▇▇▇▇▇▇▇▇▇▇▇▇▇▇▇▇▇▇▇▇

18. NURSING DIAGNOSIS

Sexual dysfunction related to:

a. burn injury to genital area;
b. fear of rejection by usual partner associated with perceived loss of sexual attractiveness;
c. decreased libido associated with altered self-concept resulting from marked changes in body image;
d. alteration in usual sexual activities associated with immobility;
e. impotence associated with depression, fear, anxiety, and disturbance in self-concept.

☐ ▇▇▇▇▇▇▇▇▇▇▇▇▇▇▇▇▇▇▇▇▇▇▇▇▇▇▇▇▇▇▇▇▇▇▇▇

DESIRED OUTCOMES	NURSING ACTIONS AND *SELECTED RATIONALES*

18. The client will demonstrate beginning acceptance of changes in sexual functioning as evidenced by:
  a. verbalization of a perception of self as sexually adequate and acceptable
  b. maintenance of relationships with significant others.
	18.a. Refer to Care Plan on Immobility, Nursing Diagnosis 15, for actions related to assessment and management of sexual dysfunction.
	   b. Implement additional measures *to promote optimal sexual functioning:*
	    1. provide accurate information about the effects of the burn injury on sexual functioning; encourage questions and clarify misconceptions
	    2. perform actions to improve self-concept (see Nursing Diagnosis 19)
	    3. if client is concerned that burn site discomfort will interfere with usual sexual activity:
	     a. assure him/her that the discomfort is temporary and will diminish as healing occurs
	     b. encourage alternatives to intercourse or use of positions that decrease pressure on affected area(s)
	    4. perform actions *to decrease possibility of rejection by partner:*
	     a. assist the partner to acknowledge both positive and negative feelings
	     b. if appropriate, involve partner in care of client (e.g. exercise sessions) *to facilitate adjustment to and integration of the change in partner's body image*
	    5. encourage client to discuss possibilities for reconstruction of genitalia with physician if appropriate.

---

19. NURSING DIAGNOSIS

Disturbance in self-concept* related to changes in appearance associated with tissue loss and scarring, alterations in motor and sensory function, dependence on others to meet basic needs, changes in usual life style and roles, and inability to participate in usual sexual activities.

---

* This diagnostic label includes the nursing diagnoses of body image disturbance and self-esteem disturbance.

DESIRED OUTCOMES	NURSING ACTIONS AND *SELECTED RATIONALES*

19. The client will demonstrate beginning adaptation to changes in appearance, body functioning, life style, and roles (see Care Plan on Immobility, Nursing Diagnosis 16, for outcome criteria).	19.a. Refer to Care Plan on Immobility, Nursing Diagnosis 16, for measures related to assessment and maintenance of a positive self-concept.
	   b. Implement additional measures *to assist client to adjust to changes in appearance, body functioning, life style, and roles:*
	    1. reinforce measures that promote optimal sexual functioning (see Nursing Diagnosis 18)
	    2. perform actions to assist client to cope with the effects of the burn injury (see Nursing Diagnosis 20, action e)
	    3. assist client with usual makeup and grooming habits; identify ways to camouflage visible scars if possible (e.g. change in hair style, particular styles of clothing)
	    4. demonstrate acceptance of client using techniques such as therapeutic touch and frequent visits; encourage significant others to do the same
	    5. encourage client contact with others *so that he/she can test and establish a new self-image*
	    6. ensure that client and significant others have similar expectations and understanding of future life style.

UNIT XVI

☐ ▬▬▬▬▬▬▬▬▬▬▬▬▬▬▬▬▬▬▬▬▬▬▬▬▬▬

20. NURSING DIAGNOSIS

Ineffective individual coping related to:

a. painful wound care procedures;
b. depression, fear, and anxiety associated with the injury, treatment, and prognosis;
c. lengthy hospitalization and rehabilitation period;
d. residual effects of burns (disfigurement and motor and sensory impairments) and their impact on body functioning and usual life style and roles;
e. increased dependence on others to meet self-care needs;
f. inadequate support system.

☐ ▬▬▬▬▬▬▬▬▬▬▬▬▬▬▬▬▬▬▬▬▬▬▬▬▬▬

DESIRED OUTCOMES	NURSING ACTIONS AND *SELECTED RATIONALES*

20. The client will demonstrate the use of effective coping skills as evidenced by:
    a. willingness to participate in treatment plan and self-care activities
    b. verbalization of ability to cope with current condition, prolonged treatment and rehabilitation, and permanent effects of the burn injury
    c. identification of stressors
    d. utilization of appropriate problem-solving techniques
    e. recognition and utilization of available support systems.

20.a. Assess effectiveness of client's coping strategies by observing behavior and noting strengths, weaknesses, ability to express feelings and concerns, and willingness to participate in treatment plan.
   b. Assess for and report signs and symptoms that may indicate ineffective coping (e.g. sleep disturbances, increasing fatigue, difficulty concentrating, irritability, decreased tolerance for pain, verbalization of inability to cope, inability to problem-solve).
   c. Determine if the circumstances associated with initial burn injury are affecting client's ability to cope.
   d. Allow time for client to adjust psychologically to the residual effects of the burn injury and anticipated life style and role changes. Recognize that the adaptation process after a burn may be lengthy depending on the severity and visibility of the injury.
   e. Implement measures *to promote effective coping:*
      1. emphasize the rationale for wound care procedures; prepare client for what he/she may feel or experience
      2. do not encourage use of a mirror until client is ready
      3. arrange for a visit with another who has successfully adjusted to a similar burn injury
      4. perform actions to reduce pain (see Nursing Diagnosis 6.A, action 5)
      5. perform actions to reduce fear and anxiety (see Nursing Diagnosis 1, action c)
      6. if client is experiencing nightmares, assure him/her that this is a common occurrence and will gradually cease
      7. include client in the planning of care, encourage maximum participation in the treatment plan, and allow choices when possible *to enable him/her to maintain a sense of control over life*
      8. instruct client in effective problem-solving techniques (e.g. accurate identification of stressors, determination of various options to solve problem)
      9. assist client to maintain usual daily routines whenever possible
      10. provide diversional activities according to client's interests
      11. assist client as he/she starts to plan for necessary life-style and role changes after discharge; provide input related to the realistic prioritization of problems that must be dealt with
      12. assist client and significant others to look at available options realistically; discuss expectations and treatment options with them
      13. assist client to identify ways to integrate follow-up care into usual daily activities
      14. assist client and significant others to identify ways that personal and family goals can be adjusted rather than abandoned
      15. assist client through methods such as role playing to prepare for negative reactions from others if extensive scarring and disfigurement have occurred
      16. assist client to identify and utilize available support systems; provide

information about available community resources that can assist client and significant others in coping with effects of the burn injury (e.g. burn injury support groups; family, individual, and/or financial counseling).

f. Encourage continued emotional support from significant others.

g. Assess for and support behaviors suggesting positive adaptation to changes experienced (e.g. increased participation in self-care activities and treatment plan, verbalization of ways to adapt to effects of the burn injury, utilization of effective problem-solving strategies).

h. Consult physician about psychological or vocational rehabilitation counseling if appropriate. Initiate a referral if necessary.

21. NURSING DIAGNOSIS

Grieving* related to:

a. alteration in appearance and body functioning;
b. changes in life style, roles, and relationships;
c. multiple losses resulting from fire (e.g. personal possessions, significant others);
d. need for long-term rehabilitation and follow-up care.

---

* This diagnostic label includes anticipatory grieving and grieving following the actual losses/changes.

DESIRED OUTCOMES	NURSING ACTIONS AND *SELECTED RATIONALES*

21. The client will demonstrate beginning progression through the grieving process and adjustment to changes and losses resulting from the burn injury as evidenced by:
   a. verbalization of feelings about changes in body image and life style
   b. expression of grief
   c. participation in treatment plan and self-care activities
   d. utilization of available support systems
   e. verbalization of a plan for integrating prescribed follow-up care into life style.

21.a. Determine the client's perception of the impact of the burn injury and related changes and losses on his/her future.
   b. Determine how client usually expresses grief.
   c. Observe for signs of grieving (e.g. changes in eating habits, insomnia, anger, noncompliance, denial).
   d. Implement measures *to facilitate the grieving process:*
      1. assist client to acknowledge the losses and changes experienced *so grief work can begin*; assess for factors that may hinder or facilitate acknowledgment
      2. discuss the grieving process and assist client to accept the stages of grieving as an expected response to actual and/or anticipated changes or losses; support the realization that grief may recur *because of the long rehabilitation process*
      3. allow time for client to progress through the stages of grieving (denial, anger, bargaining, depression, acceptance [Kübler-Ross, 1969]); be aware that not every stage is experienced or expressed by all individuals
      4. provide an atmosphere of care and concern (e.g. provide privacy, be available and nonjudgmental, display empathy and respect) *so that client will feel free to verbalize both positive and negative feelings and concerns*
      5. perform actions *to promote trust* (e.g. answer questions honestly, provide requested information)
      6. encourage the expression of anger and sadness about the losses/changes experienced; recognize displacement of anger and assist client to see actual cause of angry feelings and resentment; establish limits on abusive behavior
      7. encourage client to express his/her feelings in whatever ways are comfortable (e.g. writing, drawing, conversation)
      8. perform actions to facilitate effective coping (see Nursing Diagnosis 20, action e)
      9. support realistic hope about the prognosis and success of rehabilitative efforts.

UNIT
XVI

e. Assess for and support behaviors suggesting successful resolution of grief (e.g. verbalizing feelings about changes in body appearance and functioning and other losses, expressing sorrow, focusing on ways to adapt to changes and losses).

f. Explain the stages of the grieving process to significant others. Encourage their support and understanding.

g. Provide information regarding counseling services and support groups that might be of assistance to client in working through grief.

h. Arrange for visit from clergy if desired by client.

i. Monitor for therapeutic and nontherapeutic effects of antidepressants if administered.

j. Consult physician regarding referral for counseling if signs of dysfunctional grieving (e.g. persistent denial of losses or changes, excessive anger or sadness, hysteria, suicidal behaviors, phobias) occur.

22. NURSING DIAGNOSIS

Diversional activity deficit related to inability to participate in usual recreational or leisure activities due to pain, prescribed activity restrictions, physical limitations, and prolonged hospitalization.

DESIRED OUTCOMES	NURSING ACTIONS AND *SELECTED RATIONALES*
22. The client will have needs for diversional activity met (see Care Plan on Immobility, Nursing Diagnosis 18, for outcome criteria).	22. Refer to Care Plan on Immobility, Nursing Diagnosis 18, for actions related to assessment of diversional activity deficit and measures to prevent boredom.

23. NURSING DIAGNOSIS

Social isolation related to:

a. isolation precautions to prevent the spread of infection;
b. fear of rejection by others as a result of altered physical appearance and need to wear visible pressure garments;
c. inability of significant others to cope with drastic changes in the client's appearance and functional ability.

DESIRED OUTCOMES	NURSING ACTIONS AND *SELECTED RATIONALES*
23. The client will experience a decreased sense of isolation as evidenced by: a. maintenance of relationships with significant others and casual acquaintances	23.a. Ascertain the client's usual degree of social interaction. b. Assess for and report behaviors indicative of social isolation (e.g. decreased interaction with significant others and staff; expression of feelings of rejection, abandonment, or being different from others; hostility; sad affect). c. Encourage client to express feelings of rejection and aloneness. Provide feedback and support.

b. verbalization of decreasing loneliness and feelings of rejection.

d. Explain the rationale for isolation precautions if indicated.
e. Implement measures *to decrease social isolation:*
  1. perform actions *to facilitate significant others' acceptance of client:*
     a. encourage and assist significant others to verbalize their personal needs, fears, feelings, and concerns
     b. include significant others in decision making about client and his/her care; convey appreciation for their input and continued support of the client
     c. allow significant others to participate in physical care of client if desired by both client and significant others; provide necessary instructions
     d. explain the purpose of the client's pressure garments and the need for constant wear
  2. set up a schedule of visiting times so that client will not go for long periods without visitors
  3. encourage telephone contact with significant others, local or national support groups, and hotlines
  4. schedule time each day to sit and talk with client
  5. assist client to identify a few persons he/she feels comfortable with and encourage interactions with them
  6. support any appropriate movement away from social isolation.

---

24. NURSING DIAGNOSIS

Knowledge deficit regarding follow-up care.

DESIRED OUTCOMES	NURSING ACTIONS AND *SELECTED RATIONALES*
24.a. The client will identify ways to reduce the risk of recurrent burn injury.	24.a.1. Assist client to recognize factors that may have contributed to or caused the burn injury (e.g. smoking in bed, excessive alcohol intake, use of faulty home appliances or equipment, inappropriate use of cleaning solutions or gasoline).
	2. Instruct client in home safety measures that may be helpful in preventing future burn injuries (e.g. smoke detectors, fire extinguishers, fire drills, proper use of electrical equipment, caps on electrical outlets, close supervision of children in kitchen and bath area, use of fire resistant sleepwear for children).
24.b. The client will demonstrate the ability to care for wounds appropriately.	24.b.1. Instruct client in proper care of healed wounds:
	a. apply a lanolin cream to healed areas several times a day *to prevent dryness*
	b. avoid use of harsh soaps and detergents
	c. wear cotton garments next to skin
	d. avoid excessive sun exposure for 1 year and trauma to grafted burn areas *(increased sensitivity to sunlight and temperature extremes and decreased sensation are common in grafted areas)*
	e. use antipruritic lotions as needed *to relieve itching of healed burn and grafted areas.*
	2. Demonstrate care of healing wounds using aseptic technique if indicated. Emphasize the importance of good handwashing before wound care *to reduce risk of infection.*
	3. If pressure garments are used *to prevent hypertrophic scarring,* instruct client to:
	a. hand wash garments using mild soap and water; lay flat to dry (do not use clothes pins or clips)

UNIT XVI

       b. use only water-base creams on skin that will be covered by the elastic garment *to prevent staining and damage to the elastic*
       c. cover open areas with gauze before applying
       d. assess frequently for proper fit (should fit snugly without causing swelling of surrounding tissue, blisters, numbness, or tingling)
       e. check at least every 2 months to see if the garments need to be replaced
       f. wear continuously as ordered (usually 23 hours/day for up to 18 months following the burn injury).
  4. Demonstrate the application of pressure garments and/or elastic wraps if indicated.
  5. Allow time for questions, clarification, and return demonstration of techniques.

24.c. The client will demonstrate ways to maintain joint mobility and function.

24.c.1. If splints or braces are prescribed, instruct client to:
       a. wear as directed (e.g. 24 hours/day, during sleep only)
       b. assess frequently for proper fit (e.g. observe for reddened areas under splint or brace and changes in sensation, color, or warmth when brace or splint is in place).
  2. Reinforce instructions regarding prescribed exercise program and application of splints or braces. Allow time for questions, clarification, and return demonstration.

24.d. The client will demonstrate the ability to correctly use adaptive devices.

24.d.1. Reinforce instructions of physical and occupational therapists regarding use of adaptive devices and mobility aids. Allow time for questions, clarification, and return demonstration.
  2. Reinforce methods for maintaining maximum level of independence at home.

24.e. The client will state signs and symptoms to report to the health care provider.

24.e. Instruct client to report the following signs and symptoms:
  1. fever, chills
  2. increased redness or pain in any wound area
  3. change in odor, color, or amount of drainage from wounds
  4. opening of previously healed areas
  5. progressive limitation in range of motion
  6. weight loss
  7. increased or persistent fatigue and weakness
  8. cough productive of purulent, green, or rust-colored sputum
  9. difficulty breathing or shortness of breath
  10. swelling, redness, or pain in lower extremities
  11. excessive depression
  12. inability to accomplish wound care or adhere to exercise program.

24.f. The client will identify community resources that can assist with home management and adjustment to changes and losses resulting from the burn injury.

24.f.1. Provide information about community resources that can assist the client and significant others with home management and adjustment to changes and losses (e.g. social services; financial services; Visiting Nurse Association; city and county health departments; local service groups; individual, family, and vocational rehabilitation counselors).
  2. Initiate a referral if indicated.

24.g. The client will verbalize an understanding of and a plan for adhering to recommended follow-up care including future appointments with health care provider and physical and occupational therapists, medications prescribed, activity level, exercise regimen, dietary recommendations, and future reconstructive procedures.

24.g.1. Reinforce the importance of keeping scheduled follow-up appointments with health care provider and physical and occupational therapists.
  2. Reinforce physician's instructions regarding activity level and exercise regimen.
  3. Explain the rationale for, side effects of, and importance of taking or applying medications prescribed.
  4. Reinforce physician's explanations about future reconstructive surgery (surgery is usually delayed until the scar tissue matures and client is physically ready).
  5. Emphasize the need for continued inclusion of high-calorie and high-protein foods/fluids in diet until healing is complete.
  6. Implement measures *to improve client compliance:*
       a. include significant others in teaching sessions if possible
       b. encourage questions and allow time for reinforcement and clarification of information provided

c. provide written instructions on scheduled appointments with health care provider and occupational and physical therapists, activity level, treatment plan, medications prescribed, wound care, and signs and symptoms to report.

□ ▬▬▬▬▬▬▬▬▬▬▬▬▬▬▬▬▬▬▬▬▬

References

Carpenito, LJ. Handbook of nursing diagnosis (3rd ed.). Philadelphia: J.B. Lippincott Company, 1989.
Kübler-Ross, E. On death and dying. New York: Macmillan, 1969.

□□□

Cancer of the Breast

Cancer of the breast is a malignant neoplasm involving breast tissue and is primarily a disease of women. It is a systemic disease with metastasis occurring by embolization via the bloodstream rather than direct extension to surrounding tissue. Axillary lymph node involvement, which is a negative prognostic sign, occurs concurrently with metastasis to distant sites rather than sequentially as previously thought.

Breast tumors can be classified as noninvasive (i.e. confined to the lumen of breast ducts) or invasive. The noninvasive forms (e.g. comedocarcinoma, ductal papillary carcinoma, lobular carcinoma in situ) account for a very small percentage of breast cancers and typically have a better prognosis than do the invasive types. The invasive forms (e.g. infiltrating ductal, medullary, lobular, mucinous) vary in histological characteristics, growth rate, incidence of metastasis, and prognosis. Infiltrating ductal carcinoma is by far the most common type, accounting for over 70% of all breast cancers. Two other unusual forms of breast cancer are Paget's disease, in which the nipple contains malignant cells, and inflammatory carcinoma. With inflammatory carcinoma, the client typically presents with a reddened, painful, and possibly ulcerated breast as a result of occlusion of dermal lymphatics by tumor cells. The prognosis with this type of cancer is very poor.

The advances in knowledge about the pathophysiology of breast cancer have resulted in changes in the way the disease is treated. There are currently several treatment options to be considered by the client with breast cancer. The three primary modes of treatment (surgery, radiation therapy, and chemotherapy) may be used individually or in combination depending on the histological type of the tumor, lymph node involvement, presence of distant metastasis, menopausal status of the client, results of estrogen and progesterone receptor assays, and condition of the client on diagnosis. Clients with Stage I or II disease will usually undergo a modified radical mastectomy or lumpectomy with axillary node dissection to control local disease. Adjuvant radiation therapy may be used in these clients to reduce the incidence of local recurrence. If 1 to 3 lymph nodes are positive, adjuvant chemotherapy is usually given with the selection of drugs depending on the menopausal status of the client. Radiation therapy is also considered to be a viable primary treatment option for clients with Stage I or II disease. Following an excisional biopsy or lumpectomy, the client receives a course of external radiation to the breast followed by a radiation boost to the tumor bed using either electron or photon therapy or an interstitial implant. Clients who elect radiation as their primary mode of treatment would also receive adjuvant chemotherapy if nodal involvement is evident at diagnosis. Clients who have Stage III disease at diagnosis have a poor prognosis but may be treated with surgery, radiation therapy, and/or chemotherapy. Clients with Stage IV or disseminated disease are treated with hormonal therapy and/or cytotoxic agents depending on the estrogen and progesterone receptor assay results, menopausal status of the client, and sites of metastasis.

This care plan focuses on the adult female client hospitalized for staging and initiation of treatment following a biopsy that is positive for cancer of the breast. Goals of care are to reduce fear and anxiety, provide emotional support, relieve symptoms associated with the treatment and the disease process, and educate the client regarding follow-up care. If surgery is planned, this care plan should be used in conjunction with the Care Plan on Mastectomy.

UNIT
XVI

DISCHARGE CRITERIA

Prior to discharge, the client will:

- verbalize the importance of doing a routine breast self-examination (BSE)
- demonstrate the ability to correctly perform a BSE
- demonstrate the ability to appropriately care for malignant skin lesions if present
- identify ways to improve appetite and nutritional status
- state signs and symptoms to report to the health care provider
- share thoughts and feelings about the diagnosis of breast cancer; the prognosis; and the effects of the disease process and its treatment on self-concept, life style, and roles
- identify community resources that can assist with home management and adjustment to changes resulting from the diagnosis and the effects of treatment
- verbalize an understanding of and a plan for adhering to recommended follow-up care including future appointments with health care provider and for laboratory studies, medications prescribed, activity level, and plans for subsequent treatment.

Use in conjunction with the Care Plans on Chemotherapy, Brachytherapy, and External Radiation Therapy.

NURSING DIAGNOSES

1. Anxiety □ *972*
2. Altered nutrition: less than body requirements □ *973*
3. Pain:
   a. breast and axillary pain
   b. pain within the irradiated area
   c. esophageal pain
   d. oral pain □ *974*
4. Impaired skin integrity:
   a. irritation and breakdown
   b. insertion/presence of applicators for interstitial radioactive implant □ *975*
5. Fatigue □ *975*
6. Activity intolerance □ *976*
7. Self-care deficit □ *976*
8. Disturbance in self-concept □ *977*
9. Ineffective individual coping □ *977*
10. Grieving □ *978*
11. Knowledge deficit regarding follow-up care □ *978*

1. NURSING DIAGNOSIS

Anxiety related to unfamiliar environment; pain; lack of understanding of diagnosis, staging procedures, treatment plan, and prognosis; anticipated effects of breast cancer and its treatment on body image and functioning and usual life style and roles; and potential for premature death.

DESIRED OUTCOMES	**NURSING ACTIONS AND *SELECTED RATIONALES***

1. The client will experience a reduction in fear and anxiety as evidenced by:
   a. verbalization of feeling less anxious or fearful
   b. relaxed facial expression and body movements
   c. stable vital signs
   d. usual skin color
   e. verbalization of an understanding of hospital routines, diagnosis, staging procedures, treatment plan and its effects, and prognosis.

1.a. Assess client on admission for:
   1. fears, misconceptions, and level of understanding about cancer of the breast, tests to stage the disease, and possible treatment modes
   2. perception of anticipated results of diagnostic tests and planned treatment
   3. significance of the diagnosis of breast cancer to the client
   4. availability of an adequate support system
   5. past experiences with cancer and its treatment
   6. signs and symptoms of fear and anxiety (e.g. verbalization of fears and concerns; tenseness; tremors; irritability; restlessness; diaphoresis; tachypnea; tachycardia; elevated blood pressure; facial tension, pallor, or flushing; noncompliance with treatment plan).
   b. Ascertain effectiveness of current coping skills.
   c. Implement measures *to reduce fear and anxiety:*
      1. explain all studies that may be performed to stage cancer of the breast and determine the appropriate treatment:
         a. chest x-ray
         b. blood chemistries
         c. bone, brain, liver, and spleen scans
         d. peritoneal fluid aspiration for cytological examination
         e. computed tomography (CT) of abdomen if ascites present
         f. biopsy of axillary nodes, satellite skin nodules, and any masses in the opposite breast
         g. estrogen and progesterone receptor assays of biopsied tumor tissue
         h. mammography, thermography, xeroradiography, ultrasonography
      2. refer to Nursing Diagnosis 1, action c, in Care Plans on Chemotherapy and/or External Radiation for measures to reduce fear and anxiety associated with planned treatment
      3. perform actions to reduce pain (see Nursing Diagnosis 3, actions a and b)
      4. perform actions to assist client to cope with the diagnosis and its implications (see Nursing Diagnosis 9)
      5. initiate preoperative and/or preprocedure teaching if surgery and/or brachytherapy is planned
      6. arrange for a visit with a woman of similar age who has been successfully treated for breast cancer.
   d. Include significant others in orientation and teaching sessions and encourage their continued support of the client.
   e. Provide information based on current needs of client and significant others at a level they can understand. Encourage questions and clarification of information provided.
   f. Consult physician if above actions fail to control fear and anxiety.

□ ▬▬▬▬▬▬▬▬▬▬▬▬▬▬▬▬▬▬

2. NURSING DIAGNOSIS

Altered nutrition: less than body requirements related to:*

a. decreased oral intake associated with:
   1. anorexia resulting from:
      a. depression, fear, and anxiety
      b. fatigue and discomfort
      c. taste alteration associated with:
         1. change in the sense of smell and the threshold for bitter, sweet, sour, and salt taste (particularly red meat, coffee, tea, tomatoes, and chocolate) related to the release of tumor byproducts into the bloodstream
         2. zinc, copper, nickel, niacin, and vitamin A deficiency and increased serum levels of calcium and lactate resulting from the disease process

---

*Some of the etiologic factors presented here are currently under investigation.

    d. alteration in the metabolism of proteins, fats, and carbohydrates

    e. early satiety associated with direct stimulation of the satiety center by an-orexigenic factors (e.g. peptides) secreted by tumor cells

    f. increased concentration of neurotransmitters in the brain and/or derangements in the serotoninergic system associated with the disease process

  2. nausea

  3. dysphagia and oral, pharyngeal, and esophageal pain resulting from mucositis associated with effects of cytotoxic agents on the gastrointestinal mucosa

  4. esophageal pain resulting from mucositis due to radiation to the chest area;

b. loss of nutrients associated with persistent vomiting resulting from effects of cytotoxic drugs and/or radiation therapy on the gastrointestinal mucosa;

c. elevated metabolic rate associated with an increased and continuous energy utilization by rapidly proliferating malignant cells;

d. utilization of available nutrients by the malignant cells rather than the host;

e. failure of feeding center to induce a sufficient increase in the intake of food to match metabolic needs;

f. inefficient and accelerated metabolism of proteins, fats, and carbohydrates associated with the disease process.

DESIRED OUTCOMES	NURSING ACTIONS AND *SELECTED RATIONALES*

2. The client will maintain an adequate nutritional status (see Care Plan on Chemotherapy, Nursing Diagnosis 3, for outcome criteria).	2.a. Refer to Care Plan on Chemotherapy, Nursing Diagnosis 3, for measures related to assessment and promotion of an optimal nutritional status.
	b. Implement additional measures *to improve oral intake:*
	  1. perform actions to reduce fear and anxiety (see Nursing Diagnosis 1, action c)
	  2. perform actions to reduce pain (see Nursing Diagnosis 3, actions a and b).

3. NURSING DIAGNOSIS

Pain:

a. **breast and axillary pain** related to pressure from enlarged lymph nodes and inflammation and/or ulceration of breast tissue due to invasion of subcutaneous tissue and skin by malignant cells;

b. **pain within the irradiated area** related to a cumulative dose of 3200–3600 rads, presence of interstitial applicators, and exposed nerve endings associated with moist desquamation if it occurs;

c. **esophageal pain** related to inflammation and/or ulceration of the mucosa associated with a radiation exposure of 3000 rads and/or side effects of cytotoxic drugs;

d. **oral pain** related to stomatitis associated with side effects of cytotoxic drugs.

DESIRED OUTCOMES	NURSING ACTIONS AND *SELECTED RATIONALES*
3. The client will experience diminished pain (see Care Plan on External Radiation, Nursing Diagnosis 5.A, for outcome criteria).	3.a. Refer to Care Plan on External Radiation, Nursing Diagnosis 5.A, for measures related to assessment and management of pain. b. Implement additional measures *to reduce pain:* 1. provide adequate support to involved breast area (e.g. pillow under arm when sitting, arm sling, supportive bra)

2. perform actions *to reduce pain in inflamed or ulcerated breast tissue:*
   a. apply moist packs to involved area as ordered
   b. monitor for therapeutic and nontherapeutic effects of corticosteroids if administered
   c. prepare client for radiation to ulcerated area if indicated.
c. Consult physician if above measures fail to provide adequate pain relief.

4. NURSING DIAGNOSIS

Impaired skin integrity:

a. **irritation and breakdown** related to:
   1. increased fragility of the skin associated with:
      a. invasion of subcutaneous tissue and skin by malignant cells
      b. malnutrition
      c. tissue hypoxia resulting from anemia due to chemotherapy-induced bone marrow suppression and nutritional deficits
   2. dry or moist desquamation at entry and exit sites of radiation
   3. contact of skin with wound drainage and use of tape;
b. **insertion/presence of applicators for interstitial radioactive implant.**

DESIRED OUTCOMES	NURSING ACTIONS AND *SELECTED RATIONALES*

4. The client will maintain skin integrity as evidenced by:
a. absence of redness and irritation
b. no skin breakdown.
	4.a. Inspect the skin, especially the affected breast, for pallor, redness, and breakdown.
	b. Refer to Care Plan on External Radiation, Nursing Diagnosis 7, action c.1, for measures to maintain or regain skin integrity within the radiation treatment field(s).
	c. If client has open lesions due to invasion of skin and subcutaneous tissue by malignant cells:
	  1. perform wound care as ordered to involved chest wall areas (e.g. povidone-iodine packs, corticosteroid creams, air drying)
	  2. keep skin around lesions clean and dry
	  3. replace soiled, damp dressings as needed (moisten dressings with normal saline *to facilitate removal if necessary*); utilize Montgomery straps or elastic netting *to secure dressings and prevent further breakdown.*
	d. Maintain an optimal nutritional status (see Nursing Diagnosis 2).
	e. If areas of breakdown fail to improve or additional breakdown occurs:
	  1. notify physician
	  2. continue with above measures to prevent further irritation and breakdown
	  3. perform wound and decubitus care as ordered or per standard hospital policy
	  4. monitor client closely and report signs and symptoms of infection (e.g. elevated temperature; redness, warmth, and edema around area of breakdown; unusual drainage from site).

5. NURSING DIAGNOSIS

Fatigue related to:

a. accumulation of cellular waste products associated with rapid lysis of cancerous and normal cells exposed to cytotoxic drugs and/or radiation;

b. inability to rest and sleep associated with discomfort resulting from the disease process and side effects of radiation and/or chemotherapy and prolonged physiological and psychological stress;
c. anxiety and depression associated with the diagnosis, the treatment regimen and its effects, the need to alter usual activities, and the inability to fulfill usual roles;
d. increased energy expenditure associated with an increase in the basal metabolic rate resulting from continuous, active tumor growth.

☐ ▬▬▬▬▬▬▬▬▬▬▬▬▬▬▬▬▬▬▬▬▬

DESIRED OUTCOMES	NURSING ACTIONS AND *SELECTED RATIONALES*

5. The client will experience a reduction in fatigue (see Care Plan on Chemotherapy, Nursing Diagnosis 10, for outcome criteria).	5.a. Refer to Care Plan on Chemotherapy, Nursing Diagnosis 10, for measures related to assessment, prevention, and management of fatigue.
	b. Implement additional measures *to reduce fatigue:*
	  1. perform actions to reduce fear and anxiety (see Nursing Diagnosis 1, action c)
	  2. perform actions to reduce pain (see Nursing Diagnosis 3, actions a and b).

☐ ▬▬▬▬▬▬▬▬▬▬▬▬▬▬▬▬▬▬▬▬▬

6. NURSING DIAGNOSIS

Activity intolerance related to:

a. tissue hypoxia associated with anemia resulting from chemotherapy-induced bone marrow suppression and nutritional deficits;
b. malnutrition:
c. inability to rest and sleep associated with discomfort and prolonged physiological and psychological stress.

☐ ▬▬▬▬▬▬▬▬▬▬▬▬▬▬▬▬▬▬▬▬▬

DESIRED OUTCOMES	NURSING ACTIONS AND *SELECTED RATIONALES*

6. The client will demonstrate an increased tolerance for activity (see Care Plan on Chemotherapy, Nursing Diagnosis 11, for outcome criteria).	6.a. Refer to Care Plan on Chemotherapy, Nursing Diagnosis 11, for measures related to assessment and improvement of activity tolerance.
	b. Implement additional measures *to promote rest and increase tolerance for activity:*
	  1. perform actions to reduce fear and anxiety (see Nursing Diagnosis 1, action c)
	  2. perform actions to reduce pain (see Nursing Diagnosis 3, actions a and b).

☐ ▬▬▬▬▬▬▬▬▬▬▬▬▬▬▬▬▬▬▬▬▬

7. NURSING DIAGNOSIS

Self-care deficit related to pain, weakness, and fatigue.

☐ ▬▬▬▬▬▬▬▬▬▬▬▬▬▬▬▬▬▬▬▬▬

DESIRED OUTCOMES	NURSING ACTIONS AND *SELECTED RATIONALES*
7. The client will demonstrate increased participation in self-care activities within limitations imposed by the disease process and treatment plan.	7.a. Refer to Care Plan on Chemotherapy, Nursing Diagnosis 13, for measures related to assessment of, planning for, and meeting the client's self-care needs. b. Implement measures to reduce pain (see Nursing Diagnosis 3, actions a and b) *in order to further facilitate the client's ability to perform self-care activities.*

☐ ▇▇▇▇▇▇▇▇▇▇▇▇▇▇▇▇▇▇▇▇▇▇▇▇▇▇▇

8. NURSING DIAGNOSIS

Disturbance in self-concept* related to:

a. change in appearance (e.g. excessive weight loss or gain, hair loss associated with chemotherapy, skin changes associated with radiation therapy, disfigurement of the breast[s] associated with biopsies and/or invasion of the skin and subcutaneous tissue by malignant cells);

b. sterility associated with ovarian failure resulting from extensive treatment with cytotoxic drugs and ablative estrogen therapy (e.g. oophorectomy, adrenalectomy, hypophysectomy, antiestrogen agents);

c. changes in sexual functioning associated with weakness, fatigue, pain, anxiety, and hormone changes (due to chemotherapy);

d. dependence on others to meet self-care needs;

e. stigma associated with the diagnosis of cancer;

f. anticipated changes in life style and roles associated with the disease process and its treatment.

---

* This diagnostic label includes the nursing diagnoses of body image disturbance and self-esteem disturbance.

☐ ▇▇▇▇▇▇▇▇▇▇▇▇▇▇▇▇▇▇▇▇▇▇▇▇▇▇▇

DESIRED OUTCOMES	NURSING ACTIONS AND *SELECTED RATIONALES*
8. The client will demonstrate beginning adaptation to changes in appearance, body functioning, life style, and roles (see Care Plan on Chemotherapy, Nursing Diagnosis 21, for outcome criteria).	8. Refer to Care Plan on Chemotherapy, Nursing Diagnosis 21, for measures related to assessment and promotion of a positive self-concept.

☐ ▇▇▇▇▇▇▇▇▇▇▇▇▇▇▇▇▇▇▇▇▇▇▇▇▇▇▇

9. NURSING DIAGNOSIS

Ineffective individual coping related to:

a. inadequate support system;

b. discomfort associated with the disease process and side effects of treatment;

c. prospect of a lengthy treatment plan (chemotherapy can extend for periods of up to 2 years);

d. depression, fear, and anxiety associated with the diagnosis, prognosis, and effects of the disease process and its treatment on usual body functioning and life style.

☐ ▇▇▇▇▇▇▇▇▇▇▇▇▇▇▇▇▇▇▇▇▇▇▇▇▇▇▇

UNIT
XVI

DESIRED OUTCOMES	NURSING ACTIONS AND *SELECTED RATIONALES*
9. The client will demonstrate the use of effective coping skills (see Care Plan on Chemotherapy, Nursing Diagnosis 22, for outcome criteria).	9.a. Refer to Care Plan on Chemotherapy, Nursing Diagnosis 22, for measures related to assessment and management of ineffective coping. b. Explain that it is not uncommon to have difficulty coping for an extended period (e.g. 2 years) after the diagnosis of breast cancer. c. Implement additional measures *to promote effective coping:* 1. perform actions to reduce fear and anxiety (see Nursing Diagnosis 1, action c) 2. perform actions to reduce pain (see Nursing Diagnosis 3, actions a and b).

10. NURSING DIAGNOSIS

Grieving* related to:

a. probable loss or disfigurement of breast;
b. anticipated changes in usual life style and roles associated with disease process and its treatment;
c. diagnosis of cancer with potential for premature death.

---

* This diagnostic label includes anticipatory grieving and grieving following the actual losses/changes.

DESIRED OUTCOMES	NURSING ACTIONS AND *SELECTED RATIONALES*
10. The client will demonstrate beginning progression through the grieving process (see Care Plan on Chemotherapy, Nursing Diagnosis 23, for outcome criteria).	10. Refer to Care Plan on Chemotherapy, Nursing Diagnosis 23, for measures related to assessment and facilitation of grieving.

11. NURSING DIAGNOSIS

Knowledge deficit regarding follow-up care.

DESIRED OUTCOMES	NURSING ACTIONS AND *SELECTED RATIONALES*
11.a. The client will verbalize the importance of doing a routine breast self-examination (BSE).	11.a.1. Explain the reason for performing monthly BSE. 2. Explore with client ways to remember to carry out BSE. The examination should be done a week after the conclusion of menses or on a specific date if postmenopausal.
11.b. The client will demonstrate the ability to correctly perform a BSE.	11.b.1. Demonstrate how to perform BSE using a model, film, or chart. 2. Allow time for questions, clarification, and return demonstration.

11.c. The client will demonstrate the ability to appropriately care for malignant skin lesions if present.	11.c.1. Instruct client in care of malignant skin lesions (e.g. moist packs, exposure to air) if present. 2. Allow time for clarification, practice, and return demonstration.
11.d. The client will identify ways to improve appetite and nutritional status.	11.d. Refer to Care Plan on Chemotherapy, Nursing Diagnosis 24, action e, for instructions related to improving appetite and maintaining an adequate nutritional status.
11.e. The client will state signs and symptoms to report to the health care provider.	11.e.1. If appropriate, refer to Care Plans on Chemotherapy (Nursing Diagnosis 24, action l), Brachytherapy (Postradiation Nursing Diagnosis 4, action d), and/or External Radiation (Nursing Diagnosis 21, action j) for signs and symptoms to report. 2. Instruct client to also report: a. draining, reddened biopsy site(s) b. increase in size or number of malignant skin lesions c. signs and symptoms of calcium excess (e.g. loss of appetite, nausea, vomiting, constipation, increased thirst, increased urination, drowsiness); these signs and symptoms may occur if bone metastasis is present.
11.f. The client will identify community resources that can assist with home management and adjustment to changes resulting from the diagnosis and the effects of treatment.	11.f.1. Provide information about community resources that can assist client and significant others with home management and adjustment to the diagnosis and effects of treatment (e.g. American Cancer Society, Meals on Wheels, counselors, support groups, Hospice, Visiting Nurse Association, home health agencies, Make Today Count). 2. Initiate a referral if indicated.
11.g. The client will verbalize an understanding of and a plan for adhering to recommended follow-up care including future appointments with health care provider and for laboratory studies, medications prescribed, activity level, and plans for subsequent treatment.	11.g.1. Reinforce physician's explanation of planned radiation therapy and/or chemotherapy if appropriate. Stress importance of strictly following the prescribed protocol for chemotherapy and/or radiation therapy and keeping all appointments for follow-up supervision and laboratory work. 2. Emphasize the need for planned rest periods and for gauging activity according to tolerance. 3. Explain the rationale for, side effects of, and importance of taking medications prescribed (e.g. allopurinol, cytotoxic agents, anti-infectives, antiestrogen agents). 4. Implement measures *to improve client compliance:* a. include significant others in teaching sessions if possible b. encourage questions and allow time for reinforcement and clarification of information provided c. provide written instructions regarding scheduled appointments with health care provider and for chemotherapy, radiation therapy, and laboratory work; medications prescribed; and signs and symptoms to report.

Mammoplasty

A mammoplasty is the surgical reconstruction of the breast(s) that is performed to augment or reduce breast size or to shape and build a new breast mound following a mastectomy. It may be performed immediately following the mastectomy or delayed 4–6 months depending on physician preference, extensiveness of the tumor, lymph node status, planned treatment program, and age and desire of client.

Following a mastectomy, the technique used for reconstruction will depend on when it is performed in relation to the mastectomy; amount, condition, and laxness of the skin on the chest wall; thickness of the skin flaps; and presence of pectoralis major muscle. In some women, a subpectoral prosthetic implant is all that is necessary. In others who have extensive skin, tissue, and muscle loss or radiation-induced skin damage, reconstruction may involve the use of a myocutaneous flap such as the latissimus dorsi or the rectus abdominis flap. With the rectus abdominis flap, an additional prosthetic implant is usually unnecessary. If the client has very taut skin on the chest wall or if the reconstruction is initiated at the time of the mastectomy, the use of a tissue expander may be necessary to promote growth and facilitate stretching of the skin. With this procedure, an inflatable device is placed beneath the pectoral muscle and then gradually filled with saline over a period of several weeks. Once adequate stretching and growth has occurred, the device is replaced with a permanent prosthesis. There are tissue expanders available that can serve as the permanent implant. With this type, only the filling port is removed when adequate expansion has been achieved. The construction of a nipple-areola com-

plex may be performed concurrently or delayed for 6 months so that placement can be more accurately determined. The areola is constructed by utilizing a graft from the medial aspect of the thigh, postauricular area, labia minora, or the contralateral breast if the areola is of sufficient size. Medical tattooing can also be done to simulate an areola. The nipple prominence is created by partitioning the remaining nipple, by utilizing a small portion of the earlobe or scar tissue, or simply by using a purse string suture. The majority of women who undergo breast reconstruction following a mastectomy will also have surgery (e.g. reduction, augmentation, mastopexy) on the contralateral breast in order to achieve symmetry.

This care plan focuses on the adult female client hospitalized for breast reconstruction following a mastectomy. Preoperatively, the goal of care is to educate the client regarding postoperative expectations and management. Postoperative goals of care are to prevent complications, assist the client to adjust to her new body image, and educate her regarding follow-up care.

DISCHARGE CRITERIA

Prior to discharge, the client will:

- verbalize the importance of doing a routine breast self-examination (BSE)
- demonstrate the ability to correctly perform a BSE
- demonstrate the appropriate technique to prevent capsule formation around breast implant(s)
- state signs and symptoms of complications to report to the health care provider
- share feelings and thoughts about the change in body image
- verbalize an understanding of and a plan for adhering to recommended follow-up care including future appointments with health care provider, medications prescribed, activity restrictions, and wound care.

NURSING/COLLABORATIVE DIAGNOSES

Preoperative
1. Knowledge deficit ☐ *981*
Postoperative
1. Ineffective breathing patterns ☐ *982*
2. Self-care deficit ☐ *982*
3. Potential complications:
   a. hematoma formation
   b. extrusion of prosthesis(es)
   c. necrosis of skin flap(s) and/or grafted nipple(s) ☐ *982*
4. Knowledge deficit regarding follow-up care ☐ *983*

Preoperative

Use in conjunction with the Standardized Preoperative Care Plan.

1. NURSING DIAGNOSIS

Knowledge deficit regarding:

a. hospital routines associated with surgery;
b. physical preparation for the mammoplasty;
c. postoperative care;
d. sensation in and appearance of the breast(s) following reconstruction.

DESIRED OUTCOMES	NURSING ACTIONS AND *SELECTED RATIONALES*
1.a. The client will verbalize an understanding of usual preoperative and postoperative care and routines.	1.a. Refer to Standardized Preoperative Care Plan, Nursing Diagnosis 4, action a, for information to include in preoperative teaching.

1.b. The client will demonstrate the ability to perform techniques designed to prevent postoperative complications.	1.b.1. Refer to Standardized Preoperative Care Plan, Nursing Diagnosis 4, action b.1, for instructions on ways to prevent postoperative complications.
	2. Provide additional instructions regarding ways *to prevent postoperative complications:*
	  a. if client is to have subpectoral implant(s), inform her that a bra should not be worn for several weeks following surgery *to allow prosthesis(es) to settle into pocket(s) created in chest wall*
	  b. inform client that she will need to keep upper arm on operative side(s) close to her body for a week after surgery (length of time will vary according to physician preference) *in order to prevent tension on the suture lines.*
	3. Allow time for questions and clarification of information provided.

1.c. The client will verbalize an awareness of expected sensation in and appearance of the breast(s) after reconstruction.	1.c.1. Provide the following information on expected sensation in and appearance of the breast(s) after reconstruction:
	  a. reinforce physician's explanation that the goal of reconstructive surgery after a mastectomy is to achieve a normal appearance in clothing; emphasize that it is impossible to duplicate the size, shape, and contour of a natural breast
	  b. explain that the breast(s) will be swollen and discolored in the immediate postoperative period and will appear unusually high on the chest wall if a subpectoral implant has been done; assure client and significant others that this is temporary
	  c. inform client that when one breast is reconstructed, symmetry does not usually occur until the tissue surrounding the implant or muscle flap has stretched
	  d. explain that a loss of sensitivity in grafted nipple and skin around the suture lines is a common occurrence.
	2. Allow time for questions and clarification of information provided.
	3. Consult physician if client has unrealistic expectations about the postoperative appearance of the breast(s).

☐ ▬▬▬▬▬▬▬▬▬▬▬▬▬▬▬▬▬▬▬▬▬▬▬

Postoperative

Use in conjunction with the Standardized Postoperative Care Plan.

☐ ▬▬▬▬▬▬▬▬▬▬▬▬▬▬▬▬▬▬

1. NURSING DIAGNOSIS

Ineffective breathing patterns related to fear, anxiety, reluctance to breathe deeply associated with chest wall incisional pain, and depressant effects of anesthesia and some medications (e.g. narcotic analgesics).

☐ ▬▬▬▬▬▬▬▬▬▬▬▬▬▬▬▬▬▬

DESIRED OUTCOMES	NURSING ACTIONS AND *SELECTED RATIONALES*
1. The client will maintain an effective breathing pattern (see Standardized Postoperative Care Plan, Nursing Diagnosis 3, for outcome criteria).	1. Refer to Standardized Postoperative Care Plan, Nursing Diagnosis 3, for measures related to assessment and improvement of breathing pattern.

☐ ▬▬▬▬▬▬▬▬▬▬▬▬▬▬▬▬▬▬

2. NURSING DIAGNOSIS

Self-care deficit related to impaired physical mobility associated with pain, depressant effects of some medications (e.g. narcotic analgesics), fear of injury to surgical site, and prescribed arm movement restrictions on operative side(s).

☐ ▬▬▬▬▬▬▬▬▬▬▬▬▬▬▬▬▬▬

DESIRED OUTCOMES	NURSING ACTIONS AND *SELECTED RATIONALES*
2. The client will perform self-care activities within physical limitations and postoperative activity restrictions.	2.a. Refer to Standardized Postoperative Care Plan, Nursing Diagnosis 12, for measures related to assessment of, planning for, and meeting client's self-care needs. b. Assist client with any personal hygiene tasks that require extension and abduction of the arm on the operative side (e.g. bathing, combing and washing hair).

☐ ▬▬▬▬▬▬▬▬▬▬▬▬▬▬▬▬▬▬

3. COLLABORATIVE DIAGNOSIS

Potential complications:

a. **hematoma formation** related to bleeding into the tissues and impaired drainage from the operative area;

b. **extrusion of prosthesis(es)** related to inadequate pocket size for implant, necrosis of skin flap(s), or trauma to surgical site;

c. **necrosis of skin flap(s) and/or grafted nipple(s)** related to infection and decreased tissue perfusion in the operative area.

☐ ▭▭▭▭▭▭▭▭▭▭▭▭▭▭▭▭▭▭▭▭▭▭▭▭▭

DESIRED OUTCOMES	NURSING ACTIONS AND *SELECTED RATIONALES*

3.a. The client will not develop a hematoma at the surgical site as evidenced by:
1. expected amount of drainage from incision(s) and drain(s)
2. no unusual increase in swelling in operative area
3. no increase in skin discoloration in operative area.

3.a.1. Assess for and immediately report increased swelling and discoloration of the operative site and less than expected amount of drainage from incision(s) and drain(s).
2. Implement measures *to prevent hematoma formation:*
   a. caution client to keep elbows at sides for 3–7 days after surgery *in order to eliminate strain on the surgical site and subsequent bleeding*
   b. maintain patency of wound drain (e.g. milk or strip tubing if ordered, keep tubing free of kinks)
   c. maintain wound drain suction as ordered.
3. If signs and symptoms of hematoma formation occur:
   a. prepare client for evacuation of hematoma if indicated
   b. provide support to client and significant others.

3.b. The client will not experience extrusion of the breast prosthesis(es) as evidenced by maintenance of implant(s) under skin flap(s).

3.b.1. Assess for and report:
   a. conditions such as trauma to operative site, separation of suture line, or necrosis of skin flap that may place client at risk for extrusion of prosthesis(es)
   b. extrusion of the prosthesis(es).
2. Implement measures *to prevent extrusion of prosthesis(es):*
   a. perform actions to prevent skin flap necrosis (see action c.2 in this diagnosis)
   b. caution client to avoid placing undue pressure on reconstructed area(s) until healing has occurred.
3. If extrusion of prosthesis(es) occurs:
   a. prepare client for surgical replacement of the implant(s)
   b. provide emotional support to client and significant others.

3.c. The client will not experience necrosis of the skin flap(s) or grafted nipple(s) as evidenced by:
1. skin flap(s) and nipple(s) warm and expected color
2. approximated wound edges
3. absence of foul odor from flap area and grafted nipple(s).

3.c.1. Assess for and report signs and symptoms of:
   a. impaired blood flow in skin flap (e.g. blue, white, or red appearing skin flap; capillary refill time greater than 3 seconds)
   b. skin flap or grafted nipple necrosis (e.g. pale, cool, darkened tissue; separation of wound edges; foul odor).
2. Implement measures *to prevent necrosis of skin flap(s) and grafted nipple(s):*
   a. perform actions *to maintain adequate circulation to wound area:*
      1. implement measures to prevent hematoma formation (see action a.2 in this diagnosis)
      2. ascertain that dressings are not too tight
   b. perform actions to promote healing of surgical incision and prevent and treat wound infection (see Standardized Postoperative Care Plan, Nursing Diagnoses 9, action a.2 and 16, actions b.4 and 5)
   c. use caution when changing dressings, being careful not to disturb graft site(s).
3. If signs and symptoms of necrosis of skin flap(s) or grafted nipple(s) occur:
   a. prepare client for surgical revision of reconstructed area
   b. provide emotional support to client and significant others.

☐ ▭▭▭▭▭▭▭▭▭▭▭▭▭▭▭▭▭▭▭▭▭▭▭▭▭

4. NURSING DIAGNOSIS

Knowledge deficit regarding follow-up care.

☐ ▭▭▭▭▭▭▭▭▭▭▭▭▭▭▭▭▭▭▭▭▭▭▭▭▭

DESIRED OUTCOMES	NURSING ACTIONS AND *SELECTED RATIONALES*
4.a. The client will verbalize the importance of doing a routine breast self-examination (BSE).	4.a.1. Explain the reasons for a monthly BSE. 2. Discuss with client the importance of being familiar with what is "normal" for her breasts as a result of surgery. 3. Explore with client ways to remember to carry out BSE. The examination should be done one week after conclusion of menses or on a specific date if postmenopausal.
4.b. The client will demonstrate the ability to correctly perform BSE.	4.b.1. Demonstrate the technique for performing BSE using a model, film, or chart. 2. Allow time for questions, clarification, and return demonstration.
4.c. The client will demonstrate the appropriate technique to prevent capsule formation around breast implant(s).	4.c.1. Instruct client on massage techniques that are used to maintain mobility of the implant(s) *in order to prevent capsule formation*. 2. Emphasize the necessity of massaging and moving the implant(s) at least 4–6 times/day as soon as permitted by physician (massage should be continued for several months postoperatively).

4.d. The client will state signs and symptoms of complications to report to the health care provider.	4.d.1. Refer to Standardized Postoperative Care Plan, Nursing Diagnosis 20, action c, for signs and symptoms to report to the health care provider.
	2. Instruct client to report these additional signs and symptoms:
	  a. thinning, change of color, or breakdown of skin over implant or flap site
	  b. increasing redness or drainage of donor site if grafting was done
	  c. sudden change in position of implants.

4.e. The client will verbalize an understanding of and a plan for adhering to recommended follow-up care including future appointments with health care provider, medications prescribed, activity restrictions, and wound care.	4.e.1. Refer to Standardized Postoperative Care Plan, Nursing Diagnosis 20, for routine postoperative instructions and measures to improve client compliance.
	2. If a subpectoral implant has been performed, reinforce that a bra should not be worn for several weeks following surgery.
	3. If client had a tissue expander inserted:
	  a. emphasize importance of keeping appointments every 7–10 days to enlarge expander (in some cases, the client will eventually be taught to do the instillation at home)
	  b. explain that a sterile solution will be added until a slight feeling of tightness is felt around the expander
	  c. instruct her to report pain, change in color of tissue over expander, redness of area, and/or separation of incision edges.
	4. Caution client to limit arm movement as prescribed.
	5. Instruct client to avoid any lifting or pushing objects over 5 pounds for at least a month *in order to prevent strain on pectoral muscles*.
	6. Explain activity limitations to significant others. Encourage their help and support in meeting the client's daily needs.

Mastectomy

A mastectomy is the surgical removal of the breast and is usually performed to treat breast cancer. There are several types of mastectomies including the Halsted radical mastectomy, total mastectomy with axillary dissection (modified radical), lumpectomy (partial mastectomy, tylectomy), and subcutaneous mastectomy.

The traditional Halsted radical mastectomy, which involves removal of the breast, major and minor pectoral muscles, and all surrounding lymph nodes, fat, and fascia, is rarely done today because of changes in thinking about breast cancer and how it spreads. The most common procedure currently performed is the total mastectomy with axillary node dissection. It includes removal of the breast, some axillary nodes, and possibly the pectoralis minor muscle. The pectoralis major muscle is preserved with this procedure so that the client retains the shape of her chest wall in order to facilitate reconstructive surgery. The risk of complications such as lymphedema and shoulder dysfunction is minimized with this more conservative procedure. A lumpectomy is an option available to a woman with a small tumor. It involves removal of only the cancerous tissue and a small margin of adjacent healthy tissue. A subcutaneous mastectomy may be performed for premalignant conditions or in situations in which the woman is at high risk for developing cancer of the breast. In this procedure, the subcutaneous breast tissue is removed, leaving the skin and nipple-areola complex intact.

This care plan focuses on the adult female client hospitalized for a total mastectomy with axillary node dissection. Goals of preoperative care are to reduce fear and anxiety and prepare her for the postoperative period. Postoperatively, the goals of care are to maintain comfort, prevent complications, assist her to adjust to the change in body image, and educate her regarding follow-up care. This care plan should be used in conjunction with the Care Plans on Cancer of the Breast and Mammoplasty if appropriate.

DISCHARGE CRITERIA

Prior to discharge, the client will:

- identify ways to reduce the risk of trauma to and infection in the arm on the operative side
- identify ways to prevent and treat lymphedema in the arm on the operative side
- demonstrate the ability to perform appropriate hand, arm, and shoulder exercises
- verbalize the importance of doing a routine breast self-examination (BSE) on the remaining breast and operative site
- demonstrate the ability to correctly perform a BSE
- state the factors to consider in selecting a breast prosthesis
- state signs and symptoms of complications to report to the health care provider
- share thoughts and feelings about the change in body image
- identify community resources that can assist with home management and adjustment to the loss of a breast
- verbalize an understanding of and a plan for adhering to recommended follow-up care including future appointments with health care provider, medications prescribed, activity level, and wound care.

NURSING/COLLABORATIVE DIAGNOSES

Preoperative
1. Anxiety □ *986*
2. Knowledge deficit □ *986*

Postoperative
1. Ineffective breathing patterns □ *987*
2. Impaired physical mobility □ *988*
3. Self-care deficit □ *988*
4. Potential complications:
   a. lymphedema of arm on operative side
   b. motor and sensory impairment of arm and/or shoulder on operative side:
      1. difficulty with adduction and internal rotation of the arm
      2. numbness and loss of sensation in the arm and the hand
      3. contractures of the shoulder
   c. seroma formation
   d. necrosis of skin flap □ *989*
5. Sexual dysfunction: decreased libido □ *991*
6. Disturbance in self-concept □ *991*
7. Ineffective individual coping □ *992*
8. Grieving □ *993*
9. Knowledge deficit regarding follow-up care □ *994*

UNIT
XVI

Preoperative

Use in conjunction with the Standardized Preoperative Care Plan.

1. NURSING DIAGNOSIS

Anxiety related to:

a. unfamiliar environment and separation from significant others;
b. effects of anesthesia;
c. mutilating effects of the mastectomy;
d. possible change in relationship with significant other because of the loss of her breast;
e. anticipated postoperative discomfort and limitations.

DESIRED OUTCOMES	NURSING ACTIONS AND *SELECTED RATIONALES*
1. The client will experience a reduction in fear and anxiety (see Standardized Preoperative Care Plan, Nursing Diagnosis 1, for outcome criteria).	1.a. Refer to Standardized Preoperative Care Plan, Nursing Diagnosis 1, for measures related to assessment and reduction of preoperative fear and anxiety. b. Implement additional measures *to reduce fear and anxiety:* 1. arrange for a Reach to Recovery volunteer to visit client if appropriate 2. reinforce information from physician about the possibility of breast reconstruction if desired by client 3. reinforce physician's explanations about the positive effects of the surgery.

2. NURSING DIAGNOSIS

Knowledge deficit regarding:

a. hospital routines associated with surgery;
b. physical preparation for the mastectomy;
c. ways to prevent lymphedema postoperatively;
d. hand and arm exercises initiated in the immediate postoperative period;
e. phantom breast sensation (thought to be associated with changes in pressure and motion, stimulation of peripheral nerves at mastectomy site, and/or psychological factors [Nail et al., 1984]).

DESIRED OUTCOMES	NURSING ACTIONS AND *SELECTED RATIONALES*
2.a. The client will verbalize an understanding of usual preoperative and postoperative care and routines.	2.a. Refer to Standardized Preoperative Care Plan, Nursing Diagnosis 4, action a, for information to include in preoperative teaching.

2.b. The client will demonstrate the ability to perform techniques designed to prevent postoperative complications.

2.b.1. Refer to Standardized Preoperative Care Plan, Nursing Diagnosis 4, action b.1, for instructions on ways to prevent postoperative complications.
   2. Provide additional instructions regarding ways *to prevent postoperative complications:*
      a. inform the client that she must keep upper arm on operative side close to her body for a week after surgery (length of time will vary according to physician preference) *in order to prevent tension on the suture lines*
      b. explain that exercise of the hand, arm, and shoulder on the affected side is essential *in order to facilitate and improve lymphatic and blood circulation, maintain muscle tone, and prevent contractures*
      c. demonstrate recommended hand, arm, and shoulder exercises (e.g. flexion and extension of the fingers and wrist, wall climbing, pulley over shower rod, rope turning)
      d. explain why lymphedema might occur after surgery (a transient edema of the arm on the operative side may occur and persist for 1–3 months until collateral lymphatic channels are developed)
      e. instruct client on ways *to minimize or prevent lymphedema in the arm on operative side:*
         1. keep arm on operative side elevated on pillows with elbow at heart level and hand higher than elbow in the early postoperative period
         2. perform recommended finger, wrist, and arm exercises as soon as allowed (finger and wrist exercises are usually begun the day of surgery)
         3. inform client that no venipunctures, injections, or B/P measurements should be performed on that arm *(these procedures increase risk of infection or trauma and subsequent lymphedema).*
   3. Allow time for questions, clarification, practice, and return demonstration of exercises.

2.c. The client will verbalize an awareness of phantom sensations that may occur after a mastectomy.

2.c.1. Provide the following information on phantom sensations that may occur after a mastectomy:
      a. explain to client that it is common to experience sensations of itching, heaviness, pain, numbness, and/or "pins and needles" in the absent breast (most clients will notice it within the first week after surgery)
      b. assure client that women experience the sensation of both breasts being present most of the time; explain that a physical awareness of the loss may occur when leaning on a solid object (e.g. table) or crossing the arms
      c. explain to client that she may feel unbalanced at first, particularly if breasts are large.
   2. Allow time for questions and clarification of information provided.

Postoperative

Use in conjunction with the Standardized Postoperative Care Plan.

1. NURSING DIAGNOSIS

Ineffective breathing patterns related to fear, anxiety, reluctance to breathe deeply associated with chest wall incisional pain, depressant effects of anesthesia and some medications (e.g. narcotic analgesics), and restrictive dressings.

DESIRED OUTCOMES	NURSING ACTIONS AND *SELECTED RATIONALES*
1. The client will maintain an effective breathing pattern (see Standardized Postoperative Care Plan, Nursing Diagnosis 3, for outcome criteria).	1.a. Refer to Standardized Postoperative Care Plan, Nursing Diagnosis 3, for measures related to assessment and improvement of breathing pattern. b. Consult physician if compression dressing appears to be too restrictive and the client is having difficulty maintaining an effective breathing pattern.

□ ▮▮▮▮▮▮▮▮▮▮▮▮▮▮▮▮▮▮▮▮▮▮▮▮▮▮▮▮▮▮▮▮▮▮▮▮▮

2. NURSING DIAGNOSIS

Impaired physical mobility related to:

a. decreased activity tolerance associated with major surgery;
b. reluctance to move because of pain and nausea;
c. depressant effects of anesthesia and some medications (e.g. narcotic analgesics, antiemetics);
d. fear of falling (may have some difficulty with balance as a result of restricted or impaired arm movement), dislodging tubes, and compromising surgical wound;
e. impaired movement of the arm on the operative side associated with nerve trauma during the surgical procedure, weakness of the pectoral muscles, lymphedema, and restrictions imposed by the treatment plan.

□ ▮▮▮▮▮▮▮▮▮▮▮▮▮▮▮▮▮▮▮▮▮▮▮▮▮▮▮▮▮▮▮▮▮▮▮▮▮

DESIRED OUTCOMES	NURSING ACTIONS AND *SELECTED RATIONALES*

2. The client will achieve maximum physical mobility within the limitations imposed by the mastectomy and postoperative management.	2.a. Assess for factors that impair physical mobility (e.g. reluctance to move because of pain or nausea, fear of falling, restricted arm movement on operative side, weakness, fatigue).
	b. Refer to Standardized Postoperative Care Plan, Nursing Diagnosis 11, action b, for measures to increase mobility.
	c. Implement additional measures *to increase mobility:*
	  1. perform actions to prevent lymphedema and arm and shoulder dysfunction (see Postoperative Collaborative Diagnosis 4, actions a.2 and b.2) *in order to allow increased arm movement*
	  2. accompany client during ambulation if balance is a problem; assure her that balance will improve when increased arm movement is permitted
	  3. instruct and assist client with prescribed hand, arm, and shoulder exercises.

□ ▮▮▮▮▮▮▮▮▮▮▮▮▮▮▮▮▮▮▮▮▮▮▮▮▮▮▮▮▮▮▮▮▮▮▮▮▮

3. NURSING DIAGNOSIS

Self-care deficit related to impaired physical mobility associated with fatigue, weakness, pain, fear of injury, and restricted or impaired arm movement.

□ ▮▮▮▮▮▮▮▮▮▮▮▮▮▮▮▮▮▮▮▮▮▮▮▮▮▮▮▮▮▮▮▮▮▮▮▮▮

DESIRED OUTCOMES	NURSING ACTIONS AND *SELECTED RATIONALES*
3. The client will perform self-care activities within physical limitations and postoperative activity restrictions.	3.a. Assess for factors that interfere with the client's ability to perform self-care (e.g. pain, sensory and motor deficits in arm on operative side, arm movement restrictions imposed by treatment plan). b. Refer to Standardized Postoperative Care Plan, Nursing Diagnosis 12, actions b–d for measures related to planning for and meeting client's self-care needs. c. Implement measures to increase mobility (see Postoperative Nursing Diagnosis 2, actions b and c) *in order to further facilitate client's ability to perform self-care.* d. Assist client with personal hygiene tasks that require extension and abduction of arm on operative side (e.g. combing and washing hair, bathing).

□ ▇▇▇▇▇▇▇▇▇▇▇▇▇▇▇▇▇▇▇▇▇▇▇▇▇▇▇▇▇▇▇▇

4. COLLABORATIVE DIAGNOSIS

Potential complications:

a. **lymphedema of arm on operative side** related to obstruction of lymphatic flow associated with removal of lymph nodes (if an extensive axillary node dissection has been performed), infection, and trauma to the arm;

b. **motor and sensory impairment of the arm and/or shoulder on the operative side:**
   1. **difficulty with adduction and internal rotation of the arm** related to damage to the thoracodorsal nerve that supplies the latissimus dorsi muscle
   2. **numbness and loss of sensation in arm and hand** related to entrapment of nerves at cervical outlet or wrist associated with lymphedema
   3. **contractures of the shoulder** due to noncompliance with the prescribed exercise program;

c. **seroma formation** related to:
   1. large potential dead space beneath flap
   2. delayed or impaired flap adherence associated with irregular shape of chest wall, movement of operative site with respiration and arm and shoulder use, and impaired wound drainage;

d. **necrosis of skin flap** related to inadequate blood supply in flap and infection of surgical wound.

□ ▇▇▇▇▇▇▇▇▇▇▇▇▇▇▇▇▇▇▇▇▇▇▇▇▇▇▇▇▇▇▇▇

DESIRED OUTCOMES	NURSING ACTIONS AND *SELECTED RATIONALES*
4.a. The client will not develop lymphedema in the arm on the operative side as evidenced by: 1. normal motor and sensory function of affected arm 2. absence of pain and swelling in affected arm.	4.a.1. Assess for and report signs and symptoms of lymphedema in arm on the operative side: a. sensory and motor deficits b. pain, sensation of heaviness c. swelling (measure arm on operative side at points 6 inches above and below elbow). 2. Implement measures *to prevent lymphedema in arm on operative side:* a. place client in a semi-Fowler's position during the immediate postoperative period; elevate arm on the operative side on pillows, keeping elbow at heart level and hand higher than elbow b. avoid prolonged adduction of arm *to prevent pressure on axilla (pressure can impede lymphatic flow)*

    c. place a sign above bed to remind personnel not to use arm on operative side for venipunctures, injections, and B/P measurement *in order to decrease risk of infection or trauma and subsequent lymphedema*

    d. perform actions to prevent and treat wound infection (see Standardized Postoperative Care Plan, Nursing Diagnosis 16, actions b.4 and 5)

    e. instruct and assist client to perform mastectomy exercises as soon as allowed (usually 1st to 7th postoperative day).

3. If signs and symptoms of lymphedema occur:

    a. continue with above measures

    b. monitor for therapeutic and nontherapeutic effects of the following medications if administered:

      1. anti-infectives *to prevent or treat cellulitis and lymphangitis*

      2. diuretics *to reduce fluid accumulation in tissues*

    c. apply elastic bandages to the affected arm if ordered

    d. assist and instruct client in use of an intermittent pneumatic compression sleeve on affected arm if ordered

    e. provide emotional support to client and significant others.

4.b. The client will maintain usual motor and sensory function of the arm and shoulder on the operative side as evidenced by:
1. ability to put arm and shoulder through full range of motion
2. absence of numbness, tingling, muscle weakness.

4.b.1. Assess for and report signs and symptoms of motor and/or sensory impairment of the arm and shoulder on operative side (e.g. inability to move joints through their full range of motion, muscle weakness, numbness, tingling).

2. Implement measures *to prevent arm and shoulder dysfunction:*

    a. perform actions to prevent lymphedema (see action a.2 in this diagnosis)

    b. reinforce preoperative instructions about hand, arm, and shoulder exercises

    c. assist client with simple hand and wrist exercises as soon as possible after surgery

    d. initiate mastectomy exercises (e.g. wall climbing) as soon as allowed (usually 1st to 7th postoperative day)

    e. encourage use of arm on operative side to perform activities of daily living as soon as allowed.

3. If signs and symptoms of impaired arm and shoulder function occur:

    a. continue with above measures

    b. assist with prescribed physical therapy

    c. provide emotional support to client and significant others.

4.c. The client will not develop a seroma as evidenced by:
1. absence of continued drainage from incision
2. expected amount of wound drainage in collection device.

4.c.1. Assess for and report signs and symptoms of seroma formation (e.g. continued drainage from incision, less than expected amount of wound drainage in collection device).

2. Implement measures *to prevent seroma formation:*

    a. maintain patency of suction catheters (e.g. re-establish suction and milk tubing as necessary)

    b. place needed items within easy reach *to prevent unnecessary arm and shoulder movement*

    c. reinforce importance of adhering to prescribed arm and shoulder movement restrictions.

3. If seroma formation occurs:

    a. prepare client for needle aspiration of excessive fluid

    b. provide emotional support to client and significant others.

4.d. The client will not experience necrosis of the skin flap as evidenced by:
1. skin flap warm and expected color
2. approximated wound edges
3. absence of foul odor from flap area.

4.d.1. Assess for and report signs and symptoms of:

    a. impaired blood flow in skin flap (e.g. blue, white, or red appearing skin flap; capillary refill time greater than 3 seconds)

    b. skin flap necrosis (e.g. pale, cool, darkened tissue; separation of wound edges; foul odor).

2. Implement measures *to prevent skin flap necrosis:*

    a. perform actions *to maintain adequate circulation to wound area:*

      1. implement measures to prevent seroma formation (see action c.2 in this diagnosis)

      2. consult physician regarding loosening of compression dressing if client complains of increased tightness of dressings or if dressing appears too restrictive

    b. perform actions to promote healing of surgical incision and prevent

and treat wound infection (see Standardized Postoperative Care Plan, Nursing Diagnoses 9, action a.2 and 16, actions b.4 and 5).
3. If skin flap necrosis occurs:
    a. prepare client for surgical revision
    b. provide emotional support to client and significant others.

5. NURSING DIAGNOSIS

Sexual dysfunction: decreased libido related to:

a. altered self-concept associated with change in body image resulting from the mastectomy;
b. discomfort associated with an extensive surgical wound;
c. fear of rejection by usual partner.

DESIRED OUTCOMES	NURSING ACTIONS AND *SELECTED RATIONALES*

5. The client will perceive self as sexually adequate and acceptable as evidenced by:
a. verbalization of same
b. maintenance of relationship with partner
c. statements reflecting beginning adjustment to the effects of a mastectomy on sexuality.
	5.a. Assess for signs and symptoms of sexual dysfunction (e.g. verbalization of sexual concerns, failure to maintain relationship with significant other).
	b. Determine attitudes, knowledge, and concerns of the client and her partner about the effects of the mastectomy on sexual functioning.
	c. Communicate interest, understanding, and respect for the values of the client and her partner.
	d. Facilitate communication between the client and her partner. Assist them to identify factors that may affect their sexual relationship.
	e. Implement measures *to decrease the possibility of rejection by partner:*
	  1. assist the partner to acknowledge both positive and negative feelings
	  2. if appropriate, involve partner in care of the wound and dressing change *to facilitate adjustment to and integration of the change in client's body image.*
	f. Arrange for uninterrupted privacy during hospital stay if desired by the couple.
	g. Implement measures to improve self-concept (see Postoperative Nursing Diagnosis 6, actions c–r).
	h. If client is concerned that operative site discomfort will interfere with usual sexual activity:
	  1. assure her that the discomfort is temporary and will diminish as the incision heals
	  2. encourage alternatives to intercourse or use of positions that decrease pressure on the surgical site (e.g. side-lying).
	i. Include partner in above discussions and encourage his/her continued support of client.
	j. Consult physician if counseling appears indicated.

6. NURSING DIAGNOSIS

Disturbance in self-concept* related to a change in body image associated with the loss of a breast, dependence on others to meet self-care needs associated with restricted arm movement, and change in sexual functioning.

* This diagnostic label includes the nursing diagnoses of body image disturbance and self-esteem disturbance.

DESIRED OUTCOMES	NURSING ACTIONS AND *SELECTED RATIONALES*

6. The client will demonstrate beginning adaptation to the loss of her breast and integration of the change in body image as evidenced by:
   a. verbalization of feelings of self-worth and sexual adequacy
   b. maintenance of relationships with significant others
   c. active participation in activities of daily living
   d. active interest in personal appearance
   e. willingness to look at surgical site
   f. willingness to participate in social activities.

6.a. Determine the meaning of the loss of a breast to the client by encouraging her to verbalize feelings and by noting nonverbal responses to change experienced.
   b. Assess for signs and symptoms of a disturbance in self-concept (e.g. verbal or nonverbal cues denoting a negative response to loss of breast such as denial of or preoccupation with the loss, refusal to look at or touch mastectomy site, or withdrawal from significant others).
   c. Implement measures *to assist client to increase self-esteem* (e.g. limit negative self-criticism, encourage positive comments about self, give positive feedback about accomplishments).
   d. Assist client to identify strengths and qualities that have a positive effect on self-concept.
   e. Implement measures to assist client to cope with the effects of mastectomy (see Postoperative Nursing Diagnosis 7, action d).
   f. Implement measures to assist client to adjust to alteration in sexual functioning (see Postoperative Nursing Diagnosis 5, actions c–i).
   g. Assist client with usual grooming and makeup habits if necessary.
   h. Demonstrate acceptance of client using techniques such as therapeutic touch and frequent visits. Encourage significant others to do the same.
   i. Stay with client during first dressing change and encourage an expression of feelings about appearance of incision and change in her body.
   j. If the client is unwilling to look at the surgical site, provide support and encouragement to do so before discharge.
   k. Encourage client to discuss possibilities for reconstruction of her breast with the physician if desired.
   l. Discuss the variety of prostheses available and ways to obtain one.
   m. Assist client's and significant others' adjustment by listening, facilitating communication, and providing information.
   n. Assess for and support behaviors suggesting positive adaptation to loss of the breast (e.g. willingness to look at and care for wound, compliance with exercise program).
   o. Encourage significant others to allow client to do what she is able *so that independence can be re-established and self-esteem redeveloped.*
   p. Encourage visits and support from significant others.
   q. Encourage client to continue involvement in social activities and to pursue interests.
   r. Provide information about and encourage utilization of community agencies or support groups (e.g. Reach to Recovery; sexual, family, and individual counseling services; American Cancer Society).
   s. Consult physician about psychological counseling if client desires or if she seems unwilling or unable to adapt to the loss of her breast.

7. NURSING DIAGNOSIS

Ineffective individual coping related to:

a. perceived loss of femininity associated with loss of the breast;
b. fear of rejection by significant others;
c. embarrassment associated with the change in body image;
d. fear and anxiety associated with the diagnosis of cancer;
e. inadequate support system.

DESIRED OUTCOMES	NURSING ACTIONS AND *SELECTED RATIONALES*

7. The client will demonstrate the use of effective coping skills as evidenced by:
  a. willingness to participate in treatment plan and self-care activities
  b. verbalization of ability to cope with the loss of a breast
  c. identification of stressors
  d. utilization of appropriate problem-solving techniques
  e. recognition and utilization of available support systems.
	7.a. Assess effectiveness of client's coping strategies by observing behavior and noting strengths, weaknesses, ability to express feelings and concerns, and willingness to participate in the treatment plan.
	  b. Assess for and report signs and symptoms that may indicate ineffective coping (e.g. rejection of significant others, sleep disturbances, increasing fatigue, difficulty concentrating, irritability, decreased tolerance for pain, verbalization of inability to cope, inability to problem-solve).
	  c. Allow time for client to adjust psychologically to loss of a breast. Inform client that a period of peak emotional distress may occur several weeks after surgery.
	  d. Implement measures *to promote effective coping:*
	    1. arrange for a Reach to Recovery volunteer to visit client
	    2. perform actions to improve self-concept (see Postoperative Nursing Diagnosis 6, actions c–r)
	    3. perform actions to relieve fear and anxiety (see Standardized Postoperative Care Plan, Nursing Diagnosis 1, action c)
	    4. include client in planning of care, encourage maximum participation in treatment plan, and allow choices when possible *to enable her to maintain a sense of control*
	    5. instruct client in effective problem-solving techniques (e.g. accurate identification of stressors, determination of various options to solve problem)
	    6. assist client to maintain usual daily routines whenever possible
	    7. provide diversional activities according to client's interests
	    8. assist client to identify and utilize available support systems; provide information on available community resources to assist client to cope with mastectomy (e.g. American Cancer Society, counselors, mastectomy support groups).
	  e. Encourage continued emotional support from significant others.
	  f. Encourage the client to share with significant others the kind of support that would be most beneficial (e.g. listening, inspiring hope, providing reassurance and accurate information).
	  g. Assess for and support behaviors suggesting positive adaptation to loss of a breast (e.g. verbalization of ability to cope, willingness to look at and care for wound, utilization of effective problem-solving strategies).
	  h. Consult physician about psychological counseling if appropriate. Initiate a referral if necessary.

☐ ▐▌▐▌▐▌▐▌▐▌▐▌▐▌▐▌▐▌▐▌▐▌▐▌▐▌▐▌▐▌▐▌

8. NURSING DIAGNOSIS

Grieving* related to the loss of a breast and change in body image.

* This diagnostic label includes anticipatory grieving and grieving following the actual losses/changes.

☐ ▐▌▐▌▐▌▐▌▐▌▐▌▐▌▐▌▐▌▐▌▐▌▐▌▐▌▐▌▐▌▐▌

DESIRED OUTCOMES	NURSING ACTIONS AND *SELECTED RATIONALES*

8. The client will demonstrate beginning progression through the grieving process as evidenced by:
  a. verbalization of feelings about the loss of a breast
	8.a. Determine the client's perception of the impact of the loss of a breast on her future.
	  b. Determine how the client usually expresses grief.
	  c. Observe for signs of grieving (e.g. changes in eating habits, insomnia, anger, noncompliance, denial).
	  d. Implement measures *to facilitate the grieving process:*

b. expression of grief
c. participation in treatment plan and self-care activities
d. utilization of available support systems.

1. assist client to acknowledge the changes resulting from loss of her breast *so grief work can begin*; assess for factors that may hinder or facilitate acknowledgment
2. discuss the grieving process and assist client to accept the stages of grieving as an expected response to loss of a breast
3. allow time for client to progress through the stages of grieving (denial, anger, bargaining, depression, acceptance [Kübler-Ross, 1969]); be aware that not every stage is experienced or expressed by all individuals
4. provide an atmosphere of care and concern (e.g. provide privacy, be available and nonjudgmental, display empathy and respect) *so that client will feel free to verbalize both positive and negative feelings and concerns*
5. perform actions *to promote trust* (e.g. answer questions honestly, provide requested information)
6. encourage the expression of anger and sadness about the loss of her breast
7. encourage client to express her feelings in whatever ways are comfortable (e.g. writing, drawing, conversation)
8. perform actions to facilitate effective coping (see Postoperative Nursing Diagnosis 7, action d)
9. support realistic hope about the effect of surgery on the disease process and the possibility of breast reconstruction.

e. Assess for and support behaviors suggesting successful resolution of grief (e.g. verbalizing feelings about loss of a breast, expressing sorrow).
f. Explain the stages of the grieving process to significant others. Encourage their support and understanding.
g. Provide information regarding counseling services and support groups that might assist client in working through grief.
h. Arrange for visit from clergy if desired by client.
i. Monitor for therapeutic and nontherapeutic effects of antidepressants if administered.
j. Consult physician regarding referral for counseling if signs of dysfunctional grieving (e.g. persistent denial of losses or changes, excessive anger or sadness, hysteria, suicidal behaviors, phobias) occur.

☐ ▬▬▬▬▬▬▬▬▬▬▬▬▬▬▬▬▬▬▬▬▬▬▬▬▬▬▬▬▬

9. NURSING DIAGNOSIS

Knowledge deficit regarding follow-up care.

☐ ▬▬▬▬▬▬▬▬▬▬▬▬▬▬▬▬▬▬▬▬▬▬▬▬▬▬▬▬▬

DESIRED OUTCOMES	NURSING ACTIONS AND *SELECTED RATIONALES*

9.a. The client will identify ways to reduce risk of trauma to and infection in the arm on the operative side.

9.a.1. Provide the following instructions regarding ways *to reduce the risk of trauma to and infection in the arm on operative side* (these recommendations are based on the American Cancer Society's guidelines):
a. push cuticles back instead of cutting them
b. use heavy work gloves when gardening and rubber gloves when in contact with steel wool or water for prolonged periods
c. use insulated gloves when reaching into a hot oven
d. use a thimble when sewing *in order to avoid pinpricks*
e. avoid wearing tight jewelry or clothing on the affected arm *to prevent unnecessary pressure*
f. carry heavy objects such as purse or packages with the unaffected arm
g. offer only the unaffected arm for blood pressure readings, injections, or blood testing
h. wash any break in the skin on the affected arm with soap and water and cover the area with a protective dressing

       i. use an electric rather than a straight-edge razor when shaving underarm area

       j. apply a lanolin hand cream several times/day *to prevent drying and cracking*

      k. avoid prolonged exposure to the sun *in order to prevent burns.*

2. Instruct client to contact physician immediately should any injury to the arm on the operative side occur.

9.b. The client will identify ways to prevent and treat lymphedema in arm on operative side.	**9.b.1.** Instruct client in ways *to prevent lymphedema in arm on operative side:*
	    a. elevate the affected arm for 30 minutes every 2 hours for the first 2 weeks postoperatively and then 3 times a day for the next 6 weeks
	    b. sleep on unaffected side or back with affected arm elevated (forearm should be higher than the elbow and elbow level with or higher than the heart) for 8 weeks postoperatively
	  2. Reinforce physician's instructions regarding ways to treat *lymphedema if present:*
	    a. adhere to a diet low in sodium
	    b. take diuretics and anti-infectives as prescribed
	    c. use elastic or pressure sleeve as recommended
	    d. massage arm as instructed.

9.c. The client will demonstrate the ability to perform appropriate hand, arm, and shoulder exercises.	**9.c.1.** Reinforce preoperative and postoperative teaching about appropriate hand, arm, and shoulder exercises.
	  2. Emphasize the need to exercise affected hand, arm, and shoulder daily as ordered.
	  3. Allow time for questions, clarification, and return demonstration.

9.d. The client will verbalize the importance of doing a routine breast self-examination (BSE) on the remaining breast and operative site.	**9.d.1.** Explain the reasons for monthly BSE of the remaining breast and operative site. 2. Explore with client ways to remember to carry out BSE. The examination should be done a week after conclusion of menses or on a specific date if postmenopausal.
9.e. The client will demonstrate the ability to correctly perform a BSE.	**9.e.1.** Demonstrate, using a model, film, or chart, how to do a BSE. 2. Allow time for questions, clarification, and return demonstration.

9.f. The client will state the factors to consider in selecting a breast prosthesis.	**9.f.1.** Invite a Reach to Recovery volunteer or prosthetist to share information about the various prostheses available.
	  2. Suggest a soft, temporary prosthesis until complete healing of the incision has occurred.
	  3. Encourage the client to take a close friend with her for the initial fitting *in order to provide emotional support.*
	  4. Emphasize that it is important to select or make a prosthesis that will balance the chest *in order to avoid difficulties with posture and subsequent back, shoulder, and neck discomfort.*
	  5. Discuss ways to improvise breast forms.

9.g. The client will state signs and symptoms of complications to report to the health care provider.	**9.g.1.** Refer to Standardized Postoperative Care Plan, Nursing Diagnosis 20, action c, for signs and symptoms to report to the health care provider.
	  2. Instruct client to report these additional signs and symptoms:
	    a. tingling, stiffness, or increased numbness in hand, arm, or shoulder on operative side (explain that a residual numbness may persist in the chest wall and arm)
	    b. increasing weakness of the affected arm
	    c. warmth or redness of the affected arm
	    d. increase in size of arm on affected side (client may be instructed to measure arm circumference weekly at points 6 inches above and below elbow and compare with unaffected arm); inform client that transient edema may occur as she increases her use of affected arm and that this should subside as collateral lymphatic circulation develops
	    e. inability to move shoulder and arm on operative side through their full range of motion.

UNIT XVI

9.h. The client will identify community resources that can assist with home management and adjustment to the loss of a breast.

9.h.1. Provide information about community resources that can assist the client and significant others with home management and adjustment to the mastectomy (e.g. American Cancer Society, Reach to Recovery, mastectomy support groups, social services, Visiting Nurse Association, individual and family counselors).

2. Initiate a referral if appropriate.

9.i. The client will verbalize an understanding of and a plan for adhering to recommended follow-up care including future appointments with health care provider, medications prescribed, activity level, and wound care.

9.i.1. Refer to Standardized Postoperative Care Plan, Nursing Diagnosis 20, for routine postoperative instructions and measures to improve client compliance.

2. Reinforce physician's explanations and instructions regarding future treatment (e.g. chemotherapy, radiation therapy, breast reconstruction) if planned.

References

Kübler-Ross, E. On death and dying. New York: Macmillan, 1969.

Nail, L, Jones, L, Giuffre, M, and Johnson, J. Sensations after mastectomy. American Journal of Nursing, 84(9):1121–1124, 1984.

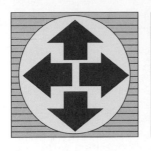
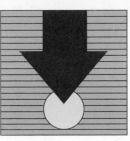
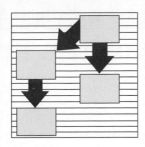
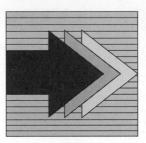
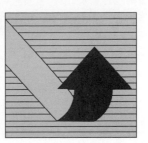

Unit XVII

Nursing Care of the Client with Disturbances of the Reproductive System

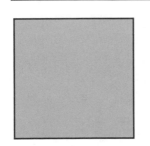
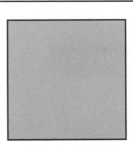

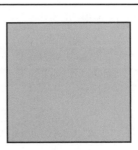
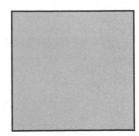

Cancer of the Prostate

Cancer of the prostate is the second most common malignancy occurring in the American male. It occurs predominantly in older men and the incidence increases significantly with age. Almost all prostatic neoplasms are adenocarcinomas, arise from the epithelium of the prostatic acini in the posterior lobe, and tend to be slow growing. The etiology is unknown, although exposure to industrial carcinogens (e.g. cadmium), infectious agents, and endocrine factors are postulated to be possible causative factors.

Lymphatic involvement appears to occur early and frequently in the natural course of the disease. Signs and symptoms of skeletal metastasis are present at the time of diagnosis in over half of the clients. The treatment selected depends on the stage and grade of the tumor and the general condition and natural life expectancy of the client. There continues to be much controversy about the optimal treatment modes for the various stages of prostatic cancer. Treatment options include close surveillance for clients with Stage A1, prostatectomy or interstitial radiation if the disease is contained within the prostatic capsule, external radiation therapy alone or in conjunction with surgery as a primary curative treatment or as a palliative measure for extensive metastatic disease, and endocrine therapy including bilateral orchiectomy and/or administration of estrogen and antiandrogens. Chemotherapy is sometimes used to treat advanced disease that is unresponsive to endocrine manipulation.

This care plan focuses on the adult client hospitalized for staging and initiation of treatment following a needle biopsy that is positive for cancer of the prostate. The goals of care are to reduce fear and anxiety, provide emotional support, relieve symptoms associated with the disease process and its treatment, and educate the client regarding follow-up care. If surgery is planned, this care plan should be used in conjunction with the Care Plan on Prostatectomy.

DISCHARGE CRITERIA

Prior to discharge, the client will:

- verbalize ways to reduce the risk of urinary retention, urinary tract infection, and urinary calculi
- identify ways to improve appetite and nutritional status
- verbalize ways to prevent pathologic fractures associated with metastasis to the bone if it has occurred
- share thoughts and feelings about the diagnosis of prostatic cancer; the prognosis; and the effects of the disease process and its treatment on self-concept, life style, and roles
- state signs and symptoms to report to the health care provider
- identify community resources that can assist with home management and adjustment to changes resulting from the diagnosis and the effects of treatment
- verbalize an understanding of and a plan for adhering to recommended follow-up care including future appointments with health care provider, medications prescribed, activity restrictions, and plans for subsequent treatment.

Use in conjunction with the Care Plans on Brachytherapy, External Radiation Therapy, Chemotherapy, and/or Immobility.

NURSING/COLLABORATIVE DIAGNOSES

1. Anxiety □ *999*
2. Altered fluid and electrolyte balance:

       a. fluid volume deficit, hyponatremia, hypokalemia, and hypochlore-
          mia
       b. metabolic acidosis
       c. metabolic alkalosis
       d. hypercalcemia ☐ *1000*
    3. Altered nutrition: less than body requirements ☐ *1001*
    4. Pain:
       a. perianal pain
       b. incisional pain
       c. back and leg pain and muscle spasms
       d. bone pain ☐ *1002*
    5. Fatigue ☐ *1003*
    6. Activity intolerance ☐ *1003*
    7. Impaired physical mobility ☐ *1004*
    8. Self-care deficit ☐ *1004*
    9. Urinary retention ☐ *1005*
   10. Potential for infection: urinary tract ☐ *1005*
   11. Potential for trauma ☐ *1006*
   12. Potential complications:
       a. renal calculi
       b. impaired renal function
       c. disseminated intravascular coagulation (DIC)
       d. pathologic fractures ☐ *1007*
   13. Sexual dysfunction:
       a. decreased libido
       b. impotence ☐ *1009*
   14. Disturbance in self-concept ☐ *1009*
   15. Ineffective individual coping ☐ *1010*
   16. Grieving ☐ *1010*
   17. Knowledge deficit regarding follow-up care ☐ *1011*

1. NURSING DIAGNOSIS

Anxiety related to unfamiliar environment; pain; lack of understanding of the diagnosis, staging procedures, treatment plan, and prognosis; anticipated effects of cancer and its treatment on body functioning and usual life style and roles; and potential for premature death.

DESIRED OUTCOMES	NURSING ACTIONS AND *SELECTED RATIONALES*
1. The client will experience a reduction in fear and anxiety as evidenced by: a. verbalization of feeling less anxious or fearful b. relaxed facial expression and body movements c. stable vital signs	1.a. Assess client on admission for: 1. fears, misconceptions, and level of understanding about cancer of the prostate, tests to stage the disease, and possible treatment modes 2. perception of anticipated results of diagnostic tests and planned treatment 3. significance of the diagnosis of cancer of the prostate 4. availability of an adequate support system 5. past experiences with cancer and its treatment

UNIT XVII

d. usual skin color
e. verbalization of an understanding of hospital routines, diagnosis, staging procedures, treatment plan and its effects, and prognosis.

6. signs and symptoms of fear and anxiety (e.g. verbalization of fears and concerns; tenseness; tremors; irritability; restlessness; diaphoresis; tachypnea; tachycardia; elevated blood pressure; facial tension, pallor, or flushing; noncompliance with treatment plan).

b. Ascertain effectiveness of current coping skills.
c. Refer to Care Plan on Immobility, Nursing Diagnosis 1, action c, for measures to reduce fear and anxiety.
d. Implement additional measures *to reduce fear and anxiety:*
 1. explain all tests performed to stage cancer of the prostate (tests will vary according to grade of the tumor and client's symptoms):
    a. cystoscopy
    b. excretory urogram
    c. total body nuclear bone scan
    d. magnetic resonance imaging (MRI)
    e. computed tomography (CT) of abdomen and pelvis
    f. chest x-ray
    g. liver-spleen nuclear scan
    h. transrectal ultrasonography
    i. CBC and blood chemistries including serum acid and alkaline phosphatase and prostate-specific antigen (PA)
    j. radioimmunoassay for prostatic acid phosphatase (PAP)
    k. lymphangiogram
    l. pelvic lymphadenectomy
 2. refer to Nursing Diagnosis 1, action c, in Care Plan on Chemotherapy or External Radiation for measures to reduce fear and anxiety associated with planned treatment
 3. perform actions to reduce pain (see Nursing Diagnosis 4)
 4. perform actions to assist client to cope with the diagnosis and its implications (see Care Plan on Chemotherapy, Nursing Diagnosis 22, action d)
 5. initiate preoperative or preprocedure teaching if surgery or interstitial radiation therapy is planned
 6. emphasize the benefits of interstitial radiation therapy if planned (e.g. no radiation-induced illness or resulting incontinence or impotence, only one application required, survival rates similar to those achieved with external radiation therapy).
e. Include significant others in orientation and teaching sessions and encourage their continued support of client.
f. Provide information based on current needs of client and significant others at a level they can understand. Encourage questions and clarification of information provided.
g. Consult physician if above actions fail to control fear and anxiety.

☐ ▉▉▉▉▉▉▉▉▉▉▉▉▉▉▉▉▉▉▉▉▉▉▉

2. NURSING/COLLABORATIVE DIAGNOSIS

Altered fluid and electrolyte balance:

a. **fluid volume deficit, hyponatremia, hypokalemia, and hypochloremia** related to:
 1. decreased oral intake associated with:
    a. anorexia
    b. dysphagia and oral, pharyngeal, and esophageal pain resulting from mucositis due to treatment with cytotoxic agents
    c. nausea
 2. excessive loss of fluid and electrolytes associated with:
    a. persistent vomiting resulting from treatment with cytotoxic drugs
    b. diarrhea resulting from side effects of chemotherapy and/or radiation therapy (if the lower bowel is included in the radiation treatment field);
b. **metabolic acidosis** related to hyponatremia and persistent diarrhea associated with the side effects of radiation therapy and/or chemotherapy;
c. **metabolic alkalosis** related to hypokalemia, hypochloremia, and persistent vomiting associated with side effects of chemotherapy;

d. **hypercalcemia** related to initiation of hormone therapy (DES) and demineralization of the bone associated with decreased activity and metastasis to the bone if it has occurred.

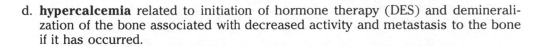

DESIRED OUTCOMES	NURSING ACTIONS AND *SELECTED RATIONALES*
2.a. The client will maintain fluid, electrolyte, and acid-base balance (see Care Plan on Chemotherapy, Nursing Diagnosis 2, outcomes a and b, for outcome criteria).	2.a. Refer to Care Plan on Chemotherapy, Nursing Diagnosis 2, actions a and b, for measures related to assessment and management of fluid, electrolyte, and acid-base balance.
2.b. The client will maintain a safe serum calcium level (see Care Plan on Immobility, Collaborative Diagnosis 5, for outcome criteria).	2.b. Refer to Care Plan on Immobility, Collaborative Diagnosis 5, for measures related to assessment, prevention, and treatment of hypercalcemia.

3. NURSING DIAGNOSIS

Altered nutrition: less than body requirements related to:*

a. decreased oral intake associated with:
   1. anorexia resulting from:
      a. depression, fear, and anxiety
      b. fatigue and discomfort
      c. taste alteration associated with:
         1. change in the sense of smell and the threshold for bitter, sweet, sour, and salt taste (particularly red meat, coffee, tea, tomatoes, and chocolate) related to the release of tumor byproducts into the bloodstream
         2. zinc, copper, nickel, niacin, and vitamin A deficiency and increased serum levels of calcium and lactate related to the disease process
      d. alteration in metabolism of proteins, fats, and carbohydrates
      e. early satiety associated with direct stimulation of the satiety center by anorexigenic factors (e.g. peptides) secreted by tumor cells
      f. increased concentration of neurotransmitters in the brain and/or derangements in the serotoninergic system associated with the disease process
   2. dysphagia and oral, pharyngeal, and esophageal pain resulting from mucositis associated with the effects of cytotoxic drugs on the gastrointestinal mucosa
   3. nausea;
b. loss of nutrients associated with:
   1. persistent vomiting resulting from administration of cytotoxic drugs;
   2. diarrhea resulting from side effects of chemotherapy and/or radiation therapy (if the lower bowel is included in the radiation treatment field);
c. elevated metabolic rate associated with an increased and continuous energy utilization by rapidly proliferating malignant cells;
d. utilization of available nutrients by the malignant cells rather than by the host;
e. failure of feeding center to induce a sufficient increase in the intake of food to match metabolic needs;
f. inefficient and accelerated metabolism of proteins, fats, and carbohydrates associated with the disease process.

* Some of the etiologic factors presented here are currently under investigation.

DESIRED OUTCOMES	NURSING ACTIONS AND *SELECTED RATIONALES*

3. The client will maintain an adequate nutritional status (see Care Plan on External Radiation, Nursing Diagnosis 3, for outcome criteria).	3.a. Refer to Care Plan on External Radiation, Nursing Diagnosis 3, for measures related to assessment and promotion of an optimal nutritional status.
	b. Implement additional measures *to improve oral intake and nutritional status:*
	  1. perform actions to reduce fear and anxiety (see Nursing Diagnosis 1, actions c and d)
	  2. perform actions to reduce pain (see Nursing Diagnosis 4).

☐ ▬▬▬▬▬▬▬▬▬▬▬▬▬▬▬▬▬▬▬▬▬▬▬

4. NURSING DIAGNOSIS

Pain:

a. **perianal pain** related to persistent diarrhea and proctitis associated with radiation therapy to rectal area;

b. **incisional pain** related to suprapubic incision utilized for interstitial implantation of ^{125}I or ^{198}Au;

c. **back and leg pain and muscle spasms** related to irritation of the sciatic nerve if tumor infiltration has occurred;

d. **bone pain** related to increased intraosseous pressure, compression or displacement of nerve roots by collapsed vertebra, and compression fractures if bone metastasis has occurred.

☐ ▬▬▬▬▬▬▬▬▬▬▬▬▬▬▬▬▬▬▬▬▬▬▬

DESIRED OUTCOMES	NURSING ACTIONS AND *SELECTED RATIONALES*

4. The client will experience diminished pain (see Care Plan on External Radiation, Nursing Diagnosis 5.A, for outcome criteria).	4.a. Refer to Care Plan on External Radiation, Nursing Diagnosis 5.A, for measures related to assessment and management of pain.
	b. Implement additional measures *to reduce pain:*
	  1. maintain activity restrictions as ordered
	  2. provide a firm mattress or place a bed board under mattress for added support
	  3. avoid jarring the bed
	  4. place alternating pressure pad, eggcrate mattress, or sheepskin on bed
	  5. consult physician about use of a kinetic bed if client is immobile
	  6. encourage and assist client to apply brace or corset if ordered and use ambulatory aids (e.g. walker with seat, cane) when up *in order to support painful limbs and back*
	  7. if bedpan is needed, use a fracture pan
	  8. utilize a bed cradle or footboard *to eliminate the weight of linens on painful areas*
	  9. keep painful limbs well supported
	  10. instruct and assist client to support affected limbs with hands or pillows when changing position
	  11. use smooth movements and allow client to move at his own pace *in order to avoid paroxysmal spasms*
	  12. instruct and assist client to keep body in good alignment
	  13. caution client to avoid sudden twisting and turning
	  14. avoid pulling and tugging on extremities and torso when positioning client
	  15. administer analgesics before planned physical activities
	  16. prepare client for radiation to involved bone areas if appropriate
	  17. consult physician about management of cough or cold *(sneezing and coughing can greatly aggravate pain)*
	  18. monitor for therapeutic and nontherapeutic effects of analgesics, muscle relaxants, anti-inflammatory agents, and/or topical anesthetics if administered.

5. NURSING DIAGNOSIS

Fatigue related to:

a. accumulation of cellular waste products associated with rapid lysis of cancerous and normal cells exposed to cytotoxic drugs and/or radiation;
b. inability to rest and sleep associated with discomfort resulting from the disease process and side effects of radiation and/or chemotherapy and prolonged physiological and psychological stress;
c. anxiety and depression associated with the diagnosis, the treatment regimen and its effects, the need to alter usual activities, and the inability to fulfill usual roles;
d. increased energy expenditure associated with an increase in the basal metabolic rate resulting from continuous, active tumor growth.

DESIRED OUTCOMES	NURSING ACTIONS AND *SELECTED RATIONALES*
5. The client will experience a reduction in fatigue (see Care Plan on External Radiation, Nursing Diagnosis 9, for outcome criteria).	5.a. Refer to Care Plan on External Radiation, Nursing Diagnosis 9, for measures related to assessment, prevention, and management of fatigue. b. Implement additional measures *to reduce fatigue:* 1. perform actions to reduce pain (see Nursing Diagnosis 4) 2. perform actions to reduce fear and anxiety (see Nursing Diagnosis 1, actions c and d).

6. NURSING DIAGNOSIS

Activity intolerance related to:

a. tissue hypoxia associated with anemia resulting from:
   1. nutritional deficits
   2. bone marrow suppression associated with chemotherapy or external radiation therapy (occurs if entire pelvis is irradiated);
b. inability to rest and sleep associated with discomfort and prolonged physiological and psychological stress;
c. malnutrition.

DESIRED OUTCOMES	NURSING ACTIONS AND *SELECTED RATIONALES*
6. The client will demonstrate an increased tolerance for activity (see Care Plan on External Radiation, Nursing Diagnosis 10, for outcome criteria).	6.a. Refer to Care Plan on External Radiation, Nursing Diagnosis 10, for measures related to assessment and improvement of activity tolerance. b. Implement additional measures *to improve activity tolerance:* 1. perform actions to reduce pain (see Nursing Diagnosis 4) 2. perform actions to reduce fear and anxiety (see Nursing Diagnosis 1, actions c and d).

UNIT
XVII

7. NURSING DIAGNOSIS

Impaired physical mobility related to:

a. fatigue and weakness associated with anemia, nutritional deficits, and inability to rest and sleep;
b. reluctance to move associated with pain and fear of falling;
c. motor deficits associated with:
1. spinal cord or nerve root compression by metastatic tumor
2. muscle weakness resulting from hypercalcemia and prolonged disuse.

DESIRED OUTCOMES	NURSING ACTIONS AND *SELECTED RATIONALES*

7.a. The client will maintain an optimal level of physical mobility within the limitations imposed by the disease process.	7.a.1. Assess for factors that impair physical mobility (e.g. weakness, fatigue, reluctance to move because of pain, loss of motor function).
	2. Implement measures *to increase mobility:*
	  a. perform actions to control pain (see Nursing Diagnosis 4)
	  b. perform actions to reduce fatigue (see Nursing Diagnosis 5)
	  c. perform actions to increase strength and improve activity tolerance (see Nursing Diagnosis 6)
	  d. perform actions to prevent falls (see Nursing Diagnosis 11, actions b and c) *in order to reduce client's fear of injury*
	  e. perform actions to prevent and treat hypercalcemia (see Care Plan on Immobility, Collaborative Diagnosis 5, action b) *in order to help maintain normal neuromuscular function*
	  f. instruct client in and assist with correct use of mobility aids (e.g. cane, walker) if appropriate
	  g. instruct client in and assist with active and/or passive range of motion exercises at least every 4 hours unless contraindicated
	  h. reinforce instructions, activities, and exercise plan recommended by physical and/or occupational therapists.
	3. Increase activity and participation in self-care activities as tolerated.
	4. Provide praise and encouragement for all efforts to increase physical mobility.
	5. Encourage the support of significant others. Allow them to assist with range of motion exercises, positioning, and activity if desired.
	6. Consult physician if client is unable to achieve expected level of mobility.

7.b. The client will not experience problems associated with immobility.	7.b. Refer to Care Plan on Immobility for actions to prevent problems associated with immobility if client remains on bedrest for longer than 48 hours.

8. NURSING DIAGNOSIS

Self-care deficit related to impaired physical mobility associated with fatigue, weakness, pain, and motor deficits.

DESIRED OUTCOMES	NURSING ACTIONS AND *SELECTED RATIONALES*
8. The client will demonstrate increased participation in self-care activities within	8.a. Refer to Care Plan on External Radiation, Nursing Diagnosis 11, for measures related to assessment of, planning for, and meeting the client's self-care needs.

limitations imposed by the disease process.

b. Implement measures to increase mobility (see Nursing Diagnosis 7, action a.2) *in order to further facilitate the client's ability to perform self-care activities.*

---

9. NURSING DIAGNOSIS

Urinary retention related to:

a. obstruction of the prostatic urethra and/or bladder outlet by the enlarged prostate, blood clots (bleeding may occur from invasion of the bladder, urethra, and adjacent structures by tumor cells), and edema (occurs during the initial phase of radiation therapy);
b. loss of bladder tone associated with prolonged distention.

DESIRED OUTCOMES	NURSING ACTIONS AND *SELECTED RATIONALES*
9. The client will experience resolution of urinary retention if it occurs as evidenced by: a. voiding adequate amounts at normal intervals b. fewer complaints of urgency, bladder fullness, and suprapubic discomfort c. absence of suprapubic distention d. balanced intake and output.	9.a. Gather baseline data regarding client's usual urinary elimination pattern. b. Assess for signs and symptoms of urinary retention: 　1. frequent voiding of small amounts (25–50 cc) of urine 　2. complaints of urgency, bladder fullness, or suprapubic discomfort 　3. suprapubic distention 　4. output less than intake. c. Catheterize client if ordered *to determine the amount of residual urine.* d. Assist with urodynamic studies (e.g. cystometrogram) if ordered. e. Implement measures *to prevent and treat urinary retention:* 　1. perform actions *to promote complete bladder emptying:* 　　a. instruct and assist client to perform Credé technique unless contraindicated 　　b. instruct client to perform Valsalva maneuver during urination 　　c. allow client to assume normal position for voiding unless contraindicated 　2. monitor for therapeutic and nontherapeutic effects of cholinergic drugs (e.g. bethanechol) if administered *to stimulate bladder contraction* 　3. if signs and symptoms of urinary retention persist: 　　a. consult physician about intermittent catheterization or insertion of an indwelling catheter (be aware that insertion may be difficult because of obstruction and a stylet or a firm, specially angled catheter may be needed) 　　b. assist with insertion of a suprapubic catheter if unable to insert urethral catheter 　4. if indwelling urinary catheter is present: 　　a. perform actions *to maintain patency of the catheter* (e.g. keep tubing free of kinks, irrigate as ordered) 　　b. monitor for therapeutic and nontherapeutic effects of continuous bladder irrigation with silver nitrate solution if performed *to stop bleeding* 　5. prepare client for surgical removal of the obstruction if indicated.

---

10. NURSING DIAGNOSIS

Potential for infection: urinary tract related to an indwelling catheter if present or urinary stasis associated with urethral obstruction, loss of bladder tone, and decreased mobility.

DESIRED OUTCOMES	NURSING ACTIONS AND *SELECTED RATIONALES*

10. The client will remain free of urinary tract infection (see Care Plan on Immobility, Nursing Diagnosis 13, outcome b, for outcome criteria).

10.a. Refer to Care Plan on Immobility, Nursing Diagnosis 13, action b, for measures related to assessment, prevention, and treatment of a urinary tract infection.
   b. Implement measures to reduce the risk of and treat urinary retention (see Nursing Diagnosis 9, action e) *in order to prevent stasis and further reduce the risk of urinary tract infection.*

☐ ▇▇▇▇▇▇▇▇▇▇▇▇▇▇▇▇▇▇▇▇▇▇▇▇▇▇▇▇▇▇▇

11. NURSING DIAGNOSIS

Potential for trauma related to:

a. falls associated with:
   1. sensory and motor impairments resulting from hypercalcemia and spinal cord and nerve root compression if the tumor has metastasized
   2. fatigue and weakness resulting from malnutrition, anemia, inability to rest and sleep, and side effects of radiation therapy and/or chemotherapy
   3. depressant effects of certain medications (e.g. narcotics, sedatives) on the central nervous system;
b. cuts and burns associated with sensory and motor deficits (may result from hypercalcemia and spinal cord and nerve root compression if the tumor has metastasized).

☐ ▇▇▇▇▇▇▇▇▇▇▇▇▇▇▇▇▇▇▇▇▇▇▇▇▇▇▇▇▇▇▇

DESIRED OUTCOMES	NURSING ACTIONS AND *SELECTED RATIONALES*

11. The client will not experience falls, burns, or cuts.

11.a. Determine whether conditions predisposing the client to falls, burns, or cuts exist:
   1. weakness and fatigue
   2. impaired body movement
   3. decreased sensation in extremities
   4. treatment with central nervous system depressants.
   b. Refer to Care Plan on External Radiation, Nursing Diagnosis 15, action b, for measures related to prevention of falls.
   c. Implement measures to maintain serum calcium within a safe range (see Care Plan on Immobility, Collaborative Diagnosis 5, action b) *in order to reduce muscle weakness and prevent falls.*
   d. Implement measures *to prevent burns:*
      1. let hot foods and fluids cool slightly before serving *to reduce risk of burns if spills occur*
      2. supervise client while smoking if indicated
      3. assess temperature of bath water and heating pad before and during use.
   e. Assist client with tasks that require fine motor skills (e.g. shaving) *in order to prevent cuts.*
   f. Administer central nervous system depressants such as narcotics and sedatives judiciously.
   g. Include client and significant others in planning and implementing measures to prevent injury.
   h. If injury does occur, initiate appropriate first aid and notify physician.

12. COLLABORATIVE DIAGNOSIS

Potential complications:

a. **renal calculi** related to:
   1. urinary stasis associated with urethral obstruction, loss of bladder tone, and decreased mobility
   2. increased renal excretion of calcium associated with administration of diethylstilbestrol (DES), disuse osteoporosis, and bone destruction due to metastasis if it has occurred
   3. increased renal excretion of uric acid associated with rapid lysis of tumor cells resulting from initiation of treatment;
b. **impaired renal function** related to the development of calculi, bilateral hydronephrosis (may result from chronic urinary retention or involvement of the ureters with tumor growth), and impaired renal blood flow associated with fluid volume deficit;
c. **disseminated intravascular coagulation (DIC)** related to:
   1. the generation of abnormal amounts of tissue thromboplastin by the tumor cells
   2. release of procoagulant substances and proteases into the circulation that activate both the intrinsic and extrinsic coagulation pathways;
d. **pathologic fractures** related to demineralization of the bone associated with bone metastasis if it has occurred and complicated further by the disuse osteoporosis that occurs with decreased activity.

DESIRED OUTCOMES	NURSING ACTIONS AND *SELECTED RATIONALES*

12.a. The client will not develop renal calculi (see Care Plan on External Radiation, Collaborative Diagnosis 16, outcome e, for outcome criteria).	12.a.1. Assess for and report signs and symptoms of renal calculi (e.g. dull, aching or severe, colicky flank pain; hematuria; urinary frequency or urgency; nausea; vomiting).
	2. Monitor serum calcium and uric acid levels and report elevations.
	3. Obtain a urine specimen for analysis if ordered. Report the presence of crystals and/or high levels of calcium and uric acid.
	4. Refer to Care Plan on Immobility, Collaborative Diagnosis 14, action c.4, for measures to prevent calcium stone formation.
	5. Refer to Care Plan on External Radiation, Collaborative Diagnosis 16, action e.4, for measures to prevent uric acid stone formation.
	6. Implement measures to prevent and treat urinary retention (see Nursing Diagnosis 9, action e) *in order to further reduce the risk of calculi formation.*
	7. If signs and symptoms of renal calculi occur:
	  a. strain all urine carefully and save any calculi for analysis; report finding to physician
	  b. encourage a minimum fluid intake of 2500 cc/day unless contraindicated
	  c. administer analgesics as ordered
	  d. refer to Care Plan on Renal Calculi for additional care measures.

12.b. The client will maintain adequate renal function as evidenced by: 1. urine output at least 30 cc/hour 2. urine specific gravity between 1.010–1.030 3. BUN and serum	12.b.1. Assess for and report signs and symptoms of impaired renal function (e.g. urine output less than 30 cc/hour, urine specific gravity fixed at or less than 1.010, elevated BUN and serum creatinine levels). 2. Collect a 24-hour urine specimen if ordered. Report decreased creatinine clearance. 3. Implement measures *to maintain adequate renal function*: a. perform actions to prevent renal calculi (see actions a.4–6 in this diagnosis)

UNIT XVII

creatinine levels within normal range.

b. perform actions to prevent fluid volume deficit (see Care Plan on Chemotherapy, Nursing Diagnosis 2, action a.3)

c. perform actions to prevent and treat urinary retention (see Nursing Diagnosis 9, action e) *in order to reduce the risk of hydronephrosis.*

4. If signs and symptoms of impaired renal function occur:
   a. continue with above actions
   b. administer diuretics as ordered
   c. monitor for and report signs of acute renal failure (e.g. oliguria or anuria; weight gain; edema; elevated B/P; lethargy and confusion; increasing BUN and serum creatinine, phosphorus, and potassium levels)
   d. prepare client for dialysis if indicated
   e. refer to Care Plan on Renal Failure for additional care measures.

12.c. The client will experience resolution of DIC if it occurs as evidenced by:
1. absence of petechiae, ecchymosis, and frank or occult bleeding
2. skin warm, dry, and usual color
3. absence of new or intensified pain
4. usual mental status
5. fibrin degradation products (FDP) and protamine sulfate test within normal range
6. fibrinogen, PT, PTT, TT, and platelet levels within normal range
7. RBC, Hct., and Hgb. levels within normal range
8. blood pressure and pulse within normal range for client
9. urine output at least 30 cc/hour.

12.c.1. Assess for and report signs and symptoms of DIC:
   a. petechiae, ecchymosis
   b. mild to severe, frank or occult bleeding from one or more sites (e.g. catheter insertion sites, urine, stool)
   c. acrocyanosis (diaphoresis and cold, mottled fingers and toes)
   d. paresthesias or dysthesias of extremities
   e. abdominal or back pain, headache
   f. restlessness, agitation, confusion.

2. Monitor for and report the following diagnostic test results (be certain that blood samples are not drawn from heparinized lines unless lines have been appropriately cleared):
   a. elevated levels of FDP
   b. positive protamine sulfate test
   c. prolonged prothrombin time (PT), partial thromboplastin time (PTT), and thrombin time (TT)
   d. reduced fibrinogen level and platelet count.

3. Assess for and report signs and symptoms of blood loss and decreased tissue perfusion:
   a. rapid or irregular pulse
   b. drop of 20 mm Hg in systolic pressure, a systolic pressure less than 80 mm Hg, or a continual drop of 5–10 mm Hg in systolic pressure with successive readings
   c. capillary refill time greater than 3 seconds
   d. below normal or decreasing RBC, Hct., and Hgb. levels
   e. urine output less than 30 cc/hour.

4. If DIC occurs:
   a. implement safety precautions *to prevent further bleeding* (e.g. use of electric rather than straight-edge razor, use of soft bristle toothbrush, avoidance of injections)
   b. maintain oxygen therapy as ordered
   c. monitor for therapeutic and nontherapeutic effects of volume expanders and/or blood products such as fresh frozen plasma (FFP), platelets, and cryoprecipitate if administered
   d. monitor for therapeutic and nontherapeutic effects of heparin if administered *to prevent further clotting and thereby free clotting factors for control of bleeding*
   e. attempt to determine amount of blood lost (e.g. weigh dressings, monitor decreases in Hct. and Hgb.)
   f. provide emotional support to client and significant others.

12.d. The client will not experience pathologic fractures (see Care Plan on Immobility, Collaborative Diagnosis 14, outcome e, for outcome criteria).

12.d. Refer to Care Plan on Immobility, Collaborative Diagnosis 14, action e, for measures related to assessment, prevention, and treatment of pathologic fractures.

13. NURSING DIAGNOSIS

Sexual dysfunction:

a. **decreased libido** related to:
1. discomfort associated with effects of chemotherapy or external radiation therapy and metastasis to the bone if it has occurred
2. altered hormone balance associated with hormone therapy or bilateral orchiectomy
3. weakness and fatigue
4. altered self-concept;
b. **impotence** related to psychological factors (e.g. anxiety, depression) and decreased testosterone and dihydroxytestosterone levels associated with hormone therapy, bilateral orchiectomy, and/or destruction of the Leydig cells if the testes are exposed to large doses of radiation.

DESIRED OUTCOMES	NURSING ACTIONS AND *SELECTED RATIONALES*
13. The client will demonstrate beginning acceptance of changes in sexual functioning (see Care Plan on External Radiation, Nursing Diagnosis 17, for outcome criteria).	13.a. Refer to Care Plan on External Radiation, Nursing Diagnosis 17, actions a–i and k–o for measures related to assessment and management of sexual dysfunction. b. Suggest alternative positions for intercourse if client has metastatic bone lesions *in order to minimize discomfort during sexual activity.*

14. NURSING DIAGNOSIS

Disturbance in self-concept* related to:

a. changes in appearance (e.g. feminization, alopecia, excessive weight loss) associated with the side effects of hormone or cytotoxic drug therapy and/or radiation therapy;
b. castration by orchiectomy (frequently performed on clients with Stage D prostatic cancer);
c. alteration in sexual functioning;
d. sterility associated with side effects of hormone or cytotoxic drug therapy, exposure of the testes to radiation, and/or castration;
e. dependence on others to meet self-care needs;
f. stigma associated with diagnosis of cancer;
g. anticipated changes in life style and roles associated with the effects of the disease process and its treatment.

---

* This diagnostic label includes the nursing diagnoses of body image disturbance and self-esteem disturbance.

DESIRED OUTCOMES	NURSING ACTIONS AND *SELECTED RATIONALES*
14. The client will demonstrate beginning adaptation to	14.a. Refer to Care Plan on Chemotherapy, Nursing Diagnosis 21, for measures related to assessment and maintenance of a positive self-concept.

UNIT · XVII

changes in appearance, body functioning, life style, and roles (see Care Plan on Chemotherapy, Nursing Diagnosis 21, for outcome criteria).

b. Implement additional measures *to assist client to adjust to changes in appearance and body functioning:*
   1. reinforce actions that may assist the client to adjust to alterations in sexual functioning (see Nursing Diagnosis 13)
   2. clarify information from physician about the possibility of testicular or penile implant if desired.
c. If estrogen therapy is planned, prepare client for radiation to breasts before initiation of treatment *in order to help prevent gynecomastia.*

15. NURSING DIAGNOSIS

Ineffective individual coping related to:

a. inadequate support system;
b. discomfort associated with the disease process and side effects of treatment;
c. depression, fear, and anxiety associated with the diagnosis, prognosis, and effects of the disease process and its treatment on usual body functioning and life style.

DESIRED OUTCOMES	NURSING ACTIONS AND *SELECTED RATIONALES*
15. The client will demonstrate the use of effective coping skills (see Care Plan on Chemotherapy, Nursing Diagnosis 22, for outcome criteria).	15.a. Refer to Care Plan on Chemotherapy, Nursing Diagnosis 22, for measures related to assessment and management of ineffective coping. b. Implement additional measures *to promote effective coping:* 1. perform actions to reduce fear and anxiety (see Nursing Diagnosis 1, actions c and d) 2. perform actions to reduce pain (see Nursing Diagnosis 4).

16. NURSING DIAGNOSIS

Grieving* related to:

a. diagnosis of cancer with potential for premature death;
b. changes in body image and usual life style and roles associated with cancer of the prostate and its treatment.

---

* This diagnostic label includes anticipatory grieving and grieving following the actual losses/changes.

DESIRED OUTCOMES	NURSING ACTIONS AND *SELECTED RATIONALES*
16. The client will demonstrate beginning progression through the grieving process (see Care Plan on External Radiation, Nursing Diagnosis 20, for outcome criteria).	16. Refer to Care Plan on External Radiation, Nursing Diagnosis 20, for measures related to assessment and facilitation of grieving.

☐ ▬▬▬▬▬▬▬▬▬▬▬▬▬▬▬▬▬▬▬▬▬▬▬

17. NURSING DIAGNOSIS

Knowledge deficit regarding follow-up care.

☐ ▬▬▬▬▬▬▬▬▬▬▬▬▬▬▬▬▬▬▬▬▬▬▬

DESIRED OUTCOMES	NURSING ACTIONS AND *SELECTED RATIONALES*

17.a. The client will verbalize ways to reduce the risk of urinary retention, urinary tract infection, and urinary calculi.

17.a.1. Provide instructions regarding ways *to prevent urinary retention:*
  a. empty bladder whenever the urge is felt
  b. avoid excessive intake of fluids (especially alcohol) over a short period
  c. limit fluids a few hours before bedtime *in order to decrease urine accumulation during sleep*
  d. if a urinary catheter is present, utilize a bedside collection bag during sleep *in order to facilitate gravity drainage.*
  2. Provide instructions on ways *to reduce risk of a urinary tract infection:*
  a. drink at least 10 glasses of liquid/day
  b. avoid urinary retention (see action a.1 in this diagnosis)
  c. maintain urine acidity by:
    1. increasing intake of foods/fluids that form an acid ash (e.g. cranberry or prune juice, meat, eggs, poultry, fish, grapes, whole grains)
    2. limiting intake of milk, citrus fruits, and carbonated beverages
    3. taking acidifying agents (e.g. ascorbic acid) as prescribed
  d. take prophylactic anti-infectives as prescribed
  e. if the client is discharged with a urinary catheter in place:
    1. demonstrate aseptic technique necessary for catheter care and changing and emptying of collection bag
    2. emphasize the importance of keeping collection bag below bladder level at all times *to prevent stasis and backflow of urine*
    3. caution client to empty bag completely at least every 8 hours *to avoid bacterial growth in collection bag*
    4. allow time for questions, clarification, and return demonstration of catheter care.
  3. Provide instructions regarding ways to prevent urinary calcium stone formation (see Care Plan on Immobility, Nursing Diagnosis 19, action a.3).
  4. Provide instructions on ways to prevent urinary uric acid stone formation (see Care Plan on External Radiation, Nursing Diagnosis 21, action e).

17.b. The client will identify ways to improve appetite and nutritional status.

17.b. Refer to Care Plan on External Radiation, Nursing Diagnosis 21, action c, for instructions related to improving appetite and maintaining an adequate nutritional status.

17.c. The client will verbalize ways to prevent pathologic fractures associated with metastasis to the bone if it has occurred.

17.c. Provide instructions regarding ways *to prevent pathologic fractures:*
  1. avoid coughing, sneezing, trauma to bones, heavy lifting, and straining to have a bowel movement
  2. apply corset, brace, or splint correctly and wear as prescribed
  3. use good body mechanics
  4. be as active as possible *in order to prevent further demineralization of bone*
  5. use ambulatory aids (e.g. cane, walker) if unsteady on feet *in order to prevent falls and further trauma to the bones.*

17.d. The client will state signs and symptoms to report to the health care provider.

17.d. Instruct the client to report:
  1. any unusual symptom such as confusion, difficulty breathing, or bone pain (may indicate metastasis)
  2. signs and symptoms of a urinary tract infection (e.g. pain or burning on urination; urinary frequency; fever; chills; cloudy, foul-smelling urine with or without sediment; burning around catheter if present)
  3. persistent blood or clots in urine

4. difficulty initiating urinary stream or decrease in force and caliber of stream
5. suprapubic distention and decrease in urine output
6. persistent incontinence of urine or stool
7. persistent bladder spasms
8. unusual odor, drainage, or pain in irradiated area
9. signs and symptoms of dehydration (e.g. dry mouth, weight loss, concentrated urine, confusion, fainting)
10. signs and symptoms of calcium excess (e.g. loss of appetite, nausea, vomiting, constipation, increased thirst, increased urination, drowsiness)
11. signs and symptoms of urinary calculi (e.g. flank pain, urinary urgency or frequency, unusual appearance of urine, nausea, vomiting)
12. side effects of hormone therapy (e.g. impotence, nausea, vomiting, loss of appetite, diarrhea, swelling of hands and feet, breast tenderness and enlargement)
13. excessive depression or difficulty coping.

17.e. The client will identify community resources that can assist with home management and adjustment to changes resulting from the diagnosis and the effects of treatment.

17.e.1. Provide information about community resources that can assist client and significant others with home management and adjustment to the diagnosis and effects of treatment (e.g. local support groups, American Cancer Society, Visiting Nurse Association, counselors, social service agencies, Meals on Wheels, Make Today Count, Hospice).
2. Initiate a referral if indicated.

17.f. The client will verbalize an understanding of and plan for adhering to recommended follow-up care including future appointments with health care provider, medications prescribed, activity restrictions, and plans for subsequent treatment.

17.f.1. Reinforce physician's explanation of planned radiation therapy or chemotherapy if appropriate. Stress importance of strictly following the prescribed protocol for radiation therapy or chemotherapy and keeping all appointments for follow-up supervision and laboratory work.
2. Emphasize the need for planned rest periods and for gauging activity according to tolerance.
3. Explain the rationale for, side effects of, and importance of taking medications prescribed (e.g. diethylstilbestrol [DES], allopurinol, urinary anesthetics).
4. Implement measures *to improve client compliance:*
   a. include significant others in teaching sessions if possible
   b. encourage questions and allow time for reinforcement and clarification of information provided
   c. provide written instructions regarding scheduled appointments with health care provider and for radiation therapy, chemotherapy, and laboratory work; medications prescribed; and signs and symptoms to report.

■ ■

Cancer of the Testis with Retroperitoneal Lymphadenectomy

Testicular cancer is the most common malignancy occurring in men between the ages of 20 and 35. The etiology of the disease is unknown but factors thought to increase the risk of its development include cryptorchidism, genetic factors, repeated testicular infection, previous history of testicular cancer, trauma to the testes, and endocrine abnormalities. Testicular cancer frequently involves only one of the testes, and metastasis, which usually involves the retroperitoneal lymph nodes or lungs, is present in approximately one third of the clients at the time of diagnosis. The 4 major types of testicular tumors arising from germ cells are seminoma, teratoma, embryonal carcinoma, and choriocarcinoma. They may appear in pure form or be a combination of the cell types. The treatment mode selected depends on the type, stage, and grade of the tumor. Inguinal orchiectomy and bilateral retroperitoneal lymphadenectomy is the treatment of choice for nonseminomas, although some centers are currently treating Stage I disease with orchiectomy and close surveillance. For Stage I and Stage II seminomas, inguinal orchiectomy and radiation therapy are indicated because of the slow growth rate and high degree of radiosensitivity of this type of tumor. Chemotherapy is indicated for seminomas or nonseminomas in advanced stages.

This care plan focuses on the adult male client who has recently undergone an orchiectomy for testicular cancer and is readmitted for staging of the disease and a bilateral retroperitoneal lymphadenectomy using the extraperitoneal thoracoabdominal approach. The goals of preoperative care are to reduce fear and anxiety and provide emotional support. Postoperatively, goals of care are to maintain comfort, prevent complications, facilitate the client's adjustment to the effects of the diagnosis and its treatment, and educate him regarding follow-up care and subsequent treatment. If chemotherapy or radiation therapy is initiated prior to discharge, refer to those care plans for specific nursing care.

DISCHARGE CRITERIA

Prior to discharge, the client will:

- verbalize the importance of doing a routine testicular self-examination
- demonstrate the ability to correctly perform a testicular self-examination
- share thoughts and feelings about the diagnosis of cancer, the prognosis, and the changes in body image resulting from the diagnosis and its treatment
- state signs and symptoms to report to the health care provider
- identify community resources that can assist with adjustment to changes resulting from the diagnosis and effects of treatment
- verbalize an understanding of and a plan for adhering to recommended follow-up care including future appointments with health care provider, medications prescribed, activity level, wound care, and plans for subsequent treatment.

NURSING/COLLABORATIVE DIAGNOSES

Preoperative
1. Anxiety □ *1014*
Postoperative
1. Ineffective breathing patterns:
   a. hypoventilation
   b. hyperventilation □ *1015*
2. Potential complication: pneumothorax □ *1015*
3. Disturbance in self-concept □ *1016*
4. Ineffective individual coping □ *1017*
5. Grieving □ *1018*
6. Knowledge deficit regarding follow-up care □ *1019*

Preoperative

Use in conjunction with the Standardized Preoperative Care Plan.

1. NURSING DIAGNOSIS

Anxiety related to unfamiliar environment; lack of understanding of diagnosis, staging procedures, planned surgery, and prognosis; and anticipated postoperative discomfort and effects of impending surgery and subsequent treatment on body image and functioning and usual life style and roles.

DESIRED OUTCOMES	NURSING ACTIONS AND *SELECTED RATIONALES*

1. The client will experience a reduction in fear and anxiety (see Standardized Preoperative Care Plan, Nursing Diagnosis 1, for outcome criteria).	1.a. Refer to Standardized Preoperative Care Plan, Nursing Diagnosis 1, for measures related to assessment and reduction of fear and anxiety.
	b. Implement additional measures *to reduce fear and anxiety:*
	  1. explain all tests used to stage cancer of the testis:
	    a. chest x-ray, chest tomography
	    b. computed tomography (CT) of retroperitoneum
	    c. excretory urogram
	    d. inferior venacavography
	    e. abdominal and pelvic ultrasound examinations
	    f. liver and bone scans if serum alkaline phosphatase is elevated
	    g. urine analysis for beta–human chorionic gonadotropin (B-HCG) and estrogens
	    h. serum analysis for elevated levels of alpha-fetoprotein (AFP) and B-HCG (the presence of AFP and B-HCG indicates that a germinal tumor is present, facilitates selection of treatment mode, and predicts prognosis)
	    i. retroperitoneal lymphadenectomy (performed for both staging and treatment)
	  2. reinforce physician's explanation about possible effects of the surgery on sexual functioning
	  3. arrange for a visit with another who has been successfully treated for cancer of the testis.

Postoperative

Use in conjunction with the Standardized Postoperative Care Plan.

1. NURSING DIAGNOSIS

Ineffective breathing patterns:

a. **hypoventilation** related to:
   1. reluctance to breathe deeply associated with pain resulting from a high abdominal and chest wall incision (symphysis pubis to xyphoid and laterally across chest wall to midaxillary line)
   2. depressant effects of anesthesia and some medications (e.g. narcotic analgesics)
   3. weakness and fatigue
   4. pressure on the diaphragm associated with abdominal distention;
b. **hyperventilation** related to pain, fear, and anxiety.

DESIRED OUTCOMES	NURSING ACTIONS AND *SELECTED RATIONALES*

1. The client will maintain an effective breathing pattern (see Standardized Postoperative Care Plan, Nursing Diagnosis 3, for outcome criteria).	1.a. Refer to Standardized Postoperative Care Plan, Nursing Diagnosis 3, for measures related to assessment and management of an ineffective breathing pattern.
	b. Implement additional measures *to improve breathing pattern:*
	  1. instruct client to bend knees while coughing and deep breathing *in order to reduce tension on abdominal muscles and incision*
	  2. instruct and assist client to splint incision with hands or pillow when coughing and deep breathing.

2. COLLABORATIVE DIAGNOSIS

Potential complication: pneumothorax related to opening the pleural cavity during surgery.

DESIRED OUTCOMES	NURSING ACTIONS AND *SELECTED RATIONALES*

2. The client will experience normal lung re-expansion as evidenced by:
a. normal breath sounds and percussion note by the 3rd or 4th postoperative day
b. unlabored respirations at 16–20/minute
	2.a. Assess for and immediately report signs and symptoms of:
	  1. malfunction of the chest drainage system (e.g. respiratory distress, sudden cessation of drainage, excessive bubbling in water seal chamber, significant increase in subcutaneous emphysema)
	  2. further lung collapse (e.g. extended area of absent breath sounds with hyperresonant percussion note, tachycardia, increased respiratory distress and chest pain, cyanosis, restlessness, confusion).
	b. Monitor blood gases. Report values that have worsened.

c. blood gases returning toward normal
d. chest x-ray showing lung re-expansion.

c. Monitor chest x-ray results. Report findings of delayed lung re-expansion.
d. Implement measures *to prevent further lung collapse and promote lung re-expansion:*
   1. perform actions *to maintain patency and integrity of chest drainage system:*
      a. maintain water seal and suction levels as ordered
      b. maintain an air occlusive dressing over chest tube insertion site
      c. tape all connections securely
      d. milk or strip tubes if ordered
      e. keep chest drainage and suction tubing free of kinks
      f. keep drainage system below level of client's chest at all times
   2. perform actions to improve breathing pattern (see Postoperative Nursing Diagnosis 1) and facilitate airway clearance (see Standardized Postoperative Care Plan, Nursing Diagnosis 4, action b).
e. If signs and symptoms of further lung collapse occur:
   1. maintain client on bedrest in a semi- to high Fowler's position
   2. maintain oxygen therapy as ordered
   3. assess for and immediately report signs and symptoms of mediastinal shift (e.g. severe dyspnea, increased restlessness and agitation, rapid and/or irregular pulse rate, cyanosis, shift in point of apical impulse and trachea toward unaffected side)
   4. assist with clearing of existing chest tube and/or insertion of a new tube
   5. provide emotional support to client and significant others.

□ ▬▬▬▬▬▬▬▬▬▬▬▬▬▬▬▬▬▬▬▬▬▬▬▬▬▬

3. NURSING DIAGNOSIS

Disturbance in self-concept* related to:

a. loss of ability to ejaculate normally;
b. possible alteration in usual sexual functioning associated with fatigue, fear, anxiety, and grieving;
c. infertility associated with:
   1. ejaculatory failure resulting from removal of the sympathetic chain from T12–L3 (depending on extent of disease process, it may be possible to preserve ejaculatory function by leaving one sympathetic chain intact)
   2. impaired spermatogenesis resulting from inadequate functioning of remaining testis and prolonged stress associated with the diagnosis, need for complex surgery, fear of disease recurrence, and change in body image;
d. recent surgical excision of the testis;
e. gynecomastia (occurs in a small percentage of clients, is thought to be due to increased production of B–HCG by the tumor [particularly nonseminoma type], and indicates a poor prognosis);
f. temporary dependence on others to meet self-care needs;
g. possible changes in life style and roles associated with the effects of the disease process and its treatment.

----

* This diagnostic label includes the nursing diagnoses of body image disturbance and self-esteem disturbance.

□ ▬▬▬▬▬▬▬▬▬▬▬▬▬▬▬▬▬▬▬▬▬▬▬▬▬▬

DESIRED OUTCOMES	NURSING ACTIONS AND *SELECTED RATIONALES*
3. The client will demonstrate beginning adaptation to changes in appearance, body	3.a. Determine the meaning of changes in appearance, body functioning, life style, and roles to the client by encouraging him to verbalize feelings and by noting nonverbal responses to the changes experienced.

functioning, life style, and roles as evidenced by:

a. verbalization of feelings of self-worth and sexual adequacy
b. maintenance of relationships with significant others
c. active participation in activities of daily living
d. active interest in personal appearance
e. willingness to participate in social activities
f. verbalization of a beginning plan for adapting life style to meet restrictions imposed by cancer of the testis and the treatment plan.

b. Assess for signs and symptoms of a disturbance in self-concept (e.g. verbal or nonverbal cues denoting a negative response to changes in body functioning or appearance such as denial of or preoccupation with changes that have occurred, refusal to look at or touch surgical area, or withdrawal from significant others).
c. Assist client to identify strengths and qualities that have a positive effect on self-concept.
d. Implement measures *to assist client to increase self-esteem* (e.g. limit negative self-criticism, encourage positive comments about self, give positive feedback about accomplishments).
e. Reinforce actions to assist the client to cope with the effects of testicular cancer and its treatment (see Postoperative Nursing Diagnosis 4, action d).
f. Clarify physician's explanation about the effects of surgery on sexual functioning and/or fertility:
   1. assure client that his ability to achieve erection and orgasm should not be affected by a retroperitoneal lymphadenectomy
   2. reiterate the likelihood of infertility after the surgery and provide further explanation about ejaculatory failure and impaired spermatogenesis if indicated
   3. discuss alternative methods of becoming a parent (e.g. adoption, artificial insemination) if of concern to client
   4. include partner in above discussions and encourage continued support of the client.
g. Encourage client to discuss the possibility of a testicular implant with the physician if desired.
h. Assist client with usual grooming if necessary.
i. Encourage maximum participation in **self-care activities** *in order to reduce feelings of dependency.*
j. Encourage significant others to allow client to do what he is able *so that independence can be re-established and/or self-esteem redeveloped.*
k. Assess for and support behaviors suggesting positive adaptation to changes experienced (e.g. willingness to participate in treatment plan, maintenance of relationships with others, interest in appearance).
l. Assist client's and significant others' adjustment by listening, facilitating communications, and providing information.
m. Ensure that client and significant others have similar expectations and understanding of future life style.
n. Assist the client and significant others to identify ways that personal and family goals can be adjusted rather than abandoned.
o. Encourage visits and support from significant others.
p. Encourage client to continue involvement in social activities and to pursue interests. If previous interests and hobbies cannot be pursued, encourage development of new ones.
q. Provide information about and encourage utilization of community agencies or support groups (e.g. American Cancer Society; sexual, family, and/or individual counseling services).
r. Consult physician about psychological counseling if client desires or if he seems unwilling or unable to adapt to changes that have occurred as a result of the disease and its treatment.

4. NURSING DIAGNOSIS

Ineffective individual coping related to:

a. inadequate support system;
b. discomfort associated with the surgical procedure, disease process, and side effects of treatments;
c. depression, fear, and anxiety associated with the diagnosis and effects of the treatment on body functioning and usual life style and roles;
d. uncertainty about the effects of treatment on the malignancy and disease prognosis.

DESIRED OUTCOMES	NURSING ACTIONS AND *SELECTED RATIONALES*

4. The client will demonstrate the use of effective coping skills as evidenced by:
   a. willingness to participate in treatment plan and self-care activities
   b. verbalization of ability to cope with cancer and its effects
   c. identification of stressors
   d. utilization of appropriate problem-solving techniques
   e. recognition and utilization of available support systems.

4.a. Assess effectiveness of client's coping strategies by observing behavior and noting strengths, weaknesses, ability to express feelings and concerns, and willingness to participate in the treatment plan.
   b. Assess for and report signs and symptoms that may indicate ineffective coping (e.g. sleep disturbances, increasing fatigue, difficulty concentrating, irritability, decreased tolerance for pain, verbalization of inability to cope, inability to problem solve).
   c. Allow time for client to adjust psychologically to the diagnosis; need for subsequent treatment; effects of surgery; and anticipated changes in future plans, life style, and roles.
   d. Implement measures *to promote effective coping:*
      1. perform actions to promote a positive self-concept and facilitate grieving (see Postoperative Nursing Diagnoses 3, actions c–q and 5, action d)
      2. perform actions to reduce fear and anxiety (see Standardized Postoperative Care Plan, Nursing Diagnosis 1, action c)
      3. perform actions to reduce postoperative discomfort (see Standardized Postoperative Care Plan, Nursing Diagnoses 7.A, action 5; 7.B, action 3; 7.C, action 2; and 7.D)
      4. arrange for a visit with another who has been successfully treated for cancer of the testis
      5. include client in the planning of care, encourage maximum participation in the treatment plan, and allow choices when possible *to enable him to maintain a sense of control*
      6. instruct client in effective problem-solving techniques (e.g. accurate identification of stressors, determination of various options to solve problem)
      7. assist client to maintain usual daily routines whenever possible
      8. encourage diversional activities according to client's interests
      9. assist client to identify and utilize available support systems; provide information about available community resources that can assist client and significant others in coping with diagnosis and treatment (e.g. American Cancer Society; local support groups; individual, family, and financial counselors).
   e. Encourage continued emotional support from significant others.
   f. Encourage client to share with significant others the kind of support that would be most beneficial (e.g. listening, inspiring hope, providing reassurance and accurate information).
   g. Assess for and support behaviors suggesting positive adaptation to changes experienced (e.g. compliance with treatment plan, increased participation in self-care activities, communication of ability to cope, utilization of effective problem-solving strategies).
   h. Consult physician about psychological counseling if appropriate. Initiate a referral if necessary.

5. NURSING DIAGNOSIS

Grieving* related to the diagnosis of cancer, loss of the testis, possible change in normal sexual functioning and reproductive ability, and possibility of premature death.

* This diagnostic label includes anticipatory grieving and grieving following the actual losses/changes.

DESIRED OUTCOMES	NURSING ACTIONS AND *SELECTED RATIONALES*

5. The client will demonstrate beginning progression through the grieving process as evidenced by:
   a. verbalization of feelings about the diagnosis of cancer and its effects
   b. expression of grief
   c. participation in treatment plan and self-care activities
   d. utilization of available support systems
   e. verbalization of a plan for integrating prescribed follow-up care into life style.

5.a. Determine the client's perception of the impact of cancer, loss of the testis, and possible change in sexual functioning and reproductive ability on his future.
 b. Determine how the client usually expresses grief.
 c. Observe for signs of grieving (e.g. changes in eating habits, insomnia, anger, noncompliance, denial).
 d. Implement measures *to facilitate the grieving process:*
    1. assist client to acknowledge the diagnosis of cancer, loss of the testis, and possible changes in sexual functioning and reproductive ability *so grief work can begin*; assess for factors that may hinder or facilitate acknowledgment
    2. discuss the grieving process and assist client to accept the stages of grieving as an expected response to actual and anticipated losses; support the realization that grief may recur *because of the extended period of treatment*
    3. allow time for client to progress through the stages of grieving (denial, anger, bargaining, depression, acceptance [Kübler-Ross, 1969]); be aware that not every stage is experienced or expressed by all individuals
    4. provide an atmosphere of care and concern (e.g. provide privacy, be available and nonjudgmental, display empathy and respect) *so that client will feel free to verbalize both positive and negative feelings and concerns*
    5. perform actions *to promote trust* (e.g. answer questions honestly, provide requested information)
    6. encourage the expression of anger and sadness about the losses and changes experienced
    7. encourage client to express his feelings in whatever ways are comfortable (e.g. writing, drawing, conversation)
    8. perform actions to facilitate effective coping (see Postoperative Nursing Diagnosis 4, action d)
    9. support realistic hope about the effects of treatment on disease process and prognosis.
 e. Assess for and support behaviors suggesting successful resolution of grief (e.g. verbalizing feelings about changes/losses, expressing sorrow, focusing on ways to adapt to changes/losses).
 f. Explain the stages of the grieving process to significant others. Encourage their support and understanding.
 g. Provide information regarding counseling services and support groups that might assist client in working through grief.
 h. Arrange for visit from clergy if desired by client.
 i. Monitor for therapeutic and nontherapeutic effects of antidepressants if administered.
 j. Consult physician about referral for counseling if signs of dysfunctional grieving (e.g. persistent denial of losses or changes, excessive anger or sadness, hysteria, suicidal behaviors, phobias) occur.

6. NURSING DIAGNOSIS

Knowledge deficit regarding follow-up care.

DESIRED OUTCOMES	NURSING ACTIONS AND *SELECTED RATIONALES*
6.a. The client will verbalize the importance of doing a routine testicular self-examination.	6.a.1. Explain the reasons for a self-examination of the testis. 2. Explore with client ways to remember to perform the testicular examination at monthly intervals.
6.b. The client will demonstrate the ability to correctly perform a testicular self-examination.	6.b.1. Demonstrate, using a model, chart, or film, how to do a testicular exam. 2. Allow time for questions, clarification, and return demonstration.

6.c. The client will state signs and symptoms to report to the health care provider.	6.c.1. Refer to Standardized Postoperative Care Plan, Nursing Diagnosis 20, action c, for signs and symptoms to report to the health care provider.
	2. Instruct client to report these additional signs and symptoms:
	  a. persistent scrotal edema
	  b. increased weakness and fatigue
	  c. excessive depression or difficulty coping with the diagnosis.

6.d. The client will identify community resources that can assist with adjustment to changes resulting from the diagnosis and effects of treatment.	6.d.1. Provide information about community resources that can assist the client and significant others with adjustment to diagnosis and effects of treatment (e.g. American Cancer Society, local support groups, Make Today Count, Hospice, social service agencies, counselors). 2. Initiate a referral if indicated.

6.e. The client will verbalize an understanding of and a plan for adhering to recommended follow-up care including future appointments with health care provider, medications prescribed, activity level, wound care, and plans for subsequent treatment.	6.e.1. Refer to Standardized Postoperative Care Plan, Nursing Diagnosis 20, for routine postoperative instructions and measures to improve client compliance.
	2. Reinforce the physician's instructions regarding:
	  a. need to avoid lifting heavy objects until healing is complete
	  b. importance of scheduling adequate rest periods
	  c. plans for subsequent radiation therapy and/or chemotherapy.

☐ ▐███▌

Reference

Kübler-Ross, E. On death and dying. New York: Macmillan, 1969.

■ ■

Colporrhaphy

Colporrhaphy is the surgical repair of the vagina and incompetent muscles and ligaments of the pelvic floor. An anterior colporrhaphy is performed to correct a cystocele, which is a protrusion or displacement of the bladder through the pubocervical fascia into the vagina. A posterior colporrhaphy is performed to repair a rectocele, which is a protrusion of part of the anterior rectal wall upward into the vagina. Cystoceles and rectoceles are caused by relaxation of the pelvic musculature and ligaments usually associated with aging and tissue damage during childbirth. They can occur alone or in conjunction with prolapse of the uterus. Surgery is indicated when conservative management (e.g. perineal exercises, insertion of a pessary) no longer controls symptoms such as back pain, stress incontinence, urinary frequency and urgency, vaginal pressure, and constipation. A procedure to elevate the urethra and restore the appropriate angle between the urethra and the posterior bladder wall (e.g. Marshall-Marchetti-Krantz, Stamey) may be performed at the same time if stress incontinence is particularly severe.

This care plan focuses on the adult female client hospitalized for an elective anterior and posterior colporrhaphy using a vaginal approach. Preoperatively, the goals of care are to reduce fear and anxiety and prepare the client for the surgical experience. The goals of postoperative care are to maintain comfort, prevent complications, and educate the client regarding follow-up care.

DISCHARGE CRITERIA

Prior to discharge, the client will:

- identify ways to prevent increased pressure on suture lines and decrease the risk of reherniation of the bladder and rectum
- identify ways to relieve surgical site discomfort
- state signs and symptoms of complications to report to the health care provider
- verbalize an understanding of and plan for adhering to recommended follow-up care including future appointments with health care provider, medications prescribed, limitations on sexual activity, and wound care.

NURSING/COLLABORATIVE DIAGNOSES

Postoperative
1. Pain: rectal and vaginal □ *1022*
2. Constipation □ *1022*
3. Potential for infection:
   a. wound infection
   b. urinary tract infection □ *1022*
4. Potential complication: reherniation of bladder and rectum □ *1023*
5. Knowledge deficit regarding follow-up care □ *1024*

Preoperative

Use in conjunction with the Standardized Preoperative Care Plan.

Postoperative

Use in conjunction with the Standardized Postoperative Care Plan.

UNIT
XVII

1. NURSING DIAGNOSIS

Pain: rectal and vaginal related to tissue trauma, pressure from vaginal packing, and reflex muscle spasm associated with the surgical procedure.

DESIRED OUTCOMES	NURSING ACTIONS AND *SELECTED RATIONALES*
1. The client will experience diminished rectal and vaginal pain as evidenced by: a. verbalization of pain relief b. relaxed facial expression and body positioning c. ability to sit and walk more comfortably d. increased participation in activities e. stable vital signs.	1.a. Refer to Standardized Postoperative Care Plan, Nursing Diagnosis 7.A, for measures related to assessment and management of postoperative pain. b. Implement additional measures *to reduce rectal and vaginal pain:* 1. apply ice packs to the perineal area for the first 24 hours postoperatively *in order to decrease edema* 2. instruct and assist client with heat lamp treatments to the perineum and sitz baths as ordered 3. encourage client to lie flat or in semi-Fowler's position when in bed *in order to minimize pressure on surgical site* 4. monitor for therapeutic and nontherapeutic effects of topical anesthetics if applied.

2. NURSING DIAGNOSIS

Constipation related to:

a. decreased gastrointestinal motility associated with anesthesia, narcotic analgesics, and decreased activity;
b. reluctance to defecate associated with fear of anorectal pain and reherniation of rectum;
c. decreased intake of fluids and foods high in fiber.

DESIRED OUTCOMES	NURSING ACTIONS AND *SELECTED RATIONALES*
2. The client will have soft, formed stool and resume usual bowel elimination pattern.	2.a. Refer to Standardized Postoperative Care Plan, Nursing Diagnosis 14, for measures related to assessment and prevention of constipation. b. Assure client that an analgesic will be given before she attempts to defecate *in order to ease the pain associated with passage of stool through the anorectal area.*

3. NURSING DIAGNOSIS

Potential for infection:

a. **wound infection** related to break in the vaginal mucosa and close proximity of the incision to the rectum and urethra;
b. **urinary tract infection** related to urinary retention and urinary catheterization.

DESIRED OUTCOMES	NURSING ACTIONS AND *SELECTED RATIONALES*

3.a. The client will remain free of wound infection (see Standardized Postoperative Care Plan, Nursing Diagnosis 16, outcome b, for outcome criteria).	3.a.1. Refer to Standardized Postoperative Care Plan, Nursing Diagnosis 16, action b, for measures related to assessment, prevention, and management of postoperative wound infection.
	    2. Implement additional measures *to reduce risk of wound infection:*
	      a. instruct client to wipe from front to back following defecation
	      b. administer perineal care 2–3 times/day and after urination and defecation
	      c. perform catheter care each shift and as necessary
	      d. avoid any invasive rectal procedure (e.g. rectal tube, suppositories, enemas, rectal temperature)
	      e. administer a heat lamp treatment 2–3 times/day for 20 minutes if ordered *to dry wound area and facilitate healing.*

3.b. The client will remain free of urinary tract infection (see Standardized Postoperative Care Plan, Nursing Diagnosis 16, outcome c, for outcome criteria).	3.b. Refer to Standardized Postoperative Care Plan, Nursing Diagnosis 16, action c, for measures related to the assessment, prevention, and management of urinary tract infection.

4. COLLABORATIVE DIAGNOSIS

Potential complication: reherniation of bladder and rectum related to pressure on suture lines associated with increased intra-abdominal, bladder, rectal, or vaginal pressure.

DESIRED OUTCOMES	NURSING ACTIONS AND *SELECTED RATIONALES*

4. The client will not experience reherniation of the bladder and rectum as evidenced by:
  a. absence of fecal and urinary stress incontinence
  b. absence of urinary frequency and urgency
  c. gradual resolution of back pain and pelvic pressure.
	4.a. Assess for signs and symptoms of reherniation of the bladder or rectum (e.g. stress incontinence of urine or stool, urinary frequency and urgency, voiding small amounts, back pain, pelvic pressure).
	  b. Implement measures *to prevent reherniation of the bladder and rectum:*
	    1. maintain patency of urinary catheter if present or encourage client to void every 4 hours *in order to prevent excessive accumulation of urine in the bladder*
	    2. avoid any invasive rectal procedures (e.g. rectal tube, suppositories, enemas, rectal temperature) *in order to reduce risk of disrupting suture line*
	    3. perform actions *to prevent increased intra-abdominal pressure and subsequent stress on suture lines:*
	      a. instruct client to lie flat or in a semi-Fowler's position while in bed
	      b. instruct client to avoid any activities that may create a Valsalva response (e.g. straining to have a bowel movement, lifting or carrying a heavy object, holding breath while moving, bending at waist, coughing)
	      c. monitor for therapeutic and nontherapeutic effects of stool softeners, laxatives, antiemetics, and antitussives if administered *to prevent straining and control nausea, vomiting, and persistent cough*
	      d. maintain dietary restrictions (may be on a liquid diet for the first week postoperatively) as ordered *to reduce bowel content*
	      e. caution client to avoid prolonged standing, sitting, or walking

UNIT
XVII

  4. if douches are ordered, slowly instill small amounts of solution and rotate
     nozzle gently.
  c. If reherniation occurs:
  1. maintain client on bedrest
  2. prepare client for surgical repair of the wound
  3. provide emotional support to client and significant others.

☐ ▓▓▓▓▓▓▓▓▓▓▓▓▓▓▓▓▓▓▓▓▓▓▓▓▓▓▓▓▓▓▓▓▓▓▓▓▓▓▓

5. NURSING DIAGNOSIS

Knowledge deficit regarding follow-up care.

☐ ▓▓▓▓▓▓▓▓▓▓▓▓▓▓▓▓▓▓▓▓▓▓▓▓▓▓▓▓▓▓▓▓▓▓▓▓▓▓▓

DESIRED OUTCOMES	NURSING ACTIONS AND *SELECTED RATIONALES*

5.a. The client will identify ways to prevent increased pressure on suture lines and decrease the risk of reherniation of the bladder and rectum.	5.a.1. Provide the following instructions on ways *to minimize pressure on the suture line and decrease the risk of reherniation of the bladder and rectum:*
	  a. instruct client to avoid any unnecessary rectal and vaginal trauma (e.g. rectal temperature, enemas, suppositories)
	  b. reinforce instructions about avoiding prolonged sitting or standing and any activity that may create a Valsalva response (e.g. straining to have a bowel movement, lifting or carrying heavy objects, holding breath while moving, bending at the waist, coughing) for at least 6 weeks
	  c. instruct client to void whenever she feels the urge or at least every 4 hours
	  d. if douches are ordered, instruct client to slowly instill small amounts of solution and rotate nozzle gently.
	  2. Encourage client to do perineal exercises (e.g. stopping and starting urinary stream, alternately contracting and relaxing the gluteal muscles) when healing is completed (usually 6 weeks) *in order to improve vaginal tone and further decrease the risk of reherniation of the bladder and rectum.*

5.b. The client will identify ways to relieve surgical site discomfort.	5.b. Provide the following instructions regarding ways *to relieve surgical site discomfort:*
	  1. take a sitz bath 2–3 times/day
	  2. apply a topical anesthetic (e.g. dibucaine, cyclomethycaine) as needed
	  3. douche if permitted by physician
	  4. avoid prolonged sitting or standing
	  5. sit on a foam pad or pillow
	  6. take analgesics as prescribed.

5.c. The client will state signs and symptoms of complications to report to the health care provider.	5.c.1. Refer to Standardized Postoperative Care Plan, Nursing Diagnosis 20, action c, for signs and symptoms to report to the health care provider.
	  2. Instruct the client to report these additional signs and symptoms:
	  a. unusual, odorous vaginal discharge
	  b. stress incontinence
	  c. vaginal leakage of urine or stool
	  d. excessive perineal edema, pain, or bleeding.

5.d. The client will verbalize an understanding of and plan for adhering to recommended follow-up care including future appointments with health care provider, medications prescribed, limitations on sexual activity, and wound care.	5.d.1. Refer to Standardized Postoperative Care Plan, Nursing Diagnosis 20, for routine postoperative instructions and measures to improve client compliance.
	  2. Instruct client not to have intercourse until permitted by physician (usually 6 weeks).
	  3. Inform client that loss of vaginal sensation is usually temporary but may persist for several months.

Hysterectomy with Salpingectomy and Oophorectomy

Hysterectomy is the surgical removal of the uterus. It is performed to treat conditions of the uterus such as benign or malignant tumors, endometriosis, dysfunctional bleeding, and prolapse. A vaginal approach may be utilized if only the uterus is to be removed or if repairs to the vaginal wall or pelvic floor are necessary. An abdominal approach is commonly used if the uterus is enlarged and/or if oophorectomy (removal of the ovaries) and salpingectomy (removal of the fallopian tubes) are performed at the same time.

This care plan focuses on the adult female client hospitalized for an elective hysterectomy with salpingectomy and oophorectomy. Preoperatively, the goals of care are to reduce fear and anxiety and prepare the client for the surgical experience. Postoperative goals are to maintain comfort, prevent and detect complications, assist the client to adjust to changes in body image, and educate her regarding follow-up care. Nursing measures will vary depending on the extensiveness of the surgery and the approach utilized.

DISCHARGE CRITERIA

Prior to discharge, the client will:

- verbalize an understanding of the effects of surgical menopause
- verbalize an understanding of medication therapy including rationale for, side effects of, schedule for taking, and importance of taking as prescribed
- state signs and symptoms of complications to report to the health care provider
- share feelings about the loss of reproductive ability
- verbalize an understanding of and a plan for adhering to recommended follow-up care including future appointments with health care provider, activity limitations, wound care, and resumption of sexual activity.

NURSING/COLLABORATIVE DIAGNOSES

Preoperative
1. Anxiety ☐ *1026*
Postoperative
1. Urinary retention ☐ *1026*
2. Potential complications:
   a. bladder or ureteral injury
   b. thromboembolism ☐ *1027*
3. Sexual dysfunction:
   a. decreased libido
   b. dyspareunia ☐ *1027*
4. Body image disturbance ☐ *1028*
5. Grieving ☐ *1029*
6. Knowledge deficit regarding follow-up care ☐ *1030*

☐ ▬▬▬▬▬▬▬▬▬▬▬▬▬▬▬▬▬▬▬▬▬▬

Preoperative

Use in conjunction with the Standardized Preoperative Care Plan.

☐ ▬▬▬▬▬▬▬▬▬▬▬▬▬▬▬▬▬▬▬▬▬▬

1. NURSING DIAGNOSIS

Anxiety related to unfamiliar environment, anticipated effects of surgery on body image and reproductive ability, effects of anesthesia, anticipated postoperative discomfort, and potential embarrassment or loss of dignity associated with exposure of genitals during surgery and preoperative and postoperative care.

☐ ▬▬▬▬▬▬▬▬▬▬▬▬▬▬▬▬▬▬▬▬▬▬

DESIRED OUTCOMES	NURSING ACTIONS AND *SELECTED RATIONALES*
1. The client will experience a reduction in fear and anxiety (see Standardized Preoperative Care Plan, Nursing Diagnosis 1, for outcome criteria).	1.a. Refer to Standardized Preoperative Care Plan, Nursing Diagnosis 1, for measures related to assessment and reduction of fear and anxiety. b. Implement additional measures *to reduce fear and anxiety:* 　1. encourage client and her partner to verbalize concerns and feelings about loss of ovarian function and reproductive ability; provide feedback 　2. assure client she will not suffer needless body exposure during surgery and preoperative and postoperative care.

☐ ▬▬▬▬▬▬▬▬▬▬▬▬▬▬▬▬▬▬▬▬▬▬

Postoperative

Use in conjunction with the Standardized Postoperative Care Plan.

☐ ▬▬▬▬▬▬▬▬▬▬▬▬▬▬▬▬▬▬▬▬▬▬

1. NURSING DIAGNOSIS

Urinary retention related to:

a. bladder atony associated with pelvic edema and nerve trauma (resulting from surgery) and depressant effects of some medications (e.g. anesthetic agents, narcotic analgesics) on bladder muscle tone;
b. stimulation of the sympathetic nervous system associated with pain, fear, and anxiety;
c. pooling of urine in kidney and bladder associated with horizontal positioning.

☐ ▬▬▬▬▬▬▬▬▬▬▬▬▬▬▬▬▬▬▬▬▬▬

DESIRED OUTCOMES	NURSING ACTIONS AND *SELECTED RATIONALES*
1. The client will not experience urinary retention (see Standardized Postoperative Care Plan, Nursing Diagnosis 13, for outcome criteria).	1. Refer to Standardized Postoperative Care Plan, Nursing Diagnosis 13, for measures related to assessment, prevention, and treatment of urinary retention (client will usually have an indwelling urinary catheter for first 24–48 hours after surgery).

□ ■■

2. COLLABORATIVE DIAGNOSIS

Potential complications:

a. **bladder or ureteral injury** related to accidental tear or ligation during the surgical procedure;
b. **thromboembolism** related to:
   1. pressure on the pelvic and calf vessels during surgery if the client was in lithotomy position
   2. trauma to the large pelvic veins associated with manipulation during surgery
   3. venous stasis associated with decreased activity and abdominal distention (the distended intestine may put pressure on the abdominal vessels)
   4. hypercoagulability associated with fluid volume deficit.

□ ■■

DESIRED OUTCOMES	NURSING ACTIONS AND *SELECTED RATIONALES*
2.a. The client will experience resolution of bladder or ureteral injury if it has occurred as evidenced by: 1. gradual resolution of hematuria and backache 2. output greater than 200 cc within 6–8 hours after surgery.	2.a.1. Assess for and report signs and symptoms of bladder or ureteral injury (e.g. hematuria, persistent or increasing backache, output less than 200 cc in first 6–8 hours after surgery). 2. If signs and symptoms of bladder or ureteral injury are present: a. continue to monitor output carefully b. prepare client for surgical repair if indicated c. provide emotional support to client and significant others.
2.b. The client will not develop a venous thrombus or pulmonary embolism (see Standardized Postoperative Care Plan, Collaborative Diagnosis 19, outcomes c.1 and 2, for outcome criteria).	2.b. Refer to Standardized Postoperative Care Plan, Collaborative Diagnosis 19, actions c.1 and 2, for measures related to assessment, prevention, and treatment of a venous thrombus and pulmonary embolism.

□ ■■

3. NURSING DIAGNOSIS

Sexual dysfunction:

a. **decreased libido** related to changes in body image, grieving, and hormone imbalance;
b. **dyspareunia** related to dryness of the vaginal mucosa associated with decreased estrogen levels.

□ ■■

DESIRED OUTCOMES	NURSING ACTIONS AND *SELECTED RATIONALES*
3. The client will demonstrate beginning acceptance of changes in sexual functioning as evidenced by: a. verbalization of a perception of self as sexually acceptable and adequate b. maintenance of relationships with significant others.	3.a. Assess for signs and symptoms of sexual dysfunction (e.g. verbalization of sexual concerns, failure to maintain relationships with significant others). b. Determine attitudes, knowledge, and concerns about removal of uterus, ovaries, and fallopian tubes in relation to sexual functioning. c. Communicate interest, understanding, and respect for the values of the client and her partner. d. Provide accurate information about the effect of loss of the uterus, ovaries, and fallopian tubes on sexual functioning. Encourage questions and clarify misconceptions. e. Implement measures to improve body image (see Postoperative Nursing Diagnosis 4, actions c–l). f. Explain that there will be a temporary loss of vaginal sensation for several weeks to months after a vaginal hysterectomy. g. Encourage the client to use a water-soluble lubricant *in order to prevent dyspareunia resulting from vaginal dryness.* h. Monitor for therapeutic and nontherapeutic effects of hormone replacements (e.g. estrogen, progesterone) if administered. i. Facilitate communication between the client and her partner. Assist them to identify issues that may affect their relationship. j. If appropriate, suggest alternative methods of sexual gratification during first 4–6 weeks postoperatively. k. Arrange for uninterrupted privacy during hospital stay if desired by the couple. l. Discuss ways to be creative in expressing sexuality (e.g. massage, fantasies, cuddling). m. Consult physician if counseling appears indicated.

□ ▬▬▬▬▬▬▬▬▬▬▬▬▬▬▬▬▬▬▬▬▬▬▬▬

4. NURSING DIAGNOSIS

Body image disturbance related to loss of reproductive organs and alteration in hormone balance.

□ ▬▬▬▬▬▬▬▬▬▬▬▬▬▬▬▬▬▬▬▬▬▬▬▬

DESIRED OUTCOMES	NURSING ACTIONS AND *SELECTED RATIONALES*
4. The client will demonstrate beginning adaptation to changes in body functioning as evidenced by: a. verbalization of feelings of self-worth and sexual adequacy b. maintenance of relationships with significant others c. active participation in activities of daily living d. active interest in personal appearance.	4.a. Determine the meaning of the loss of reproductive organs to the client by encouraging her to verbalize feelings and by noting nonverbal responses to the changes experienced. b. Assess for signs and symptoms of a disturbance in body image (e.g. verbal or nonverbal cues denoting a negative response to changes in body functioning such as denial of or preoccupation with changes that have occurred or withdrawal from significant others). c. Implement measures to facilitate the grieving process (see Postoperative Nursing Diagnosis 5, action d). d. Assist client to identify strengths and qualities that have a positive effect on body image. e. Assist client to identify and utilize coping techniques that have been helpful in the past. f. Reinforce measures that may assist the client to adjust to alteration in sexual functioning (see Postoperative Nursing Diagnosis 3, actions c–l). g. Encourage the client to verbalize her feelings about the effects of surgery on her femininity. h. Assist client with usual grooming and makeup habits if necessary. i. Assess for and support behaviors suggesting positive adaptation to loss of

reproductive organs (e.g. active interest in personal appearance, maintenance of relationships with significant others).
   j. Assist client's and significant others' adjustment by listening, facilitating communication, and providing information.
   k. Encourage visits and support from significant others.
   l. If client expresses an interest in the adoption of children, provide names of appropriate community agencies.
   m. Consult physician about psychological counseling if client desires or if she seems unwilling or unable to adapt to changes resulting from the surgery.

□ ▬▬▬▬▬▬▬▬▬▬▬▬▬▬▬▬▬▬▬▬▬▬▬▬

5. NURSING DIAGNOSIS

Grieving* related to loss of reproductive organs.

* This diagnostic label includes anticipatory grieving and grieving following the actual losses/changes.

□ ▬▬▬▬▬▬▬▬▬▬▬▬▬▬▬▬▬▬▬▬▬▬▬▬

DESIRED OUTCOMES	NURSING ACTIONS AND *SELECTED RATIONALES*

5. The client will demonstrate beginning progression through the grieving process as evidenced by:
   a. verbalization of feelings about loss of reproductive organs
   b. expression of grief
   c. participation in treatment plan and self-care activities
   d. utilization of available support systems.

5.a. Determine client's perception of the impact of loss of her reproductive organs on her future.
   b. Determine how client usually expresses grief.
   c. Observe for signs of grieving (e.g. changes in eating habits, insomnia, anger, noncompliance, denial).
   d. Implement measures *to facilitate the grieving process:*
      1. assist client to acknowledge losses and changes experienced *so grief work can begin*
      2. discuss the grieving process and assist client to accept the stages of grieving as an expected response to loss of her reproductive organs and usual body functioning
      3. allow time for client to progress through the stages of grieving (denial, anger, bargaining, depression, acceptance [Kübler-Ross, 1969]); be aware that not every stage is experienced or expressed by all individuals
      4. provide an atmosphere of care and concern (e.g. provide privacy, be available and nonjudgmental, display empathy and respect) *so that client will feel free to verbalize both positive and negative feelings and concerns*
      5. perform actions *to promote trust* (e.g. answer questions honestly, provide requested information)
      6. encourage the expression of anger and sadness about the losses and changes experienced
      7. encourage client to express her feelings in whatever ways are comfortable (e.g. writing, drawing, conversation)
      8. assist client to identify personal strengths that have helped her to cope in previous situations of loss.
   e. Assess for and support behaviors suggesting successful resolution of grief (e.g. verbalizing feelings about changes in physical functioning, expressing sorrow, focusing on ways to adapt to loss of reproductive function).
   f. Explain the stages of the grieving process to significant others. Encourage their support and understanding.
   g. Provide information about counseling services and support groups that might be of assistance to client in working through grief.
   h. Arrange for visit from clergy if desired by client.
   i. Monitor for therapeutic and nontherapeutic effects of antidepressants if administered.
   j. Consult physician about referral for counseling if signs of dysfunctional grieving (e.g. persistent denial of losses or changes, excessive anger or sadness, hysteria, suicidal behaviors, phobias) occur.

□ ▌▌▌▌▌▌▌▌▌▌▌▌▌▌▌▌▌▌▌▌▌▌▌▌▌▌▌▌▌▌▌▌▌▌▌▌▌

6. NURSING DIAGNOSIS

Knowledge deficit regarding follow-up care.

□ ▌▌▌▌▌▌▌▌▌▌▌▌▌▌▌▌▌▌▌▌▌▌▌▌▌▌▌▌▌▌▌▌▌▌▌▌▌

DESIRED OUTCOMES	NURSING ACTIONS AND *SELECTED RATIONALES*
6.a. The client will verbalize an understanding of the effects of surgical menopause.	6.a. Reinforce the physician's explanation of surgical menopause and its effects (e.g. hot flashes, facial hair growth, decrease in vaginal lubrication, insomnia, nervousness, palpitations, depression).
6.b. The client will verbalize an understanding of medication therapy including rationale for, side effects of, schedule for taking, and importance of taking as prescribed.	6.b.1. Explain the rationale for, side effects of, and importance of taking medications prescribed. 2. If client is discharged on estrogen replacement therapy, instruct her to: a. take medication with meals or at bedtime *to prevent nausea* b. be aware that headache, weight gain, acne, increased skin pigmentation, nausea, and tender breasts are potential side effects of estrogen therapy c. wear a supportive bra if breasts are tender d. report the following to the health care provider: 1. side effects that are not controlled or tolerable 2. blurring or loss of vision 3. swelling, pain, or redness of an extremity e. keep scheduled follow-up appointments with health care provider while on estrogen replacement therapy.
6.c. The client will state signs and symptoms of complications to report to the health care provider.	6.c.1. Refer to Standardized Postoperative Care Plan, Nursing Diagnosis 20, action c, for signs and symptoms to report to the health care provider. 2. Instruct the client to report these additional signs and symptoms: a. foul-smelling vaginal discharge b. heavy vaginal bleeding (slight spotting is normal 2 weeks postoperatively when internal sutures are absorbed) c. excessive depression or difficulty dealing with changes in body image d. excessive discomfort associated with effects of surgical menopause.
6.d. The client will verbalize an understanding of and a plan for adhering to recommended follow-up care including future appointments with health care provider, activity limitations, wound care, and resumption of sexual activity.	6.d.1. Refer to Standardized Postoperative Care Plan, Nursing Diagnosis 20, for routine postoperative instructions and measures to ensure client compliance. 2. Reinforce the physician's instructions regarding: a. the need to avoid lifting objects over 10 pounds, sitting for long periods, stair climbing, and strenuous activity for 6–8 weeks postoperatively b. resumption of sexual intercourse, douching, and tub bathing (usually 6 weeks postoperatively).

□ ▌▌▌▌▌▌▌▌▌▌▌▌▌▌▌▌▌▌▌▌▌▌▌▌▌▌▌▌▌▌▌▌▌▌▌▌▌

Reference

Kübler-Ross, E. On death and dying. New York: Macmillan, 1969.

Penile Implant

A penile implant is a device used to treat erectile dysfunction associated with spinal cord injury, diabetes, atherosclerosis, radical pelvic or perineal surgery, radiation therapy to the prostate and surrounding area, and other organic disorders. The device may also be used to treat impotence associated with psychological factors that has not responded to conservative treatment. Two basic types of penile prostheses are the inflatable and semi-rigid. Some of the semi-rigid models are malleable or hinged at the base to enable the client to position the penis closer to the body and conceal the permanently erect state. There are two types of inflatable prostheses. The newer type is self-contained and consists of paired cylinders each with its own pump, reservoir, and inflation chamber. With this type of unit, the length and width of the penis does not change with activation and deactivation. The other type of inflatable prosthesis is a multicomponent unit consisting of a 60 cc reservoir that is implanted in the lower abdomen under the rectus abdominis muscle, a pair of hollow cylinders that are placed in the corpora cavernosa, and a pump with a release valve that is placed in the scrotum. This type of prosthesis more closely simulates a normal erection. The prosthesis selected depends primarily on client preference, his manual dexterity, the potential for subsequent urological problems requiring transurethral instrumentation, and financial considerations (the inflatable kind is more expensive). Either type of prosthesis will enable the client to achieve the basic goal of vaginal penetration.

This care plan focuses on the adult client hospitalized for insertion of a penile prosthesis. Preoperatively, goals of care are to reduce fear and anxiety and prepare the client for the surgical experience. Postoperative goals of care are to prevent complications, provide psychological support, and educate the client regarding follow-up care.

DISCHARGE CRITERIA

Prior to discharge, the client will:

- demonstrate the ability to operate and care for an inflatable prosthesis if present
- state signs and symptoms to report to the health care provider
- verbalize an understanding of and a plan for adhering to recommended follow-up care including future appointments with health care provider, medications prescribed, wound care, activity level, and resumption of sexual activity.

NURSING DIAGNOSES

Preoperative
1. Anxiety □ *1032*
Postoperative
1. Pain: perineal and penile □ *1033*
2. Potential for infection: wound □ *1033*
3. Body image disturbance □ *1034*
4. Knowledge deficit regarding follow-up care □ *1034*

Preoperative

Use in conjunction with the Standardized Preoperative Care Plan.

1. NURSING DIAGNOSIS

Anxiety related to unfamiliar environment, lack of understanding of the prosthesis and the effects of surgery, effects of anesthesia, anticipated postoperative discomfort, embarrassment about the need for and nature of the surgical procedure, and potential loss of dignity associated with exposure of the genitals during surgery and preoperative and postoperative care.

DESIRED OUTCOMES	NURSING ACTIONS AND *SELECTED RATIONALES*

1. The client will experience a reduction in fear and anxiety (see Standardized Preoperative Care Plan, Nursing Diagnosis 1, for outcome criteria).	1.a. Refer to Standardized Preoperative Care Plan, Nursing Diagnosis 1, for measures related to assessment and reduction of fear and anxiety.
	  b. Implement additional measures *to reduce fear and anxiety:*
	  1. reinforce physician's explanation about the type of prosthesis that will be used
	  2. if an inflatable prosthesis is to be inserted, use a teaching model, diagrams, or pictures to explain how it works
	  3. provide the following information to the client and his partner *to ensure that their expectations about the effects of the prosthesis are realistic:*
	    a. explain that the erection experienced with an implant will be similar to a normal erection depending on the type of prosthesis; reinforce the fact that sexual stimulation will still be necessary *to provide the sensation of sexual arousal usually associated with erection*
	    b. explain that an existing ability to have a partial erection may be permanently lessened by surgery
	    c. reinforce physician's explanation that the insertion of the prosthesis will not restore the capacity for climax and ejaculation
	  4. explain that the incision will be very small (usually 2.5 cm [1 inch]) and will not be visible once healing has occurred (for most of the prostheses, the incision is located at the penoscrotal junction)
	  5. arrange for a visit with a person who successfully uses a penile prosthesis if client desires
	  6. suggest that sexual counseling may help the couple adapt to the implant
	  7. inform the client receiving an inflatable prosthesis that it may be left partially inflated in the immediate postoperative period *in order to control bleeding* (depends on physician preference)
	  8. display a matter-of-fact attitude in initiating discussion about the prosthesis
	  9. express an understanding of client's feelings of embarrassment; assure client that many men have an implant and that his feelings are not unusual
	  10. assure client that he will not suffer needless body exposure during surgery and preoperative and postoperative care.

☐ ▬▬▬▬▬▬▬▬▬▬▬▬▬▬▬▬▬▬▬▬▬▬▬▬▬▬▬▬▬▬▬▬▬

Postoperative

Use in conjunction with the Standardized Postoperative Care Plan.

☐ ▬▬▬▬▬▬▬▬▬▬▬▬▬▬▬▬▬▬▬▬▬▬▬▬▬▬▬▬▬▬▬▬▬

1. NURSING DIAGNOSIS

Pain: perineal and penile related to tissue trauma during surgery, edema, and displacement of tissue associated with the implant.

☐ ▬▬▬▬▬▬▬▬▬▬▬▬▬▬▬▬▬▬▬▬▬▬▬▬▬▬▬▬▬▬▬▬▬

DESIRED OUTCOMES	NURSING ACTIONS AND *SELECTED RATIONALES*
1. The client will experience diminished perineal and penile pain as evidenced by: a. verbalization of pain relief b. relaxed facial expression and body positioning c. ability to sit and ambulate comfortably d. stable vital signs.	1.a. Refer to Standardized Postoperative Care Plan, Nursing Diagnosis 7.A, for measures related to assessment and management of postoperative pain. b. Implement additional measures *to reduce pain:* 1. apply ice packs to scrotum and penis for first 24 hours postoperatively as ordered 2. elevate penis and scrotum as ordered *to help reduce edema in operative area* 3. provide a flotation pad or foam ring for client to sit on when up in chair *in order to prevent pressure on surgical site.*

☐ ▬▬▬▬▬▬▬▬▬▬▬▬▬▬▬▬▬▬▬▬▬▬▬▬▬▬▬▬▬▬▬▬▬

2. NURSING DIAGNOSIS

Potential for infection: wound related to break in skin integrity and contamination of wound site with urine or feces.

☐ ▬▬▬▬▬▬▬▬▬▬▬▬▬▬▬▬▬▬▬▬▬▬▬▬▬▬▬▬▬▬▬▬▬

DESIRED OUTCOMES	NURSING ACTIONS AND *SELECTED RATIONALES*
2. The client will remain free of wound infection (see Standardized Postoperative Care Plan, Nursing Diagnosis 16, outcome b, for outcome criteria).	2.a. Refer to Standardized Postoperative Care Plan, Nursing Diagnosis 16, action b, for measures related to assessment, prevention, and treatment of infection at the surgical site. b. Implement additional measures *to promote wound healing and prevent infection of the surgical site:* 1. instruct and assist client to cleanse rectal area well after each bowel movement *in order to prevent wound contamination with feces* 2. change dressings and linen if they become contaminated with urine or feces 3. if client has an inflatable prosthesis, instruct him not to inflate it until permitted by physician *since full inflation earlier than this could interfere with wound healing* (many urologists prefer to do the initial inflation themselves about a week after discharge *in order to minimize risk of wound disruption*).

UNIT XVII

c. If signs and symptoms of wound infection occur:
1. prepare client for surgical removal and replacement of prosthesis (the corpora cavernosa are usually irrigated well with an anti-infective solution during the surgical procedure before the prosthesis is replaced)
2. monitor for therapeutic and nontherapeutic effects of anti-infectives if administered.

☐ ▬▬▬▬▬▬▬▬▬▬▬▬▬▬▬▬▬▬▬

3. NURSING DIAGNOSIS

Body image disturbance related to penile surgery and permanent erection if semi-rigid type of prosthesis has been inserted.

☐ ▬▬▬▬▬▬▬▬▬▬▬▬▬▬▬▬▬▬▬

DESIRED OUTCOMES	NURSING ACTIONS AND *SELECTED RATIONALES*
3. The client will demonstrate beginning integration of the change in appearance and functioning of the penis into body image as evidenced by: a. verbalization of feelings of self-worth and sexual adequacy b. willingness to discuss the prosthesis and its care c. resumption of usual activities of daily living d. maintenance of relationships with significant others e. active interest in personal appearance.	3.a. Determine the meaning of the change in body image to client by encouraging him to verbalize feelings and by noting nonverbal responses to the presence of the prosthesis. b. Assess for signs and symptoms of a disturbance in body image (e.g. verbal or nonverbal cues denoting a negative response to change in penile functioning and appearance such as denial of or preoccupation with the change that has occurred, refusal to look at or touch penis, or withdrawal from significant others). c. Assist client to identify strengths and qualities that have a positive effect on body image. d. Provide privacy during assessments, treatments, and hygienic care. e. Supply pajama bottoms in addition to hospital gown as soon as feasible *in order to provide added privacy for client.* f. Include partner in teaching sessions and encourage participation in operation of the pump *to promote acceptance and successful use of the prosthesis by the client and partner.* g. If a semi-rigid prosthesis was implanted, suggest methods for concealing permanent erection (e.g. wearing snug-fitting jockey or knit shorts with penis placed upward against abdomen, loose trousers or shirts, or top segment of women's pantyhose over underwear). h. Assess for and support behaviors suggesting positive adaptation to the change experienced (e.g. willingness to discuss implant and its effect on his life, maintenance of relationships with significant others). i. Assist client's and partner's adjustment by listening, facilitating communication, and providing information. j. Encourage visits and support from partner.

☐ ▬▬▬▬▬▬▬▬▬▬▬▬▬▬▬▬▬▬▬

4. NURSING DIAGNOSIS

Knowledge deficit regarding follow-up care.

☐ ▬▬▬▬▬▬▬▬▬▬▬▬▬▬▬▬▬▬▬

DESIRED OUTCOMES	NURSING ACTIONS AND *SELECTED RATIONALES*
4.a. The client will demonstrate the ability to operate and	4.a.1. Use a model to demonstrate how to inflate and deflate the prosthesis. 2. If client has a multicomponent inflatable prosthesis:

care for an inflatable prosthesis if present.

    a. use a model to demonstrate how to locate pump and pull it to the lowest part of the scrotum (physician may want client to do this daily beginning the 2nd to 7th postoperative day for 4–6 weeks *in order to maintain proper pump position*)

    b. caution client to avoid compressing the pump too firmly (*excessive pressure can occlude fluid flow*)

    c. assure client and partner that it takes time to become proficient in operating the prosthesis, particularly the release valve *because it is small and can be difficult to locate.*

3. Inform client that he will be required to inflate and deflate the device daily for 6 weeks beginning 3–4 weeks after surgery *in order to promote formation of fibrous tissue around the implant.* Instruct client to maintain inflation for about 15 minutes.

4. Allow time for questions, clarification, practice, and return demonstration of inflation and deflation of the prosthesis on the model.

4.b. The client will state signs and symptoms to report to the health care provider.

4.b.1. Refer to Standardized Postoperative Care Plan, Nursing Diagnosis 20, action c, for signs and symptoms to report to the health care provider.

2. Instruct the client to report these additional signs and symptoms:
    a. difficulty with inflation or deflation of prosthesis
    b. inability to pull pump into lowest part of the scotum
    c. persistent or intensified perineal or penile pain
    d. persistent penile or scrotal edema
    e. breakdown of skin surrounding implant
    f. bending of the glans during vaginal penetration.

4.c. The client will verbalize an understanding of and a plan for adhering to recommended follow-up care including future appointments with health care provider, medications prescribed, wound care, activity level, and resumption of sexual activity.

4.c.1. Refer to Standardized Postoperative Care Plan, Nursing Diagnosis 20, for routine postoperative instructions and measures to improve client compliance.

2. Caution client to avoid strenuous activity for approximately 3 weeks.

3. Explain that sexual activity should be delayed until sufficient healing has occurred and permission is given by the physician (usually 3 weeks for semi-rigid and 6 weeks for inflatable prosthesis).

4. Emphasize the need for adequate lubrication during intercourse *to prevent trauma to recently healed penile tissue.*

5. Instruct client with either type of prosthesis to avoid constrictive underwear (e.g. jockey shorts, athletic support) until healing is complete (at least 3 weeks postoperatively) *in order to prevent undue pressure on the surgical site.*

6. If client has decreased sensation in penile area associated with underlying medical condition, instruct him to periodically check that excessive pressure is not being placed on penis.

Prostatectomy

A **prostatectomy** is the surgical removal of the prostate gland, although in most cases only the prostatic adenoma is removed and the true prostate and fibrous capsule are left intact. A prostatectomy may be performed to treat cancer of the prostate or, more frequently, to remove a benign prostatic neoplasm that has enlarged enough to block the bladder outlet or urethra and impede the flow of urine. The most frequent cause of a benign neoplasm is benign prostatic hypertrophy or hyperplasia (BPH).

This condition is common in men over 50 years of age and is believed to result from the changes in estrogen and androgen levels that occur with aging. Surgical treatment of BPH is indicated when signs and symptoms (e.g. urgency, frequency, hesitancy, decreased force of urinary stream, nocturia, urinary incontinence) interfere with life style or complications such as recurrent urinary tract infection, urinary retention, severe hematuria, renal calculi, or hydronephrosis occur.

UNIT XVII

The four surgical approaches that may be used to perform a prostatectomy are the suprapubic, retropubic (retrovesical), perineal, and transurethral approaches. The transurethral approach is used most frequently. The type of approach selected depends on the size of the prostate, diagnosis, and client's age and health status. A radical prostatectomy (removal of the entire prostate gland, seminal vesicles, cuff of the bladder neck, and possibly the pelvic lymph nodes) may be performed via the retropubic or perineal approach to treat cancer of the prostate.

This care plan focuses on the adult client hospitalized for a prostatectomy.* Preoperative goals of care are to reduce fear and anxiety and promote adequate urinary elimination. Postoperatively, goals of care are to maintain comfort, prevent complications, provide emotional support, and educate the client regarding follow-up care.

---

* The care plan is directed mainly at surgical removal of a benign prostatic neoplasm. If the client is having surgery as treatment for cancer of the prostate, use in conjunction with the Care Plan on Cancer of the Prostate.

DISCHARGE CRITERIA

Prior to discharge, the client will:

- identify ways to prevent bleeding in the surgical area
- identify ways to regain or maintain control of bladder emptying
- demonstrate care of urinary catheter if present
- share feelings and concerns about changes in body functioning that may occur as a result of a prostatectomy
- state signs and symptoms of complications to report to the health care provider
- verbalize an understanding of and a plan for adhering to recommended follow-up care including future appointments with health care provider, medications prescribed, activity level, and wound care.

NURSING/COLLABORATIVE DIAGNOSES

Preoperative
  1. Anxiety ☐ *1037*
  2. Urinary retention ☐ *1037*
Postoperative
  1. Altered fluid balance: fluid volume excess or water intoxication ☐ *1039*
  2. Altered comfort:
     a. pain
     b. bladder spasms ☐ *1039*
  3. Altered pattern of urinary elimination:
     a. retention
     b. incontinence following catheter removal ☐ *1040*
  4. Bowel incontinence ☐ *1042*
  5. Potential for infection:
     a. wound infection
     b. urinary tract infection ☐ *1042*
  6. Potential complications:
     a. shock
     b. thromboembolism
     c. epididymitis ☐ *1043*
  7. Sexual dysfunction:
     a. decreased libido
     b. impotence ☐ *1045*
  8. Disturbance in self-concept ☐ *1046*
  9. Grieving ☐ *1047*
  10. Knowledge deficit regarding follow-up care ☐ *1048*

Preoperative

Use in conjunction with the Standardized Preoperative Care Plan.

1. NURSING DIAGNOSIS

Anxiety related to unfamiliar environment, potential embarrassment or loss of dignity associated with exposure of genitals during surgery and preoperative and post-operative care, effects of anesthesia, and anticipated postoperative discomfort and effects of surgery on body functioning.

DESIRED OUTCOMES	NURSING ACTIONS AND *SELECTED RATIONALES*

1. The client will experience a reduction in fear and anxiety (see Standardized Preoperative Care Plan, Nursing Diagnosis 1, for outcome criteria).	1.a. Refer to Standardized Preoperative Care Plan, Nursing Diagnosis 1, for measures related to assessment and reduction of fear and anxiety.
	b. Implement additional measures *to reduce fear and anxiety*:
	   1. allow time for verbalization of concerns regarding the possible effect of surgery on body functioning (e.g. urinary incontinence after the transurethral approach; temporary or permanent infertility after the transurethral, retropubic, and suprapubic approaches; sterility, impotence, and urinary and bowel incontinence after the perineal approach and/or a radical prostatectomy)
	   2. instruct client to expect the following postoperatively *so that he is not overly concerned when they occur*:
	      a. presence of suprapubic urinary catheter (with suprapubic approach or some radical prostatectomies) and/or urethral catheter
	      b. red urine in drainage tubing
	      c. blood clots in the urine
	      d. bloody drainage around urinary catheter(s)
	      e. large amount of drainage from incisions and drains, frequent dressing changes, and/or presence of drainage collection bags over drains (if perineal, suprapubic, or retropubic approach is used)
	      f. feeling of an urgent need to urinate or defecate (may indicate bladder spasms)
	   3. explain to client that urinary symptoms such as urgency, frequency, hesitancy, dribbling, and incontinence that are present before surgery may still continue after catheter removal postoperatively *as a result of poor bladder tone and trauma from the surgery and urethral catheter*; assure client that urinary pattern usually improves with time (may take months to a year).

2. NURSING DIAGNOSIS

Urinary retention related to:

a. obstruction of the urethra and/or bladder neck by the enlarged prostate or blood clots (bleeding may occur as a result of trauma to the bladder vessels due to

client's straining to urinate and/or rapid decompression of the bladder following catheterization);
b. loss of bladder tone associated with hypertrophy of the bladder resulting from the gradual increase in residual urine as obstruction progressed.

□ ▆▆

DESIRED OUTCOMES	NURSING ACTIONS AND *SELECTED RATIONALES*

2. The client will experience resolution of urinary retention if it occurs as evidenced by:
a. no complaints of urgency, bladder fullness, and suprapubic discomfort
b. absence of suprapubic distention
c. balanced intake and output.
	2.a. Gather baseline data regarding client's usual urinary elimination pattern.
	b. Assess for signs and symptoms of urinary retention:
	  1. frequent voiding of small amounts (25–50 cc) of urine
	  2. complaints of urgency, bladder fullness, or suprapubic discomfort
	  3. suprapubic distention
	  4. output less than intake.
	c. Catheterize client if ordered *to determine the amount of residual urine.*
	d. Implement measures *to treat urinary retention:*
	  1. perform actions *to promote complete bladder emptying:*
	    a. instruct and assist client to perform the Credé technique unless contraindicated
	    b. allow client to assume normal position for voiding
	  2. monitor for therapeutic and nontherapeutic effects of cholinergic drugs (e.g. bethanechol) if administered *to stimulate bladder contraction*
	  3. if signs and symptoms of urinary retention persist:
	    a. insert a urethral catheter as ordered (if insertion is difficult because of obstruction of the prostatic urethra or bladder neck, it may be necessary to use a stylet or a firm, specially angled catheter)
	    b. assist with insertion of a suprapubic catheter if unable to insert a urethral catheter because of obstruction
	    c. after catheter insertion, gradually decompress the bladder (e.g. clamp catheter for 15 minutes after each 300 cc of urine output until decompression is complete or clamp catheter for 30 minutes after 600 cc of urine output and then unclamp to decompress bladder completely) according to hospital policy or physician's orders *in order to reduce risk of bleeding (rapid decompression can rupture blood vessels in the stretched bladder mucosa) and fluid and electrolyte imbalances (due to postobstructive diuresis)*
	  4. if indwelling catheter is present:
	    a. keep drainage tubing free of kinks
	    b. keep collection container below level of bladder
	    c. tape catheter securely to abdomen or thigh *in order to prevent inadvertent removal*
	    d. perform intermittent catheter irrigations with normal saline and/or maintain continuous bladder irrigation with normal saline *(to flush out clots)* or silver nitrate solution *(to control bleeding)* as ordered.
	e. Consult physician if signs and symptoms of urinary retention persist despite implementation of above actions.

Postoperative

Use in conjunction with the Standardized Postoperative Care Plan.

1. NURSING DIAGNOSIS

Altered fluid balance: fluid volume excess or water intoxication related to:

a. vigorous fluid therapy during and immediately after surgery;
b. increased production of antidiuretic hormone (ADH) and aldosterone associated with trauma, pain, anesthetic agents, and narcotic analgesics (especially after a radical prostatectomy, which is a more extensive surgery and has a longer recovery period);
c. excessive absorption of irrigating solution during surgery via the venous sinusoids in the prostate gland.

DESIRED OUTCOMES	NURSING ACTIONS AND *SELECTED RATIONALES*

1. The client will not experience fluid volume excess or water intoxication (see Standardized Postoperative Care Plan, Nursing Diagnosis 5, outcome b, for outcome criteria).	1.a. Refer to Standardized Postoperative Care Plan, Nursing Diagnosis 5, action b, for measures related to assessment, prevention, and treatment of fluid volume excess and water intoxication.
	 b. Implement additional measures *to prevent fluid volume excess:*
	   1. use normal saline rather than hypotonic solutions for bladder irrigations *to reduce risk of additional fluid absorption and subsequent water intoxication*
	   2. do not increase frequency of bladder irrigations or speed up continuous irrigation unless indicated *in order to decrease risk of further absorption of fluids.*

2. NURSING DIAGNOSIS

Altered comfort:*

a. **pain** related to tissue trauma and reflex muscle spasm associated with the surgical procedure (especially with retropubic, suprapubic, and perineal approaches);
b. **bladder spasms** related to:
  1. irritation of the bladder wall associated with tissue trauma during surgery (especially with transurethral and suprapubic approaches), presence of urinary catheter(s), rapid infusion of irrigation solution, and urine retention (causes overdistention of the bladder)
  2. pressure on the bladder neck and prostatic fossa when traction is applied to the urethral catheter (traction may be applied to pull the catheter balloon into the prostatic fossa in order to put pressure on bleeding vessels).

---

* In this care plan, the nursing diagnosis "pain" is included under the diagnostic label of altered comfort.

DESIRED OUTCOMES	NURSING ACTIONS AND *SELECTED RATIONALES*

2.a. The client will experience diminished pain (see Standardized Postoperative Care Plan, Nursing Diagnosis 7.A, for outcome criteria).

2.a.1. Refer to Standardized Postoperative Care Plan, Nursing Diagnosis 7.A, for measures related to assessment and management of pain.
　2. Implement additional measures *to reduce pain:*
　　a. instruct client to avoid straining to have a bowel movement *in order to prevent increased pressure on operative site*; consult physician about an order for a stool softener or laxative if indicated
　　b. if client has a perineal incision:
　　　1. provide a pillow or foam pad for him to sit on if desired
　　　2. apply warm, moist compresses to perineum and/or assist with sitz baths if ordered following removal of wound drains (some physicians will not order sitz baths until urethral catheter is also removed).

2.b. The client will experience relief of bladder spasms as evidenced by:
　1. verbalization of relief of suprapubic discomfort
　2. no complaints of an urgent need to urinate or defecate
　3. no leakage of urine around the urinary catheter(s).

2.b.1. Assess for signs and symptoms of bladder spasms:
　　a. complaints of suprapubic discomfort
　　b. statements of an urgent need to urinate or defecate
　　c. leakage of urine around the urinary catheter(s).
　2. Implement measures *to decrease risk of bladder spasms:*
　　a. maintain patency of urethral and, if present, suprapubic catheters (e.g. irrigate as needed, keep tubing free of kinks) *to prevent overdistention of bladder*
　　b. perform actions *to keep urinary catheter(s) from irritating bladder mucosa:*
　　　1. tape suprapubic catheter securely to client's abdomen and tape urethral catheter securely to his abdomen or thigh
　　　2. instruct client to avoid pulling on and twisting the urinary catheter(s)
　　c. release traction on the urethral catheter as soon as ordered *to reduce pressure on the bladder neck and prostatic fossa*
　　d. do not increase frequency of bladder irrigations or speed up continuous irrigation unless bleeding or clots are present *because irrigating solution can irritate bladder mucosa* (especially if the solution contains silver nitrate, which may be ordered *to control bleeding*).
　3. If bladder spasms occur:
　　a. encourage client to take short, frequent walks unless contraindicated *(walking seems to reduce spasms)*
　　b. decrease the rate of continuous bladder irrigation if urine is not red and clots are not present
　　c. monitor for therapeutic and nontherapeutic effects of antispasmodics (e.g. probantheline bromide) and analgesics if administered.
　4. Consult physician if above measures fail to control bladder spasms.

3. NURSING DIAGNOSIS

Altered pattern of urinary elimination:

a. **retention** related to:
　1. obstruction of the urinary catheter(s)
　2. difficulty urinating following removal of the catheter(s) associated with:
　　a. loss of bladder tone due to overdistention of bladder preoperatively
　　b. surgical site discomfort
　　c. obstruction of the urethra and bladder neck by blood clots or edema resulting from surgical trauma and irritation of the tissues by the urinary catheter(s), particularly if traction had been applied to the urethral catheter to control bleeding;

b. **incontinence following catheter removal** related to:
1. trauma to the urinary sphincter resulting from surgical instrumentation (mainly with a transurethral approach) and presence of urethral catheter
2. damage to urinary sphincter and perineal nerves and muscles (occurs primarily after a perineal approach and/or radical prostatectomy)
3. decreased bladder capacity associated with continued decompression of the bladder while the suprapubic and/or urethral catheters were in place.

DESIRED OUTCOMES	NURSING ACTIONS AND *SELECTED RATIONALES*
3.a. The client will not experience urinary retention as evidenced by: 1. no complaints of bladder fullness and suprapubic discomfort 2. absence of suprapubic distention 3. balanced intake and output within 48 hours after surgery 4. voiding adequate amounts at expected intervals after removal of catheter(s).	3.a.1. Assess for and report the following: a. urinary retention when suprapubic and/or urethral catheters are present (e.g. complaints of bladder fullness or suprapubic discomfort, suprapubic distention, absence of fluid in urinary drainage tubing [especially if continuous bladder irrigation is running], output that continues to be less than intake 48 hours after surgery) b. increasing obstruction of the urethra or bladder neck after urethral catheter removal (e.g. complaints of decreasing size of urinary stream, increasing need to strain to empty bladder, increasing frequency and urgency) c. urinary retention following removal of catheters (e.g. complaints of bladder fullness or suprapubic discomfort, frequent voiding of small amounts [25–50 cc] of urine, increasing complaints of urgency, suprapubic distention, output that continues to be less than intake 48 hours after surgery). 2. Implement measures to maintain patency of urinary catheters (see Preoperative Nursing Diagnosis 2, action d.4) *in order to prevent urinary retention when catheters are present.* 3. Following removal of urinary catheter(s), implement the following measures *to prevent urinary retention:* a. perform actions *to facilitate voiding* (e.g. provide privacy, allow client to assume normal position for voiding, run water, place client's hands in warm water, encourage client to void while relaxing in bathtub or sitz bath) b. instruct client to void whenever the urge is first felt (*bladder is still hypotonic and can easily become distended*) c. have urinal within easy reach or assist client to the bathroom every 2–3 hours d. perform actions to relieve discomfort (see Postoperative Nursing Diagnosis 2, actions a and b.2 and 3). 4. If signs and symptoms of urinary retention occur after removal of the urinary catheter(s), consult physician about intermittent catheterization or reinsertion of an indwelling catheter.
3.b. The client will experience urinary continence.	3.b.1. Assess for urinary incontinence after removal of urinary catheters. (A urethral catheter is usually removed 2–3 days after a transurethral approach, 5–7 days after a suprapubic or retropubic approach, and 10–14 days after a perineal approach and/or a radical prostatectomy. A suprapubic catheter, which may be inserted during the suprapubic approach or radical prostatectomy, is usually removed a few days before or after the urethral catheter depending on physician preference.) 2. Implement measures *to maintain urinary continence:* a. perform actions *to prevent trauma to the urinary sphincter while the urethral catheter is in place in order to reduce the risk of urinary incontinence following removal of the catheter(s):* 1. if traction is ordered to control bleeding, release it as soon as allowed (traction should not be maintained for longer than 4–6 hours without being released) *in order to reduce pressure on the urinary sphincter*

      2. tape urethral catheter securely to client's abdomen or thigh *in order to prevent excessive movement of the catheter*

  b. following removal of catheter(s):
      1. offer urinal or assist client to commode or bathroom every 2–3 hours
      2. allow client to assume normal position for voiding unless contraindicated *in order to promote complete emptying of bladder*
      3. instruct client to perform perineal exercises (e.g. stopping and starting stream during voiding; pressing buttocks together, then relaxing the muscles) *in order to improve urinary sphincter tone*
      4. limit oral fluid intake in the evening *to decrease the possibility of nighttime incontinence*
      5. instruct client to avoid drinking beverages containing caffeine *(caffeine is a mild diuretic and may make urinary control more difficult)*
      6. consult physician before administering antispasmodic agents for reduction of bladder spasms *(these drugs relax urinary sphincter and can increase the risk of incontinence)*
      7. monitor for therapeutic and nontheraeutic effects of alpha-adrenergic agonists (e.g. ephedrine) if administered *to increase tone of urinary sphincter.*

3. If urinary incontinence persists:
  a. consult physician regarding intermittent catheterization, insertion of indwelling catheter, or use of external catheter
  b. provide emotional support to client and significant others.

☐ ▬▬▬▬▬▬▬▬▬▬▬▬▬▬▬▬▬▬

4. NURSING DIAGNOSIS

Bowel incontinence related to damage to the rectal sphincter during surgery, compression of the nerves controlling the rectal sphincter (may occur during surgery and as a result of postoperative edema in the surgical area), and/or incision of perianal muscles (especially with a perineal approach and/or radical prostatectomy).

☐ ▬▬▬▬▬▬▬▬▬▬▬▬▬▬▬▬▬▬

DESIRED OUTCOMES	NURSING ACTIONS AND *SELECTED RATIONALES*

4. The client will regain usual bowel function.	4.a. Monitor for episodes of bowel incontinence.
	b. Instruct client to perform perineal exercises (e.g. stopping and starting stream during voiding; pressing buttocks together, then relaxing the muscles) *in order to improve tone of perianal muscles and subsequently reduce risk of bowel incontinence.*
	c. If bowel incontinence occurs:
	  1. instruct client to adhere to a bowel training program *in order to promote scheduled bowel evacuation and decrease risk of incontinence*
	  2. provide client with disposable liners for underwear or absorbent undergarments such as Attends if needed
	  3. provide emotional support to client and significant others.

☐ ▬▬▬▬▬▬▬▬▬▬▬▬▬▬▬▬▬▬

5. NURSING DIAGNOSIS

Potential for infection:

a. **wound infection** related to wound contamination (especially with a perineal approach because incision is close to the anus);

b. **urinary tract infection** related to instrumentation of urinary tract during surgery, presence of indwelling urinary catheter(s), frequent bladder irrigations, and urinary retention.

DESIRED OUTCOMES	NURSING ACTIONS AND *SELECTED RATIONALES*

5.a. The client will not experience wound infection (see Standardized Postoperative Care Plan, Nursing Diagnosis 16, outcome b, for outcome criteria).	5.a.1. Refer to Standardized Postoperative Care Plan, Nursing Diagnosis 16, action b, for measures related to assessment, prevention, and treatment of wound infection.
	2. If a perineal approach was used, implement additional measures *to prevent wound infection:*
	  a. instruct and assist client to perform good perineal care immediately after bowel movements
	  b. perform actions *to reduce trauma to the surgical area:*
	    1. instruct client to avoid sitting for prolonged periods
	    2. use a double-tailed T-binder, scrotal support, or jockey shorts to secure perineal dressings *(loose dressings can irritate wound)*
	    3. take oral rather than rectal temperatures
	    4. avoid use of rectal suppositories, rectal tubes, and enemas
	  c. consult physician regarding:
	    1. use of heat lamp or application of warm compresses to perineum *in order to promote healing*
	    2. order for sitz bath *to cleanse the wound and promote healing* (this will usually not be ordered until wound drains and urethral catheter are removed).

5.b. The client will not experience urinary tract infection (see Standardized Postoperative Care Plan, Nursing Diagnosis 16, outcome c, for outcome criteria).	5.b.1. Refer to Standardized Postoperative Care Plan, Nursing Diagnosis 16, action c, for measures related to assessment, prevention, and treatment of urinary tract infection.
	2. Implement additional measures *to prevent urinary tract infection:*
	  a. perform actions to prevent urinary retention (see Postoperative Nursing Diagnosis 3, actions a.2 and 3)
	  b. consult physician about removal of the urinary catheter(s) as soon as the urine is clear and free of clots *(risk of urinary tract infection increases the longer the urinary catheters are in place).*

6. COLLABORATIVE DIAGNOSIS

Potential complications:

a. **shock** related to:
　1. hypovolemia associated with hemorrhage (the prostate gland is very vascular), excessive fluid loss, and inadequate fluid replacement
　2. septicemia (septic shock) associated with infection (there is a high correlation between urinary tract infection and septicemia);
b. **thromboembolism** related to:
　1. trauma to the large pelvic veins as a result of manipulation during surgery (can occur with retropubic, suprapubic, and perineal approaches)
　2. venous stasis associated with:
　　a. pressure on the pelvic and calf vessels during surgery if the client was in lithotomy position (this position is used for the transurethral and perineal approaches)
　　b. decreased activity;
c. **epididymitis** related to reflux of urine into the vas deferens (can occur if a vasectomy is not performed before or during surgery).

DESIRED OUTCOMES	NURSING ACTIONS AND *SELECTED RATIONALES*

6.a. The client will not develop shock (see Standardized Postoperative Care Plan, Collaborative Diagnosis 19, outcome a, for outcome criteria).

6.a.1. Assess for and report the following:
    a. excessive operative site bleeding:
       1. excessive bloody drainage on dressings or from drains
       2. bright red, viscous drainage (could indicate arterial bleeding) or persistent darker drainage (venous bleeding) in urinary catheter(s)
       3. persistent redness of and blood clots in serial urines after removal of the catheter(s)
       4. significant decline in RBC, Hct., and Hgb. levels
    b. persistent vomiting
    c. difficulty maintaining intravenous or oral fluid intake as ordered
    d. signs and symptoms of septic shock:
       1. early or hyperdynamic stage (e.g. confusion; chills and fever; warm, flushed skin; lower extremity mottling; tachycardia; tachypnea)
       2. hypodynamic stage (e.g. cool, clammy skin; severe hypotension; tachycardia; thready pulse; cyanosis; low pH and CO_2 content; oliguria or anuria; respiratory insufficiency or failure)
    e. signs and symptoms of hypovolemic shock (see Standardized Postoperative Care Plan, Collaborative Diagnosis 19, action a.3).
  2. Refer to Standardized Postoperative Care Plan, Collaborative Diagnosis 19, action a.4 for measures to prevent shock.
  3. Implement additional measures *to prevent shock:*
    a. perform actions *to prevent and control hemorrhage:*
       1. implement measures *to minimize strain or pressure on the prostatic area:*
          a. tape urethral catheter tubing securely to client's abdomen or thigh *in order to minimize movement of catheter*
          b. caution client to avoid pulling on the urethral catheter; utilize wrist restraints if necessary
          c. perform actions to prevent urinary retention (see Postoperative Nursing Diagnosis 3, actions a.2 and 3) *in order to avoid overdistention of the bladder, which could create strain on the newly coagulated blood vessels*
          d. instruct client to avoid sitting or standing for long periods
          e. instruct client to avoid coughing, sneezing, and straining to have a bowel movement; consult physician regarding an order for antitussives, decongestants, stool softeners, and laxatives if indicated
       2. maintain traction on the urethral catheter as ordered *so that the catheter balloon exerts direct pressure on bleeding vessels in prostatic fossa*
       3. maintain continuous bladder irrigation of a silver nitrate solution if ordered *to cauterize the exposed vessels of the prostatic fossa*
       4. instruct client to return to bed and limit activity for a few hours if urine becomes more red when ambulating or sitting in chair
       5. monitor for therapeutic and nontherapeutic effects of hemostatic agent (e.g. aminocaproic acid) if administered
    b. perform actions to prevent and/or treat urinary tract and wound infections (see Postoperative Nursing Diagnosis 5, actions a and b) *in order to reduce the risk of septicemia.*
  4. Implement measures to treat shock if it occurs (see Standardized Postoperative Care Plan, Collaborative Diagnosis 19, action a.5).

6.b. The client will not develop a venous thrombus or pulmonary embolism (see Standardized Postoperative Care Plan, Collaborative Diagnosis 19, outcomes c.1 and 2, for outcome criteria).

6.b. Refer to Standardized Postoperative Care Plan, Collaborative Diagnosis 19, actions c.1 and 2, for measures related to assessment, prevention, and treatment of a venous thrombus and pulmonary embolism. Be aware that prophylactic anticoagulant and antiplatelet medications are usually contraindicated *because of the high risk of hemorrhage during and following surgery on the vascular prostate gland.*

6.c. The client will experience resolution of epididymitis if it occurs as evidenced by:

6.c.1. Assess for and report signs and symptoms of epididymitis (e.g. scrotal tenderness, pain, and swelling; fever and chills).
  2. If epididymitis occurs:

1. no complaints of scrotal pain and tenderness
2. resolution of scrotal edema
3. absence of chills and fever.

a. maintain activity restrictions as ordered (usually bedrest)
b. elevate scrotum on folded towel or scrotal bridge
c. apply cold compresses to scrotum intermittently during the first 24 hours after signs and symptoms appear
d. consult physician about an order for sitz bath or application of warm compresses following the period that cold compresses are applied (use heat cautiously *because excessive heat can lead to destruction of sperm cells*)
e. encourage client to wear a scrotal support when activity increases
f. monitor for therapeutic and nontherapeutic effects of anti-infectives if administered.

□ ▬▬▬▬▬▬▬▬▬▬▬▬▬▬▬▬▬▬▬▬▬▬▬

7. NURSING DIAGNOSIS

Sexual dysfunction:

a. **decreased libido** related to fear of urinary and/or bowel incontinence, alteration in self-concept, and surgical site discomfort (especially following a retropubic, suprapubic, or perineal prostatectomy);
b. **impotence** related to damage to the prostatic plexus (includes sympathetic and parasympathetic nerves) during surgery (can occur during the perineal approach and/or a radical prostatectomy).

□ ▬▬▬▬▬▬▬▬▬▬▬▬▬▬▬▬▬▬▬▬▬▬▬

DESIRED OUTCOMES	NURSING ACTIONS AND *SELECTED RATIONALES*

7. The client will demonstrate beginning acceptance of changes in sexual functioning as evidenced by:
   a. verbalization of a perception of self as sexually acceptable and adequate
   b. maintenance of relationships with significant others.

7.a. Assess for signs and symptoms of sexual dysfunction (e.g. verbalization of sexual concerns, failure to maintain relationships with significant others).
  b. Determine attitudes, knowledge, and concerns about the prostatectomy in relation to sexual functioning.
  c. Communicate interest, understanding, and respect for the values of the client and his partner.
  d. Provide accurate information about effects of prostatectomy on sexual functioning. Encourage questions and clarify misconceptions.
  e. Facilitate communication between client and partner. Assist them to identify changes that may affect their sexual relationship.
  f. Arrange for uninterrupted privacy during hospital stay if desired by the couple.
  g. Implement measures to improve self-concept (see Postoperative Nursing Diagnosis 8, actions c–p).
  h. If impotence is a problem:
    1. discuss ways to be creative in expressing sexuality (e.g. massage, fantasies, cuddling)
    2. suggest alternative methods of sexual gratification and use of assistive devices if appropriate
    3. encourage client to discuss the possibility of a penile prosthesis with physician if desired.
  i. If incontinence of urine or stool is a problem:
    1. reinforce the importance of continuing to do perineal exercises *in order to improve bowel and bladder control*
    2. encourage client to void and/or defecate just before sexual activity.
  j. If client is concerned that operative site discomfort will interfere with usual sexual activity:
    1. assure him that the discomfort is temporary and will diminish as incision heals
    2. encourage alternatives to intercourse and, when intercourse is allowed, use of positions that decrease pressure on the surgical site (e.g. side-lying).

UNIT
XVII

k. Include partner in above discussions and encourage his/her continued support.
l. Consult physician if counseling appears indicated.

☐ ▬▬▬▬▬▬▬▬▬▬▬▬▬▬▬▬▬▬▬▬▬

8. NURSING DIAGNOSIS

Disturbance in self-concept* related to:

a. urinary incontinence (usually resolves but may be permanent depending on the extensiveness of surgery);
b. bowel incontinence (especially with a perineal approach and/or radical prostatectomy);
c. infertility associated with retrograde ejaculation resulting from direct trauma to the urinary sphincter and/or surgical incision of the nerves supplying the bladder neck;
d. sterility associated with removal of the entire prostate gland and seminal vesicles during a radical prostatectomy;
e. alteration in sexual functioning.

---

* This diagnostic label includes the nursing diagnoses of body image disturbance and self-esteem disturbance.

☐ ▬▬▬▬▬▬▬▬▬▬▬▬▬▬▬▬▬▬▬▬▬

DESIRED OUTCOMES	NURSING ACTIONS AND *SELECTED RATIONALES*

8. The client will demonstrate beginning adaptation to changes in body functioning as evidenced by:
a. verbalization of feelings of self-worth and sexual adequacy
b. maintenance of relationships with significant others
c. active participation in activities of daily living
d. active interest in personal appearance
e. willingness to participate in social activities.
	8.a. Determine the meaning of changes in body functioning to the client by encouraging him to verbalize feelings and by noting nonverbal responses to the changes experienced.
	b. Assess for signs and symptoms of a disturbance in self-concept (e.g. verbal or nonverbal cues denoting a negative response to changes in body functioning such as denial of or preoccupation with changes that have occurred, refusal to look at or touch a body part, or withdrawal from significant others).
	c. Implement measures to facilitate the grieving process (see Postoperative Nursing Diagnosis 9, action d).
	d. Assist client to identify strengths and qualities that have a positive effect on self-concept.
	e. Implement measures *to assist client to improve self-esteem* (e.g. limit negative self-criticism, encourage positive comments about self, give positive feedback about accomplishments).
	f. Assist client to identify and utilize coping techniques that have been helpful in the past.
	g. Reinforce actions that may assist client to adjust to alteration in sexual functioning (see Postoperative Nursing Diagnosis 7, actions c–k).
	h. Assist client with usual grooming if necessary.
	i. Provide privacy during catheter care and dressing changes.
	j. If incontinence of urine or stool is a problem:
	  1. reinforce the importance of continuing to do perineal exercises *in order to improve bowel and bladder control*
	  2. assist client to establish a bowel training program *to reduce incidence of bowel incontinence*
	  3. reinforce proper application of external catheter if indicated
	  4. instruct client in ways to minimize incontinence *so that social interaction is possible* (e.g. placing disposable liners in underwear, wearing absorbent undergarments such as Attends).

k. If impotence, infertility, or sterility is expected, discuss alternative methods of becoming a parent (e.g. adoption, artificial insemination) if of concern to client.

l. Assess for and support behaviors suggesting positive adaptation to changes experienced (e.g. verbalization of feelings of self-worth, participation in treatment plan, maintenance of relationships with others).

m. Assist client's and significant others' adjustment by listening, facilitating communication, and providing information.

n. Encourage visits and support from significant others.

o. Encourage client to continue involvement in social activities and to pursue interests.

p. Provide information and encourage utilization of community resources (e.g. sexual, family, and individual counseling).

q. Consult physician about psychological counseling if client desires or if he seems unwilling or unable to adapt to changes that have occurred as a result of the prostatectomy.

□ ▬▬▬▬▬▬▬▬▬▬▬▬▬▬▬▬

9. NURSING DIAGNOSIS

Grieving* related to temporary or permanent loss of normal sexual functioning and bowel and/or bladder control.

_____

* This diagnostic label includes anticipatory grieving and grieving following the actual losses/changes.

□ ▬▬▬▬▬▬▬▬▬▬▬▬▬▬▬▬

DESIRED OUTCOMES	NURSING ACTIONS AND *SELECTED RATIONALES*

9. The client will demonstrate beginning progression through the grieving process as evidenced by:
a. verbalization of feelings about changes in body functioning
b. expression of grief
c. participation in self-care activities
d. utilization of available support systems.
	9.a. Determine client's perception of the impact of the loss of sexual functioning and bowel and/or bladder control on his future.
	b. Determine how client usually expresses grief.
	c. Observe for signs of grieving (e.g. changes in eating habits, insomnia, anger, noncompliance, denial).
	d. Implement measures *to facilitate the grieving process:*
	  1. assist client to acknowledge the losses and changes experienced *so grief work can begin*; assess for factors that may hinder or facilitate acknowledgment
	  2. discuss the grieving process and assist client to accept the stages of grieving as an expected response to actual and/or anticipated changes or losses
	  3. allow time for client to progress through the stages of grieving (denial, anger, bargaining, depression, acceptance [Kübler-Ross, 1969]); be aware that not every stage is experienced or expressed by all individuals
	  4. provide an atmosphere of care and concern (e.g. provide privacy, be available and nonjudgmental, display empathy and respect) *so that client will feel free to verbalize both positive and negative feelings and concerns*
	  5. perform actions *to promote trust* (e.g. answer questions honestly, provide requested information)
	  6. encourage the expression of anger and sadness about the losses and changes experienced
	  7. encourage client to express his feelings in whatever ways are comfortable (e.g. writing, drawing, conversation)
	  8. assist client to identify personal strengths that have helped him to cope in previous situations of loss or change
	  9. if appropriate, support realistic hope that bowel and/or bladder control will improve if he continues to do perineal exercises.

e. Assess for and support behaviors suggesting successful resolution of grief (e.g. verbalizing feelings about loss of sexual functioning and bowel and/or bladder control, expressing sorrow, focusing on ways to adapt to changes that have occurred).

f. Explain the stages of the grieving process to significant others. Encourage their support and understanding.

g. Provide information about counseling services and support groups that might assist client in working through grief.

h. Arrange for visit from clergy if desired by client.

i. Monitor for therapeutic and nontherapeutic effects of antidepressants if administered.

j. Consult physician regarding referral for counseling if signs of dysfunctional grieving (e.g. persistent denial of losses or changes, excessive anger or sadness, hysteria, suicidal behaviors, phobias) occur.

☐ ▐▬▬▬▬▬▬▬▬▬▬▬▬▬▬▬▬▬▬▬▬▬▬▬▬

10. NURSING DIAGNOSIS

Knowledge deficit regarding follow-up care.

☐ ▐▬▬▬▬▬▬▬▬▬▬▬▬▬▬▬▬▬▬▬▬▬▬▬▬

DESIRED OUTCOMES	NURSING ACTIONS AND *SELECTED RATIONALES*
10.a. The client will identify ways to prevent bleeding in the surgical area.	10.a. Instruct client in ways *to prevent pressure on the surgical area in order to prevent bleeding:* 1. avoid straining during bowel movements (provide instructions about increasing fluid intake and intake of foods high in fiber if client tends to be constipated) 2. perform actions to regain or maintain control of bladder emptying (see action b in this diagnosis) *in order to reduce risk of urinary retention (overdistention of the bladder can create strain on the newly coagulated blood vessels)* 3. avoid prolonged sitting or standing 4. avoid long walks, long car rides, running, strenuous exercise, sexual intercourse, and lifting objects over 10 pounds for as long as recommended by physician (usually 4–8 weeks after discharge).
10.b. The client will identify ways to regain or maintain control of bladder emptying.	10.b. Instruct client in ways *to regain or maintain control of bladder emptying:* 1. try to urinate every 2–3 hours and whenever the urge is felt 2. urinate in a standing or sitting position *to facilitate bladder emptying* 3. avoid drinking large quantities of liquids (especially alcohol) over a short period 4. avoid drinking caffeine-containing beverages (e.g. coffee, tea, colas) 5. stop drinking liquids a few hours before bedtime *(reduces risk of urine retention and nighttime incontinence)* 6. avoid activities that make it difficult to empty bladder as soon as the urge is felt (e.g. long car rides, lengthy meetings) *in order to prevent retention and incontinence* 7. perform perineal exercises (e.g. stopping and starting stream during voiding; pressing buttocks together, then relaxing the muscles) 10–20 times/hour while awake until urinary control is regained; assist client to set up a schedule that will remind him to do the exercises (e.g. before and after each meal, during television commercials, when talking on telephone).
10.c. The client will demonstrate care of urinary catheter if present.	10.c.1. Demonstrate catheter care, emptying of the collection devices, changing from the nighttime collection bag to a leg bag, and cleaning the collection devices.

2. Stress the importance of keeping urine collection bag below bladder level *to prevent backflow of urine.*
3. Allow time for questions, clarification, and return demonstration.

10.d. The client will state signs and symptoms of complications to report to the health care provider.

10.d.1. Refer to Standardized Postoperative Care Plan, Nursing Diagnosis 20, action c, for signs and symptoms to report to the health care provider.
2. Instruct client to report these additional signs and symptoms:
   a. persistent bright red urine (inform client that some blood is expected intermittently for 2–4 weeks after surgery but that this should diminish with increased rest and fluid intake)
   b. presence of large blood clots or continued passage of smaller clots
   c. increase in burning around catheter if present
   d. increase in frequency, burning, or pain when urinating
   e. decrease in urine output or force and caliber of urinary stream
   f. suprapubic distention
   g. unexpected or continued loss of bladder or bowel control
   h. persistent or increased bladder pain or spasms.

10.e. The client will verbalize an understanding of and a plan for adhering to recommended follow-up care including future appointments with health care provider, medications prescribed, activity level, and wound care.

10.e.1. Refer to Standardized Postoperative Care Plan, Nursing Diagnosis 20, for routine postoperative instructions and measures to improve client compliance.
2. Reinforce the physician's instructions regarding the importance of lying down for a few hours and increasing fluid intake if amount of blood or number of clots in the urine increases.

□ ▬▬▬▬▬▬▬▬▬▬▬▬▬▬▬▬▬▬▬▬▬▬▬▬▬▬▬▬▬▬

Reference

Kübler-Ross, E. On death and dying. New York: Macmillan, 1969.

UNIT
XVII

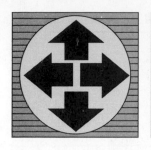
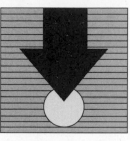
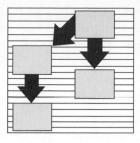
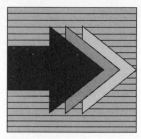
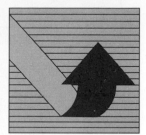

Unit XVIII

Nursing Care of the Client with Disturbances of the Ear, Nose, and Throat

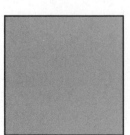

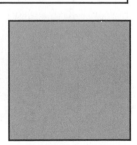

Radical Neck Surgery

Radical neck surgery (total laryngectomy with radical neck dissection) is the usual treatment for cancer of the larynx with metastasis to regional lymph nodes or adjacent neck structures. A total laryngectomy includes removal of the larynx, hyoid bone, hyoid and cricoid cartilages, pre-epiglottic space, one or more tracheal rings, and the strap muscles. The extent of metastasis dictates which additional structures will be removed during the concurrent radical neck dissection. Structures that may be removed include the sternocleidomastoid, omohyoid, stylohyoid, and digastric muscles; submaxillary gland; part of the thyroid and parathyroid glands on the affected side; cervical lymph nodes and the lymphatic channels; internal jugular vein; spinal accessory nerve; a portion of the mandible; and local subcutaneous tissue. The current trend is to spare the spinal accessory nerve, the sternocleidomastoid muscle, and the internal jugular vein if possible.

This care plan focuses on the adult client with cancer of the larynx hospitalized for radical neck surgery. Preoperatively, the goals of care are to reduce fear and anxiety and prepare the client for the postoperative period. The goals of postoperative care are to prevent complications, assist the client to cope with the change in body image and functioning, facilitate rehabilitative efforts, and educate the client regarding follow-up care. The care plan will need to be individualized according to the extensiveness of the dissection, the amount and type of skin grafting necessary, and the physiological and psychological status of the client. If the client has received a preoperative course of radiation therapy, refer to the Care Plan on External Radiation for specific nursing care measures related to side effects the client may still be experiencing.

DISCHARGE CRITERIA

Prior to discharge, the client will:

- demonstrate appropriate stomal care and suctioning, oral hygiene, and tube feeding techniques
- identify appropriate safety precautions related to the presence of a tracheostomy and nerve damage resulting from surgery
- identify signs and symptoms of complications to report to the health care provider
- share feelings and thoughts about the effects of radical neck surgery on body image and usual life style and roles
- identify community resources that can assist with home management and adjustment to the effects of surgery
- communicate an understanding of and a plan for adhering to recommended follow-up care including future appointments with health care provider and speech pathologist, medications prescribed, activity level, and wound care.

NURSING/COLLABORATIVE DIAGNOSES

Preoperative
1. Anxiety ☐ 1053
2. Knowledge deficit ☐ 1054
Postoperative
1. Ineffective breathing patterns:
   a. hyperventilation
   b. hypoventilation ☐ 1055
2. Ineffective airway clearance ☐ 1055
3. Altered nutrition: less than body requirements ☐ 1056
4. Impaired swallowing ☐ 1057

5A. Altered comfort:
    1. pain
    2. headache □ *1058*
5B. Altered comfort: nausea and vomiting □ *1059*
  6. Impaired verbal communication □ *1060*
  7. Impaired skin integrity:
    a. surgical incision, tracheostomy, and donor site (if grafting was done)
    b. impaired wound healing
    c. irritation or breakdown □ *1060*
  8. Constipation □ *1062*
  9. Potential complications:
    a. hypovolemic shock
    b. necrosis of the skin flap
    c. tracheal necrosis, ulceration, and/or fistula formation
    d. pneumothorax
    e. shoulder and neck dysfunction □ *1062*
10. Sexual dysfunction □ *1065*
11. Disturbance in self-concept □ *1066*
12. Ineffective individual coping □ *1068*
13. Impaired social interaction □ *1069*
14. Grieving □ *1070*
15. Knowledge deficit regarding follow-up care □ *1071*

Preoperative

Use in conjunction with the Standardized Preoperative Care Plan.

1. NURSING DIAGNOSIS

Anxiety related to unfamiliar environment, diagnosis of cancer, effects of anesthesia, anticipated postoperative discomfort, impending mutilating surgery that will result in loss of speech and drastic change in physical appearance, and possible death.

DESIRED OUTCOMES	NURSING ACTIONS AND *SELECTED RATIONALES*
1. The client will experience a reduction in fear and anxiety (see Standardized Preoperative Care Plan, Nursing Diagnosis 1, for outcome criteria).	1.a. Refer to Standardized Preoperative Care Plan, Nursing Diagnosis 1, for measures related to assessment and reduction of fear and anxiety. b. Implement additional measures *to reduce fear and anxiety:* 1. support client's decision to accept and endure aggressive treatment for his/her disease

UNIT
XVIII

2. discuss and plan with a speech pathologist an alternative method of communication during the postoperative period (e.g. artificial larynx, paper and pencil, pictures, magic slate, flash cards); be aware that denervation of the trapezius muscle as a result of the surgery may interfere with client's writing ability

3. reinforce instructions and information from speech pathologist about prostheses available (e.g. duckbill) and different methods of speech production that can be learned postoperatively

4. arrange for a visit with a volunteer from the Lost Chord or New Voice Club or International Association of Laryngectomees who has successfully adjusted to radical neck surgery.

☐ ▬▬▬▬▬▬▬▬▬▬▬▬▬▬▬▬▬

2. NURSING DIAGNOSIS

Knowledge deficit regarding hospital routines associated with surgery, physical preparation for radical neck surgery, and postoperative care and expectations.

☐ ▬▬▬▬▬▬▬▬▬▬▬▬▬▬▬▬▬

DESIRED OUTCOMES	NURSING ACTIONS AND *SELECTED RATIONALES*

2.a. The client will verbalize an understanding of usual preoperative and postoperative care and routines.

2.a.1. Refer to Standardized Preoperative Care Plan, Nursing Diagnosis 4, actions a.1–4, for information to include in preoperative teaching.

2. Provide additional information regarding specific expectations and care after radical neck surgery:
   a. purpose of each part of a tracheostomy tube and how it works; allow client to handle a tube or use a chart or model *in order to clarify explanation*
   b. length of time the tracheostomy tube will be in place (depends on physician preference and length of healing time)
   c. purpose, frequency, and procedure for tracheostomy care
   d. suctioning procedure and purpose and sensations (e.g. pain, choking, pressure) that client may experience during the procedure
   e. techniques that will be used to provide moisture to inspired air (e.g. nebulizer, moist curtain, humidifier)
   f. tube feedings and the reason for them; assure client that oral feedings will be initiated as soon as suture line has healed (usually around 8th postoperative day unless area has been irradiated preoperatively)
   g. self-care expectations after surgery (client may be actively involved in wound care, suctioning, and tube feeding very early in the postoperative period)
   h. the need to avoid whispering if he/she is planning to learn esophageal speech *(whispering interferes with the development of this type of speech)*.

3. Allow time for questions and clarification. Provide feedback.

2.b. The client will demonstrate the ability to perform techniques designed to prevent postoperative complications.

2.b.1. Refer to Standardized Preoperative Care Plan, Nursing Diagnosis 4, action b.1, for teaching related to prevention of postoperative complications.

2. Provide additional instructions on ways *to prevent complications associated with radical neck surgery:*
   a. demonstrate oral hygiene techniques that will be used postoperatively (e.g. power spray, irrigations with saline or hydrogen peroxide and water)
   b. demonstrate exercises (e.g. shoulder flexion, abduction, and external rotation; wall climbing with fingers; pulley exercises) that may be ordered to prevent shoulder and neck dysfunction on the affected side
   c. emphasize the need to stop smoking *in order to help prevent respiratory infection and irritation of oral mucosa*
   d. if positioning sutures will be used in conjunction with grafting, instruct

client of the need to limit head movement for about 5 days postoperatively *in order to prevent stress on sutures* (positioning sutures are used to keep the recipient site closer to the donor site *in order to maintain a good blood flow*).
3. Allow time for questions, clarification, practice, and return demonstration of exercises and oral hygiene techniques.

Postoperative

Use in conjunction with the Standardized Postoperative Care Plan.

1. NURSING DIAGNOSIS

Ineffective breathing patterns:

a. **hyperventilation** related to fear, anxiety, and pain;
b. **hypoventilation** related to depressant effects of anesthesia and some medications (e.g. narcotic analgesics), generalized weakness, fatigue, and inadequate tracheostomy cuff pressure during respiratory physiotherapy.

DESIRED OUTCOMES	NURSING ACTIONS AND *SELECTED RATIONALES*
1. The client will maintain an effective breathing pattern (see Standardized Postoperative Care Plan, Nursing Diagnosis 3, for outcome criteria).	1.a. Refer to Standardized Postoperative Care Plan, Nursing Diagnosis 3, for measures related to assessment and improvement of breathing pattern. b. Maintain adequate tracheostomy cuff pressure during respiratory physiotherapy (e.g. IPPB treatments, assisted ventilation) *to ensure adequate ventilation.*

2. NURSING DIAGNOSIS

Ineffective airway clearance related to:

a. obstruction or dislodgment of tracheostomy tube;
b. stasis of secretions associated with decreased activity and poor cough effort (resulting from depressant effects of anesthesia and some medications [e.g. narcotic analgesics], pain, weakness, fatigue, and inability to raise intrathoracic pressure as a result of removal of the larynx);
c. tenacious secretions associated with fluid loss and decreased fluid intake;
d. excessive mucus production associated with irritation of the respiratory tract resulting from inhalation anesthetics, endotracheal intubation, and inhalation of cool, dry air due to rerouting of normal air passages (the nose and mouth normally humidify and warm inspired air);
e. tracheal compression associated with edema, bleeding, and positioning of the neck (especially if large compression dressing or positioning sutures are in place).

DESIRED OUTCOMES	NURSING ACTIONS AND *SELECTED RATIONALES*

2. The client will maintain clear, open airways (see Standardized Postoperative Care Plan, Nursing Diagnosis 4, for outcome criteria).

2.a. Refer to Standardized Postoperative Care Plan, Nursing Diagnosis 4, for measures related to assessment and promotion of effective airway clearance.
  b. Implement additional measures *to promote effective airway clearance:*
    1. perform actions *to decrease risk of dislodgment of tracheostomy tube:*
       a. obtain adequate assistance when changing tracheostomy tube ties
       b. fasten tracheostomy tube ties securely; check ties frequently to be sure that they have not become loose
       c. minimize movement of outer cannula when removing or replacing inner cannula *(movement can irritate the trachea and stimulate coughing)*
       d. cover stomal area with a nonraveling material *to prevent lint from entering tracheostomy tube and stimulating coughing*
       e. discourage vigorous coughing
       f. consult physician about an order for an antitussive if client is coughing excessively
    2. if tracheostomy tube does become dislodged, perform or assist with immediate replacement according to hospital policy (proper size tracheostomy or laryngectomy tube should be kept at the bedside)
    3. perform additional measures *to liquefy tenacious pulmonary secretions:*
       a. instill small amounts (usually 3–5 cc) of sterile normal saline into tracheostomy tube before suctioning
       b. maintain humidification of inspired air:
          1. place a moist, thin 4 × 4 gauze pad over stomal opening
          2. place humidifier in room
          3. provide oxygen mist by nebulizer as ordered
    4. perform actions *to decrease risk or degree of tracheal compression:*
       a. position client with head elevated and slightly extended *to reduce pressure associated with large compression dressing*
       b. implement measures to reduce stress on the surgical site (see Postoperative Nursing Diagnosis 7, action a.2.c) *in order to reduce risk of hemorrhage*
       c. implement measures *to decrease edema in surgical area:*
          1. apply ice packs to area if ordered
          2. maintain client in semi- to high Fowler's position.

3. NURSING DIAGNOSIS

Altered nutrition: less than body requirements related to:

a. decreased oral intake associated with:
   1. prescribed dietary modifications
   2. anorexia resulting from discomfort, fatigue, depression, and an impaired sense of taste and smell (olfactory stimulation does not occur because of altered nasal airflow)
   3. difficulty eating resulting from:
      a. inability to retain food in the mouth associated with nerve damage
      b. dysphagia associated with edema, nerve damage, and removal of some muscles and structures necessary for swallowing
   4. nausea;
b. loss of nutrients associated with vomiting;
c. increased nutritional needs associated with an elevated metabolic rate, which occurs during wound healing.

DESIRED OUTCOMES	**NURSING ACTIONS AND *SELECTED RATIONALES***

3. The client will maintain an adequate nutritional status (see Standardized Postoperative Care Plan, Nursing Diagnosis 6, for outcome criteria).

3.a. Refer to Standardized Postoperative Care Plan, Nursing Diagnosis 6, for measures related to assessment and improvement of nutritional status.
  b. Implement additional measures *to improve nutritional status:*
    1. administer tube feedings as ordered (usually progress from water to a commercial formula)
    2. perform actions to reduce nausea and vomiting (see Postoperative Nursing Diagnosis 5.B)
    3. perform actions *to improve oral intake when allowed* (oral feedings are usually initiated about the 8th postoperative day):
      a. implement measures to improve client's ability to swallow (see Postoperative Nursing Diagnosis 4, action b)
      b. implement measures *to compensate for impaired taste and smell* (assure client that both senses will usually return to some degree):
        1. serve foods warm *to stimulate the sense of smell*
        2. provide extra sweeteners for foods/fluids
        3. encourage client to experiment with spices and other seasonings (e.g. lemon, garlic, onion, mint) *to enhance taste sensation*
      c. assist client with oral hygiene before meals *to eliminate unpleasant tastes*
      d. implement measures to facilitate client's psychological adjustment to the effects of the surgery (see Postoperative Nursing Diagnoses 11, actions c–w; 12, action d; and 14, action d) *in order to reduce depression and improve appetite*
      e. support client during self-feeding attempts by staying with him/her and offering encouragement
      f. provide privacy for client during early self-feeding attempts *in order to reduce the embarrassment associated with eating difficulties.*

□ ▬▬▬▬▬▬▬▬▬▬▬▬▬▬▬▬▬▬▬▬▬▬▬

4. NURSING DIAGNOSIS

Impaired swallowing related to:

a. edema of surgical area;
b. impaired tongue movement associated with damage to the hypoglossal nerve;
c. pain and fatigue;
d. structural changes in the pharynx (e.g. pseudodiverticuli at the base of the tongue and submucosal masses in the posterior pharyngeal wall resulting from contractions of detached constrictor muscles);
e. narrowing of the esophagus associated with excessive scar tissue formation;
f. xerostomia if client has had radiation therapy preoperatively;
g. fistula formation.

□ ▬▬▬▬▬▬▬▬▬▬▬▬▬▬▬▬▬▬▬▬▬▬▬

DESIRED OUTCOMES	**NURSING ACTIONS AND *SELECTED RATIONALES***

4. The client will experience an improvement in swallowing as evidenced by:
  a. communication of same
  b. absence of coughing and choking when eating and drinking.

4.a. Assess for and report signs and symptoms of impaired swallowing (e.g. coughing or choking when eating or drinking, stasis of food in oral cavity).
  b. Implement measures *to improve ability to swallow:*
    1. place client in high Fowler's position for meals and snacks; head should be erect with chin tilted forward *to facilitate posterior movement of the tongue*
    2. assist client to select foods that have a distinct texture and are easy to swallow (e.g. custard, cottage cheese, ground meat)

3. instruct client to avoid mixing foods of different texture in his/her mouth at same time
4. provide thick liquids (e.g. cream soups) or semisoft or pureed foods; blenderize food if acceptable to client
5. avoid serving foods that are sticky (e.g. peanut butter, soft bread, bananas)
6. serve foods that are hot or cold instead of room temperature *(the more extreme temperatures stimulate the sensory receptors and swallowing reflex)*
7. moisten dry foods with gravy or sauces (e.g. sour cream, salad dressings)
8. utilize adaptive devices (e.g. long-handled spoon) *to place food in back of mouth if tongue movement is impaired*
9. encourage client to concentrate on the act of swallowing; verbally prompt each step of the swallowing process
10. gently stroke client's throat when he/she is swallowing if possible
11. if client is retaining food/fluid in mouth, instruct him/her to tilt head to unaffected side when eating or drinking
12. if client has decreased lip control, instruct him/her to close lips with hand prior to swallowing
13. perform actions *to reduce discomfort associated with swallowing* (e.g. medicate before meals)
14. perform actions *to improve impaired swallowing due to xerostomia:*
    a. implement measures *to stimulate salivation:*
        1. serve foods that are visually pleasing
        2. provide oral care before meals
        3. place a piece of lemon or sour pickle on plate
        4. provide sour hard candy for client to suck just before meals unless contraindicated
    b. encourage client to use artificial saliva (e.g. Moi-stir, Salivart, Xero-Lube)
15. perform actions *to reduce and/or liquefy viscous oral secretions:*
    a. encourage a fluid intake of 2500 cc/day unless contraindicated
    b. encourage client to avoid milk and milk products (unless boiled) and chocolate *(when combined with saliva, these products produce very thick secretions)*
    c. dissolve a papain product (e.g. papase tablet, meat tenderizer made from papaya) under tongue 10 minutes before eating *(contains a proteolytic enzyme that will liquefy secretions)*
16. provide an oily liquid such as chicken or beef broth at the beginning of a meal
17. instruct client in exercises to strengthen the muscles involved with the act of swallowing.
c. Consult physician if swallowing difficulties persist or worsen.

5.A. NURSING DIAGNOSIS

Altered comfort:*

1. **pain** related to tissue trauma and reflex muscle spasm associated with the surgical procedure;
2. **headache** related to fear, anxiety, and irritation of the dura mater associated with increased cerebral pressure resulting from disruption of regional lymphatic drainage pathways and ligation of the internal jugular vein if performed.

---

* In this care plan, the nursing diagnosis "pain" is included under the diagnostic label of altered comfort.

DESIRED OUTCOMES   **NURSING ACTIONS AND *SELECTED RATIONALES***

5.A.1. The client will experience diminished pain (see Standardized Postoperative Care Plan, Nursing Diagnosis 7.A, for outcome criteria).

5.A.1. See Standardized Postoperative Care Plan, Nursing Diagnosis 7.A, for measures related to the assessment and management of postoperative pain.

5.A.2. The client will obtain relief of headache as evidenced by:
a. communication of headache relief
b. relaxed facial expression and body positioning.

5.A.2.a. Determine how client usually responds to pain.
b. Assess for nonverbal signs of headache (e.g. reluctance to move head, wrinkled brow, clenched fists, squinting, rubbing head, avoidance of bright lights and noises).
c. Assist client to communicate information about type, location, and severity of headache.
d. Implement measures *to relieve headache:*
1. perform actions to reduce fear and anxiety (see Standardized Postoperative Care Plan, Nursing Diagnosis 1, action c)
2. keep head of bed elevated 45° *to promote lymphatic and venous drainage*
3. perform actions *to minimize environmental stimuli* (e.g. provide a calm environment, restrict visitors, dim lights)
4. avoid jarring bed or startling client *to minimize the risk of sudden movements*
5. provide or assist with nonpharmacological measures for headache relief (e.g. cool cloth to forehead, relaxation techniques, diversional activities)
6. assure client that headache will gradually subside
7. monitor for therapeutic and nontherapeutic effects of analgesics if administered.
e. Consult physician if above actions fail to relieve headache.

5.B. NURSING DIAGNOSIS

Altered comfort: nausea and vomiting related to stimulation of the vomiting center associated with:

1. cortical stimulation due to pain and stress;
2. vagal and/or sympathetic stimulation resulting from visceral irritation associated with:
a. rapid administration of tube feedings
b. administration of cold tube feeding solutions
c. abdominal distention due to depressant effects of anesthesia and some medications (e.g. narcotic analgesics), decreased activity, and rapid administration of tube feedings.

DESIRED OUTCOMES   **NURSING ACTIONS AND *SELECTED RATIONALES***

5.B. The client will experience relief of nausea and vomiting (see Standardized Postoperative Care Plan, Nursing Diagnosis 7.C, for outcome criteria).

5.B.1. Refer to Standardized Postoperative Care Plan, Nursing Diagnosis 7.C, for measures related to assessment and prevention of nausea and vomiting.
2. Administer tube feedings slowly and at room temperature *in order to further reduce the risk of nausea and vomiting.*

☐

6. NURSING DIAGNOSIS

Impaired verbal communication related to the surgical removal of the larynx.

☐

DESIRED OUTCOMES	NURSING ACTIONS AND *SELECTED RATIONALES*

6. The client will develop and use an effective communication system.	6.a. Implement measures *to facilitate communication:*
	  1. maintain a patient, calm approach and allow ample time for communication
	  2. answer call signal promptly and in person rather than using the intercommunication system
	  3. make frequent rounds *to ascertain needs*
	  4. if client is frustrated or fatigued, try to anticipate needs *in order to minimize the necessity of communication attempts*
	  5. reinforce communication techniques prescribed by speech pathologist
	  6. ask questions that require short answers or nod of head
	  7. provide materials necessary for communication (e.g. magic slate, pad and pencil, flash cards); be aware that denervation of the trapezius muscle may interfere with client's ability to write
	  8. ensure that intravenous therapy does not interfere with client's ability to write
	  9. assist client to operate artificial larynx if indicated.
	  b. Post a sign on the door, intercommunication system, and above bed *to remind health care personnel that the client is nonverbal.*
	  c. Inform significant others and health care personnel of approaches being used to maximize client's ability to communicate. Encourage their use of these techniques.
	  d. Encourage client to communicate with the physician about the possibility of future surgical reconstruction of the larynx (possible in a limited number of cases) or the insertion of a Panje Voice or Bloom-Singer prosthesis *in order to allow him/her to regain the ability to speak in a more normal fashion.*

☐

7. NURSING DIAGNOSIS

Impaired skin integrity:

a. **surgical incision, tracheostomy, and donor site (if grafting was done)**;
b. **impaired wound healing** related to:
  1. preoperative radiation to tumor site (results in vascular sclerosing and compromised circulation)
  2. infection
  3. stress on wound area
  4. inadequate nutritional status
  5. increased levels of glucocorticoids (levels usually rise with stress);
c. **irritation or breakdown** related to contact of skin with wound drainage, pressure from drainage tubes, and use of tape.

☐

DESIRED OUTCOMES	NURSING ACTIONS AND *SELECTED RATIONALES*

7.a. The client will experience normal healing of surgical wounds (see Standardized Postoperative Care Plan, Nursing Diagnosis 9, outcome a, for outcome criteria).

7.a.1. Refer to Standardized Postoperative Care Plan, Nursing Diagnosis 9, action a, for measures related to assessment and promotion of normal wound healing.

2. Implement additional measures *to promote normal wound healing:*
   a. perform actions *to promote healing of tracheal stoma:*
      1. cleanse peristomal area gently with normal saline or half-strength hydrogen peroxide
      2. implement measures *to reduce risk of infection of the tracheal stoma:*
         a. perform actions to decrease the risk of wound infection (see Standardized Postoperative Care Plan, Nursing Diagnosis 16, action b.4)
         b. apply anti-infective ointment as ordered
         c. cleanse inner cannula as necessary *in order to remove excessive secretions*
   b. perform actions *to promote healing of donor site:*
      1. implement measures to prevent wound infection (see Standardized Postoperative Care Plan, Nursing Diagnosis 16, action b.4)
      2. utilize a bed cradle *to protect area from pressure of linens*
      3. if a transparent occlusive dressing (e.g. Op-Site) is applied in surgery, leave in place as ordered (usually 5–7 days); aspirate fluid collecting under dressing with a 25-gauge needle as ordered; allow to air dry after dressing removal
      4. if a gauze dressing is used, expose to air or utilize heat lamp as ordered *to facilitate drying*; when sufficient healing has occurred, dressing can be soaked off in bathtub
      5. monitor for therapeutic and nontherapeutic effects of the following medications if administered:
         a. topical anti-infectives *to reduce risk of infection*
         b. corticosteroid creams and/or antihistamines *to relieve pruritus in order to decrease the risk of trauma to donor site associated with scratching*
   c. perform actions *to reduce stress on and trauma to suture lines and/or surrounding tissue:*
      1. position client as ordered (e.g. supine, head elevated and supported with pillows) *to prevent pressure on graft site*
      2. instruct client to avoid any manipulation of nasogastric tube
      3. support client with pillows as necessary *to maintain positioning sutures* (if grafting was done, these sutures may be used to position recipient site closer to the vascular pedicle of the flap)
      4. support client's head and neck during position change until client is able to do so
      5. instruct client to support head and neck with hands when moving and to avoid turning head abruptly and hyperextending neck
      6. place personal articles and call signal within easy reach *so client does not have to turn or strain to reach them*
      7. maintain patency of wound drainage system *in order to prevent fluid accumulation under the flap*
      8. utilize an isolation mask rather than tape to secure dressings
      9. soak adherent dressings with sterile normal saline before removal
      10. change dressings as needed *to prevent maceration of tissue*
      11. implement measures to improve breathing pattern and airway clearance (see Postoperative Nursing Diagnoses 1 and 2) *in order to prevent strenuous respiratory efforts and resultant use of accessory muscles in the operative area*
      12. focus on deep breathing rather than vigorous coughing to promote effective breathing pattern and airway clearance (some physicians prefer that their clients not cough *because it increases stress on the suture line*)
      13. implement measures to prevent nausea and vomiting (see Postoperative Nursing Diagnosis 5.B)
   d. perform actions to promote an optimal nutritional status (see Postoperative Nursing Diagnosis 3).

7.b. The client will maintain skin integrity (see Standardized Postoperative Care Plan, Nursing Diagnosis 9, outcome b, for outcome criteria).

7.b.1. Refer to Standardized Postoperative Care Plan, Nursing Diagnosis 9, actions b.1 and 2, for measures related to assessment and prevention of skin irritation and breakdown resulting from contact with wound drainage, drainage tubings, and tape.
   2. Implement additional measures *to prevent skin irritation and breakdown:*
      a. secure neck dressings with an isolation mask rather than tape
      b. soak adherent dressings with sterile normal saline before removal
      c. change dressings as needed *to prevent maceration of tissue.*
   3. If skin irritation or breakdown occurs:
      a. notify physician
      b. continue with above measures to prevent further irritation and breakdown
      c. perform wound care as ordered or per standard hospital policy
      d. monitor client closely and report signs and symptoms of infection (e.g. elevated temperature; redness, warmth, and edema around incision or area of breakdown; unusual drainage from site).

8. NURSING DIAGNOSIS

Constipation related to:

a. decreased gastrointestinal motility associated with anesthesia, narcotic analgesics, and decreased activity;
b. decreased fluid intake;
c. decreased intake of foods high in fiber associated with dietary restrictions and difficulty swallowing;
d. inability to bear down or strain to have a bowel movement (client is not able to perform a Valsalva maneuver due to removal of the larynx).

DESIRED OUTCOMES	NURSING ACTIONS AND *SELECTED RATIONALES*

8. The client will resume usual bowel elimination pattern.

8.a. Refer to Standardized Postoperative Care Plan, Nursing Diagnosis 14, for measures related to assessment, prevention, and management of constipation.
   b. Establish a routine time for defecation based on client's usual bowel elimination pattern.
   c. Implement measures to improve oral intake (see Postoperative Nursing Diagnosis 3, action b.3).
   d. Consult physician if signs and symptoms of constipation persist.

9. COLLABORATIVE DIAGNOSIS

Potential complications:

a. **hypovolemic shock** related to:
   1. hemorrhage associated with carotid artery erosion and subsequent rupture resulting from:
      a. prolonged exposure of vessel to atmospheric air during surgery (causes drying and destruction of the blood supply to vessel wall)
      b. wound site infection, necrosis, and tissue sloughing
      c. weakening of the vessel wall as a result of preoperative radiation to tumor site

2. fluid volume deficit associated with excessive fluid loss and inadequate fluid replacement;

b. **necrosis of the skin flap** related to:
1. inadequate blood supply associated with mechanical obstruction of blood flow within the flap
2. vascular congestion associated with pressure differences in blood flow to and from the flap
3. wound infection;

c. **tracheal necrosis, ulceration, and/or fistula formation** related to excessive cuff or ventilation pressures; inappropriate cannula size; and impaired wound healing associated with preoperative radiation therapy, postoperative infection, an inadequate nutritional status, and high levels of glucocorticoids (occurs with pain and stress);

d. **pneumothorax** related to injury to the pleura during surgery (if this occurs, client will return from surgery with chest tube);

e. **shoulder and neck dysfunction** related to removal of or damage to the spinal accessory nerve during surgery.

□ ▌▌

DESIRED OUTCOMES	NURSING ACTIONS AND *SELECTED RATIONALES*

9.a. The client will not develop hypovolemic shock (see Standardized Postoperative Care Plan, Collaborative Diagnosis 19, outcome a, for outcome criteria).

9.a.1. Assess for and report:
  a. signs and symptoms of conditions that could lead to carotid artery rupture:
    1. impaired circulation to wound and surrounding skin (e.g. change in color from red to pale or black, coolness, increased edema)
    2. impaired wound healing (e.g. increase in size and altered shape of wound, delayed wound closure)
    3. wound infection (e.g. change in type, odor, and volume of drainage; increased redness and tenderness of site)
    4. carotid artery exposure
  b. signs and symptoms of impending carotid artery rupture (e.g. "herald bleed" [slight amount of bright red blood on packing or from margins of wound] 24–48 hours before rupture, sternal or high epigastric pain a few hours before rupture)
  c. frank, profuse bleeding from wound, tracheostomy, or oropharynx
  d. declining RBC, Hct., and Hgb. levels
  e. signs and symptoms of hypovolemic shock (see Standardized Postoperative Care Plan, Collaborative Diagnosis 19, action a.3, for signs and symptoms).
2. Have suction equipment, gloves, and absorbent dressings at bedside in case of carotid artery rupture.
3. Refer to Standardized Postoperative Care Plan, Collaborative Diagnosis 19, action a.4, for measures to prevent hypovolemic shock.
4. Implement measures *to prevent carotid artery rupture in order to further reduce the risk of shock:*
  a. perform actions to promote healing of the surgical incision (see Standardized Postoperative Care Plan, Nursing Diagnosis 9, action a) and prevent and treat wound infection (see Standardized Postoperative Care Plan, Nursing Diagnosis 16, actions b.4 and 5) *in order to prevent tissue sloughing and subsequent drying and erosion of the carotid artery*
  b. perform actions to reduce stress on and trauma to the suture lines and surrounding tissue (see Postoperative Nursing Diagnosis 7, action a.2.c)
  c. assess for pulsation of tracheostomy tube (*indicates tip is in close proximity to carotid artery and may be causing undue pressure*)
  d. maintain tracheostomy tube in midtracheal alignment at all times.
5. If carotid artery rupture occurs:
  a. apply firm, prolonged, continuous pressure to area using absorbent materials

UNIT XVIII

b. position client with head turned to side or in side-lying position and ensure that tracheostomy cuff is inflated *to prevent aspiration*
c. suction as necessary *to clear airway and oral cavity*
d. prepare for surgical intervention
e. provide emotional support to client and significant others if decision not to resuscitate has been made
f. remain with client and administer medications such as intravenous morphine sulfate and diazepam *to allay anxiety.*

6. Implement measures to treat hypovolemic shock if it occurs (see Standardized Postoperative Care Plan, Collaborative Diagnosis 19, action a.5).

9.b. The client will not experience necrosis of skin flap as evidenced by:
1. skin flap warm and expected color
2. approximated wound edges
3. absence of foul odor from flap area.

9.b.1. Assess for and report:
a. signs and symptoms of impaired blood flow in skin flap (e.g. blue, white, or red appearing skin flap; capillary refill time greater than 3 seconds)
b. signs and symptoms of skin flap necrosis (e.g. pale, cool, darkened tissue; separation of wound edges; foul odor).

2. Implement measures *to prevent skin flap necrosis:*
a. perform actions to reduce stress on and trauma to suture lines and surrounding tissue (see Postoperative Nursing Diagnosis 7, action a.2.c)
b. perform actions to promote healing of surgical incision (see Standardized Postoperative Care Plan, Nursing Diagnosis 9, action a) and prevent and treat wound infection (see Standardized Postoperative Care Plan, Nursing Diagnosis 16, actions b.4 and 5).

3. If skin flap necrosis occurs:
a. prepare client for surgical revision or replacement of graft
b. provide emotional support to client and significant others.

9.c. The client will not experience tracheal necrosis, ulceration, and/or fistula formation as evidenced by:
1. usual drainage from tracheostomy and neck wounds
2. expected improvement in swallowing ability.

9.c.1. Assess for and report signs and symptoms of tracheal necrosis, ulceration, and/or fistula formation (e.g. evidence of food or ingested fluids in tracheal secretions; blood-tinged, purulent drainage from trachea or neck wounds; choking on food and fluids).

2. Implement measures *to prevent tracheal necrosis, ulceration, and/or fistula formation:*
a. perform actions *to prevent pressure on tracheal mucosa:*
   1. do not overinflate tracheostomy cuff (cuff pressure should be high enough to prevent air leak but should not be higher than 20 mm Hg)
   2. deflate tracheostomy tube cuff for 1–5 minutes every hour unless contraindicated (if client is on a ventilator, cuff deflation may be tolerated for only 10–15 seconds at a time)
b. perform actions to prevent and treat wound infection (see Standardized Postoperative Care Plan, Nursing Diagnosis 16, actions b.4 and 5)
c. perform actions to improve nutritional status (see Postoperative Nursing Diagnosis 3).

3. If tracheal necrosis, ulceration, and/or fistula develop:
a. continue with above actions
b. withhold oral food and fluid as ordered
c. maintain intravenous therapy and nasogastric or gastrostomy tube feedings as ordered
d. perform wound care as ordered
e. monitor for therapeutic and nontherapeutic effects of anti-infectives if administered
f. prepare client for surgical intervention if indicated
g. provide emotional support to client and significant others.

9.d. The client will experience normal lung re-expansion as evidenced by:
1. normal breath sounds and percussion note for client by 3rd–4th postoperative day
2. unlabored respirations at 16–20/minute

9.d.1. Assess for and immediately report signs and symptoms of:
a. malfunction of the chest drainage system (e.g. respiratory distress, sudden cessation of drainage, excessive bubbling in water seal chamber, significant increase in subcutaneous emphysema)
b. further lung collapse (e.g. extended area of absent breath sounds and hyperresonant percussion note, further increase in pulse rate or respiratory distress, chest pain, cyanosis, restlessness, confusion).

2. Monitor blood gases. Report values that have worsened.
3. Monitor chest x-ray results. Report findings of delayed lung re-expansion.

3. blood gases returning toward normal
4. chest x-ray showing lung re-expansion.

4. Implement measures *to prevent further lung collapse and promote lung re-expansion:*
   a. perform actions *to maintain patency and integrity of chest drainage system if present:*
      1. maintain water seal and suction levels as ordered
      2. maintain an air occlusive dressing over chest tube insertion site
      3. tape all connections securely
      4. milk or strip chest tubes if ordered
      5. keep chest drainage and suction tubing free of kinks
      6. keep drainage system below level of client's chest at all times
   b. perform actions to improve breathing pattern and facilitate airway clearance (see Postoperative Nursing Diagnoses 1 and 2).
5. If signs and symptoms of further lung collapse occur:
   a. maintain client on bedrest in a semi- to high Fowler's position
   b. maintain oxygen therapy as ordered
   c. assess for and immediately report signs and symptoms of mediastinal shift (e.g. severe dyspnea, increased restlessness and agitation, rapid and/or irregular pulse rate, cyanosis, shift in point of apical impulse and trachea toward unaffected side)
   d. assist with clearing of existing chest tube and/or insertion of a new tube
   e. provide emotional support to client and significant others.

9.e. The client will regain optimal shoulder and neck function as evidenced by:
1. improved range of motion of shoulder and neck
2. ability to maintain shoulder in near-normal position
3. gradual resolution of pain in shoulder and neck.

9.e.1. Assess for and report signs and symptoms of spinal accessory nerve damage (e.g. inability to abduct arm on affected side, drooping shoulder, continued pain in neck and shoulder).
   2. If shoulder and neck dysfunction occur:
     a. instruct client to support affected arm in a sling when ambulating and rest it on a chair arm, table, or pillow when sitting *in order to prevent overstretching of the trapezius muscle*
     b. assist with self-care activities he/she is unable to perform independently
     c. reinforce the need to begin neck and shoulder exercises (e.g. wall climbing with fingers, shoulder swing, pulley exercises, range of motion of neck) as soon as allowed *in order to improve tone and strength of affected muscles* (exercises are usually started 10 days to 3 months postoperatively depending on extensiveness of surgery)
     d. assure client that partial neck and shoulder function may be regained if exercise program and physical therapy schedule are adhered to.

10. NURSING DIAGNOSIS

Sexual dysfunction related to:

a. fear of rejection by partner associated with perceived loss of sexual appeal resulting from the loss of ability to communicate verbally, changes in physical appearance, and neck breathing;
b. fear that rapid breathing during climax will result in a coughing episode;
c. discomfort associated with an extensive surgical wound;
d. inability to assume those positions for sexual activity that necessitate supporting one's body weight and performing Valsalva maneuver (e.g. "missionary position" if male);
e. depression and ineffective coping.

DESIRED OUTCOMES	NURSING ACTIONS AND *SELECTED RATIONALES*

10. The client will communicate a perception of self as sexually acceptable and

10.a. Assess for signs and symptoms of sexual dysfunction (e.g. communication of sexual difficulties, limitations, and/or changes in sexual behavior or activities; failure to maintain relationships with significant others).

adequate as evidenced by:
a. maintenance of relationships with significant others
b. behaviors reflecting adjustment to effects of radical neck surgery on sexual functioning.

b. Determine attitudes, knowledge, and concerns about radical neck surgery on sexual functioning.
c. Communicate interest, understanding, and respect for the values of the client and his/her partner.
d. Provide accurate information about the effects of radical neck surgery on sexual functioning. Encourage questions and clarify misconceptions.
e. Facilitate communication between client and his/her partner. Assist them to identify issues that may affect their sexual relationship.
f. Implement measures to facilitate client's psychological adjustment to the effects of radical neck surgery (see Postoperative Nursing Diagnoses 11, actions c–w; 12, action d; and 14, action d).
g. Implement measures *to decrease possibility of rejection by partner:*
 1. assist partner to acknowledge both positive and negative feelings
 2. if appropriate, involve partner in care of the wound, dressing change, and suctioning *to facilitate adjustment to and integration of the change in the partner's body image*
 3. instruct client to suction and cleanse stoma and cover it with a porous shield just before sexual activity.
h. Instruct client in ways to compensate for loss of larynx and resultant inability to perform a Valsalva maneuver during intercourse (e.g. experimenting with positions other than the "missionary position" such as rear entry or leg over leg side entry, using exaggerated pelvic thrust).
i. If client is concerned that operative site discomfort will interfere with usual sexual activity, assure him/her that discomfort is temporary and will diminish as incision heals.
j. Reinforce physician's instructions regarding when client can resume sexual activity.
k. Arrange for uninterrupted privacy during hospital stay if desired by couple.
l. Include partner in above discussions and encourage his/her continued support of the client.
m. Consult physician if counseling appears indicated.

11. NURSING DIAGNOSIS

Disturbance in self-concept* related to:

a. changes in appearance:
 1. obvious mutilation of face and neck structures
 2. drooling and paralysis of the muscles controlling facial expression associated with damage to the facial nerve
 3. drooping of the shoulder associated with removal of or damage to the spinal accessory nerve
 4. persistent facial edema associated with disruption of lymphatic channels;
b. alteration in usual body functioning:
 1. loss of ability to speak, sing, produce audible crying and laughing sounds, and whistle
 2. loss of sense of taste and smell and ability to blow nose
 3. loss of normal shoulder, neck, and arm movement associated with removal of or damage to the spinal accessory nerve and removal of sternocleidomastoid muscle if performed
 4. impaired swallowing ability and tongue movement associated with damage to the hypoglossal nerve
 5. loss of ability to perform activities such as coughing effectively, straining to have a bowel movement, and lifting heavy objects associated with inability to perform a Valsalva maneuver resulting from loss of the larynx;
c. dependence on others to meet self-care needs;
d. possible life-style, career, and role changes.

---

* This diagnostic label includes the nursing diagnoses of body image disturbance and self-esteem disturbance.

DESIRED OUTCOMES	NURSING ACTIONS AND *SELECTED RATIONALES*

11. The client will demonstrate beginning adaptation to and integration of the changes in appearance, body functioning, life style, and roles as evidenced by:
   a. communication of feelings of self-worth and sexual adequacy
   b. maintenance of relationships with significant others
   c. interest and participation in tracheostomy care and speech techniques
   d. active participation in activities of daily living
   e. active interest in personal appearance
   f. willingness to participate in social activities
   g. communication of a beginning plan for adapting life style to meet restrictions imposed by the residual effects of radical neck dissection
   h. willingness to participate in or seek vocational rehabilitation if appropriate.

11.a. Determine the meaning of the changes in appearance, body functioning, life style, and roles to the client by encouraging him/her to communicate feelings and by noting nonverbal responses to the changes experienced.
   b. Assess for signs and symptoms of a disturbance in self-concept (e.g. nonverbal cues denoting a negative response to changes in body functioning and appearance such as preoccupation with changes that have occurred, refusal to look at or touch neck area, refusal to participate in self-care activities, or withdrawal from significant others).
   c. Assist the client to identify strengths and qualities that have a positive effect on self-concept.
   d. Implement measures *to assist client to increase self-esteem* (e.g. limit negative self-criticism, encourage positive communication about self, give positive feedback about accomplishments).
   e. Reinforce actions to assist client to cope with effects of radical neck surgery (see Postoperative Nursing Diagnosis 12, action d).
   f. Implement measures *to reduce drooling:*
      1. instruct client to wipe mouth or suction oral cavity frequently (if circumoral paresthesias are present, he/she may be unaware of drooling)
      2. place a wick with one end in corner of mouth and other end in an emesis basin when client is resting in bed
      3. perform actions to improve client's ability to swallow (see Postoperative Nursing Diagnosis 4, action b).
   g. Provide privacy when eating *to reduce embarrassment associated with eating difficulties.*
   h. Remain with client for the first look at his/her appearance after removal of dressings. Explain that some of the physical changes will not be as severe once edema and redness have subsided and the tracheostomy tube is out.
   i. Assure client that neck and shoulder function will usually improve if exercise and physical therapy regimens are adhered to.
   j. Encourage client to pursue available options in relation to regaining speech (e.g. voice prosthesis, esophageal speech, artificial larynges).
   k. Assist client with usual grooming and makeup habits if necessary.
   l. Demonstrate acceptance of client using techniques such as therapeutic touch and frequent visits. Encourage significant others to do the same.
   m. Assist significant others to verbalize feelings about physical changes in the client and the care he/she requires (recognize that they may be repulsed by client's appearance or wound care). Assure them that their responses are normal but caution them not to show distaste in front of the client.
   n. Encourage significant others to allow client to do what he/she is able *so that independence can be re-established and/or self-esteem redeveloped.*
   o. Assist client to identify ways to provide support to significant others *in order to increase their comfort level in dealing with changes in client.*
   p. Encourage client contact with others *so that he/she can test and establish a new body image.*
   q. Assess for and support behaviors suggesting positive adaptation to changes experienced (e.g. willingness to participate in wound/stomal care, tube feedings, and suctioning).
   r. Assist client's and significant others' adjustment by listening, facilitating communication, and providing information.
   s. Instruct significant others to allow client to communicate and attempt to express his/her needs.
   t. If client appears to be rejecting significant others, explain that this is a common occurrence (client rejects family and/or spouse before they have a chance to reject him/her). Encourage them to visit often and persist in offering support and love for the client.
   u. Ensure that client and significant others have similar expectations and understanding of future life style; assist them to identify ways that personal and family goals can be adjusted rather than abandoned.
   v. Encourage client to continue involvement in social activities and to pursue interests. If previous interests and hobbies cannot be pursued, encourage development of new ones.
   w. Provide information about and encourage utilization of community resources or support groups (e.g. Lost Chord Club; vocational rehabilitation; family, individual, and/or financial counseling).

x. Consult physician about psychological counseling if client desires or if he/she seems unwilling or unable to adapt to changes resulting from radical neck surgery.

☐ ▬▬▬▬▬▬▬▬▬▬▬▬▬▬▬▬▬▬▬▬▬▬▬

12. NURSING DIAGNOSIS

Ineffective individual coping related to:

a. visible changes in appearance;
b. loss of ability to speak and audibly laugh and cry;
c. difficulty mastering new speaking techniques;
d. fear, anxiety, and depression;
e. self-care expectations regarding tube feeding and wound and tracheostomy care;
f. inadequate support system.

☐ ▬▬▬▬▬▬▬▬▬▬▬▬▬▬▬▬▬▬▬▬▬▬▬

DESIRED OUTCOMES	NURSING ACTIONS AND *SELECTED RATIONALES*

12. The client will demonstrate the use of effective coping skills as evidenced by:
a. willingness to participate in treatment plan and self-care activities
b. communication of ability to cope with the effects of radical neck surgery
c. identification of stressors
d. utilization of appropriate problem-solving techniques
e. recognition and utilization of available support sytems.
	12.a. Assess effectiveness of client's coping strategies by observing behavior and noting strengths, weaknesses, ability to express feelings and concerns, and willingness to participate in treatment plan.
	b. Assess for and report signs and symptoms that may indicate ineffective coping (e.g. sleep disturbances, increasing fatigue, difficulty concentrating, irritability, decreased tolerance for pain, communication of inability to cope, inability to problem-solve).
	c. Allow time for the client to adjust psychologically to the self-care required of him/her, the residual effects of the surgery, and anticipated life-style and role changes. However, expect and encourage client to participate in stomal and wound care, tube feeding, and suctioning as soon as possible.
	d. Implement measures *to promote effective coping:*
	  1. arrange for a visit with another who has successfully adjusted to loss of larynx
	  2. perform actions to reduce fear and anxiety (see Standardized Postoperative Care Plan, Nursing Diagnosis 1, action c)
	  3. perform actions to assist the client to adapt to changes in appearance, body functioning, life style, and roles (see Postoperative Nursing Diagnosis 11, actions c–w)
	  4. include client in the planning of care, encourage maximum participation in the treatment plan, and allow choices when possible *to enable him/her to maintain a sense of control*
	  5. perform actions to improve social interaction (see Postoperative Nursing Diagnosis 13, action c)
	  6. instruct client in effective problem-solving techniques (e.g. accurate identification of stressors, determination of various options to solve problem)
	  7. assist client to maintain usual daily routines whenever possible
	  8. provide diversional activities according to client's interests and abilities
	  9. assist client as he/she starts to plan for necessary life-style and role changes after discharge; provide input related to realistic prioritization of problems that need to be dealt with
	  10. assist client through methods such as role playing to prepare for negative reactions from others because of changes in appearance and inability to speak normally
	  11. assist client to identify and utilize available support systems; provide

information about available community resources that can assist client and significant others in coping with effects of surgery (e.g. New Voice and Lost Chord Clubs, American Cancer Society, vocational rehabilitation, International Association of Laryngectomees).

e. Encourage continued emotional support from significant others.

f. Encourage client to share with significant others the kind of support that would be most beneficial (e.g. being there, inspiring hope, providing reassurance and accurate information).

g. Assess for and support behaviors suggesting positive adaptation to changes experienced (e.g. willingness to participate in care, communication of ability to cope, recognition and utilization of available support systems and effective problem-solving strategies).

h. Consult physician about psychological or vocational rehabilitation counseling if appropriate. Initiate a referral if necessary.

13. NURSING DIAGNOSIS

Impaired social interaction related to inability to communicate verbally, changes in physical appearance, ineffective coping, and depression.

DESIRED OUTCOMES	NURSING ACTIONS AND *SELECTED RATIONALES*

13. The client will experience an improvement in the quantity and quality of social interaction as evidenced by:
a. communication of same
b. maintenance of relationships with significant others and casual acquaintances
c. use of appropriate social interaction behaviors
d. communication of decreasing loneliness and feelings of rejection.
	13.a. Ascertain client's usual degree of social interaction.
	b. Assess for and report behaviors indicative of impaired social interaction (e.g. communication of or observed discomfort in social situations, inability to maintain relationships with significant others and casual acquaintances, use of inappropriate social interaction behaviors, communication of loneliness and feelings of rejection).
	c. Implement measures *to improve social interaction:*
	  1. perform actions to facilitate communication (see Postoperative Nursing Diagnosis 6, action a)
	  2. perform actions to facilitate client's psychological adjustment to the effects of radical neck surgery (see Postoperative Nursing Diagnoses 11, actions c–w; 12, action d; and 14, action d)
	  3. encourage client to express feelings of rejection and aloneness; provide feedback and support
	  4. assist client to identify a few persons he/she feels comfortable with and encourage interactions with them
	  5. encourage client to communicate his/her feelings but set limits on inappropriate behavior or responses
	  6. explain to significant others that client may be rejecting them because he/she fears rejection by them; encourage them to visit frequently and continue to demonstrate support of the client
	  7. encourage client to initiate communication with others and focus on them rather than him/herself
	  8. use role playing to assist client to develop appropriate social interaction skills
	  9. give positive reinforcement for attempts to interact with others in a positive way.
	d. Consult physician regarding referral for counseling if signs of impaired social interaction persist.

14. NURSING DIAGNOSIS

Grieving* related to:

a. changes in appearance;
b. loss of ability to speak normally and audibly laugh and cry associated with removal of larynx;
c. possible changes in life style and roles.

---

* This diagnostic label includes anticipatory grieving and grieving following the actual losses/changes.

DESIRED OUTCOMES	NURSING ACTIONS AND *SELECTED RATIONALES*

14. The client will demonstrate beginning progression through the grieving process as evidenced by:
    a. communication of feelings about the radical neck dissection and its effects on appearance, body functioning, life style, and roles
    b. expression of grief
    c. participation in treatment plan and self-care activities
    d. utilization of available support systems.

14.a. Determine client's perception of the impact of the radical neck dissection on his/her future.
   b. Determine how client usually expresses grief.
   c. Observe for signs of grieving (e.g. changes in eating habits, insomnia, anger, noncompliance, denial).
   d. Implement measures *to facilitate the grieving process:*
      1. assist client to acknowledge the losses and changes experienced *so grief work can begin;* assess for factors that may hinder or facilitate acknowledgment
      2. discuss the grieving process and assist client to accept the stages of grieving as an expected response to actual and/or anticipated changes or losses
      3. allow time for client to progress through the stages of grieving (denial, anger, bargaining, depression, acceptance [Kübler-Ross, 1969]); be aware that not every stage is experienced or expressed by all individuals
      4. provide an atmosphere of care and concern (e.g. provide privacy, be available and nonjudgmental, display empathy and respect) *so that client will feel free to communicate both positive and negative feelings and concerns*
      5. perform actions *to promote trust* (e.g. answer questions honestly, provide requested information)
      6. encourage the expression of anger and sadness about the losses/changes experienced
      7. encourage client to express his/her feelings in whatever ways are comfortable (e.g. writing, drawing)
      8. perform actions to facilitate effective coping (see Postoperative Nursing Diagnosis 12, action d)
      9. support realistic hope regarding ability to resume usual activities and regain speech
      10. encourage client to pursue all options for regaining speech (e.g. esophageal speech, artificial larynges, voice prosthesis, reconstruction).
   e. Assess for and support behaviors suggesting successful resolution of grief (e.g. communicating feelings about the loss of speech, expressing sorrow, focusing on ways to adapt to loss of speech).
   f. Explain the stages of the grieving process to significant others. Encourage their support and understanding.
   g. Provide information regarding counseling services and support groups that might assist client in working through grief.
   h. Arrange for a visit from clergy if desired by client.
   i. Monitor for therapeutic and nontherapeutic effects of antidepressants if administered.
   j. Consult physician regarding referral for counseling if signs of dysfunctional grieving (e.g. persistent denial of loss and necessary changes in life style, excessive anger or sadness, hysteria, suicidal behaviors, phobias) occur.

15. NURSING DIAGNOSIS

Knowledge deficit regarding follow-up care.

DESIRED OUTCOMES	NURSING ACTIONS AND *SELECTED RATIONALES*
15.a. The client will demonstrate appropriate stomal care and suctioning, oral hygiene, and tube feeding techniques.	15.a.1. Reinforce instructions and demonstrate the following if appropriate: a. procedure for insertion of new tracheostomy tube in an emergency situation b. procedure for cleansing stoma and changing tracheostomy tube ties and stoma dressing c. methods for maintaining skin integrity around stoma (e.g. keep skin clean, dry, and well lubricated) d. removal and cleansing of the inner cannula (clean technique is used) e. oral and tracheal suctioning f. ways to increase moisture content of inspired air (e.g. use humidifier, wear a moist bib, place pans of water around the home) g. administration of tube feedings h. oral care (e.g. irrigation with normal saline or 1:4 solution of hydrogen peroxide and water). 2. Allow time for questions, clarification, practice, and return demonstration.
15.b. The client will identify appropriate safety precautions related to the presence of a tracheostomy and nerve damage resulting from surgery.	15.b. Provide the following instructions regarding appropriate safety precautions related to the presence of a tracheostomy and nerve damage resulting from surgery: 1. always keep an obturator and outer cannula available for an emergency situation 2. always wear a Medic-Alert tag indicating neck breather status 3. reduce the risk of injury in surgical area (the area will remain numb for several months after surgery): a. use an electric rather than a straight-edge razor *in order to decrease risk of cuts in surgical area* b. avoid extremely hot foods/fluids *to decrease risk of burning the oral cavity or esophagus* 4. have smoke detectors installed in home if ability to smell is impaired 5. prevent blockage of and entrance of foreign particles into stoma: a. do not wear constrictive clothing around neck b. wear a protective shield over stoma (e.g. crocheted bib, moistened 4 × 4 gauze pad, scarf, cravat) at all times c. prevent water from entering stoma (e.g. do not swim, direct shower nozzle well below stoma, use stoma guard or shield while bathing) d. use nonaerosol shaving cream *to avoid getting cream into stoma* 6. do not drive if shoulder and neck movement is impaired.
15.c. The client will identify signs and symptoms of complications to report to the health care provider.	15.c.1. Refer to Standardized Postoperative Care Plan, Nursing Diagnosis 20, action c, for signs and symptoms to report to the health care provider. 2. Instruct client to report these additional signs and symptoms: a. persistent choking or difficulty swallowing b. bloody sputum c. presence of food or formula in secretions from stoma d. darkening of skin flap site or separation of skin edges e. increased weakness of arm on affected side f. persistent painful, drooping shoulder g. persistent nausea, vomiting, diarrhea, cramping, and/or feeling of fullness associated with tube feeding.
15.d. The client will identify community resources that	15.d.1. Provide information about community resources that can assist the client and significant others with home management and adjustment to the

can assist with home management and adjustment to the effects of surgery.

surgery (e.g. American Cancer Society, Visiting Nurse Association, home health agencies, counselors, social service agencies, Make Today Count, Lost Chord Club, vocational rehabilitation, International Association of Laryngectomees, church groups, American Speech and Hearing Association).
2. Initiate a referral if indicated.

15.e. The client will communicate an understanding of and a plan for adhering to recommended follow-up care including future appointments with health care provider and speech pathologist, medications prescribed, activity level, and wound care.

15.e.1. Refer to Standardized Postoperative Care Plan, Nursing Diagnosis 20, for routine postoperative instructions and measures to improve client compliance.
2. Caution client not to lift heavy objects.
3. Encourage client to pursue speech rehabilitation when he/she is physically ready.

Reference

Kübler-Ross, E. On death and dying. New York, Macmillan, 1969.

Stapedectomy

Stapedectomy is a surgical procedure performed to restore hearing loss that has resulted from otosclerosis (fixation of the footplate of the stapes by abnormal bone growth). The surgery is performed through an endaural incision and involves detaching and removing a portion or all of the stapes. The opening that has been created in the oval window of the ear is sealed with a piece of fascia, vein, perichondrium, or Gelfoam. A wire or prosthetic device is then attached between the incus and repaired oval window to re-establish the normal sound pathway. The surgery is usually performed under local anesthesia.

This care plan focuses on the adult client hospitalized for a stapedectomy in one ear. Preoperatively, goals of care are to reduce fear and anxiety and prepare the client for the postoperative period. The goals of postoperative care are to maintain comfort, prevent complications, and educate the client regarding follow-up care.

DISCHARGE CRITERIA

Prior to discharge, the client will:

- identify ways to prevent dislodgment of the prosthesis
- identify ways to prevent infection in the operative ear
- state signs and symptoms of complications to report to the health care provider
- verbalize an understanding of and a plan for adhering to recommended follow-up care including future appointments with health care provider, medications prescribed, activity level, and wound care.

NURSING/COLLABORATIVE DIAGNOSES

Preoperative
1. Sensory-perceptual alteration: auditory: hearing loss □ *1073*
2. Knowledge deficit □ *1074*
Postoperative
1. Altered comfort: nausea and vomiting □ *1075*
2. Sensory-perceptual alteration: auditory: hearing loss □ *1075*
3. Potential for infection: external, middle, or inner ear □ *1076*
4. Potential for trauma □ *1076*
5. Potential complications:
   a. facial nerve injury
   b. dislodgment of the prosthesis
   c. leakage of perilymph □ *1077*
6. Knowledge deficit regarding follow-up care □ *1078*

Preoperative

Use in conjunction with the Standardized Preoperative Care Plan.

1. NURSING DIAGNOSIS

Sensory-perceptual alteration: auditory: hearing loss related to otosclerosis.

DESIRED OUTCOMES	NURSING ACTIONS AND *SELECTED RATIONALES*

1. The client will be able to comprehend others as evidenced by:
a. appropriate responses
b. cooperation with treatment regimen.
	1.a. Assess client's ability to hear by:
	  1. observing for cues indicative of decreased hearing ability (e.g. speaking loudly, staring at other person's lips during conversation, moving closer to others when they speak, acts of frustration, nodding yes with subsequent inappropriate response)
	  2. noting client's verbal complaints of not being able to hear or understand what others are saying.
	b. Determine from significant others what techniques have been effective in communicating with client.
	c. Implement measures *to facilitate communication:*
	  1. provide adequate lighting in room *so client can read lips*
	  2. reduce environmental noise
	  3. speak slightly louder and more slowly than usual; avoid lowering voice at end of sentences
	  4. use simple sentences
	  5. avoid overenunciation of words
	  6. face client while speaking
	  7. avoid chewing gum or eating while talking to client

8. talk into the less impaired ear
9. rephrase sentences when client does not understand
10. employ related nonverbal cues such as facial expressions or pointing when appropriate
11. use alternative forms of communication (e.g. flash cards, paper and pencil, magic slate) if indicated
12. respond to client's call signal in person rather than over intercommunication system
13. remind client to use his/her hearing aid.

    d. Instruct significant others regarding communication techniques that are effective with the client.

□ ▬▬▬▬▬▬▬▬▬▬▬▬▬▬▬▬▬▬▬▬▬▬▬▬▬▬▬▬▬▬▬▬▬▬

2. NURSING DIAGNOSIS

Knowledge deficit regarding hospital routines associated with surgery, physical preparation for the stapedectomy, postoperative care, precautions necessary to prevent dislodgment of the prosthesis and infection in the operative ear, and effects of surgery on hearing.

□ ▬▬▬▬▬▬▬▬▬▬▬▬▬▬▬▬▬▬▬▬▬▬▬▬▬▬▬▬▬▬▬▬▬▬

DESIRED OUTCOMES	NURSING ACTIONS AND *SELECTED RATIONALES*
2.a. The client will verbalize an understanding of usual preoperative and postoperative care and routines.	2.a.1. Refer to Standardized Preoperative Care Plan, Nursing Diagnosis 4, actions a.1–4, for information to include in preoperative teaching. 2. Inform client that movement may cause dizziness and disequilibrium for 2–4 days after surgery. Instruct client that he/she will need to change positions slowly, move head and upper torso in unison, and avoid watching fast-moving objects on television after surgery *in order to reduce dizziness and disequilibrium.* 3. Allow time for questions and clarification of information provided.
2.b. The client will demonstrate the ability to perform techniques designed to prevent postoperative complications.	2.b. Refer to Standardized Preoperative Care Plan, Nursing Diagnosis 4, action b, for instructions on ways to prevent postoperative complications.

2.c. The client will verbalize an understanding of precautions necessary to prevent infection, an increase in middle ear pressure, and dislodgment of the prosthesis.	2.c.1. Inform client that he/she will not be allowed to shampoo hair for 10–14 days after surgery *in order to reduce the risk of infection.*
	2. Explain to client that he/she will be expected to lie quietly in bed for 24 hours after surgery (specific position in relation to lying on operative or unoperative side varies according to physician preference) and, following that period, to avoid any sudden, rapid movements *in order to prevent dislodgment of the prosthesis.*
	3. Instruct client on precautions necessary postoperatively *to prevent an increase in middle ear pressure and subsequent dislodgment of the prosthesis:*
	  a. avoid coughing and sneezing; if unavoidable, open mouth and cough and sneeze as gently as possible
	  b. do not blow nose for a week after surgery
	  c. avoid bending at the waist or straining to have a bowel movement
	  d. request an antiemetic or antivertigo medication if nauseated *so that vomiting is avoided.*

2.d. The client will verbalize an understanding of the expected effects of stapedectomy on hearing.	2.d.1. Reinforce physician's explanation of the expected effects of stapedectomy on hearing. 2. Inform client that hearing in the operative ear will continue to be diminished for several weeks after surgery *as a result of edema and blood accumulation in the ear and the presence of ear packing or a dressing.*

☐ ▬▬▬▬▬▬▬▬▬▬▬▬▬▬▬▬▬▬▬▬▬▬▬▬▬▬▬▬▬▬▬▬▬▬▬▬▬▬

Postoperative

Use in conjunction with the Standardized Postoperative Care Plan.

☐ ▬▬▬▬▬▬▬▬▬▬▬▬▬▬▬▬▬▬▬▬▬▬▬▬▬▬▬▬▬▬▬▬▬▬▬▬▬▬

1. NURSING DIAGNOSIS

Altered comfort: nausea and vomiting related to stimulation of the vomiting center associated with:

a. trauma to the vagal nerve (some vagal fibers are close to the middle ear) during surgery;
b. vestibulocerebellar and chemoreceptor trigger zone stimulation resulting from possible changes in inner ear pressure due to leakage of perilymph and/or labyrinthitis;
c. cortical stimulation due to pain and stress.

☐ ▬▬▬▬▬▬▬▬▬▬▬▬▬▬▬▬▬▬▬▬▬▬▬▬▬▬▬▬▬▬▬▬▬▬▬▬▬▬

DESIRED OUTCOMES	NURSING ACTIONS AND *SELECTED RATIONALES*

1. The client will experience relief of nausea and vomiting (see Standardized Postoperative Care Plan, Nursing Diagnosis 7.C, for outcome criteria).	1.a. Refer to Standardized Postoperative Care Plan, Nursing Diagnosis 7.C, for measures related to assessment and prevention of nausea and vomiting.
	b. Implement additional measures *to prevent nausea and vomiting:*
	  1. remind client to change positions slowly, move head and upper torso in unison, and avoid watching quick-moving objects *(movement stimulates the chemoreceptor trigger zone)*
	  2. perform actions *to minimize changes in inner ear pressure:*
	    a. implement measures to prevent and treat ear infection (see Postoperative Nursing Diagnosis 3, actions d and e)
	    b. implement measures to prevent dislodgment of the prosthesis (see Postoperative Collaborative Diagnosis 5, action b.2) *in order to prevent subsequent leakage of perilymph*
	  3. monitor for therapeutic and nontherapeutic effects of antiemetics and antivertigo medications (e.g. dimenhydrinate, meclizine hydrochloride, scopolamine) if administered.

☐ ▬▬▬▬▬▬▬▬▬▬▬▬▬▬▬▬▬▬▬▬▬▬▬▬▬▬▬▬▬▬▬▬▬▬▬▬▬▬

2. NURSING DIAGNOSIS

Sensory-perceptual alteration: auditory: hearing loss related to blood accumulation or edema in the operative ear and the presence of ear packing or a dressing.

☐ ▬▬▬▬▬▬▬▬▬▬▬▬▬▬▬▬▬▬▬▬▬▬▬▬▬▬▬▬▬▬▬▬▬▬▬▬▬▬

DESIRED OUTCOMES	NURSING ACTIONS AND *SELECTED RATIONALES*
2. The client will be able to comprehend others (see Preoperative Nursing Diagnosis 1 for outcome criteria).	2. Refer to Preoperative Nursing Diagnosis 1 for measures related to assessment of hearing loss and measures to facilitate communication.

3. NURSING DIAGNOSIS

Potential for infection: external, middle, or inner ear related to intraoperative or postoperative wound contamination.

DESIRED OUTCOMES	NURSING ACTIONS AND *SELECTED RATIONALES*

3. The client will not develop an infection in the operative ear as evidenced by:
a. gradual resolution of ear pressure and pain
b. expected drainage from ear
c. afebrile status
d. resolution of vertigo and tinnitus
e. absence of nystagmus
f. WBC count declining toward normal
g. negative cultures of drainage from ear.
	3.a. Assess for and report signs and symptoms of infection in the operative ear (e.g. persistent or increased pain and pressure in ear; purulent, yellow-green, or foul-smelling drainage on ear dressing; persistent temperature elevation; persistent or increased vertigo and tinnitus; nystagmus).
	b. Monitor WBC count. Report persistent elevation of or an increasing WBC count.
	c. Obtain ear drainage specimen for culture as ordered. Report positive results.
	d. Implement measures *to prevent infection in operative ear:*
	  1. maintain aseptic technique when reinforcing or changing dressing
	  2. instruct client to keep hands away from dressing
	  3. remind client to avoid blowing nose, coughing, and sneezing (*these activities force air and organisms up the eustachian tube into the middle ear*)
	  4. avoid getting operative ear wet
	  5. do not shampoo client's hair (can use rinseless shampoo)
	  6. protect client from persons known to have respiratory infection
	  7. monitor for therapeutic and nontherapeutic effects of anti-infectives if administered prophylactically.
	e. If signs and symptoms of ear infection occur:
	  1. continue with above actions
	  2. assess closely for and report signs and symptoms of meningitis (e.g. nuchal rigidity, headache, photophobia, inability to straighten knee when hip is flexed, flexion of hip and knee in response to forward flexion of the neck)
	  3. monitor for therapeutic and nontherapeutic effects of anti-infectives if administered.

4. NURSING DIAGNOSIS

Potential for trauma related to falls associated with vertigo resulting from:

a. leakage of perilymph around the prosthesis;
b. labyrinthitis associated with trauma to the labyrinth during surgery and/or development of infection in the labyrinth.

DESIRED OUTCOMES	NURSING ACTIONS AND *SELECTED RATIONALES*
4. The client will not experience falls.	4.a. Refer to Standardized Postoperative Care Plan, Nursing Diagnosis 17, action b, for measures to prevent falls. b. Implement measures *to reduce vertigo in order to further reduce risk of falls:* 1. reinforce preoperative teaching on the need to change positions slowly,

move head and upper torso in unison, and avoid watching quick-moving objects

2. caution client to avoid looking down when ambulating
3. monitor for therapeutic and nontherapeutic effects of antivertigo medications (e.g. dimenhydrinate, meclizine hydrochloride, scopolamine) if administered.

□ ▇▇▇▇▇▇▇▇▇▇▇▇▇▇▇▇▇▇▇▇▇▇▇▇▇▇▇▇

5. COLLABORATIVE DIAGNOSIS:

Potential complications:

a. **facial nerve injury** related to damage during injection of local anesthetic, surgical trauma to the nerve, or pressure on the nerve due to postoperative edema (the facial nerve passes through the middle ear);
b. **dislodgment of the prosthesis** related to improper movement and increased pressure in the eustachian tube and middle or inner ear;
c. **leakage of perilymph** related to incomplete closure of the oval window, fistula formation, and/or dislodgment of the prosthesis.

□ ▇▇▇▇▇▇▇▇▇▇▇▇▇▇▇▇▇▇▇▇▇▇▇▇▇▇▇▇

DESIRED OUTCOMES	NURSING ACTIONS AND *SELECTED RATIONALES*

5.a. The client will have resolution of facial nerve damage if it occurs as evidenced by:
1. gradual improvement of any facial motor weakness
2. gradual return of normal taste sensation.

5.a.1. Assess for signs and symptoms of facial nerve damage (e.g. inability to wrinkle forehead or close eyelids tightly, drooping of mouth on operative side, drooling when drinking fluids from a cup or glass, statements of diminished taste sensation).
2. If signs and symptoms of facial nerve damage occur:
   a. instruct client to avoid hot foods/fluids *in order to decrease the risk of mouth and lip burns*
   b. if drooling when drinking fluids is a problem, encourage client to use a straw
   c. if client has diminished taste sensation, encourage him/her to use additional seasonings on food
   d. reassure client that the signs and symptoms usually resolve within a few months
   e. assess for and report an increase in the severity of signs and symptoms.

5.b. The client will not experience dislodgment of the prosthesis or leakage of perilymph as evidenced by:
1. gradual resolution of ear pain
2. resolution of vertigo and tinnitus
3. continued improvement in hearing
4. absence of nystagmus.

5.b.1. Assess for and report signs and symptoms of loosening of the prosthesis and/or leakage of perilymph (e.g. increased pain or pressure in ear, recurrent or increased vertigo or tinnitus, fluctuation in ability to hear, nystagmus).
2. Implement measures *to prevent dislodgment of the prosthesis:*
   a. maintain activity and position restrictions as ordered (usually on strict bedrest for first 24 hours after surgery)
   b. remind client to avoid any sudden, rapid movements
   c. reinforce preoperative teaching about ways to prevent increasing pressure in the middle ear (see Preoperative Nursing Diagnosis 2, action c.3)
   d. administer antiemetics or antivertigo medications at first indication of nausea *in order to prevent vomiting*
   e. perform actions to prevent and treat infection in the operative ear (see Postoperative Nursing Diagnosis 3, actions d and e) *in order to reduce inflammation and additional pressure in the ear.*
3. If signs and symptoms of dislodgment of the prosthesis or leakage of perilymph occur:
   a. continue with above measures
   b. prepare client for surgical revision if planned
   c. provide emotional support to client and significant others.

6. NURSING DIAGNOSIS

Knowledge deficit regarding follow-up care.

DESIRED OUTCOMES	NURSING ACTIONS AND *SELECTED RATIONALES*
6.a. The client will identify ways to prevent dislodgment of the prosthesis.	6.a. Instruct client regarding ways *to reduce risk of dislodging the prosthesis:* 1. avoid coughing and sneezing for at least a week after surgery; if coughing and sneezing are unavoidable, open mouth and cough and sneeze gently 2. do not blow nose for a week after surgery; after this period, blow nose gently with nostrils unobstructed 3. avoid lifting heavy objects for at least 2 months 4. avoid straining to have a bowel movement; consult physician if constipation occurs 5. avoid sudden, rapid movements and activities that create changes in ear pressure (e.g. diving, flying, riding in elevators) until physician allows.
6.b. The client will identify ways to prevent infection in the operative ear.	6.b. Instruct client regarding ways *to prevent infection in the operative ear:* 1. avoid touching ear dressing unnecessarily 2. use clean technique when changing dressings 3. do not wash hair for 10–14 days after surgery and then avoid getting water in ear while washing hair for an additional 4 weeks 4. avoid showering or swimming for at least 6 weeks after surgery *to reduce risk of water entering ear* 5. keep operative ear covered when outside until healing is complete 6. avoid persons known to have a respiratory infection.

6.c. The client will state signs and symptoms of complications to report to the health care provider.	6.c.1. Refer to Standardized Postoperative Care Plan, Nursing Diagnosis 20, action c, for signs and symptoms to report to the health care provider.
	2. Instruct client to report these additional signs and symptoms:
	  a. persistent or increased pain or pressure in operative ear
	  b. fluctuation in hearing ability in operative ear
	  c. persistent or recurrent dizziness or ringing in operative ear
	  d. unexplained nausea and vomiting
	  e. headache, stiff neck, unusual sensitivity to light.

6.d. The client will verbalize an understanding of and a plan for adhering to recommended follow-up care including future appointments with health care provider, medications prescribed, activity level, and wound care.	6.d.1. Refer to Standardized Postoperative Care Plan, Nursing Diagnosis 20, for routine postoperative instructions and measures to improve client compliance. 2. Reinforce teaching on the need to change positions slowly, move head and upper torso in unison, and avoid watching fast-moving objects on television for 2–4 days after surgery. 3. Reinforce physician's instructions about changing the ear dressing.

APPENDIX
Nursing Diagnoses Approved by NANDA* Through 1988†

ACTIVITY INTOLERANCE

Definition

A state in which an individual has insufficient physiological or psychological energy to endure or complete required or desired daily activities.

Defining Characteristics

*Verbal report of fatigue or weakness; abnormal heart rate or blood pressure response to activity; exertional discomfort or dyspnea; electrocardiographic changes reflecting arrhythmias or ischemia.

Related Factors

Bedrest/immobility; generalized weakness; sedentary life style; imbalance between oxygen supply/demand.

---

* Critical defining characteristic.

ACTIVITY INTOLERANCE, POTENTIAL

Definition

A state in which an individual is at risk of experiencing insufficient physiological or psychological energy to endure or complete required or desired daily activities.

Defining Characteristics

Presence of risk factors such as:

History of previous intolerance; deconditioned status; presence of circulatory/respiratory problems; inexperience with the activity.

Related Factors

See risk factors.

---

* North American Nursing Diagnosis Association.

† These diagnostic labels with definitions, defining characteristics, and related factors are reprinted from *Taxonomy I: revised 1989* published by NANDA, 3525 Caroline St., St. Louis, MO 63104.

ADJUSTMENT, IMPAIRED

Definition

The state in which the individual is unable to modify his/her life style/behavior in a manner consistent with a change in health status.

Defining Characteristics

Major

Verbalization of nonacceptance of health status change; nonexistent or unsuccessful ability to be involved in problem-solving or goal-setting.

Minor

Lack of movement toward independence; extended period of shock, disbelief, or anger regarding health status change; lack of future-oriented thinking.

Related Factors

Disability requiring change in life style; inadequate support systems; impaired cognition; sensory overload; assault to self-esteem; altered locus of control; incomplete grieving.

AIRWAY CLEARANCE, INEFFECTIVE

Definition

A state in which an individual is unable to clear secretions or obstructions from the respiratory tract to maintain airway patency.

Defining Characteristics

Abnormal breath sounds (rales [crackles], rhonchi [wheezes]); changes in rate or depth of respiration; tachypnea; cough, effective/ineffective, with or without sputum; cyanosis; dyspnea.

Related Factors

Decreased energy/fatigue; tracheobronchial infection, obstruction, secretion; perceptual/cognitive impairment; trauma.

ANXIETY

Definition

A vague uneasy feeling whose source is often nonspecific or unknown to the individual.

Defining Characteristics

Subjective: increased tension; apprehension; painful and persistent increased helplessness; uncertainty; fearful; scared; regretful; overexcited; rattled; distressed; jittery; feelings of inadequacy; shakiness; fear of unspecific consequences; expressed concerns about change in life events; worried; anxious.

Objective: *sympathetic stimulation–cardiovascular excitation, superficial vasoconstriction, pupil dilation; restlessness; insomnia; glancing about; poor eye contact; trembling/hand tremors; extraneous movement (foot shuffling, hand/arm movements); facial tension; voice quivering; focus "self"; increased wariness; increased perspiration.

Related Factors

Unconscious conflict about essential values/goals of life; threat to self-concept; threat of death; threat to or change in health status; threat to or change in role functioning; threat to or change in environment; threat to or change in interaction patterns; situational/maturational crises; interpersonal transmission/contagion; unmet needs.

---

* Critical defining characteristic.

ASPIRATION, POTENTIAL FOR

Definition

The state in which an individual is at risk for entry of gastrointestinal secretions, oropharyngeal secretions, or solids or fluids into tracheobronchial passages.

Defining Characteristics

Presence of risk factors such as:

Reduced level of consciousness; depressed cough and gag reflexes; presence of tracheostomy or endotracheal tube; incompetent lower esophageal sphincter; gastroin-

testinal tubes; tube feedings; medication administration; situations hindering elevation of upper body; increased intragastric pressure; increased gastric residual; decreased gastrointestinal motility; delayed gastric emptying; impaired swallowing; facial/oral/neck surgery or trauma; wired jaws.

Related Factors

See risk factors.

BODY IMAGE DISTURBANCE

Definition

Disruption in the way one perceives one's body image.

Defining Characteristics

A *or* B must be present to justify the diagnosis of body image disturbance. *A = verbal response to actual or perceived change in structure and/or function; *B = nonverbal response to actual or perceived change in structure and/or function. The following clinical manifestations may be used to validate the presence of A *or* B.

Objective: missing body part; actual change in structure and/or function; not looking at body part; not touching body part; hiding or overexposing body part (intentional or unintentional); trauma to nonfunctioning part; change in social involvement; change in ability to estimate spatial relationship of body to environment.

Subjective: verbalization of: change in life style; fear of rejection or of reaction by others; focus on past strength, function, or appearance; negative feelings about body; and feelings of helplessness, hopelessness, or powerlessness; preoccupation with change or loss; emphasis on remaining strengths, heightened achievement; extension of body boundary to incorporate environmental objects; personalization of part or loss by name; depersonalization of part or loss by impersonal pronouns; refusal to verify actual change.

Related Factors

Biophysical; cognitive/perceptual; psychosocial; cultural or spiritual.

---

* Critical defining characteristics.

BODY TEMPERATURE, POTENTIAL, ALTERED

Definition

The state in which the individual is at risk for failure to maintain body temperature within normal range.

Defining Characteristics

Presence of risk factors such as:

Extremes of age; extremes of weight; exposure to cold/cool or warm/hot environments; dehydration; inactivity or vigorous activity; medications causing vasoconstriction/vasodilation; altered metabolic rate; sedation; inappropriate clothing for environmental temperature; illness or trauma affecting temperature regulation.

Related Factors

See risk factors.

BOWEL INCONTINENCE

Definition

A state in which an individual experiences a change in normal bowel habits characterized by involuntary passage of stool.

Defining Characteristics

Involuntary passage of stool.

Related Factors

To be developed.

BREASTFEEDING, INEFFECTIVE

Definition

The state in which a mother, infant, or child experiences dissatisfaction or difficulty with the breastfeeding process.

Defining Characteristics

Major

Unsatisfactory breastfeeding process.

Minor

Actual or perceived inadequate milk supply; infant inability to attach onto maternal breast correctly; no observable signs of oxytocin release; observable signs of inadequate infant intake; nonsustained suckling at the breast; insufficient emptying of each breast per feeding; persistence of sore nipples beyond the first week of breastfeeding; insufficient opportunity for suckling at the breast; infant exhibiting fussiness and crying within the first hour after breastfeeding; unresponsive to other comfort measures; infant arching and crying at the breast; resisting latching on.

Related Factors

Prematurity; infant anomaly; maternal breast anomaly; previous breast surgery; previous history of breastfeeding failure; infant receiving supplemental feedings with artificial nipple; poor infant sucking reflex; nonsupportive partner/family; knowledge deficit; interruption in breastfeeding; maternal anxiety or ambivalence.

BREATHING PATTERN, INEFFECTIVE

Definition

The state in which an individual's inhalation and/or exhalation pattern does not enable adequate pulmonary inflation or emptying.

Defining Characteristics

Dyspnea, shortness of breath, tachypnea, fremitus, abnormal arterial blood gas, cyanosis, cough, nasal flaring, respiratory depth changes, assumption of 3-point position, pursed-lip breathing/prolonged expiratory phase, increased anteroposterior diameter, use of accessory muscles, altered chest excursion.

Related Factors

Neuromuscular impairment; pain; musculoskeletal impairment; perception/cognitive impairment; anxiety; decreased energy/fatigue.

CARDIAC OUTPUT, DECREASED

Definition

A state in which the blood pumped by an individual's heart is sufficiently reduced that it is inadequate to meet the needs of the body's tissues.

Defining Characteristics

Variations in blood pressure readings; arrhythmias; fatigue; jugular vein distention; color changes, skin and mucous membranes; oliguria; decreased peripheral pulses; cold, clammy skin; rales; dyspnea, orthopnea; restlessness.

Other Possible Characteristics

Change in mental status; shortness of breath; syncope; vertigo; edema; cough; frothy sputum; gallop rhythm; weakness.

Related Factors

To be developed.

COMMUNICATION, IMPAIRED VERBAL

Definition

The state in which an individual experiences a decreased or absent ability to use or understand language in human interaction.

Defining Characteristics

*Unable to speak dominant language; *speaks or verbalizes with difficulty; *does not or cannot speak; stuttering; slurring; difficulty forming words or sentences; difficulty expressing thought verbally; inappropriate verbalization; dyspnea; disorientation.

Related Factors

Decrease in circulation to brain; brain tumor; physical barrier (tracheostomy, intubation); anatomical defect, cleft palate; psychological barriers (psychosis, lack of stimuli); cultural difference; developmental or age-related.

---

* Critical defining characteristics.

CONSTIPATION

Definition

A state in which an individual experiences a change in normal bowel habits characterized by a decrease in frequency and/or passage of hard, dry stools.

Defining Characteristics

Decreased activity level; frequency less than usual pattern; hard, formed stools; palpable mass; reported feeling of pressure in rectum; reported feeling of rectal fullness; straining at stool.

Other Possible Characteristics

Abdominal pain; appetite impairment; back pain; headache; interference with daily living; use of laxatives.

Related Factors

To be developed.

CONSTIPATION, COLONIC

Definition

The state in which an individual's pattern of elimination is characterized by hard, dry stool that results from a delay in passage of food residue.

Defining Characteristics

Major

Decreased frequency; hard, dry stool; straining at stool; painful defecation; abdominal distention; palpable mass.

Minor

Rectal pressure; headache; appetite impairment; abdominal pain.

Related Factors

Less than adequate fluid intake; less than adequate dietary intake; less than adequate fiber; less than adequate physical activity; immobility; lack of privacy; emotional disturbances; chronic use of medication and enemas; stress; change in daily routine; metabolic problems, e.g. hypothyroidism, hypocalcemia, hypokalemia.

CONSTIPATION, PERCEIVED

Definition

The state in which an individual makes a self-diagnosis of constipation and ensures a daily bowel movement through abuse of laxatives, enemas, and suppositories.

Defining Characteristics

Major

Expectation of a daily bowel movement with the resulting overuse of laxatives, enemas, and suppositories; expected passage of stool at same time every day.

Related Factors

Cultural/family health beliefs; faulty appraisal; impaired thought processes.

COPING, DEFENSIVE

Definition

The state in which an individual repeatedly projects falsely positive self-evaluation based on a self-protective pattern that defends against underlying perceived threats to positive self-regard.

Defining Characteristics

Major

Denial of obvious problems/weaknesses; projection of blame/responsibility; rationalizes failures; hypersensitive to slight criticism; grandiosity.

Minor

Superior attitude toward others; difficulty establishing/ maintaining relationships; hostile laughter or ridicule of others; difficulty in reality testing perceptions; lack of follow-through or participation in treatment or therapy.

COPING, FAMILY: POTENTIAL FOR GROWTH

Definition

Effective managing of adaptive tasks by family member involved with the client's health challenge, who now is exhibiting desire and readiness for enhanced health and growth in regard to self and in relation to the client.

Defining Characteristics

Family member attempting to describe growth impact of crisis on his/her own values, priorities, goal, or relationships; family member moving in direction of health-promoting and enriching life style that supports and monitors maturational processes, audits and negotiates treatment programs, and generally chooses experiences that optimize wellness; individual expressing interest in making contact on a one-to-one basis or on a mutual-aid group basis with another person who has experienced a similar situation.

Related Factors

Needs sufficiently gratified and adaptive tasks effectively addressed to enable goals of self-actualization to surface.

COPING, FAMILY: INEFFECTIVE, COMPROMISED

Definition

A usually supportive primary person (family member or close friend) is providing insufficient, ineffective, or compromised support, comfort, assistance, or encouragement that may be needed by the client to manage or master adaptive tasks related to his/her health challenge.

Defining Characteristics

Subjective: client expresses or confirms a concern or complaint about significant other's response to his/her health problem; significant person describes preoccupation with personal reaction (e.g. fear, anticipatory grief, guilt, anxiety to client's illness, disability, or other situational or developmental crises); significant person describes or confirms an inadequate understanding or knowledge base that interferes with effective assistive or supportive behaviors.
Objective: significant person attempts assistive or supportive behaviors with less than satisfactory results; significant person withdraws or enters into limited or temporary personal communication with the client at the time of need; significant person displays protective behavior disproportionate (too little or too much) to the client's abilities or need for autonomy.

Related Factors

Inadequate or incorrect information or understanding by a primary person; temporary preoccupation by a significant person who is trying to manage emotional conflicts and personal suffering and is unable to perceive or act effectively in regard to client's needs; temporary family disorganization and role changes; other situational or developmental crises or situations the significant person may be facing; little support provided by client, in turn, for primary person; prolonged disease or disability progression that exhausts supportive capacity of significant people.

COPING, FAMILY: INEFFECTIVE, DISABLING

Definition

Behavior of significant person (family member or other primary person) that disables his/her own capacities and the client's capacities to effectively address tasks essential to either person's adaptation to the health challenge.

Defining Characteristics

Neglectful care of the client in regard to basic human needs and/or illness treatment; distortion of reality regarding the client's health problem, including extreme denial about its existence or severity; intolerance; rejection; abandonment; desertion; carrying on usual routines, disregarding client's needs; psychosomaticism; taking on illness signs of client; decisions and actions by family that are detrimental to economic or social well-being; agitation, depression, aggression, hostility; impaired restructuring of a meaningful life for self, impaired individualization, prolonged overconcern for client; neglectful relationships with other family members; client's development of helpless, inactive dependence.

Related Factors

Significant person with chronically unexpressed feelings of guilt, anxiety, hostility, despair, etc.; dissonant discrepancy of coping styles for dealing with adaptive tasks by the significant person and client or among significant people; highly ambivalent family relationships; arbitrary handling of family's resistance to treatment, which tends to solidify defensiveness since it fails to deal adequately with underlying anxiety.

COPING, INDIVIDUAL: INEFFECTIVE

Definition

Impairment of adaptive behaviors and problem-solving abilities of a person in meeting life's demands and roles.

Defining Characteristics

*Verbalization of inability to cope or inability to ask for help; inability to meet role expectations; inability to meet basic needs; *inability to problem-solve; alteration in societal participation; destructive behavior toward self or others; inappropriate use of defense mechanisms; change in usual communication patterns; verbal manipulation; high illness rate; high rate of accidents.

Related Factors

Situational crises; maturational crises; personal vulnerability.

---

* Critical defining characteristics.

DECISIONAL CONFLICT (SPECIFY)

Definition

The state of uncertainty about course of action to be taken when choice among competing actions involves risk, loss, or challenge to personal life values.

Defining Characteristics

Major

Verbalized uncertainty about choices; verbalization of undesired consequences of alternative actions being considered; vacillation between alternative choices; delayed decision making.

Minor

Verbalized feeling of distress while attempting a decision; self-focusing; physical signs of distress or tension (increased heart rate, increased muscle tension, restlessness, etc.); questioning personal values and beliefs while attempting a decision.

Related Factors

Unclear personal values/beliefs; perceived threat to value system; lack of experience or interference with decision making; lack of relevant information; support system deficit; multiple or divergent sources of information.

DENIAL, INEFFECTIVE

Definition

The state of a conscious or unconscious attempt to disavow the knowledge or meaning of an event to reduce anxiety/fear to the detriment of health.

Defining Characteristics

Major

Delays seeking or refuses health care attention to the detriment of health; does not perceive personal relevance of symptoms or danger.

Minor

Uses home remedies (self-treatment) to relieve symptoms; does not admit fear of death or invalidism; minimizes symptoms; displaces source of symptoms to other organs; unable to admit impact of disease on life pattern; makes dismissive gestures or comments when speaking of distressing events; displaces fear of impact of the condition; displays inappropriate affect.

DIARRHEA

Definition

A state in which an individual experiences a change in normal bowel habits characterized by the frequent passage of loose, fluid, unformed stools.

Defining Characteristics

Abdominal pain; cramping; increased frequency; increased frequency of bowel sounds; loose, liquid stools; urgency.

Other Possible Characteristics

Change in color.

Related Factors

To be developed.

DISUSE SYNDROME, POTENTIAL FOR

Definition

A state in which an individual is at risk for deterioration of body systems as the result of prescribed or unavoidable musculoskeletal inactivity.*

Defining Characteristics

Presence of risk factors such as:

Paralysis; mechanical immobilization; prescribed immobilization; severe pain; altered level of consciousness.

Related Factors

See risk factors.

---

* Complications from immobility can include pressure ulcer, constipation, stasis of pulmonary secretions, thrombosis, urinary tract infection/retention, decreased strength/endurance, orthostatic hypotension, decreased range of joint motion, disorientation, body image disturbance, and powerlessness.

DIVERSIONAL ACTIVITY DEFICIT

Definition

The state in which an individual experiences a decreased stimulation from or interest or engagement in recreational or leisure activities.

Defining Characteristics

Patient's statements regarding: boredom, wish there was something to do, to read, etc.; usual hobbies cannot be undertaken in hospital.

Related Factors

Environmental lack of diversional activity, as in: long-term hospitalization, frequent lengthy treatments.

DYSREFLEXIA

Definition

The state in which an individual with a spinal cord injury at T7 or above experiences a life-threatening uninhibited sympathetic response of the nervous system to a noxious stimulus.

Defining Characteristics

Major: Individual with spinal cord injury (T7 or above) with:

Paroxysmal hypertension (sudden periodic elevated blood pressure where systolic pressure is over 140 mm Hg and diastolic is above 90 mm Hg); bradycardia or tachycardia (pulse rate of less than 60 or over 100 beats/minute); diaphoresis (above the injury); red splotches on skin (above the injury); pallor (below the injury); headache (a diffuse pain in different portions of the head and not confined to any nerve distribution area).

Minor

Chilling; conjunctival congestion; Horner's syndrome (contraction of the pupil, partial ptosis of the eyelid, enophthalmos and sometimes loss of sweating over the affected side of the face); paresthesia; pilomotor reflex (gooseflesh formation when skin is cooled); blurred vision; chest pain; metallic taste in mouth; nasal congestion.

Related Factors

Bladder distention; bowel distention; skin irritation; lack of patient and caregiver knowledge.

FAMILY PROCESSES, ALTERED

Definition

The state in which a family that normally functions effectively experiences a dysfunction.

Defining Characteristics

Family system unable to meet physical needs of its members; family system unable to meet emotional needs of its members; family system unable to meet spiritual needs of its members; parents do not demonstrate respect for each other's views on child-rearing practices; inability to express/accept wide range of feelings; inability to express/accept feelings of members; family unable to meet security needs of its members; inability of the family members to relate to each other for mutual growth and maturation; family uninvolved in community activities; inability to accept/receive help appropriately; rigidity in function and roles; family not demonstrating respect for individuality and autonomy of its members; family unable to adapt to change/deal with traumatic experience constructively; family failing to accomplish current/past developmental task; unhealthy family decision-making process; failure to send and receive clear messages; inappropriate boundary maintenance; inappropriate/poorly communicated family rules, rituals, symbols; unexamined family myths; inappropriate level and direction of energy.

Related Factors

Situation transition and/or crisis; developmental transition and/or crisis.

FATIGUE

Definition

An overwhelming sustained sense of exhaustion and decreased capacity for physical and mental work.

Defining Characteristics

Major

Verbalization of an unremitting and overwhelming lack of energy; inability to maintain usual routines.

Minor

Perceived need for additional energy to accomplish routine tasks; increase in physical complaints; emotionally labile or irritable; impaired ability to concentrate; decreased performance; lethargic or listless; disinterest in surroundings/introspection; decreased libido; accident prone.

Related Factors

Decreased/increased metabolic energy production; overwhelming psychological or emotional demands; increased energy requirements to perform activity of daily living; excessive social and/or role demands; states of discomfort; altered body chemistry (e.g. medications, drug withdrawal, chemotherapy).

FEAR

Definition

Feeling of dread related to an identifiable source that the person validates.

Defining Characteristics

Ability to identify object of fear.

Related Factors

To be developed.

FLUID VOLUME DEFICIT

Definition

The state in which an individual experiences vascular, cellular, or intracellular dehydration.

Defining Characteristics

Change in urine output; change in urine concentration; sudden weight loss or gain; decreased venous filling; hemoconcentration; change in serum sodium.

Other Possible Characteristics

Hypotension; thirst; increased pulse rate; decreased skin turgor; decreased pulse volume/pressure; change in mental state; increased body temperature; dry skin; dry mucous membranes; weakness.

Related Factors

Active fluid volume loss; failure of regulatory mechanisms.

FLUID VOLUME DEFICIT, POTENTIAL

Definition

The state in which an individual is at risk of experiencing vascular, cellular, or intracellular dehydration.

Defining Characteristics

Presence of risk factors such as:

Extremes of age; extremes of weight; excessive losses through normal routes, e.g. diarrhea; loss of fluid through abnormal routes, e.g. indwelling tubes; deviations affecting access to or intake or absorption of fluids, e.g. physical immobility; factors influencing fluid needs, e.g. hypermetabolic state; knowledge deficiency related to fluid volume; medications, e.g. diuretics.

Related Factors

See risk factors.

FLUID VOLUME EXCESS

Definition

The state in which an individual experiences increased fluid retention and edema.

Defining Characteristics

Edema; effusion; anasarca; weight gain; shortness of breath, orthopnea; intake greater than output; S_3 heart sound; pulmonary congestion (chest x-ray); abnormal breath sounds, rales (crackles); change in respiratory pattern; change in mental status; decreased hemoglobin and hematocrit; blood pressure changes; central venous pressure changes; pulmonary artery pressure changes; jugular vein distention; positive hepatojugular reflex; oliguria; specific gravity changes; azotemia; altered electrolytes; restlessness and anxiety.

Related Factors

Compromised regulatory mechanism; excess fluid intake; excess sodium intake.

GAS EXCHANGE, IMPAIRED

Definition

The state in which the individual experiences a decreased passage of oxygen and/or carbon dioxide between the alveoli of the lungs and the vascular system.

Defining Characteristics

Confusion; somnolence; restlessness; irritability; inability to move secretions; hypercapnea; hypoxia.

Related Factors

Ventilation-perfusion imbalance.

GRIEVING, ANTICIPATORY

Defining Characteristics

Potential loss of significant object; expression of distress at potential loss; denial of potential loss; guilt; anger; sorrow, choked feelings; changes in eating habits; alterations in sleep patterns; alterations in activity level; altered libido; altered communication patterns.

Related Factors

To be developed.

GRIEVING, DYSFUNCTIONAL

Defining Characteristics

Verbal expression of distress at loss; denial of loss; expression of guilt; expression of unresolved issues; anger; sadness; crying; difficulty in expressing loss; alterations in: eating habits, sleep patterns, dream patterns, activity level, libido; idealization of lost object; reliving of past experiences; interference with life functioning; developmental regression; labile affect; alterations in concentration and/or pursuit of tasks.

Related Factors

Actual or perceived object loss (object loss is used in the broadest sense); objects may include: people, possessions, a job, status, home, ideals, parts and processes of the body.

GROWTH AND DEVELOPMENT, ALTERED

Definition

The state in which an individual demonstrates deviations in norms from his/her age group.

Defining Characteristics

Major

Delay or difficulty in performing skills (motor, social, or expressive) typical of age group; altered physical growth; inability to perform self-care or self-control activities appropriate for age.

Minor

Flat affect; listlessness, decreased responses.

Related Factors

Inadequate caretaking: indifference, inconsistent responsiveness, multiple caretakers; separation from significant others; environmental and stimulation deficiencies; effects of physical disability; prescribed dependence.

HEALTH MAINTENANCE, ALTERED

Definition

Inability to identify, manage, and/or seek out help to maintain health.

Defining Characteristics

Demonstrated lack of knowledge regarding basic health practices; demonstrated lack of adaptive behaviors to internal/external environmental changes; reported or observed inability to take responsibility for meeting basic health practices in any or all functional pattern areas; history of lack of health seeking behavior; expressed interest in improving health behaviors; reported or observed lack of equipment, financial, and/or other resources; reported or observed impairment of personal support systems.

Related Factors

Lack of or significant alteration in communication skills (written, verbal, and/or gestural); lack of ability to make deliberate and thoughtful judgments; perceptual/cognitive impairment (complete/partial lack of gross and/or fine motor skills); ineffective individual coping; dysfunctional grieving; unachieved developmental tasks; ineffective family coping; disabling spiritual distress; lack of material resources.

HEALTH SEEKING BEHAVIORS

Definition

A state in which an individual in stable health is actively seeking ways to alter personal health habits and/or the environment in order to move toward a higher level of health.*

Defining Characteristics

Major

Expressed or observed desire to seek a higher level of wellness.

---

* Stable health status is defined as age-appropriate illness prevention measures are achieved; client reports good or excellent health; and signs and symptoms of disease, if present, are controlled.

Minor

Expressed or observed desire for increased control of health practice; expression of concern about current environmental conditions on health status; stated or observed unfamiliarity with wellness community resources; demonstrated or observed lack of knowledge in health promotion behaviors.

HOME MAINTENANCE MANAGEMENT, IMPAIRED

Definition

Inability to independently maintain a safe growth-promoting immediate environment.

Defining Characteristics

Subjective: *household members express difficulty in maintaining their home in a comfortable fashion; *household members request assistance with home maintenance; *household members describe outstanding debts or financial crises.

Objective: disorderly surroundings; *unwashed or unavailable cooking equipment, clothes, or linen; *accumulation of dirt, food wastes, or hygienic wastes; offensive odors; inappropriate household temperature; *overtaxed family members, e.g. exhausted, anxious; lack of necessary equipment or aids; presence of vermin or rodents; *repeated hygienic disorders, infestations, or infections.

Related Factors

Individual/family member disease or injury; insufficient family organization or planning; insufficient finances; unfamiliarity with neighborhood resources; impaired cognitive or emotional functioning; lack of knowledge; lack of role modeling; inadequate support systems.

---

* Critical defining characteristics.

HOPELESSNESS

Definition

A subjective state in which an individual sees limited or no alternatives or personal choices available and is unable to mobilize energy on own behalf.

Defining Characteristics

Major

Passivity, decreased verbalization; decreased affect; verbal cues (despondent content, "I can't," sighing).

Minor

Lack of initiative; decreased response to stimuli; decreased affect; turning away from speaker; closing eyes; shrugging in response to speaker; decreased appetite; increased/decreased sleep; lack of involvement in care/passively allowing care.

Related Factors

Prolonged activity restriction creating isolation; failing or deteriorating physiological condition; long-term stress; abandonment; lost belief in transcendent values/God.

HYPERTHERMIA

Definition

A state in which an individual's body temperature is elevated above his/her normal range.

Defining Characteristics

Major

Increase in body temperature above normal range.

Minor

Flushed skin; warm to touch; increased respiratory rate; tachycardia; seizures/convulsions.

Related Factors

Exposure to hot environment; vigorous activity; medications/anesthesia; inappropriate clothing; increased metabolic rate; illness or trauma; dehydration; inability or decreased ability to perspire.

HYPOTHERMIA

Definition

The state in which an individual's body temperature is reduced below normal range.

Defining Characteristics

Major

Reduction in body temperature below normal range; shivering (mild); cool skin; pallor (moderate).

Minor

Slow capillary refill; tachycardia; cyanotic nail beds; hypertension; piloerection.

Related Factors

Exposure to cool or cold environment; illness or trauma; damage to hypothalamus; inability or decreased ability to shiver; malnutrition; inadequate clothing; consumption of alcohol; medications causing vasodilation; evaporation from skin in cool environment; decreased metabolic rate; inactivity; aging.

INCONTINENCE, FUNCTIONAL

Definition

The state in which an individual experiences an involuntary, unpredictable passage of urine.

Defining Characteristics

Major

Urge to void or bladder contractions sufficiently strong to result in loss of urine before reaching an appropriate receptacle.

Related Factors

Altered environment; sensory, cognitive, or mobility deficits.

INCONTINENCE, REFLEX

Definition

The state in which an individual experiences an involuntary loss of urine, occurring at somewhat predictable intervals when a specific bladder volume is reached.

Defining Characteristics

Major

No awareness of bladder filling; no urge to void or feelings of bladder fullness; uninhibited bladder contraction/spasm at regular intervals.

Related Factors

Neurological impairment (e.g. spinal cord lesion that interferes with conduction of cerebral messages above the level of the reflex arc).

INCONTINENCE, STRESS

Definition

The state in which an individual experiences a loss of urine of less than 50 cc occurring with increased abdominal pressure.

Defining Characteristics

Major

Reported or observed dribbling with increased abdominal pressure.

Minor

Urinary urgency; urinary frequency (more often than every 2 hours).

Related Factors

Degenerative changes in pelvic muscles and structural supports associated with increased age; high intra-abdominal pressure (e.g. obesity, gravid uterus); incompetent bladder outlet; overdistention between voidings; weak pelvic muscles and structural supports.

INCONTINENCE, TOTAL

Definition

The state in which an individual experiences a continuous and unpredictable loss of urine.

Defining Characteristics

Major

Constant flow of urine occurs at unpredictable times without distention or uninhibited bladder contractions/spasm; unsuccessful incontinence refractory to treatments; nocturia.

Minor

Lack of perineal or bladder filling awareness; unawareness of incontinence.

Related Factors

Neuropathy preventing transmission of reflex indicating bladder fullness; neurological dysfunction causing triggering of micturition at unpredictable times; independent contraction of detrusor reflex due to surgery; trauma or disease affecting spinal cord nerves; anatomical (fistula).

INCONTINENCE, URGE

Definition

The state in which an individual experiences involuntary passage of urine occurring soon after a strong sense of urgency to void.

Defining Characteristics

Major

Urinary urgency; frequency (voiding more often than every 2 hours); bladder contracture/spasm.

Minor

Nocturia (more than 2 times per night); voiding in small amounts (less than 100 cc) or in large amounts (more than 550 cc); inability to reach toilet in time.

Related Factors

Decreased bladder capacity (e.g. history of PID, abdominal surgeries, indwelling urinary catheter); irritation of bladder stretch receptors causing spasm (e.g. bladder infection); alcohol; caffeine; increased fluids; increased urine concentration; overdistention of bladder.

INFECTION, POTENTIAL FOR

Definition

The state in which an individual is at increased risk for being invaded by pathogenic organisms.

Defining Characteristics

Presence of risk factors such as:

Inadequate primary defenses (broken skin, traumatized tissue, decrease in ciliary action, stasis of body fluids, change in pH secretions, altered peristalsis); inadequate secondary defenses (e.g. decreased hemoglobin, leukopenia, suppressed inflammatory response) and immunosuppression; inadequate acquired immunity; tissue destruction and increased environmental exposure; chronic disease; invasive procedures; malnutrition; pharmaceutical agents; trauma; rupture of amniotic membranes; insufficient knowledge to avoid exposure to pathogens.

Related Factors

See risk factors.

INJURY, POTENTIAL FOR

Definition

A state in which the individual is at risk of injury as a result of environmental conditions interacting with the individual's adaptive and defensive resources.

Defining Characteristics

Presence of risk factors such as:

Internal: biochemical, regulatory function (sensory dysfunction, integrative dysfunction, effector dysfunction); tissue hypoxia; malnutrition; immunoautoimmune; abnormal blood profile (leukocytosis/leukopenia; altered clotting factors; thrombocytopenia; sickle cell, thalassemia; decreased hemoglobin); physical (broken skin, altered mobility); developmental age (physiological, psychosocial); psychological (affective, orientation).
External: biological (immunization level of community, microorganism); chemical (pollutants, poisons, drugs, pharmaceutical agents, alcohol, caffeine, nicotine, preservatives, cosmetics and dyes); nutrients (vitamins, food types); physical (design, structure, and arrangement of community, building, and/or equipment); mode of transport/transportation; people/provider (nosocomial agents; staffing patterns; cognitive, affective, and psychomotor factors).

Related Factors

See risk factors.

KNOWLEDGE DEFICIT (SPECIFY)

Defining Characteristics

Verbalization of the problem; inaccurate follow-through of instruction; inaccurate performance of test; inappropriate or exaggerated behaviors, e.g. hysterical, hostile, agitated, apathetic.

Related Factors

Lack of exposure; lack of recall; information misinterpretation; cognitive limitation; lack of interest in learning; unfamiliarity with information resources.

NONCOMPLIANCE (SPECIFY)

Definition

A person's informed decision not to adhere to a therapeutic recommendation.

Defining Characteristics

*Behavior indicative of failure to adhere (by direct observation or by statements of patient or significant others); objective tests (physiological measures, detection of markers); evidence of development of complications; evidence of exacerbation of symptoms; failure to keep appointments; failure to progress.

Related Factors

Patient value system: health beliefs, cultural influences, spiritual values; client-provider relationships.

---

* Critical defining characteristic.

NUTRITION: LESS THAN BODY REQUIREMENTS, ALTERED

Definition

The state in which an individual experiences an intake of nutrients insufficient to meet metabolic needs.

Defining Characteristics

Loss of weight with adequate food intake; body weight 20% or more under ideal; reported inadequate food intake less than RDA (recommended daily allowance); weakness of muscles required for swallowing or mastication; reported or evidence of lack of food; aversion to eating; reported altered taste sensation; satiety immediately after ingesting food; abdominal pain with or without pathology; sore, inflamed buccal cavity; capillary fragility; abdominal cramping; diarrhea and/or steatorrhea; hyperactive bowel sounds; lack of interest in food; perceived inability to ingest food; pale conjunctiva and mucous membranes; poor muscle tone; excessive loss of hair; lack of information, misinformation; misconceptions.

Related Factors

Inability to ingest or digest food or absorb nutrients due to biological, psychological, or economic factors.

NUTRITION: MORE THAN BODY REQUIREMENTS, ALTERED

Definition

The state in which an individual is experiencing an intake of nutrients that exceeds metabolic needs.

Defining Characteristics

Weight 10% over ideal for height and frame; *weight 20% over ideal for height and frame; *triceps skinfold greater than 15 mm in men, 25 mm in women; sedentary activity level; reported or observed dysfunctional eating pattern: pairing food with other activities; concentrating food intake at the end of day; eating in response to external cues such as time of day, social situation; eating in response to internal cues other than hunger, e.g. anxiety.

Related Factors

Excessive intake in relation to metabolic need.

---

* Critical defining characteristics.

NUTRITION: POTENTIAL FOR MORE THAN BODY REQUIREMENTS, ALTERED

Definition

The state in which an individual is at risk of experiencing an intake of nutrients that exceeds metabolic needs.

Defining Characteristics

Presence of risk factors such as:

*Reported or observed obesity in one or both parents; *rapid transition across growth percentiles in infants or children; reported use of solid food as major food source before 5 months of age; observed use of food as reward or comfort measure; reported or observed higher baseline weight at beginning of each pregnancy; dysfunctional eating patterns: pairing food with other activities; concentrating food intake at end of day; eating in response to external cues such as time of day, social situation; eating in response to internal cues other than hunger such as anxiety.

Related Factors

See risk factors.

---

* Critical defining characteristics.

ORAL MUCOUS MEMBRANE, ALTERED

Definition

The state in which an individual experiences disruptions in the tissue layers of the oral cavity.

Defining Characteristics

Oral pain/discomfort; coated tongue; xerostomia (dry mouth); stomatitis; oral lesions or ulcers; lack of or decreased salivation; leukoplakia; edema; hyperemia; oral plaque; desquamation; vesicles; hemorrhagic gingivitis; carious teeth; halitosis.

Related Factors

Pathological conditions—oral cavity (radiation to head or neck); dehydration; trauma (chemical, e.g. acidic foods, drugs, noxious agents, alcohol; mechanical, e.g. ill-fitting dentures, braces, tubes [endotracheal/nasogastric], surgery in oral cavity); NPO for more than 24 hours; ineffective oral hygiene; mouth breathing; malnutrition; infection; lack of or decreased salivation; medication.

PAIN

Definition

A state in which an individual experiences and reports the presence of severe discomfort or an uncomfortable sensation.

Defining Characteristics

Subjective: communication (verbal or coded) of pain descriptors.
Objective: guarding behavior, protective; self-focusing; narrowed focus (altered time perception, withdrawal from social contact, impaired thought process); distraction behavior (moaning, crying, pacing, seeking out other people and/or activities, restlessness); facial mask of pain (eyes lack luster, "beaten look," fixed or scattered movement, grimace); alteration in muscle tone (may span from listless to rigid); autonomic responses not seen in chronic stable pain (diaphoresis, blood pressure and pulse change, pupillary dilation, increased or decreased respiratory rate).

Related Factors

Injury agents (biological, chemical, physical, psychological).

PAIN, CHRONIC

Definition

A state in which the individual experiences pain that continues for more than 6 months in duration.

Defining Characteristics

Major

Verbal report or observed evidence of pain experienced for more than 6 months.

Minor

Fear of reinjury; physical and social withdrawal; altered ability to continue previous activities; anorexia; weight changes; changes in sleep patterns; facial mask; guarded movement.

Related Factors

Chronic physical/psychosocial disability.

PARENTAL ROLE CONFLICT

Definition

The state in which a parent experiences role confusion and conflict in response to crisis.

Defining Characteristics

Major

Parent(s) expresses concerns/feelings of inadequacy to provide for child's physical and emotional needs during hospitalization or in the home; demonstrated disruption in caretaking routines; parent(s) expresses concerns about changes in parental role, family functioning, family communication, family health.

Minor

Expresses concern about perceived loss of control over decisions relating to child; reluctant to participate in usual caretaking activities even with encouragement and support; verbalizes/demonstrates feelings of guilt, anger, fear, anxiety, and/or frustrations about effect of child's illness on family process.

Related Factors

Separation from child due to chronic illness; intimidation with invasive or restrictive modalities (e.g. isolation, in-tubation), specialized care centers, policies; home care of a child with special needs (e.g. apnea monitoring, postural drainage, hyperalimentation); change in marital status; interruptions of family life due to home care regimen (treatments, caregivers, lack of respite).

PARENTING, ALTERED

Definition

The state in which a nurturing figure experiences an inability to create an environment that promotes the optimal growth and development of another human being.†

Defining Characteristics

Abandonment; runaway; verbalization cannot control child; incidence of physical and psychological trauma; lack of parental attachment behaviors; inappropriate visual, tactile, auditory stimulation; negative identification of infant's/child's characteristics; negative attachment of meanings to infant's/child's characteristics; constant verbalization of disappointment in gender or physical characteristics of the infant/child; verbalization of resentment toward the infant/child; verbalization of role inadequacy; *inattentive to infant's/child's needs; verbal disgust at body functions of infant/child; noncompliance with health appointments for self and/or infant/child; *inappropriate caretaking behavior (toilet training, sleep/rest, feeding); inappropriate or inconsistent discipline practices; frequent accidents; frequent illness; growth and development lag in the child; *history of child abuse or abandonment by primary caretaker; verbalizes desire to have child call him/herself by first name versus traditional cultural tendencies; child receives care from multiple caretakers without consideration for the needs of the infant/child; compulsively seeking role approval from others.

Related Factors

Lack of available role model; ineffective role model; physical and psychosocial abuse of nurturing figure; lack of support between/from significant other(s); unmet social/emotional maturation needs of parenting figures; interruption in bonding process, i.e. maternal, paternal, other; unrealistic expectation for self, infant, partner; perceives threat to own survival, physical and emotional; mental and/or physical illness; presence of stress (financial, legal, recent crisis, cultural move); lack of knowledge; limited cognitive functioning; lack of role identity;

---

† It is important to state as a preface to this diagnosis that adjustment to parenting in general is a normal maturational process that elicits nursing behaviors of prevention of potential problems and health promotion.

* Critical defining characteristics.

lack or inappropriate response of child to relationship; multiple pregnancies.

PARENTING, POTENTIAL ALTERED

Definition

The state in which a nurturing figure is at risk to experience an inability to create an environment that promotes the optimal growth and development of another human being.†

Defining Characteristics

Presence of risk factors such as:

Lack of parental attachment behaviors; inappropriate visual, tactile, auditory stimulation; negative identification of infant's/child's characteristics; negative attachment of meanings to infant's/child's characteristics; constant verbalization of disappointment in gender or physical characteristics of the infant/child; verbalization of resentment toward the infant/child; verbalization of role inadequacy; *inattentive to infant's/child's needs; verbal disgust at body functions of infant/child; noncompliance with health appointments for self and/or infant/child; *inappropriate caretaking behaviors (toilet training, sleep/rest, feeding); inappropriate or inconsistent discipline practices; frequent accidents; frequent illness; growth and development lag in the child; *history of child abuse or abandonment by primary caretaker; verbalizes desire to have child call him/herself by first name versus traditional cultural tendencies; child receives care from multiple caretakers without consideration for the needs of the infant/child; compulsively seeking role approval from others.

Related Factors

Lack of available role model; ineffective role model; physical and psychosocial abuse of nurturing figure; lack of support between/from significant other(s); unmet social/emotional maturation needs of parenting figures; interruption in bonding process, i.e., maternal, paternal, other; unrealistic expectation for self, infant, partner; perceive threat to own survival, physical and emotional; mental and/or physical illness; presence of stress (financial, legal, recent crisis, cultural move); lack of knowledge; limited cognitive functioning; lack of role identity; lack or inappropriate response of child to relationship; multiple pregnancies.

---

† It is important to state as a preface to this diagnosis that adjustment to parenting in general is a normal maturational process that elicits nursing behaviors of prevention of potential problems and health promotion.

* Critical defining characteristics.

PERSONAL IDENTITY DISTURBANCE

Definition

Inability to distinguish between self and nonself.

Defining Characteristics

To be developed.

PHYSICAL MOBILITY, IMPAIRED

Definition

A state in which the individual experiences a limitation of ability for independent physical movement.

Defining Characteristics

Inability to purposefully move within the physical environment, including bed mobility, transfer, and ambulation; reluctance to attempt movement; limited range of motion; decreased muscle strength, control, and/or mass; imposed restrictions of movement, including mechanical, medical protocol; impaired coordination.

Related Factors

Intolerance to activity/decreased strength and endurance; pain/discomfort; perceptual/cognitive impairment; neuromuscular impairment; musculoskeletal impairment; depression/severe anxiety.

Suggested Functional Level Classification†

0 = Completely independent.
1 = Requires use of equipment or device.
2 = Requires help from another person, for assistance, supervision, or teaching.
3 = Requires help from another person and equipment device.
4 = Dependent, does not participate in activity.

---

† Code adapted from Jones, E., et al. Patient classification for long-term care: users' manual. HEW, Publication No. HRA–74–3107, November, 1974.

POISONING, POTENTIAL FOR

Definition

Accentuated risk of accidental exposure to or ingestion of drugs or dangerous products in doses sufficient to cause poisoning.

Defining Characteristics

Presence of risk factors such as:

Internal (individual): reduced vision; verbalization of occupational setting without adequate safeguards; lack of safety or drug education; lack of proper precaution; cognitive or emotional difficulties; insufficient finances.

External (environmental): large supplies of drugs in house; medicines stored in unlocked cabinets accessible to children or confused persons; dangerous products placed or stored within the reach of children or confused persons; availability of illicit drugs potentially contaminated by poisonous additives; flaking, peeling paint or plaster in presence of young children; chemical contamination of food and water; unprotected contact with heavy metals or chemicals; paint, lacquer, etc. in poorly ventilated areas or without effective protection; presence of poisonous vegetation; presence of atmospheric pollutants.

Related Factors

See risk factors.

POST-TRAUMA RESPONSE

Definition

The state of an individual experiencing a sustained painful response to an overwhelming traumatic event.

Defining Characteristics

Major

Re-experience of the traumatic event that may be identified in cognitive, affective, and/or sensory motor activities (flashbacks, intrusive thoughts, repetitive dreams or nightmares, excessive verbalization of the traumatic event, verbalization of survival guilt or guilt about behavior required for survival).

Minor

Psychic/emotional numbness (impaired interpretation of reality, confusion, dissociation or amnesia, vagueness about traumatic event, constricted affect); altered life style (self-destructiveness such as substance abuse, suicide attempt or other acting out behavior; difficulty with interpersonal relationship; development of phobia regarding trauma; poor impulse control/irritability and explosiveness).

Related Factors

Disasters, wars, epidemics, rape, assault, torture, catastrophic illness or accident.

POWERLESSNESS

Definition

Perception that one's own action will not significantly affect an outcome; a perceived lack of control over a current situation or immediate happening.

Defining Characteristics

Severe: verbal expressions of having no control or influence over situation; verbal expressions of having no control or influence over outcome; verbal expressions of having no control over self-care; depression over physical deterioration that occurs despite patient compliance with regimens; apathy.

Moderate: nonparticipation in care or decision making when opportunities are provided; expressions of dissatisfaction and frustration over inability to perform previous tasks and/or activities; does not monitor progress; expression of doubt regarding role performance; reluctance to express true feelings; fearing alienation from caregivers; passivity; inability to seek information regarding care; dependence on others that may result in irritability, resentment, anger, and guilt; does not defend self-care practices when challenged.

Low: expressions of uncertainty about fluctuating energy levels; passivity.

Related Factors

Health care environment; interpersonal interaction; illness-related regimen; life style of helplessness.

RAPE-TRAUMA SYNDROME

Definition

Forced, violent sexual penetration against the victim's will and consent. The trauma syndrome that develops from this attack or attempted attack includes an acute phase of disorganization of the victim's life style and a long-term process of reorganization of life style.*

Defining Characteristics

Acute phase: emotional reactions (anger, embarrassment, fear of physical violence and death, humiliation, revenge, self-blame); multiple physical symptoms (gastrointestinal irritability, genitourinary discomfort, muscle tension, sleep pattern disturbance).

---

* This syndrome includes three subcomponents: rape-trauma, compound reaction, and silent reaction. In this text, each appears as a separate diagnosis.

Long-term phase: changes in life style (change in residence; dealing with repetitive nightmares and phobias; seeking family support; seeking social network support).

RAPE-TRAUMA SYNDROME: COMPOUND REACTION

Definition

Forced, violent sexual penetration against the victim's will and consent. The trauma syndrome that develops from this attack or attempted attack includes an acute phase of disorganization of the victim's life style and a long-term process of reorganization of life style.*

Defining Characteristics

Acute phase: emotional reaction (anger, embarrassment, fear of physical violence and death, humiliation, revenge, self-blame); multiple physical symptoms (gastrointestinal irritability, genitourinary discomfort, muscle tension, sleep pattern disturbance); reactivated symptoms of such previous conditions, i.e. physical illness, psychiatric illness; reliance on alcohol and/or drugs.

Long-term phase: change in life style (changes in residence; dealing with repetitive nightmares and phobias; seeking family support; seeking social network support).

---

* This syndrome includes three subcomponents: rape-trauma, compound reaction, and silent reaction. In this text, each appears as a separate diagnosis.

RAPE-TRAUMA SYNDROME: SILENT REACTION

Definition

Forced, violent sexual penetration against the victim's will and consent. The trauma syndrome that develops from this attack or attempted attack includes an acute phase of disorganization of the victim's life style and a long-term process of reorganization of life style.*

Defining Characteristics

Abrupt changes in relationships with men; increase in nightmares; increased anxiety during interview, i.e. blocking of associations, long periods of silence, minor stuttering, physical distress; pronounced changes in sexual behavior; no verbalization of the occurrence of rape; sudden onset of phobic reactions.

---

* This syndrome includes three subcomponents: rape-trauma, compound reaction, and silent reaction. In this text, each appears as a separate diagnosis.

ROLE PERFORMANCE, ALTERED

Definition

Disruption in the way one perceives one's role performance.

Defining Characteristics

Change in self-perception of role; denial of role; change in others' perception of role; conflict in roles; change in physical capacity to resume role; lack of knowledge of role; change in usual patterns of responsibility.

Related Factors

To be developed.

SELF-CARE DEFICIT: BATHING/ HYGIENE

Definition

A state in which the individual experiences an impaired ability to perform or complete bathing/hygiene activities for oneself.

Defining Characteristics

*Inability to wash body or body parts; inability to obtain or get to water source; inability to regulate temperature or flow.

Related Factors

Intolerance to activity, decreased strength and endurance; pain, discomfort; perceptual or cognitive impairment; neuromuscular impairment; musculoskeletal impairment; depression, severe anxiety.

---

* Critical defining characteristic.

SELF-CARE DEFICIT: DRESSING/ GROOMING

Definition

A state in which the individual experiences an impaired ability to perform or complete dressing and grooming activities for oneself.

Defining Characteristics

*Impaired ability to put on or take off necessary items of clothing; impaired ability to obtain or replace articles of clothing; impaired ability to fasten clothing; inability to maintain appearance at a satisfactory level.

Related Factors

Intolerance to activity, decreased strength and endurance; pain, discomfort; perceptual or cognitive impairment; neuromuscular impairment; musculoskeletal impairment; depression, severe anxiety.

---

* Critical defining characteristic.

SELF-CARE DEFICIT: FEEDING

Definition

A state in which the individual experiences an impaired ability to perform or complete feeding activities for oneself.

Defining Characteristics

Inability to bring food from a receptacle to the mouth.

Related Factors

Intolerance to activity, decreased strength and endurance; pain, discomfort; perceptual or cognitive impairment; neuromuscular impairment; musculoskeletal impairment; depression, severe anxiety.

SELF-CARE DEFICIT: TOILETING

Definition

A state in which the individual experiences an impaired ability to perform or complete toileting activities for oneself.

Defining Characteristics

*Unable to get to toilet or commode; *unable to sit on or rise from toilet or commode; *unable to manipulate clothing for toileting; *unable to carry out proper toilet hygiene; unable to flush toilet or commode.

Related Factors

Impaired transfer ability; impaired mobility status; intolerance to activity, decreased strength and endurance;

---

* Critical defining characteristics.

pain, discomfort; perceptual or cognitive impairment; neuromuscular impairment; musculoskeletal impairment; depression, severe anxiety.

SELF-ESTEEM, CHRONIC LOW

Definition

Long-standing negative self-evaluation/feelings about self or self-capabilities.

Defining Characteristics

Major: long-standing or chronic:

Self-negating verbalization; expressions of shame/guilt; evaluates self as unable to deal with events; rationalizes away/rejects positive feedback and exaggerates negative feedback about self; hesitant to try new things/situations.

Minor

Frequent lack of success in work or other life events; overly conforming, dependent on others' opinions; lack of eye contact; nonassertive/passive; indecisive; excessively seeks reassurance.

SELF-ESTEEM, SITUATIONAL LOW

Definition

Negative self-evaluation/feelings about self that develop in response to a loss or change in an individual who previously had a positive self-evaluation.

Defining Characteristics

Major

Episodic occurrence of negative self-appraisal in response to life events in a person with a previous positive self-evaluation; verbalization of negative feelings about self (helplessness, uselessness).

Minor

Self-negating verbalizations; expressions of shame/guilt; evaluates self as unable to handle situations/events; difficulty making decisions.

SELF-ESTEEM DISTURBANCE

Definition

Negative self-evaluation/feelings about self or self-capabilities, which may be directly or indirectly expressed.

Defining Characteristics

Self-negating verbalization; expressions of shame/guilt; evaluates self as unable to deal with events; rationalizes away/rejects positive feedback and exaggerates negative feedback about self; hesitant to try new things/situations; denial of problems obvious to others; projection of blame/responsibility for problems; rationalizing personal failures; hypersensitive to slight criticism; grandiosity.

SENSORY/PERCEPTUAL ALTERATIONS (SPECIFY) (VISUAL, AUDITORY, KINESTHETIC, GUSTATORY, TACTILE, OLFACTORY)

Definition

A state in which an individual experiences a change in the amount or patterning of oncoming stimuli accompanied by a diminished, exaggerated, distorted, or impaired response to such stimuli.

Defining Characteristics

Disoriented in time, in place, or with persons; altered abstraction; altered conceptualization; change in problem-solving abilities; reported or measured change in sensory acuity; change in behavior pattern; anxiety; apathy; change in usual response to stimuli; indication of body image alteration; restlessness; irritability; altered communication patterns.

Other Possible Characteristics

Complaints of fatigue; alteration in posture; change in muscular tension; inappropriate responses; hallucinations.

Related Factors

Altered environmental stimuli, excessive or insufficient; altered sensory reception, transmission, and/or integration; chemical alterations, endogenous (electrolyte), exogenous (drugs, etc.); psychological stress.

SEXUAL DYSFUNCTION

Definition

The state in which an individual experiences a change in sexual function that is viewed as unsatisfying, unrewarding, inadequate.

Defining Characteristics

Verbalization of problem; alterations in achieving perceived sex role; actual or perceived limitation imposed by disease and/or therapy; conflicts involving values; alteration in achieving sexual satisfaction; inability to achieve desired satisfaction; seeking confirmation of desirability; alteration in relationship with significant other; change of interest in self and others.

Related Factors

Biopsychosocial alteration of sexuality: ineffectual or absent role models; physical abuse; psychosocial abuse, e.g. harmful relationships; vulnerability; values conflict; lack of privacy; lack of significant other; altered body structure or function (pregnancy, recent childbirth, drugs, surgery, anomalies, disease process, trauma, radiation); misinformation or lack of knowledge.

SEXUALITY PATTERNS, ALTERED

Definition

The state in which an individual expresses concern regarding his/her sexuality.

Defining Characteristics

Major

Reported difficulties, limitations, or changes in sexual behaviors or activities.

Related Factors

Knowledge/skill deficit about alternative responses to health-related transitions, altered body function or structure, illness or medical treatment; lack of privacy; lack of significant other; ineffective or absent role models; conflicts with sexual orientation or variant preferences; fear of pregnancy or of acquiring a sexually transmitted disease; impaired relationship with a significant other.

SKIN INTEGRITY, IMPAIRED

Definition

A state in which the individual's skin is adversely altered.

Defining Characteristics

Disruption of skin surface; destruction of skin layers; invasion of body structures.

Related Factors

External (environmental): hyper- or hypothermia; chemical substance; mechanical factors (shearing forces, pressure, restraint); radiation; physical immobilization; humidity.

Internal (somatic): medication; altered nutritional state (obesity, emaciation); altered metabolic state; altered circulation; altered sensation; altered pigmentation; skeletal prominence; developmental factors; immunological deficit; alterations in turgor (change in elasticity).

SKIN INTEGRITY, POTENTIAL IMPAIRED

Definition

A state in which the individual's skin is at risk of being adversely altered.

Defining Characteristics

Presence of risk factors such as:

External (environmental): hypo- or hyperthermia; chemical substance; mechanical factors (shearing forces, pressure, restraint); radiation; physical immobilization; excretions/secretions; humidity.

Internal (somatic): medication; alterations in nutritional state (obesity, emaciation); altered metabolic state; altered circulation; altered sensation; altered pigmentation; skeletal prominence; developmental factors; alterations in skin turgor (change in elasticity); psychogenic; immunological.

Related Factors

See risk factors.

SLEEP PATTERN DISTURBANCE

Definition

Disruption of sleep time causes discomfort or interferes with desired life style.

Defining Characteristics

*Verbal complaints of difficulty falling asleep; *awakening earlier or later than desired; *interrupted sleep; *verbal complaints of not feeling well rested; changes in

---

* Critical defining characteristics.

---

behavior and performance (increasing irritability, restlessness, disorientation, lethargy, listlessness); physical signs (mild fleeting nystagmus, slight hand tremor, ptosis of eyelid, expressionless face, dark circles under eyes, frequent yawning, changes in posture); thick speech with mispronunciation and incorrect words.

Related Factors

Sensory alterations: internal (illness, psychological stress); external (environmental changes, social cues).

SOCIAL INTERACTION, IMPAIRED

Definition

The state in which an individual participates in an insufficient or excessive quantity or ineffective quality of social exchange.

Defining Characteristics

Major

Verbalized or observed discomfort in social situations; verbalized or observed inability to receive or communicate a satisfying sense of belonging, caring, interest, or shared history; observed use of unsuccessful social interaction behaviors; dysfunctional interaction with peers, family, and/or others.

Minor

Family report of change of style or pattern of interaction.

Related Factors

Knowledge/skill deficit about ways to enhance mutuality; communication barriers; self-concept disturbance; absence of available significant others or peers; limited physical mobility; therapeutic isolation; sociocultural dissonance; environmental barriers; altered thought processes.

SOCIAL ISOLATION

Definition

Aloneness experienced by the individual and perceived as imposed by others and as a negative or threatened state.

Defining Characteristics

Objective: *absence of supportive significant other(s) [family, friends, group]; sad, dull affect; inappropriate or immature interests/activities for development age/stage; uncommunicative, withdrawn, no eye contact; preoccupation with own thoughts, repetitive meaningless actions; projects hostility in voice, behavior; seeks to be alone, or exists in a subculture; evidence of physical/mental handicap or altered state of wellness; shows behavior unaccepted by dominant cultural group.

Subjective: *expresses feelings of aloneness imposed by others; *expresses feelings of rejection; experiences feelings of difference from others; inadequacy in or absence of significant purpose in life; inability to meet expectations of others; insecurity in public; expresses values acceptable to the subculture but unacceptable to the dominant cultural group; expresses interests inappropriate to the developmental age/stage.

Related Factors

Factors contributing to the absence of satisfying personal relationships, such as: delay in accomplishing developmental tasks; immature interests; alterations in physical appearance; alterations in mental status; unaccepted social behavior; unaccepted social values; altered state of wellness; inadequate personal resources; inability to engage in satisfying personal relationships.

---

* Critical defining characteristics.

SPIRITUAL DISTRESS (DISTRESS OF THE HUMAN SPIRIT)

Definition

Disruption in the life principle that pervades a person's entire being and that integrates and transcends one's biological and psychosocial nature.

Defining Characteristics

*Expresses concern with meaning of life/death and/or belief systems; anger toward God; questions meaning of suffering; verbalizes inner conflict about beliefs; verbalizes concern about relationship with deity; questions meaning of own existence; unable to participate in usual religious practices; seeks spiritual assistance; questions moral/ethical implications of therapeutic regimen; gallows humor; displacement of anger toward religious representatives; description of nightmares/sleep disturbances; alteration in behavior/mood evidenced by anger, crying, withdrawal, preoccupation, anxiety, hostility, apathy, and so forth.

---

* Critical defining characteristic.

Related Factors

Separation from religious/cultural ties; challenged belief and value system, e.g. due to moral/ethical implications of therapy, due to intense suffering.

SUFFOCATION, POTENTIAL FOR

Definition

Accentuated risk of accidental suffocation (inadequate air available for inhalation).

Defining Characteristics

Presence of risk factors such as:

Internal (individual): reduced olfactory sensation; reduced motor abilities; lack of safety education; lack of safety precautions; cognitive or emotional difficulties; disease or injury process.

External (environmental): pillow placed in an infant's crib; propped bottle placed in an infant's crib; vehicle warming in closed garage; children playing with plastic bags or inserting small objects into their mouths or noses; discarded or unused refrigerators or freezers without removed doors; children left unattended in bathtubs or pools; household gas leaks; smoking in bed; use of fuel-burning heaters not vented to outside; low-strung clothesline; pacifier hung around infant's head; person who eats large mouthfuls of food.

Related Factors

See risk factors.

SWALLOWING, IMPAIRED

Definition

The state in which an individual has decreased ability to voluntarily pass fluids and/or solids from the mouth to the stomach.

Defining Characteristics

Major

Observed evidence of difficulty in swallowing, e.g. stasis of food in oral cavity, coughing/choking.

Minor

Evidence of aspiration.

Related Factors

Neuromuscular impairment (e.g. decreased or absent gag reflex, decreased strength or excursion of muscles involved in mastication, perceptual impairment, facial paralysis); mechanical obstruction (e.g. edema, tracheostomy tube, tumor); fatigue; limited awareness; reddened, irritated oropharyngeal cavity.

THERMOREGULATION, INEFFECTIVE

Definition

The state in which the individual's temperature fluctuates between hypothermia and hyperthermia.

Defining Characteristics

Major

Fluctuations in body temperature above or below the normal range. See also major and minor characteristics present in hypothermia and hyperthermia.

Related Factors

Trauma or illness; immaturity; aging; fluctuating environmental temperature.

THOUGHT PROCESSES, ALTERED

Definition

A state in which an individual experiences a disruption in cognitive operations and activities.

Defining Characteristics

Inaccurate interpretation of environment; cognitive dissonance; distractibility; memory deficit/problems; egocentricity; hyper- or hypovigilance.

Other Possible Characteristics

Inappropriate nonreality-based thinking.

Related Factors

To be developed.

TISSUE INTEGRITY, IMPAIRED

Definition

A state in which an individual experiences damage to mucous membrane, corneal, integumentary, or subcutaneous tissue.

Defining Characteristics

Major

Damaged or destroyed tissue (cornea, mucous membrane, integumentary, or subcutaneous).

Related Factors

Altered circulation; nutritional deficit/excess; fluid deficit/excess; knowledge deficit; impaired physical mobility; irritants, chemical (including body excretions, secretions, medications); thermal (temperature extremes); mechanical (pressure, shear, friction); radiation (including therapeutic radiation).

TISSUE PERFUSION, ALTERED (SPECIFY TYPE) (RENAL, CEREBRAL, CARDIOPULMONARY, GASTROINTESTINAL, PERIPHERAL)†

Definition

The state is which an individual experiences a decrease in nutrition and oxygenation at the cellular level due to a deficit in capillary blood supply.

Defining Characteristics

	Estimated sensitivities and specificities	
	Chances that characteristic will be present in given diagnosis.	Chances that characteristic will not be explained by any other diagnosis.
Skin temperature cold extremities	High	Low
Skin color		
dependent blue or purple	Moderate	Low
*Pale on elevation, color does not return on lowering of leg	High	High

---

† Further work and development are required for the subcomponents, specifically cerebral, renal, and gastrointestinal.

* Critical defining characteristics.

*Diminished arterial pulsations	High	High
Skin quality: shining	High	Low
Lack of lanugo	High	Moderate
Round scars covered with atrophied skin		
Gangrene	Low	High
Slow-growing, dry brittle nails	High	Moderate
Claudication	Moderate	High
Blood pressure changes in extremities		
Bruits	Moderate	Moderate
Slow healing of lesions	High	Low

Related Factors

Interruption of flow, arterial; interruption of flow, venous; exchange problems; hypovolemia; hypervolemia.

---

* Critical defining characteristic.

TRAUMA, POTENTIAL FOR

Definition

Accentuated risk of accidental tissue injury, e.g. wound, burn, fracture.

Defining Characteristics

Presence of risk factors such as:

Internal (individual): weakness; poor vision; balancing difficulties; reduced temperature and/or tactile sensation; reduced large or small muscle coordination; reduced hand-eye coordination; lack of safety education; lack of safety precautions; insufficient finances to purchase safety equipment or effect repairs; cognitive or emotional difficulties; history of previous trauma.

External (environmental): slippery floors, e.g. wet or highly waxed; snow or ice collected on stairs, walkways; unanchored rugs; bathtub without hand grip or antislip equipment; use of unsteady ladders or chairs; entering unlighted rooms; unsturdy or absent stair rails; unanchored electric wires; litter or liquid spills on floors or stairways; high beds; children playing without gates at the top of the stairs; obstructed passageways; unsafe window protection in homes with young children; inappropriate call-for-aid mechanisms for bedresting client; pot handles facing toward front of stove; bathing in very hot water, e.g. unsupervised bathing of young children; potential igniting gas leaks; delayed lighting of gas burner or oven; experimenting with chemical or gasoline; un-

screened fires or heaters; wearing plastic apron or flowing clothes around open flame; children playing with matches, candles, cigarettes; inadequately stored combustible or corrosives, e.g. matches, oily rags, lye; highly flammable children's toys or clothing; overloaded fuse boxes; contact with rapidly moving machinery, industrial belts, or pulleys; sliding on coarse bed linen or struggling within bed restraints; faulty electric plugs, frayed wires, or defective appliances; contact with acids or alkalies; playing with fireworks or gunpowder; contact with intense cold; overexposure to sun, sun lamps, radiotherapy; use of cracked dishware or glasses; knives stored uncovered; guns or ammunition stored unlocked; large icicles hanging from the roof; exposure to dangerous machinery; children playing with sharp-edged toys; high crime neighborhood and vulnerable clients; driving a mechanically unsafe vehicle; driving after partaking of alcoholic beverages or drugs; driving at excessive speeds; driving without necessary visual aids; children riding in the front seat in car; smoking in bed or near oxygen; overloaded electrical outlets; grease waste collected on stoves; use of thin or worn potholders or misuse of necessary headgear for motorized cyclists or young children carried on adult bicycles; unsafe road or road-crossing conditions; play or work near vehicle pathways, e.g. driveways, laneways, railroad tracks; nonuse or misuse of seat restraints.

Related Factors

See risk factors.

UNILATERAL NEGLECT

Definition

A state in which an individual is perceptually unaware of and inattentive to one side of the body.

Defining Characteristics

Major

Consistent inattention to stimuli on an affected side.

Minor

Inadequate self-care; positioning and/or safety precautions in regard to the affected side; does not look toward affected side; leaves food on plate on the affected side.

Related Factors

Effects of disturbed perceptual abilities, e.g. hemianopsia; one-sided blindness; neurological illness or trauma.

URINARY ELIMINATION, ALTERED

Definition

The state in which the individual experiences a disturbance in urine elimination.

Defining Characteristics

Dysuria; frequency; hesitancy; incontinence; nocturia; retention; urgency.

Related Factors

Multiple causality, including: anatomical obstruction, sensory motor impairment, urinary tract infection.

URINARY RETENTION

Definition

The state in which the individual experiences incomplete emptying of the bladder.

Defining Characteristics

Major

Bladder distention; small, frequent voiding or absence of urine output.

Minor

Sensation of bladder fullness; dribbling; residual urine; dysuria; overflow incontinence.

Related Factors

High urethral pressure caused by weak detrusor; inhibition of reflex arc; strong sphincter; blockage.

VIOLENCE, POTENTIAL FOR: SELF-DIRECTED OR DIRECTED AT OTHERS

Definition

A state in which an individual experiences behaviors that can be physically harmful to either the self or others.

Defining Characteristics

Presence of risk factors such as:

Body language (clenched fists, tense facial expression, rigid posture, tautness indicating effort to control); hostile, threatening verbalizations (boasting to or prior abuse of others); increased motor activity (pacing, excitement, irritability, agitation); overt and aggressive acts (goal-directed destruction of objects in environment); possession of destructive means (gun, knife, weapon); rage, self-destructive behavior, active aggressive suicidal acts; suspicion of others, paranoid ideation, delusions, hallucinations; substance abuse/withdrawal.

Other Possible Characteristics

Increasing anxiety levels; fear of self or others; inability to verbalize feelings; repetition of verbalizations (continued complaints, requests, and demands); anger; provocative behavior (argumentative, dissatisfied, overreactive, hypersensitive); vulnerable self-esteem; depression (specifically active, aggressive, suicidal acts).

Related Factors

Antisocial character; battered women; catatonic excitement; child abuse; manic excitement; organic brain syndrome; panic states; rage reactions; suicidal behavior; temporal lobe epilepsy; toxic reactions to medication.

Bibliography

General Bibliography

Abrams, AC. Clinical drug therapy: rationales for nursing practice (2nd ed.). Philadelphia: J.B. Lippincott Company, 1987.

Aistars, J. Fatigue in the cancer patient: a conceptual approach to a clinical problem. Oncology Nursing Forum, 14(6): 25–35, 1987.

Alspach, JG, & Williams, SM. Core curriculum for critical care nursing (3rd ed.). Philadelphia: W.B. Saunders Company, 1985.

Anderson, JL. Nursing management of the cancer patient in pain: a review of the literature. Cancer Nursing, 5(1): 33–41, 1982.

Ayres, T. Sexuality and fertility after cancer. Proceedings of the fourth national conference on human values and cancer—1984, pp. 127–133.

Bahnson, CB. Psychological aspects of cancer. In Pilch, YH (Ed.), Surgical oncology. New York: McGraw-Hill, 1984, pp. 231–253.

Baer, CL, & Williams, BR. Clinical pharmacology and nursing. Springhouse, PA: Springhouse Publishing Company, 1988.

Baldonado, AA, & Stahl, DA. Cancer nursing: a holistic multidisciplinary approach (2nd ed.). Garden City, NY: Medical Examination Publishing Company, 1982.

Barry, PD. Psychosocial nursing assessment and intervention. Philadelphia: J.B. Lippincott Company, 1984.

Basch, A. Changes in elimination. Seminars in Oncology Nursing, 3(4): 287–292, 1987.

Bates, B. A guide to physical examination (4th ed.). Philadelphia: J.B. Lippincott Company, 1987.

Billings, DM, & Stokes, LG. Medical-surgical nursing: common health problems of adults and children across the life span. St. Louis: C.V. Mosby, 1987.

Bouchard-Kurtz, R, & Speese-Owens, N. Nursing care of the cancer patient (4th ed.). St. Louis: C.V. Mosby, 1981.

Braunwald, E, Isselbacher, KJ, Petersdorf, RG, et al. (Eds.). Harrison's principles of internal medicine (11th ed.). New York: McGraw-Hill, 1987.

Brill, EL, & Kilts, DF. Foundations for nursing (2nd ed.). New York: Appleton-Century-Crofts, 1986.

Brown, MH, Kiss, ME, Outlaw, EM, & Viamontes, CM. Standards of oncology nursing practice. New York: John Wiley & Sons, 1986.

Brunner, LS, & Suddarth, DS. The Lippincott manual of nursing practice (4th ed.). Philadelphia: J.B. Lippincott Company, 1986.

Brunner, LS, & Suddarth, DS. Textbook of medical-surgical nursing (6th ed.). Philadelphia: J.B. Lippincott Company, 1988.

Burns, N. Nursing and cancer. Philadelphia: W.B. Saunders Company, 1982.

Byrne, CJ, Saxton, DF, Pelikan, PK, & Nugent, PM. Laboratory tests: implications for nurses and allied health professionals (2nd ed.). Menlo Park, CA: Addison-Wesley, 1986.

Carpenito, LJ. Handbook of nursing diagnosis 1989–1990. Philadelphia: J.B. Lippincott Company, 1989.

Carrieri, VK, Lindsey, AM, & West, CM. Pathophysiological phenomena in nursing. Philadelphia: W.B. Saunders Company, 1986.

Chambers, JK. Metabolic bone disorders: imbalances of calcium and phosphorus. Nursing Clinics of North America, 22(4): 861–872, 1987.

Chenevey, B. Overview of fluids and electrolytes. Nursing Clinics of North America, 22(4): 749–759, 1987.

Chlebowski, RT, & Heber, D. Metabolic abnormalities in cancer patients: carbohydrate metabolism. Surgical Clinics of North America, 66(5): 957–968, 1986.

Clark, JB, Queener, SF, & Karb, VB. Pharmacological basis of nursing practice (2nd ed.). St. Louis: C.V. Mosby, 1986.

Corbett, JV. Laboratory tests and diagnostic procedures with nursing diagnoses (2nd ed.). Norwalk, CT: Appleton & Lange, 1987.

Coyle, N, & Foley, K. Pain in patients with cancer: profile of patients and common pain syndromes. Seminars in Oncology Nursing, 1(2): 93–99, 1985.

Cushman, KE. Symptom management: a comprehensive approach to increasing nutritional status in the cancer patient. Seminars in Oncology Nursing, 2(1): 30–35, 1986.

D'Agostino, NS. Managing nutrition problems in advanced cancer. American Journal of Nursing, 89(1): 50–56, 1989.

Dangel, RB. Pruritus and cancer. Oncology Nursing Forum, 13(1): 17–21, 1986.

DeVita, VT, Jr, Hellman, S, & Rosenberg, SA (Eds.). Cancer: principles and practice of oncology (2nd ed.). Philadelphia: J.B. Lippincott Company, 1985.

Doenges, ME, Moorhouse, MF, & Geissler, AC. Nursing care plans: guidelines for planning patient care (2nd ed.). Philadelphia: F.A. Davis Company, 1989.

Ellis, JR, & Nowlis, EA. Nursing: a human needs approach (3rd ed.). Boston: Houghton Mifflin Company, 1985.

Foley, KM. The treatment of pain in the patient with cancer. CA—A Cancer Journal for Clinicians, 36(4): 194–215, 1986.

Folz, AT. The influence of cancer on self-concept and life quality. Seminars in Oncology Nursing, 3(4): 303–312, 1987.

Germino, BB. Symptom distress and quality of life. Seminars in Oncology Nursing, 3(4): 299–302, 1987.

Glasgow, M, Halfin, V, & Althausen, AF. Sexual response and cancer. CA—A Cancer Journal for Clinicians, 37(6): 322–333, 1987.

Gobel, BH, & Donovan, MI. Depression and anxiety. Seminars in Oncology Nursing, *3*(4): 267–276, 1987.

Gordon, M. Manual of nursing diagnosis. New York: McGraw-Hill, 1987.

Govoni, LE, & Hayes, JE. Drugs and nursing implications (6th ed.). Norwalk, CT: Appleton-Century-Crofts, 1989.

Grady, C. Host defense mechanisms: an overview. Seminars in Oncology Nursing, *4*(2): 86–94, 1988.

Grant, M. Nausea, vomiting, and anorexia. Seminars in Oncology Nursing, *3*(4): 277–286, 1987.

Grant, MM. Nutritional interventions: increasing oral intake. Seminars in Oncology Nursing, *2*(1): 36–43, 1986.

Groenwald, SL (Ed.). Cancer nursing. Boston: Jones and Bartlett Publishers, 1987.

Groer, MW, & Shekleton, ME. Basic pathophysiology: a holistic approach (3rd ed.). St. Louis: C.V. Mosby, 1989.

Gurevich, I, & Tafuro, P. The compromised host—deficit-specific infection and the spectrum of prevention. Cancer Nursing, *9*(5): 263–275, 1986.

Guyton, AC. Textbook of medical physiology (7th ed.). Philadelphia: W.B. Saunders Company, 1986.

Haylock, PJ. Breathing difficulty: changes in respiratory function. Seminars in Oncology Nursing, *3*(4): 293–298, 1987.

Hickey, JV. The clinical practice of neurological and neurosurgical nursing (2nd ed.). Philadelphia: J.B. Lippincott Company, 1986.

Holloway, NM. Medical surgical care plans. Springhouse, PA: Springhouse Corporation, 1988.

Holroyde, CP, & Reichard, GA, Jr. General metabolic abnormalities in cancer patients: anorexia and cachexia. Surgical Clinics of North America, *66*(5): 947–956, 1986.

Hone, MM, & Swearingen, PL. Pocket guide to fluid and electrolytes. St. Louis: C.V. Mosby, 1989.

Iverson-Carpenter, MS. Impaired skin integrity. Journal of Gerontological Nursing, *14*(3): 25–29, 1988.

Jeejeebhoy, KN, & Meguid, MM. Assessment of nutritional status in the oncologic patient. Surgical Clinics of North America, *66*(6): 1077–1090, 1986.

Kim, MJ, McFarland, GK, & McLane, AM (Eds.). Pocket guide to nursing diagnosis (3rd ed.). St. Louis: C.V. Mosby, 1989.

Kissane, JM (Ed.). Anderson's pathology (8th ed.). St. Louis: C.V. Mosby, 1985.

Kneisel, CN, & Ames, SW. Adult health nursing: a biopsychosocial approach. Menlo Park, CA: Addison-Wesley, 1986.

Kozier, B, & Erb, G. Fundamentals of nursing (3rd ed.). Menlo Park, CA: Addison-Wesley, 1987.

Kübler-Ross, E. On death and dying. New York: Macmillan, 1969.

Kurzer, M, & Meguid, MM. Cancer and protein metabolism. Surgical Clinics of North America, *66*(5): 969–1001, 1986.

Lambert, CE, Jr, & Lambert, VA. Psychosocial impacts created by chronic illness. Nursing Clinics of North America, *22*(3): 527–533, 1987.

Lancaster, LE. Renal and endocrine regulation of water and electrolyte balance. Nursing Clinics of North America, *22*(4): 761–772, 1987.

Lederer, JR, Marculescu, GL, Gallagher, J, & Mills, P. Care planning pocket guide: a nursing diagnosis approach. Menlo Park, CA: Addison-Wesley, 1986.

Lewis, SM, & Collier, IC. Medical-surgical nursing: assessment and management of clinical problems (2nd ed.). New York: McGraw-Hill, 1987.

Lindsey, AM. Cancer cachexia: effects of the disease and its treatment. Seminars in Oncology Nursing, *2*(1): 19–29, 1986.

Loebl, S, & Spratto, GR. The nurse's drug handbook. New York: John Wiley & Sons, 1986.

Long, BC, & Phipps, WJ. Medical-surgical nursing: a nursing process approach (2nd ed.). St. Louis: C.V. Mosby, 1989.

Luckmann, J, & Sorensen, KC. Medical-surgical nursing: a psychophysiological approach (3rd ed.). Philadelphia: W.B. Saunders Company, 1987.

Marino, LB. Cancer nursing. St. Louis: C.V. Mosby, 1981.

Martocchio, BC. Family coping: helping families help themselves. Seminars in Oncology Nursing, *1*(4): 292–297, 1985.

McAndrew, PF. Fat metabolism and cancer. Surgical clinics of North America, *66*(5): 1003–1012, 1986.

McAnena, OJ, & Daly, JM. Impact of antitumor therapy on nutrition. Surgical Clinics of North America, *66*(6): 1213–1228, 1986.

McCaffery, M, & Beebe, A. Pain: clinical manual for nursing practice. St. Louis: C.V. Mosby, 1989.

McEvoy, GK (Ed.). Drug information '88. Bethesda, MD: American Society of Hospital Pharmacists, 1988.

McFarland, GK, & McFarlane, EA. Nursing diagnosis and intervention: planning for patient care. St. Louis: C.V. Mosby, 1989.

McGee, RF, & Clark, JC. Hope: a vital component in cancer care and coping. Proceedings of the fourth national conference on human values and cancer—1984, pp. 134–139.

McNally, JC, Stair, JC, & Somerville, ET (Eds.). Guidelines for cancer nursing practice. New York: Grune & Stratton, 1985.

Metheny, NM. Fluid and electrolyte balance. Philadelphia: J.B. Lippincott Company, 1987.

Miller, BF, & Keane, CB. Encyclopedia and dictionary of medicine, nursing, and allied health (4th ed.). Philadelphia: W.B. Saunders Company, 1987.

Miller, JF. Inspiring hope. American Journal of Nursing, *85*(1): 22–25, 1985.

Morrissey, BG. Therapeutic nutrition. Philadelphia: J.B. Lippincott Company, 1984.

Muir, BL. Pathophysiology (2nd ed.). New York: John Wiley & Sons, 1988.

Nail, LM, & King, KB. Fatigue. Seminars in Oncology Nursing, *3*(4): 257–262, 1987.

Nurse's Clinical Library. Respiratory disorders. Springhouse, PA: Springhouse Corporation, 1984.

Nurses Reference Library. Patient teaching. Springhouse, PA: Springhouse Corporation, 1986.

Padilla, GV. Psychological aspects of nutrition and cancer. Surgical Clinics of North America, *66*(6): 1121–1135, 1986.

Pallett, PJ, & O'Brien, MT. Textbook of neurological nursing. Boston: Little, Brown & Company, 1985.

Patrick, ML, Woods, SL, Craven, RF, Rokosky, JS, & Bruno, PM. Medical-surgical nursing: pathophysiological concepts. Philadelphia: J.B. Lippincott Company, 1986.

Piper, BF, Lindsay, AM, & Dodd, MJ. Fatigue mechanisms in cancer patients: developing nursing theory. Oncology Nursing Forum, *14*(6): 17–23, 1987.

Portenoy, RK. Practical aspects of pain control in the patient with cancer. CA—A Cancer Journal for Clinicians, *38*(6): 327–352, 1988.

Porth, CM. Pathophysiology: concepts of altered health states (2nd ed.). Philadelphia: J.B. Lippincott Company, 1986.

Poyss, AS. Assessment and nursing diagnosis in fluid and electrolyte disorders. Nursing Clinics of North America, *22*(4): 773–783, 1987.

Price, SA, & Wilson, LM. Pathophysiology: clinical concepts of disease processes (3rd ed.). New York: McGraw-Hill, 1986.

Raffensperger, EB, Zusy, ML, & Marchesseault, LC. Clinical nursing handbook. Philadelphia: J.B. Lippincott Company, 1986.

Rakel, RE (Ed.). Conn's current therapy. Philadelphia: W.B. Saunders Company, 1989.

Raucheisen, ML. Therapeutic touch: maybe there's something to it after all. RN, *47*(12): 49–51, 1984.

Sabiston, DC (Ed.). Textbook of surgery (13th ed.). Philadelphia: W.B. Saunders Company, 1986.

Schroeder, SA, Krupp, MA, & Tierney, LM (Eds.). Current medical diagnosis and treatment 1988. Norwalk, CT: Appleton & Lange, 1988.

Schultz, MC, & Dark, SL. Manual of psychiatric nursing care plans (2nd ed.). Boston: Little, Brown & Company, 1986.

Schwartz, SI (Ed.). Principles of surgery (5th ed.). New York: McGraw-Hill, 1989.

Smith, DB. Sexual rehabilitation of the cancer patient. Cancer Nursing, *12*(1): 10–15, 1989.

Smith, K., & Lesko, LM. Psychosocial problems in cancer survivors. Oncology, *2*(1): 33–40, 1988.

Smith, SAN. Theories and intervention of nutritional deficits in neoplastic disease. Oncology Nursing Forum, *9*(2): 43–46, 1982.

Snyder, CC. Oncology nursing. Boston: Little, Brown & Company, 1986.

Soeken, KL, & Carson, VJ. Responding to the spiritual needs of the chronically ill. Nursing Clinics of North America, *22*(3): 603–610, 1987.

Sorensen, KC, & Luckmann, J. Basic nursing: a psychophysiologic approach (2nd ed.). Philadelphia: W.B. Saunders Company, 1986.

Spencer, RT, Nichols, LW, Lipkin, GB, et al. Clinical pharmacology and nursing management (2nd ed.). Philadelphia: J.B. Lippincott Company, 1986.

Stein, JH (Ed.). Internal medicine (2nd ed.). Boston: Little, Brown & Company, 1987.

Swartz, MH. Textbook of physical diagnosis. Philadelphia: W.B. Saunders Company, 1989.

Swearingen, PL. The photo-atlas of nursing procedures. Menlo Park, CA: Addison-Wesley, 1984.

Taylor, C, Lillis, C, & LeMone, P. Fundamentals of nursing. Philadelphia: J.B. Lippincott Company, 1989.

Thomas, CD. Insomnia: identification and management. Seminars in Oncology Nursing, *3*(4): 263–266, 1987.

Thomas, CL (Ed.). Taber's cyclopedic medical dictionary (16th ed.). Philadelphia: F.A. Davis Company, 1989.

Thompson, JM, McFarland, GK, Hirsch, JE, Tucker, SM, & Bowers, AC. Mosby's manual of clinical nursing (2nd ed.). St. Louis: C.V. Mosby, 1989.

Townsend, MC. Nursing diagnoses in psychiatric nursing. Philadelphia: F.A. Davis Company, 1988.

Treseler, KM. Clinical laboratory and diagnostic tests: significance and implications (2nd ed.). Norwalk, CT: Appleton & Lange, 1988.

United States Pharmacopeial Convention. Drug information for the health care professional (9th ed.). Harrisonburg, VA: Banta Company, 1989.

Vredevoe, DL. Concepts of oncology nursing. Englewood Cliffs, NJ: Prentice-Hall, 1981.

Wahl, SC. Septic shock—how to detect it early. Nursing '89, *19*(1): 52–59, 1989.

Way, LW (Ed.). Current surgical diagnosis and treatment (8th ed.). Norwalk, CT: Appleton & Lange, 1988.

Weatherall, DJ, Ledingham, JGG, & Warrell, DA (Eds.). Oxford textbook of medicine (2nd ed.). Oxford: Oxford University Press, 1987.

Woods, ME. Assessment of the adult with cancer. Nursing Clinics of North America, *17*(4): 539–556, 1982.

Woods, NF, Lewis, FM, & Ellison, ES. Living with cancer: family experiences. Cancer Nursing, *12*(1): 28–33, 1989.

Wurtman, RJ, & Wurtman, JJ. Carbohydrates and depression. Scientific American, *260*(1): 68–75, 1989.

Wyngaarden, JB, & Smith, LH (Eds.). Cecil textbook of medicine (18th ed.). Philadelphia: W.B. Saunders Company, 1988.

Yasko, JM. Guidelines for cancer care: symptom management. Reston, VA: Reston Publishing Company, 1983.

UNIT 1. Nursing Care of the Elderly Client

Bachman, GA. Sexual dysfunction in postmenopausal women: the role of medical management. Geriatrics, *43*(11): 79–83, 1988.

Bellantoni, MF, & Blackman, MR. Osteoporosis: diagnostic screening and its place in current care. Geriatrics, *43*(2): 63–66, 69–70, 1988.

Berman, R, Haxby, JV, & Pomerantz, RS. Physiology of aging. part I: normal changes. Patient Care, *22*(1): 20, 26, 31–32, 34–36, 1988.

Branch, LG, & Meyers, AR. Assessing physical function in the elderly. Clinics in Geriatric Medicine, *3*(1): 29–52, 1987.

Campbell, EB, Williams, MA, & Ynarczyk, SM. After the

fall—confusion. American Journal of Nursing, *86*(2): 151–154, 1986.

Carnevali, DL, & Patrick, M. Nursing management for the elderly (2nd ed.). Philadelphia: J.B. Lippincott Company, 1986.

Ciocon, JO, & Potter, JF. Age-related changes in human memory: normal and abnormal. Geriatrics, *43*(10): 43–48, 1988.

Dychtwald, K (Ed.). Wellness and health promotion for the elderly. Rockville, MD: Aspen Publication, 1986.

Eliopoulos, C. Gerontological nursing (2nd ed.). Philadelphia: J.B. Lippincott Company, 1987.

Forman, MD. Acute confusional states in hospitalized elderly: a research dilemma. Nursing Research, *35*(1): 34–38, 1986.

Frank-Stromberg, M. Sexuality and the elderly cancer patient. Seminars in Oncology Nursing, *1*(1): 49–55, 1985.

Gallagher, D. Assessing affect in the elderly. Clinics in Geriatric Medicine, *3*(1): 65–86, 1987.

Gioelli, EC, & Bevil, CW. Nursing care of the aging client. Norwalk, CT: Appleton-Century-Crofts, 1985.

Gray-Vickrey, M. Color them special—a sensible, sensitive guide to caring for elderly patients. Nursing '87, *17*(5): 59–62, 1987.

Gurland, BJ, Coté, LJ, Cross, PS, & Toner, JA. The assessment of cognitive function in the elderly. Clinics in Geriatric Medicine, *3*(1): 53–64, 1987.

Hall, GH. Alterations in thought process. Journal of Gerontological Nursing, *14*(3): 30–37, 1988.

Jirovec, MM, Brink, CA, & Wells, TJ. Nursing assessments in the inpatient geriatric population. Nursing Clinics of North America, *23*(1): 219–230, 1988.

Lonergan, ET. Aging and the kidney: adjusting treatment to physiologic change. Geriatrics, *43*(3): 27–30, 32–33, 1988.

Masoro, EJ. Biology of aging, current state of knowledge. Archives of Internal Medicine, *147*(1): 166–169, 1987.

Matteson, MA, & McConnell, ES. Gerontological Nursing. Philadelphia: W.B. Saunders Company, 1988.

McCormick, KA, Scheve, AAS, & Leahy, E. Nursing management of urinary incontinence in geriatric inpatients. Nursing Clinics of North America, *23*(1): 231–264, 1988.

Milde, FK. Impaired physical mobility. Journal of Gerontological Nursing, *14*(3): 20–24, 1988.

Ouslander, JG, & Bruskewitz, R. Disorders of micturition in the aging patient. Advances in Internal Medicine, *34*: 165–190, 1989.

Nesbitt, B. Nursing diagnosis in age-related changes. Journal of Gerontological Nursing, *14*(7): 7–12, 1988.

Palmer, MH. Incontinence: the magnitude of the problem. Nursing Clinics of North America, *23*(1): 139–157, 1988.

Pritchard, V. Geriatric infections: the gastrointestinal tract. RN, *51*(4): 58–60, 1988.

Ramsey, R. Adjusting drug dosages for critically ill elderly patients. Nursing '88, *18*(7): 47–49, 1988.

Richey, ML, Richey, HK, & Fenske, NA. Aging-related skin changes: development and clinical meaning. Geriatrics, *43*(4): 49–52, 57–59, 63–64, 1988.

Rossman, I (Ed.). Clinical geriatrics (3rd ed.). Philadelphia: J.B. Lippincott Company, 1986.

Santo-Novak, DA. Seven keys to assessing the elderly. American Journal of Nursing, *88*(8): 60–63, 1988.

Schwab, R, Walters, CA, & Weksler, ME. Host defense mechanisms and aging. Seminars in Oncology, *16*(1): 20–27, 1989.

Thienhaus, OJ. Practical overview of sexual function and advancing age. Geriatrics, *43*(8): 63–67, 1988.

Trulock, EP. Approaches to deep venous thrombosis and pulmonary embolism in aging patients. Geriatrics, *43*(2): 101–102, 104, 106, 108, 1988.

Welch-McCaffrey, D, & Dodge, J. Acute confusional states in elderly cancer patients. Seminars in Oncology Nursing, *4*(3): 208–216, 1988.

Westfall, LK, & Pavlis, RW. Why the elderly are so vulnerable to drug reactions. RN, *50*(11): 39–43, 1987.

Wyman, JF. Nursing assessment of the incontinent geriatric outpatient population. Nursing Clinics of North America, *23*(1): 169–187, 1988.

UNIT II. Nursing Care of the Client Having Surgery

II.2. Postoperative Care

Burden, N. Post-anesthesia: when the patient wakes up. RN, *51*(4): 40–44, 1988.

Conti, MT, & Eutropius, L. Preventing UTI's: what works. American Journal of Nursing, *87*(3): 307–309, 1987.

Hull, RD, Raskob, GE, & Hirsch, J. Prophylaxis of venous thromboembolism: an overview. Chest (supplement), *89*(5): 374S–383S, 1986.

Kearns, PC. Exercises to ease pain after abdominal surgery. RN, *49*(7): 45–48, 1986.

Oster, G, Tuden, RL, & Colditz, GA. Prevention of venous thromboembolism after general surgery. American Journal of Medicine, *82*(5): 889–899, 1987.

Patwell, T. Postoperative care of the elderly surgical patient. Journal of Practical Nursing, *37*(3): 34–37, 1987.

Sarsany, SL. Are you ready for this bedside emergency? . . . wound dehiscence and evisceration. RN, *50*(12): 32–34, 1987.

Vaughn, JB, & Nemcek, MA. Postoperative flatulence: causes and remedies. Today's OR Nurse, *8*(10): 19–23, 1986.

Vaughn, JB, & Taylor, K. Homeward bound—discharge following surgery. Nursing Times, *84*(15): 28–33, 1988.

Young, ME, & Flynn, KT. Third spacing: when the body conceals fluid loss. RN, *51*(8): 46–48, 1988.

UNIT III. Nursing Care of the Immobile Client (Immobility)

Maynard, FM. Immobilization hypercalcemia following spinal cord injury. Archives of Physical Medicine and Rehabilitation, *67*(1): 41–44, 1986.

Moser, KM. The therapeutic focus in pulmonary embolism. Emergency Medicine, *19*(20): 67–79, 81, 82–83, 1987.

Rubin, M. The physiology of bed rest. American Journal of Nursing, *88*(1): 50–56, 1988.

Teitelbaum, SL. Metabolic and other nontumorous disorders of bone. In Kissane, JM (Ed.), Anderson's pathology (8th ed.) (Vol. 2). St. Louis: C.V. Mosby, 1985, pp. 1748–1749.

Trulock, EP. Approaches to deep venous thrombosis and pulmonary embolism in aging patients. Geriatrics, *43*(2): 101–102, 104, 106, 108, 1988.

Tyler, M. The respiratory effects of body positioning and immobilization. Respiratory Care, *29*(5): 472–483, 1984.

Winslow, EH. Cardiovascular consequences of bed rest. Heart and Lung, *14*(3): 236–246, 1985.

UNIT IV. Nursing Care of the Client Who is Dying (Terminal Care)

Alexander, J, & Kiely, J. Working with the bereaved. Geriatric Nursing, *7*(2): 85–86, 1986.

Amenta, MO, & Bohnet, NL. Nursing care of the terminally ill. Boston: Little, Brown & Company, 1986.

Archer, DN, & Smith, AC. Sorrow has many faces: helping families cope with grief. Nursing '88, *18*(5): 43–45, 1988.

Benoliel, JQ. Loss and terminal illness. Nursing Clinics of North America, *20*(2): 439–448, 1985.

Benoliel, JQ, & McCorkle, R. A holistic approach to terminal illness. Cancer Nursing, *1*(2): 143–149, 1978.

Benton, RG. Death and dying: principles and practices in patient care. New York: D. Van Nostrand Company, 1978.

Bledsoe, AS, & Krueger, NJ. Dying patients: caring makes the difference. Nursing '87, *17*(6): 44–45, 1987.

Blues, AG, & Zerwekh, JV. Hospice and palliative nursing care. Orlando, FL.: Grune & Stratton, 1984.

Conrad, NL. Spiritual support for the dying. Nursing Clinics of North America, *20*(2): 415–426, 1985.

Dufault, K, & Martocchio, BC. Hope: its spheres and dimensions. Nursing Clinics of North America, *20*(2): 379–391, 1985.

Epstein, C. Nursing the dying patient. Reston, VA: Reston Publishing Company, 1975.

Evans, MA, Esbenson, M, & Jaffe, C. Expect the unexpected when you care for a dying patient. Nursing '81, *11*(12): 55–56, 1981.

Franks, LC. "Does that mean I'm dying?" RN, *47*(2): 25–28, 1984.

Geltman, RL, & Paige, RL. Symptom management in hospice care. American Journal of Nursing, *83*(1): 78–85, 1983.

Granstrom, S. Spiritual nursing care for oncology patients. Topics in Clinical Nursing, *7*(1): 39–45, 1985.

Holtz, M (Ed.). Symptom management program: for the adult patient with end stage cancer. Seattle, WA: Community Home Health Care, 1981.

Kübler-Ross, E. Death: the final stage of growth. Englewood Cliffs, NJ: Prentice-Hall, 1975.

Lerner, J, & Khan, J. Mosby's manual of urologic nursing. St. Louis: C.V. Mosby, 1982.

Lipman, AG. Drug therapy in cancer pain. Cancer Nursing, *3*(1): 39–46, 1980.

Martocchio, BC. Living while dying. Bowie, MD: R.J. Brady Company, 1982.

Martocchio, BC. Grief and bereavement. Nursing Clinics of North America, *20*(2): 327–341, 1985.

McGivney, WT, & Crooks, GM. The care of patients with severe chronic pain in terminal illness. Journal of the American Medical Association, *251*(9)): 1182–1188, 1984.

Megerle, JS. Surviving. American Journal of Nursing, *83*(6): 892–894, 1983.

Miller, JF. Inspiring hope. American Journal of Nursing, *85*(1): 23–25, 1985.

Moseley, JR. Alterations in comfort. Nursing Clinics of North America, *20*(2): 427–438, 1985.

Murphy, P. Studies of loss and grief. American Journal of Hospice Care, *2*(2): 10–14, 1985.

Murphy, P. Pastoral care and persons with AIDS—a means to alleviate physical, emotional, social, and spiritual suffering. American Journal of Hospice Care, *3*(2): 38–40, 1986.

Niland, M., & Atwood, J. Care of the hospitalized dying patient. Topics in Clinical Nursing, *3*(3): 17–27, 1981.

Peterson, EA. How to meet your client's spiritual needs. Journal of Psychosocial Nursing, *25*(5): 34–39, 1987.

Reuben, D, & Mor, V. Dyspnea in terminally ill cancer patients. Chest, *89*(2): 234–236, 1986.

Taylor, PB, & Gideon, MD. Holding out hope to your dying patient: paradoxical but possible. Nursing '82, *12*(2): 42–45, 1982.

Twycross, RG. The management of pain in cancer: a guide to drugs and dosages. Oncology, *2*(4): 35–43, 1988.

Tyner, R. Elements of empathic care for dying patients and their families. Nursing Clinics of North America, *20*(2): 393–401, 1985.

Ufema, J. Grieving families: let your heart do the talking. Nursing '81, *11*(11): 80–83, 1981.

Ufema, JK. How to talk to dying patients. Nursing '87, *17*(8): 43–46, 1987.

Vastiyan, EA. Spiritual aspects of the care of cancer patients. Cancer, *36*(2): 110–114, 1986.

Whelan, E. Support for the survivor. Geriatric Nursing, *6*(1): 21–23, 1985.

Zack, MV. Loneliness: a concept relevant to the care of dying persons. Nursing Clinics of North America, *20*(2): 403–414, 1985.

Zerwekh, JV. The dehydration question. Nursing '83 *13*(1): 47–51, 1983.

Zerwekh, JV. Comforting the dying, dyspneic patient. Nursing '87, *17*(11): 66–69, 1987.

UNIT V. Nursing Care of the Client Receiving Treatment for Neoplastic Disorders

V.1. Brachytherapy

Becker, DV, & Siegel, BA. Guidelines for patients receiving radioiodine treatment. The Society of Nuclear Medicine, 1983.

Dudjak, LA. Future directions of brachytherapy. Seminars in Oncology Nursing, *3*(1): 74–77, 1987.

Fletcher, GH. Textbook of radiotherapy (3rd ed.). Philadelphia: Lea & Febiger, 1980.

Hassey, K. Radiation alternative to mastectomy. American Journal of Nursing, *83*(11): 1567–1569, 1983.

Hassey, K. Demystifying care of patients with radioactive implants. American Journal of Nursing, *85*(7): 788–792, 1985.

Haylock, P, & Hart, L. Fatigue in patients receiving localized radiation. Cancer Nursing, *2*(6): 461–467, 1979.

Jenkins, B. Sexual healing after pelvic irradiation. American Journal of Nursing, *83*(11): 920–922, 1986.

Kreamer, K, Aquila, K, Haller, M, Pelliccia, E, & Perrone, J. Information about radiation therapy. Oncology Nursing Forum, *11*(4): 67–71, 1984.

Lamb, S. Interstitial radiation for the treatment of brain tumors using the stereotactic method. Journal of Neurosurgical Nursing, *12*(3): 138–144, 1980.

Leahy, IM, St. Germain, JM, & Varricchio, CG. The nurse and radiotherapy: a manual for daily care. St. Louis: C.V. Mosby, 1979.

Maddock, PG. Brachytherapy sources and applicators. Seminars in Oncology Nursing, *3*(1): 15–22, 1987.

Marinari, B. Stereotaxis. Journal of Neurosurgical Nursing, *16*(3): 140–143, 1984.

Randall, TM, Drake, DK, & Sewchand, W. Neuro-oncology update: radiation safety and nursing care during interstitial brachytherapy. Journal of Neuroscience Nursing, *19*(6): 315–320, 1987.

Richards, S, & Hiratzka, S. Vaginal dilatation post pelvic irradiation: a patient education tool. Oncology Nursing Forum, *13*(4): 89–91, 1986.

Shell, JA, & Carter, J. The gynecological implant patient. Seminars in Oncology Nursing, *3*(1): 54–66, 1987.

Siebel, J. Playing it safe around cesium implants. RN, *46*(10): 42–43, 1983.

Strohl, RA. Head and neck implants. Seminars in Oncology Nursing, *3*(1): 30–46, 1987.

Witt, ME, McDonald-Lynch, A, & Grimmer, D. Adjuvant radiotherapy to the colorectum. Oncology Nursing Forum, *14*(3): 17–21, 1987.

V.2. Chemotherapy

Abrahm, J. Management of the immunocompromised host. Medical Clinics of North America, *68*(3): 617–637, 1984.

Bahnson, CB. Psychological aspects of cancer. In Pilch, YH (Ed.), Surgical oncology. New York: McGraw-Hill, 1984, pp. 231–253.

Barry, SA. Septic shock: special needs of patients with cancer. Oncology Nursing Forum, *16*(1): 31–35, 1989.

Bender, CM, Bast, JF, Drapac, D, & Kray, C. Patient teaching in hepatic artery infusion. Oncology Nursing Forum, *11*(2): 61–65, 1984.

Bersani, G, & Carl, W. Oral care for cancer patients. American Journal of Nursing, *83*(4): 533–536, 1983.

Black, ML, Gallucci, BB, & Katakkar, SB. The nutritional

assessment of patients receiving cancer chemotherapy. Oncology Nursing Forum, *10*(2): 53–58, 1983.

Brant, B. A nursing protocol for the client with neutropenia. Oncology Nursing Forum, *11*(2): 24–28, 1984.

Butler, JH. Nutrition and cancer: a review of the literature. Cancer Nursing, *3*(2): 131–136, 1980.

Camp, LD. Care of the Groshong catheter. Oncology Nursing Forum, *15*(6): 745–749, 1988.

Carter, SK, Bakowski, MT, & Hellmann, K. Chemotherapy of cancer (2nd ed.). New York: John Wiley & Sons, 1987.

Cline, BW. Prevention of chemotherapy-induced alopecia: a review of the literature. Cancer Nursing, *7*(3): 221–228, 1984.

Cobb, SC. Teaching relaxation techniques to cancer patients. Cancer Nursing, *7*(2): 157–161, April, 1984.

Cohen, MR. Action stat! Drug-induced anaphylaxis. Nursing '85, *15*(2): 43, 1985.

Cotanch, PM, & Strum, S. Progressive muscle relaxation for antiemetic therapy for cancer therapy. Oncology Nursing Forum, *14*(1): 3–37, 1987.

Couillard-Getreuer, DL. Herpes zoster in the immunocompromised patient. Cancer Nursing, *5*(5): 361–370, 1982.

Cozzi, E, Hagle, M, McGregor, ML, & Woodhouse, D. Nursing management of patients receiving hepatic arterial chemotherapy through an implanted infusion pump. Cancer Nursing, *7*(3): 229–234, 1984.

Cunningham, SG. Fluid and electrolyte disturbances associated with cancer and its treatment. Nursing Clinics of North America, *17*(4): 579–593, 1982.

Daeffler, R. Oral hygiene measures for patients with cancer, I. Cancer Nursing, *3*(5): 347–356, 1980.

Daeffler, R. Oral hygiene measures for patients with cancer, II. Cancer Nursing, *3*(6): 427–432, 1980.

Daeffler, R. Oral hygiene measures for patients with cancer, III. Cancer Nursing, *4*(1): 29–35, 1981.

Daeffler, R, & Lewinski, J. Hickman/Broviac catheter. Oncology Nursing Forum, *9*(4): 61–63, 1982.

Daniels, M, & Belt, RJ. High dose metoclopramide as an antiemetic for patients receiving chemotherapy with cis-platinum. Oncology Nursing Forum, *9*(3): 20–22, 1982.

Donaldson, SS, & Lenon, RA. Alterations of nutritional status: impact of chemotherapy and radiation therapy. Cancer, *43*(5): 2036–2052, 1979.

Donoghue, M. Anorexia. In Nursing care of the cancer patient with nutritional problems. Report of the Ross Roundtable on Oncology Nursing, pp. 27–33. August, 1981.

Donaghue, M, Nunnally, C, & Yasko, JM. Nutritional aspects of cancer care. Reston, VA: Reston Publishing Company, 1982.

Duigon, A. Anticipatory nausea and vomiting associated with cancer chemotherapy. Oncology Nursing Forum, *13*(1): 35–40, 1986.

Dunagin, W. Clinical toxicity of chemotherapeutic agents: dermatologic toxicity. Seminars in Oncology, *9*(1): 14–22, 1982.

Ellerhorst-Ryan, JM. Complications of the myeloproliferative system: infection and sepsis. Seminars in Oncology Nursing, *1*(4): 244–250, 1985.

Engelking, CH, & Steele, NE. A model for pretreatment nursing assessment of patients receiving cancer chemotherapy. Cancer Nursing, *7*(3): 203–212, 1984.

Eriksson, JH, & Swenson, KK. Your guide to intraperitoneal chemotherapy. Oncology Nursing Forum, *13*(5): 77–81, 1986.

Esparza, DM, & Weyland, JB. Nursing care for the patient with an Ommaya reservoir. Oncology Nursing Forum, *9*(4): 17–20, 1982.

Fanslow, J. Guidelines for nursing care of patients with a knowledge deficit. Oncology Nursing Forum, *10*(3): 99–100, 1983.

Frank-Stromberg, M, Wright, PS, Segalla, M, & Diekmann, J. Psychological impact of the "cancer" diagnosis. Oncology Nursing Forum, *11*(3): 16–22, 1984.

Friedman, BD. Coping with cancer: a guide for health professionals. Cancer Nursing, *3*(2): 105–110, 1980.

Garvey, E, & Kramer, R. Improving cancer patients' adjustment to infusion chemotherapy: evaluation of a patient education program. Cancer Nursing, *6*(5): 373–378, 1983.

Goodman, M. External venous catheters: home management. Oncology Nursing Forum, *15*(3): 357–360, 1988.

Groër, M, & Pierce, M. Guarding against cancer's hidden killer: anorexia-cachexia. Nursing '81. *11*(6): 39–43, 1981.

Hagle, M. Implantable devices for chemotherapy: access and delivery. Seminars in Oncology Nursing, *3*(2): 96–105, 1987.

Hoagland, HC. Hematologic complications of cancer chemotherapy. Seminars in Oncology, *9*(1): 95–102, 1982.

Hoff, S. Concepts in intraperitoneal chemotherapy. Seminars in Oncology Nursing, *3*(2): 112–117, 1987.

Holden, S, & Felde, G. Nursing care of patients experiencing cisplatin-related peripheral neuropathy. Oncology Nursing Forum *14*(1): 13–19, 1987.

Hubbard, SM. Chemotherapy and the cancer nurse. In Marino, LB (Ed.), Cancer nursing. St. Louis: C.V. Mosby, 1981, pp. 287–343.

Hughes, CB. Giving cancer drugs: some guidelines. American Journal of Nursing, *86*(1): 34–38, 1986.

Hunt, JM, Anderson, JE, & Smith, IE. Scalp hypothermia to prevent Adriamycin-induced hair loss. Cancer Nursing, *5*(1): 25–31, 1982.

Itri, LM. The effects of chemotherapy on gonadal function. Your Patient and Cancer, March, 1983, pp. 45–49.

Kaempfer, SH. The effects of cancer chemotherapy on reproduction: a review of the literature. Oncology Nursing Forum, *8*(1): 11–17, 1981.

Kaplan, R, & Wiernik, P. Neurotoxicity of antineoplastic drugs. Seminars in Oncology, *9*(1): 103–130, 1982.

Kaszyk, LK. Cardiac toxicity associated with cancer therapy. Oncology Nursing Forum, *13*(4): 81–88, 1986.

Keller, JF, & Blausey, LA. Nursing issues and management in chemotherapy-induced alopecia. Oncology Nursing Forum, *15*(5): 603–607, 1988.

Kennedy, M, Packard, R, Grant, MM, & Padilla, CV. Che-

motherapy-related nausea and vomiting: a survey to identify problems and interventions. Oncology Nursing Forum, *8*(1): 19–22, 1981.

Kirchner, CW, & Reheis, CE. Two serious complications of neoplasia: sepsis and disseminated intravascular coagulation. Nursing Clinics of North America, *17*(4): 595–606, 1982.

Knobf, MKT. Intravenous therapy guidelines for oncology practice. Oncology Nursing Forum, *9*(2): 30–44, 1982.

Lamb, MA, & Woods, NF. Sexuality and the cancer patient. Cancer Nursing, *4*(2): 137–144, 1981.

Lindsey, AM, Piper, BF, & Stotts, N. The phenomenon of cancer cachexia: a review. Oncology Nursing Forum, *9*(2): 38–42, 1982.

Livingstone, RB. Principles of cancer chemotherapy. In Pilch, YH (Ed.), Surgical oncology: New York: McGraw-Hill, 1984, pp. 124–141.

Lydon, J. Nephrotoxicity of cancer treatment. Oncology Nursing Forum, *13*(2): 68–77, 1986.

Malamud, SC, & Haubenstock, A. Complications of antineoplastic treatment. Topics in Emergency Medicine, *8*(2): 59–74, 1986.

Malseed, RT. Pharmacology: drug therapy and nursing considerations (2nd ed.). Philadelphia: J.B. Lippincott Company, 1985.

McDevitt, B. Standards of clinical practice: the side effects of chemotherapy in the treatment of leukemia. Cancer Nursing, *5*(4): 317–323, 1982.

Miller, SA. Nursing actions in cancer chemotherapy administration. Oncology Nursing Forum, *7*(4): 8–16, 1980.

Montrose, P. Extravasation management. Seminars in Oncology Nursing, *3*(2): 128–132, 1987.

Morrow, GR. Chemotherapy-related nausea and vomiting: etiology and management. CA—Cancer Journal for Clinicians, *39*(2): 89–104, 1989.

Nunnally, C, Donoghue, M, & Yasko, J. Nutritional needs of cancer patients. Nursing Clinics of North America, *17*(4): 557–578, 1982.

Ogriniz, M. Sensory/perceptual alterations related to peripheral neuropathy. In McNally, JC, Stair, JC, & Sommerville, ET (Eds.), Guidelines for cancer nursing practice. New York: Grune & Stratton, 1985, pp. 185–188.

Oncology Nursing Society. Cancer Chemotherapy Guidelines, Modules 1 & 2. Pittsburgh, PA.: Oncology Nursing Society, 1988.

O'Rourke, ME. Enhanced cutaneous effects in combined modality therapy. Oncology Nursing Forum, *14*(6): 31–35, 1987.

Ostchega, Y. Cancer chemotherapy's oral complications. Nursing '80, *10*(8): 47–52, 1980.

Ostchega, Y, & Jacob. J. Providing "safe conduct": helping your patient cope with cancer. Nursing '84, *14*(4): 42–47, 1984.

Perry, NC (Ed.). Toxicity of chemotherapy. Seminars in Oncology, *9*(1): 1–154, 1982.

Petton, S. Easing the complications of chemotherapy: a matter of little victories. Nursing '84, *14*(2): 58–63, 1984.

Reheis, C. Neutropenia—causes, complications, treatment, and resulting nursing care. Nursing Clinics of North America, *20*(1): 219–225, 1985.

Sarno, LP. Concepts in nursing management of patients receiving cancer chemotherapy and immunotherapy. In Vredevoe DL, et al. (Eds.), Concepts of oncology nursing. Englewood Cliffs, NJ: Prentice-Hall, 1981, pp. 81–153.

Schilsky, RL. Renal and metabolic toxicities of cancer chemotherapy. Seminars in Oncology, *9*(1): 75–83, 1982.

Schlesselman, SM. Helping your cancer patient cope with alopecia. Nursing '88, *18*(12): 43–45, 1988.

See-Lasley, K, & Ignoffo, RJ (Eds.). Manual of oncology therapeutics. St. Louis: C.V. Mosby, 1981.

Shapiro, T. How to help patients get through chemotherapy. RN, *50*(3): 58–60, 1987.

Simonson, GM. Caring for patients with acute myelocytic leukemia. American Journal of Nursing, *88*(3): 304–309, 1988.

Spiegel, RJ. The acute toxicites of chemotherapy. Cancer Treatment Review, *81*(8): 197–207, 1981.

Spross, J. (Ed.). Issues in chemotherapy administration. Oncology Nursing Forum, *9*(1): 50–54, 1982.

Strohl, R. Nursing management of the patient with cancer experiencing taste changes. Cancer Nursing, *6*(5): 353–359, 1983.

Strohl, R. Understanding taste changes. Oncology Nursing Forum, *11*(3): 81–84, 1984.

Swenson, KK, & Eriksson, JH. Nursing management of intraperitoneal chemotherapy. Oncology Nursing Forum, *13*(5): 33–39, 1986.

Theologides, A. Pathogenesis of cachexia in cancer: a review and a hypothesis. Cancer, *29*: 484, 1972.

Trester, AK. Nursing management of patients receiving cancer chemotherapy. Cancer Nursing, *5*(3): 201–210, 1982.

Watson, PM. Patient education: the adult with cancer. Nursing Clinics of North America, *17*(4): 739–752, 1982.

Weiss, RB. Hypersensitivity reactions to cancer chemotherapy. Seminars in Oncology, *9*(1): 5–13, 1982.

Weiss, RB, & Trush, DM. A review of the pulmonary toxicity of cancer chemotherapeutic agents. Oncology Nursing Forum, *9*(1): 16–21, 1982.

Weltman, R, & Shupack, J. Pruritus in the cancer patient. Your Patient & Cancer (special edition for oncology nurses), pp. 10–24, Fall, 1984.

Wickham, R. Pulmonary toxicity secondary to cancer treatment. Oncology Nursing Forum, *13*(5): 69–76, 1986.

Wilding, G, Caruso, R, Lawrence, T, Ostchega, Y, Ballintine, EJ, Young, RC, & Ozols, RJ. Retinal toxicity after high-dose cisplatinum therapy. Journal of Clinical Oncology, *3*(12): 1683–1689, 1985.

Winters, V. Implantable vascular access devices. Oncology Nursing Forum, *11*(6): 25–31, 1984.

Wroblewski, SS, & Wroblewski, SH. Caring for the patient with chemotherapy-induced thrombocytopenia. American Journal of Nursing, *81*(4): 746–749, 1981.

Yasko, JM (Ed.). Nursing management of symptoms associated with chemotherapy, (rev. ed.) Adria Laboratories, 1986.

Yasko, JM. Holistic management of nausea and vomiting caused by chemotherapy. Topics in Clinical Nursing, *7*(1): 26–38, 1985.

V.3. External Radiation Therapy

Abraham, J. Management of the immunocompromised host. Medical Clinics of North America, *68*(3): 617–637, 1984.

Bersani, G, & Carl, W. Oral care for cancer patients. American Journal of Nursing, *83*(4): 533–536, 1983.

Butler, JH. Nutrition and cancer: a review of the literature. Cancer Nursing, *3*(2): 131–136, 1980.

Cobb, SC. Teaching relaxation techniques to cancer patients. Cancer Nursing, *7*(2): 157–161, April, 1984.

Cunningham, SG. Fluid and electrolyte disturbances associated with cancer and its treatment. Nursing Clinics of North America, *17*(4): 579–593, 1982.

Daeffler, R. Oral hygiene measures for patients with cancer, I. Cancer Nursing, *3*(5): 347–356, 1980.

Daeffler, R. Oral hygiene measures for patients with cancer, II. Cancer Nursing, *3*(6): 427–432, 1980.

Daeffler, R. Oral hygiene measures for patients with cancer, III. Cancer Nursing, *4*(1): 29–35, 1981.

Dangel, RB. Pruritus and cancer. Oncology Nursing Forum, *13*(1): 17–21, 1986.

Dodd, MJ. Patterns of self care in cancer patients receiving radiation therapy. Oncology Nursing Forum, *11*(3): 23–27, 1984.

Donoghue, M. Anorexia. In Nursing care of the cancer patient with nutritional problems. Report of the Ross Roundtable on Oncology Nursing, pp. 27–33, August, 1981.

Donoghue, M, Nunnally, C, & Yasko, JM. Nutritional aspects of cancer care. Reston, VA: Reston Publishing Company, 1982.

Ellerhorst-Ryan, JM. Complications of the myeloproliferative system: infection and sepsis. Seminars in Oncology Nursing, *1*(4): 244–250, 1985.

Fanslow, J. Guidelines for nursing care of patients with a knowledge deficit. Oncology Nursing Forum, *10*(3): 99–100, 1983.

Fletcher, GH. Textbook of radiotherapy (3rd ed.). Philadelphia: Lea & Febiger, 1980.

Frank-Stromberg, M, Wright, PS, Segalla, M, & Diekmann, J. Psychological impact of the "cancer" diagnosis. Oncology Nursing Forum, *11*(3): 16–22, 1984.

Friedman, BD. Coping with cancer: a guide for health professionals. Cancer Nursing, *3*(2): 105–110, 1980.

Gallucci, BB, & Iwamoto, RR. Taste alterations in patients with cancer. In Nursing care of the cancer patient with nutritional problems. Report of the Ross Roundtable on Oncology Nursing. Columbus, Ohio: Ross Laboratories, 1981.

Goldstein, I, Feldman, MI, Deckers, PJ, Babayan, RK, & Krane, RJ. Radiation-associated impotence. Journal of American Medical Association, *251*(7): 903–910, 1984.

Hassey, KM. Radiation therapy for rectal cancer and the implications for nursing. Cancer Nursing, *10*(6): 311–318, 1987.

Hassey, KM, & Rose, CM. Altered skin integrity in patients receiving radiation therapy. Oncology Nursing Forum, *9*(4): 44–50, 1982.

Haylock, PJ, & Hart, LK. Fatigue in patients receiving localized radiation. Cancer Nursing, *2*(6): 461–467, 1979.

Hilderley, L. Skin care in radiation therapy: a review of the literature. Oncology Nursing Forum, *10*(1): 51–56, 1983.

Hilderley, LJ. The role of the nurse in radiation oncology. Seminars in Oncology, *7*(1): 39–47, 1980.

Jenkins, B. Sexual healing after pelvic irradiation. American Journal of Nursing, *86*(8): 920–922, 1986.

Johnson, C. Nutritional care of cancer patients receiving radiotherapy. In Fletcher, GH (Ed.), Textbook of radiotherapy. Philadelphia: Lea & Febiger, 1980, pp. 92–103.

Kelly, PP, & Tinsley, C. Planning care for the patient receiving external radiation. American Journal of Nursing, *81*(2): 338–342, 1981.

King, KB, Nail, LM, Kreamer, K, Strohl, RA, & Johnson, JE. Patients' descriptions of the experience of receiving radiation therapy. Oncology Nursing Forum, *12*(4): 55–61, 1985.

Kreamer, K, Aquila, K, Haller, M, Pelliccia, E, & Perrone, J. Information about radiation therapy. Oncology Nursing Forum, *11*(4): 67–71, 1984.

Lamb, MA, & Woods, NF. Sexuality and the cancer patient. Cancer Nursing, *4*(2): 137–144, 1981.

Leahy, IM, St. Germain, JM, & Varricchio, CG. The nurse and radiotherapy—a manual for daily care. St. Louis: C.V. Mosby, 1979.

Lewis, FL, & Levita, M. Understanding radiotherapy. Cancer Nursing, *11*(3): 174–185, 1988.

Lindsey, AM, Piper, BF, & Stotts, N. The phenomenon of cancer cachexia: a review. Oncology Nursing Forum *9*(2): 38–42, 1982.

Lydon, J. Nephrotoxicity of cancer treatment. Oncology Nursing Forum, *13*(2): 68–77, 1986.

O'Rourke, ME. Enhanced cutaneous effects in combined modality therapy. Oncology Nursing Forum, *14*(6): 31–35, 1987.

Ostchega, Y, & Jacob, J. Providing "safe conduct": helping your patient cope with cancer. Nursing '84, *14*(4): 42–47, 1984.

Richards, S, & Hiratzka, S. Vaginal dilatation post pelvic irradiation: a patient education tool. Oncology Nursing Forum, *13*(4): 89–91, 1986.

Smith, DS, & Chamorro, TP. Nursing care of patients undergoing combination chemotherapy and radiotherapy. Cancer Nursing, *1*(2): 129–134, 1978.

Strohl, R. Nursing management of the patient with cancer experiencing taste changes. Cancer Nursing, *6*(5): 353–359, 1983.

Strohl, R. Understanding taste changes. Oncology Nursing Forum, *11*(3): 81–84, 1984.

Strohl, RA. The nursing role in radiation oncology: symptom management of acute and chronic reactions. Oncology Nursing Forum, *15*(4): 429–434, 1988.

Strohl, RA, & Salazar, OM. Management of the patient receiving hemibody irradiation. Oncology Nursing Forum, *9*(4): 13–16, 1982.

Theologides, A. Pathogenesis of cachexia in cancer: a review and a hypothesis. Cancer, *29*: 484, 1972.

Trowbridge, JE, & Carl, W. Oral care of the patient having head and neck irradiation. American Journal of Nursing, *75*(12): 2146–2149, 1975.

Varricchio, C. The patient on radiation therapy. American Journal of Nursing, *81*(2): 334–337, 1981.

Welch, DA. Assessment of nausea and vomiting in cancer patients undergoing external beam radiotherapy. Cancer Nursing *3*(5): 365–371, 1980.

Welch, D. Radiation-related nausea and vomiting: a review of the literature. Oncology Nursing Forum, *6*(4): 8–11, 1979.

Weltman, R, & Shupack, J. Pruritus in the cancer patient. Your Patient & Cancer (special edition for oncology nurses), pp. 10–24, Fall, 1984.

Witt, ME. Questions on colon and rectum radiation therapy. Oncology Nursing Forum, *14*(3): 79–82, 1987.

Witt, ME, McDonald-Lynch, A, & Grimmer, D. Adjuvant radiotherapy to the colorectum: nursing implications. Oncology Nursing Forum, *14*(3): 17–21, 1987.

Yasko, JM. Care of the client receiving external radiation therapy. Reston, VA: Reston Publishing Company, 1982.

Yasko, JM. Care of the patient receiving radiation therapy. Nursing Clinics of North America, *17*(4): 631–648, 1982.

UNIT VI. Nursing Care of the Client with Disturbances of Neurological Function

VI.1. Cerebrovascular Accident

American Association of Neuroscience Nurses. Core curriculum for neurosurgical nursing (2nd ed.). Park Ridge, IL: Author, 1984.

Edelman, AS, & Weiss, MH. Cerebral edema—techniques for monitoring and options for management. Consultant, *25*(6): 58–60, 63–64, 66–68, 1985.

Gardner, S. Caring for the stroke patient: a guide for LP/VN's. Journal of Practical Nursing, *37*(3): 38–41, 1987.

Gary, R, Jermier, B, & Hickey, A. Stroke: how to contain the damage. RN, *49*(5): 36–41, 1986.

Goetter, W. Nursing diagnoses and interventions with the acute stroke patient. Nursing Clinics of North America, *21*(2): 309–319, 1986.

Gorelick, PB. Cerebrovascular disease: pathophysiology and diagnosis. Nursing Clinics of North America, *21*(2): 275–288, 1986.

Hahn, K. Left vs right: what a difference the side makes in a stroke. Nursing '87, *17*(9): 44–47, 1987.

Jess, LW. Assessing your patient for increased I.C.P. Nursing '87, *17*(6): 34–41, 1987.

Konopad, E, & Noseworthy, T. Stress ulceration: a serious complication in critically ill patients. Heart and Lung, *17*(4): 339–348, 1988.

Loustav, A, & Lee, KA. Dealing with the dangers of dysphagia. Nursing '85, *15*(2): 47–50, 1985.

Passarella, P, & Gee, Z. Starting right after stroke. American Journal of Nursing, *87*(6): 802–805, 1987.

Stevens, SA. A simple, step-by-step approach to neurologic assessment (part 2). Nursing '88, *18*(10): 51–58, 1988.

Vogt, G, Miller, M, & Esluer, M. Mosby's manual of neurological care. St. Louis: C.V. Mosby, 1985.

VI.2. Craniocerebral Trauma

American Association of Neuroscience Nurses. Core curriculum for neurosurgical nursing (2nd ed.). Park Ridge, IL: Author, 1984.

Baggerly, J. Rehabilitation of the adult with head trauma. Nursing Clinics of North America, *21*(4): 577–587, 1986.

Carpenter, R. Infections and head injury: a potentially lethal combination. Critical Care Nursing Quarterly, *10*(3): 1–11, 1987.

Decker, SI. The life-threatening consequences of a GI bleed. RN, *48*(10): 18–25, 1985.

Edelman, AS, & Weiss, MH. Cerebral edema—techniques for monitoring and options for management. Consultant, *25*(6): 58–60, 63–64, 66–68, 1985.

Germon, K. Fluid and electrolyte problems associated with diabetes insipidus and syndrome of inappropriate antidiuretic hormone. Nursing Clinics of North America, *22*(4): 785–796, 1987.

Grinspun, DR. Nursing intervention in the cognitive retraining of the traumatic brain injury client. Rehabilitation Nursing, *12*(6): 323–330, 1987.

Grinspun, DR. Teaching families of traumatic brain-injured adults. Critical Care Nursing Quarterly, *10*(3): 61–72, 1987.

Guentz, SJ. Cognitive rehabilitation of the head-injured patient. Critical Care Nursing Quarterly, *10*(3): 51–60, 1987.

Hinkle, J. Nursing care of patients with minor head injury. Journal of Neuroscience Nursing, *20*(1): 8–16, 1988.

Hugo, M. Alleviating the effects of care on the intracranial pressure (ICP) of head injured patients by manipulating nursing care activities. Intensive Care Nursing, *3*(2): 78–82, 1987.

Jess, LW. Assessing your patient for increased I.C.P. Nursing '87, *17*(6): 34–41, 1987.

Konopad, E, & Noseworthy, T. Stress ulceration: a serious complication in critically ill patients. Heart and Lung, *17*(4): 339–348, 1988.

Lovely, MP. Severe head injury: a case study. Critical Care Nursing Quarterly, *10*(3): 43–50, 1987.

Palmer, M, & Wyness, MA. Positioning and handling: important considerations in the care of the severely head-injured patient. Journal of Neuroscience Nursing, *20*(1): 42–49, 1988.

Reimer, M. Head-injured patients: how to detect early signs of trouble. Nursing '89, *19*(3): 34–41, 1989.

Stavros, MK. Family issues in moderate to severe head injury. Critical Care Nursing Quarterly, *10*(3): 73–82, 1987.

VI.3. Intracranial Surgery

American Association of Neuroscience Nurses. Core curriculum for neurosurgical nursing (2nd ed.). Park Ridge, IL: Author, 1984.

Edelman, AS, & Weiss, MH. Cerebral edema—techniques for monitoring and options for management. Consultant, *25*(6): 58–60, 63–64, 66–68, 1985.

Germon, K. Fluid and electrolyte problems associated with diabetes insipidus and syndrome of inappropriate antidiuretic hormone. Nursing Clinics of North America, *22*(4): 785–796, 1987.

Jess, LW. Assessing your patient for increased I.C.P. Nursing '87, *17*(6): 34–41, 1987.

Konopad, E, & Noseworthy, T. Stress ulceration; a serious complication in critically ill patients. Heart and Lung, *17*(4): 339–348, 1988.

Savoy, SM. The craniotomy patient: identifying the patient's neurological status. AORN Journal, *40*(5): 716–724, 1984.

Vogt, G, Miller, M, & Esluer, M. Mosby's manual of neurological care. St. Louis: C.V. Mosby, 1985.

VI.4. Multiple Sclerosis

American Association of Neuroscience Nurses. Core curriculum for neurosurgical nursing (2nd ed.). Park Ridge, IL: Author, 1984.

Csesko, PA. Sexuality and multiple sclerosis. Journal of Neuroscience Nursing, *20*(6): 353–355, 1988.

Ferguson, JM. Helping an MS patient live a better life. RN, *50*(12): 22–27, 1987.

Kassirer, MR, & Osterberg, DH. Pain in multiple sclerosis. American Journal of Nursing, *87*(7): 968–969, 1987.

Kelly, B, et al. Nursing care of the patient with multiple sclerosis. Rehabilitation Nursing, *13*(5): 238–242, 1988.

McBride, EV, & Distefano, K. Explaining diagnostic tests for M.S. Nursing '88, *18*(2): 68–72, 1988.

Samonds, RJ, & Cammermeyer, M. The patient with multiple sclerosis. Nursing '85, *15*(9): 60–64, 1985.

Schapiro, RT. Symptom management in multiple sclerosis. New York: Demos Publications, 1987.

Vogt, G, Miller, M, & Esluer, M. Mosby's manual of neurological care. St. Louis: C.V. Mosby, 1985.

VI.5. Spinal Cord Injury

American Association of Neuroscience Nurses. Core curriculum for neurosurgical nursing (2nd ed.). Park Ridge, IL: Author, 1984.

Bourdon, SE. Psychological impact of neurotrauma in the acute care setting. Nursing Clinics of North America, *21*(4): 629–640, 1987.

Decker, SI. The life-threatening consequences of a GI bleed. RN, *48*(10): 18–25, 1985.

Drayton-Hargrove, S, & Reddy, MA. Rehabilitation and long-term management of the spinal cord injured adult. Nursing Clinics of North America, *21*(4): 599–610, 1986.

Goddard, LR. Sexuality and spinal cord injury. Journal of Neuroscience Nursing, *20*(4): 240–244, 1988.

Konopad, E, & Noseworthy, T. Stress ulceration: a serious complication in critically ill patients. Heart and Lung, *17*(4): 339–348, 1988.

Metcalf, JA. Acute phase management of persons with spinal injury: a nursing diagnosis perspective. Nursing Clinics of North America, *21*(4): 589–598, 1986.

Pettibone, KA. Management of spasticity in spinal cord injury: nursing concerns. Journal of Neuroscience Nursing, *20*(4): 217–222, 1988.

Romeo, JH. Spinal cord injury: nursing the patient toward a new life. RN, *51*(5): 31–35, 1988.

Spica, MM. Sexual counseling standards for the spinal cord–injured. Journal of Neuroscience Nursing, *21*(1): 56–60, 1989.

Stevens, SA. A simple, step-by-step approach to neurological assessment (part 2). Nursing '88, *18*(10): 51–58, 1988.

Vogt, G, Miller, M, & Esluer, M. Mosby's manual of neurological care. St. Louis: C.V. Mosby, 1985.

Waters, JD. Learning needs of spinal cord–injured patients. Rehabilitation Nursing, *12*(6): 309–312, 1987.

UNIT VII. Nursing Care of the Client with Disturbances of Cardiovascular Function

VII.1. Angina Pectoris

Amsterdam, E. Unstable angina: ischemic chest pain that mimics MI. Consultant, *28*(4): 127–130, 1988.

Barkett, PA. Cardiac MUGA scan. Nursing '88, *18*(10): 76–79, 1988.

Bealehole, R. Diet, serum cholesterol and prevention of coronary artery disease. New Zealand Medical Journal, *101*(848): 415–418, 1988.

Braunwald, E (Ed.). Heart disease: a textbook of cardiovascular medicine (3rd ed.). Philadelphia: W.B. Saunders Company, 1988.

Cooke, DH. When angina destabilizes. Emergency Medicine, *20*(9): 142–144, 147, 151–154, 1988.

Elizardi, DJ. Angina pectoris: special considerations in treating elderly patients. Consultant, *28*(1): 115–116, 118–120, 129, 1988.

Norsen, L, Telfair, M, & Wagner, AL. Detecting dysrhythmias. Nursing '86 *16*(11): 34–40, 1986.

Position statement: dietary guidelines for healthy American adults. Circulation, *72*(3): 721A–723A, 1988.

Roberts, A. Senior systems: cardiovascular system . . . ischemic heart disease . . . angina. Nursing Times, *84*(12): 59–62, 1988.

Roberts, A. Senior systems: cardiovascular system. Nursing Times, *84*(14): 43–46, 1988.

Smith, WM, & Wallace, AG. Drugs used to treat cardiac arrhythmias. In Hurst, JW (Ed.), The heart (6th ed.) (Vol. 2). New York: McGraw-Hill, 1986, pp. 1593–1605.

Thompson, VL. Chest pain: your response to a classic warning. RN, *52*(4): 32–37, 1989.

Yacone, LA. The nurse's guide to cardiovascular drugs. RN, *51*(9): 40–47, 1988.

VII.2. Congestive Heart Failure

Bernhard, R. Heart failure: can earlier diagnosis and vasodilators boost survival? Emergency Medicine, *20*(5): 2–3, 21, 1988.

Braunwald, E. (Ed.). Heart disease: a textbook of cardiovascular medicine (3rd ed.). Philadelphia: W.B. Saunders Company, 1988.

Cheng, TO. International textbook of cardiology. New York: Pergamon Press, 1986.

Franciosa, JA, Jelliffe, R, Levine, B, et al. CHF: when vasodilators are indicated. Patient Care, *21*(3): 22–34, 1987.

Franciosa, JA, Jelliffe, R, Levine, B, et al. Intervening effectively in early CHF. Patient Care, *21*(2): 39–46, 1987.

Franciosa, JA, Jelliffe, R, Levine, B, et al. Management options in progressive CHF. Patient Care, *21*(5): 101–105, 1987.

Hurst, JW (Ed.). The heart (6th ed.). New York: McGraw-Hill, 1986.

Knorr, C. Early clues to chronic CHF. Patient Care, *21*(1): 22–25, 28, 30, 1987.

Parmley, WW, & Chatterjee, K. Cardiology (Vols. 1 & 2). Philadelphia: J.B. Lippincott Company, 1987.

Roberts, R. Inotropic therapy for cardiac failure associated with acute myocardial infarction. Chest, *93*(1): 22S–24S, 1988.

Van Parys, E. Assessing the failing state of the heart. Nursing '87, *17*(2): 42–49, 1987.

Zema, MJ. Left ventricular failure: clinical recognition and management. Hospital Medicine, *22*(5): 63–65, 68, 70, 79, 1986.

VII.3. Heart Surgery: Coronary Artery Bypass Grafting (CABG) or Valve Replacement

Bohachick, P, & Eldridge, R. Chest pain after cardiac surgery. Critical Care Nurse, *8*(1): 16–18, 20–22, 1988.

Dudley, H, & Carter, D. (Eds.). Operative surgery: cardiac surgery (4th ed.). St. Louis: C.V. Mosby, 1986.

Duncan, CR, Erickson, RS, & Weigel, RM. Effect of chest tube management on drainage after cardiac surgery. Heart and Lung, *16*(1): 9–13, 1987.

Estes, MEZ. Management of the cardiac tamponade patient: a nursing framework. Critical Care Nurse, *5*(5): 17–26, 1985.

Gordon, HS. Action STAT! cardiac tamponade. Nursing '86, *16*(8): 33, 1986.

King, KB. Measurement of coping strategies, concerns, and emotional response in patients undergoing coronary artery bypass grafting. Heart and Lung, *14*(6): 579–586, 1985.

Kirklin, JW, & Barratt-Boyes, BG. Cardiac surgery. New York: John Wiley & Sons, 1986.

Ley, SJ. Fluid therapy following intracardiac operation. Critical Care Nurse, *8*(1): 26–36, 1988.

Lim-Levy, F, Babler, SA, DeGroot-Kosolcharoen, J, et al. Is milking and stripping chest tubes really necessary? Annals of Thoracic Surgery, *42*(1): 77–80, 1986.

Norsen, L, Telfair, M, & Wagner, AL. Detecting dysrhythmias. Nursing '86, *16*(11): 34–40, 1986.

Swithers, CM. Tools for teaching about anticoagulants. RN, *51*(1): 57–58, 1988.

Yacone, LA. The nurse's guide to cardiovascular drugs. RN, *51*(9): 40–47, 1988.

VII.4. Hypertension

Black, HR. A new approach to mild hypertension. Diagnosis, *10*(9): 20–21, 24, 26–32, 35, 1988.

Cerrato, P. Some diet surprises for hypertensive patients. RN, *51*(4): 85–86, 1988.

Cressman, MD. New approaches to therapy of mild hypertension. Practical Cardiology, *12*(5): 83–92, 1986.

Cressman, MD, & Gifford, RW. Use of calcium-channel blockers in antihypertensive therapy. Practical Cardiology, *12*(5): 95–103, 1986.

Gonzalez, DG, & Ram, CV. New approaches for the treatment of hypertensive urgencies and emergencies. Chest, *93*(1): 193–195, 1988.

Goodman, RP. What to look for when a good regimen doesn't work. Consultant, *27*(9): 65–70, 1987.

Hurst, JW. (Ed.). The heart (6th ed.). New York: McGraw-Hill, 1986.

Kaplan, NM. Arterial hypertension. In Stein, JH (Ed.), Internal Medicine (2nd ed.). Boston: Little, Brown & Company, 1987, pp. 550–566.

McEntee, MA, & Peddicord, K. Coping with hypertension. Nursing Clinics of North America, *22*(3): 583–591, 1987.

Ram, CV. Management of resistant hypertension. Chest, *92*(6): 1096–1097, 1987.

Ram, CV. Management of refractory hypertension. Diagnosis, *10*(9): 83–90, 1988.

The 1988 report of Joint National Committee on detection, evaluation, and treatment of high blood pressure. U.S. Department of Health and Human Services, 1988.

Wollam, GL, & Hall, WD. Hypertension management: clinical practice and therapeutic dilemmas. Chicago: Year Book Medical Publishers, 1988.

VII.5. Myocardial Infarction

Barkett, PA. Cardiac MUGA scan. Nursing '88, *18*(10): 76–79, 1988.

Bealehole, R. Diet, serum cholesterol and prevention of coronary artery disease. New Zealand Medical Journal, *101*(848): 415–418, 1988.

Burgess, AW. Patients' perceptions of the cardiac crisis:

key to recovery. American Journal of Nursing, *86*(5): 568–571, 1986.

Braunwald, E. (Ed.). Heart disease: a textbook of cardiovascular medicine (3rd ed.). Philadelphia: W.B. Saunders Company, 1988.

Caplan, M, & Ranieri, C. What's his EKG telling you? A guide for nurses. RN, *52*(2): 42–50, 1989.

Chung, EK. Arrhythmias associated with acute myocardial infarction. Physician Assistant, *12*(4): 53–55, 58, 1988.

Conover, MB. Understanding electrocardiography. St. Louis: C.V. Mosby, 1988.

Croft, CH. Newer modes of therapy for myocardial infarction. Hospital Medicine, *22*(3): 55–56, 59, 63, 1986.

Dubin, D. Rapid interpretation of EKG's. Tampa, FL: Cover Publishing Company, 1988.

Estes, MEZ. Management of the cardiac tamponade patient: a nursing framework. Critical Care Nurse, *5*(5): 17–26, 1985.

Floch, MH. Dietary fiber: rational recommendations. Hospital Medicine, *21*(10): 142–158, 1985.

Gordon, HS. Action STAT! cardiac tamponade. Nursing '86, *16*(8): 33, 1986.

Hurst, JW (Ed.). The heart (6th ed.). New York: McGraw-Hill, 1986.

Milligan, KS. Tissue-type plasminogen activator: a new fibrinolytic agent. Heart and Lung, *16*(1): 69–73, 1987.

Miracle, VA. Understanding the different types of MI. Nursing '88, *18*(1): 53–56, 1988.

Mutnick, AH, & Fecitt, S. Cardiac drugs: inotropic and chronotropic agents. Nursing '87, *17*(10): 58–61, 1987.

Norsen, L, Telfair, M. & Wagner, AL. Detecting dysrhythmias. Nursing '86, *16*(11): 34–40, 1986.

Nyamath, AM. The coping responses of female spouses of patients with myocardial infarction. Heart and Lung, *16*(1): 86–92, 1987.

Olson, AR. What you should know about thrombolytic therapy. Nursing '87, *17*(12): 52–55, 1987.

Parmley, WW, & Chatterjee, K. Cardiology (Vols. 1 & 2). Philadelphia: J.B. Lippincott Company, 1987.

Position statement: dietary guidelines for healthy American adults. Circulation, *72*(3): 721A–723A, 1988.

Robert, EW. Complications of acute myocardial infarction. Hospital Medicine, *21*(11): 39–41, 45–46, 1985.

Roberts, R. Enzymatic diagnosis of acute myocardial infarction. Chest, *93*(1): 3S–6S, 1988.

Roberts, R. Inotropic therapy for cardiac failure associated with acute myocardial infarction. Chest, *93*(1): 22S–24S, 1988.

Sakallaris, BR. Laser therapy for cardiovascular disease. Heart and Lung, *16*(5): 465–471, 1987.

Strauss, E. Tissue plasminogen activator: a new drug in reperfusion therapy. Critical Care Nurse, *6*(3): 30, 32–35, 38, 43, 1986.

Weinberg, LA. Buying time with an intra-aortic balloon pump. Nursing '88, *18*(9): 44–49, 1988.

Wilerson, JT. Radionuclide assessment and diagnosis of acute myocardial infarction. Chest, *93*(1): 7S–9S, 1988.

Yacone, LA. The nurse's guide to cardiovascular drugs. RN, *51*(9): 40–47, 1988.

Yusuf, S. The use of beta-adrenergic blocking agents, IV nitrates, and calcium channel blocking agents following acute myocardial infarction. Chest, *93*(1): 25S–28S, 1988.

VII.6. Pacemaker Insertion

Bayless, WA. The elements of permanent cardiac pacing. Critical Care Nurse, *8*(7): 31–33, 37, 39–41, 1988.

Hurst, JW (Ed.). The heart (6th ed.). New York: McGraw-Hill, 1986.

Mickus, D, Monahan, KJ, & Brown, C. Exciting external pacemakers. American Journal of Nursing, *86*(4): 403–405, 1986.

Murdock, DK, Moran, JF, Stafford, M, et al. Pacemaker malfunction: fact or artifact? Heart and Lung, *15*(2): 150–154, 1986.

Stafford, MJ. Monitoring patients with permanent cardiac pacemakers. Nursing Clinics of North America, *22*(2): 503–519, 1987.

UNIT VIII. Nursing Care of the Client with Disturbances of Peripheral Vascular Function

VIII.1. Abdominal Aortic Aneurysm Repair

Czapinski, N, Antig, P, Beloria, D, et al. Nursing plan for abdominal aortic aneurysms. AORN Journal, *37*(2): 205–208, 210, 1983.

Hotter, AN. Preventing cardiovascular complications following abdominal aortic aneurysm surgery. Dimensions of Critical Care Nursing, *6*(1): 10–19, 1987.

Lamberth, WC, & Doty, DB. Peripheral vascular surgery. Chicago: Year Book Medical Publishers, 1987.

Teaching Rounds. Abdominal aortic aneurysm. Hospital Medicine, *23*(7): 112, 115–117, 1987.

Zimmerman, TA, & Ruplinger, J. Thoracoabdominal aortic aneurysms: treatment and nursing interventions. Critical Care Nurse, *3*(6): 54–63, 1983.

VIII.2. Carotid Endarterectomy

American Association of Neuroscience Nurses. Core curriculum for neurosurgical nursing (2nd ed.). Park Ridge, IL: Author, 1984.

Brown, SL. Practical points in the assessment and care of the patient having a carotid endarterectomy. Journal of Post Anesthesia Nursing, *2*(1): 41–42, 1987.

Loftus, CM. Carotid endarterectomy: current indications for elective and emergency surgery. Postgraduate Medicine, *82*(5): 241–248, 1987.

Lusby, RJ, & Wylie, EJ. Complications of carotid endarterectomy. Surgical Clinics of North America, *63*(6): 1293–1302, 1983.

Maran, JN, & Franklin, D. Carotid endarterectomy: restoring cerebral circulation. Today's OR Nurse, *7*(9): 26–28, 30–32, 1985.

Sanchez, F. Carotid endarterectomy: a comprehensive approach to care. Journal of Post Anesthesia Nursing, *1*(2): 97–106, 1986.

Sundt, TM, Piepgras, DB, Ebersold, MJ, & Walsh, WR. Carotid artery surgery: postoperative evaluation and management of complications with illustrative cases. In Sundt, TM (Ed.), Occlusive cerebrovascular disease: diagnosis and surgical management. Philadelphia: W.B. Saunders Company, 1987, pp. 243–260.

Theodotou, B, & Mahaley, MS, Jr. Complications following carotid endarterectomy for all indications: report of 192 operations. Surgical Neurology, *24*(5): 484–489, 1985.

VIII.3. Femoropopliteal Bypass

Lamberth, WC, & Doty, DB. Peripheral vascular surgery. Chicago: Year Book Medical Publishers, 1987.

Lavin, RJ. The high-pressure demands of compartment syndrome. RN, *52*(2): 22–25, 1989.

Massey, JA. Diagnostic testing for peripheral vascular disease. Nursing Clinics of North America, *21*(2): 207–218, 1986.

VIII.4. Thrombophlebitis

Bernstein, EF. Operative management of acute venous thromboembolism. In Rutherford, RB (Ed.), Vascular surgery (2nd ed.). Philadelphia: W.B. Saunders Company, 1984.

Colman, RW, Hirsh, J, Marder, VJ, & Salzman, EW (Eds.). Hemostasis and thrombosis: basic principles and clinical practice (2nd ed.). Philadelphia: J.B. Lippincott Company, 1987.

Coon, WW, Hirsh, J, & Rubin, LJ. Preventing deep vein thrombosis. Patient Care, *21*(3): 82–90, 1987.

Fahey, VA. Vascular nursing. Philadelphia: W.B. Saunders Company, 1988.

Fahey, VA. An in-depth look at deep vein thrombosis. Nursing '89, *19*(1): 56–93, 1989.

Gerdes, L. Recognizing multisystemic effects of embolism. Nursing '87, *17*(12): 34–41, 1987.

McMahan, BE. Why deep vein thrombosis is so dangerous. RN, *50*(1): 20–23, 1987.

Moser, KM. The therapeutic focus in pulmonary embolism. Emergency Medicine, *19*(20): 67–79, 81, 82–83, 1987.

Silver, D. Nonoperative management of acute venous thromboembolism. In Rutherford, RB (Ed.), Vascular surgery (2nd ed.). Philadelphia: W.B. Saunders Company, 1984.

Swithers, CM. Tools for teaching about anticoagulants. RN, *51*(1): 57–58, 1988.

Wilson, SE, Veith, FJ, Hobson, RW, & Williams, RA. Vascular surgery: principles and practice. New York: McGraw-Hill, 1987.

VIII.5. Vein Ligation

Fahey, VA. Vascular nursing. Philadelphia: W.B. Saunders Company, 1988.

Lamberth, WC, & Doty, DB. Peripheral vascular surgery. Chicago: Year Book Medical Publishers, 1987.

Wilson, SE, Veith, FJ, Hobson, RW, & Williams, RA. Vascular surgery: principles and practice. New York: McGraw-Hill, 1987.

UNIT IX. Nursing Care of the Client with Disturbances of Respiratory Function

IX.1. Asthma

Aberman, A. Managing asthmatics. Emergency Medicine, *18*(8): 26–30, 32, 37–38, 1986.

Bailey, WC, Keens, TG, & Tinstman, TC. Plotting a course for asthma therapy. Patient Care, *21*(9): 62–65, 68, 71–73, 75, 77, 80–82, 1987.

Brandstetter, RD. The adult respiratory distress syndrome. Heart and Lung, *15*(3): 155–164, 1986.

Carroll, PF. A.R.D.S.: pathophysiology—and the resulting signs and symptoms. Nursing '88, *18*(10): 74–75, 1988.

Cherniack, RM. Continuity of care in asthma management. Hospital Practice, *22*(9): 119–126, 135–136, 141–143, 1987.

Donohue, JF. Status asthmaticus. Consultant, *26*(7): 43–48, 50, 53, 1986.

Hudson, LD. Respiratory failure: etiology and mortality. Respiratory Care, *32*(7): 584–593, 1987.

Krohmer, JR. Asthma out of control. Emergency Medicine, *20*(9): 96–100, 105, 109, 1988.

Reed, CE. Basic mechanisms of asthma: role of inflammation. Chest, *94*(1): 175–177, 1988.

Reynolds, HY. Asthma: unusual presentations and causative mechanisms. Consultant, *27*(9): 29–34, 39, 44–45, 1987.

Weinberg, H. Long-term management of asthma. Physician Assistant, *12*(6): 30–31, 35–36, 41–42, 1988.

IX.2. Cancer of the Lung

Armstrong, DA. Lung cancer: the diagnostic workup. American Journal of Nursing, *87*(11): 1433, 1987.

Brown, ML, Carrieri, V, Janson-Bjerklie, S, & Dodd, M. Lung cancer and dyspnea: the patient's perception. Oncology Nursing Forum, *13*(5): 19–24, 1986.

Bull, FE. Hypercalcemia in cancer. In Yarbro, JW, & Bornstein, RS (Eds.), Oncologic emergencies. New York: Grune & Stratton, 1981, pp. 197–214.

Cohen, MH. Signs and symptoms of bronchogenic carcinoma. Seminars in Oncology, *1*(3): 183–189, 1984.

Comis, RL, & Martin, G. Small cell carcinoma of the lung: an overview. Seminars in Oncology Nursing, *3*(3): 174–182, 1987.

Doogan, RA. Hypercalcemia of malignancy. Cancer Nursing, *4*(4): 299–304, 1981.

Elbaum, N. With cancer patients, be alert for hypercalcemia. Nursing '84, *14*(8): 58–59, 1984.

Engelking, C. Lung cancer: teaching, counseling, and caring. American Journal of Nursing, *87*(11): 1439–1441, 1987.

Engelking, C. Lung cancer: chemotherapy. American Journal of Nursing, *87*(11): 1438–1439, 1987.

Engelking, C. Lung cancer: the language of staging. American Journal of Nursing, *87*(11): 1434–1437, 1987.

Foote, M, Sexton, DL, & Pawlik, L. Dyspnea: a distressing sensation in lung cancer. Oncology Nursing Forum, *13*(5): 25–31, 1986.

Gobel, BH, & Lawler, PE. Malignant pleural effusions. Oncology Nursing Forum, *12*(4): 49–54, 1985.

Harwood, KVS. Non–small cell lung cancer: issues in diagnosis, staging and treatment. Seminars in Oncology Nursing, *3*(3): 183–193, 1987.

Haskell, CM. Paraneoplastic syndromes. In Pilch, YH (Ed.), Surgical oncology. New York: McGraw-Hill, 1984, pp. 1025–1040.

Haylock, PJ. Lung cancer: radiation therapy. American Journal of Nursing, *87*(11): 1441–1446, 1987.

Holmes, EC. Pulmonary neoplasms. In Pilch, YH (Ed.), Surgical oncology. New York: McGraw-Hill, 1984, pp. 433–447.

Jones, LA. Superior vena cava syndrome: an oncologic complication. Seminars in Oncology Nursing, *3*(3): 221–215, 1987.

Lind, JM. Ectopic hormonal production: nursing implications. Seminars in Oncology Nursing, *1*(4): 251–258, 1985.

Lindsey, AM, Piper, BF, & Carrieri, VL. Malignant cells and ectopic hormone production. Oncology Nursing Forum, *8*(3): 13–15, 1981.

Maran, JN, & Gray, MA. Pulmonary laser therapy. American Journal of Nursing, *88*(6): 828–831, 1988.

McNaull, FW. Radiation therapy for lung cancer: nursing considerations. Seminars in Oncology Nursing, *3*(3): 194–201, 1987.

McNaull, FW. Lung cancer: what are the odds? American Journal of Nursing, *87*(11): 1428–1429, 1987.

Minna, JD, Higgins, GA, & Glatstein, EJ. Cancer of the lung. In Devita, VT, Hellman, S, & Rosenberg, SA (Eds.), Cancer principles and practice of oncology (2nd ed.). Philadelphia: J.B. Lippincott Company, 1985, pp. 507–596.

Moseley, JR. Nursing management of toxicities associated with chemotherapy for lung cancer. Seminars in Oncology Nursing, *3*(3): 202–210, 1987.

Odell, WD. Paraendocrine syndromes of cancer. Advances in Internal Medicine, *34:* 325–352, 1989.

O'Mara, SR. Lung carcinoma. Critical Care Quarterly, *9*(3): 1–11, 1986.

Oleske, DM. The epidemiology of lung cancer: an overview. Seminars in Oncology Nursing, *3*(3): 165–173, 1987.

Raffin, TA. Pancoast syndrome. Hospital Medicine, *22*(5): 218–221, 1986.

Ryan, LS. Lung cancer: psychosocial implications. Seminars in Oncology Nursing, *3*(3): 222–227, 1987.

Simpson, JR, Perez, CA, Presant, CA, & VanAmburg, AL. Superior vena cava syndrome. In Yarbro, JW, & Bornstein, RS (Eds.), Oncologic emergencies. New York: Grune & Stratton, 1981, pp. 43–72.

Stanford, W, & Doty, DB. The role of venography and surgery in the management of patients with superior vena cava obstruction. Annals of Thoracic Surgery, *41*(2): 158–163, 1986.

Theologides, A. Cancer cachexia. Cancer, *43:* 2004–2012, 1979.

Turrisi, AT, III. Limited small cell lung cancer—the role of radiotherapy. Oncology, *2*(7): 19–25, 1988.

Valentine, AS, & Stewart, JA. Oncologic emergencies. American Journal of Nursing, *83*(9): 1282–1285, 1983.

Varricchio, C. Clinical management of superior vena cava syndrome. Heart and Lung, *14*(4): 411–416, 1985.

Varricchio, C, & Jassak, PF. Acute pulmonary disorders associated with cancer. Seminars in Oncology Nursing, *1*(4): 269–277, 1985.

Weisenberger, TH. Superior vena caval syndrome. In Haskell, CM (Ed.), Cancer treatment. Philadelphia: W.B. Saunders Company, 1985, pp. 925–927.

IX.3. Chronic Obstructive Pulmonary Disease

Baigelman, W. Exacerbation of chronic obstructive pulmonary disease. Emergency Medicine, *19*(19): 79–80, 82–83, 86, 1987.

Brandstetter, RD. The adult respiratory distress syndrome. Heart and Lung, *15*(3): 155–164, 1986.

Carroll, PF. A.R.D.S.: pathophysiology—and the resulting signs and symptoms. Nursing '88, *18*(10): 74–75, 1988.

Davis, AL. Managing the patient with advanced chronic obstructive pulmonary disease (part 1). Hospital Medicine, *22*(1): 127, 131, 134, 137–139, 143–144, 146–148, 150–151, 1986.

Davis, AL. Managing the patient with advanced chronic obstructive pulmonary disease (part 2). Hospital Medicine, *22*(2): 70–72, 82, 84–86, 88, 91, 94, 1986.

Decker, SI. The life-threatening consequences of a GI bleed. RN, *48*(10): 18–25, 1985.

Downie, RL. Obstructive airway disease. Topics in Emergency Medicine, *8*(4): 13–31, 1987.

Eggland, ET. Teaching the ABCs of C.O.P.D. Nursing '87, *17*(1): 60–64, 1987.

Hahn, K. Slow-teaching the C.O.P.D. patient. Nursing '87, *17*(4): 34–41, 1987.

Hudson, LD. Respiratory failure: etiology and mortality. Respiratory Care, *32*(7): 584–593, 1987.

Lareau, S, & Larson, JL. Ineffective breathing pattern related to airflow limitation. Nursing Clinics of North America, *22*(1): 179–191, 1987.

Petty, TL. COPD in the setting of "multidimensional" illness. Hospital Practice, *23*(1): 39–50, 1988.

Shekleton, ME. Coping with chronic respiratory difficulty. Nursing Clinics of North America, *22*(3): 569–581, 1987.

Taylor, JD. Helping your patient cope with COPD. Nursing Life, *6*(3): 33–40, 1986.

IX.4. Lung Surgery

Burkhart, C. Pneumonectomy. American Journal of Nursing, *83*(11): 1562–1565, 1983.

Harper, RW. A guide to respiratory care: physiology and clinical applications. Philadelphia: J.B. Lippincott Company, 1981.

Mims, BC. Helping your patient breathe easier after chest surgery. RN, *47*(12): 24–31, 1984.

IX.5. Pneumonia

Coleman, DA. Pneumonia: where nursing really counts. RN, *49*(2): 22–29, 1986.

Harper, RW. A guide to respiratory care: physiology and clinical applications. Philadelphia: J.B. Lippincott Company, 1981.

Niederman, MS, & Fein, AM. Pneumonia in the elderly. Clinics in Geriatric Medicine, *2*(2): 241–268, 1986.

Ryan, AM. Pneumonia: aggressive treatment is the key. RN, *45*(8): 44–50, 1982.

Stratton, CW. Bacterial pneumonias—an overview with emphasis on pathogenesis, diagnosis, and treatment. Heart Lung, *15*(3): 226–244, 1986.

IX.6. Pneumothorax

Carroll, PF. Action stat! Tension pneumothorax. Nursing '85, *15*(9): 41, 1985.

Idell, S. Management of pneumothorax. Emergency Medicine, *19*(17): 39–49, 1987.

IX.7. Pulmonary Embolism

Bohachick, P, & Eldridge, R. Chest pain after cardiac surgery. Critical Care Nurse, *8*(1): 16–18, 20–22, 24–25, 1988.

Daeschner, SA. Action STAT: pulmonary embolism. Nursing '88, *18*(9): 33, 1988.

Dickinson, SP, & Bury, GM. Pulmonary embolism: anatomy of a crisis. Nursing '89, *19*(4): 34–41, 1989.

Gerdes, L. Recognizing the multisystemic effects of embolism. Nursing '87, *17*(12): 34, 1987.

Hull, RD, Raskob, GE, & Hirsch, J. Prophylaxis of venous thromboembolism: an overview. Chest (supplement), *89*(5): 374S–383S, 1986.

Hyers, TM, McMullen, WR, Ravin, CE, & Salzman, EW. Pulmonary embolism. Patient Care, *21*(3): 24–27, 31, 34, 39–41, 45, 1987.

Meloche, AT. PE: pulmonary embolism. Canadian Nurse, *82*(7): 23–26, 1986.

Moser, KM. The therapeutic focus in pulmonary embolism. Emergency Medicine, *19*(20): 66–70, 75, 79, 81–83, 1987.

Roberts, SL. Pulmonary tissue perfusion altered: emboli. Heart and Lung, *16*(2): 128–138, 1987.

West, JW. Pulmonary embolism. Medical Clinics of North America, *70*(4): 877–894, 1986.

UNIT X. Nursing Care of the Client with Disturbances of the Kidney and Urinary Tract

X.1. Cystectomy

Broadwell, DC. Peristomal skin integrity. Nursing Clinics of North America, *22*(2): 321–332, 1987.

Broadwell, DC, & Jackson, BS. Principles of ostomy care. St. Louis: C.V. Mosby, 1982.

Brubacher, LL, & Beard, P. A helpful new handout for your ostomy patients. RN, *46*(8): 34–37, 1983.

Doering, KJ, & LaMountain, P. Flowcharts to facilitate

caring for ostomy patients: part 1: preop assessment. Nursing '84, *14*(9): 47–49, 1984.

Doering, KJ, & LaMountain, P. Flowcharts to facilitate caring for ostomy patients: part 2: immediate postop care. Nursing '84, *14*(10): 47–49, 1984.

Doering, KJ, & LaMountain, P. Flowcharts to facilitate caring for ostomy patients: part 3: recuperative care. Nursing '84, *14*(11): 54–57, 1984.

Doering, KJ, & LaMountain, P. Flowcharts to facilitate caring for ostomy patients: part 4: discharge outcome assessment. Nursing '84, *14*(12): 47–49, 1984.

Erickson, PJ. The art of pouching. Nursing Clinics of North America, *22*(2): 311–320, 1987.

Gerber, A. The Kock continent urostomy. Journal of Enterostomal Therapy, *9*(5): 6–7, 1982.

Killeen, KP, & Libertino, JA. Management of bowel and urinary tract complications after urinary diversion. Urologic Clinics of North America, *15*(2): 183–194, 1988.

Lamb, MA, & Woods, NF. Sexuality and the cancer patient. Cancer Nursing, *4*(2): 137–144, 1981.

Lerner, J, & Khan, Z. Mosby's manual of urologic nursing. St. Louis: C.V. Mosby, 1982.

Mandell, J, Bauer, SB, Colodny, AH, & Retik, AB. Complications of urinary tract diversion. Urologic Clinics of North America, *15*(2): 207–217, 1988.

Montie, JE, MacGregor, PS, Fazio, VW, & Lavery, I. Continent ileal urinary reservoir (Kock pouch). Urologic Clinics of North America, *13*(2): 251–260, 1986.

Petillo, MH. The patient with a urinary stoma. Nursing Clinics of North America, *22*(2): 263–279, 1987.

Rolstad, BS. Innovative surgical procedures and stoma care in the future. Nursing Clinics of North America, *22*(2): 341–356, 1987.

Rowland, RG. Continent urinary reservoirs. Surgical Clinics of North America, *68*(5): 891–907, 1988.

Shipes, E. Psychosocial issues: the person with an ostomy. Nursing Clinics of North America, *22*(2): 291–302, 1987.

Simmons, KN. Sexuality and the female ostomate. American Journal of Nursing, *83*(3): 409–411, 1983.

Smith, DB, & Johnson, DE (Eds.). Ostomy care and the cancer patient. New York: Grune & Stratton, 1986.

Toth, JM. When your patient faces a urostomy. RN, *48*(11): 50–55, 1985.

Watt, RC. Nursing management of a patient with a urinary diversion. Seminars in Oncology Nursing, *2*(4): 265–269, 1986.

X.2. Nephrectomy

Lerner, J, & Khan, Z. Mosby's manual of urologic nursing. St. Louis: C.V. Mosby, 1982.

Richard, CJ. Comprehensive nephrology nursing. Boston: Little, Brown & Company, 1986.

Walsh, PC, Gittes, RF, Perlmutter, AD, & Stamey, TA. Campbell's urology. Philadelphia: W.B. Saunders Company, 1986.

X.3. Renal Calculi with Lithotomy

Andriani, RT, & Carson, CC. Urolithiasis. Clinical Symposia, *38*(3): 5–32, 1986.

Coe, FL, & Favus, MJ. Disorders of stone formation. In Brenner, BM, & Rector, FC (Eds.), The kidney (3rd ed.) (Vol. 2.). Philadelphia: W.B. Saunders Company, 1986, pp. 1403–1442.

Coe, FL, & Parks, JH. Pathophysiology of kidney stones and strategies for treatment. Hospital Practice, *23*(3): 185–189, 193–195, 199–200, 1988.

Ghiotto, DL. A full range of care for nephrostomy patients. RN, *51*(4): 72–74, 76–77, 1988.

Parker-Cohen, PD. Extracorporeal shock-wave lithotripsy treatment for kidney stones. Nurse Practitioner, *13*(3): 32, 37–38, 40–42, 1988.

Reilly, NJ, & Torosian, LC. The new wave in lithotripsy: implications for nursing. RN, *51*(3): 44–50, 1988.

Rotolo, JE, O'Brien, WM, & Pahira, JJ. Urinary tract calculi: part 2: update on evaluation and medical management. Consultant, *29*(2): 143–147, 151–152, 1989.

Wasserman, AG. Kidney stones: advice on preventing first episodes and recurrences. Consultant, *26*(5): 81–84, 87–88, 91–92, 1986.

X.4. Renal Failure

Chambers, JK. Fluid and electrolyte problems in renal and urological disorders. Nursing Clinics of North America, *22*(4): 815–826, 1987.

Fallon, K. Chronic renal failure. Journal of Medical Technology, *4*(6): 230–233, 1987.

Fine, LG. The uremic syndrome: adaptive mechanisms and therapy. Hospital Practice, *22*(9): 63–73, 1987.

Hahn, D. The many signs of renal failure. Nursing '87, *17*(8): 34–42, 1987.

Hine, J, & Daines, MA. Sexuality and the renal patient. Nursing Times, *83*(20): 35–36, 1987.

Kaye, WA. Understanding kidney disease. Diabetes Forecast, *40*(11): 24–29, 1987.

Kokko, J. Chronic renal failure. In Brenner, MM, & Rector, FC (Eds.), The kidney (3rd ed.) (Vol. 2). Philadelphia: W.B. Saunders Company, 1986, pp. 549–558.

Maxwell, MG, Kleeman, CR, & Narins, RG. Clinical disorders of fluid and electrolyte metabolism (4th ed.). New York: McGraw-Hill, 1987.

Richard, CJ. Comprehensive nephrology nursing. Boston: Little, Brown & Company, 1986.

Schrier, RW, & Gottschalk, CW (Eds.). Diseases of the kidney (4th ed.) (Vol. 2.). Boston: Little, Brown & Company, 1988.

UNIT XI.

XI.1. Acquired Immune Deficiency Syndrome: Human Immunodeficiency Virus Infection

Barrick, B. Caring for AIDS patients: a challenge you can meet. Nursing '88, *18*(11): 50–59, 1988.

Beckham, M, & Rudy, E. Acquired immunodeficiency syndrome: impact and implication for the neurological system. Journal of Neuroscience Nursing, *18*(1): 5–10, 1986.

Bennett, JA. Helping people with AIDS live well at home. Nursing Clinics of North America, *23*(4): 731–748, 1988.

Carpenter, CCJ, & Mayer, KH. Advances in AIDS and HIV infection. Advances in Internal Medicine, *33:* 45–80, 1988.

Clark, CC, Curley, A, Hughes, A, & James, R. Hospice care: a model for caring for the person with AIDS. Nursing Clinics of North America, *23*(4): 851–862, 1988.

Coleman, DA. How to care for an AIDS patient. RN, *49*(7): 16–21, 1986.

Donehower, MG. Malignant complications of AIDS. Oncology Nursing Forum, *14*(1): 57–64, 1987.

Durham, J, & Cohen, F (Eds.). The person with AIDS: nursing perspectives. New York: Springer, 1987.

Fauci, AS. The human immunodeficiency virus: infectivity and mechanisms of pathogenesis. Science, *239*(4840): 617–622, 1988.

Fears, JK. A review of immune defects in AIDS. Topics in Emergency Medicine, *9*(2): 13–17, 1987.

Felberbaum, MJ, & Salzberg, MR. Epidemiology and risk factors associated with AIDS. Topics in Emergency Medicine, *9*(2): 1–12, 1987.

Fineberg, HV. The social dimension of AIDS. Scientific American, *259*(4): 128–134, 1988.

Fiumara, NJ. Acquired immune deficiency syndrome (AIDS). Medical Aspects of Human Sexuality, *20*(3): 58–61, 1986.

Gallo, RC, & Montagnier, L. AIDS in 1988. Scientific American, *259*(4): 40–48, 1988.

Garett, JE. The AIDS patient: helping him and his parents cope. Nursing '88, *18*(9): 50–52, 1988.

Gee, G, Moran, T, & Wong, R. Current strategies in the treatment of HIV infection. Seminars in Oncology Nursing, *4*(2): 126–131, 1988.

Govoni, LA. Psychosocial issues of AIDS in the nursing care of homosexual men and their significant others. Nursing Clinics of North America, *23*(4): 749–765, 1988.

Grady, C. HIV: epidemiology, immunopathogenesis, and clinical consequences. Nursing Clinics of North America, *23*(4): 683–696, 1988.

Haines, J. AIDS: new consideration in caring. Canadian Nurse, *83*(6): 11–12, 1987.

Haseltine, WA, & Wong-Staal, F. The molecular biology of the AIDS virus. Scientific American, *259*(4): 52–62, 1988.

Hilton, G. AIDS dementia. Journal of Neuroscience Nursing, *21*(1): 24–29, 1989.

Kotler, DP. Intestinal and hepatic manifestations of AIDS. Advances in Internal Medicine, *34:* 43–72, 1989.

LaCharite, CL, & Meisenhelder, JB. Zidovudine: flawed champion against AIDS. RN, *52*(1): 35–38, 1989.

Lamke, C, & Marquardt, D. Management of human immunodeficiency virus in the emergency department. Topics in Emergency Medicine, *9*(2): 43–59, 1987.

Lewis, A (Ed.). Nursing care of the person with AIDS/ARC. Rockville, MD: Aspen Publishers, 1988.

Lovejoy, NC. The pathophysiology of AIDS. Oncology Nursing Forum, *15*(5): 563–571, 1988.

Loveless, MO. The emergency medical management of patients with AIDS-related complex. Topics in Emergency Medicine, *9*(2): 19–25, 1987.

Lusby, G, Martin, JP, & Schietinger, H. Infection control at home: a guideline for caregivers to follow. American Journal of Hospice Care, *3*(2): 24–27, 1986.

McArthur, JH, & McArthur, JC. Neurological manifestations of acquired immunodeficiency syndrome. Journal of Neuroscience Nursing, *18*(5): 241–249, 1986.

McArthur, JH, Palenicek, JG, & Bowersox, LL. Human immunodeficiency virus and the nervous system. Nursing Clinics of North America, *23*(4): 823–841, 1988.

Moran, TA, Lovejoy, N, Viele, CS, Dodd, M, & Abrams, DI. Informational needs of homosexual men diagnosed with AIDS or AIDS-related complex. Oncology Nursing Forum, *15*(3): 311–314, 1988.

Perlstein, LM. AIDS: an overview for the neuroscience nurse. Journal of Neuroscience Nursing, *19*(6): 296–299, 1987.

Price, RW, Brew, B, Sidtis, J, Rosenblum, M, Scheck, AC, & Cleary, P. The brain in AIDS: central nervous system HIV-1 infection and AIDS dementia complex. Science, *239*(4840): 586–592, 1988.

Redfield, RR, & Burke, DS. HIV infection: the clinical picture. Scientific American, *259*(4): 90–98, 1988.

Robertson, S. Drugs that keep AIDS patients alive. RN, *52*(2): 35–41, 1989.

Rosenblum, ML, Levy, RM, & Bredesen, DE. AIDS and the nervous system. New York: Raven Press, 1988.

Rosenthal, Y, & Haneiwich, S. Nursing management of adults in the hospital. Nursing Clinics of North America, *23*(4): 707–718, 1988.

Sande, M, and Volberding, P (Eds.). The medical management of AIDS. Philadelphia: W.B. Saunders Company, 1988.

Schietinger, H. A home care plan for AIDS. American Journal of Nursing, *86*(9): 1021–1028, 1986.

Segal, M. A progress report on AIDS research. FDA Consumer, *21*(8): 8–12, 1987.

Selwyn, PA. AIDS: what is now known: history and immunovirology. Hospital Practice, *21*(5): 67–82, 1986.

Selwyn, PA. AIDS: what is now known: clinical aspects. Hospital Practice, *21*(9): 119–153, 1986.

Selwyn, PA. AIDS: what is now known: psychosocial aspects, treatment prospects. Hospital Practice, *21*(10): 125–164, 1986.

Truax, AB. Psychosocial aspects of AIDS: Topics in Emergency Medicine, *9*(2): 61–69, 1987.

Ungvarski, P. Assessment: the key to nursing the AIDS patient. RN, *51*(9): 28–33, 1988.

Ungvarski, P. Coping with infections that AIDS patients develop. RN, *51*(11): 53–58, 1988.

Weber, JN, & Weiss, JN. HIV infection: the cellular picture. *259*(4): 100–109, 1988.

Yancovitz, SR. Opportunistic infections in AIDS. Topics in Emergency Medicine, *9*(2): 27–35, 1987.

Yarchoan, R, Mitsuya, H, & Broder, S. AIDS therapies. Scientific American, *259*(4): 110–119, 1988.

Young, LS. Management of opportunistic infections complicating the acquired immunodeficiency syndrome. Medical Clinics of North America, *70*(3): 677–692, 1986.

XI.2. Anemia

Beck, WS (Ed.). Hematology. Cambridge, MS: MIT Press, 1985.

Froberg, JH. The anemias: causes and courses of action. RN, *52*(1): 24–29, 1989.

Jandyl, JH. Blood: textbook of hematology. Boston: Little, Brown & Company, 1987.

XI.3. Multiple Myeloma

Abrahm, J. Management of the immunocompromised host. Medical Clinics of North America, *68*(3): 617–637, 1984.

Barry, SA. Septic shock: special needs of patients with cancer. Oncology Nursing Forum, *16*(1): 31–35, 1989.

Bull, FE. Hypercalcemia in cancer. In Yarbo, JW, & Bornstein, RS (Eds.), Oncologic emergencies. New York: Grune & Stratton, 1981, pp. 197–214.

Carlson, A. Infection prophylaxis in the patient with cancer. Oncology Nursing Forum, *12*(3): 56–64, 1985.

Donoghue, M, Nunnally, C, & Yasko, J. Nutritional aspects of cancer care. Reston, VA: Reston Publishing Company, 1982.

Farrant, C. Multiple myeloma. RN, *50*(1): 38–42, 1987.

Fer, MF, McKinney, TD, Richardson, RL, Hande, KR, Oldham, RK, & Greco, FA. Cancer and the kidney: renal complications of neoplasms. American Journal of Medicine, *71*(10): 704–718, 1981.

Jacobsen, DR, & Zolla-Pazner, S. Immunosuppression and infection in multiple myeloma. Seminars in Oncology, *13*(3): 282–290, 1986.

Krakusis, P. Considerations in the therapy of septic shock. Medical Clinics of North America, *70*(4): 933–942, 1986.

Mundy, GR, & Bertolini, DR. Bone destruction and hypercalcemia in plasma cell myeloma. Seminars in Oncology, *13*(3): 291–299, 1986.

Oken, MM. Multiple myeloma. Medical Clinics of North America, *68*(3): 757–787, 1984.

Poe, CM, & Radford, AI. The challenge of hypercalcemia in cancer. Oncology Nursing Forum, *12*(6): 29–34, 1985.

Reheis, C. Neutropenia—causes, complications, treatment, and resulting nursing care. Nursing Clinics of North America, *20*(1): 219–225, 1985.

Trotta, P, & Knobf, MT. Nursing assessment of symptoms associated with hyperviscosity syndrome. Oncology Nursing Forum, *14*(1): 21–25, 1987.

Zimmerman, J, & Dietrich, C. Current perspectives on septic shock. Pediatric Clinics of North America, *34*(1): 131–156, 1987.

XI.4. Splenectomy

Deters, GE. Managing complications after abdominal surgery. RN, *50*(3): 27–32, 1987.

Ellison, EC, & Fabri, PJ. Complications of splenectomy: etiology, prevention, and management. Surgical Clinics of North America, *63*(6): 1313–1330, 1983.

Gold, E. Postsplenectomy infection: assessing risk, planning management. Consultant, *24*(1): 301–305, 1984.

Schwartz, SI. The spleen. In Schwartz, SI, & Ellis, H (Eds.), Maingot's abdominal operations (8th ed.) (Vol. 2). Norwalk, CT: Appleton-Century-Crofts, 1985, pp. 2253–2289.

UNIT XII. Nursing Care of the Client with Disturbances of the Gastrointestinal Tract

XII.2. Bowel Diversion: Ileostomy

Broadwell, DC, & Jackson, BS. Principles of ostomy care. St. Louis: C.V. Mosby, 1982.

Deters, GE. Managing complications after abdominal surgery. RN, *50*(3): 27–32, 1987.

Kelly, M. Adjusting to ileostomy. Nursing Times, *83*(33): 29–31, 1987.

McConnell, EA. Fluid and electrolyte concerns in intestinal surgical procedures. Nursing Clinics of North America, *22*(4): 853–860, 1987.

Pearl, RK. Complications of ileostomy. In Nelson, RL, & Nyhus, LM, Surgery of the small intestine. Norwalk, CT: Appleton & Lange, 1987, pp. 499–509.

Phillips, SF. Conventional and alternative ileostomies. In Sleisenger, MG, & Fordtran, JS (Eds.), Gastrointestinal disease: pathophysiology, diagnosis, management (4th ed.). Philadelphia: W.B. Saunders Company, 1989, pp. 1477–1482.

Rolstad, BS. Innovative surgical procedures and stoma care in the future. Nursing Clinics of North America, *22*(2):341–356, 1987.

Tan, AB, & Prasad, ML. Stoma care. In Nelson, RL, & Nyhus, LM, Surgery of the small intestine. Norwalk, CT: Appleton & Lange, 1987, pp. 485–497.

Watson, P. Meeting the needs of patients undergoing ostomy surgery. Journal of Enterostomal Therapy, *12*(4): 121–124, 1985.

XII.3. Gastrectomy

Deters, GE. Managing complications after abdominal surgery. RN, *50*(3): 27–32, 1987.

Given, BA, & Simmons, SJ. Gastroenterology in clinical nursing (4th ed.). St. Louis: C.V. Mosby, 1984.

Jordan, PH. Operations for peptic ulcer disease and early postoperative complications. In Sleisenger, MG, & Fordtran, JS (Eds.), Gastrointestinal disease: pathophysiology, diagnosis, management (4th ed.). Philadelphia: W.B. Saunders Company, 1989, pp. 939–952.

Kirkham, JS. Partial and total gastrectomy. In Schwartz, SI, & Ellis, H (Eds.), Maingot's abdominal operations

(8th ed.). Norwalk, CT: Appleton-Century-Crofts, 1985, pp. 839–895.

Thirlby, RC, & Feldman, M. Postoperative recurrent ulcer. In Sleisenger, MG, & Fordtran, JS (Eds.), Gastrointestinal disease: pathophysiology, diagnosis, management (4th ed.). Philadelphia: W.B. Saunders Company, 1989, pp. 952–962.

Zollinger, RM. What the nonsurgeon should know about gastrectomy. Hospital Medicine, *22*(9): 118, 120–122, 125, 128–137, 1986.

XII.4. Gastric Partitioning

Deters, GE. Managing complications after abdominal surgery. RN, *50*(3): 27–32, 1987.

Feickert, DM. Gastric surgery: your crucial pre- and postop role. RN, *50*(1): 24–35, 1987.

Kennedy-Caldwell, C. The morbidly obese surgical patient. Critical Care Nurse, *7*(5): 87–89, 1987.

Kral, JG. Surgical treatment of obesity. Medical Clinics of North America, *73*(1): 251–264, 1989.

Menguy, R. Morbid obesity. In Schwartz, SI, & Ellis, H (Eds.), Maingot's abdominal operations (8th ed.). Norwalk, CT: Appleton-Century-Crofts, 1985, pp. 1003–1024.

Williams, RM, McMahon, LC, & Macgregor, AMC. Gastric bypass with Roux en Y: surgical treatment for morbid obesity. AORN Journal, *43*(5): 1094, 1096, 1098–1103, 1986.

XII.5. Hemorrhoidectomy

Birkett, DH. Hemorrhoids—diagnosis and treatment options. Hospital Practice, *23*(1A): 99–102, 105, 108, 1988.

Goligher, J. Surgery of the anus, rectum, and colon. London: Bailliere-Tindall, 1984.

Sleisenger, MH, & Fordtran, JS. Gastrointestinal disease: pathophysiology, diagnosis, management. Philadelphia: W.B. Saunders Company, 1989.

XII.6. Hiatal Hernia Repair

Deters, DE. Managing complications after abdominal surgery. RN, *50*(3): 27–32, 1987.

Ellis, FH, Jr. Hiatus hernia. Clinical Symposia, *38*(5): 2–31, 1986.

Given, BA, & Simmons, SJ. Gastroenterology in clinical nursing (4th ed.). St. Louis: C.V. Mosby, 1984.

Hogan, WJ, & Dodds, WJ. Gastroesophageal reflux disease. In Sleisenger, MG, & Fordtran, JS (Eds.), Gastrointestinal disease: pathophysiology, diagnosis, management (4th ed.). Philadelphia: W.B. Saunders Company, 1989, pp. 594–619.

XII.7. Inflammatory Bowel Disease: Ulcerative Colitis and Crohn's Disease

Berk, JE (Ed.). Gastroenterology (4th ed.) (Vol. 4). Philadelphia: W.B. Saunders Company, 1985.

Farraye, FA, & Peppercorn, MA. Inflammatory bowel disease: advances in the management of ulcerative colitis and Crohn's disease. Consultant, *28*(10): 39–43, 46–47, 1988.

Given, BA, & Simmons, SJ. Gastroenterology in clinical nursing (4th ed.). St. Louis: C.V. Mosby, 1984.

Kinash, RG. IBD: implications for patients, challenges for nurses. Rehabilitation Nursing, *12*(2): 82, 86–87, 89, 1987.

Neufeldt, J. Helping the IBD patient cope with the unpredictable. Nursing '87, *17*(8): 47–49, 1987.

Nord, HJ. Complications of inflammatory bowel disease. Hospital Practice, *22*(11A): 65–67, 70–72, 75, 78, 80, 82, 1987.

Sleisenger, MH, & Fordtran, JS. Gastrointestinal disease: pathophysiology, diagnosis, management. Philadelphia: W.B. Saunders Company, 1989.

XII.8. Jaw Reconstruction

Donovan, S. When your patient faces jaw reconstruction. RN, *50*(1): 43–44, 46, 1987.

Freedman, SD, & Devine, BA. A clean break: postop oral care. American Journal of Nursing, *87*(4): 474–475, 1987.

Holt, SR. Maxillofacial trauma. In Cummings, CS, Fredrickson, JM, Harker, LA, et al. (Eds.), Otolaryngology: head and neck surgery. St. Louis: C.V. Mosby, 1986, pp. 313–344.

Newbould, M. Improving appearance. Nursing Times, *83*(6): 30, 32, 1987.

Roberts, PA. Arthroscopic surgery of the temporomandibular joint. Today's OR Nurse, *9*(11): 24–32, 44–46, 1987.

Watts, V, Madick, S, Pepperney, J, & Petras, C. When your patient has jaw surgery. RN, *48*(10): 44–47, 1985.

XII.9. Peptic Ulcer

Brasitus, TA, & Foster, ES. Peptic ulcer update: approaches to treatment. Physician Assistant, *12*(4): 71–72, 77–78, 83+, 1988.

Bruckstein, AH. Peptic ulcer disease: new concepts, new and current therapeutics. Consultant, *26*(4): 157–161, 164–166, 1986.

Decker, SI. The life-threatening consequences of a GI bleed. RN, *48*(10): 18–25, 1985.

Deters, GE. Managing complications after abdominal surgery. RN, *50*(3): 27–32, 1987.

Given, BA, & Simmons, SJ. Gastroenterology in clinical nursing (4th ed.). St. Louis: C.V. Mosby, 1984.

Graham, DY. Complications of peptic ulcer disease and indications for surgery. In Sleisenger, MG, & Fordtran, JS (Eds.), Gastrointestinal disease: pathophysiology, diagnosis, management (4th ed.). Philadelphia: W.B. Saunders Company, 1989, pp. 925–938.

Koch, MJ. How to detect and heal lesions and relieve pain. Consultant, *27*(5): 21–24, 27, 1987.

Lewis, JH, & London, JF. Peptic ulcer and reflux esophagitis: management for the long term. Consultant, *29*(2): 91–94, 97–98, 102–103, 1989.

Olsen, KM, & Barton, CL. Peptic ulcer disease. Journal of Practical Nursing, *37*(4): 20–27, 1987.

Roberts, A. Senior systems: the stomach and duodenum (part 8). Nursing Times, *82*(47): 19–25, 1986.

Sebesin, SM. Guidelines to counseling patients with peptic ulcer disease. Physician Assistant, *8*(10): 76, 81–84, 88, 1984.

Smith, S. How drugs act: drugs and the GI tract (part 6). Nursing Times, *83*(26): 50–52, 1987.

Soll, AH. Duodenal ulcer and drug therapy. In Sleisenger, MG, & Fordtran, JS (Eds.). Gastrointestinal disease: pathophysiology, diagnosis, management (4th ed.). Philadelphia: W.B. Saunders Company, 1989, pp. 814–879.

UNIT XIII. Nursing Care of the Client with Disturbances of the Liver, Biliary Tract, and Pancreas

XIII.1. Cholecystectomy

Berk, JE (Ed.). Gastroenterology (4th ed.) (Vol. 6). Philadelphia: W.B. Saunders Company, 1985.

Given, BA, & Simmons, SJ. Gastroenterology in clinical nursing (4th ed.). St. Louis: C.V. Mosby, 1984.

Ransohoff, DF, Schoenfield, LJ, & Thistle, JL. What's new in the blitz on gallstones. Patient Care, *22*(3): 111–114, 117–119, 122–123, 1988.

Schwartz, SI, & Ellis, H (Eds.). Maingot's abdominal operations (8th ed.) (Vol. 2). Norwalk, CT: Appleton-Century-Crofts, 1985.

Sleisenger, MH, & Fordtran, JS. Gastrointestinal disease: pathophysiology, diagnosis, management. Philadelphia: W.B. Saunders Company, 1989.

XIII.2. Cholelithiasis/Cholecystitis

Berk, JE (Ed.). Gastroenterology (4th ed.) (Vol. 6). Philadelphia: W.B. Saunders Company, 1985.

Given, BA, & Simmons, SJ. Gastroenterology in clinical nursing (4th ed.). St. Louis: C.V. Mosby, 1984.

Grant, G, White, EM, & Zeman, RK. Clinical and cost advantages of the newer techniques. Consultant, *27*(3): 30–34, 37–38, 1987.

Hauser, SC. Answers to questions on gallbladder disease. Hospital Medicine, *23*(6): 44–45, 48, 50–55, 58, 60–62, 68, 72, 1987.

Ransohoff, DF, Schoenfield, LJ, & Thistle, JL. What's new in the blitz on gallstones. Patient Care, *22*(3): 111–114, 117–119, 122–123, 1988.

Roberts, A. Senior systems . . . gallstones. Nursing Times, *83*(43): 55–58, 1987.

Sherlock, S. Diseases of the liver and biliary system (7th ed.). Oxford: Blackwell Scientific Publications, 1985.

Sleisenger, MH, & Fordtran, JS. Gastrointestinal disease: pathophysiology, diagnosis, management. Philadelphia: W.B. Saunders Company, 1989.

XIII.3. Cirrhosis

Adinaro, D. Liver failure and pancreatitis: fluid and electrolyte concerns. Nursing Clinics of North America, *22*(4): 843–852, 1987.

Berk, JE (Ed.). Gastroenterology (4th ed.). (Vol. 5). Philadelphia: W.B. Saunders Company, 1985.

Dickson, ER, Koff, RS, Sabesin, SM, et al. Toxic liver disease: alcohol? drugs? Patient Care, *21*(11): 153–159, 162–163, 1987.

Dickson, ER, Koff, RS, Sabesin, SM, et al. Which tests for liver disease? Patient Care, *21*(7): 124–132, 1987.

Given, BA, & Simmons, SJ. Gastroenterology in clinical nursing (4th ed.). St. Louis: C.V. Mosby, 1984.

Pimstone, NR. The spectrum of alcoholic liver disease. Hospital Medicine, *22*(10): 23–25, 29, 32+, 1986.

Roberts, A. Senior systems . . . chronic liver disease. Nursing Times, *84*(5): 45–48, 1988.

Schiff, L, & Schiff, ER (Eds.). Diseases of the liver (6th ed.). Philadelphia: J.B. Lippincott Company, 1987.

Sherlock, S. Diseases of the liver and biliary system (7th ed.). Oxford: Blackwell Scientific Publications, 1985.

Witkin, GB, Chapman, JF, & Lesesne, HR. Choosing liver function tests. Emergency Medicine, *19*(20): 23–38, 40–41, 45–46, 1987.

XIII.4. Hepatitis

Berk, JE (Ed.). Gastroenterology (4th ed.) (Vol. 5). Philadelphia: W.B. Saunders Company, 1985.

Dickson, ER, Koff, RS, Sabesin, SM, et al. Toxic liver disease: alcohol? drugs? Patient Care, *21*(11): 153–159, 162–163, 1987.

Given, BA, & Simmons, SJ. Gastroenterology in clinical nursing (4th ed.). St. Louis: C.V. Mosby, 1984.

Hollinger, FB. Serologic evaluation of viral hepatitis. Hospital Practice, *22*(2): 101–114, 1987.

Koff, RS. Fulminant hepatitis due to HBV/HDV coinfection. Hospital Practice, *22*(11): 123–130, 145–150, 154, 1987.

Koff, RS, & Galambos, JT. Viral hepatitis. In Schiff, L, & Schiff, ER (Eds.), Diseases of the liver (6th ed.). Philadelphia: J.B. Lippincott Company, 1987.

Sherlock, S. Diseases of the liver and biliary system (7th ed.). Oxford: Blackwell Scientific Publications, 1985.

Witkin, GB, Chapman, JF, & Lesesne, HR. Choosing liver function tests. Emergency Medicine, *19*(20): 23–38, 40–41, 45–46, 1987.

XIII.5. Pancreatitis

Adinaro, D. Liver failure and pancreatitis: fluid and electrolyte concerns. Nursing Clinics of North America, *22*(4): 843–852, 1987.

Berger, HG, & Büchler, M (Eds.). Acute pancreatitis: research and clinical management. Berlin: Springer-Verlag, 1987.

Brandstetter, RD. The adult respiratory distress syndrome. Heart and Lung, *15*(3): 155–164, 1986.

Carroll, PF. A.R.D.S.: pathophysiology—and the resulting signs and symptoms. Nursing '88, *18*(10): 74–75, 1988.

Geokas, MC, Baltaxe, HA, Banks, PA, et al. Acute pancreatitis. Annals of Internal Medicine, *103*(1): 86–100, 1985.

Given, BA, & Simmons, SJ. Gastroenterology in clinical nursing (4th ed.). St. Louis: C.V. Mosby, 1984.

Moorehouse, MF, Geissler, AC, & Doenges, ME. Acute pancreatitis. Journal of Emergency Nursing, *14*(6): 387–391, 1988.

Soergel, KH. Acute pancreatitis. In Sleisenger, MG, & Fordtran, JS (Eds.), Gastrointestinal disease: pathophysiology, diagnosis, management (4th ed.). Philadelphia: W.B. Saunders Company, 1989, pp. 1814–1842.

Teaching Rounds. Pancreatic pseudocyst: a complication of pancreatitis. Hospital Medicine, *23*(9): 45, 46, 49, 53, 1987.

Toskes, PP. Recurrent acute pancreatitis (part 4). Hospital Practice, *20*(7): 85–88, 90–92, 1985.

Welch, JP. Recognizing and treating acute pancreatitis. Hospital Medicine, *21*(9): 91–95, 98, 103–104, 1985.

UNIT XIV. Nursing Care of the Client with Disturbances of Metabolic Function

XIV.1. Diabetes Mellitus

Armstrong, N. Coping with diabetes mellitus. Nursing Clinics of North America, *22*(3): 559–569, 1987.

Bell, DSH, & Clements, RS. Diabetes and the digestive system. Diabetes Forecast, *40*(12): 43–46, 1987.

Butts, DE. Fluid and electrolyte disorders associated with diabetic ketoacidosis and hyperglycemic hyperosmolar nonketotic coma. Nursing Clinics of North America, *22*(4): 827–836, 1987.

Christman, C, & Bennett, J. Diabetes: new names, new test, new diet. Nursing '87, *17*(1): 34–41, 1987.

deTejada, IS, & Goldstein, I. Diabetic penile neuropathy. Urologic Clinics of North America, *15*(1): 17–21, 1988.

Dyck, PJ, Thomas, PK, Asbury, AK, et al. (Eds.). Diabetic neuropathy. Philadelphia: W.B. Saunders Company, 1987.

Felig, P, Baxter, JD, Broadus, AE, & Frohman, LA (Eds.). Endocrinology and metabolism (2nd ed.). New York: McGraw-Hill, 1987.

Freinkel, RK. Caring for your skin. Diabetes Forecast, *41*(7): 76–78, 81, 1988.

Gavin, J. Diabetes and exercise. American Journal of Nursing, *88*(2): 178–180, 1988.

Huzar, JG, & Cerrato, PL. The role of diet and drugs. RN, *52*(4): 46–50, 1989.

Levin, ME, & O'Neal, LW (Eds.). The diabetic foot (4th ed.). St. Louis: C.V. Mosby, 1988.

Lumley, W. Hypoglycemia and hyperglycemia. Nursing '88, *18*(10): 34, 36–41, 1988.

Marble, A, Krall, LP, Bradley, RF, et al. (Eds.). Joslin's diabetes mellitus (12th ed.). Philadelphia: Lea & Febiger, 1985.

Mendelsohn, G. Diagnosis and pathology of endocrine diseases. Philadelphia: J.B. Lippincott Company, 1988.

Morrison, SRN. Diabetic impotence. Nursing Times, *84*(32): 35–37, 1988.

Nath, C, Murray, S, & Ponte, C. Lessons in living with type II diabetes mellitus. Nursing '88, *18*(8): 45–49, 1988.

Pankey, GA. Diabetic foot and leg ulcers: therapy must be prompt and aggressive. Consultant, *28*(3): 43–45, 48, 53–54, 1988.

Ramsey, PW. Hyperglycemia at dawn. American Journal of Nursing, *87*(11): 1424–1426, 1987.

Sabo, CE. Managing DKA and preventing a recurrence. Nursing '89, *19*(2): 50–56, 1989.

Schatz, PE. An evaluation of the components of compliance in patients with diabetes. Journal of the American Dietetic Association, *88*(6): 708–712, 1988.

Shinbarger, NI. Limited joint mobility in adults with diabetes mellitus. Physical Therapy, *67*(2): 215–218, 1987.

Tomky, D. A three-pronged approach to monitoring. RN, *52*(3); 24–29, 1989.

Unger, RH, & Foster, DW. Diabetes mellitus. In Wilson, JD, & Foster, DW (Eds.), Williams' textbook of endocrinology (7th ed.). Philadelphia: W.B. Saunders Company, 1985, pp. 1018–1067.

Whitehead, ED. Diabetes-related impotence: putting new knowledge to use. Geriatrics, *43*(2): 114, 116, 120, 1988.

Wozniak, L. Your teaching plan: the key to controlling type II diabetes. RN, *51*(8): 29–33, 1988.

XIV.2. Hypophysectomy

American Association of Neuroscience Nurses. Core curriculum for neurosurgical nursing (2nd ed.). Park Ridge, IL: Author, 1984.

Eitel, DM. Nursing care for hypophysectomy. AORN Journal, *33*(2): 256–260, 1981.

Germon, K. Fluid and electrolyte problems associated with diabetes insipidus and syndrome of inappropriate antidiuretic hormone. Nursing Clinics of North America, *22*(4): 785–796, 1987.

Resio, MJ. Nursing diagnosis: alteration in oral/nasal mucous membranes related to trauma of transsphenoidal surgery. Journal of Neuroscience Nursing, *18*(3): 112–115, 1986.

Stillman, MJ. Transsphenoidal hypophysectomy for pituitary tumors. Journal of Neurosurgical Nursing, *13*(3): 117–122, 1981.

Vogt, G, Miller, M, & Esluer, M. Mosby's manual of neurological care. St. Louis: C.V. Mosby, 1985.

XIV.3. Hypothyroidism

Bybee, DE. Saving lives in thyroid crisis. Emergency Medicine, *19*(16): 20–23, 27, 31, 1987.

Felig, P, Baxter, P, Broadus, AE, et al. (Eds.). Endocrinology and metabolism (2nd ed.). New York: McGraw-Hill, 1987.

Hare, JW. Signs and symptoms in endocrine and metabolic disorders. Philadelphia: J.B. Lippincott Company, 1986.

Ingbar, SH, & Braverman, LE (Eds.). Werner's The thyroid (5th ed.). Philadelphia: J.B. Lippincott Company, 1986.

Labhart, A. Clinical endocrinology (2nd ed.). New York: Springer-Verlag, 1986.

Mendelsohn, G. Diagnosis and pathology of endocrine diseases. Philadelphia: J.B. Lippincott Company, 1988.

Wilson, JD, & Foster, DW (Eds.). Williams' textbook of endocrinology (7th ed.). Philadelphia: W.B. Saunders Company, 1985.

XIV.4. Thyroidectomy

Bybee, DE. Saving lives in thyroid crisis. Emergency Medicine, *19*(16): 20–23, 27, 31, 1987.

Lockhart, JS. Postthyroidectomy: respiratory distress. Nursing '87, *17*(7): 33, 1987.

Lockhart, JS. Tetany. Nursing '88, *18*(8): 33, 1988.

UNIT XV. Nursing Care of the Client with Disturbances of Musculoskeletal Function

XV.1. Amputation

Bourne, BA, & Kutcher, JL. Amputation: helping the patient face loss of a limb. RN, *48*(2): 38–44, 1985.

Ceccio, CM, & Horosz, JE. Teaching the elderly amputee to meet the world. RN, *51*(9): 70–77, 1988.

Engstrand, JL. Rehabilitation of the patient with a lower extremity amputation. Nursing Clinics of North America, *11*(4): 659–669, 1976.

Farrell, J. Illustrated guide to orthopedic nursing (3rd ed.). Philadelphia: J.B. Lippincott Company, 1986.

Frazier, D. Advances in prostheses. RN, *51*(9): 73, 1988.

Pasnau, RO, & Pfefferbaum. B. Post-amputation grief. Nursing Clinics of North America, *11*(4): 687–690, 1976.

Pasnau, RO, & Pfefferbaum, B. Psychologic aspects of post-amputation pain. Nursing Clinics of North America, *11*(4): 679–685, 1976.

Smith, AG. Common problems of lower extremity amputees. Orthopedic Clinics of North America, *13*(3): 569–578, 1982.

Walters, J. Coping with a leg amputation. American Journal of Nursing, *81*(7): 1349–1352, 1981.

XV.2. Fractured Femur with Skeletal Traction

Batra, P. Fat embolism syndrome. Journal of Thoracic Imaging, *2*(3): 12–17, 1987.

Chapman, MW (Ed.). Operative orthopaedics (Vol. 1). Philadelphia: J.B. Lippincott Company, 1988.

Farrell, J. Orthopedic pain: what does it mean? American Journal of Nursing, *84*(4): 466–469, 1984.

Gerdes, L. Recognizing multisystemic effects of embolism. Nursing '87, *17*(12): 34–41, 1987.

Morris, L, Kraft, S, Tessem, S, & Reinisch, S. Special care for skeletal traction. RN, *51*(2): 24–29, 1988.

Resnick, D, & Niwayama, G. Diagnosis of bone and joint disorders (2nd ed.). Philadelphia: W.B. Saunders Company, 1988.

Rockwood, CA, & Green, DP (Eds.). Fractures in adults (2nd ed.) (Vol. 2). Philadelphia: J.B. Lippincott Company, 1984.

Sisk, TD. Fractures of the lower extremity. In Crenshaw, AH (Ed.), Campbell's operative orthopaedics (7th ed.) (Vol. 3). St. Louis: C.V. Mosby, 1987, pp. 1607–1718.

Stevenson, CK. Take no chances with fat embolism. Nursing '85, *15*(6): 58–63, 1985.

Walton, PJ. Effects of pin care on pin reactions in adults with extremity fracture treated with skeletal traction and external fixation. Orthopaedic Nursing, *7*(4): 29–33, 1988.

XV.3. Fractured Hip with Internal Fixation or Prosthesis Insertion

Krug, BM. The hip: nursing fracture patients to full recovery. RN, *52*(4): 56–61, 1989.

Rockwood, CA, & Green, DP (Eds.). Fractures in adults (2nd ed.) (Vol. 2). Philadelphia: J.B. Lippincott Company, 1984.

Schoen, DG. Assessing a fractured hip. Nursing '87, *17*(3): 97–98, 1987.

Sisk, TD. Fractures of the lower extremity. In Crenshaw, AH (Ed.), Campbell's operative orthopaedics (7th ed.) (Vol. 3). St. Louis: C.V. Mosby, 1987, pp. 1607–1718.

XV.4. Laminectomy/Discectomy with or without Fusion

American Association of Neuroscience Nurses. Core curriculum for neurosurgical nursing (4th ed.). Park Ridge, IL: Author, 1989.

Burnand, J. Back payment . . . a prolapsed intervertebral disc. Nursing Mirror, *159*(8): 37–39, 1984.

Devoti, AL. Lumbar laminectomy: diagnosis to discharge. Journal of Neurosurgical Nursing, *15*(3): 140–143, 1983.

Farrell, J. Illustrated guide to orthopedic nursing (3rd ed.). Philadelphia: J.B. Lippincott Company, 1986.

Gates, SJ. Update: nursing care following percutaneous posterolateral discectomy. Orthopaedic Nursing, *6*(5): 37–41, 1987.

Larson, C, & Gould, M. Orthopedic nursing (9th ed.). St. Louis: C.V. Mosby, 1987.

Nagler, W, & vonEstorff, I. Rehabilitation of the patient with low back pain, pre- and postoperatively. In Camins, MB, & O'Leary, PE (Eds.), The lumbar spine. New York: Raven Press, 1987, pp. 357–371.

Reilly, JP, & O'Leary, PF. Complications of lumbar spine surgery. In Camins, MB, & O'Leary, PE (Eds.), The lumbar spine. New York: Raven Press, 1987, pp. 357–371.

Schlegel, M. Helping your patient recover from a lumbar laminectomy. NursingLife, *6*(5): 31–32, 1986.

Stevens, SA. A simple, step-by-step approach to neurologic assessment (part 2). Nursing '88, *18*(10): 51–58, 1988.

XV.5. Total Hip Replacement

Batra, P. Fat embolism syndrome. Journal of Thoracic Imaging, *2*(3): 12–17, 1987.

Calandruccio, RA. Arthroplasty of hip. In Crenshaw, AH (Ed.), Campbell's operative orthopaedics (7th ed.) (Vol. 2). St. Louis: C.V. Mosby, 1987, pp. 1213–1491.

Coon, WW, Hirsch, J, & Rubin, LJ. Preventing deep vein thrombosis. Patient Care, *21*(3): 82–86, 89–90, 1987.

Enis, JE. Total hip arthroplasty in the geriatric patient. Hospital Medicine, *23*(4): 41–42, 44, 46–48, 51, 54, 56, 1987.

Gerdes, L. Recognizing multisystemic effects of embolism. Nursing '87, *17*(12): 34–41, 1987.

Gever, LN. Embolex: to prevent a double postop danger . . . DVT and pulmonary embolism. Nursing '86, *16*(5): 73, 1986.

Gill, KP. New hope for a permanent, biologically compatible joint prosthesis. Canadian Nurse, *83*(9): 19–20, 1987.

Moser, KM. The therapeutic focus in pulmonary embolism. Emergency Medicine, *19*(20): 67–79, 81–83, 1987.

Putnam, J. Total hip replacement: helping your patient avoid complications. Nursing Life, *6*(2): 31–32, 1986.

Rockwood, CA, & Green, DP (Eds.). Fractures in adults (2nd ed.) (Vol. 2). Philadelphia: J.B. Lippincott Company, 1984.

Stevenson, CK. Take no chances with fat embolism. Nursing '85, *15*(6): 58–63, 1985.

Total hip replacement. Orthopaedic Nursing, *6*(1): 35–37, 1987.

Turke, SL. Orthopaedics: principles and their application (4th ed.) (Vol. 2). Philadelphia: J.B. Lippincott Company, 1984.

XV.6. Total Knee Replacement

Batra, P. Fat embolism syndrome. Journal of Thoracic Imaging, *2*(3): 12–17, 1987.

Gerdes, L. Recognizing multisystemic effects of embolism. Nursing '87, *17*(12): 34–41, 1987.

Haug, J, & Wood, LT. Efficacy of neuromuscular stimulation of the quadriceps femoris during continuous passive motion following total knee arthroplasty. Archives of Physical Medicine and Rehabilitation, *69*(6): 423–424, 1988.

Moser, KM. The therapeutic focus in pulmonary embolism. Emergency Medicine, *19*(20): 67–79, 81–83, 1987.

Stevenson, CK. Take no chances with fat embolism. Nursing '85, *15*(6): 58–63, 1985.

Tooms, RE. Arthroplasty of ankle and knee. In Crenshaw, AH (Ed.), Campbell's operative orthopaedics (7th ed.) (Vol. 2). St. Louis: C.V. Mosby, 1987, pp. 1145–1211.

Total knee arthroplasty. Orthopaedic Nursing, *7*(4): 56–57, 1988.

Total knee replacement. Orthopaedic Nursing, *6*(3): 37–39, 1987.

UNIT XVI. Nursing Care of the Client with Disturbances of the Integumentary System

XVI.1. Burns

Archambeault-Jones, & Feller, I. Burn nursing is nursing. Critical Care Quarterly, *1*(3): 77–92, 1978.

Bayley, EW, & Smith, GA. The three degrees of burn care. Nursing 87, *17*(3): 34–41, 1987.

Demling, RH. Fluid replacement in burned patients. Surgical Clinics of North America, *67*(1): 15–30, 1987.

Desai, MH. Inhalation injuries in burn victims. Critical Care Quarterly, *7*(3): 1–6, 1984.

Eskridge, RA. Septic shock. Critical Care Quarterly, *2*(4): 55–75, 1980.

Gaston, S, & Schumann, LL. Inhalation injury: smoke inhalation. American Journal of Nursing, *80*(1): 94–97, 1980.

Hansbrough, JF, Zapata-Sirvent, RL, & Peterson, VM. Immunomodulation following burn injury. Surgical Clinics of North America, *67*(1): 69–92, 1987.

Heimbach, DM. Early burn excision and grafting. Surgical Clinics of North America, *67*(1): 93–107, 1987.

Helm, PA, Head, MD, Pullium, G, O'Brien, M, & Cromes, GF, Jr. Burn rehabilitation— a team approach. Surgical Clinics of North America, *58*(6): 1263–1277, 1978.

Herndon, DN, Langner, F, Thompson, P, Linares, HA, Stein, M, & Traber, DL. Pulmonary injury in burned patients. Surgical Clinics of North America, *67*(1), 31–46, 1987.

Hurt, RA. More than skin deep: guidelines on caring for the burn patient. Nursing '85, *15*(6): 52–57, 1985.

Jackson, S. Dealing with burns. RN, *47*(10): 35–39, 1984.

Jacoby, F. Care of the massive burn wound. Critical Care Quarterly, *7*(3): 44–53, 1984.

Johnson, CL, & Cain, VJ. The rehab guide. American Journal of Nursing, *85*(1): 48–50, 1985.

Kibbee, E. Burn pain management. Critical Care Quarterly, *7*(3): 54–62, 1984.

Long, CL. Energy and protein requirements in stress and trauma (part 1). Ross Laboratories Critical Care Nursing Currents, *2*(1): 1–5, 1984.

Luterman, A, Adams, M, & Curreri, PW. Nutritional management of the burn patient. Critical Care Quarterly, *7*(3): 34–42, 1984.

Marvin, JA, Planning home care for burn patients. Nursing '83, *13*(8): 65–67, 1983.

Mieszala, P. Postburn psychological adaptation: an overview. Critical Care Quarterly, *1*(3): 93–111, 1978.

Monafo, WW, & Freedman, B. Topical therapy for burns. Surgical Clinics of North America, *67*(1): 133–145, 1987.

Moran, K, & Munster, AM. Alterations of the host defense mechanism in burned patients. Surgical Clinics of North America, *67*(1): 47–55, 1987.

Nadel, E, & Kozerefski, PM. Rehabilitation of the critically ill burn patient. Critical Care Quarterly, *7*(3): 19–33, 1984.

Pasulka, PS, & Wachtel, TL. Nutritional considerations for the burned patient. Nursing Clinics of North America, *67*(1): 109–131, 1987.

Robertson, KE, Cross, PJ, & Terry, JC. The crucial first days. American Journal of Nursing, *85*(1): 30–44, 1985.

Rosequist, CC, & Shepp, PH. The nutrition factor. American Journal of Nursing, *85*(1): 45–47, 1985.

Surveyer, JA, & Clougherty, IM. Burn scars: fighting the effects. American Journal of Nursing, *83*(5): 746–751, 1983.

Van Oss, S. Emergency burn care: those crucial first minutes. RN, *45*(10): 45–49, 1982.

West, DA, & Shuck, JM. Emotional problems of the severely burned patient. Surgical Clinics of North America, *58*(6): 1189–1204, 1978.

XVI.2. Cancer of the Breast

Abeloff, MD, & Beveridge, RA. Adjuvant chemotherapy of breast cancer—the consensus development conference revisited. Oncology, *2*(4): 21–29, 1988.

Allegra, JC. Rational approaches to the hormonal treatment of breast cancer. Seminars in Oncology, *10*(4), Supplement 4:1–10, 1983.

Gates, CC. The "most-significant-other" in the care of the breast cancer patient. CA—A Cancer Journal for Clinicians, *38*(3): 146–153, 1988.

Goodman, M. Concepts of hormonal manipulation in the treatment of cancer. Oncology Nursing Forum, *15*(5): 639–647, 1988.

Graydon, JE. Stress points. American Journal of Nursing, *84*(9): 1124–1125, 1984.

Greifzu, S. Breast cancer: the risks and the options. RN, *49*(10): 26–31, 1986.

Hardesty, I. Helping breast cancer patients help themselves. Innovations in Oncology, *3*(3): 8–9, 1987.

Hassey, K. Radiation therapy for breast cancer. Seminars in Oncology Nursing, *1*(3): 181–185, 1985.

Holland, JC, & Mastrovito, R. Psychological adaptation to breast cancer. Cancer, *46*(4): 1045–1052, 1980.

Knobf, MKT. Breast cancer: the treatment evolution. American Journal of Nursing, *84*(9): 1110–1119, 1984.

Lamb, MA, & Woods, NF. Sexuality and the cancer patient. Cancer Nursing, *4*(2): 137–144, 1981.

Lewis, F, Ellison, E, & Woods, N. The impact of breast cancer on the family. Seminars in Oncology Nursing, *1*(3): 206–213, 1985.

Lierman, LM. Phantom breast experiences after mastectomy. Oncology Nursing Forum, *15*(1): 41–44, 1988.

McCarthy, CP. The role of interstitial implantation in the treatment of primary breast cancer. Seminars in Oncology Nursing, *3*(1): 47–53, 1987.

Nail L, Jones, LS, Guiffre, M, & Johnson, JE. Sensations after mastectomy. American Journal of Nursing, *84*(9): 1121–1124, 1984.

Nash, JA. Cancer prevention and detection: breast cancer. Cancer Nursing, *7*(2): 163–178, 1984.

Pilch, YH. Breast cancer. In Pilch, YH (Ed.), Surgical oncology. New York: McGraw-Hill, 1984, pp. 491–540.

Rice, MA, & Szopa, TJ. Group intervention for reinforcing self-worth following mastectomy. Oncology Nursing Forum, *15*(1): 33–37, 1988.

Schain, W. Breast cancer surgeries and psychosexual sequelae: implications for remediation. Seminars in Oncology Nursing *1*(3): 200–205, 1985.

Schain, WS. The sexual and intimate consequences of breast cancer treatment. CA—A Cancer Journal of Clinicians, *38*(3): 154–161, 1988.

Schwarz-Appelbaum, J, Dedrick, J, Jusenuis, K, & Kirchner, CW. Nursing care plans: sexuality and treatment of breast cancer. Oncology Nursing Forum, *11*(6): 16–24, 1984.

Scott, DW. Quality of life following the diagnosis of breast cancer. Topics in Clinical Nursing, *4*(4): 20–37, 1983.

Scott, DW, Eisendrath, SJ. Dynamics of the recovery process following initial diagnosis of breast cancer. Journal of Psychosocial Oncology, *3*(4): 53–66, 1986.

Sheth, SP, & Allegra, JC. What role for concurrent chemohormonal therapy. Oncology, *1*(8): 19–24, 1987.

Simmons, CC. The relationship between life changes, losses and stress levels for females with breast cancer. Oncology Nursing Forum, *11*(2): 37–41, 1984.

Sinsheimer, LM, & Holland, JC. Psychological issues in breast cancer. Seminars in Oncology, *14*(1): 75–82, 1987.

Swain, SM. Noninvasive breast cancer: ductal carcinoma in situ—incidence, presentation, guidelines to treatment. Oncology, *3*(3): 25–31, 1989.

Swain, SM. Lobular carcinoma in situ—incidence, presentation, guidelines to treatment. Oncology, *3*(3): 35–40, 1989.

Theologides. A. Cancer cachexia. Cancer, *43*: 2004–2012, 1979.

Townsend, CM, Jr. Management of breast cancer. Clinical Symposia. Summit, NJ: Pharmaceuticals Division, CIBA-GEIGY Corp., 1987.

Wellisch, D. The psychologic impact of breast cancer on relationships. Seminars in Oncology Nursing, *1*(3): 195–199, 1985.

Worden, JW, & Weisman, AD. The fallacy in postmastectomy depression. American Journal of Medical Science, *273*: 169–175, March-April, 1977.

XVI.3. Mammoplasty

Austad, E, & Rose, A. A self-inflating tissue expansion. Plastic and Reconstructive Surgery, *70*(5): 588–593, 1982.

d'Angelo, TM, & Gorrell, CR. Breast reconstruction using tissue expanders. Oncology Nursing Forum, *16*(1): 23–27, 1989.

Dowden, RV. The current approach to breast reconstruction. Oncology, *1*(10): 29–36, 1987.

Goldberg, P, Stolzman, M, & Goldberg, HM. Psychological considerations in breast reconstruction. Annals of Plastic Surgery, *13*(1): 38–43, 1984.

Hutcheson, HA. TAIF: new option for breast reconstruction. Nursing '86, *16*(2): 52–53, 1986.

Knobf, MKT. Breast cancer: the treatment evolution. American Journal of Nursing, *84*(9): 1110–1119, 1984.

McDonald, H. Reconstruction of the breast. In Lippman, M, Lichter, A, & Danforth, D (Eds.), Diagnosis and management of breast cancer. Philadelphia: W.B. Saunders Company, 1988, pp. 468–485.

Radovan, C. Tissue expansion in soft-tissue reconstruction. Plastic and Reconstructive Surgery, *74*(4): 482–490, 1984.

Strohecker, BA, Moore, L, Tepsich, J, et al. Soft tissue expansion. American Journal of Nursing, *88*(5): 668–671, 1988.

XVI.4. Mastectomy

Aitken, DR, & Minton, JP. Complications associated with mastectomy. Surgical Clinics of North America, *63*(6): 1331–1352, 1983.

Carroll, R. The impact of mastectomy on body image. Oncology Nursing Forum, *8*(4): 29–32, 1981.

Dowden, RV. The current approach to breast reconstruction. Oncology, *1*(10): 29–36, 1987.

Goldberg, P, Stolzman, M, & Goldberg, HM. Psychological considerations in breast reconstruction. Annals of Plastic Surgery, *13*(1): 38–43, 1984.

Hutcheson, HA. TAIF: new option for breast reconstruction. Nursing '86, *16*(2): 52–53, 1986.

Lierman, LM. Phantom breast experiences after mastectomy. Oncology Nursing Forum, *15*(1): 41–48, 1988.

Nail, L, Jones, LS, Giuffre, M, & Johnson, JE. Sensations after mastectomy. American Journal of Nursing, *84*(9): 1121–1123, 1984.

Rice, MA, & Szopa, TJ. Group intervention for reinforcing self-worth following mastectomy. Oncology Nursing Forum, *15*(1): 33–37, 1988.

Schain, W. Breast cancer surgeries and psychosexual sequelae: implications for remediation. Seminars in Oncology Nursing, *1*(3): 200–205, 1985.

Strohecker, BA, Moore, L, Tepsich, J, et al. Soft tissue expansion. American Journal of Nursing, *88*(5): 668–671, 1988.

Tarrier, N. Coping after a mastectomy. Nursing Mirror, *158*(2): 29–30, 1984.

Thomas, SG, & Yates, MM. Breast reconstruction after mastectomy. American Journal of Nursing, *77*(9): 1438–1442, 1977.

Wellisch, D. The psychologic impact of breast cancer on relationships. Seminars in Oncology Nursing, *1*(3): 195–199, 1985.

UNIT XVII. Nursing Care of the Client with Disturbances of the Reproductive System

XVII.1. Cancer of the Prostate

Andriole, GL, & Catalona, WJ. Early diagnosis of prostate cancer. Urologic Clinics of North America, *14*(4): 657–661, 1987.

Bachers, ES. Sexual dysfunction after treatment for genitourinary cancers. Seminars in Oncology Nursing, *1*(1): 18–24, 1985.

Bahnson, RR, & Catalona, WJ. Current management of prostatic carcinoma. Primary Care, *12*(4): 795–812, 1985.

Bull, FE. Hypercalcemia in cancer. In Yarbro, JW, & Bornstein, RS (Eds.), Oncologic emergencies. New York: Grune & Stratton, 1981, pp. 197–214.

Champagne, EE, & Kane, NE. Teaching program for patients receiving interstitial radioactive iodine[125] for cancer of the prostate. Oncology Nursing Forum, *7*(1): 12–15, 1980.

Dutcher, JP. Nonhematologic malignancies. Hematology/

Oncology Clinics of North America, *1*(2): 281–299, 1987.

Feinstein, D. Diagnosis and management of disseminated intravascular coagulation: the role of heparin therapy. Blood, *60*(2): 284–287, 1982.

Frank-Stromberg, M. Sexuality and the elderly cancer patient. Seminars in Oncology Nursing, *1*(1): 49–55, 1985.

Garnick, MB. Current status of endocrine therapy for prostate cancer. Oncology, *1*(7): 19–25, 1987.

Goodman, M. Concepts of hormonal manipulation in the treatment of cancer. Oncology Nursing Forum, *15*(5): 639–647, 1988.

Hasegawa, DK, & Bloomfield, CD. Thrombotic and hemorrhagic manifestations of malignancy. In Yarbro, JW, & Bornstein, RS (Eds.), Oncologic emergencies. New York: Grune & Stratton, 1981, pp. 141–196.

Heinrich-Rynning, T. Prostatic cancer treatments and their effects on sexual functioning. Oncology Nursing Forum, *14*(6): 37–41, 1987.

Huben, RP, & Murphy, GP. Prostate cancer: an update. CA—A Journal for Cancer Clinicians, *36*(5): 274–290, 1986.

Jones, AG, & Hoeft, RT. Cancer of the prostate. American Journal of Nursing, *82*(5): 826–828, 1982.

Lamb, MA, & Woods, NF. Sexuality and the cancer patient. Cancer Nursing, *4*(2): 137–144, 1981.

Lerner, J, & Khan, Z. Mosby's manual of urologic nursing. St. Louis: C.V. Mosby, 1982.

MacElveen-Hoehn, P. Sexual assessment and counseling. Seminars in Oncology Nursing, *1*(1): 69–75, 1985.

McGillick, K. DIC: the deadly paradox, RN, *45*(8): 41–43, 1982.

Murphy, GP, & Slack, NH. Prostate cancer: what chemotherapy can accomplish. Your Patient and Care (special edition for oncology nurses), Fall, 1984, pp. 25–31.

NIH Consensus Development Conference. Management of clinically localized prostate cancer. Oncology, *1*(9): 46–49, 1987.

Paulson, DF. Radiotherapy versus surgery for localized prostatic cancer. Urologic Clinics of North America, *14*(4): 675–684, 1987.

Pollen, JJ, & Schmidt, JD. Tumors of the prostate. In Pilch, YH, (Ed.), Surgical oncology. New York: McGraw-Hill, 1984, pp. 698–728.

Raghavan, D. Non-hormone chemotherapy for prostate cancer: principles of treatment and application to the testing of new drugs. Seminars in Oncology, *15*(4): 371–389, 1988.

Rooney, A, & Haviley, C. Nursing management of disseminated intravascular coagulation. Oncology Nursing Forum, *12*(1): 15–22, 1985.

Siegrist, CW, & Jones, JA. Disseminated intravascular coagulopathy and nursing implications. Seminars in Oncology Nursing, *1*(4): 237–243, 1985.

Strohl, R. Nursing management of the patient with cancer experiencing taste changes. Cancer Nursing, *6*(5): 353–359, 1983.

Tansey, LA, Shanberg, AM, Nisar Syed, AM, & Puthawala, A. Treatment of prostatic carcinoma by pelvic lymphadenectomy, temporary iridium-192 implant, and external radiation. Urology, *21*(6): 594–598, 1983.

Trachtenberg, J. Hormonal management of stage D carcinoma of the prostate. Urologic Clinics of North America, *14*(4): 685–692, 1987.

Walsh, PC. Nerve sparing radical prostatectomy for early stage prostate cancer. Seminars in Oncology, *15*(4): 351–358, 1988.

Walsh, PC, Jewett, HJ. Radical surgery for prostatic cancer. Cancer, *45*(7): 1906–1911, 1980.

XVII.2. Cancer of the Testis with Retroperitoneal Lymphadenectomy

Bachers, ES. Sexual dysfunction after treatment for genitourinary cancers. Seminars in Oncology Nursing, *1*(1): 18–24, 1985.

Bihrle, RB, Donohue, JP, & Foster, RS. Complications of retroperitoneal lymph node dissection. Urologic Clinics of North America, *15*(2): 237–242, 1988.

Casey, MP. Testicular cancer: the worst disease at the worst time. RN, *50*(2): 36–40, 1987.

Fisher, S. The psychosexual effects of cancer and cancer treatment. Oncology Nursing Forum, *10*(2): 63–68, 1983.

Giannone, L, & Wolfe, SN. Recent progress in the treatment of seminoma. Oncology, *2*(10): 21–26, 1988.

Hubbard, SM, & Jenkins, J. An overview of current concepts in the management of patients with testicular tumors of germ cell origin—part I: pathophysiology, diagnoses and staging. Cancer Nursing, *6*(1): 39–47, 1983.

Hubbard, SM, & Jenkins, J. An overview of current concepts in the management of patients with testicular tumors of germ cell origin—part II: treatment strategies by histology and stage. Cancer Nursing, *6*(2): 125–139, 1983.

Javadpour, N. Testicular cancer. In Pilch, YH (Ed.), Surgical oncology. New York: McGraw-Hill, 1984, pp. 729–740.

Lamb, MA, & Woods, NF. Sexuality and the cancer patient. Cancer Nursing, *4*(2): 137–144, 1981.

Lange, PH, & Fraley, EE. Controversies in the management of low volume stage II nonseminomatous germ cell testicular cancer. Seminars in Oncology, *15*(4): 324–334, 1988.

Lange, PH, Chang, WY, & Fraley, EE. Fertility issues in the therapy of nonseminomatous testicular tumors. Urologic Clinics of North America, *14*(4): 731–747, 1987.

Loehrer, PJ, Sr., Williams, SD, & Einhorn, LH. Status of chemotherapy for testis cancer. Urologic Clinics of North America, *14*(4): 713–720, 1987.

Peters, PC. Selective surgery for testicular cancer (surveillance). Seminars in Oncology, *15*(4): 321–323, 1988.

Roth, BJ, Einhorn, LH, & Greist, A. Long-term complications of cisplatin-based chemotherapy for testis cancer. Seminars in Oncology, *15*(4): 345–350, 1988.

Whitmore, WF, Jr., & Morse, MJ. Surgery of testicular neoplasms. In Walsh, PC, Gittes, RF, et al., Campbell's Urology (5th ed.). Philadelphia: W.B. Saunders Company, 1986, pp. 2933–2954.

XVII.4. Hysterectomy with Salpingectomy and Oophorectomy

Droegemueller, W, Herbst, AL, Mishell, DR, Jr., & Stenchever, MA. Comprehensive gynecology. St. Louis: C.V. Mosby, 1987.

Holden, LS. Helping your patient through her hysterectomy. RN, *46*(9): 42–46, 1983.

Lerner, J, & Khan, Z. Mosby's manual of urologic nursing. St. Louis: C.V. Mosby, 1982.

Pearson, L. Climacteric. American Journal of Nursing, *82*(7): 1098–1102, 1982.

XVII.5. Penile Implant

Furlow, W (Ed.). Symposium on male sexual dysfunction. Urology Clinics of North America, *8*(1): 1–202, 1981.

Googe, MCS, & Mook, TM. The inflatable penile prosthesis: new developments. American Journal of Nursing, *83*(7): 1044–1047, 1983.

Krane, RJ. Penile prostheses. Urologic Clinics of North America, *15*(1): 103–109, 1988.

Lerner, J, & Khan, Z. Mosby's manual of urologic nursing. St. Louis: C.V. Mosby, 1982.

Merrill, DC. Mentor inflatable penile prostheses. Urologic Clinics of North America, *16*(1): 51–66, 1989.

Montague, DK. Penile prostheses: an overview. Urologic Clinics of North America, *16*(1): 7–12, 1989.

Mulcahy, JJ. The hydroflex penile prosthesis. Urologic Clinics of North America, *16*(1): 33–38, 1989.

Mulcahy, JJ. The OmniPhase and DuraPhase penile prostheses. Urologic Clinics of North America, *16*(1): 25–32, 1989.

Nielsen, KT, & Bruskewitz, RC. Semirigid and malleable rod penile prostheses. Urologic Clinics of North America, *16*(10): 13–24, 1989.

Schover, LR. Sex therapy for the penile prosthesis recipient. Urologic Clinics of North America, *16*(1): 91–98, 1989.

XVII.6. Prostatectomy

Ashby, D. Hyponatremia after transurethral resection of the prostate. Journal of Post Anesthesia Nursing, *3*(2): 121–122, 1988.

Bates, P. Three post-op perils of prostate surgery. RN, *47*(2): 40–43, 1984.

Blandy, JP, & Lytton, B (Eds.). The prostate. London: Butterworths, 1986.

LaFollett, SS. Radical retropubic prostatectomy. AORN Journal, *45*(1): 57–63, 66–67, 69–71, 1987.

Lawler, PE. Benign prostatic hyperplasia: knowing pathophysiology aids assessment. AORN Journal, *40*(5): 745–748, 750, 1984.

Learner, J, & Azfar, K. Mosby's manual of urological nursing. St. Louis: C.V. Mosby, 1982.

Libman, E, Creti, L, & Fichten, CS. Determining what patients should know about transurethral prostatectomy. Patient Education and Counseling, *9*(2): 145–153, 1987.

Littleton, MT. Pathophysiology and assessment of sepsis and septic shock. Critical Care Nursing Quarterly, *11*(1): 30–47, 1988.

Molitor, P. Transurethral resection. Nursing Mirror, *157*(14): 22–27, 1983.

Turner, A. Post-prostatectomy incontinence. Nursing Mirror, *157*(14): 27–31, 1983.

UNIT XVIII. Nursing Care of the Client with Disturbances of the Ear, Nose, and Throat

XVIII.1. Radical Neck Surgery

Ariyan, S. Radical neck dissection. Surgical Clinics of North America, *66*(1): 133–148, 1986.

Baker, BM, & Cunningham, CA. Vocal rehabilitation of the patient with a laryngectomy. Oncology Nursing Forum, *7*(4): 23–36, 1980.

Bayer, LM, Scholl, DE, & Ford, EG. Tube feeding at home. American Journal of Nursing, *83*(9): 1321–1325, 1983.

Biggs, CB. The cancer that cost a patient his voice. RN, *50*(4): 44–51, 1987.

Blues, K. A framework for nurses providing care to laryngectomy patients. Cancer Nursing, *1*(6): 441–446, 1978.

Coleman, JJ, III. Complications in head and neck surgery. Surgical Clinics of North America, *66*(1): 149–167, 1986.

Denning, DC. Head and neck cancer: our reactions. Cancer Nursing, *5*(4): 269–273, 1982.

Dropkin, MJ. Changes in body image associated with head and neck cancer. In Marino, LB (Ed.), Cancer Nursing. St. Louis: C.V. Mosby, 1981, pp. 560–581.

Dropkin, MJ. Development of a self-care teaching program for postoperative head and neck patients. Cancer Nursing, *4*(2): 103–106, 1981.

Dunavant, MK. Wound and fistula management. In Broadwell, DC, & Jackson, BS (Eds.), Principles of ostomy care. St. Louis: C.V. Mosby, 1982, pp. 658–686.

Feinstein, D. What to teach the patient who's had a total laryngectomy. RN, *50*(4): 53–57, 1987.

Hufler, DR. Helping your dysphagic patient eat. RN, *50*(4): 36–38, 1987.

Kane, KK. Carotid artery rupture in advanced head and neck cancer patients. Oncology Nursing Forum, *10*(1): 14–18, 1983.

Kashima, H, & Kalinowski, B. Taste impairment following laryngectomy. Ear, Nose & Throat, *58*: 88–92, 1979.

Knapp, BA, & Panje, WR. A voice button for laryngectomees. AORN Journal, *36*(2): 183–192, 1982.

Konstantinides, NN, & Shronts, E. Tube feeding: managing the basics. American Journal of Nursing, *83*(9): 1311–1320, 1983.

Metcalfe, MC, & Fischman, SH. Factors affecting the sexuality of patients with head and neck cancer. Oncology Nursing Forum, *12*(2): 21–25, 1985.

Oermann, MH, McHugh, NG, Dietrich, J, & Boyll, R. After a tracheostomy: patients describe their sensations. Cancer Nursing. *6*(5): 361–366, 1983.

Panje, WR. Musculocutaneous and free flaps: physiology and practical considerations. Otolaryngologic Clinics of North America, *17*(2): 401–412, 1984.

Rodzwic, D, & Donnard, J. The use of myocutaneous flaps in reconstructive surgery for head and neck cancer: guidelines for nursing care. Oncology Nursing Forum, *13*(3): 29–34, 1986.

Schneider, W. Nutrition in head and neck cancer. Oncology Nursing Forum, *6*(1): 5–11, 1979.

Sigler, BA. Nursing care of the head and neck cancer patient. Oncology, *2*(12): 49–53, 1988.

XVIII.2. Stapedectomy

Ballenger, JJ. Diseases of the nose, throat, ear, head, and neck (13th ed.). Philadelphia: Lea & Febiger, 1985.

DeWeese, DD. Otolaryngology—head and neck surgery (7th ed.). St. Louis: C.V. Mosby, 1988.

Houck, JR, & Harker, LA. Otosclerosis. In Cummings, CW (Ed.), Otolaryngology—head and neck surgery (Vol. 4). St. Louis: C.V. Mosby, 1986, pp. 3102–3111.

Miglets, AW. Paparella, MM, & Saunders, WH. Atlas of ear surgery (4th ed.). St. Louis: C.V. Mosby, 1986.

INDEX